MANUAL OF CLINICAL PROBLEMS IN PULMONARY MEDICINE

SIXTH EDITION

MANUAL OF CLINICAL PROBLEMS IN PULMONARY MEDICINE

SIXTH EDITION

Editors

Richard A. Bordow, M.D.
Associate Director, Pulmonary Function Lab, Doctors' Hospital,
San Pablo, California

Andrew L. Ries, M.D., M.P.H.
Associate Dean for Academic Affairs, Professor of Medicine and Family
and Preventive Medicine, University of California, San Diego, School of
Medicine, La Jolla, California; Director, Pulmonary Rehabilitation,
University of California, San Diego, Medical Center, San Diego, California

Timothy A. Morris, M.D.
Associate Professor of Medicine, Division of Pulmonary and Critical Care
Medicine, University of California, San Diego, School of Medicine, La Jolla,
California; Medical Director, Respiratory Care Department, University of
California, San Diego, Medical Center, San Diego, California

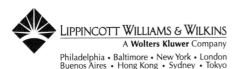

LIPPINCOTT WILLIAMS & WILKINS
A **Wolters Kluwer** Company
Philadelphia • Baltimore • New York • London
Buenos Aires • Hong Kong • Sydney • Tokyo

Acquisitions Editor : Sonya Seigafuse
Developmental Editor : Scott Scheidt
Production Editor : Bridgett Dougherty
Senior Manufacturing Manager : Benjamin Rivera
Marketing Manager : Kathy Neely
Design Coordinator : Terry Mallon
Compositor : TechBooks
Printer : RR Donnelley

**WF
39
M2943
2005**

Library of Congress Cataloging-in-Publication Data

Manual of clinical problems in pulmonary medicine / editors, Richard A.
  Bordow, Andrew L. Ries, Timothy A. Morris.—6th ed.
    p. ; cm.
    Includes bibliographical references and index.
    ISBN 0-7817-5277-9 (alk. paper)
    1. Lungs—Diseases—Handbooks, manuals, etc.   I. Bordow, Richard A.
  II. Ries, Andrew L.   III. Morris, Timothy A.
    [DNLM: 1. Lung Diseases—Handbooks.
  WF 39 M2943 2005]
  RC756.M26   2005
  616.2′4—dc22

                                                                        2005007831

Care has been taken to confirm the accuracy of the information presented and to describe generally accepted practices. However, the authors and publisher are not responsible for errors or omissions or for any consequences from application of the information in this book and make no warranty, expressed or implied, with respect to the currency, completeness, or accuracy of the contents of the publication. Application of this information in a particular situation remains the professional responsibility of the practitioner.

The authors and publisher have exerted every effort to ensure that drug selection and dosage set forth in this text are in accordance with current recommendations and practice at the time of publication. However, in view of ongoing research, changes in government regulations, and the constant flow of information relating to drug therapy and drug reactions, the reader is urged to check the package insert for each drug for any change in indications and dosage and for added warnings and precautions. This is particularly important when the recommended agent is a new or infrequently employed drug.

Some drugs and medical devices presented in this publication have Food and Drug Administration (FDA) clearance for limited use in restricted research settings. It is the responsibility of the health care provider to ascertain the FDA status of each drug or device planned for use in their clinical practice.

10 9 8 7 6 5 4 3 2 1

To

Liz, Vivian, and Prudy

You have played a pivotal role in nurturing our compassion and knowledge and compelling us to always pursue the high road. Without you, our lives would not be the same and our passions unrequited. We are grateful for your enduring support throughout our careers.

CONTENTS

I. PULMONARY DIAGNOSTIC TECHNIQUES

II. SPECIAL PROBLEMS

III. PULMONARY INFECTION

IV. AIRWAYS DISEASE

V. ACUTE RESPIRATORY FAILURE

VI. CARDIOVASCULAR AND THROMBOEMBOLIC DISEASE

VII. CONGENITAL AND PEDIATRIC LUNG DISEASE

VIII. CHEST WALL AND NEUROMUSCULAR DISORDERS

IX. ENVIRONMENTAL AND OCCUPATIONAL DISEASES

X.   IDIOPATHIC, IMMUNOLOGIC, AND GRANULOMATOUS DISEASES

XI. NEOPLASTIC DISEASES

CONTRIBUTING AUTHORS

Dennis E. Amundson, D.O.
Associate Professor of Medicine
Internal Medicine
Uniformed Service University of the
  Health Sciences
Bethesda, Maryland
Program Director
Pulmonary and Critical Care
Naval Medical Center
Pulmonary Medicine
San Diego, California

William R. Auger, M.D.
Professor of Clinical Medicine
Internal Medicine
University of California, San Diego,
  School of Medicine
La Jolla, California
Director, Thorton ICU
University of California, San Diego,
  Medical Center
San Diego, California

Colleen L. Bailey, M.D.
Clinical Instructor of Medicine
Pulmonary / Critical Care
  Medicine
University of California, San Diego,
  Medical Center
San Diego, California

John E. Barkley, M.D., F.C.C.P.
Medical Director
Palliative Care Consultants
Hospice at Charlotte
Charlotte, North Carolina

Frank D. Bender, M.D.
Medical Director of
  Respiratory Therapy
Respiratory Therapy
Palomar Medical Center
Escondido, California

Timothy D. Bigby, M.D.
Professor of Medicine
Department of Medicine
University of California, San Diego,
  School of Medicine
Chief, Pulmonary and
  Critical Care
Medicine Service Department
VA San Diego Healthcare System
La Jolla, California

Richard A. Bordow, M.D.
Associate Director
Pulmonary Function Lab
Doctors' Hospital
San Pablo, California

Stephen Bradley, M.D.
ICU Director
Chest and Critical Care Division
Scripps Clinic
La Jolla, California

David A. Bradshaw, M.D.
Head, Pulmonary Division
Naval Medical Research Center
San Diego, California

Shari A. Brazinsky, M.D., F.C.C.P.
Clinical Instructor of Medicine
Pulmonary and Critical
  Care Division
University of California, San Diego,
  School of Medicine
San Diego, California

David M. Burns, M.D.
Professor
Department of Family and Preventative
  Medicine
University of California, San Diego
San Diego, California

Antonio Catanzaro, M.D.
Professor of Medicine
University of California, San Diego,
  School of Medicine
La Jolla, California
Attending Physician
University of California, San Diego,
  Medical Center
San Diego, California

Paul Cianci, M.D.
Medical Director
Department of Hyperbaric Medicine
John Muir Medical Center
Walnut Creek, California
Saint Francis Memorial Hospital
San Francisco, California

Jack L. Clausen, M.D.
Clinical Professor of Medicine
University of California, San Diego,
  School of Medicine

La Jolla, California
University of California, San Diego,
    Medical Center
San Diego, California

Henri Colt, M.D.
Professor of Medicine
Department of Pulmonary
    Critical Care
University of California, Irvine
Orange, California

Douglas J. Conrad, M.D.
Associate Professor of
    Clinical Medicine
Department of Medicine
University of California, San Diego
San Diego, California
Director, Adult CF Clinic
Department of Medicine
University of California, San Diego,
    School of Medicine
La Jolla, California

Jana R. Cooke, M.D.
Fellow
Division of Pulmonary Critical Care
    Medicine
University of California, San Diego,
    School of Medicine
La Jolla, California
University of California, San Diego,
    Medical Center
San Diego, California

Asha Vyas Devereaux, M.D., M.P.H.
Clinical Staff
Pulmonary / Critical Care Medicine
Sharp-Coronado Hospital
Coronado, California

David W. Dockweiler, M.D.
Chief
Department of Anesthesia
Scripps Memorial Hospital
La Jolla, California

Richard D. Drucker, M.D.
Assistant Clinical Professor
Department of Medicine
University of California,
    Los Angeles
Los Angeles, California

Peter F. Fedullo, M.D.
Professor of Pulmonary and Critical
    Care Medicine
University of California, San Diego
    School of Medicine

La Jolla, California
Director, Medical Intensive
    Care Unit
University of California, San Diego
    Medical Center
San Diego, California

Richard M. Ford, B.S., R.R.T., F.A.A.R.C.
Administrative Director
Respiratory Services
University of California, San Diego,
    Medical Center
San Diego, California

Paul J. Friedman, M.D., F.A.C.R., F.C.C.P.
Emeritus Professor
Radiology Department
University of California, San Diego,
    School of Medicine
La Jolla, California
University of California, San Diego,
    Medical Center
San Diego, California

Mark Fuster, M.D.
Clinical Instructor of Medicine
Department of Medicine
Division of Pulmonary and
    Critical Care
University of California, San Diego
San Diego, California
Staff Physician
Pulmonary & Critical Care Section
VA San Diego Healthcare System
La Jolla, California

Frank T. Grassi, M.D.
Fellow
Pulmonary and Critical Care
Naval Medical Center
San Diego, California

Ian R. Grover, M.D.
Assistant Clinical Professor
    of Medicine
Department of Emergency Medicine
University of California, San Diego
Attending Physician
Department of Emergency Medicine
Hillcrest Hospital / Thorton
    Hospital
San Diego, California

Tony S. Han, M.D.
Fellow
Internal Medicine / Pulmonary / Critical
    Care
Naval Medical Center
San Diego, California

James H. Harrell, II, M.D.
Professor of Medicine
Department of Medicine
University of California, San Diego,
  School of Medicine
Director
Pulmonary Diagnostic & Nd: Yag Laser
  Unit
University of California, San Diego,
  Medical Center
San Diego, California

Gale S. Haydock, M.D.
Physician
Wang Ambulatory Care Center
Massachusetts General Hospital
Boston, Massachusetts

William G. Hughson, M.D., Ph.D.
Clinical Professor of Medicine, Director
Center for Occupational and
  Environmental Medicine
University of California, San Diego
San Diego, California

Shazia M. Jamil, M.D., F.C.C.P.
Assistant Clinical Professor
Department of Medicine
University of California, San Diego
Pulmonary and Critical Care Attending
  Physician
Scripps Green Hospital
La Jolla, California

Stuart M. Jasmer, M.D.
Assistant Professor of Medicine
Department of Medicine
University of California,
  San Francisco
Co-Director, Medical Intensive
  Care Unit
Department of Medicine
San Francisco General Hospital
San Francisco, California

Kim M. Kerr, M.D.
Associate Professor
Division of Pulmonary and Critical
  Care Medicine
University of California, San Diego,
  School of Medicine
La Jolla, California

David H. Kupferberg, M.D., M.P.H.
Assistant Clinical Professor
Pulmonary and Critical Care
University of California,
  San Diego
Associate Physician

Pulmonary and Critical Care
Kaiser Pemanente
San Diego, California

Judd Warren Landsberg, M.D.
Clinical Instructor
Department of Medicine
University of California, San Diego,
  School of Medicine
La Jolla, California
Attending Physician
Pulmonary and Critical
  Care Medicine
University of California, San Diego,
  Medical Center
San Diego, California

Thomas E. Lawrie, M.D.
Research Fellow
Division of Pulmonary / Critical
  Care Medicine
University of California, San Diego
San Diego, California

Stephen H. Lee, M.D.
Clinical Instructor
Division of Pulmonary and Critical
  Care Medicine
University of California, San Diego,
  School of Medicine
La Jolla, California

Julian P. Lichter, M.D.
Associate Clinical Professor
Department of Medicine
University of California, San Diego
La Jolla, California
Medical Director
Respiratory Care Departments
Scripps Mercy Hospital
San Diego, California

Philip A. LoBue, M.D., F.A.C.P., F.C.C.P.
Team Leader, Medical Consultant
  Team
Division of Tuberculosis Elimination
Centers for Disease Control and
  Prevention
Atlanta, Georgia

Mark R. Looney, M.D.
Fellow
Division of Pulmonary and Critical Care
  Medicine
University of California, San Francisco,
  School of Medicine
University of California, San Francisco,
  Medical Center
San Francisco, California

Jose S. Loredo, M.D., M.S., F.C.C.P.
Associate Professor of Clinical Medicine
Department of Medicine
University of California, San Diego,
    School of Medicine
Medical Director UCSD Sleep
    Medicine Center
University of California, San Diego,
    Medical Center
San Diego, California

Bao Quoc Luu, M.D.
Pulminologist / Intensivist
Pulmonary and Critical Care
John Muir Medical Center
Walnut Creek, California

Mehran Mandegar, M.D.
Associate Physician
Pulmonary and Critical Care Medicine
University of California, San Diego,
    Medical Center
San Diego, California

Timothy A. Morris, M.D.
Associate Professor of Medicine
Division of Pulmonary and Critical
    Care Medicine
University of California, San Diego,
    School of Medicine
La Jolla, California
Medical Director
Respiratory Care Department
University of California,
    San Diego, Medical Center
San Diego, California

Dominic A. Munafo, Jr., M.D.
Assistant Clinical Professor of Medicine
University of California, San Diego,
    School of Medicine
La Jolla, California
Medical Director
Sleep Data, Inc.
San Diego, California

Kevin M. Murray, M.D.
Staff Physician
Pulmonary Division
Kaiser Permanente
San Diego, California

Tom S. Neuman, M.D., F.A.C.P., F.A.C.P.M.
Professor of Medicine and Surgery
Department of Emergency Medicine
University of California, San Diego
Associate Director
Department of Emergency Medicine

Hillcrest Hospital / Thornton Hospital
San Diego, California

John Scott Parrish, M.D.
Chairman
Critical Care Medicine
Naval Medical Center
San Diego, California

Andrew L. Ries, M.D., M.P.H.
Associate Dean for Academic Affairs
Professor of Medicine and Family and
    Preventive Medicine
University of California, San Diego,
    School of Medicine
La Jolla, California
Director, Pulmonary
    Rehabilitation
University of California, San Diego,
    Medical Center
San Diego, California

Ann M. Romaker, M.D.
Clinical Associate Professor
Department of Internal Medicine
University of Missouri, Kansas City
St. Lukes Hospital
Kansas City, Missouri

Gregory A. Ruff, M.D.
Fellow
Pulmonary / Critical Care Medicine
Naval Medical Center
San Diego, California

Kenneth J. Serio, M.D.
Assistant Professor
Department of Medicine
Division of Pulmonary and
    Critical Care
University of California, San Diego
Staff Physician
VA San Diego Healthcare System
San Diego, California

David M. Shaw, M.D.
Fellow
Pulmonary / Critical Care Medicine
University of California, San Diego
San Diego, California

Cecilia M. Smith, D.O.
Professor of Medicine
Division of Pulmonary and Critical Care
    Medicine
Medical Director
Medical Director's Office
University of California, San Diego,
    Medical Center
San Diego, California

Robert M. Smith, M.D.
Professor
Department of Medicine
Division of Pulmonary and Critical
  Care
University of California, San Diego,
  Medical Center
San Diego, California
Associate Chief of Staff
Director, Critical Care Services
VA San Diego Healthcare System
La Jolla, California

Christopher M. Stafford, M.D.
Pulmonary and Critical Care
  Department
Naval Medical Center
San Diego, California

Antine E. Stenbit, M.D., Ph.D.
Fellow
Department of Medicine / Pulmonary
  Critical Care
University of California, San Diego
San Diego, California

Donna Tigno, M.D.
Fellow
Division of Pulmonary and
  Critical Care
University of California, San Diego
San Diego, California

Angela C. Wang, M.D.
Associate Clinical Professor
  of Medicine

Department of Medicine
University of California, San Diego,
  School of Medicine
Staff Physician and Research Scientist
Department of Medicine
VA San Diego Healthcare System
San Diego, California

James H. Williams, Jr., M.D.
Adjunct Professor
Department of Medicine
University of California, Irvine
Irvine, California
Hospitalist / Intensivist, Pulmonary
  Consultant
Internal Medicine, Pulmonary and
  Critical Care
University of California, Irvine Medical
  Center
Orange, California

Gordon L. Yung, M.D.
Associate Clinical Professor
Department of Surgery
University of California, San Diego,
  School of Medicine
Director, Advanced Lung Diseases
  Program
Medical Director, Lung Transplant
  Program
Department of Medicine
University of California, San Diego,
  Medical Center
San Diego, California

PREFACE

For the last 27 years, I have spent nearly 1 year in 4, together with my co-editors, creating six editions of this manual. It is a process that includes many steps: thoroughly reviewing prior chapters; deciding to add and delete chapters; developing contracts, author lists, and schedules; editing each chapter and references; creating fresh front matter; and approving the final manuscript. I will miss this process, but I am delighted to place it into the highly competent hands of Andy Ries and Tim Morris.

In 1976, fresh out of the U.S. Army Medical Corps, I began my fellowship in pulmonary medicine at the University of California, San Diego (UCSD) Medical Center and sought a project that would further my goal of becoming a clinician. As a medical student in Baltimore, I had been inspired by the likes of T.E. Woodward and M.S. Al-Ibrahim, and as an intern and resident at Mt. Sinai Hospital in New York, I was inspired by such luminaries as the Bader brothers, S. Berson, R. Sherwin, M. Korstin, and F. Swerdlow. Yet, "never did I breathe its pure serene" until, at UCSD, I met Dr. Kenneth Moser (a.k.a. "K.M."), a superb clinician and researcher, and a man beloved by his staff and students. K.M. became my principal teacher, inspiration, lifelong friend, and co-editor of the first four editions of the *Manual of Clinical Problems in Pulmonary Medicine* until his untimely death. Dr. Moser and I labored over every word, each paragraph, and every reference in each edition. He was as passionate about his prose as he was about clinical medicine and research. Dr. Ries and Dr. Morris joined *Clinical Problems* for the fifth edition and immediately contributed their considerable skills, knowledge, and dedication to this project.

Now, we have completed the sixth edition and present a compendium of the most current, authoritative, and well-referenced chapters pertaining to 110 topics. As has been our practice since the first edition, we have removed some of the older chapters and added new ones. Once again, we thank our dedicated group of contributors who have helped to produce this version. As in the previous edition, all proceeds from the sale of this manual will be donated to the Kenneth M. Moser Fellowship Endowment established at UCSD.

Finally, I thank my co-editors, Dr. Andy Ries and Dr. Tim Morris, for the vast quantity of plain hard work that it took to organize and produce this manual. I am sure that K.M. would be proud of the result and comforted that future editions are in good and caring hands that will capture the spirit and quality of this manual—and this man.

RAB

ACKNOWLEDGMENTS

This book would not have been possible without the generous support and hard work of members and friends of the Division of Pulmonary and Critical Care Medicine at the University of California, San Diego (UCSD). Their commitment to this process has been unflagging since its inception. Our editor, Scott Scheidt of Lippincott Williams & Wilkins, has quite simply been a delight to work with; his support, understanding, and, when necessary, gentle prodding helped us to find equilibrium and keep going during what at times seemed like an overwhelming task. We thank him for his guidance and patience. The Web site that Lippincott developed for this project made the task much easier for us and more seamless for the many authors. To Barbara Tipton, who assisted with the myriad administrative details and organized our regular phone conferences, we owe a debt of gratitude. Most of all, we are indebted to and thank all of the contributors—old and new—who provided the background work and, for the most part, helped us meet our deadlines. For all that is good, they deserve the praise. For any shortcomings, we accept the blame.

I. PULMONARY DIAGNOSTIC TECHNIQUES

1. RADIOGRAPHIC EVALUATION OF LUNG DISEASE

Paul J. Friedman and Paul Stark

Chest radiography has provided noninvasive information about patient anatomy and pathology for more than 100 years. The traditional technique uses a cassette or dedicated chest unit with intensifying screens to record the x-ray image and lightboxes for viewing the films. Traditional methods are rapidly being replaced by electronic imaging, computer manipulation, distribution of data via networks, and viewing of images and reports on computer workstations. (Newer imaging modalities such as computed tomography [CT] and magnetic resonance imaging are discussed in Chapter 2.)

Radiography is invaluable in the assessment of lung, pleural, mediastinal, cardiovascular, and chest wall diseases. The effective use of imaging modalities in general, and chest radiography in particular, depends on integrating clinical information with the imaging findings. Knowledge of the limitations and costs of imaging modalities is also essential.

When a patient is considered for a chest radiograph, the clinician should have in mind a specific question and should convey it to the radiologist to get the most constructive and useful interpretation. Supplementary views offer advantages that are rarely appreciated. Selection of such studies requires communication between the chest physician and radiologist. Chest physicians should be aware that the most valuable study to complement an abnormal chest film is comparison to prior chest films.

TECHNIQUE

Standard chest films are made at a 6-foot distance (from x-ray tube focus to film), in posteroanterior (PA) and left lateral projections (left side against the film cassette). The patient is instructed to take a maximal inspiration and hold it; normally, no attempt is made to control whether the patient maintains total lung capacity with the glottis open or closed. The film-screen combination should have a wide latitude and high sensitivity to limit the contrast of the image and the required radiation dose. Using kilovoltage above 120 kilovolt peak (kVp) makes it possible to show findings in the lungs and the mediastinum on the same radiographic film. A fixed grid is used to absorb x-ray scatter. Supplementary methods, such as beam-shaping filters (to intensify mediastinal penetration), asymmetric intensifying screens or film emulsions with high and low sensitivity, as well as anticrossover film base are available.

Portable or bedside examinations, despite their greater cost and lesser quality, account for a large proportion of chest radiographs. They are more difficult to interpret because of shallow inspiration, which crowds normal parenchymal structures together to simulate lung parenchymal abnormalities, and low kilovoltage technique, which can result in overexposed lungs and an underpenetrated mediastinum. Because of the apical lordotic angle of the x-ray beam in the bedridden patient, the diaphragm obscures a considerable portion of the lower lobes. The anteroposterior projection and short tube-film distance geometrically magnify the heart, which also obscures part of the lungs. On supine radiographs, pleural effusions and pneumothorax are more difficult to detect. It is important to avoid overinterpretation of bedside studies, particularly those of poor quality.

Fluoroscopy of the chest serves mainly as a guide to special procedures or as a means of localizing a lesion seen on only one radiographic view. However, diaphragmatic paralysis, mediastinal shift resulting from air trapping, or tracheobronchial collapse can be detected with fluoroscopy.

NONROUTINE RADIOGRAPHIC STUDIES

Apical lordotic views are used in the assessment of lesions obscured by the clavicle and first rib. Tilting the thorax or the x-ray tube to project those anterior structures upward enhances visibility of lesions in the posterior segments of the upper lobes. The apical lordotic projection is not useful for lesions above the level of the clavicle or for anterior pathology. With the high-kilovoltage technique, the bones are much less opaque than they would be with old-fashioned nongrid techniques (70–100 kVp). Hence, this view is now seldom used.

Oblique views were used formerly to assess cardiac chambers, but are now useful mainly to provide additional tangential projection of the pleura, as in screening for asbestos plaques. Localization of pulmonary nodules and differentiation of lung from chest wall pathology can be facilitated. Oblique views also can be useful when abnormalities are in the costophrenic sulcus or superimposed on the hilar shadows.

The lung bases are frequently seen best on supine views of the abdomen, owing to better penetration and more favorable orientation of the central x-ray beam.

Lateral decubitus views are probably overused. In the case of pleural disease, they have a dual function: to show that an effusion is free (not loculated or organized) by layering when it is dependent, and to reveal whether the otherwise obscured lung expands normally when it is nondependent. The decubitus view is named according to the dependent side. The study is often misused to see if large effusions are free (or *layer out*). The real clinical issue with large effusions is whether and where to put the needle or chest tube, not whether the effusion is free. It may require special studies, such as ultrasound or CT to determine the optimal site for drainage. In the bedridden patient, gas-liquid levels in lung abscesses or pleural pockets can be shown best with the decubitus position, because it requires a horizontal x-ray beam to show a gas-liquid level. This position is also effective in the detection of pneumothorax on the nondependent side in patients who cannot assume the upright position. The decubitus position also makes it possible to test for diaphragmatic mobility by producing a deep inspiration on the nondependent side, even in an uncooperative patient.

Frontal chest radiography in the prone position is an underused examination that expands the posterior lung and shifts pleural effusions, resulting in unobstructed views of the lung base.

An expiratory film is traditionally used to detect a small pneumothorax, because the trapped pleural gas will appear larger in a smaller hemithorax. This procedure is not recommended for several reasons: (1) a pneumothorax so small as to be visible only on an expiratory film is not clinically significant; (2) prospective studies have shown that virtually every pneumothorax detected on expiratory films also can be identified on an accompanying inspiratory film; and (3) the expiratory film cannot be compared with prior or subsequent inspiratory studies to see if the patient is getting better or worse. A dynamic expiratory film to test for mediastinal shift or more subtle findings caused by air trapping requires an x-ray exposure before the end of full expiration and restoration of equilibrium. Similarly, a forced expiration, or Valsalva maneuver, will cause a reduction in the size of systemic veins compared to an inspiratory study, and can be used to help distinguish them from nodes.

Conventional tomography is no longer used in facilities that have CT, because both mediastinal and hilar abnormalities are better displayed and diagnosed with CT (Chapter 2).

DIGITAL CHEST RADIOGRAPHY

The pattern of x-rays that emerges from the body has traditionally been captured by intensifying screens whose light directly exposed film. The developed film negative is what we look at on a light box. Since 1980, there has been increasing use of phosphor plates to receive the x-ray image, with electronic readout (CR, or computed radiography), effectively replacing the detection, display, and storage functions of conventional film. The image can be printed on film (hard copy) using a laser printer or, alternatively, can be read from a video screen (soft copy). Detail resolution has improved such that it is now almost comparable to conventional radiography. The wide latitude of CR leads to marked reduction in over- or underpenetrated films.

This technique has been most useful for bedside radiography. Bedside exposures are often technically poor and the computer interface allows correction of image density. Because bedside films are already limited in resolution, no significant degradation of quality is seen with digitized images.

For situations in which a dedicated chest unit can be used, direct digital radiography (DR) has been introduced. The image is formed on a radiation-sensitive selenium- or silicone-based detector, scanned, processed, and sent to a video workstation. In general, nodule detection is superior because of computer enhancement of the image.

One interesting feature is the ability to make images at different x-ray energies, so that it is possible to identify the high atomic number (i.e., calcium) materials in the image by calculation. Bone and soft tissue images can be separated, enhancing the opportunity to show lung lesions without superimposed ribs, or to detect calcium in pulmonary nodules.

PACS (picture archiving and communications system) is an important advance in making images accessible to all, eliminating lost films, improving retrieval of comparison films, and speeding up the radiographic interpretation of current images. All digital images can be viewed simultaneously at multiple sites, eliminating delays.

Computer-Aided Diagnosis

Computer-aided diagnosis (CAD) relies on computerized schemes for automated detection of lung nodules and interstitial lung disease. Automated nodule detection can be implemented as an advanced PACS application. The location of possible nodules can be indicated as overlays on images. Temporal subtraction techniques subtract a previous from a current chest radiograph in order to enhance interval changes. These algorithms have the potential to improve performance and efficacy, and enhance diagnostic accuracy and work flow.

SCREENING

The exception to the concept of carefully planned radiography is the screening examination. Large screening surveys for tuberculosis have been shown to be ineffective with current prevalence rates, although institutions still use routine films for pregnant women who have positive tuberculin skin tests or have not been tested before delivery, and some states require films for teachers or food handlers. Screening films for tuberculosis can be justified in patients in whom skin tests are unreliable (e.g., those with AIDS). Usually, just a frontal view is sufficient.

Screening for occupational lung disease is a well-established practice and has epidemiologic and clinical utility. An elaborate system of classification of pneumoconiosis-related changes in the lungs and pleura has been developed for the International Labour Organization (ILO). A network of readers qualified by examination is maintained by the National Institute of Occupational Safety and Health (NIOSH).

Screening for lung cancer has been studied extensively; its efficacy can be expressed in terms of cost per resectable lung cancer discovered, or by decrease of disease-specific mortality in the population, or by a favorable stage-shift in detected cancers. Recent studies have raised the question of whether early detection of lung cancer actually increases survival or merely brings the patient to care earlier in the course of the disease without lengthening the patient's lifespan. This means that 5-year survival after detection may not be a meaningful measure. Whereas systematic screening of high-risk groups is of debatable but measurable utility, a routine annual chest film, as part of an annual physical examination, is of limited value. See Chapter 2 for further discussion of chest CT in lung cancer screening.

Another controversial screening application is the routine admission chest film. Patients with no history or findings related to the heart or lungs are not likely to show abnormalities. Similarly, a routine preoperative screening chest film has low efficacy in patients without clinical evidence of heart or lung abnormalities, but in patients older than age 60, there is a high likelihood of confirming significant pathology. Preoperative films also can play an important role as reference films in the postoperative period.

Error

Radiologic evaluation of the chest is accompanied by a significant rate of error. Studies dealing with detection of well-defined abnormalities (e.g., lung cancer) have shown an average false-negative rate of 30 to 40%. Part of the error may be attributed to failure to detect lesions against the background complexity of normal anatomy and, in part, to errors in interpreting whether shadows are significant. It has been shown that the likelihood of making a correct diagnosis from the film is enhanced by having an appropriate clinical history and by independent double reading of relevant studies. For these reasons, to maximize accuracy, the primary physician and radiologist should study chest films both independently and in consultation.

1. Fraser RS, Muller NL, Colman N, Pare PD, et al. and Pare's Diagnosis of Diseases of the Chest. 4th Ed. Philadelphia: WB Saunders; 1999.
   Comprehensive review of the subject. Encyclopedic reference source.
2. Reed JC. *Chest Radiology: Plain Film Patterns and Differential Diagnosis.* Philadelphia: Mosby, 2003.
   Practical approach to differential diagnosis and interpretation of chest radiographs.
3. Milne ENC, Pistolesi M. *Reading the Chest Radiograph—A Physiologic Approach.* Philadelphia, Mosby; 1993.
   Detailed review of cardiopulmonary physiology as it pertains to the interpretation of chest radiographs.
4. Friedman PJ. Practical radiology of the hila and mediastinum. *Postgrad Radiol.* 1981;1:269.
   Practical approach to radiographic anatomy as it pertains to interpreting the chest radiograph.
5. International Labour Office. *Guidelines for the Use of the ILO International Classification of Radiographs of Pneumoconiosis.* 2000 Ed. Geneva, ILO, 2002.
6. Schaefer-Prokop C, Uffmann M, Eisenhuber E, et al. Digital radiography of the chest: Detector techniques and performance parameters. *J Thoracic Imag.* 2003; 18:124–137.
   Practical review of physics and equipment used in digital radiography.
7. Mac Mahon H. Digital chest radiography: practical issues. *J Thoracic Imag.* 2003;18:139–147.
   Review of clinical applications of digital chest radiography.
8. Kakeda S, Moriya J, Sato H, et al. Improved detection of lung nodules on chest radiographs using a commercial computer-aided diagnosis system. *AJR* 2004;182: 505–510.
   Describes advantages of computer-aided diagnosis.
9. Mendelson DS, Khilnani N, Wagner LD, et al. Preoperative chest radiography: value as a baseline examination for comparison. *Radiology.* 1987;165:341–343.
   Preoperative chest radiographs may have an important role to play when used as reference films for postoperative imaging.

2. ADVANCED IMAGING AND IMAGE-GUIDED INTERVENTION IN CHEST RADIOLOGY

Paul J. Friedman and Paul Stark

Imaging-based procedures include computed tomography (CT), high-resolution CT (HRCT), magnetic resonance imaging (MRI), diagnostic and interventional ultrasonography, bronchography, bronchial arteriography and embolization, aortography, and percutaneous biopsy or drainage of effusions under image guidance.

COMPUTED TOMOGRAPHY

CT is a reliable way to study nearly all abnormalities of the lungs, pleura, and mediastinum. Because CT displays cross-sectional anatomy with high-contrast resolution, it has inherent advantages over conventional radiographic techniques (1) in showing structures without superimposition and (2) in distinguishing fat, cystic, or solid tissues. Its sensitivity for pulmonary nodules or parenchymal disease is much greater than that of conventional radiography. Intravenous contrast material helps distinguish vessels from other soft tissue structures in the hila and mediastinum (e.g., lymph nodes, tumors). CT has replaced conventional tomography of the lungs and mediastinum, as well as bronchography.

New helical or spiral scanners can acquire data continuously while the patient is moved, allowing a complete scan during the arterial phase of an intravenous injection. It can capture the entire lung without the respiratory misregistration inherent in multiple breath-holds. These scanners use multiple rows of detectors to allow collection of four to 64 simultaneous images. This makes CT screening of the entire lung on a single inspiration possible. Multislice scanning produces volumetric datasets that can be reformatted in any plane, producing two- or even three-dimensional displays (volume rendering). Special applications are CT angiography, including coronary angiography, CT pulmonary arteriography and CT aortography.

Computed tomography can be used to explain abnormal mediastinal contours seen on chest radiography and to detect enlarged lymph nodes in the staging of lung cancer. No significant attenuation differences are seen between lymph nodes enlarged by inflammation or by tumor. CT angiography of the pulmonary arteries has largely replaced ventilation/perfusion scanning for pulmonary embolism in patients without contraindication to intravenous contrast agent, especially in those with an abnormal chest radiograph.

CT is unsurpassed for studying the pleural space. Pleural effusions are readily distinguished from solid masses or consolidated lung. Pleural gas collections can be distinguished from lung abscess cavities more easily than on chest films. Pleural fibrosis or plaques can be readily detected and distinguished from extrapleural fat.

HIGH-RESOLUTION CT

HRCT of the lungs is a well-established procedure. It uses narrow collimation and an edge-enhancing high spatial frequency algorithm. Instead of contiguous 5- to 7-mm thick slices of the lungs, HRCT uses 1-mm thick slices, usually every 10 to 20 mm, to produce spacing appropriate to sampling. The thinner slice reduces volume averaging that obscures fine detail on conventional slices.

Inflammatory changes that are invisible on chest radiographs can be seen with HRCT, including bronchitis, bronchiectasis, early interstitial disease, miliary disease, or minimal alveolar filling. HRCT findings are often more diagnostically specific than those of chest radiography. Emphysema can be detected with greater sensitivity than is reflected in abnormal pulmonary function tests and can be quantified for comparative studies.

MAGNETIC RESONANCE IMAGING

MRI is used only in selected patients with disease of the heart, lungs, and mediastinum. Technically, it should be understood that MRI does not depend on ionizing radiation, but on the magnetic properties of atoms, notably the most abundant—hydrogen. The molecular environment of these atoms affects the rate at which they can dissipate energy, and this energy is converted into a spatial distribution of image densities, using mathematical reconstruction techniques similar to those used in CT. Successful use of MRI in the chest is optimized with cardiac gating when image acquisition time is more than one cardiac cycle, because heart motion shakes the nearby lung and mediastinum.

MRI has lost its advantage over CT in the production of sagittal and coronal (or oblique) images, because multislice CT scanning is widespread and can duplicate these features. CT angiography now competes directly with MR angiography, both usually using contrast material, but otherwise being noninvasive. MRI is still regarded as the gold standard for cardiac chamber volume measurements, especially for the geometrically irregular right ventricle. It is the most accurate, although complex, method of measuring ventricular ejection fraction.

Determination of myocardial viability by measuring delayed gadolinium enhancement is a recent important application. Calcium is invisible on MR scans, so radiographic techniques (including CT) cannot be completely replaced in studying the mediastinum. The soft tissue specificity of MRI is greater than that of CT, however, so that MRI has an important application in the assessment of direct invasion of the chest wall, mediastinum, and diaphragm by lung cancer or malignant mesothelioma.

FLUORODEOXYGLUCOSE POSITRON EMISSION TOMOGRAPHY

Fluorodeoxyglucose positron emission tomography (FDG-PET) is a nuclear medicine technique that labels the glycolytic pathway of tumor cells or other metabolically active cells to identify glucose-avid tissue. This method has a high sensitivity for malignant solitary pulmonary nodules, but because active granulomata can also display high FDG-PET activity, solitary nodules with high activity are indeterminate. Conversely, pulmonary nodules measuring 1 cm or more with no or weak activity can be safely followed with sequential chest radiographs or CT scans to ascertain size stability.

Another application of FDG-PET is staging of bronchogenic carcinoma. Metastatic hilar and mediastinal lymph nodes with high activity can be detected. Unexpected extrathoracic metastases can be detected as well with FDG-PET.

ULTRASONOGRAPHY

Ultrasonography has been used for many years by radiologists and chest physicians to localize pleural effusions and to guide drainage procedures. Less widely used applications include suprasternal, transbronchial, or transesophageal examination of the mediastinum to localize lymph nodes (for biopsy), and transthoracic detection of pulmonary nodules at the time of thoracoscopic biopsy or excision. Transesophageal ultrasound also provides excellent delineation of cardiac valves and flow velocities.

The physical principle of ultrasound imaging is the production of echoes from the vibrations of a piezoelectric crystal transducer by orthogonal tissue planes; the delay in the echo is converted into a distance, and the data are transformed into a cross-section of anatomy. Three-dimensional ultrasound is a new technique that has not been used in chest disease except for experimental work in the fetal heart.

BRONCHOGRAPHY

Bronchography is an archaic technique for evaluating the morphology of the bronchial tree. Its major indication was in the preoperative assessment of bronchiectasis, but HRCT has become the standard for this purpose and in the workup of hemoptysis. Evaluation of central bronchial abnormalities is more directly performed by fiberoptic bronchoscopy, although *virtual bronchoscopy* by three-dimensional reconstruction of multislice CT images is a limited diagnostic alternative.

SELECTIVE BRONCHIAL ARTERIOGRAPHY

Selective bronchial arteriography is useful to identify and treat by embolization enlarged bronchial arteries causing hemorrhage in patients with chronic infection. This is a very specialized procedure, requiring knowledge of anatomic variations of the bronchial and spinal arteries. The principal complication of embolization, aside from failure to control bleeding, is accidental embolization of a spinal artery, with spinal cord damage.

AORTOGRAPHY

Aortography has been used to diagnose aneurysms, pseudoaneurysms and dissections. CT aortography with multislice CT scanners can replace catheter aortography for the diagnosis of acute and chronic aortic diseases, including traumatic aortic rupture.

PERCUTANEOUS LUNG BIOPSY

Percutaneous lung biopsy under fluoroscopic control is discussed in Chapter 8, but lesions too small or too central to be safely needled under the fluoroscope can be biopsied successfully using CT control. CT is now the method of choice for most image-guided biopsy procedures in the chest. Mediastinal nodes can be approached percutaneously with the help of CT and transbronchially or transesophageally with ultrasound. New, faster multidetector row CT scanners offer a *fluoroscopic* mode of several axial views per second, which greatly simplifies the procedure.

The subspecialty of *interventional radiology* is used routinely for percutaneous catheter drainage of pus from various body sites, including the pleural space. Most pleural collections can be drained with the use of ultrasound guidance, but complex cases often require CT, both to establish the anatomic location of the effusion and to help direct the catheter safely. Loculations in a liquid collection can be detected only by sonography. Percutaneous drainage of lung abscess may be considered for patients who cannot control their secretions, to avoid soiling other parts of the lung when the abscess is contiguous to an empyema or thickened pleura.

1. Naidich DP, Muller NL, Zerhouni EA, et al. *Computed Tomography and Magnetic Resonance of the Thorax*. 3rd ed. New York: Lippincott, Williams & Wilkins Publications; 1999.
   Comprehensive reference to CT and MR findings in the chest.
2. Stern EJ, Swensen SJ. *High Resolution CT of the Chest: Atlas*. Philadelphia: Lippincott Williams & Wilkins Publishers; 2001.
   Recent atlas with numerous high resolution images.
3. Remy-Jardin M, Remy J. *Spiral CT of the Chest*. Brooklyn, NY: Springer-Verlag New York; 1996.
   Recent text with a wide range of CT images.
4. Webb WR, Muller NL, Naidich DP. *High Resolution CT of the Lung*. 3rd ed. Philadelphia: Lippincott Williams & Wilkins Publishers; 2001.
   Comprehensive review of the subject.
5. Schoepf UJ, Costello P. CT angiography for diagnosis of pulmonary embolism: state of the art. *Radiology*. 2004;230:329–337.
   Timely review on utility of CT pulmonary angiography.
6. Swensen SJ, Jett JR, Hartman TE, et al. Lung cancer screening with CT: Mayo Clinic experience. *Radiology*. 2003;226:757–761.
   This paper emphasizes problems and challenges of lung cancer screening.
7. Henschke CI, Yankelevitz DF, Naidich DP, et al. CT screening for lung cancer: suspiciousness of nodules according to size on baseline scans. *Radiology*. 2004;231:164–168.
   Helpful stratification of nodules according to size and strategy for follow-up examinations.
8. Kavanagh EC, O'Hare A, Hargaden G, et al. Risk of pulmonary embolism after negative MDCT pulmonary angiography findings. *AJR*. 2004;182:499–504.
   Report emphasizes negative predictive value of CT pulmonary angiography.

9. Worthy SA, Muller NL, Hartman TE, et al. Mosaic attenuation pattern on thin-section CT scans of the lung: differentiation among infiltrative lung, airway, and vascular diseases as a cause. *Radiology*. 1997;205:465.
10. Cartier Y, Kavanagh PV, Johkoh T, et al. Bronchiectasis: accuracy of high-resolution CT in the differentiation of specific diseases. *AJR*. 1999;173:47.
11. Johkoh T, Muller NL, Cartier Y, et al. Idiopathic interstitial pneumonias: diagnostic accuracy of thin-section CT in 129 patients. *Radiology*. 1999;211:555.
   9.-11. Recent reports on the utility of HRCT in diffuse lung disease and small airways disease.
12. Yoon W, Kim JK, Kim YH, et al. Bronchial and nonbronchial systemic artery embolism for life-threatening hemoptysis: a comprehensive review. *RadioGraphics*. 2002;22:1395–1409.
   Review of anatomy, pathology, and interventional procedures in patients with massive hemoptysis.
13. Rubens DJ, Strang JG, Fulz PJ, et al. Sonographic guidance of mediastinal biopsy: an effective alternative to CT guidance. *AJR*. 1997;169:1605.
14. Gould MK, Kuschner WG, Rydzak CE. Test performance of positron emission tomography and computed tomography for mediastinal staging in patients with non–small-cell lung cancer: a meta-analysis. *Ann Intern Med*. 2003;139:879.
   Comprehensive review of FDG-PET utility in staging lung cancer.
15. Lardinois D, Weder W, Hany TF. Staging of non–small-cell lung cancer with integrated positron-emission in tomography and computed tomography. *N Engl J Med*. 2003;348:2500.
16. Macura KJ, Corl FM, Fishman EK, et al. Pathogenesis in acute aortic syndromes. *AJR*. 2003;181:303–316.
   Well-illustrated review of aortic aneurysms, dissections, penetrating ulcers, intramural hematomas, and lacerations.

3. PULMONARY FUNCTION TESTING

Jack L. Clausen

The pulmonary function laboratory is a valuable resource for the diagnosis and management of patients with respiratory disorders. Pulmonary function tests (PFTs) serve multiple clinical purposes: (1) uncover clinically undetected dysfunction and disease, (2) diagnose and characterize type of dysfunction, (3) evaluate objectively physiologic severity of disease; and (4) monitor response to therapeutic interventions. The utility of PFTs varies according to the technical and clinical expertise of the personnel performing the studies. In addition, optimal equipment, testing techniques, accurate measurements, data reduction, and selection of appropriate normal predictive data are essential.

Because of the wide range of normal values observed for most PFTs, it is essential to narrow the predicted *normal* range for a given patient, if *normal* is to be distinguished from *abnormal* with any degree of precision. This distinction may be achieved by using regression equations based on parameters such as age, height, and sex. For some PFTs, weight, race, and altitude of the laboratory can also be important. Published series for predicted normal values are numerous. Suggested references are listed in Table 3-1.

Predicted values for some pulmonary function parameters differ by race which, in part, may be secondary to differences in nutrition. Optimal correction factors are controversial and not well defined. For African Americans, the American Thoracic Society recommends reducing Caucasian predicted values for vital capacity (VC),

Table 3-1. Suggested references for normal values

Test	References[a]
Spirometry	6, 7, 10
Flow-volume	8
Lung volumes (RV, FRC, TLC)	9, 10, 22
DLCO	13, 14
PaO_2, $PaCO_2$, pH	12
MIP/MEP	11

RV, Residual volume; *FRC,* Functional residual capacity; *TLC,* Total lung capacity; *PaO₂,* Arterial oxygen tension; *PaCO₂,* Partial pressure of carbon dioxide in arterial blood; *DLCO,* Carbon monoxide, diffusing capacity; *MIP,* Maximum inspiratory pressure.
[a] Numbers refer to references at the end of this chapter.

total lung capacity (TLC), and forced expiratory volume in one second (FEV_1) by 12%. Predictive values for residual volume (RV), functional residual capacity (FRC), and instantaneous flows (e.g., forced expiratory flow [FEF] 50%) are reduced by 7%. For Asians, the issue of race correction is more complex and is affected by the subject's nutritional history; in our laboratory, we use a 7% reduction for VC, TLC, and FEV_1.

For many PFT parameters (e.g., VC and FEV_1), predictive values for a given patient calculated from equations from different published studies are generally similar. For other tests (e.g., single-breath diffusing capacity for carbon monoxide [DLCO], instantaneous maximal expiratory flows, partial pressure of oxygen in arterial blood [PaO_2]), predictive values derived from different equations can differ significantly. For such parameters, it is important that each laboratory evaluate its testing methodology and choice of predicted values by comparing measured values in normal subjects (n = 10–20) with the predicted ones. If more normal subjects than expected have test results outside normal limits, then both the testing methodology and choice of predictive values need to be reevaluated. The optimal prediction equations can then be identified from the study that produces the lowest sum of residuals.

The clinical significance of PFT results for an individual patient often requires an appreciation of the lower limits of normalcy. Although the mean minus 1.96 times SD (two-tailed *t* test, *P* <.05) is a commonly used statistical criterion, the mean minus 1.65 times SD (one-tailed *t* test, *P* <.05) is a more appropriate lower or upper limit of normal when extreme values in one direction are not considered to be clinically abnormal (e.g., high flow rates or VC). For parameters in which the data are not distributed normally, the lower limits must be defined either by normalizing the regression equation or by observing the actual upper and lower percentile values taken from a large population. Exact identification of the limits of normalcy for a specific patient is most readily accomplished using computer-developed reports that use the specific limits of normalcy from each prediction equation. Approximate lower limits of normal (95th percentile) are presented in Table 3-2.

Because results from patients with mild disease can widely overlap the range of predicted normal values, for borderline-low results (e.g., 90th percentile), it is often best to interpret such results as being consistent with either mild disease or normal function (*low-normal*). Such a conclusion may suggest the need for further testing if clinically indicated.

Despite rigorous efforts to predict optimal normal values, a relatively wide range of normalcy is still found for most PFT parameters. Hence, the most useful predictive values in an individual patient are baseline measurements made when the patient was free of disease.

Logical selection of appropriate PFTs is essential for obtaining the maximal clinical information without unnecessary overuse of healthcare resources. A variety of tests are available; selection should be based on the clinical problem being evaluated. A survey of the available tests and their potential applications follows.

Table 3-2. Approximate upper and lower limits of normal at the fifth percentile level

Parameter	Limits of normal (% of predicted)
VC, FVC	75
FRC	70, 130
RV	65, 135
TLC	80, 120
FEV_1	75
FEV_1/FVC (%)	85
FEF 25/75	65
MIP	65

VC, Vital capacity; *FVC*, Forced vital capacity; *FRC*, Functional residual capacity; *RV*, Residual volume; *TLC*, Total lung capacity; *FEV_1*, One-second forced expiratory volume; *FEF*, Forced expiratory flow; *MIP*, Maximum inspiratory pressure.

Spirometry can be used to measure the inspiratory and expiratory flow rates (Fig. 3-1). It allows assessment of certain lung volumes (e.g., tidal volume, expiratory reserve volume, inspiratory capacity, and VC) (Fig. 3-2). Simple spirometry can usually differentiate obstructive from restrictive pulmonary disorders by measuring VC and expiratory flow rates. In obstructive disorders, spirometry demonstrates a decrease in flow rates and a normal or decreased VC. Asthma, chronic bronchitis, and emphysema are the most common obstructive diseases; obstruction can also result from a localized lesion (e.g., a tumor, foreign body, granulation tissue, or scarring) anywhere in the tracheobronchial tree.

A large number of processes cause restrictive lung diseases (conditions that reduce TLC). This complicated differential diagnosis can be simplified into five basic pathophysiologic categories (summarized by the mnemonic PAINT): Pleural disease, Alveolar, Interstitial, Neuromuscular weakness involving ventilatory muscles, and Thoracic cage abnormalities (e.g., kyphoscoliosis, obesity).

In restrictive diseases, spirometry demonstrates a decrease in VC and normal or increased ratio of FEV_1 to forced vital capacity (FVC). Flow rates may be reduced solely because of the reduction of absolute lung volumes in the absence of any identifiable causes of obstructive airway disease (Fig. 3-3). Spirometry alone, however, cannot identify the presence of restriction when a patient has combined obstructive and restrictive disorders; in such patients, direct measurements of TLC are needed to identify and quantify the degree of restriction.

The FEV_1 is the most reproducible flow parameter and is particularly useful in diagnosing and monitoring response to therapy in patients with obstructive disease. The FEF measured during expiration of 25 to 75% of the VC ($FEF_{25-75\%}$), previously called *maximum mid-expiratory flow rate*, may be more sensitive than the FEV_1 in detecting mild dysfunction of the small airways, but the long-term clinical significance of this finding is uncertain. The broader range of normal values for $FEF_{25-75\%}$ and instantaneous flows such as $FEF_{50\%}$ and $FEF_{75\%}$ also limits the clinical usefulness of these parameters.

In an effort to obviate the need for prolonged forced expiration in patients with obstructive lung disease, the FEV expired in the first 6.0 seconds (FEV_6) has been proposed as a surrogate for FVC. Analyses indicate that the FEV_1/FEV_6 is comparable to the FEV_1/FVC ratio for identifying obstructive lung disease, is reasonably comparable to FVC for diagnosing restrictive disease, and that its reproducibility is superior to FVC. Volume-based flow parameters (e.g., $FEF_{25-75\%}$), however, may differ significantly if based on the FEV_6 rather than the FVC, necessitating new reference values based on the FEV_6.

Spirometry performed before and after exercise is useful for confirming the diagnosis of exercise-induced asthma. In patients undergoing evaluation for hypersensitivity lung disease (bronchospastic or restrictive), physiologic testing after inhalation of

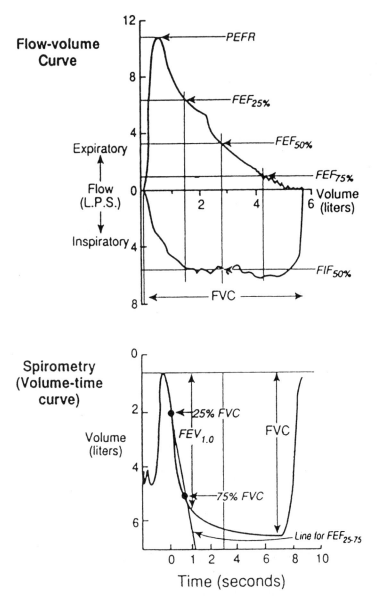

FIG. 3-1. Illustrations of measurements of forced vital capacity and maximal inspiratory and expiratory flow parameters from either flow-volume curves or volume-time curves. (Reproduced with permission from Clausen J. Pulmonary function testing, In: Kelley's *Textbook of Internal Medicine,* 4th edition. Editors: Humes HD. (Editor-in-Chief), DuPont HL, Gardner LB, Griffin JW, Harris JR ED, Hazzard WR, et al. Lippincott Williams & Wilkins, Philadelphia, 2000. [From: Slonim NB, Hamilton LH. *Respiratory Physiology.* 3rd ed. St. Louis: Mosby; 1976.])

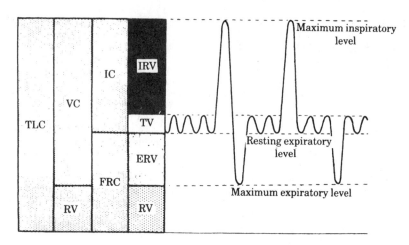

FIG. 3-2. The static lung volumes are derived from standard spirometry and from a measurement of functional residual capacity, either by body plethysmography or by gas dilution or washout. They include TLC (total lung capacity), VC (vital capacity), RV (residual volume), FRC (functional residual capacity), TV (tidal volume), IRV (inspiratory reserve volume), ERV (expiratory reserve volume), and IC (inspiratory capacity). (Reproduced with permission from Comroe Jr JH. *Physiology of Respiratory*, 2nd ed. Chicago: Year Book; 1974.)

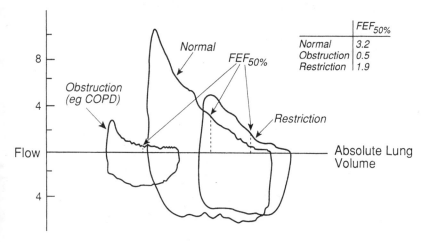

FIG. 3-3. Examples of flow-volume curves in obstructive and restrictive disease (flow-volume loops demonstrating normal, obstructive, and restrictive patterns). Although representing the same respiratory maneuver as the standard volume-time plot, the flow-volume loop provides a more graphic demonstration of the relationship of flow rates to lung volumes. Although flow rates referenced to forced vital capacity (FVC) are lower than normal in the patient with restriction, when referenced to the absolute lung volumes, the flows are actually higher than in a normal subject. (Reproduced with permission from Clausen J. Pulmonary function testing. In: Kelley's *Textbook of Internal Medicine,* 4th edition. Editors: Humes HD. (Editor-in-Chief), DuPont HL, Gardner LB, Griffin JW, Harris JR ED, Hazzard WR, et al. Lippincott Williams & Wilkins, Philadelphia, 2000. [From Slonim NB, Hamilton LH. *Respiratory Physiology.* 3rd ed. St. Louis: Mosby; 1976.])

cholinergic agents or of the suspected antigenic material is often useful in identifying a specific cause. In addition to serial measurements of VC and expiratory flow rates (and airway resistance or specific conductance, if available), temperature and white blood cell count should be monitored after antigen inhalation.

In contrast to the spirogram, which measures volume versus time, the flow-volume loop (Figs. 3-1 and 3-3) displays flow rates in relation to lung volume during maximum inspiration from RV and maximum expiration from TLC. The principal advantage of the flow-volume loop is that the relationship of flows to lung volume is more readily recognized. Although marked blunting of peak flows and the resultant square loop shape of flow-volume curves are commonly taught to be characteristic of localized upper airway obstruction (e.g., tracheal stenosis), it is important to note that these are relatively insensitive signs of localized obstruction and usually signify severe localized airway narrowing (Fig. 3-4).

Gas dilution (or washout) techniques, body plethysmography, and radiographic planimetry can be used to measure the absolute volumes of the lung (i.e., TLC, FRC, RV). In normal subjects, all three techniques give comparable results, but this is

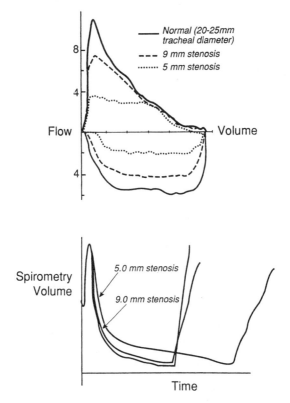

FIG. 3-4. Effects of different degrees of tracheal obstruction on volume-time and flow-volume displays. The squared loop characteristic of localized fixed obstruction of central airways (e.g., tracheal stenosis) is not apparent until the stenosis approaches a 9-mm diameter opening, and it is even more difficult to appreciate from volume-time displays. (Reproduced with permission from Clausen J. Pulmonary function testing. In: Kelley's *Textbook of Internal Medicine*, 4th edition. Editors: Humes HD. (Editor-in-Chief), DuPont HL, Gardner LB, Griffin JW, Harris JR ED, Hazzard WR, et al. Lippincott Williams & Wilkins, Philadelphia, 2000. [From Slonim NB, Hamilton LH. *Respiratory Physiology*. 3rd ed. St. Louis: Mosby; 1976.])

frequently not the case in patients with certain lung diseases. Gas dilution techniques (e.g., helium dilution, nitrogen washout) are the most commonly available methods for measuring absolute lung volume but often underestimate the true TLC in patients with obstructive disease, because they measure only the lung volume that communicates freely with the upper airways. Body plethysmography measures the compressible gas volume within the thorax and gives more accurate TLC measurements in chronic obstructive pulmonary disease, although under some conditions plethysmography may overestimate lung volumes in patients with severe obstruction. TLC can also be measured from conventional posteroanterior chest radiographs using planimetric or ellipsoid techniques; although averages of radiographic volumes from groups of normal subjects have shown remarkable correspondence to plethysmographically measured TLC, the accuracy of the measurements in individual patients can limit the clinical usefulness of these measurements to serial studies. In patients with severe reduction in lung volumes from space-occupying abnormalities, radiographic TLC can be significantly larger than plethysmographic measurements. Assuming the patient has made an adequate effort (an oft-overlooked assumption), a reduced TLC indicates the presence of a restrictive disorder.

Measurements of DLCO by either the single-breath or the steady-state method are relatively sensitive, but nonspecific, indicators of respiratory dysfunction and loss of alveolar-capillary surface area. Decreases in the single-breath DLCO correlate well with loss of lung tissue secondary to emphysema; however, in contrast to the steady-state method, the single-breath method occasionally gives false-negative results. Because of the wide range of normal values, both the single-breath and steady-state techniques are of limited usefulness for early detection of emphysema. The DLCO is also reduced in a variety of restrictive diseases involving the lung parenchyma such as sarcoidosis, interstitial fibrosis, and drug toxicity. It can also be low in pulmonary vascular diseases such as pulmonary emboli; hence, the specificity of the DLCO is low. The test may be most useful in the evaluation of a patient complaining of dyspnea who has normal spirometry and arterial blood gases. In such patients, a low DLCO strongly suggests the presence of significant lung disease, although a normal DLCO does not exclude the presence of disease. Recent data also indicate that serial measurements of DLCO are useful in treating patients with Goodpasture's syndrome, in which an occult pulmonary hemorrhage is mirrored by an increase in DLCO.

Measurements of the elastic recoil (ER) and static compliance (SC) of the lung require measuring changes in esophageal pressure obtained via an esophageal balloon and plotting these changes versus the corresponding changes in lung volume. The SC measures the ratio of the change in lung volume to the change in transpulmonary pressure—pressure required for lung inflation, or alveolar minus pleural pressure—during periods of no gas flow. The transpulmonary pressure measured at TLC reflects the ER of the lung and is useful for physiologically documenting pathologic alterations in lung elasticity in diseases such as sarcoidosis (increased ER) or emphysema (decreased ER). The wide range of reported normal values, however, significantly limits the sensitivity of the ER or SC for early detection of disease. The time and technical expertise required for these measurements, as well as limited patient acceptance, prevent their use as routine or screening procedures.

Closing volume, phase III slope, helium-oxygen studies, and assessments of dynamic compliance are tests that may be sensitive indicators of early small airways dysfunction. However, because these tests generally do not identify the patients whose disease will progress to clinically disabling obstructive lung disease, they now play a limited role in clinical practice.

Maximum inspiratory pressure is determined during maximum inspiratory effort against a closed system, usually at RV. It is a useful direct test of inspiratory muscle strength and should be evaluated in all patients with suspected neuromuscular disease or in those with dyspnea, restricted lung volumes, and an absence of parenchymal or thoracic cage abnormalities on chest roentgenograms.

Maximum inspiratory pressure is nonspecific in that it cannot distinguish among lack of effort, muscle weakness or dysfunction, and neural disease. Nonetheless, the test is useful for following the course of the disease. Tests to assess respiratory muscle fatigue have improved but are too complex for widespread clinical use. The contributions of respiratory muscle fatigue to dyspnea and respiratory failure remain poorly defined.

Exercise testing is useful for diagnosis and assessment of dysfunction in patients with lung and heart disease (see Chapter 4). Its measured parameters include respiratory rate and tidal volumes, arterial blood gases, expired gas concentrations, and, frequently, heart rate and blood pressure. Abnormalities in gas exchange (e.g., hypoxemia or hypercapnia) can occur in patients who are normal at rest. Exercise testing can be valuable in detecting lung disease, assessing the impact on exercise, establishing the need for supplementary oxygen, and assessing the impact of therapy, including rehabilitation programs for patients with chronic lung diseases.

Assessments of changes in FRC and flow limitation of tidal volumes during exercise can help to identify causes of dyspnea during exercise and exercise limitation not otherwise detected during conventional exercise testing. Such testing is currently available in relatively few centers, and its clinical usefulness remains to be fully defined. Assessing changes in tidal breathing flow-volume curves during the application of negative pressures can be useful also in identifying patients for whom airway collapse may play an important role in the genesis of dyspnea at rest or during exercise.

The development of pulse oximeters has clearly expanded the ability to monitor arterial oxygenation in a variety of situations (e.g., during general anesthesia or bronchoscopy, and in intensive care units). However, the absolute accuracy of these devices for measuring oxygen saturation (± 3-5%) limits their usefulness when accurate assessments of oxygenation are needed (e.g., prescribing long-term ambulatory oxygen therapy, detecting changes in arterial oxygenation with exercise).

Causes of hypoxemia include hypoventilation, diffusion abnormalities, ventilation-perfusion mismatches, right-to-left shunts, and decreased oxygen in inspired gases. Gas exchange abnormalities leading to hypoxemia and hypercapnia occur as a result of (1) wasted ventilation, when lung units are ventilated but not perfused, (2) shunted pulmonary blood flow when lung units are perfused but not ventilated, and, more commonly, (3) other less extreme forms of ventilation-perfusion ($\dot{V}/\dot{Q}$) mismatch. The alveolar-arterial oxygen difference (P[A-a]O_2) estimates the degree of shunt and *low* ($\dot{V}/\dot{Q}$) mismatch. More specific tests are available to quantify and define the topography of such mismatching within the lungs. Wasted ventilation can be calculated by determining the percentage of alveolar dead space ($\dot{V}_D$) per unit of tidal ventilation ($\dot{V}_T$) using the Bohr equation:

$$\dot{V}_D/\dot{V}_T = \frac{Pa_{CO_2} - P_E{CO_2}}{Pa_{CO_2}}$$

where $P_E{CO_2}$ is the end-tidal expiratory concentration of carbon dioxide and Pa_{CO_2} is the arterial carbon dioxide concentration. An elevated $\dot{V}_D/\dot{V}_T$ (>0.45), in the absence of restrictive or obstructive lung disease, may suggest pulmonary vascular disease.

The degree of right to left shunt can be assessed by determining the arterial oxygen tension (Pa_{O_2}) while the patient breathes 100% oxygen; this technique does not distinguish between intracardiac and intrapulmonary shunts. A Pa_{O_2} of less than 550 mmHg suggests the presence of a shunt. However, resorptive atelectasis induced by breathing 100% oxygen may convert areas of low ($\dot{V}/\dot{Q}$) to apparent shunt. Quantitative information regarding the spectrum of ($\dot{V}/\dot{Q}$) mismatch can be derived by elegant but complicated multiple inert gas methods. So far, these methods remain a tool of the research laboratory. The topography of ($\dot{V}/\dot{Q}$) relationships can be displayed in a semiquantitative fashion by ventilation and perfusion scintiphotography.

The importance of disturbances of respiration during sleep has been increasingly recognized. Comprehensive sleep studies, including electromyographically and electroencephalographically defined stages of sleep and arousals, are important for understanding the relationship between disturbances of respiration and sleep, daytime fatigue, and excessive daytime sleepiness. The increasing availability of miniaturized, portable multichannel recorders has made available options much less expensive than full polysomnography for the detection of nocturnal desaturation, alterations in inspiratory airflow and ventilatory effort, and cardiac arrhythmias that may occur only during sleep, with resultant impact on daytime function (see Chapter 77).

1. American Thoracic Society. Lung function testing: selection of reference values and interpretative strategies. *Am Rev Respir Dis*. 1991;144:1202.
   Consensus document contains recommendations regarding the use of predicted values and the interpretation of PFT.
2. Clausen JL. *Pulmonary Function Testing Guidelines and Controversies: Equipment, Methods, and Normal Values.* New York: Academic Press; 1983.
   Detailed guidelines for methods of clinical pulmonary function testing.
3. Coates JE. *Lung Function: Assessment and Application in Medicine.* 5th ed. Oxford: Blackwell Scientific Publications; 1993.
   An enduring and comprehensive guide to pulmonary function testing.
4. Cerveri I, Dore R, Corsico A, et al. Assessment of emphysema in COPD: a functional and radiologic study. *Chest*. 2004;125:1714–1718.
   One of a couple of recent articles comparing PFTs and high resolution CT (HRCT)scans for assessing the extent of emphysema. FRC, $FEV_{50\%}/FIV_{50\%}$ ratio, and $DLCO/V_A$correlated with extent of emphysema as determined by HRCT.
5. Coates AL, Peslin R, Rodenstein D, et al. Measurement of lung volumes by plethysmography. *Eur Respir J*. 1997;10:1415.
   Comprehensive review of these demanding measurements by experts experienced withboth pediatric and adult applications.
6. Hankinson JL, Odencrantz JR, Fedan KB. Spirometric reference values from a sample of the general U.S. population. *Am J Respir Crit Care Med*. 1999;159:179–187.
   An important contribution because of the inclusion of significant numbers of Blacks and Hispanics in the subjects.
7. Crapo RO, Morris AH, Gardner RM. Reference spirometric values using techniques and equipment that meet ATS recommendations. *Am Rev Respir Dis*. 1981;123:659.
   Sophisticated statistical analyses and comparisons with other published studies.
8. Bass H. The flow volume loop: normal standards and abnormalities in chronic obstructive pulmonary disease. *Chest*. 1973;63:171.
   Contains predictive equations for both inspiratory and expiratory flow rates derived from 247 nonsmoking adults.
9. Crapo RO, Morris AH, Clayton PD, et al. Lung volumes in healthy nonsmoking adults. *Bull Eur Physiopathol Respir*. 1982;18:419.
   Although measured by the single-breath helium dilution technique, which may result in volumes in healthy subjects slightly (e.g., 0.3 L) smaller than plethysmography, the predicted values from these equations were among the best when testing normals and equations in our laboratory.
10. European Respiratory Society. Standardized lung function testing. *Eur Respir J*. 1993;6(suppl 16):1.
    Includes reference values for spirometry, lung volumes, and DLCO developed by merging data from a number of different studies.
11. Black LF, Hyatt RE. Maximal static respiratory pressures in generalized neuromuscular disease. *Am Rev Respir Dis*. 1971;102:641.
    Includes references for normal values.
12. Crapo RO, Jensen RL, Hegewald M, et al. Arterial blood gas reference values for sea level and an altitude of 1,400 meters. *Am J Respir Crit Care Med*. 1999;160:1525.
    A meticulous and comprehensive contribution that includes well-defined confidence limits. The predicted values for PaO_2 are significantly higher than those of Sorbini, et al., Respiration 1968;25:3, a reference used commonly in the past.

13. Crapo RO, Morris AH. Standardized single breath normal values for carbon monoxide diffusing capacity. *Am Rev Respir Dis.* 1981;123:185.

Although widely used for predictive values for DLCO, for many laboratories the values are inappropriately high, perhaps related to the 1400 meter elevation of the study sample.

14. Miller A, Thornton JC, Warshaw R, et al. Single breath diffusing capacity in a representative of the population of Michigan, a large industrial state. *Am Rev Respir Dis.* 1983;127:270.

An important source because it includes predictive equations for both nonsmokers and smokers and represents data from adults living at sea level altitudes.

15. ATS Statement. Single breath carbon monoxide diffusing capacity (transfer factor): recommendations for a standard technique—1995 update. *Am J Respir Crit Care Med.* 1995;152:2185.

Recommendations approved by the American Thoracic Society, which, if followed, should reduce interlaboratory differences for measurements of DLCO.

16. ATS Statement. Standardization of spirometry—1994 update. *Am J Respir Crit Care Med.* 1995;152:1107.

American Thoracic Society recommendations on standards for instrumentation and methods of spirometry; widespread adoption of these standards should reduce interlaboratory differences of spirometry results.

17. Shade DRJ, Cordova F, Lando Y, et al. Relationship between resting hypercapnia and physiologic parameters before and after lung volume reduction surgery in severe chronic obstructive pulmonary disease. *Am J Respir Crit Care Med.* 1999;159:1405.

In addition to illustrating the important role that PFT is playing in selecting patients for and assessing the benefits of lung volume reduction surgery, this article challenges the convention of labeling patients with CO_2 retention as high risk for thoracic surgery.

18. Crapo RO, Casaburi R, Coates AL, et al. Guidelines for methacholine and exercise challenge testing-1999. *Am J Respir Crit Care Med.* 2000;161:309–329.

Guidelines adopted by the ATS in 1999. Standardization of these complex tests is long overdue. However, the usefulness of these guidelines is diluted somewhat by a number of the controversial issues being resolved by approving alternative methods for which scientific evidence of equivalency is not always available.

19. Carlin BW, Clausen JL, Ries AL. The use of cutaneous oximetry in the prescription of long-term oxygen therapy. *Chest.* 1988;94:239.

An important example of the limitations of cutaneous oximetry. More than 80% of patients who would qualify for home oxygen therapy based on measurement of PaO_2 did not qualify based on pulse oximetry.

20. Hart N, Kearney MT, Pride NB, et al. Inspiratory muscle load and capacity in chronic heart failure. *Thorax.* 2004;59:477–482.

Illustrates current methodology for assessing inspiratory muscle strength and endurance.

21. Babb TG, Rodarte JR. Exercise capacity and breathing mechanics in patients with airflow limitation. *Med Sci Sports Exerc.* 1992;24:967.

Illustrates the greater sensitivity of analyses of tidal breathing flow limitation duringexercise to limitations in exercise when compared with the expired volume per unit time:maximumvoluntary ventilation ratio.

22. Clausen JL and Wanger JS, for the Workshop Participants, ATS/NHLBI Consensus Document 12 Nov 03, Consensus Statement on Measurements of Lung Volumes in Humans. 2003; *http://www.thoracic.org/adobe/lungvolume.pdf.*

The complete final report from the ATS and ERS on measurements of lung volumes in humans and includes sections on methodology, reference values, pathophysiology, and clinical significance.

23. Swanney MP, Jensen RL, Crichton DA, et al. FEV(6) is an acceptable surrogate for FVC in the spirometric diagnosis of airway obstruction and restriction. *Am J Respir Crit Care Med.* 2000;162(3 pt 1):917–919.

This study supports the termination of FVC efforts after 6.0 seconds, thereby obviating the need for prolonged maximal expiratory efforts in patients with obstructive lung disease. Normal values for the FEV_6 are being published.

24. Eltayara L, Becklake MR, Volta CA, et al. Relationship between chronic dyspnea and expiratory flow limitation in patients with chronic obstructive pulmonary disease. *Am J Respir Crit Care Med.* 1996;154:1726.

    One of a number of papers on the application of negative pressures at the mouth during tidal expiration to identify and assess the consequences of airway collapse during mechanical ventilation, spontaneous breathing, and exercise.

4. EXERCISE

Andrew L. Ries

Exercise is a physiologic stimulus that stresses the body's reserves for increased metabolic activity and gas transport necessary to produce energy to meet this work demand. Diseases that reduce reserves in organ function will produce exertional symptoms not present at rest. Physiologic evaluation in clinical medicine, however, generally has been limited to the resting state. Dyspnea on exertion is among the most common complaints leading patients to seek medical advice. Because dyspnea is a subjective symptom, with multiple potential origins, evaluation during exercise can be used to reproduce the patient's symptoms and to characterize the physiologic responses. In recent years, exercise testing has become more widely used in evaluating pulmonary patients.

Exercise testing may have several objectives:

1. Measure an individual's work capacity (e.g., to guide exercise training, follow the course of disease, prognostic indicator of risk)
2. Assess the factors limiting exercise tolerance (e.g., evaluation of unexplained dyspnea, assess respiratory disability)
3. Evaluate changes in gas exchange with physical activity (e.g., detect exercise-induced hypoxemia, prescribe supplemental oxygen)
4. Evaluate exercise-induced bronchospasm-asthma (e.g., assess changes with disease or the effects of therapeutic interventions)
5. Determine the need for certain forms of therapy (e.g., supplemental oxygen).

There are differences in the physiologic principles and appropriate techniques used for exercise testing of different populations, such as normal individuals, cardiac patients, and patients with pulmonary disease. These differences reflect the reason(s) for exercise limitation in each of these groups. Therefore, to be safe and informative, exercise testing should be planned with consideration of these limiting factors.

In the normal individual, maximum exercise capacity is limited by the level to which cardiac output can be elevated and by the ability of the muscles to generate sufficient metabolic energy. No limitations are imposed by ventilatory reserves or pulmonary gas exchange, except with extreme exercise levels.

In normal subjects, low-level exercise results in an increase in cardiac output (primarily due to an increase in heart rate), widening of the arterial-mixed venous oxygen difference (a-vO_2), and increase in oxygen consumption ($\dot{V}O_2$) and carbon dioxide production ($\dot{V}CO_2$). Minute ventilation increases sufficiently to maintain the alveolar ventilation at a level sufficient to remove all the carbon dioxide produced; therefore, the PaCO_2 remains normal. The P(A-a)O_2 gradient may decrease slightly with exercise because of improvement in ventilation-perfusion ($\dot{V}/\dot{Q}$) relationships as pulmonary blood flow increases and pulmonary perfusion becomes more evenly distributed.

As the exercise level is increased further, the blood flow to the exercising muscles ultimately becomes inadequate to provide sufficient oxygen to maintain pure aerobic metabolism. At that point, anaerobic glycolytic metabolism occurs (anaerobic threshold). Lactic acid enters the venous circulation, is buffered by bicarbonate, and an additional amount of carbon dioxide is produced. In response to this nonoxidative carbon dioxide production, minute ventilation ($\dot{V}_E$) rises disproportionately to the $\dot{V}O_2$—a signal that the anaerobic threshold has been reached. At higher exercise levels, lactic acidosis decreases the pH level sufficiently to drive $\dot{V}_E$ higher, out of proportion to carbon dioxide production, causing a fall in $PaCO_2$. This classic sequence of response to exercise has been characterized carefully in normal subjects. For example, at lower "aerobic" levels of exercise, the physiologic variables reflecting increased metabolic demand are related closely, e.g., $\dot{V}O_2$, $\dot{V}CO_2$, $\dot{V}_E$, heart rate, cardiac output, and a-vO_2. The patterns of response to exercise stress can be used to detect abnormalities in patients with cardiac or pulmonary dysfunction. In patients with left ventricular failure and reduced stroke volume, for instance, the heart rate increases and the a-vO_2 difference widens more at a given level of $\dot{V}O_2$ than in normal subjects.

In many patients with lung diseases, the classic physiologic principles described in normals are not followed during exercise, because pulmonary patients generally are not limited by hemodynamic capabilities but rather, by ventilatory function limitations, pulmonary gas exchange compromise, or both. Recent evidence suggests that peripheral muscle dysfunction also may contribute to the limitations in maximum exercise tolerance in patients with chronic lung disease. Ventilatory limitations are imposed by factors such as disordered respiratory mechanics, an increase in the work of breathing, disturbances of $\dot{V}/\dot{Q}$ relationships (e.g., large dead space ventilation), and respiratory muscle fatigue. Recent work emphasizes the important role of dynamic hyperinflation in end-tidal lung volume in patients with chronic obstructive pulmonary disease (COPD) as a cause of exertional dyspnea and exercise limitation. Gas exchange limitations may be a consequence of alveolar hypoventilation, shunting, and right heart failure, or $\dot{V}/\dot{Q}$ mismatch. Because the limitation to exercise in many pulmonary patients is not of hemodynamic origin, the use of heart rate, for example, to guide "maximum exercise" or training targets is often not useful. Furthermore, many patients with moderate to severe lung disease may not achieve a definable anaerobic threshold because they are forced by dyspnea to discontinue exercise before this point is reached.

Thus, it is characteristic in pulmonary patients for exercise limitation to occur at $\dot{V}O_2$ and heart rate levels well below those predicted from nomograms developed in normal populations. Furthermore, to test exercise tolerance safely in pulmonary patients, it is important to monitor arterial oxygenation; hypoxemia is not a consequence of exercise in normal subjects, except at extreme levels of exertion.

The practical details of exercise testing in the pulmonary patient depend on the purpose for which such testing is done. For example, if the exercise testing is a prelude to developing an exercise training program for a patient with chronic lung disease, testing is best accomplished on an apparatus (e.g., treadmill) that requires exercise comparable to that used during training (e.g., walking). This is because muscle conditioning is most specific for the type of exercise used in training and may not be transferable directly to another form of exercise. For example, tolerance for walking is not improved by training on a supine bicycle or by arm exercises.

The specific measurements made also depend on the purposes of the test. For instance, if the question relates to whether the patient requires supplemental oxygen during exercise, then measurement of arterial blood gases (or cutaneous oximetry) at rest and during exercise is necessary, and the exercise level should be appropriate to the patient's daily activities. Furthermore, if arterial hypoxemia appears with exercise, the test may be repeated with supplemental oxygen provided at known flow rates, to ensure that the flow rate selected prevents hypoxemia.

Laboratory exercise testing is most commonly performed using either (1) rapid, progressive, incremental levels to a symptom-limited maximum or (2) defined steady-state levels. The former is most useful for determining exercise tolerance and the limitations to maximum performance. The latter may be preferred for assessing training prescriptions (e.g., heart rate target for endurance exercise) or for accurately measuring physiologic variables requiring a steady state (e.g., arterial blood gases, cardiac output, or dead space ventilation). Simpler exercise tests, such as the 6-minute walk test, have been used increasingly in recent years to measure exercise tolerance outside of a laboratory setting. These timed distance walk tests measure the maximum distance a person can walk within a defined period (e.g., 6 minutes). Such tests have the advantage of requiring less equipment and technical expertise; however, attention must be paid to the details of testing procedures because variations in factors such as the walking course, patient instructions, encouragement during tests, use of oxygen or monitoring devices, and number of tests performed will influence the results. If these tests are to be used widely, then better standardization of procedures is needed. Also, these tests do not provide the detailed physiologic data typically included in more formal laboratory exercise tests.

Two common errors in the use of exercise tests in pulmonary patients are to assume that (1) normal arterial blood gas (ABG) values at rest obviate the need for exercise measurements and (2) one can judge from resting pulmonary function and ABG testing that the patient will or will not have serious gas exchange deterioration with exercise. Neither of these assumptions is correct. Also, it is often difficult to relate a patient's report of dyspnea on exertion to his or her actual physiologic performance during exercise—not a surprising fact, as dyspnea, like pain, is a largely subjective sensation.

In exercise training for the pulmonary patient, another common error is to select target training levels that are too low. In normal subjects or cardiac patients, training levels typically are chosen at submaximum percentages (e.g., 60 to 70%) of maximum $\dot{V}O_2$ or heart rate. Many patients with chronic lung disease, however, are often ventilatory limited at low levels of exercise, which may be below their anaerobic threshold. Such individuals are able to sustain exercise levels at higher percentages of maximum (e.g., 90% or above), even though the absolute levels are low.

Exercise testing has become an increasingly important component of the diagnostic-management approach to the patient with pulmonary disease. Familiarity with the techniques used and with the utility of the data derived is essential to proper patient care.

---

1. American Thoracic Society/American College of Chest Physicians. ATS/ACCP Statement on cardiopulmonary exercise testing. *Am J Respir Crit Care Med.* 2003; 167:211.
    Comprehensive review of current state of exercise testing, including sections on Indications, Methodology, Physiologic Basis of Measurements, Reference Values, Normal Response, Limitation in Cardiopulmonary Patients, and Interpretation.
2. Jones NL. Clinical Exercise Testing. 4th ed. Philadelphia: W. B. Saunders; 1997.
    A practical guide to clinical exercise testing. Discussion of physiologic basis, clinical uses, methods, and interpretation including normal standards.
3. Kelley's Textbook of Internal Medicine, 4th edition. Editors: Humes HD. (Editor-in-Chief), DuPont HL, Gardner LB, Griffin JW, Harris JR ED, Hazzard WR, et al. Lippincott Williams & Wilkins, Philadelphia, 2000.
    Comprehensive text including physiologic principles, measurement techniques, protocols, normal values, and interpretations with case examples.
4. Ries AL. The role of exercise testing in pulmonary diagnosis. *Clin Chest Med.* 1987;8:81.
    Review of principles of exercise testing for pulmonary patients including discussion of methods, protocols, and indications.
5. Hansen J. Exercise testing. In: Clausen JL, ed. *Pulmonary Function Testing Guidelines and Controversies.* New York: Academic Press; 1982:259–279.

Guidelines of the California Thoracic Society including recommended methods, normal values, and controversies for exercise testing in pulmonary laboratories.

6. O'Donnell DE, Revill SM, Webb KA. Dynamic hyperinflation and exercise intolerance in chronic obstructive pulmonary disease. *Am J Respir Crit Care Med.* 2001;164:770.

   Demonstration of the key role of dynamic hyperinflation of end-tidal lung volume as a determinant of exercise intolerance in patients with COPD.

7. Mahler DA. The measurement of dyspnea during exercise in patients with lung disease. *Chest.* 1992;101:242S.

   Review of techniques of measuring dyspnea during exercise in pulmonary patients. The Borg and visual analog scales are used most commonly. Breathlessness ratings are generally reliable over time and sensitive to change with interventions.

8. American Thoracic Society. Guidelines for the six-minute walk test. *Am J Respir Crit Care Med.* 2002;166:111.

9. Sciurba FC, Slivka WA. Six-minute walk testing. *Sem Respir Crit Care Med.* 1998;9:383.

10. Steele B. Timed walking tests of exercise capacity in chronic cardiopulmonary illness. *J Cardiopulm Rehabil.* 1996;6:25.

    References 8, 9, and 10 provide a review of the use of timed distance walk tests for evaluating exercise tolerance. Emphasize details of testing procedures and discuss advantages and disadvantages.

11. American Thoracic Society/European Respiratory Society. Skeletal muscle dysfunction in chronic obstructive pulmonary disease. *Am J Respir Crit Care Med.* 1999;159:S1.

    Comprehensive summary of skeletal muscle dysfunction in patients with chronic lung disease, including discussion of principles of normal muscle function, skeletal muscle abnormalities in COPD, and effects of interventions on muscle dysfunction.

12. Casaburi R. Exercise training in chronic obstructive lung disease. In: Casaburi R, Petty TL, eds. *Principles and Practice of Pulmonary Rehabilitation*. Philadelphia: Saunders; 1993:204–224.

    Review of principles and benefits of exercise training in patients with COPD. Comprehensive table summarizing 37 published studies in 933 patients with overwhelmingly positive results.

13. Ries AL, Farrow JT, Clausen JL. Pulmonary function tests cannot predict exercise-induced hypoxemia in chronic obstructive pulmonary disease. *Chest.* 1988;93:454.

14. Owens GR, Rogers RM, Pennock BE, et al. The diffusing capacity as a predictor of arterial oxygen desaturation during exercise in patients with chronic obstructive pulmonary disease. *New Engl J Med.* 1984;310:1218.

    References 11 and 12 highlight the variability of changes of arterial oxygenation with exercise in patients with COPD. Although titles and focus of the two articles differ, both demonstrate that in patients with mild obstructive disease, oxygenation does not worsen with exercise (tends to improve or stay the same), whereas in those with moderate to severe disease, it changes unpredictably (ie, worsens, improves or is unchanged).

15. Ries AL, Farrow JT, Clausen JL. Accuracy of two ear oximeters at rest and during exercise in pulmonary patients. *Am Rev Respir Dis.* 1985;132:685.

    Accuracy of ear oximeters (95% confidence limits) +/– 4–5% compared to direct measurement of Sao_2. More accurate in measuring change in Sao_2 (+/– 2.5–3.5%).

16. Storms WW. Review of exercise-induced asthma. *Med Sci Sports Exerc.* 2003; 35:1464.

    Succinct review of exercise-induced asthma.

5. RADIOISOTOPIC TECHNIQUES

Timothy A. Morris

Lung ventilation and perfusion ($\dot{V}/\dot{Q}$) scanning is a powerful tool for assessing regional pulmonary blood flow and ventilation. Its most common use is for the diagnosis of pulmonary embolism, which is represented as a focal perfusion defect without a matching ventilation defect. Although contrast-enhanced computed tomographic (CT) scanning is becoming more frequently used for this purpose, nuclear medicine lung scanning remains the most affordable, reliable, and noninvasive diagnostic option for pulmonary embolism. In addition, $\dot{V}/\dot{Q}$ scanning has unique diagnostic properties that make it useful in several other clinical situations.

Perfusion scans are performed after injection of the radioisotope technetium 99m (99mTc), incorporated into particles of macroaggregated albumin (MAA) or human albumin microspheres (HAM). A typical dose of 99mTc MAA for a Q scan contains 100,000 particles and 1 to 2 mCi of radioactivity. Because the individual particles are larger than the pulmonary capillary lumen, they become trapped in the lungs on the "first pass." The focal 99-Tc radioactivity intensity therefore reflects the proportional distribution (but not the absolute amount) of blood flow to each lung region. The capillary obstruction from the scan is harmless, as only 0.3% of the capillaries are affected and the albumin particles disintegrate by 8 hours.

Because the distribution of pulmonary blood flow is gravity-dependent, the radioisotope should, ideally, be injected half in the supine and half in the prone position. Injecting in the sitting or standing position can lead to artifactual apical "defects" on the scan. Optimally, the perfusion scan should include at least six views: anterior, posterior, right and left lateral, and two oblique views.

Ventilation scanning can be performed with several different radiopharmaceuticals, either as a gas or as an aerosol. The most commonly used isotopic gas is xenon 133 (133Xe). For ventilation scans, 133Xe is mixed with air or with a suitable concentration of oxygen to obtain a dose of approximately 5 mCi/L. After several deep breaths of air, the patient is connected to a shielded spirometer containing the radioactive gas. Usually, an initial breath is taken to total lung capacity and recorded (single-breath scan). Next, the patient breathes tidally while the distribution of gas is recorded (wash-in phase). After the concentration of radioactivity has equilibrated between the patient's lung and spirometer (equilibrium phase), the patient resumes breathing room air (washout phase). Retention of the gas locally during the washout phase is the most sensitive finding for detecting ventilation abnormalities; this phase should be used for interpretation.

Aerosolized radio-labeled particles have become popular alternative agents for ventilation scans. The most widely used of these is 99mTc DTPA. Because it is an aerosol rather than a gas, 99mTc DTPA distribution is determined by the mass and inertial properties of the particles as well as by the patterns of regional ventilation. Turbulent airflow in large airways can lead to deposition on bronchial walls, causing localized "hot spots" that complicate scan interpretation. Although they have some practical advantages, some ventilation scans performed with aerosolized 99-Tc particles yield different results than 133Xe scans. Pertechnegas, consisting of very small (<1 μm) aerosolized 99mTc-labeled carbon particles, avoids some of the disadvantages inherent in other radiolabeled particle ventilation scans. The small Pertechnegas particles travel to the alveoli without depositing on airway walls. Thus, there is less residual radioactivity superimposed on perfusion images. It has yet to be determined whether the theoretical advantages of Pertechnegas will translate into improved diagnostic accuracy over more conventional (and less expensive) methods.

While cost and efficiency considerations have led to wide use of aerosols, we prefer 133Xe for diagnostic ventilation studies. In addition to the improved image characteristics, there are practical advantages to this method. Because of the differences in gamma emission "windows" between the two isotopes, the (133Xe) ventilation scan can follow the (99-Tc) perfusion scan without significant degradation of the ventilation images. The ventilation scan can, in this sequence, be performed in the view that optimally displays the perfusion defects; also, a normal perfusion scan makes ventilation scanning unnecessary, minimizing scanning cost and radiation exposure. Finally, aerosols do not provide a washout phase, and we have found that phase to be of diagnostic value in several clinical contexts.

The major application of perfusion and ventilation scans has been to exclude or confirm the diagnosis of pulmonary embolism. Multiple clinical trials defining the sensitivity and specificity of lung scans for pulmonary embolism make clear that the perfusion and ventilation tests should be considered separately. Interpreted alone, the *sensitivity* of the perfusion scan is extremely high. Indeed, a normal perfusion scan excludes the diagnosis of clinically significant embolism; that is, outcome studies have shown that withholding treatment in patients with a normal scan (and no venous thrombosis) is safe. However, abnormal perfusion scans are nonspecific. To enhance specificity, three key collateral considerations can be invoked: (1) the size of the perfusion defect, (2) matching chest x-ray findings, and, if necessary, (3) corresponding ventilation scan findings. If the perfusion defects are in areas with infiltrates by chest radiograph or if all defects are subsegmental in size, the study is nondiagnostic and ventilation scanning will add little of diagnostic value. If one or more defects are segmental or larger, without corresponding chest x-ray findings, a ventilation scan is done. If the areas with perfusion defect(s) ventilate normally, the scan is diagnostic for pulmonary arterial occlusion. If they ventilate abnormally, the scan is nondiagnostic.

Depending on the patient population, normal perfusion scans will be found in 10 to 20% of embolic suspects, diagnostic scans in 15 to 20%, and nondiagnostic studies in the remainder. Nondiagnostic studies, however, are associated with a significant incidence of embolism. Calling such nondiagnostic studies "intermediate" or "low" probability, unfortunately, may lull the physician into complacency and lead to serious management errors.

In patients with acute symptoms, the $\dot{V}/\dot{Q}$ scan indicating "pulmonary arterial obstruction" means acute pulmonary embolism in the overwhelming majority of patients. However, any process that blocks flow through pulmonary arteries can produce this pattern. Among such processes are chronic pulmonary thromboembolic disease (where the obstruction is due, at least in part, to fibroblastic organization of a once-active thrombus), Takayasu's arteritis, fibrosing mediastinitis, primary tumors of the pulmonary arteries, pulmonary artery agenesis, and, rarely, invasion or compression of pulmonary arteries by tumors or other mediastinal components (eg, aorta, lymph nodes).

Another application of $\dot{V}/\dot{Q}$ scans pertains to the decision to perform lung surgery in a patient with limited lung reserve. For example, in a patient being considered for lung resection for cancer or bronchiectasis or for bullectomy, the lung scan provides important regional information that spirometry and other function tests cannot. Specifically, it can define whether the proposed area of resection/bullectomy is a major contributor to the patient's overall ventilation and pulmonary blood flow. In these situations, it is helpful to perform "quantitative" scans, in which the proportion of counts from various lung regions (relative to the entire lung) are measured to determine their contribution to the total lung ventilation and perfusion. If, for example, a right lower lobe site of bronchiectasis is poorly ventilated and barely perfused, its removal won't significantly impair gas exchange function; indeed, it may even improve it. If, however, the lobe carries a large percentage of the total blood flow, its resection may have serious hemodynamic and gas exchange consequences. Thus, quantitative $\dot{V}/\dot{Q}$ scans provide topographic data that, along with indicators of global function such as spirometry, help complete the pulmonary assessment of the surgical candidate.

$\dot{V}/\dot{Q}$ scanning also offers a means of noninvasively differentiating primary pulmonary hypertension (PPH) from large-vessel, chronic thromboembolic pulmonary hypertension (CTEPH). In PPH, perfusion scans are normal or demonstrate a "mottled" appearance; in CTEPH, multiple, segmental or larger perfusion defects are invariably present. It should be noted, however, that $\dot{Q}$ scan results in CTEPH often significantly underestimate the actual degree of angiographic obstruction. Patients with unexplained pulmonary hypertension and one or more segmental perfusion defects should undergo further workup, especially if the perfusion defects are mismatched (see Chapter 66).

Radioisotope techniques using thrombus-specific targeting agents have also been used, or are under study, for the detection of venous thrombi and pulmonary emboli. The prototype of such approaches, radiolabeled fibrinogen (RLF), is no longer available but was of great value in prior epidemiologic studies of deep venous thrombosis. Of potentially greater diagnostic value are radiolabeled antibodies and other radiolabeled agents with high affinity for fibrin, platelet receptors, and other components of active thrombi. Radiolabeled antifibrin antibodies, for example, bind to sites on the surface of acute thrombi and allow them to be detected by gamma camera imaging. An important advantage these agents may have over other imaging modalities is the ability to distinguish *acute* thrombi from other causes of vascular obstruction. For example, intravascular "scars" in the deep veins or pulmonary arteries resulting from prior (inactive) thromboembolic disease may be confused with acute thrombi on more conventional "anatomic" tests, such as ultrasound imaging, $\dot{V}/\dot{Q}$ scanning, helical CT, and even contrast angiography. However, radiolabeled antibodies will bind to vascular lesions only if biological components of thrombosis are present. In addition, because the antibodies bind equally well to both deep vein thrombi and pulmonary emboli, both lesions may be imaged with a single test. Gallium-67 (67Ga) lung scanning has limited usefulness in pulmonary medicine. After intravenous injection, 67Ga accumulates in tissues with increased metabolic activity (eg, neoplasm, inflammation). Although capable of detecting roentgenographically inapparent foci of disease, the clinical application of 67Ga scanning is limited by its nonspecificity. Certain "niches" for 67Ga lung scanning are still used by some clinicians. For example, in sarcoidosis, 67Ga scanning is frequently positive and is used in some centers to follow the progression of this condition. Whether 67Ga scanning can predict functional deterioration or response to therapy more accurately than more standard tests (eg, chest roentgenogram, spirometry) remains inconclusive.

Finally, radiolabeled white blood cells have been used widely to detect the presence of abscesses in the lungs and solid organs. The technique is imprecise and typically used only if other means of diagnosing infection have failed.

---

1. Alderson PO, Lee H, Summer WR, et al. Comparison of Xe-133 washout and single breath imaging for the detection of ventilation abnormalities. *J Nucl Med.* 1979;20:917.
   Demonstrates the superiority of Xe-133 washout imaging over single-breath imaging in the diagnosis of pulmonary embolism.
2. Baughman RP, Shipley R, Eisentrout CE. Predictive value of gallium scan, angiotensin-converting enzyme level, and bronchoalveolar lavage in two-year follow-up of pulmonary sarcoidosis. *Lung.* 1987;165:371.
   The finding of a negative gallium scan suggests a small likelihood that disease activity will worsen after 2 years.
3. Fishmann A, et al. The role of perfusion scanning versus pulmonary angiography in the evaluation of suspected primary pulmonary hypertension. *Chest.* 1983;84:679.
   Patients with primary pulmonary hypertension had normal or "mottled" perfusion scan patterns; those with chronic thromboembolic pulmonary hypertension had scans characterized by multiple, mismatched segmental defects.
4. Heyes JW. Three dimensional display of SPECT images: Advantages and problems. *J Nucl Med.* 1990;31:1428.
   A good discussion of the problems and promise of SPECT.
5. Hull RD, Hirsh J, Carter CJ, et al. Diagnostic value of ventilation-perfusion lung

scanning in patients with suspected pulmonary embolism. *Chest*. 1985;88:819.
The frequency of angiographically documented pulmonary embolism in scans classified as "low probability" ranged from 25 to 40%.

6. Hull RD, Raskob G. Low probability lung scan findings: a need for change. *Ann Intern Med*. 1991;114:142.
The term "low probability," or even "intermediate," is potentially harmful to proper assessment of embolic suspects. The term "nondiagnostic" is preferable.

7. Kahn D, Bushnell DL, Dean R, et al. Clinical outcome of patients with a "low probability" of pulmonary embolism on ventilation-perfusion lung scan. *Arch Intern Med*. 1989;149:377.
None of 90 patients with a "low probability" perfusion scan demonstrated clinical evidence of pulmonary embolism subsequent to the V̇/Q scan.

8. Knight LC. Do we finally have a radiopharmaceutical for rapid, specific imaging of venous thrombosis? *J Nuc Med*. 1991;32:791–795. Editorial.
Review of the various approaches, with a good reference list. Seems to favor antifibrin antibodies over other agents.

9. Kanke M, Matsueda GR, Strauss HW, et al. Localization and visualization of pulmonary emboli with radiolabeled fibrin-specific monoclonal antibody. *J Nucl Med*. 1991;32:1254.
One of multiple papers describing similar approaches to the diagnosis of venous thromboembolism.

10. Kipper MS, Moser KM, Kortman KE, et al. Longterm follow-up of patients with suspected embolism and a normal lung scan. Perfusion scans in embolic suspects. *Chest*. 1982;82:411.
This report describes long-term follow-up of embolic suspects who had normal perfusion scans and were not treated with anticoagulant drugs. Excellent outcomes indicate that, in the absence of venous thrombosis, anticoagulant therapy can be withheld on the basis of a normal scan.

11. Kipper MS, Alazraki N. The feasibility of performing Xe-133 ventilation imaging following the perfusion study. *Radiology*. 1982;144:581.
Demonstrates that the ventilation scan can follow the perfusion scan without significant image degradation.

12. Miniati M, Pistolesi M, Marini C, et al. Value of perfusion lung scan in the diagnosis of pulmonary embolism: results of the Prospective Investigative Study of Acute Pulmonary Embolism Diagnosis (PISA-PED). *Am J Respir Crit Care Med*. 1996;154:1387–1393.
Perfusion scans alone were assessed, without ventilation, for patients suspected of having PE. Characteristic wedge-shaped defects were highly associated with the presence of PE on angiogram, particularly if the clinical suspicion was high prior to the scan itself.

13. Oster ZH, Sum P. Of monoclonal antibodies and thrombus specific imaging. *J Nucl Med*. 1990;31:1055.
A good review of the past, present, and future of this approach.

14. Pantin CF, Valind SO, Sweatman M, et al. Measures of the inflammatory response in cryptogenic fibrosing alveolitis. *Am Rev Respir Dis*. 1988;138:1234.
The initial level of gallium-67 uptake did not predict response to therapy.

15. Peters AM. Imaging inflammation: current role of labeled autologous leukocytes. *J Nucl Med*. 1992;33:65.
The authors review the use of radiolabeled leukocytes in diagnosing inflammatory states.

16. Ramanna L, Alderson PO, Waxman AD, et al. Regional comparison of technetium-99m DTPA aerosol and radioactive gas ventilation (Xenon and Krypton) studies in patients with suspected pulmonary embolism. *J Nucl Med*. 1986;27:1391.
Discrepancies existed between gas and aerosol ventilation scan findings but did not impact on the final scintigraphic probability of pulmonary embolism.

17. Ryan KL, Fedullo PF, Davis GB. Perfusion scan findings understate the severity of angiographic and hemodynamic compromise in chronic thromboembolic pulmonary hypertension. *Chest*. 1988;93:1180.

Perfusion scanning can suggest the diagnosis of thromboembolic pulmonary hypertension but cannot provide information regarding its severity or surgical accessibility.

18. Sulavik SB, Spencer RP, Weed DA, et al. Recognition of distinctive patterns of gallium-67 distribution in sarcoidosis. *J Nucl Med.* 1990;31:1901.

    The authors describe useful patterns of 67Ga in patients with different distributions of sarcoidosis.

---

6. EVALUATION OF ARTERIAL BLOOD GASES AND ACID–BASE HOMEOSTASIS

Robert M. Smith

Arterial blood gas (ABG) measurements are invaluable in assessing the adequacy of pulmonary gas exchange and the presence and severity of acid–base disturbances. However, these values cannot be interpreted in a vacuum. Proper interpretation of arterial oxygen and carbon dioxide tension (PaO_2 and $PaCO_2$) and pH values requires knowledge of the clinical state, the therapy being applied, and frequently other data such as mixed venous oxygen saturation, hemoglobin concentration, and cardiac output.

Scrupulous attention must be paid to sample collection, handling, and the actual analysis of an arterial blood gas specimen. Direct radial artery puncture with a 20-gauge (or smaller) needle and a heparinized syringe is the technique of choice for routine analysis. When repeated sampling is necessary, an indwelling arterial catheter may be used but must be carefully monitored for local complications including infection, thrombus formation, occlusion of arterial flow, or distal microemboli. The radial or dorsalis pedis arteries are the preferred sites for monitoring, as the ulnar or posterior tibial arteries provide redundant circulation. The brachial and femoral arteries are less desirable, but can be used when circumstances warrant.

The specimen should be collected without exposure to ambient air, usually by allowing arterial pressure to force blood into the syringe. Many devices have been designed specifically for this purpose and facilitate good sampling technique. Any bubbles introduced into the syringe during collection should be promptly expelled; the sample should be mixed to ensure complete anticoagulation and placed in ice water. Analysis should take place within minutes using an instrument system that has been recently calibrated against commercially available standards for each blood gas electrode (PO_2, PCO_2, and pH). The electrodes and sampling chambers are maintained at 37°C, and the results must be corrected to the patient's body temperature if it is abnormal. PaO_2 and $PaCO_2$ are expressed in terms of pressure, typically as mmHg or kilopascal (kPa) (1 torr = 1 mmHg = 7.5 kPa).

The blood gas results often include oxygen saturation, bicarbonate, base excess or deficit, and alveolar-arterial oxygen difference. Accurate knowledge of the inspired oxygen (FIO_2) and an estimate of the respiratory exchange ratio (R or RER) are necessary for this latter calculation. All of these are calculated values and depend on the accurate measurement of PO_2, PCO_2, and pH. The electrodes are extremely accurate when calibrated correctly (PO_2 and PCO_2 ± 2 torr, pH ± 0.01 units) and the calculated values are equally precise. A common misconception is that the $[HCO_3^-]$ value calculated from ABG analysis is less accurate than that measured in the chemistry laboratory. However, the assumptions about $PaCO_2$ when $[HCO_3^-]$ is measured from a sample of venous blood in a chemistry analyzer render that latter measurement less accurate in the presence of a respiratory disturbance.

The initial evaluation of an ABG should include a consideration of its technical adequacy. A few simple rules can help: (1) a PO_2 above 48 is unlikely to have been collected from a venous sample; (2) the sum of the PaO_2 and $PaCO_2$ should be less than 140 mmHg if the patient is breathing room air; and (3) a rapid large change in the calculated bicarbonate by more than 5 mEq suggests an error in the $PaCO_2$ or pH, or the presence of excessive amounts of heparin (an acid) in the collection syringe in the absence of a primary metabolic disturbance.

OXYGEN

The normal value of PaO_2 decreases with age and is influenced by barometric pressure (PB) and, therefore, by altitude. A PaO_2 less than 80 mmHg should always be considered abnormal at sea level. However, the predicted value for PaO_2 in Denver (where ambient barometric pressure is 625 mm) for a young person is only 80 mmHg and lower for elderly persons (60 to 65 mmHg).

Only small amounts of oxygen are transported in solution in the plasma. The bulk of the oxygen-carrying capacity of blood resides in hemoglobin contained in red blood cells. The relationship between the PaO_2 and hemoglobin oxygen saturation (SaO_2) is depicted in a sigmoidal oxyhemoglobin dissociation curve in which a decrease in PaO_2 corresponds to a minimal decline in SaO_2 until the PaO_2 drops to 60 mmHg (corresponding to an SaO_2 of 90%), and then SaO_2 falls more rapidly with further drops in PaO_2. For this reason, efforts to elevate the PaO_2 above 60 to 65 mmHg rarely provide significant clinical benefit in the management of hypoxemic patients. The dissociation curve is shifted to the right in acidosis and to the left in alkalosis, so that a PaO_2 of 60 and a pH of 7.30 will yield a saturation of 87.7%, whereas PaO_2 of 60 and pH of 7.50 lead to an oxygen saturation of 93.4%.

The classification of hypoxemia severity is based on PaO_2 and is arbitrary. A reduced value to 60 mmHg is usually considered mild hypoxemia, 45 to 59 mmHg is moderate, and below 45 mmHg is severe. The major causes of hypoxemia are: (1) a decrease in the oxygen content of the inhaled gas (eg, from reduced barometric pressure with altitude, or a hypoxemic gas mixture); (2) global hypoventilation; (3) ventilation-perfusion ($\dot{V}/\dot{Q}$) imbalance; and (4) right-to-left shunt (intrapulmonary or intracardiac). A decreased mixed venous oxygen content, as can occur when cardiac output is severely reduced does not typically cause hypoxemia, but will markedly worsen the effects of shunt or $\dot{V}/\dot{Q}$ imbalance. These mechanisms can be differentiated by calculation of the alveolar-arterial oxygen difference (A-a)DO_2 using the simplified alveolar gas equation:

$$P_AO_2 = P_IO_2 - \frac{PaCO_2}{R} \tag{6.1}$$

where $R = \dfrac{\dot{V}CO_2}{\dot{V}O_2}$ and (A-a) $DO_2 = P_AO_2 - P_aO_2$

The (A–a)DO_2 (also known as the [A–a] gradient or the [A-a] PO_2 difference) is normally less than 20 mmHg. Patients with hypoxemia resulting from a decreased FIO_2 (eg, altitude) or from hypoventilation (elevated $PaCO_2$) have a normal $P(A-a)O_2$, whereas the other processes lead to a widened $P(A-a)O_2$. Characteristically, patients with hypoventilation or $\dot{V}/\dot{Q}$ mismatch show a 3 to 5 mmHg rise in $PaCO_2$ for each 1% increment in F_IO_2; those with a shunt show a less than 2 mmHg rise for each 1% increment in F_IO_2. Alternatives to the (A-a)DO_2 calculation are the PaO_2/PaO_2 or PaO_2/F_IO_2 ratios; these values are easier to compute but are not entirely independent of changes in F_IO_2.

The pulse oximeter is a popular and relatively low-cost method for monitoring patients and can reduce the number of ABG analyses required when treating a patient on a ventilator or with respiratory failure. The accuracy of oximetry is reasonably good if one assumes no significant carboxyhemoglobin or methemoglobin. However, oximetry gives no information about alveolar ventilation or about the acid-base status.

CARBON DIOXIDE

The $Paco_2$ reflects the balance between carbon dioxide production and carbon dioxide elimination by ventilation. This is stated by the equation:

$$Paco_2 = \frac{k \times \dot{V}co_2}{\dot{V}_A} \tag{6.2}$$

Where $\dot{V}co_2$ = carbon dioxide production per minute, $\dot{V}_A$ = alveolar ventilation, and k is a constant. If $\dot{V}_A$ decreases, $Paco_2$ will rise (hypercapnia), whereas a rise in $\dot{V}_A$ will result in a fall in $Paco_2$ (hypocapnia).

The normal range for $Paco_2$ is 37 to 43 mmHg, regardless of age. $Paco_2$ values of 30 to 37 mmHg are regarded as mild hypocapnia, 26 to 29 mmHg as moderate, and below 25 mmHg as severe. Mild hypercapnia is in the 44 to 50 mm Hg range; moderate, 51 to 60 mmHg; and severe, above 60 mmHg. These numbers should also be compared to baseline values, as any sudden change of baseline CO_2 may portend a serious change in pulmonary function. It is helpful to distinguish hypercapnic conditions in which total ventilation is normal or increased and there is increased dead space ventilation (eg, chronic obstructive airway disease) from those with diminished total ventilation (eg, sedative overdose or neuromuscular disease).

ARTERIAL pH AND ACID–BASE HOMEOSTASIS

Two major principles of physical chemistry govern our understanding of acid–base balance. The first principle is that dissociation constants describe the equilibrium between a weak acid (HA) and its conjugate base:

$$HA \leftrightarrow H^+ + HA^-$$

or expressed mathematically $K_A = \dfrac{[H^+][A^-]}{[HA]}$ $\hspace{2em}$ (6.3)

The primary buffer in blood is the carbonate-bicarbonate base pair. Carbon dioxide is hydrated to carbonic acid and this dissociates to bicarbonate and $[H^+]$, according to the relationship:

$$CO_2 + H_2O \leftrightarrow H_2CO_3 \leftrightarrow H^+ + HCO_3^-$$

$$pK = 6.1 \tag{6.4}$$

Mathematically, this is expressed as:

$$K = \frac{[H^+][HCO_3^-]}{[H_2CO_3]} \quad \text{or} \quad K = \frac{[H^+][HCO_3^-]}{[CO_2]} \tag{6.5}$$

Rearranging and supplying the correct constants gives the Henderson Equation, whereas taking the negative log of each side and rearranging gives the Henderson-Hasselbach Equation:

$$[H^+] = \frac{24[Pco_2]}{[HCO_3^-]} \hspace{3em} pH = 6.1 + \log \frac{[HCO_3^-]}{[0.03 \times Pco_2]} \tag{6.6}$$

Henderson Equation $\hspace{2em}$ Henderson-Hasselbach Equation

Although pH is the usual form of reporting the ABG, it is useful to be able to readily convert logarithm-based pH units to $[H^+]$ in nanoequivalents per liter (nEq/L). A normal pH (between 7.37 and 7.43) converts to $[H^+]$ of 43 to 37 nEq/L. A change in pH of 1 unit corresponds to a tenfold. change in concentration, and a 0.3-unit pH change corresponds to a twofold concentration change ($\log[10] = 1$, and $\log[2] = 0.3$). On this basis, it is easy to construct a conversion table even when a scientific calculator is not available (Table 6-2) This conversion permits easier calculation of

Table 6-1. Guidelines for assessing hypoxemia

Status	(A-a)Do$_2$	Pao$_2$/P$_{AO_2}$	
Normal	5–20	>0.80	>5υ
Low V̇/Q̇	30–50	0.65–0.70	300–4υ
Shunt	>60	<0.55	<250

acid–base relationships using the simplified Henderson formula. An elevation of blood pH (decrease in blood [H$^+$]) is called alkalemia, whereas a decrease in pH (increase in [H$^+$]) is called acidemia. A condition that leads to acidemia or alkalemia is an acidosis or alkalosis, respectively, but compensatory mechanisms may actually leave the patient with a normal pH.

The second principle that governs acid–base homeostasis is that a solution must contain equal numbers of positively and negatively charged ions. For biologic systems, this can be expressed as:

Total cations − total anions = 0, or

$$[Na^+] + [K^+] - [Cl^-] - [Hco_3^-] - [A^-] - [\text{unmeasured anions}] = 0$$
$$140 + 4 - 102 - 25 - 15 - 2 = 0 \tag{6.7}$$

The concentration of the unmeasured anions that are normally present (eg, So_4^{2-} or Po_4^{2-}) is only 1 to 3 mEq/L, and the [H$^+$] concentration is so low relative to other charged species that it can be neglected. [A$^-$] represents the base pairs of other weak acids in blood. These consist predominantly of charged amino acid residues on plasma proteins. The pK of these charged groups is typically 6.6 to 6.8, and so they are 90% dissociated at pH 7.4. The total concentration of these protein-based weak acids in blood (A$_{TOT}$ in mEq/L) is 2.4 times the protein concentration (g/dl). Thus:

$$A^- = A_{TOT} \times 0.90 = [\text{protein g/dl}] \times 2.4 \times 0.90 \ (\text{normal} = 11 - 16) \tag{6.8}$$

This equation allows calculation of [A$^-$] and fosters an understanding of the effect of hypoproteinemia on its magnitude. This concept is also the basis for the more common calculation of the "anion gap" in which [A$^-$] and [K$^+$] are assumed to be constant. With that assumption, a shortened version of the equation is:

$$\text{Anion gap} = [Na^+] - [Cl^-] - [Hco_3^-] \ (\text{normal range} = 10 - 15) \tag{6.9}$$

Table 6-2. Conversion between pH and hydrogen ion concentration

Alkalemia		Acidemia	
pH	[H$^+$] (nEq/L)	pH	[H$^+$] (nEq/L)
8.00	10	7.30	50
7.90	12.5	7.20	63
7.80	16	7.10	79
7.70	20	7.00	100
7.60	25	6.90	125
7.50	32	6.80	160
Normal		6.70	200
7.40	40		

re, increases in the anion gap above the normal range reflect the presence of ...asured anions, but there is no provision for changes resulting from hypopro- ...nemia or for changes in [A⁻] caused by pH (which changes the dissociation state of ...e buffer groups). Correct estimation of the amount of unmeasured anions in solution is essential, as an elevation indicates the presence of a metabolic acidosis.

As noted, the hydrogen ion concentration $[H^+]$ is controlled to a very narrow concentration range between 10 and 100 nEq/L. To maintain the $[H^+]$ within this range, acid generation must closely match acid elimination. This extremely low concentration range (six orders of magnitude less than that of most other electrolytes) is even more remarkable relative to those overall rates of acid production. More than 100 mEq of "fixed" nonvolatile acids (eg, sulfates or phosphates) and approximately 13,000 mEq of volatile acid are generated daily as byproducts of metabolism. The kidney excretes nonvolatile acids while the lungs eliminate the volatile acid load as CO_2 (equivalent to 200 mL/min).

Disorders that alter CO_2 elimination (e.g., ventilatory changes that affect $Paco_2$) are reflected in the numerator of the Henderson Equation. These are referred to as respiratory derangements of acid–base balance. Conversely, if the excretion of fixed acids slows or accelerates in relationship to production, or if there is abnormal intake of acid or alkali, a metabolic disturbance in acid–base balance is said to develop. These changes are largely reflected in the denominator of the Henderson Equation.

If the bicarbonate-carbonate system were the only buffer in blood, then changes in pH as a result of acute changes in $Paco_2$ should not cause any change in bicarbonate levels. However, the presence of other blood buffers with a pK that is different from

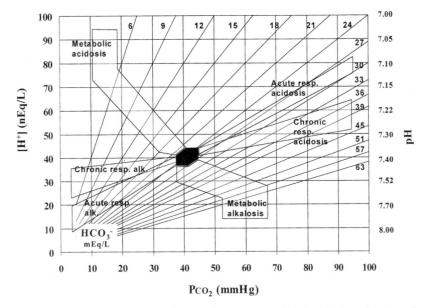

FIG. 6-1. Acid–base nomogram. The acid–base map provides insight into the type of acid–base disturbance (metabolic vs respiratory) and its duration (acute vs chronic). The dark lines represent the "95 percent confidence" bands for the predicted $Paco_2$, pH, and H^+; concentration in each simple disturbance. A point falling outside the confidence bands implies that the arterial blood gases cannot be explained by a simple disturbance alone (see text). *Resp.* = respiratory; *alk.* = alkalosis; *N* = normal. (Adapted from McCurdy, DK. Mixed metabolic and respiratory acid–base disturbances: diagnosis and management. *Chest.* 1972;62[suppl]:35s.)

that of bicarbonate means that changes in pH will generate or use $[H^+]$ with a resulting small change in $[HCO_3^-]$. The magnitude of these changes in pH and in bicarbonate as a result of acute changes in ventilation can be shown graphically (Fig. 6-1) or can be estimated from prediction equations (Table 6-3). For example, elevation of $PaCO_2$ from 40 to 60 mmHg (an acute respiratory acidosis) produces a fall in pH (20×0.008) of 0.16 unit to 7.24 and a 2-mEq rise (0.1×20) in $[HCO_3^-]$. An acute respiratory alkalosis, characterized by a decrease in $PaCO_2$, produces a rise in pH of the same magnitude as that in acute respiratory acidosis, but bicarbonate falls 0.2 mEq for every 1-mmHg decrease in $PaCO_2$. The ability to predict pH and bicarbonate changes in response to ventilation is the basis for the concept of "base excess" and "base deficit." Base excess (or deficit) is the difference between the measured bicarbonate and the bicarbonate level that would be predicted on the basis of the measured PCO_2 change alone. Base excess is often reported with the directly measured ABG results and can be useful as a means of estimating the metabolic processes that are present in combination with respiratory changes. However, the calculations assume normal values for electrolytes and serum protein that may not be valid. Thus, uncritical use of base excess or deficit values can lead to error.

The response to a chronic (more than several days) change in $PaCO_2$ is compensation through increased elimination or retention of bicarbonate by the kidney. These compensatory mechanisms act to restore the pH toward, but not quite to, normal values. The magnitudes of these compensatory metabolic changes are well established from clinical observation (Table 6-3 and Fig. 6-1). For every 10 mmHg elevation of $PaCO_2$ in chronic CO_2 retention, bicarbonate retention results in an increase in levels by 4 mEq/L, blunting the pH change to 0.003 units for every 1-mmHg change in $PaCO_2$. With chronic hyperventilation, there is renal bicarbonate elimination until levels fall by 0.5 mEq for every 1-mmHg fall in $PaCO_2$ with full compensation.

Table 6-3. Predicted changes in response to processes causing acidosis or alkalosis

Respiratory acidosis: (primary disorder: ↑ $PaCO_2$ compensation: ↑ $[HCO_3^-]$)

	Acute	Chronic
ΔpH	$-0.008 \times \Delta PCO_2$[a]	$-0.003 \times \Delta PCO_2$
ΔH^+	$0.8 \times \Delta PCO_2$	$0.3 \times \Delta PCO_2$
ΔHCO_3^-	$0.1 \times \Delta PCO_2$	$0.4 \times \Delta PCO_2$
H^+	$0.8 \times PCO_2 + 8$	$0.3 \times PCO_2 + 27$

Respiratory alkalosis: (primary disorder: ↓ $PaCO_2$ compensation: ↓ $[HCO_3^-]$)

	Acute	Chronic
$\Delta pH =$	$-0.01 \times \Delta PCO_2$[a]	$-0.003 \times \Delta PCO_2$
$\Delta H^+ =$	$0.75 \times \Delta PCO_2$	$0.3 \times \Delta PCO_2$
$\Delta HCO_3^- =$	$0.2 \times PCO_2$	$0.5 \times \Delta PCO_2$
$H^+ =$	$0.75 \times PCO_2 + 10$	$0.3 \times PCO_2 + 28$

Metabolic acidosis: (primary disorder: ↓ $[HCO_3^-]$, compensation: ↓ $PaCO_2$)

$\Delta PCO_2 = 1.1–1.3 \times \Delta HCO_3$
$PCO_2 = 1.5 \times [HCO_3] + 8$
$PCO_2 =$ last 2 digits of the pH

Metabolic alkalosis: (primary disorder: ↑ $[HCO_3^-]$, compensation: ↑ $PaCO_2$)

$\Delta PCO_2 = 0.6–0.8 \times \Delta HCO_3$
$PCO_2 = 0.7 \times [HCO_3] + 21$

[a]Applicable for PCO_2 between 40 and 80 mmHg

Metabolic acidosis and alkalosis occur when there is a primary disturbance in the bicarbonate concentration of the blood. Respiratory responses occur to moderate the acidemia or alkalemia (Table 6-3 and Fig. 6-1). A quick rule of thumb is that the $Paco_2$ in response to a metabolic acidosis should equal the last two digits of the pH, although maximum respiratory compensation will only reduce the $Paco_2$ to 12 to 15 mmHg. If significant underlying respiratory disease is present, adequate compensation may not occur, and the pH will be lower than anticipated. For example, a $Paco_2$ of 35 mmHg in the presence of a pH of 7.20 suggests an inadequate respiratory compensation caused either by underlying respiratory disease or by altered respiratory drive from a central nervous system (CNS) process. An individual with normal lungs would reduce his $Paco_2$ to approximately 20 mmHg. Significant hypoventilation ($Paco_2 > 45$) resulting from metabolic alkalosis also occurs, but less consistently. The best "rule of thumb" in metabolic alkalosis is that $Paco_2$ rises by 0.7 for every 1-mEq rise in $[HCO_3^-]$.

When metabolic and respiratory processes have similar effects on pH, a mixed acid–base disturbance is said to exist. For instance, during cardiac arrest, respiratory acidosis and metabolic acidosis coexist in a combined acid–base disturbance and result in a greater reduction in pH than expected from the $Paco_2$ elevation alone. Combined

Table 6-4. Common causes of disturbances of acid–base balance

Respiratory acidosis	Respiratory alkalosis
–Diminished ventilatory drive	–Catastrophic CNS event
–Sedatives	–Drug with direct stimulation of
–Central hypoventilation syndromes	respiration (salicylates,
–Severe CNS depression or injury	progesterone)
–Diminished respiratory muscle	–Sepsis (early)
function	–Cirrhosis
–Guillain-Barré syndrome	–Pregnancy (third trimester)
–Myasthenia gravis	–Decreased lung compliance
–Severe hypokalemia	(J receptor)
–Diminished pulmonary function	–Anxiety
–Chronic obstructive pulmonary	
disease	
–Status asthmaticus	
–Severe restrictive disease	

Metabolic acidosis	Metabolic alkalosis
With normal anion "gap"	–Hypochloremia (often with
–GI bicarbonate loss	volume contraction)
–Renal tubular acidosis	–Hypokalemia
–Ureteral diversion	–Mineralocorticoid excess
–NH_4Cl or HCl infusion	–Bartter's syndrome
–Rehydration	–Administration of alkali
–Hyperalimentation	–Compensation for respiratory
–Compensation for respiratory,	acidosis
alkalosis	
With elevated anion "gap"	
–Ketoacidosis	
–Lactic acidosis	
–Salicylate intoxication	
–Methanol ingestion	
–Ethylene glycol ingestion	

CNS, central nervous system.

metabolic and respiratory alkalosis can lead to marked elevation of pH with cardiac arrhythmia, fall in cardiac output, or seizures. In contrast, a mixed metabolic and respiratory disturbance exists when a process leading to acidosis is superimposed on an alkalosis, or vice versa. These are common in clinical practice and tend to be of somewhat less immediate clinical impact because the pH tends to be more normal. For instance, patients with chronic respiratory acidosis from obstructive pulmonary disease will develop a compensatory metabolic alkalosis. If treated with corticosteroids or diuretics, they may develop a further metabolic alkalosis resulting in a normal or slightly alkalemic pH. One condition to be aware of is the mixed metabolic acidosis and respiratory alkalosis of salicylate intoxication. The characteristic pattern of low pH, elevated anion gap, and a lower $Paco_2$ than predicted from the compensation rules points to such a diagnosis.

Common conditions leading to acid–base derangements are listed in Table 6-4. In general, therapy should be directed at the underlying condition and not simply at correcting the pH toward a normal value.

To understand fully acid–base derangements, it is valuable to use a systematic approach to the analyses of the ABG results (Table 6-5). Most approaches begin by identifying any respiratory component to the derangement. If the entire abnormality is explained on the basis of acute respiratory changes, then a primary respiratory

Table 6-5. Approaches to the interpretation of blood gases

Step-by-step	"Quick and Dirty"
1. Is the patient acidemic or alkalemic?	1. Determine the predicted pH if all of the abnormality were due to changes in ventilation (i.e., if the Pco_2 were corrected to 40).
2. If the Pco_2 is abnormal, estimate whether an **acute** change in Pco_2 is sufficient to explain the pH change. If so, then the disturbance is predominantly a respiratory disturbance in acid–base balance.	
	2. Determine the difference between the measured and predicted pH.
3. If an acute change in Pco_2 is insufficient to explain all of the pH change, evaluate the nature of the additional metabolic disorder. Is the metabolic disturbance consistent with the predicted compensation for a chronic respiratory change?	3. Estimate the base deficit or excess: multiply the difference between the measured and predicted pH and move the decimal point two places to the right (answer is in mEq/L).
	4. Calculate the anion gap to estimate the contribution of strong ions to any base deficit.
4. If the disturbance appears primarily metabolic, evaluate the adequacy of respiratory compensation. The absence of complete respiratory compensation or of excessive respiratory compensation for a metabolic disturbance implies a secondary respiratory disturbance.	
5. If a metabolic acidosis is present, ascertain the presence or absence of unmeasured anions using the anion gap or charge neutrality equations.	
6. Identify other metabolic disturbances present in the patient with an anion gap metabolic acidosis.	

disorder is said to be present. If there is change in [Hco_3^-] beyond that predicted for an acute respiratory disturbance, is the change an appropriate compensation for a chronic respiratory disturbance? Metabolic compensation that is greater than the predicted value suggests a combined acid–base disturbance, whereas compensation that is less that the predicted range indicates either a mixed disorder or incomplete compensation. A similar analytic approach should be used if the primary disorder is metabolic. Finally, the presence of increased amounts of unmeasured anions determines the presence of a metabolic acidosis even when [Hco_3^-] is normal.

---

1. Albert MS, Dell RB, Winters RW. Quantitative displacement of acid–base equilibrium in metabolic acidosis. *Ann Intern Med.* 1967;66:312.
   Classic article that establishes confidence limits for metabolic acidosis.
2. Adrogue HJ, Madias NE. Management of life-threatening acid–base disorders. Part one. *N Engl J Med.* 1998;338:26–34; and Adrogue HJ, Madias NE. Management of life-threatening acid–base disorders. Part two. *N Engl J Med.* 1998;338:107–111.
   A two-part comprehensive review of acid–base homeostasis (153 references).
3. Forsythe SM, Schmidt GA. Sodium bicarbonate for the treatment of lactic acidosis. *Chest.* 2000;117:260–267.
   A review of the literature supporting bicarbonate administration in lactic acidosis. The absence of evidence suggesting improved outcomes prompts the authors to recommend that it not be used (91 references).
4. Gilfix BM, Bique M, Magder S. A physical chemical approach to the analysis of acid–base balance in the clinical setting. *J Crit Care.* 1993;8:187–197.
   A discussion of an alternative approach to estimating unmeasured anions and comparing with the classical anion "gap" approach.
5. Inman KJ, Sibbald WJ, Rutledge FS, et al. Does implementing pulse oximetry in a critical care unit result in substantial arterial blood gas savings? *Chest.* 1993;104:543.
   Compares the practice relating to obtaining ABG on 300 patients in the critical care unit, before and after the availability of oximetry.
6. McCurdy DK. Mixed metabolic and respiratory acid base disturbances: diagnosis and treatment. *Chest.* 1972;63:355S.
   One of the best reviews of metabolic acid-base disorders with the classic graphic relationship of $Paco_2$ to $[H^+]$.
7. Morris LR, Murphy MB, Kitabchi AE. Bicarbonate therapy in severe diabetic ketoacidosis. *Ann Intern Med.* 1986;105:836.
   This article sparked a controversy on the use of bicarbonate in metabolic acid–base disturbances.
8. Narins RG. Diagnostic strategies in disorders of fluid, electrolyte, and acid–base homeostasis. *Am J Med.* 1982;72:496.
   An excellent review with clinical case studies.
9. Palmer BF, Alpern RJ. Metabolic alkalosis. *J Am Soc Nephrol.* 1997;8:1462–1469.
   A review of the manifestations and approach to the management of metabolic alkalosis in the critical care environment.
10. Peris LV, Boix JH, Salom JV, et al. Clinical use of the arterial/alveolar oxygen tension ratio. *Crit Care Med.* 1983;11:881.
    Review of the use of the Pao_2/Pao_2 ratio and how it also can be used to predict the Fio_2 level needed to provide desired Pao_2.

7. BRONCHOSCOPIC PROCEDURES

Priscilla Madsen and James H. Harrell II

The history of bronchoscopy dates to 1887 when a German laryngologist, Gustov Killian, used a rigid esophagoscope to remove a pork bone from the right main stem bronchus of a patient who aspirated while dining. Chavalier Jackson is credited with establishing the field of bronchoscopy and developing numerous bronchoscopic techniques, safety protocols, and training courses. Rigid bronchoscopy remained the only way to visualize the airways until Ikeda introduced the flexible fiberoptic bronchoscope (FFB) in the 1960s.

The introduction of the FFB has substantially advanced the diagnostic and therapeutic possibilities in pulmonary medicine and has replaced the rigid bronchoscope in many situations. Currently, 97% of all airway interventions performed by pulmonologists use the FFB. The principal advantages of flexible bronchoscopy include (1) a more extensive view of the tracheobronchial tree, (2) ease of performance, and (3) no requirement for general anesthesia or an operating room. FFBs are available in various sizes and differ in external diameter, size of the working channel, and degree of flexion and extension of the tip. The optimal choice of bronchoscope depends on the specific purpose. The largest diameter bronchoscopes with a 6.5-mm outside diameter and an inside working channel of 2.5 mm are most useful if hemoptysis exists or might develop. Newer ultrathin FFBs with an outside diameter of 2.8 mm and inside working channel of 1.2 mm can sample peripheral lesions with some success and bypass a central airway obstruction to assess the peripheral bronchial tree without compromising the airway. The main drawback of the ultrathin FFB is intrinsic floppiness that makes it difficult to control. The standard FFB has an outside diameter of approximately 5.0 mm, an inside working channel of 2.0 mm and remains the "workhorse" for most bronchoscopies.

The most common indications for flexible bronchoscopy are lung masses, lung cancer staging, undiagnosed pulmonary infiltrates, mediastinal lymphadenopathy, hemoptysis, disorders affecting the central airways, endobronchial lesions, endotracheal tube placement, and therapeutic suctioning. The decision to perform bronchoscopy requires a careful risk/benefit analysis for each patient. There are few absolute contraindications. Contraindications include unstable bronchospasm, severe blood gases abnormalities (not correctable by bronchoscopy), unstable cardiac conditions, severe hypertension, increased intracranial pressure, uncontrolled seizures, and thrombocytopenia. Biopsies are contraindicated in uncontrolled bleeding disorders, thrombocytopenia, uremia, cirrhosis, severe pulmonary hypertension, and in some cases of severe anemia.

Fortunately, flexible bronchoscopy is a safe procedure with a strikingly low complication rate. Mortality has been reported to be less than 0.04%, with deaths resulting hemorrhage, a cardiovascular event, bronchospasm, aspiration pneumonia, or a medication reaction. Major complications are reported in approximately 0.1%, and include pneumothorax, bleeding (most often from biopsy), bronchospasm, fever, hypoxemia, cardiac dysrhythmias, and medication reactions.

Most of the complications reported involve reactions to premedication or topical anesthesia; consequently, we do not routinely use premedication or sedation and rely solely on topical anesthesia. If sedation is needed, we use midazolam because of its short half-life and amnestic effects. A short-acting narcotic also can be used to control coughing.

Bronchoscopy often is associated with modest hypoxemia (mean decrease in PaO_2 of 20 mmHg): The use of bronchoalveolar lavage (BAL) can worsen hypoxia. For this reason, patients with significant hypoxemia (e.g., PaO_2 <70 mmHg) should not undergo elective bronchoscopy unless absolutely necessary. To ensure adequate oxygenation, an oxygen mask with a fenestrated diaphragm for insertion of the bronchoscope can be used. Mechanically ventilated patients should be oxygenated with 100% oxygen before and during the procedure. After the procedure, oxygen supplementation should be weaned gradually, as tolerated.

Significant bleeding occurs in 1% to 4% of bronchoscopies, usually related to transbronchial biopsies, brushings, or endobronchial biopsies. For this reason, it is recommended that a patient's platelet count be above 50,000 for bronchoscopy and 75,000 for transbronchial biopsy. Patients who are immunocompromised, uremic, or have a chest malignancy have a higher incidence of bleeding. Attention should also be paid to medications that increase the risk of bleeding. Aspirin has been shown not to increase the risk of bleeding after transbronchial biopsy when there are no other risk factors. There are no studies of the safety of bronchoscopy in patients taking Coumadin or antiplatelet agents. For these reasons, we do not delay bronchoscopy if the patient has used aspirin, but we will delay elective bronchoscopy until antiplatelet agents have been discontinued for 7 to 10 days. For patients taking Coumadin, we routinely switch them to low-molecular-weight heparin and delay biopsy until the patient's INR normalizes.

Cardiac ischemia and dysrhythmias during bronchoscopy can occur even without a history of heart disease. Likewise, bronchospasm can occur in patients without a history of asthma; smokers have the highest risk. Fever within the first 24 hours after bronchoscopy is common and has been related to the volume of liquid instilled into the airways during the procedure. Bacteremia after flexible bronchoscopy, however, is very unusual. Antibiotic prophylaxis is optional for flexible bronchoscopy with or without biopsy, but it is recommended before rigid bronchoscopy in patients at moderate or high risk of endocarditis. Prophylaxis is also recommended in immunocompromised patients and those at risk for hematogenous joint infections.

Infection control in the bronchoscopy suite is an important aspect of ensuring the safety of the procedure. Transmission can be airborne or by contaminated instruments, including the bronchoscope itself or ancillary equipment. General guidelines to prevent infections in bronchoscopy suites have been published.

Patient preparation for elective bronchoscopy includes (1) fasting before the procedure to reduce the risk of aspiration (>8 hours preferable); (2) informed consent; (3) optional premedication (e.g., 0.5 mg atropine, intramuscularly, to reduce secretions); and (4) topical anesthesia (e.g., 0.45% tetracaine). Routine monitoring during bronchoscopy should include continuous pulse oximetry, blood pressure, heart rate, and a continuous electrocardiogram. All patients should receive supplemental oxygen during and after the procedure.

The flexible bronchoscope can be inserted either transnasally or transorally. We prefer the transnasal approach because it is simpler. The oral route may be necessary if significant nasal pathology or hemostatic disorders exist. When using the transnasal approach, the nasal fossa and nasopharynx should be carefully examined before the flexible bronchoscope is passed into the larynx. Once the larynx is reached, advancement of the bronchoscope is halted. At this point, the vocal cords can be anesthetized, examined for normal abduction and adduction, and assessed for pathology (polyps, lesions, erythema). Next, the flexible bronchoscope is passed through the cords, and the circumference of the trachea is carefully examined for mucosal changes and lesions, external compression, and abnormalities of the cartilaginous rings. Then the carina is examined for splaying, position, and mucosal abnormalities. All segmental bronchial orifices are inspected systematically with careful attention paid to their color, texture, position, relative size, patency, and the presence of splaying. The bronchial mucosa should be assessed carefully to identify submucosal infiltration, degree of acute or chronic inflammation, and nature and quantity of secretions.

A variety of sampling techniques, including bronchial washing, bronchial brushing (protected or nonprotected), bronchoalveolar lavage (protected or nonprotected), endobronchial or transbronchial forceps biopsy, and endobronchial or transbronchial needle aspiration, allows the operator to collect specimens from the respiratory tract. Selected peritracheal or peribronchial lymph nodes or other lesions also can be sampled by transbronchial needle aspiration techniques. The samples should be submitted for cytologic, histologic, microbiologic, biochemical, immunologic, and molecular laboratory analyses.

Flexible bronchoscopy plays a major role in determining the three most important considerations for managing patients with a lung mass or lung cancer: (1) tissue diagnosis, (2) staging, and (3) surgical options. Obtaining a tissue diagnosis is first and foremost in the evaluation of a patient with a lung mass. Because of its low risk and high yield, bronchoscopy, combined with computed tomography (CT) generally is the first step. The diagnostic yield for directly visible lesions when a variety of sampling techniques are used is approximately 72% to 94%. Reported yields for peripheral lesions not visible endoscopically range from 44% to 86%. Transbronchial biopsy techniques can be helpful, depending on the location of the lesion. The yield of transbronchial needle aspiration in the presence of mediastinal adenopathy detected by CT is 50%. In peripheral nodules, size is important: for lesions less than 2 cm in diameter, the yield can be as low as 23%.

Staging and evaluation of surgical options are important considerations. A second radiologically inapparent endobronchial tumor can be present in up to 7% of patients with lung cancer. In addition, endobronchial tumors should be evaluated before surgery, as the length of healthy bronchus and absence of lymphatic disease are important considerations in planning surgical technique during resection. In general, at least 2 cm of disease-free bronchus is required to create an adequate stump after a pneumonectomy.

Bronchoscopy is an important component of management after medical or surgical treatment for lung cancer. Endobronchial disease often can be radiographically silent; therefore, any patient with a prior history of lung cancer, lateralizing clinical signs, or new onset of hemoptysis should be considered for bronchoscopy.

The most frequent causes of hemoptysis include bronchitis, bronchiectasis, lung cancer, pneumonia, and tuberculosis. Bronchoscopy and CT are often complementary in evaluating hemoptysis. Bronchoscopy can be used to: (1) establish the cause; (2) determine the anatomic source of bleeding; and (3) apply therapeutic intervention(s). The diagnostic yield of bronchoscopy in hemoptysis is highest when the chest radiograph demonstrates focal findings. In this circumstance, bronchoscopy can help to determine the cause (72%) or source (10%) of bleeding in up to 82% of patients; approximately 30% of patients will prove to have a malignancy. However, with a normal or nonlocalizing chest radiograph, the detection of malignancy is much lower, averaging 6% (range of 0% to 16%). Risk factors that increase the likelihood of cancer with hemoptysis include male gender, age younger than age 50, and a smoking history of more than 40 pack-years.

When the chest radiograph is normal or nonlocalizing and the bronchoscopic examination is normal, the prognosis in patients with hemoptysis is generally good. Hemoptysis resolves in most patients within 6 months. During follow-up, lung cancer is identified rarely; 1% and 6% of patients were subsequently found to have cancer at 38 and 32 months, respectively, in two studies. Localizing the source of bleeding may be especially important with massive hemoptysis (>600 mL within 24 hours) when angiography, surgical interventions, or both are being considered. Potential therapeutic options for hemoptysis that can be applied through the bronchoscope include: (1) iced saline lavage; (2) topical vasoconstrictors (e.g., epinephrine); (3) endobronchial tamponade using the bronchoscope itself or a balloon catheter (e.g., a Fogarty balloon catheter can be introduced alongside the bronchoscope, whereas a 200-cm pulmonary tamponade balloon can be inserted through the bronchoscope); or (4) laser photocoagulation.

The specific diagnostic yield of transbronchial lung biopsy in diffuse lung disease in nonimmunocompromised patients is approximately 38%, but the yield depends on the patient population. For example, bronchoscopic diagnosis is relatively easy in sarcoidosis, lymphangitic cancer, alveolar proteinosis, and eosinophilic granuloma.

Bronchoscopy may be very valuable in the management of lower respiratory tract infections. In community-acquired pneumonia, most patients are treated effectively with empiric therapy. Bronchoscopic techniques may be useful if a patient responds incompletely or only transiently. A similar approach has been suggested in nonventilated patients with hospital-acquired pneumonia. In ventilator-associated pneumonia, the optimal use of bronchoscopic techniques and an invasive diagnostic procedure is unclear. Multiple studies have not clearly established better outcome measures such as mortality, cost-effectiveness, and antibiotic use. In nonimmunocompromised patients with smear-negative tuberculosis, bronchoscopy may increase the immediate diagnostic yield when smears of washings and bronchoalveolar lavage fluid are combined with stains of transbronchial biopsies. Postbronchoscopy sputum specimens may produce the highest diagnostic yield. In immunocompromised patients (e.g., transplant recipients and those with the human immunodeficiency virus [HIV] infection), bronchoscopy often proves helpful in evaluating a variety of infectious and noninfectious pulmonary complications. Such patients often present with nonspecific pulmonary infiltrates. Bronchoscopy plays a central role in the diagnosis of tuberculosis, *Pneumocystis carinii* pneumonia, and Kaposi's sarcoma in HIV-positive patients, and is frequently used early in the diagnosis of HIV-positive patients with chest infiltrates thought not to be due to community-acquired pneumonia.

In patients undergoing organ transplantation, bronchoscopic evaluation with bronchoalveolar lavage may be useful in diagnosing a variety of bacterial, mycobacterial, parasitic, and fungal infections. In addition to infectious complications, bone marrow and lung transplant recipients experience unique noninfectious problems in which bronchoscopy may be important in diagnosis. In bone marrow transplant recipients, the diagnosis of diffuse alveolar hemorrhage, idiopathic pneumonia syndrome, and secondary alveolar proteinosis can be facilitated by bronchoscopy. In lung transplant recipients, bronchoscopy is useful in assessing airway complications such as anastomotic ischemia, stenosis, dehiscence, and bronchomalacia. Rejection can be diagnosed by transbronchial biopsies with a sensitivity of 72 to 94% for acute rejection and 15 to 38% for chronic rejection with a single bronchoscopic examination. Routine surveillance transbronchial biopsies are used to monitor for acute rejection in some centers.

Bronchoscopic examination also plays an important role in intensive and special care units and anesthesia. Flexible bronchoscopy is both sensitive and specific in the diagnosis of inhalation injury and tracheal and bronchial rupture after blunt chest trauma. In anesthesia and intensive care units, flexible bronchoscopy can help manage endotracheal intubation, particularly if double lumen endotracheal tubes are needed. Indications for bronchoscopic-guided endotracheal intubation include patients at high risk for aspiration, patients in whom cervical movement is limited or undesirable (ankylosing spondylitis, Down syndrome, cervical spine injury) and patients with difficult airways. In addition, bronchoscopic intubation techniques are frequently used in the context of a difficult airway (difficulty with mask ventilation or laryngoscopic intubation, and obese sleep apnea patients). Endotracheal tube placement can be achieved in both the awake and the anesthetized patient using either a nasal or oral approach. The nasal route generally allows for easier access to the larynx. However, factors such as endotracheal tube size and sinusitis or bleeding risk need to be considered when choosing a nasal versus an oral approach.

In the awake patient, pharyngeal muscle tone is better maintained. Consequently, visualization of the larynx is easier than in a sedated or anesthetized patient. Once the bronchoscope enters the trachea and is passed into the mainstem bronchus, a premounted, well-lubricated endotracheal tube is advanced over the bronchoscope into the trachea. Proper placement 4 cm above the carina is verified and the tube is secured. When using the flexible bronchoscope for elective or emergent intubation, we prefer using only topical anesthesia with the patient awake and sitting upright. Under these circumstances, tracheal intubation with a flexible bronchoscope is safe and almost always successful and well tolerated. Emergent bronchoscopic intubation has a higher failure rate. Reasons for failure of bronchoscopic intubation include the inability to adequately visualize the larynx and impediments to advancing the endotracheal tube.

Bronchoscopy can be invaluable in assessing and managing upper airway injury, particularly during extubation. Bronchoscopy in patients at risk for upper airway obstruction (burn or cervical spine repair patients) can produce valuable information and suggest the optimal timing of extubation. High-risk patients may be extubated with bronchoscopic assistance. The FFB is passed through the endotracheal tube and initially maintained at the main carina. The endotracheal tube is pulled over the FFB and the patient is observed for stridor. The upper airway is carefully inspected as the bronchoscope is slowly withdrawn. If respiratory compromise occurs, the endotracheal tube is advanced over the bronchoscope and immediately replaced.

Tracheostomy tube placement is often necessary for long-term ventilation. Flexible bronchoscopy plays a role in the evaluation of posttracheostomy airway complications such as granulation tissue formation (frequently located on the anterior tracheal wall superior to the tracheostomy tube), tracheal stenosis, and tracheomalacia. Tracheal stenosis related to tracheostomy can present as failure to wean from mechanical ventilatory support. Other disorders that present in a similar manner include tracheomalacia and herpetic tracheobronchitis. Bronchoscopy is essential in establishing these diagnoses. Percutaneous dilatational tracheostomy is an alternative to surgical tracheostomy. Monitoring tube placement with bronchoscopy improves the safety of this procedure.

Bronchoscopy is of great value in removing secretions and foreign bodies. Retained or impacted secretions are associated with atelectasis, pneumonia, lung abscess, cystic fibrosis, and middle lobe syndrome. Bronchoscopy is performed when conservative measures fail and may be combined with saline lavage to clear impacted secretions. In pulmonary alveolar proteinosis, large-volume bronchoalveolar lavage (10 to 12 L of warm saline) through a double lumen endotracheal tube is the therapeutic procedure of choice. A variety of special techniques and instruments (grasping forceps, baskets, and Fogarty balloons) are available to facilitate foreign body removal.

Rigid bronchoscopy plays a special role in managing diseases of the central airways. The rigid bronchoscope offers several advantages over the flexible bronchoscope: (1) it provides improved airway control and ventilation, (2) it allows larger tissue pieces and blood clots to be removed and can be used to "core out" lesions, (3) it can be used to dilate stenotic airways, (4) it allows placement of silicone stents, and (5) it offers an improved safety profile of certain procedures (i.e., less risk of endobronchial fire when used for endobronchial ablative therapy). The flexible bronchoscope is frequently used through a rigid bronchoscope; in fact, the rigid bronchoscope is rarely used *without* a flexible bronchoscope.

Obstruction of the central airways can be from benign or malignant causes. Benign airway stenosis is associated with a wide variety of disorders, including sarcoidosis, amyloidosis, broncholithiasis, relapsing polychondritis, Wegener's granulomatosis, lung transplantation, pill aspiration, and postintubation tracheal stenosis. Bronchoscopic techniques applied to these conditions include the Nd:YAG laser (neodymium:yttrium-aluminum-garnet), dilatational therapy, and stents.

Malignant obstruction of the central airways is a common indication for rigid bronchoscopy. Malignant airway obstruction comes in three forms: (1) endobronchial tumor, (2) pure extrinsic tumors with external compression, or (3) a combination of the above. Patients with malignant central airway obstruction usually have inoperable malignancy, are elderly, have accompanying medical problems, or have failed other therapeutic interventions. The therapeutic goal is usually palliation, as cure is rare. The modality used depends on the form of obstruction and tumor type. In general, techniques available include:

1. Endobronchial ablative techniques
   (a) Nd:YAG laser therapy
   (b) Argon plasma coagulation (APC)
   (c) Electrocautery
   (d) Cryotherapy
2. Dilatational therapy using the rigid bronchoscope or balloons
3. Airway stents
4. Brachytherapy
5. Photodynamic therapy

Endobronchial ablative therapies are used to destroy endobronchial disease. Of the ablative techniques, the Nd:YAG laser is a key instrument. It provides a variety of tissue effects, including coagulation, carbonization, and vaporization. Tissue penetration is approximately 4 mm. Favorable conditions for Nd:YAG laser therapy include short endobronchial obstructing lesions with patent airways and functional lung distal to the obstruction. The best results are achieved in the large central airways (trachea, main bronchi, bronchus intermedius). Airway patency can be established in approximately 80 to 90% of patients. Besides palliation from a variety of symptoms, improvement in functional status usually results. It should be emphasized that airway obstruction from extrinsic compression is a contraindication to all the endobronchial ablative methods, including Nd:YAG laser therapy. Major complications are rare (~1%) and include perforations (tracheobronchial wall, blood vessels), arrhythmia, myocardial infarction, air embolism, and death. Safety and training guidelines for laser therapy have been published.

The remainder of endobronchial ablative techniques are relatively new in interventional pulmonology, including APC, a form of electrocautery using argon gas. The advantage of APC is the ability to treat lesions at right angles to the probe, which makes it amenable to therapy directed at the upper lobes. Tissue penetration is generally limited to 3 mm and complications are rare. A disadvantage of APC is that it is time consuming, making it unsuitable for debulking large tumors. Standard electrocautery can be used in most situations in which laser is used. Its main advantage is a cost savings for the institution; however, the risk of endotracheal fire is higher whenever flexible techniques are used. Cryotherapy uses cold temperature to destroy tissue. It requires successive freezing cycles during the same treatment session. Unfortunately, depth of tissue destruction is hard to predict and cell death happens progressively over a 1- to 2-week period. This requires a second "clean-up" bronchoscopy after the initial treatment to remove necrotic debris. It is not suitable for emergency management of central airway obstruction.

Dilatational therapy for benign airway stenosis is performed with either the rigid bronchoscope itself or with different angioplasty or valvuloplasty balloons. Typically, sequentially larger diameter scopes or balloons are introduced into the airways. The risk of tracheobronchial tears is minimized by experience, and several treatment sessions may be necessary to achieve the desired airway diameter.

The use of endobronchial stents has enhanced the methods available to interventional bronchologists by providing a means to maintain airway patency. Indications include (1) extrinsic compression from benign or malignant causes; (2) preparation for subsequent therapy in patients with malignancy (e.g., radiation therapy after tumor debulking by laser); (3) benign airway obstruction, including tracheobronchomalacia; and (4) management of tracheoesophageal fistula. A variety of different silicone stents are available, and custom-made stents can be requested from some companies. Important features of Silastic^{TM} stents include external studs that impede migration and smooth edges. Placement and removal of Silastic stents requires rigid bronchoscopy. Complications include migration, the development of granulation tissue at the stent margins, and impacted secretions. Stent migration in the subglottic space is a particularly difficult problem that can be prevented by a percutaneous suturing technique. For tracheoesophageal fistulas, successful double stenting of the trachea or left main bronchus and the esophagus has been performed.

Metal stents can be placed under bronchoscopic or fluoroscopic guidance and may not require rigid bronchoscopy. However, granulation tissue formation, migration, and stent fracture is common. A major disadvantage of metal stents is that they can be difficult to remove, and there are case reports of patients exsanguinating during attempted removal. In our view, this property makes silicone stents vastly superior to metal stents, especially when airway stenting may be needed transiently. Metal stents have a complication rate of 4 to 30%, depending on the population studied and, in our opinion, should never be placed for benign disease. Brachytherapy (endoluminal radiotherapy) is another treatment option for malignant airway lesions. The procedure is used mainly for palliation, although cure is possible for certain lesions (e.g., carcinoma in situ).

Brachytherapy is commonly used in patients with malignant recurrences after external beam radiation. A number of different treatment regimens have been described in the literature. We prefer the high-dose rate technique using a bronchoscopically placed afterloading catheter. Dosages given at a 10-mm distance from the source (iridium 192) are either 1000 cGy (one fraction) or 660 cGy (three to five fractions at weekly intervals), depending on the indication. Response rates reported in the literature vary from 71 to 100%. Complications include necrosis, hemorrhage, and fistula formation.

Photodynamic therapy refers to treatment of tumors with sensitizers and light in the presence of oxygen. Hematoporphyrin derivatives and porfimer sodium are the sensitizers predominantly used. Following intravenous injection, they are preferentially retained by neoplastic tissue. A light source using a laser is introduced endoscopically to activate the sensitizer approximately 48 hours after injection. In the presence of oxygen, tumor necrosis is produced and normal tissue regenerates. Photodynamic therapy is approved for treating both advanced and early lung cancer. Preliminary studies suggest that photodynamic therapy allows selected patients with early lung cancer to be spared surgical resection. In our institution, we have been using photodynamic therapy for the treatment of airway papilloma. The major complication of this intervention is photosensitivity. The patient needs to avoid direct sun exposure for several weeks after the injection of sensitizers. In the earlier literature, complications included massive hemorrhage and fistula formation. New sensitizing drugs and treatment regimens are being studied that may result in a more widespread use of photodynamic therapy.

One potential new technique for early detection of lung cancer is *fluorescent bronchoscopy*. This technique is based on the optical properties of tissue. Normal and neoplastic tissues fluoresce differently when illuminated by light of certain wavelengths. Normal tissue will fluoresce apple green, whereas abnormal tissue appears a deep maroon red. This helps guide biopsies and is useful in detecting precancerous squamous cell lesions. Whether fluorescent bronchoscopy becomes clinically useful remains to be seen, as it is only capable of screening the surface of the proximal airways and it is unclear how many preneoplastic lesions will progress to frank, invasive lung cancer. However, its usefulness as a research tool in the morphogenesis of predysplastic lesions to frank cancer is promising.

Endobronchial ultrasound is a promising new modality. It has been described for a variety of indications, including defining tumor depth before brachytherapy and assisting in central and peripheral transbronchial needle aspiration. A newly developed convex probe, EBUS, allows transbronchial needle aspiration with real-time ultrasound, which allows for direct visualization of the needle as it enters a lymph node. This newer technique uses Doppler technology to avoid vascular structures. Other advances include using a miniature EBUS probe to guide biopsy of peripheral nodules.

Virtual bronchoscopy is a new imaging technique that simulated bronchoscopy. It represents one form of three-dimensional reconstruction of the airways made possible by recent advances in processing volumetric (helical) CT data. Further studies and developments are needed to examine the impact of these new imaging techniques on diagnostic and therapeutic bronchoscopic procedures.

1. Wang KP, Mehta AC. *Flexible Bronchoscopy.* Cambridge: Blackwell Scientific; 1995.
   This text covers all the clinical aspects of flexible bronchoscopy.
2. Borchers SD, Beamis JF Jr. Flexible bronchoscopy. *Chest Surg Clin N Am.* 1996;6:169.
   References 2 to 38 are almost exclusively review articles.
3. Arroliga AC, Matthay RA. The role of bronchoscopy in lung cancer. *Clin Chest Med.* 1993;14:87.
4. Dasgupta A, Mehta AC. Transbronchial needle aspiration. An underused diagnostic technique. *Clin Chest Med.* 1999;20:39.
   This entire issue of Clinics in Chest Medicine *is devoted to aspects of flexible bronchoscopy.*
5. Sharafkhaneh A, Baaklini W, Gorin AB, et al. Yield of transbronchial needle aspiration in diagnosis of mediastinal lesions. *Chest.* 2003;24:2131–2135.
6. Herth F, Becker HD, Ernst A. Aspirin does not increase bleeding complications after transbronchial biopsy. *Chest.* 2002;122:1461–1464.

7. Mares DC, Wilkes DS. Bronchoscopy in the diagnosis of respiratory infections. *Curr Opin Pulm Med*. 1998;4:123.

    A brief review.
8. Ewig S, Torres A. Flexible bronchoscopy in nosocomial pneumonia. *Clin Chest Med*. 2001:22:263–279.
9. Narayanswami G, Salzman SH. Bronchoscopy in the human immunodeficiency virus-infected patient. *Semin Respir Infect*. 2003;18:80–86.
10. Chan KM, Allan SA. Infectious pulmonary complications in lung transplant recipients. *Semin Respir Infect*. 2002;14:291–302.
11. Soubani AO, Miller KB, Hassoun PM. Pulmonary complications in bone marrow transplantation: a practical approach to diagnosis and treatment. *Clin Chest Med*. 2004;25:189–201.

    A general review.
12. Shorr AF, Susla GM, O'Grady NP. Pulmonary infiltrates in the non-HIV-infected immunocompromised patient: etiologies, diagnostic strategies, and outcomes. *Chest*. 2004;125:260–271.
13. Paul S, Bueno R. The burned trachea. *Chest Surg Clin N Am*. 2003;10:343–348.

    A concise review covering acute and chronic management.
14. Davies D, Hopkins JS. Patterns in traumatic rupture of the bronchus. *Injury*. 1973;4:261.

    Useful description of the two types of tracheobronchial rupture.
15. Blosser SA, Stauffer JL. Intubation of critically ill patients. *Clin Chest Med*. 1996;17:355.

    References 15 and 16 are well-illustrated reviews.
16. Blando M, Gallo UE. Emergency airway management. *Emerg Clin North Am*. 2003;21:80–85.
17. Fulling PD, Roberts JT. Fiberoptic intubation. *Int Anesthesiol Clin*. 2000:38:189–217.
18. Guidelines for competency and training in fiberoptic bronchoscopy. Section on Bronchoscopy, American College of Chest Physicians. *Chest*. 1982;81:739.
19. Guidelines for fiberoptic bronchoscopy in adults. American Thoracic Society. Medical Section of the American Lung Association. *Am Rev Respir Dis*. 1987;136:1066.
20. Culver DA, Gordon SM, Mehta AC. Infection control in the bronchoscopy suite. A review of outbreaks and guidelines for prevention. *Am J Respir Crit Care Med*. 2003;167:1050–1056.

    A well written review.
21. Martin MA, Reichelderfer M. APIC guidelines for infection prevention and control in flexible endoscopy. Association for Professionals in Infection Control and Epidemiology, Inc. 1991, 1992, and 1993 APIC Guidelines Committee. *Am J Infect Control*. 1994;22:19.
22. Dajani AS, Taubert KA, Wilson W, et al. Prevention of bacterial endocarditis: recommendations by the American Heart Association. *Clin Infect Dis*. 1997;25:1448.
23. Prakash UBS. Prophylactic antibacterial therapy for bronchoscopy: indications. *J Bronchol*. 1997;4:281.
24. Karmy-Jones R, Cuschieri J, Vallieres E. Role of bronchoscopy in massive hemoptysis. *Chest Surg Clin N Am*. 2001;11:873–906.
25. Ernst A, Silvestri GA, Johnstone D, et al. Interventional pulmonary procedures: guidelines from the American College of Chest Physicians. *Chest*. 2003;123:1693–1717.
26. Wain JC. Rigid bronchoscopy: the value of a venerable procedure *Chest Surg Clin N Am*. 2001;11:735–748.

    A concise review.
27. Duhamel DR, Harrell JH II. Laser bronchoscopy. *Chest Surg Clin N Am*. 2001;11:769–789.

    A concise review.
28. Ciccone AM, De Giacomo T, Venuta F. Operative and non-operative treatment of benign subglottic laryngotracheal stenosis. *Eur J Cardiothorac Surg*. 2004;26:818–922.

A comparison of surgical and nonsurgical therapies for subglottic stenosis with a discussion of complications.

29. Wood DE. Airway stenting. *Chest Surg Clin N Am*. 2001;11:841–860.
    A general review of airway stents.
30. Unger M. Endobronchial therapy of neoplasms. *Chest Surg Clin N Am*. 2003;13:129–147.
    Review of interventional techniques in the management of endobronchial neoplasms.
31. Dweik RA, Stoller JK. Role of bronchoscopy in massive hemoptysis. *Clin Chest Med*. 1999;20:89.
32. Swanson KL, Edell ES. Tracheobronchial foreign bodies. *Chest Surg Clin N Am*. 2001;11:861–872.
33. Yasufuku K, Chiyo M, Sekine Y, et al. Real-time endobronchial ultrasound guided transbronchial needle aspiration of mediastinal and hilar lymph nodes. *Chest*. 2004;126:122–128.
34. Kurimoto N, Miyazawa T, Okimasa S. Endobronchial ultrasonography using a guide sheath increases the ability to diagnose peripheral pulmonary lesions endoscopically. *Chest*. 2004;126:959–965.
35. Escobar-Sacristan JA, Granda-Orive JI, Gutierrez Jimenez T, et al. Endobronchial brachytherapy in the treatment of malignant lung tumors. *Eur Respir J*. 2004;24:348–352.
36. Moghissi K, Dixon K. Is bronchoscopic photodynamic therapy a therapeutic option in lung cancer? *Eur Respir J*. 2003;22:535–541.
    A comprehensive review of the evidence supporting photodynamic therapy in early and advanced lung cancer.
37. Steiner RM, Liu JB, Goldberg BB, et al. The value of ultrasound-guided fiberoptic bronchoscopy. *Clin Chest Med*. 1995;16:519.
38. Gilbert S, Luketich JD, Christie NA. Fluorescence bronchoscopy. *Thoracic Surg Clin*. 2004;14:71–77.
    A review of fluorescence bronchoscopy.
39. Lacasse Y, Martel S, Hebert A, et al. Accuracy of virtual bronchoscopy to detect endobronchial lesions. *Ann Thorac Surg*. 2004;77:1774–1780.
    A prospective evaluation of the sensitivity, specificity, positive predictive value, and negative predictive value, and a review of prior studies evaluating virtual bronchoscopy.

8. LUNG BIOPSY AND THORACOSCOPY

Henri G. Colt

The tissue diagnosis of an infectious, neoplastic, or interstitial process responsible for a focal, nodular, or diffuse pulmonary infiltrate requires sampling of lung parenchyma. Bronchoscopy and bronchoalveolar lavage (BAL) are clearly beneficial for diagnosis of tuberculosis or *Pneumocystis carinii* pneumonia (PCP); however, lung biopsy often is indicated when BAL or other less-invasive procedures do not provide a diagnosis. Standard methods for lung biopsy include transbronchial biopsy (TBB), transbronchial needle aspiration (TBNA), percutaneous or transthoracic needle aspiration (TTNA), and open lung biopsy by thoracotomy (OLB).

Diagnostic strategies evolve continually and are affected by new technologies, concerns regarding resource allocation, and established outcome criteria. One such example is the resurgence of *thoracoscopy*. This procedure allows visualization of the lung, pleura, and mediastinum by a rigid telescope and pleural trocars through single or multiple small intercostal incisions. Thoracoscopy has been performed safely by some chest physicians and thoracic surgeons for many years, mainly for pleural biopsies and pleurodesis.

Recent improvements in instrumentation and video equipment have led to an increased use of thoracoscopic lung biopsy (TLB) and development of many video-assisted thoracic surgical techniques. TLB specimens are essentially wedge resections of lung parenchyma obtained using a disposable stapler and are similar in size (3–6 cm) to specimens obtained during thoracotomy. Diagnostic yield is also similar, making TLB an effective alternative to formal thoracotomy for many patients. Duration of hospitalization and patient morbidity are less than after thoracotomy. Relative contraindications to TLB include a history of a bleeding diathesis (because bleeding can be difficult to control using 5- and 7-mm instruments through small pleural trocars) and a history of intolerance to general anesthesia and selective single lung ventilation (e.g., intubated and mechanically ventilated patients with profound hypoxemia and poor lung compliance). Whether TLB using reusable forceps (instead of a stapling device) provides satisfactory parenchymal sampling, lower costs, and identical low morbidity requires further investigation.

Flexible fiberoptic bronchoscopy is probably the least invasive and most cost-effective means of obtaining specimens from the lung. Bronchoscopy allows (1) inspection of the central airways, (2) washings and brushings, and (3) biopsies of endobronchial lesions and lung parenchyma.

Transbronchial biopsy provides samples that range from 1.5 to 2.5 mm in size. Alveolar architecture (ideally bronchioles as well) should be present for specimens to be considered adequate or representative. This is especially true in patients with interstitial lung disease and in lung transplant recipients. Diagnostic yield is probably increased when four or more specimens are obtained. In lung transplant recipients, for example, most centers advocate six to eight specimens from different lung areas because of the nonuniform nature of lung rejection. Separate specimens should be obtained for microbiology and pathology. Fluoroscopic guidance is suggested for biopsy of parenchymal nodules, masses, and localized infiltrates. In lung cancer, when lesions are greater than 3 cm in diameter, diagnostic yield is greater than 80%; with peripheral nodules less than 2 cm in diameter, yield is less than 40%. The addition of washings, brushings, BAL, and TBNA, however, can increase diagnostic yield to 60% or more.

Also, TBB is helpful in diagnosing infection in both normal and immunocompromised hosts. TBB usually is not indicated when bacterial pneumonia is suspected, but is extremely helpful for the diagnosis of smear-negative tuberculosis, PCP, and fungal or viral infections (biopsy specimens confirm tissue invasion with organisms), especially when BAL is negative. With diffuse bilateral infiltrates on chest radiographs, specimens are obtained from multiple segments of one lung only because of the risk of complications.

Diseases with peribronchial predominance (e.g., sarcoidosis, lymphoma, or lymphangitic spread of cancer) are more likely to be diagnosed by TBB than are other diffuse processes. Other diseases commonly diagnosed by TBB, however, include alveolar proteinosis, pulmonary hemosiderosis, Goodpasture's syndrome, and eosinophilic granuloma. Less commonly diagnosed are Kaposi's sarcoma, lymphomatoid granulomatosis, hypersensitivity pneumonitis, Wegener's granulomatosis, bronchiolitis obliterans, and other specific causes of alveolitis or interstitial pulmonary fibrosis. Possible reasons for a less-than-satisfactory diagnostic yield in these instances are small specimen size, loss of tissue architecture, and collapse or crushing of biopsy samples by forceps that makes pattern recognition difficult for the pathologist. A diagnosis of inflammation or fibrosis should probably be considered nonspecific, prompting a more aggressive diagnostic approach, if clinically indicated.

Transbronchial needle aspiration is performed during bronchoscopy, principally for diagnosis and staging of lung cancer. Diagnostic yield is a function of instrumentation, operator experience, technique, perseverance, and lesion accessibility. TBNA can provide samples from mediastinal lymph nodes or tumors adjacent to the major airways. Depending on the needle, specimens may be obtained for cytology or histology. Needles vary in size from 18 gauge to smaller 22 gauge and are usually retractable into a protective sheath designed to prevent laceration of the bronchoscope during insertion and withdrawal. Some needles have inner stylets to improve rigidity. The addition of fluoroscopically guided TBNA to TBB may improve diagnostic yield in peripheral lesions. TBNA also enables sampling of mediastinal lymph nodes, especially in the paratracheal (group 4), subcarinal (group 7), and perihilar regions (group 10). A thorough knowledge of thoracic and mediastinal anatomy is essential. Computed tomography (CT) scans of the chest are helpful in guiding bronchoscopic sampling. Histology specimens are less likely to yield false-positive results than cytology specimens. Positive aspiration, however, in patients without evidence of nodal enlargement on imaging studies should be interpreted with caution. In general, experts agree that the diagnostic yield of TBNA is increased as operators acquire experience, perform more aspirates (although a plateau in yield has been noted after seven aspirates), and, most importantly, use rapid onsite examination (ROSE) by an experienced cytopathologist. Currently there is considerable interest about the potential use of endoscopic bronchial ultrasound (EBUS) to perform ultrasound guided biopsy in real time to increase yield. Decisions regarding unresectability should be based on firm evidence of mediastinal extension. Mediastinoscopy or mediastinotomy may be indicated, and a multidisciplinary approach to cancer therapy is advocated.

Complications of TBB and TBNA include pneumothorax in up to 3% of patients and bleeding. Risk of pneumothorax probably increases with forceps size, number of specimens, and whether patients have hyperinflated lung or cystic disease such as bullous emphysema, cystic fibrosis, or acquired immune deficiency syndrome (AIDS) with a history of PCP or pneumothorax. Fluoroscopic guidance increases diagnostic yield and decreases incidence of pneumothorax. Scant, transient hemoptysis often occurs after TBB and is of no consequence. Frank bleeding (>50 mL) can occur, especially if pulmonary or bronchial arteries are inadvertently biopsied or in patients with cavitating lesions. Complications can be avoided by performing a careful history and physical examination and obtaining a coagulation profile before the procedure. Patients with pulmonary hypertension, uremia, or known coagulopathy and individuals taking anticoagulants are at higher risk.

Procedures should be performed by trained personnel in a bronchoscopy suite fully equipped for emergency resuscitation. Bronchoscopists should be familiar with laryngoscopic or bronchoscopic endotracheal intubation techniques, chest tube insertion, and endoscopic techniques used to stop bleeding.

Transthoracic needle aspiration is especially helpful for lesions inaccessible to bronchoscopy (e.g., central masses, peripheral lesions abutting the pleura or chest wall) or when bronchoscopy is nondiagnostic. TTNA using biplane fluoroscopic guidance is less costly and time-consuming than CT-guided TTNA, which is usually reserved for lesions that cannot be well visualized fluoroscopically or those adjacent to vascular structures. Ultrasound guidance is promising, but can be used only in lesions abutting the pleural surface.

Large-bore cutting needles have been used for TTNA, but result in a greater number of complications, including potentially fatal air embolism. With smaller needles (18 to 22 gauge), complications are less frequent and sensitivity for diagnosis of malignancy in peripheral lesions is greater than 85%. The specific yield in benign lesions, however, ranges from 12 to 68%. A nondiagnostic aspirate, therefore, cannot exclude malignancy. A false-negative TTNA finding usually results from inadequate sampling or tissue necrosis. For these reasons, multiple samples from the lesion's center and periphery are advocated. Specimens should always be processed for cytology and microbiology, including Gram stain, fungal stains, and culture, because TTNA is particularly helpful in diagnosing granulomatous infection.

Complications of TTNA include pneumothorax and, occasionally, bleeding. Malignant seeding of the needle tract, although described, is extremely infrequent. Pneumothorax can occur in 5% to 60% of instances, but chest tubes are necessary in less than 20% of cases. Pneumothoraces have been related to extent of operator experience, needle size, number of passes, depth of the lesion from the skin, and presence of obstructive lung disease. Most occur immediately or within 1 hour after the procedure, so chest radiographs should be obtained after TTNA.

Open lung biopsy is the standard to which all lung biopsy techniques are compared. Diagnostic yield can vary, however, depending on whether the radiographically most involved lobe is sampled. Usually, at least two separate specimens are obtained. CT assessment of abnormalities helps to determine areas that should be sampled. The indications for surgical lung biopsies remain controversial; however, it appears that many healthcare providers are more inclined to proceed to lung biopsy with thoracoscopic wedge resections. In the presence of diffuse infiltrates and suspected infection, particularly in patients with AIDS or malignancy, investigators have suggested a limited role for OLB. In selected patient populations, however, such as when vasculitis, active interstitial pneumonitis, bronchiolitis, or infectious (aspergillosis, cytomegalovirus, or other viral pneumonias) lung disease is suspected, lung biopsy results, even when negative, help guide therapy. On occasion, specific causes altering medical therapy may not be identified, and biopsy results may not affect outcome. Most agree that when less-invasive procedures are nondiagnostic, appropriate timing of OLB or TLB requires careful consideration of clinical status, potential causes, therapeutic options, a planned management strategy based on biopsy findings, and an overall assessment of outcome probabilities and prognosis.

---

1. Anderson CL, Acevedo Crespo JC, et al. Risk of pneumothorax is not increased by obstructive lung disease in percutaneous needle biopsy. *Chest.* 1994;105:1705.
   Questions previous reports suggesting a linear correlation between degree of obstructive ventilatory impairment and risk of pneumothorax.
2. Anders GT, Linville KC, Johnson JE, et al. Evaluation of the float sign for determining adequacy of specimens obtained with transbronchial biopsy. *Am Rev Respir Dis.* 1991;144:1406.
   Specimens containing greater amounts of alveolar tissue float more often than sink.
3. Chin R Jr, McCain TW, Lucia MA, et al. Transbronchial needle aspiration in diagnosing and staging lung cancer: how many aspirates are needed? *Am J Respir Crit Care Med.* 2002;166:377–381.
   Maximum yield at about seven aspirates was noted. Also notes the importance of ROSE.
4. DeCamp MM Jr, Jaklitsch MT, Mentzer SJ, et al. The safety and versatility of video-thoracoscopy: a prospective analysis of 895 consecutive cases [see comments]. *J Am Coll Surg.* 1995;181:113.
   With videothoracoscopy, morbidity was often less than 2%, even in the elderly.
5. Ferson PF, Landreneau RJ, Dowling RD, et al. Comparison of open versus thoracoscopic lung biopsy for diffuse infiltrative pulmonary disease. *J Thorac Cardiovasc Surg.* 1993;106:194.
   Diagnostic yield of TLB was similar to that of OLB. Thoracoscopy resulted in a significant decrease in hospital stay.
6. Glaspole IN, Wells AU, duBois RM. Lung biopsy in diffuse parenchymal lung disease. *Monaldi Arch Chest Dis.* 2001;56:225–232.
7. Krasnik M, Vilmann P, Jacobsen GK. Preliminary experience with a new method of endoscopic transbronchial real time ultrasound guided biopsy for diagnosis of mediastinal or hilar lesions. *Thorax.* 2003;58:1083–1086.
   Excellent yield described in 15 patients under general anesthesia.
8. Kurimoto N, Murayama M, Yoshioka S, et al. Assessment of usefulness of endobronchial ultrasonography in determination of depth of tracheobronchial invasion. *Chest.* 1999;115:1500–1506.
   The beginning of a new science: the bronchoscopic ultrasonographic mapping of airway wall and tumor penetration. Such studies might help determine appropriate roles for various bronchoscopic modalities being proposed for therapy of early lung cancers.
9. Lee P, Colt HG. Using diagnostic thoracoscopy to optimal effect. *J Resp Illness.* 2003;24:503–509.
   A review of indications and techniques for pleuroscopy and thoracoscopy.

10. Lee P, Lan RS, Colt HG. Survey of pulmonologists' perspectives on thoracoscopy. *J Bronchol.* 2003;10:99–106.

Pulmonologists feel that this procedure is probably underutilized.

11. Loube DI, Johnson JE, Wiener D, et al. The effect of forceps size on the adequacy of specimens obtained by transbronchial biopsy. *Am Rev Respir Dis.* 1993;148:1411.

Large forceps used for TBB overall yielded more tissue, including more alveolar tissue, than did a small forceps. Subsequent studies by other investigators refute this hypothesis.

12. Robbin ED, Burke CM. Lung biopsy in immunosuppressed patients. *Chest.* 1986;89:276.

A clinical commentary regarding risks, benefits, and outcome of OLB. A review of the role of VATS also addressing role of CT scanning.

13. Ravini M, Ferraro G, Barbieri B, et al. Changing strategies of lung biopsies in diffuse lung diseases: the impact of video-assisted thoracoscopy. *Eur Respir J.* 1998;11:99.

Many clinicians are proposing the use of thoracoscopy earlier in the course of the evaluative process in patients with lung diseases.

14. Roviaro GC, Varoli F, Vergani C, et al. State of the art in thoracoscopic surgery: a personal experience of 2000 videothoracoscopic procedures and an overview of the literature. *Surg Endosc.* 2002;16:881–892.

Despite relatively frequent usage, VATS is still far from achieving the scientific and operational maturity attained by laparoscopy.

15. Schenk DA, Strollo PJ, Pickard JS, et al. Utility of the Wang 18 gauge transbronchial histology needle and the staging of bronchogenic carcinoma. *Chest.* 1989;96:272.

Transbronchial needle aspiration yielded malignant diagnosis in 20 of 29 (69%) patients with bronchogenic carcinoma and mediastinal adenopathy demonstrated by chest CT scan.

16. Shure D. Transbronchial biopsy and needle aspiration. *Chest.* 1989;95:1130.

An older but classic review covering the equipment, techniques, indications, results, and complications of TBB and TBNA.

17. Shure D, Fedullo PF. Transbronchial needle aspiration of peripheral masses. *Am Rev Respir Dis.* 1983;128:1090.

The addition of TBNA to TBB, brushings, and washings significantly increases diagnostic yield of flexible fiberoptic bronchoscopy. One of the first, yet major, studies demonstrating the utility of TBNA.

9. MEDIASTINAL EXPLORATION

John E. Barkley

Surgical exploration of the mediastinum is useful for staging bronchogenic carcinoma prior to thoracotomy and for evaluating other causes of mediastinal lymphadenopathy, such as lymphoma, sarcoidosis, and tuberculosis. The terms *mediastinoscopy, mediastinotomy,* and *extended cervical mediastinoscopy* are often used interchangeably, but they are very different procedures with different indications and risks.

Mediastinoscopy was first introduced by Carlens in 1959 as a staging technique to assess the operability of bronchogenic carcinoma. The procedure is performed by making a 3-cm transverse incision between the thyroid cartilage and the suprasternal notch. The dissection is carried down through the pretracheal fascia, and a plane is developed between the trachea and the innominate artery, aorta, and pulmonary artery by blunt dissection. The mediastinoscope, similar in design to a Jackson straight laryngoscope, is introduced into the incision, using the anterior tracheal and bronchial cartilaginous rings as reference points. Lymph nodes accessible at mediastinoscopy include the right and left upper paratracheal (AJCC stations 2R and 2L), the right and left lower paratracheal (AJCC stations 4R and 4L), and the anterior subcarinal (AJCC station 7) nodes. Tracheobronchial angle nodes (AJCC stations 10R and 10L) are within the pleural reflection; they are now designated as N1 (hilar) and therefore cannot be biopsied without creating a pneumothorax. The subaortic (AJCC station 5), para-aortic (AJCC station 6), paraesophageal (AJCC station 8), and inferior pulmonary ligament (AJCC station 9) nodes cannot be biopsied by cervical mediastinoscopy. In experienced hands, reported complications are infrequent, occurring in approximately 3% of cases. The most frequent complication is right-sided pneumothorax resulting from inadvertent transmediastinal pleural biopsy of the lung. Other reported complications include hemorrhage, recurrent laryngeal nerve damage, injuries to the trachea and esophagus, and wound infections. Mortality is exceedingly rare; no deaths were reported in two series that analyzed results from 2,259 procedures.

Anterior (parasternal) mediastinotomy was originally introduced by McNeill and Chamberlain in 1966 as an alternative to cervical mediastinoscopy. It is currently used to evaluate anterior mediastinal lymph nodes in cases of left upper lobe carcinoma and as a means of biopsy of anterior mediastinal masses. Nodal groups unreachable by traditional cervical mediastinoscopy—aortopulmonary nodes and anterior mediastinal nodes (AJCC stations 5 and 6)—are approachable by this technique.

Many modifications of McNeill and Chamberlain's initial procedure have been reported. An incision can be made either over the seccond costal cartilage, which is then excised, or in an intercostal location without any cartilage excision. An intrapleural or extrapleural approach may be used. After blunt dissection and digital palpation, a mediastinoscope is then inserted to identify and biopsy lymph nodes in the involved chains. Experience with anterior mediastinotomy is considerably less than that with cervical mediastinoscopy; nonetheless, the complication rate appears similar.

Ginsberg and colleagues have reported results with extended *cervical mediastinoscopy*, which allows access to superior and anterior mediastinal lymph nodes in a single procedure. Following traditional cervical mediastinoscopy, the pretracheal fascia is broken down digitally and the mediastinoscope is passed over the aortic arch, between the left carotid and innominate arteries and posterior to the left innominate vein, to sample subaortic and para-aortic lymph nodes. A single superficial wound infection was the only complication in a series of 100 consecutive cases. More experience with this procedure must be obtained prior to its widespread use because of the potential for injury to so many major vascular structures.

Transbronchial needle aspiration (TBNA) has proved to be a valuable and less invasive means of evaluating the status of mediastinal lymph nodes prior to thoracotomy. Bronchoscopically, there is excellent access to the paratracheal and subcarinal lymph nodes. However, it is a blind biopsy procedure leading to false negatives. False-positive aspirates, although rare, have been reported as well. Additionally, there is increasing evidence that a number of variables may influence the resectability rate of bronchogenic carcinoma. These include the site and extent of mediastinal extension and whether this extension is intranodal or extranodal in nature—data that cannot be obtained by a blind transbronchial approach. Several new modalities for mediastinal exploration may help increase the yield of TBNA and are being studied.

Endoscopic ultrasound-guided needle aspiration (EUS-NA) uses an endoscope with an ultrasound probe on the end and a working channel through which a catheter with a needle can be passed. EUS-NA performed from the gastrointestinal side provides access to nodal levels 2R/L, 4R/L, 5, 7, 8, 9, the left adrenal gland and portions of the liver. *Endobronchial ultrasound-guided needle aspiration (EBUS-NA)* from the tracheobronchial side also allows direct visualization of the lesion being sampled. EUS-NA and EBUS-NA require additional equipment and operator expertise that are not yet widely available.

Less well-studied but emerging adjunctive imaging techniques are *CT fluoroscopy* and *virtual bronchoscopy*. Further investigation is required to determine their roles in mediastinal exploration.

Exactly which patients with bronchogenic carcinoma should undergo or, more precisely, not undergo mediastinal lymph node biopsy before thoracotomy remains controversial. No patient should be denied the opportunity of surgical cure based on imaging techniques alone. Neither should a patient undergo the risk of a needless thoracotomy if a less invasive technique will establish unresectability. Although CT scanning of the chest is considered a standard part of the preoperative assessment of patients with bronchogenic carcinoma, the sensitivity and specificity are poor at approximately 65%. Positron emission tomography (PET) has better sensitivity and specificity for detecting lymph node metastases and can help direct the surgeon toward particular lymph node groups that show increased activity on PET scanning. The roles of CT scanning, PET, bronchoscopy, EUS-NA, EBUS-NA, CT fluoroscopy, virtual bronchoscopy, mediastinoscopy, and mediastinotomy will continue to evolve with advancements in the molecular biology, immunohistochemistry, prognostication, and therapy of bronchogenic carcinoma.

---

1. Coughlin M, Deslauriers J, Beaulieu M, et al. Role of mediastinoscopy in pretreatment staging of patients with primary lung cancer. *Ann Thorac Surg.* 1985;40:556.
   No deaths were attributed to mediastinoscopy in a series of 1,259 cases. Abnormal mediastinal lymph nodes were found at mediastinoscopy in 27% of cases.
2. Daly BD Jr, Faling LJ, Bite G, et al. Mediastinal lymph node evaluation by computed tomography in lung cancer. An analysis of 345 patients grouped by TNM staging, tumor size, and tumor location. *J Thorac Cardiovasc Surg.* 1987;94:664.
   No true positive CT scans were obtained in 59 patients with peripheral lesions less than 2 cm in diameter.
3. Dasgupta A, Mehta AC. Transbronchial needle aspiration: an underused diagnostic technique. *Clin Chest Med.* 1999;20:39.
   Excellent review of the role of transbronchial needle aspiration in lung cancer. Excellent bibliography.
4. Ginsberg RJ, Rice TW, Goldberg M, et al. Extended cervical mediastinoscopy. *J Thorac Cardiovasc Surg.* 1987;94:673.
   After extended cervical mediastinoscopy, only one of 75 patients could not undergo a complete resection.
5. Goldstraw P. Mediastinal exploration by mediastinoscopy and mediastinotomy. *Br J Dis Chest.* 1988;82:111.
   Concise, well-referenced review of indications, limitations, and surgical techniques.
6. Luke WP, Pearson FG, Todd TR, et al. Prospective evaluation of mediastinoscopy for assessment of carcinoma of the lung. *J Thorac Cardiovasc Surg.* 1986;91:53.
   No deaths were attributable to mediastinoscopy in a series of 1,000 patients. Abnormal mediastinal lymph nodes were found at mediastinoscopy in 30% of patients; at thoracotomy, 52 of 596 patients had abnormal mediastinal nodes.
7. McLoud TC, Bourgouin PM, Greenberg RW, et al. Bronchogenic carcinoma: analysis of staging in the mediastinum with CT by correlative lymph node imaging and sampling. *Radiology.* 1992;182:319.
   Using lymph node size greater than 10 mm (short-axis diameter), CT scanning had sensitivity and specificity of 64% and 62%, respectively.
8. Mountain CF. Revisions in the International System for Staging Lung Cancer. *Chest.* 1997;111:1710.
   Revised AJCC staging system for non–small-cell lung cancer.
9. Mountain CF, Dresler CM. Regional lymph node classification for lung cancer staging. *Chest.* 1997;111:1718.
   Revised AJCC staging system for non–small-cell lung cancer. Updated mediastinal lymph node map.

10. Patterson GA, Piazza D, Pearson FG, et al. Significance of metastatic disease in subaortic lymph nodes. *Ann Thorac Surg.* 1987;43:155.
    Patients with left upper lobe or left main stem tumors and subaortic (AJCC station 5) lymph node involvement as the only site of metastasis had a 5-year survival of 28%.
11. Ratto GB, Mereu C, Motta G. The prognostic significance of preoperative assessment of mediastinal lymph nodes in patients with lung cancer. *Chest.* 1988;93: 807.
    Mediastinoscopy was more sensitive and specific in detecting mediastinal metastases than two-plane tomography, CT, and transbronchial needle aspiration.
12. Requet M, Hedden G, Debesse P. Direct lymphatic drainage of lung segments to the mediastinal nodes: an anatomic study on 260 patients. *J Thorac Cardiovasc Surg.* 1987;94:673.
    Detailed discussion of lymphatic spread of bronchogenic carcinoma.
13. Schreinemakers HH, Joosten HJ, Mravunac M, et al. Parasternal mediastinoscopy. Assessment of operability in left upper lobe lung cancer: a prospective analysis. *J Thorac Cardiovasc Surg.* 1988;95:298.
    The addition of parasternal mediastinoscopy to cervical mediastinoscopy proved useful in identifying mediastinal metastases in patients with left upper lobe bronchogenic carcinoma.
14. Seely JM, Mayo JR, Miller RR, Muller NL. T1 Lung cancer: prevalence of mediastinal nodal metastases and diagnostic accuracy of CT. *Radiology.* 1993;186: 129.
    Twenty-one percent of 104 patients with T1 lesions had mediastinal nodal metastases.
15. Vansteenkiste JF, Stroobants SG, De Leyn PR, et al. Lymph node staging in non-small-cell lung cancer with FDG-PET scan: a prospective study on 690 lymph node stations from 68 patients. *J Clin Oncol.* 1998;16:2142.
    Combination of PET and CT scanning dramatically improved the accuracy of staging the mediastinum.
16. Vansteenkiste JF, De Leyn PR, Deneffe GJ, et al. Survival and prognostic factors in resected N2 non-small-cell lung cancer: a study of 140 cases. *Ann Thorac Surg.* 1997;63:1441.
    Excellent discussion section with nice review of the literature on surgical treatment of N2 disease.
17. Wallace MB, Silvestri GA, Sahai AV, et al. Endoscopic ultrasound-guided fine needle aspiration for staging patients with carcinoma of the lung. *Ann Thorac Surg.* 2001;72:1861.
    Sensitivity and specificity of EUS-NA 87 and 100%, respectively.
18. Okamoto H, Watanabe K, Nagatomo A, et al. Endobronchial ultrasonography for mediastinal and hilar lymph node metastases of lung cancer. *Chest.* 2002;121: 1498.
    Overall accuracy of EBUS 94% in 37 patient studies. Good discussion of technique.
19. Toloza EM, Harpole L, Detterbeck F, et al. Invasive staging of non-small-cell lung cancer: a review of the current evidence. *Chest.* 2003;123:157S.
    Excellent review of current state of invasive staging of the mediastinum. Excellent bibliography.

10. PREOPERATIVE PULMONARY EVALUATION

Stephen H. Lee

The goal of preoperative pulmonary evaluation (PPE) is to identify individuals who are at increased risk for pulmonary-related morbidity and mortality due to surgery. The risk assessment is accomplished by carefully reviewing the specific characteristics of the patient and the details of the operative procedure. Some risk factors may be attenuated by preoperative measures.

The major postoperative pulmonary complications (PPCs) are pneumonia, atelectasis, bronchospasm, hypoxemia, and ventilatory failure. Other complications include pneumothorax, bronchitis, and pleural effusions. The reported incidence of PPCs varies widely, depending on the patient population, type of surgery, and criteria used to define PPCs. No one standard exists. Most published studies are retrospective, but prospective studies and randomized trials are beginning to appear.

The most important patient-related risk factors for PPCs are general health status, underlying chronic obstructive pulmonary disease (COPD), and smoking. The general health status reflects the patient's overall function and the presence of comorbidities. The American Society of Anesthesiologists "class," originally formulated to stratify perioperative mortality risk, strongly correlates with risk for PPC. Preoperative exercise capacity (stair climbing, stationary bike, walk test) and functional dependence also accurately predict either PPCs alone or combined cardiopulmonary endpoints. Other markers of general health, such as nutritional status, recent weight loss, central neurologic deficits, and albumin level, also may be important.

COPD is a strong, consistent risk factor for PPCs in many studies. In one study of patients with severe COPD undergoing nonthoracic surgery, the odds of a PPC were 14 times higher for those in ASA class 4 or 5 compared with ASA class 1, 2, or 3. The incidence of PPCs increases with the severity of the underlying disease and is likely the result of perioperative changes in lung volumes, diaphragmatic function, chest wall mechanics, and effects of anesthesia. Acute exacerbations should be treated before any elective or nonemergent surgery. For those with chronic, stable COPD, lung function should be optimized to the best level possible. Prophylactic antibiotics are not recommended. It may be necessary to delay surgery to achieve these goals. The data on asthma as a risk factor are less clear. Those with active, symptomatic asthma are prone to more PPCs; therefore, like COPD, asthma should be treated appropriately before surgery. If needed, a short course of preoperative corticosteroids does not appear to increase the incidence of postoperative complications. During induction of anesthesia, the use of thiobarbiturates and oxybarbiturates is associated with a much higher incidence of wheezing in asthmatics compared with nonasthmatics. Propofol does not appear to cause wheezing in either population.

Finally, smoking history, particularly current smoking and prior heavy smoking, is an important risk factor for PPCs and increases the risk twofold to sixfold, as compared with never-smokers. Although quitting should be a goal for any smoker, the timing of smoking cessation or reduction in relation to surgery appears to be very important. Several studies have shown significantly greater risk of PPCs in those who reduce or stop smoking less than 8 weeks before surgery compared with never smokers or those who reduce or quit smoking more than 4 to 8 weeks before surgery. Clearly, smoking cessation should be encouraged as early as possible and, whenever possible, at least 8 weeks before surgery.

Other factors also should be considered during the preoperative evaluation. Although older age is likely a weak risk factor, obesity does not appear to increase the risk of PPCs when confounding variables are considered. Obstructive sleep apnea (OSA) is associated with increased postoperative complications, but it is unclear whether pulmonary complications are increased. Certainly, careful clinical monitoring is warranted in patients with OSA, given the potential impact that pain, diaphragmatic and chest wall dysfunction, sedatives, and analgesics may have on upper and lower airway respiratory function during the postoperative period. Continuous positive airway pressure or noninvasive ventilation may be needed.

The most important operative risk factor for PPCs is the anatomic location of the procedure. Surgery close to the diaphragm (ie, thoracic and upper abdominal) is associated with a much higher risk of PPCs than for surgery outside of these areas. PPCs are rare in extremity surgery. The exceptions are for neurosurgical or head and neck operations, in which the risk of aspiration pneumonia appears to be higher. In chest and upper abdominal surgeries, there are significant decreases in both vital capacity and functional residual capacity (FRC). FRC decreases by about 30% after upper abdominal surgery and by 35% after thoracotomy, compared to about 10 to 15% reduction in FRC for lower abdominal surgery. Diaphragmatic dysfunction for up to 1 week that is not mitigated by analgesics may play a significant role in postoperative restrictive physiology. Maintaining an adequate FRC is important to prevent atelectasis and subsequent ventilation-perfusion mismatch.

Laparoscopic techniques appear to have a lower PPC rate than open techniques. In a meta-analysis of open (OS) versus laparoscopic splenectomy (LS), the PPC rate was three times higher in the OS group (9.0% vs 3.1%, respectively, for the OS and LS groups). In another study, the incidence of PPC was 6.4 times higher from open cholecystectomy compared with laparoscopic surgery (17.2% vs 2.7%, respectively).

General anesthesia can lead to pulmonary complications by several mechanisms. Endotracheal intubation may be complicated by aspiration or bronchospasm. Anesthetic gases attenuate hypoxic vasoconstriction, impair mucociliary function and clearance of secretions, abolish the cough reflex and periodic sighs, and impair diaphragmatic function. The consequences are ventilation-perfusion mismatch, atelectasis, and decrease in FRC. There is some evidence that regional neuraxial (spinal, epidural) anesthesia results in less PPCs than general anesthesia. A comprehensive meta-analysis of randomized trials showed that the odds of postoperative pneumonia are reduced by 37% with use of regional anesthesia as opposed to general anesthesia. When comparing procedures in which a combination of regional and general anesthesia was used versus general anesthesia alone, the odds of respiratory depression are reduced by 57% and pneumonia by 47%. Thus, the use of regional anesthesia, with or without general anesthesia, appears to be associated with less risk for PPCs.

The preoperative evaluation should include a thorough history and physical examination to identify risk factors for PPCs. In otherwise healthy patients, routine, preoperative chest radiographs to detect occult disease are not indicated, as they rarely alter the choice of anesthetic technique or surgical approach. For those with evidence of cardiopulmonary disease, a chest radiograph before high-risk surgery may be helpful as a baseline for comparative purposes. Routine arterial blood gas (ABG) studies also are not recommended. Although several older case series identify $PaCO_2$ higher than 45 mmHg as a significant risk factor for PPCs, a recent review of blinded trials did not find hypercarbia to be a significant risk factor in either univariate or multivariate analyses. Furthermore, hypercarbia is usually found in patients with severe underlying lung disease that can be suspected on clinical grounds and confirmed by pulmonary function testing. It may be reasonable to obtain a preoperative ABG in patients with chronic lung disease, especially those who are undergoing high-risk procedures, and is recommended for all who are undergoing lung resection. Although not an absolute contraindication for surgery, the finding of hypercarbia should increase one's clinical vigilance for providing meticulous perioperative care.

Methodologic differences in studies about preoperative pulmonary function testing (PFT) make it difficult to make a single statement about the value of these tests. The most useful spirometric parameters are the forced vital capacity (FVC), forced expiratory volume during the first second of the FVC maneuver (FEV_1), and the FEV_1/FVC ratio. Several reviews suggest that the information from the clinical evaluation (eg, history, physical examination, functional/ASA class) is just as informative as that derived from PFTs for purposes of preoperative evaluation. Nevertheless, in patients undergoing high-risk surgery, PFTs are recommended in those with a history of unexplained dyspnea, chronic lung disease, or significant smoking. In such patients, the PFT data may influence preoperative pulmonary care and other perioperative management strategies.

The preoperative evaluation of patients undergoing lung resection surgery differs from the recommendations outlined above. In addition to assessing the usual factors, patients should undergo a thorough evaluation to determine whether they can withstand the loss of resected lung tissue without significantly increasing morbidity or mortality risk. In one retrospective review of patients undergoing pneumonectomy, lobectomy, or wedge resection, 25% of patients had a PPC and the mortality rate was 7.5%. All patients who are candidates for lung resection surgery should undergo PFTs, particularly the FEV_1 and diffusing capacity for carbon monoxide. This evaluation may be supplemented with additional tests including exercise capacity (e.g., cardiopulmonary exercise testing, stair climbing, or 6-minute walk) and/or estimation of predicted postoperative (PPO) lung function to calculate the anticipated pulmonary reserve remaining after resection. PPO FEV_1 after pneumonectomy may be calculated based on the results of quantitative perfusion scanning: preoperative FEV_1 × (1-fraction of total perfusion for the resected lung). In a similar manner, PPO FEV_1 after lobectomy may be calculated using the results of the quantitative perfusion scan, or by using the following formula: preoperative FEV_1 × (# of segments remaining/total # of segments). There are a total of 19 bronchopulmonary segments: RUL (3), RML (2), RLL (5), LUL (5), LLL (4). Several recent, evidence-based algorithms for the evaluation of the lung resection candidate have been published and are listed in the reference section.

1. Powell CA, Caplan CE. Pulmonary function tests in preoperative pulmonary evaluation. *Clin Chest Med.* 2001;22:703–714.
   A thorough review article on preoperative pulmonary evaluation, including a section on lung resection surgery.
2. Smetana GW. Preoperative pulmonary evaluation. *N Engl J Med.* 1999;340:937–944.
   A short but thorough general review on risk factors, evaluation, and management strategies.
3. Arozullah AM, Daley J, Henderson WG, et al. Multifactorial risk index for predicting postoperative respiratory failure in men after major noncardiac surgery. *Ann Surg.* 2000;232:242–253.
   This paper presents a point scoring system to stratify patients into five groups based on risk of postoperative pneumonia. The model performed well when tested against the validation sample. A major strength of this study lies in the huge sample sizes of both the derivation (n = 160,805) and validation (n = 155,266) cohorts.
4. Arozullah AM, Khuri SF, Henderson WG, et al. Development and validation of a multifactorial risk index for predicting postoperative pneumonia after major noncardiac surgery. *Ann Intern Med.* 2001;135:847–857.
   This paper presents a point–scoring system to stratify patients into five groups based on risk of postoperative respiratory failure. The model performed well when tested against the validation sample. A major strength of this study lies in the huge sample sizes of both the derivation (n = 81,719) and validation (n = 99,390) cohorts.
5. Wong DH, Weber EC, Schell MJ, et al. Factors associated with postoperative pulmonary complications in patients with severe chronic obstructive pulmonary disease. *Anesth Analg.* 1995;80:276–284.
   In this retrospective review of patients with severe underlying COPD undergoing nonthoracic surgery, the odds of a PPC were 14 times higher for those in ASA class IV or higher compared with those in ASA class III or lower (multivariate analysis).
6. Girish M, Trayner E Jr, Dammann O, et al. Symptom-limited stair climbing as a predictor of postoperative complications after high-risk surgery. *Chest.* 2001;120:1147–1151.
   In this prospective study of patients undergoing high-risk surgeries (thoracotomy, sternotomy, upper abdominal), the positive predictive values for a postoperative cardiopulmonary complication were 89%, 80%, 63%, 52%, and 32% for those unable to climb at least one, two, three, four, and five flights of stairs, respectively.

Overall, pulmonary complications were nearly three times as common as cardiac complications (30% vs 11%, respectively).

7. Kroenke K, Lawrence VA, Theroux JF, et al. Postoperative complications after thoracic and major abdominal surgery in patients with and without obstructive lung disease. *Chest.* 1993;104:1445–1451.

The incidence of serious, postoperative pulmonary complications increased with increasing severity of the underlying COPD. For those with no, mild–moderate, and severe COPD, the incidence of severe PPCs was 4% versus 10% versus 23 percent, respectively.

8. Ferguson MK. Preoperative assessment of pulmonary risk. *Chest.* 1999;115:58S–63S.

A concise review of PPCs related to different types of surgeries with a particular focus on the pathophysiology underlying the increased risk.

9. Kabalin CS, Yarnold PR, Grammer LC. Low complication rate of corticosteroid-treated asthmatics undergoing surgical procedures. *Arch Intern Med.* 1995; 155:1379–1384.

Preoperative treatment with corticosteroids in asthmatics does not increase the risk of postoperative infection.

10. Pizov R, Brown RH, Weiss YS, et al. Wheezing during induction of general anesthesia in patients with and without asthma: a randomized, blinded trial. *Anesthesiology.* 1995;82:1111–1116.

Wheezing during induction of anesthesia occurred in 45% versus 26% of asthmatics receiving thiobarbiturates and oxybarbiturates, respectively, compared with 16% versus 3% of nonasthmatics, respectively. There was no wheezing in either group when propofol was used as the induction agent.

11. Nagagawa M, Tanaka H, Tsukuma H, et al. Relationship between the duration of the preoperative smoke-free period and the incidence of postoperative pulmonary complications after pulmonary surgery. *Chest.* 2001;120:705–710.

Among patients who quit smoking before surgery, the incidence of PPCs does not start to decline until the smoke-free period is at least 5 to 8 weeks, and reaches the incidence of never-smokers with 8 to 11 weeks of a smoke-free period.

12. Warner MA, Offord KP, Warner ME, et al. Role of preoperative cessation of smoking and other factors in postoperative pulmonary complications: a blinded prospective study of coronary artery bypass patients. *Mayo Clin Proc.* 1989;64:609–616.

The PPC rate was four times greater for those patients who stopped smoking for 2 months or less compared with those who stopped for more than 2 months. With 6 months of smoking cessation, the PPC rate was similar to that of nonsmokers.

13. Simonneau G, Vivien A, Sartene R, et al. Diaphragm dysfunction induced by upper abdominal surgery. Role of postoperative pain. *Am Rev Respir Dis.* 1983;128:899–903.

Small study on five patients showing marked diaphragmatic dysfunction lasting 1 week after upper abdominal surgery that is not mitigated by postoperative analgesics. The result is restrictive physiology.

14. Winslow ER, Brunt ML. Perioperative outcomes of laparoscopic versus open splenectomy: a meta-analysis with an emphasis on complications. *Surgery.* 2003; 134:647–655.

Laparoscopic splenectomy is associated with a threefold decreased risk of PPCs compared with open splenectomy (3.1% vs 9.0%, respectively).

15. Hall JC, Tarala RA, Hall JL. A case-control study of postoperative pulmonary complications after laparoscopic and open cholecystectomy. *J Laparoendosc Surg.* 1996;6:87–92.

Open cholecystectomy is associated with a 6.4 times higher risk of PPCs compared with laparoscopic cholecystectomy (17.2% vs 2.7%, respectively).

16. Rodgers A, Walker N, Schug S, et al. Reduction of postoperative mortality and morbidity with epidural or spinal anaesthesia: results from overview of randomized trials. *BMJ.* 2000;321:1–12.

The use of regional, neuraxial (spinal, epidural) anesthesia, with or without general anesthesia, is associated with decreased risk of postoperative pneumonia and respiratory depression.

17. Fisher BW, Majumdar SR, McAlister FA. Predicting pulmonary complications after nonthoracic surgery: a systematic review of blinded studies. *Am J Med.* 2002; 112:219–225.

   A review of all blinded trials between 1966–2001 (n = 7) that reported comparisons of preoperative or operative factors with PPCs.

18. Stephan F, Boucheseiche S, Hollande J, et al. Pulmonary complications following lung resection. A comprehensive analysis of incidence and possible risk factors. *Chest.* 2000;118:1263–1270.

   Of those undergoing pneumonectomy, lobectomy, or wedge resection, the mortality rate was 7.5% and the PPC rate was 25%. The most common PPCs were prolonged air leak, bacterial pneumonia, and acute respiratory failure.

19. Beckles MA, Spiro SG, Colice GL, et al. The physiologic evaluation of patients with lung cancer being considered for resectional surgery. *Chest.* 2003;123:105S–114S.

   An evidence-based guideline on the physiologic evaluation of lung resection candidates.

20. Wyser C, Stulz P, Soler M, et al. Prospective evaluation of an algorithm for the functional assessment of lung resection candidates. *Am J Respir Care Med.* 1999;159:1450–1456.

   Utilization of the proposed algorithm led to a 50% reduction in complications, down to 11%, whereas the percentage of inoperable candidates remained unchanged, compared with a historical control group.

11. RIGHT HEART CATHETERIZATION AND MONITORING OF ARTERIAL PRESSURE

Nick H. S. Kim

The first human cardiac and right heart catheterization was performed by Dr. Wermer Forssmann in 1929—on himself. After inserting a catheter into his antecubital vein and advancing it 65 cm into his heart, the surgical trainee walked to the radiology department and took a radiograph to confirm its location. Disproving the then popular theory that such a procedure would be fatal, and despite strong criticism, Dr. Forssmann continued to perform numerous such procedures. He would later practice rural medicine and share the 1956 Nobel Prize with Drs. Cournand and Richards for their contributions in advancing the field of cardiac catheterization.

Dr. Dexter made an important contribution when he recorded pressures after advancing the catheter distally into the pulmonary arteries until it "wedged." The idea of placing a flotation balloon on the end of the pulmonary artery catheter (PAC) came later, inspired by Dr. Swan's observation of sailboats off the California coast. The flow-directed catheter revolutionized right heart catheterization, allowing for bedside insertions without the aid of fluoroscopy. Teamed with Dr. Ganz's work on hemodynamic measurements, the modern right heart catheterization was realized. With its ability to measure central pressures and hemoglobin saturations, estimate intravascular volume, and evaluate perturbations in cardiac output, the PAC has been a valuable diagnostic tool in cardiopulmonary medicine and critical care.

The utility and benefit of PAC in critically ill patients, however, have come under scrutiny in recent years since publication of a report in 1996 by Connors et al. that PAC was associated with a higher mortality rate and resource utilization in the intensive care unit. This report sparked numerous debates and other studies on the risk and usefulness of PAC. These studies have noted conflicting observations, including two randomized, controlled trials that reported no mortality difference or benefit with PAC in either critically ill or high-risk surgical patients. Another byproduct of the

Connors report was multiple expert conferences on PAC, each with its own consensus statements. These statements, in addition to summarizing the data regarding PAC, offer guidelines for current use and future research directions.

The PAC is typically inserted through an internal jugular, subclavian, or femoral vein using percutaneous guide-wire dilatation (Seldinger) technique. Each venous access site has its unique set of advantages and disadvantages. As with other procedures, the choice in access site depends on both patient-related factors and operator preference and experience. The typical PAC requires the placement of an introducer sheath (usually 8Fr for a 7Fr PAC). The transducer is zeroed at the level of the left atrium—approximated at the fourth intercostal space at the midaxillary line. The fluid-filled catheter is adequately flushed to clear any air bubbles that can dampen and degrade the signal. Under most conditions, the flotation catheter can be positioned without fluoroscopic guidance. Patients with significant cardiomegaly, low output states, or severe pulmonary hypertension may require fluoroscopy for proper PAC placement. The right internal jugular and the left subclavian approaches facilitate PAC insertion into the pulmonary artery, but are not required for successful placement, even in potentially difficult cases.

The complications related to right heart catheterization can be divided into immediate and delayed. Immediate complications such as pneumothorax, arterial puncture or dilatation, air embolism, and arrhythmias (including right bundle branch block and vagal episodes), occur during the initial procedure. Delayed complications include catheter-related infection, thrombosis, air embolism, pulmonary infarction or arterial

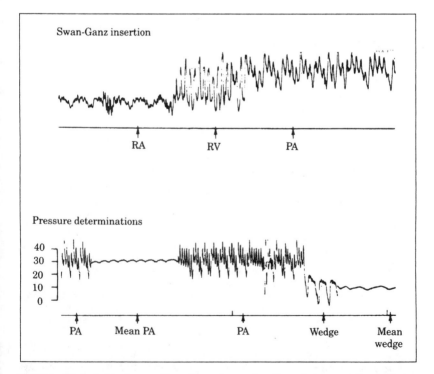

FIG. 11-1. Typical pressure configurations observed as the pulmonary artery catheter (Swan-Ganz) passes through the right atrium (RA), right ventricle (RV), pulmonary artery (PA), and into the pulmonary wedge position. (Courtesy of Stuart J. Menn, MD, Veterans Administration Hospital, San Diego, California.)

rupture, arterial–venous fistula, and pseudoaneurysm. A review of PAC-related complications reported a rate of less than 5% for serious (mostly nonlethal) complications. The complication with the highest mortality (40–70%) is pulmonary artery rupture. Fortunately, this serious complication occurs rarely (0.03–0.2%). This complication can be reduced by repositioning the catheter if the occlusion occurs with insufflation of 1 mL or less. The balloon should not be insufflated with more than 1.5 mL.

Another critical, iatrogenic complication stems from inaccurate interpretation of the data. A typical set of PAC waveforms are shown in Figure 11.1 The zero should be reconfirmed when interpreting pressures. The "wedge" pressure, more appropriately termed *pulmonary artery occluded pressure* (PAOP), estimates the pressure in the similarly sized pulmonary vein after balloon occlusion. Under most conditions, PAOP estimates left atrial pressure, which then estimates left ventricular end-diastolic pressure (LVEDP). PAOP tends to overestimate LVEDP under circumstances such as incomplete occlusion, mitral valve disorders, left atrial myxoma, and in intubated patients with high alveolar pressures. The ideal PAC placement for reading PAOP is in zone 3 lung, where the arterial pressure exceeds venous pressure that exceeds alveolar pressure. Once the PAC has been inserted, a chest radiograph should be obtained to confirm position and guide catheter repositioning, if required. The PAC should be removed once the indication for its placement and any other new indications are no longer present.

ARTERIAL CATHETERIZATION

Arterial cannulation for the purposes of directly monitoring systemic blood pressure and sampling blood gases is performed routinely in the intensive care unit. Risks include bleeding, line-related infections, arterial thrombosis, and ischemic injury. The radial artery is often the first choice and should be performed after a modified Allen test confirms intact collateral circulation. A heparin flush system has been shown to reduce the incidence of thrombosis and is routinely used except in patients with suspected heparin-induced thrombocytopenia. Temporary occlusion is the most common, but usually benign, complication of radial artery cannulation. Permanent occlusion with distal ischemia or necrosis is rare (<0.1%). The risk of line related infection increases with duration (longer than 4 days). Femoral cannulation has not been shown to cause higher rates of infectious complications compared with radial artery cannulation. The reported rates of sepsis caused by arterial catheters are generally less than 1%.

1. Grossman W. Cardiac catheterization: historical perspective and present practice. In: Grossman W, ed. *Cardiac Catheterization and Angiography.* 2nd ed. Philadelphia: Lea & Febiger; 1980:3.
2. Swan HJ, Ganz W, Forrester J, et al. Catheterization of the heart in man with use of a flow-directed balloon-tipped catheter. *N Engl J Med.* 1970;283:447.
3. Connors AF Jr, Speroff T, Dawson NV, et al. The effectiveness of right heart catheterization in the initial care of critically ill patients. SUPPORT Investigators. *JAMA.* 1996;276:889.
   Retrospective study found PAC associated with higher mortality and resource utilization from a cohort of 5,735 critically ill patients treated among five teaching hospitals.
4. Rhodes A, Cusack RJ, Newman PJ, et al. A randomised, controlled trial of the pulmonary artery catheter in critically ill patients. *Intensive Care Med.* 2002;28:256.
   A randomized, controlled trial (RCT) of 201 critically ill patients found no difference in mortality between PAC and control groups.
5. Sandham JD, Hull RD, Brant RF, et al. A randomized, controlled trial of the use of pulmonary-artery catheters in high-risk surgical patients. *N Engl J Med.* 2003;348:5.
   RCT of 1,994 high-risk surgical patients found no benefit in PAC group over standard care group.

6. Pulmonary Artery Catheter Consensus Conference: consensus statement. *Crit Care Med.* 1997;25:910.

Addresses PAC controversy and makes future recommendations.

7. Mueller HS, Chatterjee K, Davis KB, et al. ACC expert consensus document. Present use of bedside right heart catheterization in patients with cardiac disease. *J Am Coll Cardiol.* 1998;32:840.

Thorough review of PAC data and indications guidelines.

8. Bernard GR, Sopko G, Cerra F, et al. Pulmonary artery catheterization and clinical outcomes: National Heart, Lung, and Blood Institute and Food and Drug Administration Workshop Report. Consensus Statement. *JAMA.* 2000;283:2568.

NIH consensus statement on PAC. Focus on areas of future investigations.

9. Abreu AR, Campos MA, Krieger BP. Pulmonary artery rupture induced by a pulmonary artery catheter: a case report and review of the literature. *J Intensive Care Med.* 2004;19:291.

Overviews reported major complications associated with PAC.

10. Scheer B, Perel A, Pfeiffer UJ. Clinical review: complications and risk factors of peripheral arterial catheters used for haemodynamic monitoring in anaesthesia and intensive care medicine. *Crit Care.* 2002;6:198.

Review of the literature on complications of arterial catheters from 1978 to 2001.

II. SPECIAL PROBLEMS

12. PLEURAL EFFUSION

Henri G. Colt

A few milliliters of pleural fluid are present normally within the pleural space, serving as a lubricating film between the visceral and parietal pleural surfaces. In normal individuals, thoracentesis generally yields less than 1 mL of fluid, although quantities of 3 to 20 mL have been obtained in as many as 10% of healthy individuals in some series. Normally, the protein content of pleural fluid is below 1.5 g/dL; the protein electrophoretic pattern is qualitatively similar to plasma, although the content of albumin is slightly higher and that of fibrinogen slightly lower.

The volume and composition of pleural fluid are maintained virtually constant in healthy individuals by an intricate balance of hydrostatic and oncotic pressures and by the relative permeabilities of the pleural capillaries and lymphatics. Systemic arteries supply the parietal pleura, whereas the visceral pleura is supplied by the bronchial arterial circulation. Fluid and protein exchange in the pleural space is almost exclusively achieved through the parietal pleura.

Pleural effusion is defined as the abnormal accumulation of fluid within the pleural space. It may be caused by either excess fluid production or decreased absorption; in some conditions, both mechanisms may be operative. Effusions are a common manifestation of both systemic and intrathoracic diseases. Factors that determine whether pleural fluid accumulates include (1) oncotic pressure in the pleural fluid, pleural microcirculation, and lymphatics; (2) permeability of the pleural microcirculation; and (3) pressures in the systemic and pulmonary veins. These factors are reflected in Starling's equation (Fig. 12-1). However, this balance can also be altered, favoring fluid accumulation, by any process that obstructs lymphatic drainage. Also, peritoneal fluid can gain access to the pleural space via both diaphragmatic defects and transdiaphragmatic lymphatics. Thus, pleural fluid exchange can be compromised by a diverse range of circumstances, leading to the development of a pleural effusion.

The most common cause of a pleural effusion is congestive heart failure with elevation of the pulmonary venous pressure. Whether elevation of systemic venous pressure alone (pure right heart failure) prompts pleural effusions remains controversial, but elevations of both venous pressures appear to result in larger effusions.

Increased negative pressure in the pleural space also encourages fluid accumulation and this can occur in patients with atelectasis. Decreased plasma oncotic pressure favors pleural fluid accumulation; however, it is unlikely that this mechanism acts alone because effusions are rare in congenitally hypoalbuminemic individuals.

Increased capillary permeability caused by local inflammation, circulating toxins, or vasoactive substances also plays a role in fluid accumulation associated with collagen-vascular diseases, pancreatitis, pulmonary emboli, and pneumonitis. An increase in pleural oncotic pressure as a consequence of (1) enhanced capillary protein leak, (2) protein exudation from local pleural inflammation or tumor, or (3) defective lymphatic resorption contributes to some effusions. As pleural space oncotic pressure approaches that of plasma (32 cm H_2O), fluid resorption is impaired.

Simple transfer of ascitic fluid across diaphragmatic defects has been invoked as a mechanism for pleural effusions accompanying ascites, as in cirrhosis and Meig's syndrome (i.e., benign ovarian fibroma, ascites, and pleural effusion). A similar mechanism has been proposed for fluid accumulation in pancreatitis or subdiaphragmatic abscess, although enhanced transdiaphragmatic lymph flow also can play a role.

On physical examination, patients with pleural effusions can have dullness to percussion, diminished breath sounds, and reduced tactile and vocal fremitus over the involved hemithorax. Altering the patient's position will occasionally *shift* these physical findings to dependent regions. Large effusions (>1500 mL) are frequently associated with an appreciable inspiratory lag, bulging intercostal margins, contralateral mediastinal shift, or atelectasis (e.g., egophony, bronchial breath sounds). A search

$$\dot{Q}_f = K_f[(P_{MV} - P_{PMV}) - \sigma(\pi_{MV} - \pi_{PMV})]$$

where $\dot{Q}_f$ is the net transvascular flow;

K_f is the fluid filtration coefficient, reflecting the permeability of the membrane to fluid;

σ is the apparent reflection coefficient, which takes into account the effect of protein permeability in determining the effective transvascular osmotic pressure difference;

P_{MV} and P_{PMV} are the hydrostatic pressures of the microvascular and perimicrovascular spaces; and

π_{MV} and π_{PMV} are the microvascular and perimicrovascular protein osmotic pressures.

FIG. 12-1. Starling's equation.

should always be made for nonthoracic signs suggesting the cause of fluid accumulation (e.g., pedal edema, distended neck veins, and an S_3 gallop indicating congestive heart failure).

Often, the chest roentgenogram is the only clue to the presence of an effusion and may suggest its cause (e.g., cardiomegaly and redistribution of pulmonary veins in heart failure, lung or pleural-based masses, atelectasis, rib erosions signifying metastatic carcinoma, or an elevated hemidiaphragm suggesting subdiaphragmatic abscess, volume loss, or bronchial obstruction). At least 150 mL of fluid is required to detect an effusion on a standard posteroanterior and lateral chest roentgenogram. Classically, fluid initially collects between the anteroinferior lung surface and the diaphragm. It then obliterates the costophrenic angle on the frontal view or creates a triangular density that obscures the ipsilateral diaphragm and posterior costophrenic sulcus on a lateral film. Further accumulation obliterates the hemidiaphragm and opacifies the hemithorax with an upward concavity that extends higher laterally than medially. On the lateral view, pleural fluid ascends obliquely along the posterior chest wall. Significantly smaller quantities of pleural fluid are detectable on lateral decubitus views, but these often are not necessary because fluid (both loculated and free flowing) can be easily detected by pleural ultrasonography before thoracentesis. On lateral decubitus films, fluid layers along the dependent chest wall. On the opposite decubitus view, fluid shift allows examination of underlying parenchyma. A very large effusion should cause a contralateral mediastinal shift. When this shift does not occur, parenchymal collapse or mediastinal fixation, often from a tumor, is suggested.

When underlying parenchymal abnormalities or adhesions between pleural layers exist, atypical patterns of fluid accumulation result. A subpulmonic effusion can harbor more than 1,000 mL of fluid and may appear only as an elevated hemidiaphragm. The *diaphragmatic* contour is often more horizontal than usual, with a steep angulation laterally, creating a shallow costophrenic angle. A lateral decubitus film may layer the fluid and reveal the true diaphragmatic shadow. When pleural fluid becomes loculated (or entrapped) within an interlobar fissure, it can create the appearance of an elliptic opacity, or *pseudotumor*, on the posteroanterior film and a spindle-shaped opacity tapering into fissure lines on the lateral film. For unknown reasons, this appearance is especially common with congestive heart failure and resolves as hemodynamics improve. Fluid that is loculated laterally can result in a smooth, contoured, semicircular opacity abutting a pleural surface, which can simulate a mass lesion on a posteroanterior film. Loculations are frequently seen in patients with evolving parapneumonic effusions or empyema after either thoracic surgery or pleurodesis. It is noteworthy that computed tomography scans often exaggerate the amount of fluid actually present.

The differential diagnosis of pleural effusion should reflect the clinical context and ancillary findings, but thoracentesis and careful examination of the pleural fluid are indicated in virtually every instance. Thoracentesis is a safe procedure with limited morbidity in experienced hands. Precautions should be used in patients with a bleeding diathesis, very small effusions, or an obliterated pleural space, as well as in those using anticoagulant drugs, in patients who are uncooperative, or if conditions are present that make even a small pneumothorax extremely hazardous. In these circumstances, the risk-to-benefit ratio of any procedure must be weighed carefully, then experienced personnel should perform the procedure, probably using ultrasound guidance. It is traditionally suggested that no more than 1,000 mL of fluid be removed at any one sitting to avoid reexpansion pulmonary edema, but this is usually not the case. The procedure should probably be halted, however, if the patient begins to cough, has chest pain, or other possible signs of increasingly negative pleural pressure. Regardless, fluid should be removed slowly.

Numerous laboratory examinations can be performed on pleural fluid; those required are largely dictated by the clinical context. If foul-smelling pus is obtained, for example, extensive biochemical analysis is not required; only Gram's stain and culture are needed. In most situations, however, fluid analysis is needed to distinguish transudates from exudates, an important distinction for differential diagnosis. The key measures are lactate dehydrogenase (LDH), total protein, white blood count and differential, glucose, and pleural pH. An exudate is defined by any one of the following: ratio of pleural fluid to serum protein greater than 0.5; LDH ratio greater than 0.6; or LDH greater than two thirds of the normal serum value.

Exudates are characteristic of malignancy, parapneumonic effusions, and a variety of infectious and noninfectious inflammatory states. Acidosis (pH <7.30) and reduced glucose (<60 μg/dL) are characteristic of empyema and rheumatoid pleurisy, but can occur in other conditions, such as pleural carcinomatosis and evolving parapneumonic effusions. Occasionally, elevated pleural fluid amylase suggests conditions such as esophageal rupture, pancreatitis, pancreatic pseudocyst, and, rarely, certain malignancies. The use of pleural cholesterol levels is still investigative, and no set of measures has yet replaced Light's criteria (LDH, protein) to differentiate exudates from transudates. If chylothorax is suspected, triglycerides and chylomicron analysis (by lipoprotein electrophoresis) should be requested; fluid is not always turbid or milky in these instances. Pleural fluid cytologic examination is indicated whenever neoplasm is suspected.

One point of particular interest has been the differentiation between a benign parapneumonic effusion that requires no chest tube drainage and one that does (increasingly referred to as a *complicated parapneumonic effusion*). The need for drainage, in addition to antibiotic therapy, is indicated by a positive Gram's stain, culture, or the presence of pus in the pleural space (empyema). Drainage also should be considered if pleural fluid pH is below 7.10 or if pleural glucose is low and LDH is greater than 1000 g/L after excluding other diagnoses for these abnormalities (e.g., tuberculosis, rheumatoid arthritis, and pleural carcinomatosis).

The procedures described above, along with the results of cultures for bacteria, fungi, and tuberculosis, will yield a diagnosis for most pleural effusions. In some instances, however, additional evaluation is warranted. A closed needle biopsy of the pleura should be considered in cases in which granulomatous diseases or a neoplasm are suspected. Fiberoptic bronchoscopy can be considered but is of no demonstrated value unless the chest x-ray study demonstrates some parenchymal or nodal abnormality or is suggestive of bronchial obstruction.

In patients with an undiagnosed effusion, especially if exudative, or if malignancy is suspected, thoracoscopy is a remarkably safe and commonly used diagnostic procedure. Thoracoscopy can be performed through a single access site, often under local anesthesia and using spontaneous ventilation and intravenous sedation, although the operating room setting, general anesthesia, and tracheal intubation are desirable in some cases in which adhesions, loculations, or infection are suspected. Thoracoscopy permits direct visualization of the pleura and external surface of the lung, as well as biopsy of pleura and lung, pleural fluid removal, and pleurodesis. In cases of loculated effusions, the adhesions can be lysed. Thoracoscopy is associated with less morbidity than open procedures. Operator experience is, as always, a key consideration.

Beyond thoracoscopy, open pleural biopsy under general anesthesia is required for patients in whom other procedures have failed to provide a diagnosis or when contemplated lung biopsy poses special risk (e.g., pulmonary hypertension) and open exposure is required to assure hemostasis. Despite proceeding to thoracoscopy or open biopsy, a small number of effusions remain undiagnosed and either resolve or, subsequently, express themselves as neoplasm.

Treatment of pleural effusions is usually that of the underlying disease. Therapeutic thoracenteses, however, are often necessary in cases of a large effusion or when the patient has significant underlying parenchymal lung disease. Always note whether symptoms such as dyspnea, chest pain, or cough resolve after evacuation of the effusion. Patients with symptoms that coincide with recurrent fluid accumulation should be considered for pleurodesis. Only patients with a very limited survival (<2 to 3 months) should continue to be treated by multiple large-volume thoracentesis. Special therapeutic approaches, which might include indwelling of tunneled percutaneous pleural catheter insertion and periodic drainage, may be necessary in patients with malignant effusions, malignant mesothelioma, empyema, tuberculosis, hemothorax, or trapped lung.

---

1. Alexandrakis MG, Passam FH, Kyriakou DS, et al. Pleural effusions in hematologic malignancies. *Chest*. 2004;125:1546–1555.

   Hodgkin and non-Hodgkin lymphoma are the most frequent, but also 10 to 20% of patients status post bone marrow transplant develop effusions. In all patients, drug toxicity should be considered.

2. Assi Z, Caruso JL, Herndon J, et al. Cytologically proved malignant pleural effusions: distribution of transudates and exudates. *Chest*. 1998;113:1302–1304.

   A retrospective review of 98 patients with malignant pleural effusion; only one had a transudate.

3. Azoulay E. Pleural effusions in the intensive care unit. *Current Opin Pulm Med*. 2003;9:291–297.

   Incidence of effusions depends on screening methods (8% for physical examination to 60% using ultrasonography). This article reviews etiologies and workup strategies.

4. Brown NE, Zamel N, Aberman A. Changes in pulmonary mechanics and gas exchange following thoracocentesis. *Chest*. 1978;74:540.

   The changes in pulmonary mechanics and gas exchange, which occurred in the first 3 hours after removal of 600 to 1800 mL in nine patients, did correlate with subjective improvement by the patients.

5. Burgess LJ, Maritz FJ, Taljaard JJF. Comparative analysis of the biochemical parameters used to distinguish between pleural transudates and exudates. *Chest*. 1995;107:1604.

   A reaffirmation of what is known, and a discussion of the potential role for serum-effusion albumin gradient.

6. Burrows CM, Mathews WC, Colt HG. Predicting survival in patients with recurrent symptomatic malignant pleural effusions: an assessment of the prognostic values of physiologic, morphologic, and quality of life measures of extent of disease. *Chest*. 2000;117:73–78.

   A study that questions the predictive value of pH and demonstrates the importance of quality of life assessment.

7. Bynum LJ, Wilson JE. Characteristics of pleural effusions associated with pulmonary embolism. *Arch Intern Med*. 1976;136:159.

   Most patients with pulmonary embolism have bloody effusions, but with a wide range of findings.

8. Cheng DS, Rodriguez RM, Rogers J, et al. Comparison of pleural fluid pH values obtained using blood gas machine, pH meter, and pH indicator strip. *Chest*. 1998;114:1368.

When patient-care decisions must be made, only those values provided by the blood gas machine are sufficiently accurate.

9. Cugell DW, Kamp DW. Asbestos and the pleura. *Chest.* 2004;125:1103–1117.

    A great recent review of history, mineralogy, and clinical significance of asbestos-related pleural disease.

10. Colt HG, Brewer N, Barbur E. Evaluation of patient-related and procedure-related factors contributing to pneumothorax following thoracentesis. *Chest.* 1999;116:134.

    Pneumothorax is rare and not easily predictable, even when procedures are performed by experienced operators.

11. Colt HG. Thoracoscopy: a prospective study of safety and outcome. *Chest.* 1995;108:324.

    One of only a few early studies designed to prospectively evaluate the safety of this minimally invasive procedure.

12. Colt HG, Mathur PN. *Manual of Pleural Procedures.* Philadelphia: Lippincott Williams and Williams, published 1999.

    A 200-page guide to performing procedures, including ultrasound, chest tubes pleurodesis, and thoracoscopy (with useful hints and many black and white photos).

13. Colt HG. Emerging technology: thoracoscopy, window to the pleura. Philadelphia. *Chest.* 1999;116:1409–1415.

    A review of various modalities of thoracoscopy, as well as of indications and therapeutic utility.

14. Doyle JJ, Hnatiuk OW, Torrington KG, et al. Necessity of routine chest roentgenography after thoracentesis. *Ann Intern Med.* 1996;124:816.

    Answers an age-old question: Are chest films needed in patients, even though the risk of thoracentesis-related pneumothorax is low in experienced hands?

15. Flatley ME, Schapira RM. Hydropneumomediastinum and bilateral hydropneumothorax as delayed complications of central venous catheterization. *Chest.* 1993;103:1914.

    A central venous catheter used for alimentation caused these complications. The widespread use of these devices may induce more effusions on this basis. Surprisingly, hemothorax is usually absent despite catheter perforation of a central vein.

16. Garcia-Pachon E, Padilla-Navas I, Sanchez JF, et al. Pleural fluid to serum cholinesterase ratio for the separation of transudates and exudates. *Chest.* 1996;110:97.

    Potential value of this ratio if Light's criteria are not indicative.

17. Goto M, Noguchi Y, Koyama H. Diagnostic value of adenosine deaminase in tuberculous pleural effusions: a meta-analysis. *Am Clin Biochem.* 2003;40:374–381.

    Adenosine deaminase may be useful and could allow avoidance of pleural biopsy, especially in countries where tuberculosis prevalence is high.

18. Griner PF. Bloody pleural fluid following pulmonary infarction. *JAMA.* 1967; 202:947.

    Only 14 of 43 patients (33%) had effusions that were bloody; of these, six likely resulted from other causes (i.e., congestive failure).

19. Halla JT, Schrohenloher RE, Volanakis JE. Immune complexes and other laboratory features of pleural effusions: a comparison of rheumatoid arthritis, systemic lupus erythematosus and other diseases. *Ann Intern Med.* 1980;92:748.

    Certain laboratory features may provide clues to the etiology of pleural effusions caused by collagen diseases.

20. Heffner JE, Highland K, Brown LK. A meta-analysis derivation of continuous likelihood ratios for diagnosing pleural fluid exudates. *Am J Respir Crit Care Med.* 2003;167:1591–1599.

    Logistic regression of a multicenter registry of pleural effusions demonstrates that diagnostic accuracy for Light's criteria decreased to as low as 65 to 86% as any one of the criteria reached its binary cutoff point.

21. Hirsch A, Ruffie P, Nebut M, et al. Pleural effusion: laboratory tests in 300 cases. *Thorax.* 1979;34:106.

    Clinical and laboratory findings are provided in this large series.

22. Joseph J, Viney S, Beck P, et al. A prospective study of amylase-rich pleural effusions with special reference to amylase isoenzyme analysis. *Chest*. 1992;102:1455.

    An elevated amylase in pleural fluid can have many causes; but in pancreatitis, pancreatic amylase isoenzyme is present, whereas in other conditions (infections, tumors), salivary amylase isoenzyme is present.

23. Jones PW, Moyers JP, Rogers JT, et al. Ultrasound-guided thoracentesis: is it a safer method? *Chest*. 2003;123:418–423.

    Prospective descriptive study of 941 thoracenteses performed by interventional radiologists using ultrasound guidance resulted in fewer complications that those reported with non–image-guided thoracentesis. Where were the pulmonologists?

24. Kaye MD. Pleuropulmonary complications of pancreatitis. *Thorax*. 1968;23:297.

    Of 38 pleural effusions associated with pancreatitis, 37 had elevated amylase exceeding plasma values. Pleural fluid was frequently hemorrhagic in severe cases.

25. Lee P, Colt HG. Using diagnostic thoracoscopy to optimal effect. *J Resp Illness*. 2003;24:503–509.

    A review of therapeutic modalities and indications, especially geared to no surgeon thoracoscopists.

26. Light RW, Erozan YS, Ball WC Jr. Cells in pleural fluid. *Arch Intern Med*. 1973;132:854.

    Of 31 exudative effusions with a predominance of lymphocytes, 30 were caused by tuberculous or a neoplasm. Also suggests that an absence of mesothelial cells (<1%) is indicative of a tuberculous cause.

27. Light RW, MacGregor MI, Ball WC Jr, et al. Diagnostic significance of pleural fluid pH and Pco_2. *Chest*. 1973;64:591.

    Parapneumonic effusions with a pH less than 7.20 required chest tube drainage, whereas those with a pH greater than 7.20 resolved with antibiotics alone.

28. Light RW, MacGregor I, Luchsinger PC. Pleural effusions: the diagnostic separation of transudates and exudates. *Ann Intern Med*. 1972;77:507.

    A prospective study of 150 pleural effusions, exploring the utility of cell counts, protein, and LDH determinations in pleural fluid. A CLASSIC!

29. Lillington GA, Carr DT, Mayne JG. Rheumatoid pleurisy with effusion. *Arch Intern Med*. 1971;128:764.

    Good review; glucose frequently below 10 mg/dL in pleural fluid.

30. Mahon RT, Colt HG. Bedside thoracentesis in critically ill patients: The "rolled bedsheet" technique. *J Bronchol*. 2000;7:340–342.

    Description of a technique that facilitates thoracentesis in mechanically ventilated patients.

31. Mares DC, Mathur PM. Medical thoracoscopic talc pleurodesis for chylothorax due to lymphoma. *Chest*. 1998;114:731.

    A 100% success rate in this series of 24 cases.

32. McCartney JP, Adams JW, Hazard PB. Safety of thoracentesis in mechanically ventilated patients. *Chest*. 1993;103:1920.

    The authors suggest that thoracentesis in the lateral decubitus position limits the risk of complications in patients being mechanically ventilated with positive end-expiratory pressure.

33. Morelock SY, Sahn SA. Drugs and the pleura. *Chest*. 1999;116:212.

    Small numbers of drugs cause effusions when compared with the large number of drugs that can cause pulmonary parenchymal abnormalities. A concise, relatively recent review.

34. Maskell NA, Butland RJA. BTS guidelines for the investigation of a unilateral pleural effusion in adults. *Thorax*. 2003;58:8–17.

    An incredibly informative recent "state of the art" review of pleural effusions: clinical workup, algorithms, differential diagnosis.

35. Pien GW, Gant MJ, Washam CL. Use of an implantable pleural catheter for trapped lung syndrome in patients with malignant pleural effusion. *Chest*. 2001;119:1641–1646.

    A series of patients with trapped lung treated successfully using the PleurRx pleural catheter, a 15.5 F silicone catheter that allows periodic drainage.

36. Poe RH, Marin MG, Israel RH, et al. Utility of pleural fluid analysis in predicting tube thoracostomy/decortication in parapneumonic effusions. *Chest.* 1991; 100:963.
    One view of pleural fluid characteristics useful in guiding the therapeutic approach.
37. Roper WH, Waring JJ. Primary serofibrinous pleural effusion in military personnel. *Am Rev Tuberc.* 1955;71:616.
    Most young adults (141) with positive purified protein derivative (PPD) and serofibrinous effusion developed evidence of active tuberculosis within 5 years, regardless of whether a mycobacterial cause of effusion was proved. A classic.
38. Ryan CJ, Rodgers RF, Unni KK, et al. The outcome of patients with pleural effusion of indeterminate cause at thoracotomy. *Mayo Clin Proc.* 1981;56:145.
    Even after thoracotomy, a number of conditions escape diagnosis; most (60%) follow a benign course.
39. Sallach SM, Sallach JA, Vasquez E, et al. Volume of pleural fluid required for diagnosis of pleural malignancy. *Chest.* 2002;122:1913–1917.
    Retrospective review of 282 patients showed that the sensitivity for diagnosis of pleural malignancy was not dependent on volume of fluid removed by thoracentesis.
40. Strange C, Sahn SA. The clinician's perspective on parapneumonic effusions and empyema. *Chest.* 1993;103:259.
    A survey of physicians and surgeons who care for patients with pleural effusions finds limited agreement with regard to management. See also the ATS statement on parapneumonic effusions.
41. Yang PC, Luh KT, Chang DB, et al. Value of sonography in determining the nature of pleural effusion: analysis of 320 cases. *AJR* 1992;159:1145.
    An excellent description of sonographic findings in patients with pleural disease. Although 12 years old, not much has changed.

---

13. PNEUMOTHORAX

Henri G. Colt

The pleural space is located between the visceral pleura surrounding the lung and the parietal pleura lining the inside of the rib cage and is occupied by a small amount of lubricating pleural fluid. Pleural pressure is negative compared with atmospheric pressure, which helps maintain lung inflation. If the parietal or visceral pleura is breached and the pleural space is exposed to atmospheric (positive) pressure, air enters the pleural space (i.e., pneumothorax occurs), and the lung collapses inward toward the mediastinum. Any condition that impairs the structural integrity of either pleural membrane can produce a pneumothorax. This entity presents a true healthcare problem, affecting more than 20,000 individuals each year in the United States and costing more than $130 million in healthcare expenditures. The prognosis and management depend on the underlying cause. Pneumothorax is often categorized as (1) idiopathic or spontaneous, (2) iatrogenic, or (3) traumatic. Within each category, pneumothoraces can be either uncomplicated (usually unaccompanied by symptoms or prolonged air leak) or complicated (accompanied by symptoms, radiographic evidence of mediastinal shift, bleeding, or prolonged air leak). Pneumothorax can also be categorized as "primary" (no underlying lung disease, estimated to occur in 18 to 28 per 100,000 men each year in Great Britain), and "secondary" (presence of underlying lung disease).

Spontaneous (idiopathic) pneumothorax (SP) occurs in patients without a history of any event known to cause pneumothorax (e.g., trauma or intervention). It generally occurs unexpectedly in an apparently healthy individual. Patients usually have no evidence of bullous lung disease on radiographic, thoracoscopic, or open surgical examination. Spontaneous pneumothoraces should be categorized as secondary, however, when abnormal lung parenchyma is noted, either from underlying lung disease or by identifying bulla or blebs during radiographic or direct examination.

At least two different mechanisms can lead to spontaneous pneumothorax. One is a visceral pleural *tear* (i.e., a bronchopleural fistula) caused by rupture of a subpleural bleb or bulla or by a parenchymal process that erodes through the visceral pleura (e.g., necrotizing pneumonia). Blebs are frequently found in up to 90% of patients with presumed primary pneumothorax. Another mechanism is partial bronchial obstruction that acts as a *check valve*. Subsequent progressive hyperinflation of distal air spaces occurs until air eventually dissects along bronchovascular spaces into the hilus and mediastinum, leading to pneumomediastinum. From there, air can also dissect through fascial planes in the neck, resulting in subcutaneous emphysema, or through visceral pleura into one (usually the right) or both pleural cavities, resulting in pneumothorax.

In a young, otherwise healthy individual without radiographic evidence of lung disease, SP usually results from the rupture of subpleural apical blebs or bullae. The peak incidence is between the ages of 20 and 30 with a 4:1 male predominance and a predilection for tall, thin individuals. The incidence of SP has been reported to be increased in cigarette smokers, but this is a controversial issue. Interestingly, most patients who smoke continue to do so after a first episode of pneumothorax, even though the recurrence rate is more than 50% during the first 4 years after a first episode.

In most cases, symptoms develop at rest; however, onset can be associated with strenuous activity in up to 20% of cases and with a forceful cough or sneeze in at least 5%. Spontaneous pneumothorax should always convey a high index of suspicion for the presence of intrinsic lung disease, particularly if pneumomediastinum also is present. Among the lung conditions often associated with pneumothorax are emphysema (particularly bullous emphysema), diffuse interstitial processes (e.g., eosinophilic granuloma, sarcoidosis, usual interstitial pneumonia, desquamative interstitial pneumonia, and the pneumoconioses), necrotizing pneumonias (including tuberculosis), endometriosis (catamenial pneumothorax in women during menses), and acquired immune deficiency syndrome (related to malnutrition or *Pneumocystis carinii* pneumonia and associated with prolonged air leaks and decreased survival).

Iatrogenic pneumothorax most commonly occurs after invasive thoracic procedures, such as thoracentesis, transbronchial lung biopsy, and subclavian vein catheterization; however, it also can complicate virtually any invasive procedure involving the neck or abdomen (e.g., liver biopsy, transtracheal aspiration, intercostal nerve block, and even acupuncture). A very infrequent cause may be tracheotomy, where iatrogenic tracheal laceration should be suspected in the presence of otherwise unexplained pneumothorax, pneumomediastinum, or even pneumoperitoneum. Iatrogenic pneumothorax can complicate positive pressure ventilation and, in this setting, can be life threatening. The mechanism is usually a combination of partial bronchial obstruction caused by edema, secretions, and check-valve air entry leading to progressive alveolar expansion and rupture.

Traumatic pneumothorax can occur in the setting of penetrating or nonpenetrating chest trauma. The former generally presents no diagnostic problem; however, the latter should prompt a careful search for rib fracture, bronchial rupture, and esophageal injury. Rib fractures are associated with tears of the visceral pleura and pneumothorax; bronchial rupture is associated with deceleration injury; and esophageal rupture is often associated with mediastinal air entry. Pneumothorax can also result from abdominal trauma (e.g., abdominal stab wound, bullet wound) and diaphragmatic tears.

The clinical manifestations of pneumothorax depend on its size, the clinical context in which it occurs, and the mechanism(s) involved. In tall, thin individuals with spontaneous rupture of apical pleural blebs, chest pain and dyspnea are common presenting symptoms. The pain is usually of sudden onset and initially pleuritic in character. After a few hours, it often changes to a dull ache, and spontaneous resolution of the pain can occur within 2 to 3 days. At least 10% of patients do not experience pain. Dyspnea occurs in 80%, often with spontaneous resolution within 24 hours despite persistence of the pneumothorax. Prominent coughing occurs in 10%; occasionally, it is the major or only symptom. Less than 5% of patients are asymptomatic. Symptoms can be transient and do not always correlate well with the radiographic size of the pneumothorax.

The most common physical findings are tachypnea, splinting, and decreased inspiratory expansion of the involved hemithorax, a tympanitic percussion note, decreased fremitus, and decreased breath sounds on the involved side. In patients with a check-valve mechanism, the initial complaint of substernal pressure or discomfort is often interpreted as cardiac in origin. Subsequently, the patient can experience chest pain, dyspnea, and relief of the substernal symptoms if pneumothorax or decompression into cervical subcutaneous tissues occurs. Mediastinal emphysema can be detected on auscultation by the presence of a mediastinal *crunch* (Hamman sign) coincident with cardiac systole and diastole. Similarly, subcutaneous emphysema may be noted on palpation of the anterior chest, axilla, shoulders, and neck. Subcutaneous infiltration of air may not always be readily visible, but can often be felt. Dyspnea can be exaggerated and persistent when underlying lung disease is present. In severely traumatized or mechanically ventilated patients, symptoms and signs can be obscured or difficult to interpret. This also is the case in patients with emphysema who have severe hyperinflation and diminished breath sounds. An electrocardiogram may show nonspecific ST-T wave changes and axis shifts, suggesting myocardial or thromboembolic disease.

The diagnosis of pneumothorax is usually made on clinical history and review of chest radiographs. In some cases, it may be necessary to obtain end-expiratory chest films to visualize the pleural reflection of the collapsed lung. The diagnosis is usually made easily by careful inspection of chest radiographs and comparisons with previous films; however, in some cases detection may be difficult, such as in patients with small, loculated pneumothoraces; on mechanical ventilation; and with known bullous lung disease. In some cases, computed tomographic (CT) scanning may be necessary for diagnosis. CT scans can be used to document or identify unilateral or bilateral bullous abnormalities during or after episodes of pneumothorax. CT scans also can be helpful to guide chest tube drainage in patients with complex, uniloculated, or multiloculated pneumothoraces, and to help differentiate pleural from bullous air collections. This is important to avoid inadvertently inserting chest tubes into lung bullae. An American College of Chest Physicians (ACCP) consensus report did not recommend routine CT scanning after a first episode of pneumothorax and did not achieve consensus regarding the role of CT scanning for recurrent pneumothorax or for planning surgical intervention.

Complications of pneumothorax are classified as *acute* and *long term* and can occur in all types. Acute complications include tension pneumothorax, acute respiratory failure, bilateral pneumothorax, hemothorax, and pyothorax. Long-term complications include failure to reexpand (i.e., persistent pneumothorax) and recurrence.

Tension pneumothorax, which can appear rapidly and, if untreated, result in death, is caused by continued air entry into the pleural space. The persistent accumulation of positive pressure within the pleural cavity results in substantial lung collapse, mediastinal shift toward the contralateral side, and even compression of the uninvolved lung. This situation can occur after rupture of an apical bleb if the visceral pleural tear forms a *flap* (i.e., opening with inspiration and closing with expiration). Tension pneumothorax also can occur after rupture of the mediastinal pleura caused by an intrapulmonary check valve if air continues to be pumped into the mediastinum. This situation is made worse if the patient is on mechanical ventilation and in some cases of cardiopulmonary resuscitation. It can also occur after penetrating chest wounds when air continues to enter the chest with each inspiration, especially if check-valving at the site of chest wall injury prevents expulsion of air during expiration. Patients with indwelling chest tubes for pneumothorax with acute deterioration also may have suspected tension. In these cases, the chest tube may not be communicating adequately with the area of air leakage (because of adhesions, plugging of the chest tube itself, or chest tube malfunction).

A diagnosis of tension pneumothorax should be considered in the setting of (1) progressive dyspnea and tachycardia, (2) shift of the trachea and mediastinal structures away from the involved side, and (3) increasing tympany of the involved side. Roentgenograms can confirm those events, but, if suspected, immediate decompression by transthoracic insertion of a needle attached to a syringe may be indicated. If a patient has a chest tube in place already and the development of a tension pneumothorax is suspected, all bandages should be removed and the tube carefully inspected. Waiting for radiographic confirmation may be fatal.

Bilateral pneumothorax is a rare event that usually is not detected without a chest roentgenogram. Reinflating one lung with a chest tube usually maintains patient stability until this complication is recognized.

Pneumothorax can be accompanied by hemothorax and pyothorax. In these cases, patients are said to have a *hydropneumothorax*. Evacuation of the pneumothorax and evaluation of the pleural effusion are mandatory. Hemothorax, often caused by adhesion rupture, lung parenchyma, or vascular structures, is potentially lethal because the pleural space easily accommodates a large amount of blood and because tamponade of the bleeding site may not occur. In the presumably healthy individual who develops an SP, discovery of pleural effusion is an indication for diagnostic thoracentesis to exclude bleeding. Effusions occur in about 20% of patients and are nonbloody; however, radiographic obscuring (i.e., blunting) of the costophrenic angle requires at least 100 mL of fluid. In the otherwise healthy individual, bleeding is more common with recurrent pneumothorax and is caused by rupture of vascular adhesions between visceral and parietal pleura. If tamponade does not occur, a patient can exsanguinate rapidly from such a benign source. Bleeding sites in other forms of pneumothorax are much more variable, but the same rule applies—thoracentesis should be performed on all effusions to exclude hemothorax.

Pyothorax, on the other hand, usually results from the entry of organisms along with air. Remember that a persistent pneumothorax noted radiographically, particularly in the presence of a thick visceral pleural peel, suggests chronic bronchopleural fistula, which may require special procedures (such as interposed muscle flaps) for surgical correction. Rare in SP not associated with preexisting lung disease, it is much more common with lung rupture caused by necrotizing pneumonia or penetrating trauma. The symptoms and findings are the same as those of an empyema.

The management of pneumothorax depends on the setting in which it occurs. Patients with uncomplicated SP and no underlying lung disease have four reasonable treatment options: (1) observation (inpatient or outpatient); (2) aspiration by needle or by a small-lumen catheter; (3) insertion of a small chest tube or catheter attached to a one-way flutter valve; or (4) insertion of a chest tube attached to water seal (*closed*) or suction drainage. Of these, aspiration is the least effective and may lacerate the lung and introduce infection. The traditional practice in the United States is either to hospitalize for observation of complications or to insert a chest tube for 1 to 3 days, or both. Both large- and small-bore chest tubes are readily attached to one-way flutter devices (Heimlich valves) that allow ambulation and discharge. Patients with hydropneumothorax, however, should probably not be treated with one-way valves because of the risk of obstruction from viscous fluid or blood. Careful exclusion of patients at risk for developing significant complications (e.g., the presence of underlying lung disease, heart disease, and advanced age) is essential for the safety of such outpatient approaches.

Insertion of a small catheter followed by aspiration may be all that is needed for therapy of a pneumothorax attributed to introduction of air during a procedure involving the chest wall (e.g., thoracentesis, central venous pressure insertion). In most other categories of pneumothorax, prompt chest tube insertion and closed drainage of the abnormal air collection is indicated. The more severe the underlying lung disease and clinical dysfunction, the more urgent the need for tube drainage. None of the usual treatments for primary spontaneous pneumothorax attempts to eradicate the cause of the pneumothorax or help determine its cause.

Patients with unexplained recurrent spontaneous pneumothoraces, persistent bleeding into the pleural space, or unsuccessful chest tube drainage (not resulting in reexpansion of the lung), warrant thoracoscopic examination of the pleura and lung. This procedure allows complete inspection of underlying lung parenchyma, identification of air leaks, and closure using endoscopic stapling devices, loop ligation, or electrocauterization of blebs and bullae. Pleurodesis also can be performed using talc insufflation, chemicals, or pleural abrasion. Most experts agree that chest tube drainage is warranted before referral for thoracoscopy, regardless of whether a patient is clinically stable or unstable. Large-bore chest tubes (28 Fr) are warranted in patients who are clinically unstable, have large air leaks, or are on mechanical ventilation with a high risk of large air leaks. In general, both the British Thoracic Society (BTS) and ACCP guidelines recommend treatment decisions based on severity of clinical symptoms and the degree of lung collapse on chest radiographs.

Thoracotomy may be necessary for some patients with pneumothorax. In these cases, a muscle-sparing axillary thoracotomy is usually possible. Hemothorax may also require exploration or repair of the bleeding site. Failure to reexpand the collapsed lung with tube drainage is another indication for thoracoscopy or thoracotomy. The length of time necessary for a visceral pleural tear to heal and for lung reexpansion to occur during tube drainage depends on the particular patient and the severity of underlying disease. For example, patients with the human immunodeficiency virus, active *P. carinii* pneumonia, and those on corticosteroids may be at increased risk for prolonged air leak with its associated increased risk for morbidity and mortality. In general, leaks persisting for more than 7 to 10 days rarely seal without surgical intervention.

Recurrence rates in otherwise healthy patients range from 10 to 50%. Approximately 60% of patients with a second recurrence will develop a third episode; after three episodes, recurrence exceeds 85%. Therefore, thoracoscopy or thoracotomy usually is recommended after the first recurrence and, increasingly, in patients with air leaks persisting for more than 3 to 5 days. The 2001 ACCP and 2003 BTS guidelines provide an excellent discussion of problems surrounding management decisions in patients with primary and secondary pneumothorax.

---

1. Bense L, Eklund G, Wiman LG. Smoking and the increased risk of contracting spontaneous pneumothorax. *Chest*. 1987;92:1009.

   Smoking increased the relative risk of SP approximately nine times among women and 22 times among men. A dose-response relationship between number of cigarettes smoked per day and risk of SP was also noted.

2. Baumann MH, Strange C, Heffner JE, et al. Management of spontaneous pneumothorax: an American College of Chest Physicians Delphi consensus statement. *Chest*. 2001;119:590–602.

   Agreement exists for general principles of care, with observation of small pneumothoraces being appropriate only for primary pneumothoraces.

3. Baumann MH, Strange C. Treatment of spontaneous pneumothorax: a more aggressive approach? *Chest*. 1997;112:789.

   An excellent review of treatment modalities as well as specific responses to the commonly asked questions, "Do chest tubes alone provide recurrence prevention, and what are the risks for developing reexpansion pulmonary edema by using a chest tube?" A must read for anyone caring for patients with pneumothorax!

4. Bauman MH. Do blebs cause primary spontaneous pneumothorax? Pro–con debate. *J Bronchol*. 2002;9:313–318.

   A debate with Dr. Noppen that reviews pathogenesis of SP.

5. Colt HG, Mathur PN. *Manual of Pleural Procedures*. Philadelphia: Lippincott Williams & Wilkins; 1999:127.

   Practical, pocket-size reference manual with photographs and text that walks readers through diagnostic and therapeutic pleural procedures, such as chest tube insertion, bedside pleurodesis, chest drainage devices, and thoracoscopy.

6. Colt HG. Thoracoscopic management of pneumothorax. In: Beamis JF, Mathur PN, eds. *Interventional Pulmonology*. New York: McGraw-Hill Publishers; 1999:207.

   Descriptive and critical analysis of thoracoscopic management strategies for patients with primary and secondary pneumothoraces, in addition to a discussion of available treatments for patients with prolonged air leaks.

7. Conces DJ, Tarver RD, Gray WC, et al. Treatment of pneumothoraces utilizing small caliber chest tubes. *Chest.* 1988;94:55.

   Use of a number 9 French catheter, usually attached to a flutter valve (in some suction alone was used), resulted in definitive treatment, without complications, in 87% of patients.

8. Green R, McLoud TC, Stark P. Pneumothorax. *Semin Roentgenol.* 1977;12:313.

   An excellent review of roentgenographic manifestations of pneumothorax.

9. Heffner JH, Huggins JT. Management of secondary spontaneous pneumothorax: there's confusion in the air. *Chest.* 2004;125:1190–1192.

   An editorial that explicitly describes many controversial areas pertaining to pneumothorax management and differences between the ACCP and BTS guidelines.

10. Henry M, Arnold T, Harvey J. BTS guidelines for the management of spontaneous pneumothorax. *Thorax.* 2003;58:39–60.

    A great review with management guidelines, including aspects such as role of CT scans in diagnosis, which patients to refer for surgery, surgical techniques, choice of chest tube size, and roles for suction and various pleurodesis modalities. on steroids.

11. Janssen JP, van Mourik J, Cuesta Valentin M, et al. Treatment of patients with spontaneous pneumothorax during videothoracoscopy. *Eur Respir J.* 1994;7: 1281.

    Of patients examined, 34% had normal thoracoscopic inspections, with bullae larger than 2 cm noted in 54% of cases.

12. Lee P, Yap WS, Pek WY, et al. An audit of medical thoracoscopy and talc poudrage for pneumothorax in advanced COPD. *Chest.* 2004;125:1315–1320.

    A study of 41 patients showing 95% success after a median follow-up of 35 months, although mortality was 10% at 30 days (each in a patient with baseline forced expiratory volume in 1 second [FEV_1] < 40% predicted).

13. Metersky ML, Colt HG, Olson LK, et al. AIDS-related spontaneous pneumothorax: risk factors and treatment. *Chest.* 1995;108:946.

    Patients with acquired immune deficiency syndrome, particularly if oncorticosteroids, have a poor prognosis. Pneumothorax is usually associated with P. carinii pneumonia. Large-bore chest tube drainage and early thoracoscopic exploration and pleurodesis may be warranted in these individuals.

14. Munnell ER. Thoracic drainage. *Ann Thorac Surg.* 1997;63:1497.

    Reviews the advantages and disadvantages of various chest tube insertion techniques and drainage devices.

15. Noppen M. Management of primary spontaneous pneumothorax. *Curr Opin Pulm Med.* 2003;9:272–275.

    Also includes an excellent discussion of management guidelines and whether they are actually being followed.

16. Noppen M, Alexander P, Driesen P, et al. Manual aspiration versus chest tube drainage in first episodes of primary spontaneous pneumothorax. *Am J Respir Crit Care Med.* 2002;165:1240–1244.

    A prospective randomized study in a homogenous population.

17. Peatfield RC, Edwards PR, Johnson NM. Two unexpected deaths from pneumothorax. *Lancet.* 1979;1:356.

    Illustrates and discusses three potentially lethal complications—unilateral pulmonary edema, tension pneumothorax, and mediastinal emphysema.

18. Roviaro GC, Varoli F, Vergani C, et al. State of the art in thoracoscopic surgery. A personal experience of 2000 video-assisted procedures. *Surg Endosc.* 2002;16: 881–892.

    Also includes an overview of the literature as well as a careful description of techniques and personal results.

19. Samelson SL, Goldberg EM, Ferguson MK. The thoracic vent. Clinical experience with a new device for treating simple pneumothorax. *Chest.* 1991;100:880.

    Describes the use of a one-way valve device that is particularly useful for ambulatory treatment of iatrogenic or simple spontaneous pneumothoraces.

20. Sewell RW, Fewel JG, Grover FL, et al. Experimental evaluation of reexpansion pulmonary edema. *Ann Thorac Surg.* 1978;26:126.

 Anatomic and functional changes were seen in the reexpanded lung after relief of pneumothorax. The longer the time of collapse, the greater the pulmonary intravascular water volume after reexpansion.

21. Tschopp JM, Brutsche M, Frey JG. Treatment of complicated spontaneous pneumothorax by simple talc pleurodesis under thoracoscopy and local anesthesia. *Thorax.* 1997;52:329.

 In this study of 93 patients undergoing thoracoscopic talc pleurodesis under local anesthesia, the major predictor for treatment failure was the presence of bullae larger than 2 cm.

22. Tschopp JM, Boutin C, Astoul P, et al. Talcage by medical thoracoscopy for primary spontaneous pneumothorax is more cost-effective than drainage: a randomized study. *Eur Respir J.* 2002;1003–1009.

 Multinational international study that warrants consideration as an example of international collaboration.

23. van de Brekel JA, Duurkens VAM, Vanderschueren RGJ. Pneumothorax: results of thoracoscopy and pleurodesis with talc poudrage and thoracotomy. *Chest.* 1993;103:345.

 Results of thoracoscopy in 622 patients with spontaneous pneumothorax.

24. Wagaruddin M, Bernstein A. Reexpansion pulmonary edema. *Thorax.* 1975;30:54.

 A good discussion of the mechanisms and clinical manifestations of pulmonary edema occurring after reexpansion of pneumothoraces.

25. Yim APC, Ho JKS. 100 consecutive cases of video-assisted thoracoscopic surgery for spontaneous pneumothorax. *Surg Endosc.* 1995;9:332.

 Recurrence rates of only 3% after follow-up of 17 months.

14. HEMOPTYSIS

Henri G. Colt

Hemoptysis (i.e., coughing up blood) is a frightening event for both healthcare providers and patients and occurs in a variety of clinical conditions. The amount and quality can range from blood-streaked sputum to several cups of blood or even massive exsanguination. Death is rare, usually resulting from asphyxiation and respiratory arrest associated with flooding of the tracheobronchial tree. Massive hemoptysis, however, is a life-threatening medical emergency that may not be controllable by endotracheal intubation and mechanical ventilation.

The incidence of hemoptysis reflects the type of patient population studied (e.g., surgical vs medical or cancer center vs tuberculosis clinic). In the United States, the most common causes are chronic bronchitis, bronchiectasis, and bronchogenic carcinoma, followed by tuberculosis, fungal infections (especially aspergillosis or aspergilloma), bacterial pneumonia and abscess, and pulmonary infarction. Less common causes of hemoptysis include mitral stenosis, Goodpasture's syndrome, endobronchial foreign bodies, bronchial adenoma, pulmonary arteriovenous (AV) fistulas, Behçet's disease, lung parasites (ascariasis, paragonimiasis, and schistosomiasis), Wegener's granulomatosis, drugs (cocaine, anticoagulants, penicillamine), cystic fibrosis, lymphangioleiomyomatosis, laceration of the pulmonary artery by balloon-tipped catheter, coagulopathies, and even bioterrorism (pneumonic plague, tularemia, and tricothecene mycotoxin). Recent data also suggest an increased risk for hemoptysis in patients with indwelling airway stents who can develop airway inflammation, granulation tissue overgrowth, and erosion of tracheobronchial mucosa.

The approach to diagnosis and initial management compels the clinician to answer the following questions:

1. What is the origin of the bleeding (lungs, the airways, nasopharynx, or digestive tract)?
2. Can the bleeding be stopped?
3. Will the bleeding recur at some time in the future?
4. Does the patient have a systemic disease that predisposes to bleeding?
5. Is emergency intervention needed and what kind of surveillance should be instituted?

The anatomic source of bleeding depends on the specific pathologic process. Data from bronchial artery embolization studies indicate that bronchial arteries and collaterals from axillary, intercostal, diaphragmatic, and other systemic arteries of the thorax are the source of bleeding in most cases. Inflammation associated with infection and carcinoma can cause reactive hypervascularity of bronchial arteries and stimulation of collaterals. Localized inflammation also can result in erosion of these hypervascular networks of vessels and bleeding. Pulmonary arteries, capillaries, and veins are the source of hemoptysis in fewer than 10% of cases.

The hemoptysis found in chronic bronchitis (accounting for more than 50% of hemoptysis cases in the United States) arises from superficial vessels in the bronchial mucosa. Hemoptysis associated with chronic fibrocavitary disorders, such as tuberculosis, is caused by rupture or erosion of enlarged bronchial arteries and bronchopulmonary anastomoses. Development of pulmonary artery aneurysms and rupture from vessel wall invasion also can occur. In mitral stenosis, the primary sites of bleeding are bronchial veins with blood supplied from both bronchial arteries and reversed blood flow from pulmonary veins.

Recent world events warrant special emphasis on potential bioterrorist causes of hemoptysis. These are the pneumonic plague caused by *Yersinia pestis,* a gram-negative bacillus easily weaponized and spread by aerosolized droplets, which would cause rapidly progressive pneumonia, chest pain, and hemoptysis. Treatment would include oral doxycycline or ciprofloxacin. Tularemia, caused by *Francisella tularensis,* an aerobic gram-negative coccobacillus, also has been weaponized through aerosolization and would cause influenzae-like symptoms with rapidly progressive pneumonia and possible hemoptysis. The treatment of choice is intravenous gentamicin. Finally, tricothecene mycotoxin, also known as "yellow rain" in its aerosolized form, can cause sore throat, skin necrosis, and hemoptysis. An oily residue on the facial skin of victims of biologic attacks might lead one to suspect the diagnosis. Treatment is, for the most part, supportive.

All instances of hemoptysis require careful evaluation to determine the cause and site of bleeding. The history often is invaluable and establishes the duration and extent of bleeding, prior episodes, and the presence of known cardiopulmonary or other diseases. It is extremely important to differentiate hemoptysis from hematemesis and nasopharyngeal bleeding. The physical examination provides specific clues to the diagnosis (e.g., oronasopharyngeal bleeding site, microtelangiectasia, pulmonary or cardiac findings). The chest radiograph may suggest the cause and location of the hemoptysis. The characteristic finding of blood in the air spaces is a confluent or patchy alveolar filling pattern that becomes reticular over days and clears in 3 to 10 days. However, an infiltrate may represent blood aspirated from another bleeding site elsewhere in the lungs, making precise localization of a bleeding site problematic. A negative chest radiograph is common, and computed tomography (CT) scans generally are not helpful, although recent studies suggest that high resolution spiral (1- to 2-mm cuts) CT with contrast may be more helpful than previously thought, especially if the chest radiograph is normal. CT will certainly assist in the diagnosis and mapping of bronchiectasis, usually precluding surgical resection if bronchiectasis is bilateral or diffused, but also directing surgical interventions in case focal pulmonary or vascular abnormalities are identified.

Other relevant laboratory studies include a complete blood count; smear, culture, and cytologic examination of the sputum; and, when appropriate, arterial blood gas analysis, as well as perfusion ($\dot{Q}$) and ventilation ($\dot{V}$) lung scans if pulmonary emboli are suspected. Perfusion scans are not useful in localizing a bleeding site. Several studies have found an elevated single-breath diffusion capacity (DLCO) in patients with intrapulmonary bleeding, although it does not appear that DLCO plays a useful role in the diagnosis or care of most patients (except, possibly, in patients with suspected Goodpasture's syndrome).

Fiberoptic bronchoscopy (FOB), the most valuable diagnostic technique, should be used for all patients with hemoptysis of uncertain cause, although it is unclear still whether diagnostic flexible bronchoscopy should be performed emergently or after bleeding has ceased. Bronchogenic carcinoma has been detected in 2 to 13% of patients with hemoptysis and a normal chest radiograph. Foreign bodies, bronchial adenoma, and other causes of bleeding can be identified readily and the site of the bleeding usually can be determined, especially if patients have previously undergone biopsy of endobronchial abnormalities.

The need for FOB in evaluating hemoptysis is clear, but the timing of the procedure in the face of active bleeding is controversial. Although early bronchoscopy is desirable because it minimizes the likelihood that the site will go undiscovered when bleeding has stopped, no evidence indicates that delaying FOB for 24 or 48 hours will adversely affect the ultimate outcome (e.g., detection of operable carcinoma). FOB should be performed carefully, however, and operators should be ready to handle massive bleeding by having large-channel bronchoscopes available for suctioning; equipment for emergency intubation, sedation, and ventilation; and, preferably, the capacity and ability to perform rigid bronchoscopy. Operators also should be familiar with the use of tamponade balloons and endobronchial blockade balloon devices. Operators should recognize that cough induced by the procedure can promote more bleeding and that blood can spread through the tracheobronchial tree during the procedure, completely filling the central airway and obscuring the bleeding site.

Arteriography and embolization of bronchial and related collateral vasculature (e.g., intercostal, axillary, and subclavian arteries) are increasingly useful in the treatment of hemoptysis that is not responsive to conservative measures. Initially, this technique was only a temporizing measure until patients could undergo lung resection; now many experienced clinicians believe it plays a primary role for long-term control of recurrent or persistent hemoptysis (e.g., recurrent episodes of more than 200 mL/day) even in patients who might be candidates for resectional surgery. Patients who are particularly suitable include those with diffuse lung disease in whom bleeding can arise from more than one site, and those who are not candidates for surgery. Actual visualization of a *bleeding blush* during arteriography is rare. Localization is inferential from the visualization of the abnormal vascularity of reactive bronchial arterial networks; hence, previous specific localization by FOB is important. Inadvertent embolization of spinal arteries is a significant complication, but uncommon if care is exercised in identifying possible spinal arteries branching from vessels considered for embolization. A number of investigators have reported initial control in 80 to 90% of cases, with long-term recurrences in 10 to 25%. Recanalization or growth of new bronchial vessels can limit the permanence of this therapeutic procedure in some patients. Embolization materials include Gelfoam, steel coils, and isobutyl-2-cyanoacrylate. Although infusion of sclerosing liquids or small embolic particles is appealing because of the theoretic advantages of occlusion of flow distal to collateral feeder vessels, the incidence of bronchial wall necrosis, spinal artery occlusion, and intense acute chest pain sometimes precludes the use of these agents.

Therapy for hemoptysis varies with bleeding severity, the specific cause of bleeding, and the patient's overall condition. The three goals of therapy are to prevent asphyxiation (protect the contralateral airway), stop the bleeding, and treat the primary cause. If the volume of hemoptysis is large (>200 mL/day), or if the patient has minimal respiratory reserve, an emergency situation exists. The first goal of therapy is to identify the bleeding site, stop the bleeding, and prevent aspiration of blood into other major airways. In experienced hands, FOB will identify the bleeding site. In some cases of massive bleeding, rigid bronchoscopy is warranted. If necessary, tamponade balloons or endobronchial balloon blockade devices can be inserted and left in place for hours or days while the patient is stabilized and readied for resectional therapy, although coughing can dislodge the balloon. If therapeutic embolization of bronchial arteries is contemplated (see below), placing a Fogarty balloon may allow time for the prerequisite angiographic studies. Bronchoscopists should avoid removing newly formed clot from the secured segmental bronchial airway once bleeding has ceased. Clot removal in these instances may lead to recurrent bleeding.

Another approach to protecting functional airways involves placing a special endotracheal tube with an inflatable distal cuff into the nonbleeding right or left main stem bronchus. The use of a double-lumen tube permits adequate suctioning of blood. However, placement of the tube requires experienced personnel. When available, bronchial arteriography with embolization is increasingly being used for patients with massive hemoptysis who do not respond to more conservative measures. Recent improvements in angiographic techniques have minimized the potential complications of spinal artery occlusions. The efficacy of temporizing measures such as iced saline lavage and Fogarty balloon placement is dependent on local expertise. The role of intravascular infusions or topical applications of vasoconstrictor agents (e.g., vasopressin) has not been established. Reports of successful treatment of bleeding pulmonary aspergilloma by percutaneous intracavitary infusion of amphotericin are anecdotal.

Surgical resection of any bleeding site requires its identification and a patient able to tolerate thoracotomy. Occasionally, patients require emergency surgery before a diagnosis has been established, particularly in some patients with massive hemoptysis. In an often-quoted older study, Crocco et al. found that the mortality of patients with massive hemoptysis (i.e., 600 mL of blood/16-hour period) treated medically was 75%. Among similar patients treated by surgical resection, the mortality was 23%. An especially high mortality rate in patients treated medically was also observed in the setting of massive hemoptysis associated with lung abscesses. The high mortality rate associated with conservative medical therapy may reflect the bias of a nonrandomized study and a patient population with advanced tuberculosis and multiple disease processes. Other studies have found comparable mortality rates between conservative medical management and surgical resection. Nevertheless, experience supports the role for surgical resection if all efforts to control bleeding medically (e.g., strict bed rest, no chest percussion or spirometric testing, aggressive cough suppression) are unsuccessful and embolization of bronchial artery and related vessels is either not available or unsuccessful in controlling bleeding.

1. Auerback O. Pathology and pathogenesis of pulmonary arterial aneurysms in tuberculous cavities. *Am Rev Tuberculosis.* 1939;40:99.
   One of the classic pathologic descriptions of Rasmussen's aneurysms as a cause of pulmonary hemorrhage in tuberculosis.
2. Bobrowitz ID, Ramakrishna S, Shim YS. Comparison of medical versus surgical treatment of major hemoptysis. *Arch Intern Med.* 1983;143:1343.
   This classic article reviews the course of 113 patients with substantial hemoptysis and argues the case for conservative management.
3. Bookstein JJ, Moser KM, Kalafer ME, et al. The role of bronchial arteriography and therapeutic embolization in hemoptysis. *Chest.* 1977;72:658.
   An excellent, detailed discussion of the risks and usefulness of this technique.
4. Colby TV. Diffuse pulmonary hemorrhage in Wegener's granulomatosis. *Semin Respir Med.* 1989;10:136.
   Although microscopic evidence of hemorrhage is common in Wegener's granulomatosis, massive alveolar hemorrhage is unusual and is discussed in this review.
5. Colice GL. Detecting lung cancer as a cause of hemoptysis in patients with normal chest radiograph: bronchoscopy versus CT. *Chest.* 1997;111:877.
   Proposes using sputum cytology first or repeat chest radiographs to select patients for bronchoscopy.
6. Colice GL. Hemoptysis. Three questions that can direct management. *Postgrad Med.* 1996;100:227.

An easy-to-understand review article describing the three steps of diagnosis (make sure bleeding is from the lower respiratory tract, identify life-threatening cases, and consider both the systemic and pulmonary circulation as a source for the bleed).

7. Corder R. Hemoptysis. *Emer Med Clin North Am.* 2003;21:421–435.
   A great review of current differential diagnosis and the role of the emergency room physician facing the patient coughing up blood.

8. Crocco JA, Rooney JJ, Fankushen DS, et al. Massive hemoptysis. *Arch Intern Med.* 1968;121:495.
   Compares medical and surgical therapy of 67 patients with massive hemoptysis.

9. DiLeo MD, Amedee RG, Butcher RB. Hemoptysis and pseudohemoptysis: the patient expectorating blood. *Ear Nose Throat J* 1995;74:822.
   The evaluation of patients coughing up blood is usually devoted to excluding a pulmonary source, but in this retrospective review of 471 cases, 10% had an upper airway cause and 2% had an upper airway malignancy as the site of their bleeding (from the primary tumor or from metastases).

10. Eddy JB. Clinical assessment and management of massive hemoptysis. *Crit Care Med.* 2000;28:1642–1647.
    Another recent review well worth reading that argues the need for CT scanning AND flexible bronchoscopy. Also presents an algorithm for managing massive bleeding.

11. Freitag L, Tekolf E, Stamatis G, et al. Three year experience with a new balloon catheter for the management of hemoptysis. *Eur Respir J* 1994;7:2033–2037.
    Another careful description of interventional techniques.

12. Gong Jr. H, Salvatierra C. Clinical efficacy of early and delayed fiberoptic bronchoscopy in patients with hemoptysis. *Am Rev Respir Dis.* 1981;124:221.
    A review of 129 patients, focusing on the pros and cons of early versus late bronchoscopy.

13. Gourin A, Garzon AA. Control of hemorrhage in emergency pulmonary resection for massive hemoptysis. *Chest.* 1975;68:120.
    A classic description of the successful use of balloon-tipped catheters to control bleeding and selective placement of a cuffed endotracheal tube for protection of the nonbleeding lung in 15 patients.

14. Gourin D, Garzon AA. Operative treatment of massive hemoptysis. *Ann Thorac Surg.* 1974;18:52.
    An update on original report by Crocco et al. that also describes cavernostomy and packing to control bleeding in patients unable to undergo resection of lung.

15. Greening AP, Hughes JMB. Serial estimations of carbon monoxide diffusing capacity in intrapulmonary haemorrhage. *Clin Sci (Lond).* 1981;60:507.
    Serial measurements were much more sensitive than requiring a single measurement to be above the upper limit of predicted. Of intrapulmonary blood, 200 mL may be the sensitivity for serial measurements of DLCO.

16. Haponik EF, Chin R. Hemoptysis: clinicians' perspectives. *Chest.* 1990;97:469–475.
    Pulmonary physicians surveyed prefer radiologic intervention to surgical intervention!

17. Haponik EF, Fein A, Chin R. Managing life-threatening hemoptysis: has anything really changed? *Chest.* 2000;118:1431–1435.
    Well, not much has really changed, but many interventional bronchoscopists can successfully palliate bleeding through a variety of airway interventions.

18. Johnston H, Reisz G. Changing spectrum of hemoptysis. *Arch Intern Med.* 1989;149:1666.
    Older study demonstrating that hemoptysis is more frequently caused by bronchitis and lung cancer than by tuberculosis.

19. Jolliet P, Soccal P, Chevrolet JC. Control of massive hemoptysis by endobronchial tamponade with a pulmonary artery balloon catheter. *Crit Care Med.* 1992;20:1730–1732
    Careful description of interventional technique.

20. Katoh O, Kishikawa T, Yamada H, et al. Recurrent bleeding after arterial embolization in patients with hemoptysis. *Chest*. 1990;97:541.

   Examines the anatomic basis for recurrent bleeding after an initially successful embolization. Major reasons for failure included bilateral disease, technical inability to position the catheter, and pulmonary artery origin of bleeding.

21. Katoh O, Yamada H, Hiura K, et al. Bronchoscopic and angiographic comparison of bronchial arterial lesions in patients with hemoptysis. *Chest*. 1987;91:486.

   Presents bronchoscopic appearances of vascular lesions noted on bronchial artery angiography.

22. Keller FS, Rosch J, Loflin TG, et al. Nonbronchial systemic collateral arteries: significance in percutaneous embolotherapy for hemoptysis. *Radiology*. 1987;164:687.

   In 45% of their cases, nonbronchial systemic collateral arteries were important sources of bleeding.

23. Kvale P, Simoff M, Prakash UBS. Palliative care. Lung cancer guidelines. *Chest*. 2003;123:284S–311S.

   10 to 20% of patients with lung cancer may actually present with symptoms of hemoptysis. This is an excellent overview of palliative care in patients with lung cancer, also addressing treatment of chest pain, dyspnea, cough, and distal metastases.

24. Liebow AA, Hales MR, Lindshog GE. Enlargement of the bronchial arteries and their anastomoses with the pulmonary arteries in bronchiectasis. *Am J Pathol*. 1949;25:211.

   An excellent pathologic study of the changes in vasculature of the lung in bronchiectasis.

25. Lordan JL, Gascoigne A, Corris PA. The pulmonary physician in critical care. *Thorax*. 2003;58:814–819.

   Excellent recent review based on single case report. Excellent images and description of therapeutic modalities, including Fogarty catheter placement and endotracheal intubation.

26. Mal H, Rullon I, Mellot F, et al. Immediate and long-term results of bronchial artery embolization for life-threatening hemoptysis. *Chest*. 1999;115:996–1001.

   Original investigation and review of results of embolization for potentially fatal hemoptysis.

27. McGuinness G, Naidich DP. CT of airways disease and bronchiectasis. *Radiol Clin N Am*. 2002;40:1–19.

   A careful description of radiographic findings with numerous examples.

28. Stern RC, Boat TF, Orenstein DM, et al. Treatment and prognosis of massive hemoptysis in cystic fibrosis. *Am Rev Respir Dis*. 1978;117:825.

   Massive hemoptysis occurred in 68 of 718 patients with cystic fibrosis with volumes as large as 2,500 mL.

29. Swanson KL, Johnson CM, Prakash UB, et al. Bronchial artery embolization: experience with 54 patients. *Chest*. 2002;121:789–795.

   A recent example of greater than 85% immediate response with cessation of bleeding for up to 30 days or more, and a 10% recurrence rate.

30. Taylor JR, Ryu J, Colby TV, et al. Lymphangioleiomyomatosis. *N Engl J Med*. 1990;323:1254.

   Of 32 patients, 44% had hemoptysis during the course of their lymphangioleiomyomatosis. The actual prevalence is probably much higher; infiltrates from hemorrhage are often misdiagnosed as pneumonia, as they can occur without hemoptysis.

15. ASPIRATION PNEUMONIA

Shazia M. Jamil

Aspiration is defined as the misdirection of oropharyngeal secretions or gastric contents into the larynx, trachea, or the lower respiratory tract. The aspirate may be characterized into three distinct entities: oropharyngeal secretions colonized with bacterial pathogens, acidified gastric contents, and particulate material. Aspiration pneumonia refers to the development of pneumonia after aspiration and is generally found in patients with risk factor(s) and predisposition(s). The reported prevalence varies reflecting differences in study populations. Mortality is as high as 70% in some groups; for example, it is the most common cause of death in advanced Alzheimer's disease.

Not all patients with aspiration develop pneumonia or suffer significant clinical morbidity. Other clinical consequences include acute airway obstruction, chemical (acid) pneumonitis, acute lung injury/acute respiratory distress syndrome (ALI/ARDS), empyema, and lung abscess. Half of all healthy adults aspirate some amount of oropharyngeal secretions while asleep. However, this is of minimal consequence because of the low virulence of bacteria in normal secretions, cough reflex, active ciliary transport, and normal cellular and humoral immune mechanisms. Aspiration of gastric contents also can occur without demonstrable sequelae in healthy persons during general anesthesia (7 to 16%) and endoscopy of the upper gastrointestinal tract (25%).

The most common risk factors for aspiration pneumonia are: (1) impaired consciousness; (2) dysphagia; (3) impaired cough reflex; (4) impaired swallowing or cough reflex secondary to medications; (5) use of nasogastric or endotracheal tubes; (6) sustained supine position as in critically ill, mechanically ventilated, or debilitated patients; (7) trauma; (8) emergency surgery and anesthesia in the absence of preoperative starvation; and (9) anatomic abnormalities, such as tracheoesophageal fistula, gastroesophageal reflux, and gastric outlet obstruction. The most important defense mechanisms preventing aspiration are intact swallowing function and cough reflex. It is not surprising that most of the risk factors associated with aspiration reflect impairment of one or both of these defenses. Nasogastric and endotracheal tubes predispose to aspiration owing to compromise of upper aerodigestive protective mechanisms. The presence of a nasogastric feeding tube also has been associated with pathogen colonization and aspiration leading to a high incidence of gram-negative pneumonia in patients on enteral nutrition. Sedatives impair consciousness, diminish protective airway reflexes, and increase the risk of pneumonia in residents of long-term facilities. Phenothiazines and haloperidol can reduce oropharyngeal swallowing coordination and cause dysphagia; medications that decrease saliva such as anticholinergics and antihistamines make swallowing more difficult and should be used carefully in the elderly. Aspiration occurs in approximately 40 to 50% of stroke patients with dysphagia leading to increased risk for aspiration pneumonia.

Aspiration of microorganisms from a previously colonized oropharynx is one of the major pathogenic mechanisms. The bacterial pathogens generally reflect the patient's location (i.e., community-acquired vs nosocomial aspiration pneumonia). The most frequently isolated organisms found in community-dwelling patients are anaerobic bacteria resembling mouth flora (e.g., *Fusobacterium nucleatum, Peptostreptococcus* spp., and *Prevotella melaninogenicus*), *Streptococcus pneumoniae,* and *Haemophilus influenzae.* Among hospitalized and nursing home patients, anaerobes, nosocomially acquired pathogens such as *Staphylococcus aureus,* and mixed aerobic and facultative gram-negative bacilli, particularly *Klebsiella pneumoniae,* are common. Patients with acid aspiration can develop secondary bacterial infections caused by aerobic gram-positive and gram-negative organisms, such as *S. aureus* and *Pseudomonas aeruginosa.*

The classic form of acid (chemical) aspiration pneumonia is Mendelson's syndrome, which was first described in pregnant women. The major risk for morbidity and mortality is obstetric surgery and general anesthesia. The degree of pulmonary injury varies; aspiration is more extensive with greater gastric volumes, and mortality rates are higher with a gastric acid pH of less than 2.5. Early pathologic examination reveals hemorrhagic pulmonary edema and patchy microatelectasis free of bacterial contamination. The diagnosis is suspected if either the aspiration is witnessed or gastric contents are visualized directly in the airway or suctioned from an endotracheal tube. Management is supportive and similar to that of ARDS: patients require immediate supplemental oxygen and hemodynamic stabilization. Tracheal intubation and mechanical ventilation generally are necessary and, in conjunction with the use of positive end-expiratory pressure, may moderate lung injury. Fiberoptic bronchoscopy should be performed if particulate aspiration is visualized or suspected. Bronchial lavage is of no benefit, because the effect of acid is immediate and its absorption occurs within minutes. Prophylactic antibiotics are not recommended; however, if evidence of infection supervenes (e.g., persistent fever, purulent sputum, progressive abnormality on chest roentgenogram), appropriate antibiotics should be administered. The value of corticosteroid administration remains controversial; the prevalent attitude is that steroids are of no benefit and may predispose to more serious infection or other complications. Pulmonary aspiration during labor can be prevented by relatively simple measures: (1) at-risk parturients should limit oral intake; (2) anesthesia should be administered with the assumption of a full stomach; (3) conduction anesthesia is preferred over general anesthesia; and (4) administration of prophylactic agents (e.g., antacids, histamine$_2$ receptor antagonists, dopamine antagonists) should be considered to raise the pH and decrease the volume of gastric contents.

Aspiration of mineral and vegetable oils can lead to a chronic form of lipoid pneumonia. Patients are frequently elderly individuals who use oil-containing agents or children with constipation who have been treated with mineral oil. These agents may not elicit a normal protective cough reflex and can impair mucociliary transport. A thorough history regarding the use of nose drops and laxatives may suggest the diagnosis. The chest roentgenogram reveals interstitial infiltrates or solitary or multiple mass lesions suggesting tumor. Pathologic examination may demonstrate oil- or fat-laden macrophages, but these are nonspecific findings. Bronchoalveolar lavage (BAL) and gas chromatography, mass spectrometry, or both can demonstrate the exogenous origin of the lipid. Appropriate therapy includes withdrawal of the offending agent and treatment of secondary infection. Aspiration of particulate material can obstruct airways, depending on the particle size, and lead to necrotizing pneumonia. Large particles can obstruct airways and cause rapid suffocation and death. The Heimlich maneuver has been widely publicized as an effective method to dislodge foreign material. Smaller particles (teeth, peanuts, food particles) can occlude smaller bronchi and result in an acute pneumonia or a chronic inflammatory process simulating a lung tumor, distal to the obstruction. Early bronchoscopy by either flexible or rigid instrumentation is indicated for removal of the foreign body; after a few days, inflammation and fibrotic organization make these procedures less successful.

Aspiration pneumonia is common in critically ill patients and deserves special mention. Such patients often have multiple factors predisposing them to aspiration and aspiration pneumonia, including sustained supine position, use of nasogastric and endotracheal tubes, use of sedatives and narcotics, impaired consciousness, exposure to nosocomial environment, and increased risk of bacterial colonization of oropharynx. Several types of bedside swallowing assessments can be used to evaluate patients suspected of aspiration, including observation during swallowing of food of various consistencies and videofluoroscopy. Many patients with dysphagia have a normal gag reflex, whereas others with absent gag reflex have normal swallowing function. Therefore, gag reflex is a poor indicator of swallow function and its absence does not predict aspiration. Coloring enteral feedings with blue dyes and glucose detection by glucose oxidase strips are no longer recommended to detect aspiration of gastric contents in hospitalized patients.

Aspiration pneumonia may be acute or chronic, depending on the time of onset, nature of aspirated material, and individual host responses. Common clinical features are dyspnea, fever, wheezing, crackles, rhonchi, hypoxia, tachycardia, leukocytosis, and respiratory failure. Severe hypoxemia is common, occurring in association with a normal or low arterial partial pressure of carbon dioxide in alveolar gas ($Paco_2$), a wide alveolar-arterial oxygen difference, and a significant reduction in chest compliance. Chest roentgenograms early in the course may be entirely normal or may reveal either localized or diffuse (multilobar) alveolar or interstitial infiltrates. All forms of aspiration pneumonia are more common in the dependent portions of the lung, as might be predicted; however, exact body position at the time of aspiration determines the exact location of the infiltrates. A pattern of pulmonary edema may be seen, but the absence of cardiac enlargement and pulmonary venous hypertension should suggest ALI/ARDS occurring as a result of aspiration. Pleural effusion is rare. The diagnosis is considered when clinical features and radiographic evidence of pneumonia are seen in individuals at risk of or in witnessed aspiration.

The treatment of aspiration pneumonias is largely supportive; therefore, recognition of risk factors and prevention is of paramount importance. Patients should receive aggressive pulmonary toilet to enhance lung volume and clear secretions. Bronchodilators should be used in patients with bronchospasm. Those with a depressed state of consciousness should not be fed through the mouth or placed in supine position. Sedatives and narcotics should be avoided or used with caution. Nasogastric tubes should not be placed without good airway control. Patients with gastroparesis (e.g., diabetics) or intestinal ileus should either be continuously drained through nasogastric tubes or started on promotility agents. Oral and dental hygiene is especially important in elderly, hospitalized, debilitated, and nursing home patients who are dependent on caregivers to provide this care. Chronic infections in the gingivodental crevice increase the concentration of anaerobic bacteria and other pathogens in the mouth. Nasogastric and endotracheal tubes should be removed as soon as possible. Frequent subglottic suctioning of secretions (in patients with nasogastric and endotracheal tubes) and aggressive oral hygiene have been indicated as additional prevention tools in this group of patients. When suspected, dysphagia should be confirmed with swallow studies. Sputum should be sent for Gram's stain and culture. Bronchoscopy is needed occasionally when diagnosis is not certain. Antibiotic use should be guided by appropriate bacteriologic studies; however, in clinical practice they are often started empirically, especially in the critically ill and those with severe pneumonia. The most common antibiotic regimens are penicillin, clindamycin, and the combination of metronidazole plus penicillin; in addition, gram-negative coverage may be added in hospitalized patients and those residing in long-term facilities. Antibiotic coverage should be narrowed once sputum culture results become available. Narcotic antagonists, frequently used in drug overdose, can induce vomiting; consequently, airway control should be secured before their administration in comatose patients. Substance P, a neurotransmitter, is believed to play a major role in both the swallow and cough sensory pathways. Lower levels of substance P are observed in patients with dysphagia. Angiotensin-converting enzyme (ACE) inhibitors prevent breakdown of substance P, and studies are underway to evaluate their usefulness in patients with aspiration pneumonia.

---

1. DePaso WJ. Aspiration pneumonia. *Clin Chest Med.* 1991;12:269.
2. Bartlett J, Gorbach S. The triple threat of aspiration pneumonia. *Chest.* 1975;68:560.
3. Wynne J, Modell J. Respiratory aspiration of stomach contents. *Ann Intern Med.* 1977;87:466.

   References 1–3 provide excellent reviews of the subject and recommendations regarding prevention and treatment.
4. Mendelson C. The aspiration of stomach contents into the lung during obstetric anesthesia. *Am J Obstet Gynecol.* 1946;52:191.

   Reference 4 is the classic description of acid aspiration as seen in obstetric patients.

5. Addington WR, Stephens RE, Gilliland KA. Assessing the laryngeal cough reflex and the risk of developing pneumonia after stroke: an interhospital comparison. *Stroke*. 1999;30:1203.

   In a high-risk group of 604 acute stroke patients (prospectively studied), a normal reflex cough test was associated with a low risk for developing aspiration pneumonia with oral feeding.

6. Marik P, Kaplan D. Aspiration pneumonia and dysphagia in the elderly. *Chest*. 2003;124:328.

   A comprehensive review article that impresses upon us the magnitude of problem that pneumonia poses in the elderly population, and discusses various ways to diagnose and treat dysphagia with the potential of preventing aspiration pneumonia.

7. Bynum L, Pierce A. Pulmonary aspiration of gastric contents. *Am Rev Respir Dis*. 1976;114:1129.

   A study concluding that prophylactic antibiotics and corticosteroids are not beneficial.

8. Stoschus B, Allescher IIB. Drug-induced dysphagia. *Dysphagia*. 1993;8:154.

   Article reviews different drug mechanisms leading to reduced swallowing function.

9. Kalia M. Dysphagia and aspiration pneumonia in patients with Alzheimer's disease. *Metabolism*. 2003;52:36.

   An excellent review article that discusses etiology of dysphagia and factors predisposing to high prevalence of aspiration pneumonia in Alzheimer's patients.

10. Loeb M, McGeer A, McArthur M, et al. Risk factors for pneumonia and other lower respiratory tract infections in elderly residents of long-term care facilities. *Arch Intern Med*. 1999;159:2058.

11. Johnson LF, Rajagopal KR. Aspiration resulting from gastroesophageal reflux: a cause of bronchopulmonary disease. *Chest*. 1988;93:676.

   The above article and an editorial pertaining to it discusses the importance of gastroesophageal reflux and pulmonary aspiration in perpetuating or initiating chronic lung disease.

12. Matsuse T, Oka T, Kida K, et al. Importance of diffuse aspiration bronchiolitis caused by chronic occult aspiration in the elderly. *Chest*. 1996;110:1289.

   The authors review chronic inflammation of bronchioles caused by recurrent aspiration.

13. Spickard A 3rd, Hirschmann JV. Exogenous lipoid pneumonia. *Arch Intern Med*. 1994;154:686.

   The authors emphasize the importance of history and discuss diagnostic tests and treatment.

14. Kallar SK, Everett LL. Potential risks and preventive measures for pulmonary aspiration: new concepts in preoperative fasting guidelines. *Anesth Analg*. 1993;77:171.

   A review with recommendations from a preoperative perspective.

15. Arai T, Yasuda Y, Takaya T, et al. ACE inhibitors and symptomless dysphagia. *Lancet*. 1998;352:1937.

   This study compared the risk of pneumonia in 576 elderly hypertensive patients who were treated with either an ACEI or calcium channel blocker and found a statically significant lower rate of pneumonia in those treated with ACEI.

16. Ramsey DJ, Smithard DG, Kalra L. Early assessments of dysphagia and aspiration risk in acute stroke patients. *Stroke*. 2003;34:1252.

   A comprehensive review of existing swallowing assessment methods, including sensitivity, specificity and limitations in the diagnosis of aspiration.

17. Yoneyama T, Yoshida M, Matsui T, et al. Oral care and pneumonia. Letter. *Lancet*. 1999;354:515.

   Article demonstrates that aggressive oral care lowered the risk of pneumonia in institutionalized elderly patients.

18. Moore FA. Treatment of aspiration in intensive care unit patients. *J Parenter Enteral Nutr*. 2002;26:S69.

19. Scolapio JS. Methods for decreasing risk of aspiration pneumonia in critically ill patients. *J Parenter Enteral Nutr.* 2002;26:S58.
20. McClave SA, DeMeo MT, DeLegge MH, et al. North American summit on aspiration in the critically ill patient: consensus statement. *J Parenter Enteral Nutr.* 2002;26:S80.

References 18–20 are a series of articles that provide excellent reviews and guidance into managing risk factors of aspiration and aspiration pneumonia in critically ill patients.

16. MIDDLE LOBE SYNDROME

Colleen L. Bailey and James H. Harrell II

The term middle lobe syndrome (MLS), coined in 1948 by Graham and colleagues, initially described patients with right middle lobe (RML) atelectasis secondary to bronchial compression by enlarged nontuberculous lymph nodes. Since then, the definition of MLS has evolved to include all types of recurrent or chronic atelectasis of the RML. MLS occurs in both genders and among all age groups.

MLS can be divided pathophysiologically into obstructive, extraluminal or intraluminal, and nonobstructive types. Intraluminal lesions include endobronchial tumors, aspirated foreign material, inspissated mucus (often associated with cystic fibrosis [CF] and allergic bronchopulmonary aspergillosis [ABPA]), broncholiths, amyloidosis, esophageal diverticulum, sarcoid granulomas, silicosis, postinflammatory granulation tissue, and mucosal edema, and scarring. The most common causes of extraluminal RML obstruction are compression by benign and malignant tumors and lymphadenopathy resulting from neoplasm, sarcoidosis, tuberculosis, atypical mycobacteria, and fungal infections. Factors that contribute to the susceptibility of the RML to extraluminal obstruction and collapse include its small luminal diameter, relatively long length before dividing into segmental bronchi, poor drainage because of its angular takeoff from the intermediate bronchus, and increased compressibility.

In nonobstructive MLS, also known as peripheral middle lobe syndrome, the RML bronchus is patent on bronchoscopy. Disorders associated with nonobstructive MLS include asthma, recurrent pneumonia, bronchitis, and bronchiectasis. The most widely accepted theory explaining nonobstructive MLS is the relative isolation of the middle lobe with resultant loss of collateral ventilation from the other lobes. It has been theorized that complete fissures surrounding the RML result in impairment or absence of collateral ventilation, resulting in impaired secretion clearance and subsequent atelectasis, chronic inflammation, and fibrosis. The most frequent causes of MLS in 933 patients collected from a series of reports were benign inflammation (47%) and malignant tumors (22%). The incidence of malignant involvement causing MLS ranges from 15 to 43%.

Symptoms associated with MLS are often nonspecific and include cough, wheezing, dyspnea, fevers, chills, chest pain, fatigue, and hemoptysis. A study of 99 patients with RML atelectasis noted recurrent episodes of pneumonitis in 77%, recurrent hemoptysis in 42%, and pleuritic pain in the right inframammary area in 52%. Some patients with MLS are asymptomatic, and the diagnosis is based on routine chest imaging. The physical examination may be normal or may reveal wheezes, crackles, rhonchi, and decreased breath sounds and dullness to percussion over the involved area. Clubbing has been reported in advanced cases.

The diagnosis of RML disease usually requires frontal and lateral chest radiographs. On the frontal view, ill-defined opacities may be visible that often obscure the adjacent right heart border (ie, "silhouette sign"). On the lateral view, a triangular density overlying the heart shadow with the apex pointing toward the hilum is most commonly seen. RML collapse may be difficult to detect on the frontal chest radiograph because this lobe is thin and lies obliquely in the superoinferior plane. The chest radiograph may be normal in patients with intermittent collapse. Earlier use of bronchography to aid in the diagnosis of middle lobe obstruction and bronchiectasis has now been supplanted by computed tomography (CT), which allows the assessment of both bronchial patency and causes of extrinsic bronchial compression (eg, lymph node enlargement). High-resolution CT is useful in assessing endobronchial and parenchymal abnormalities, as well as distal bronchiectasis.

Bronchoscopy plays an important diagnostic and therapeutic role in MLS. Direct visualization of the RML bronchus allows evaluation of obstructive etiologies such as inflammation, tumors, foreign bodies, and stenosis. In one review of 613 patients, bronchoscopy was reported to show bronchial stenosis or tumor in 38%, abnormal but nonspecific changes in 17%, and no abnormalities in 45% of cases. Bronchial secretions should be routinely collected from the RML for pathologic and microbiologic studies. The therapeutic role of bronchoscopy in MLS includes removal of secretions, tumors, broncholiths, and foreign bodies; balloon dilation of the RML bronchus; and laser therapy to remove obstructing lesions.

Both medical and surgical treatment options have been advocated since this syndrome was originally described more than 50 years ago. Lobectomy was initially considered the treatment of choice when a high proportion of cases were the result of compression by enlarged lymph nodes. The trend in the management of MLS has shifted toward medical therapy with treatment aimed at the underlying cause. In one series of 98 patients with MLS, 65 had complete resolution of MLS with medical management after bronchoscopy, whereas 31 required lobectomy. If the cause of MLS is an obstructing neoplasm, treatment often includes surgical resection with radiation and chemotherapy as deemed necessary. Nonobstructing MLS caused by chronic infection and bronchiectasis may require prolonged antibiotic treatment. Postural drainage, bronchodilators, and avoidance of bronchial irritants such as tobacco may also be beneficial. Lobectomy is generally reserved for patients with persistent, debilitating symptoms that have not responded to prolonged medical therapy.

1. Graham EA, Burford TH, Mayer JH. Middle lobe syndrome. *Postgrad Med.* 1948;4:29.

   These authors first used the term middle lobe syndrome *to describe 12 patients with RML atelectasis resulting from compression of the bronchus by enlarged nontuberculous lymph nodes.*

2. Culiner MM. The right middle lobe syndrome, a nonobstructive complex. *Dis Chest.* 1966;50:57.

   This paper challenged the hypothesis that MLS was only caused by bronchial compression by presenting nine patients with RML atelectasis and patency of the RML bronchus. It postulated that isolation of the RML and loss of collateral ventilation from adjacent lobes was the cause of RML atelectasis.

3. Inners CR, Terry PB, Traystman RJ, et al. Collateral ventilation and the middle lobe syndrome. *Am Rev Respir Dis.* 1978;118:305.

   Compared the mechanics of collateral ventilation in the RML versus the upper lobe of five normal volunteers and found higher resistance and longer time-constants in the RML. Concluded that lack of collateral ventilation plays an important role in the pathophysiology of MLS.

4. Bertelsen S, Struve-Christensen E, Aasted A, et al. Isolated middle lobe atelectasis: etiology, pathogenesis, and treatment of the so-called middle lobe syndrome. *Thorax.* 1980;35:449.

   A 10-year study of 135 patients with isolated RML atelectasis. 58 of 135 patients were found to have malignant tumors as a cause of MLS.

5. Saha SP, Mayo P, Long GA, et al. Middle lobe syndrome: diagnosis and management. *Ann Thorac Surg.* 1982;33:28.

Of 98 patients with MLS, 65 had a full recovery after intensive medical therapy, whereas 31 underwent lobectomy for persistent disease.

6. Wagner RB, Johnston MR. Middle lobe syndrome. *Ann Thorac Surg.* 1983;35:679.

   A collective review of the literature on RML syndrome.

7. Rosenbloom SA, Ravin CE, Putman CE, et al. Peripheral middle lobe syndrome. *Radiology.* 1983;149:17.

   A review of clinical and radiographic findings in 129 patients with chronic disease of the RML and/or lingula; 58 patients had no evidence of central airway obstruction.

8. Livingston GL, Holinger LD, Luck SR. Right middle lobe syndrome in children. *Int J Pediatr Otorhinolaryngol.* 1987;13:11.

   In this series of 21 patients with MLS, most had asthma or a family history of atopic disorders. Resolution of RML atelectasis occurred promptly after bronchoscopy in one third of cases and eventually in another third.

9. Springer C, Avital A, Noviski N, et al. Role of infection in the middle lobe syndrome in asthma. *Arch Dis Child.* 1992;67:592.

   This study evaluated the incidence of bacterial infection in RML or lingula collapse in asthmatic children. Of the 21 children studied, nine grew pathogenic bacteria from BAL cultures. With appropriate antibiotic therapy, all but one of the nine children had complete resolution of MLS in a few weeks.

10. Albo RJ, Grimes OF. The middle lobe syndrome: a clinical study. *Dis Chest.* 1966;50:509.

    A review of 99 patients that characterizes the etiology and symptoms associated with MLS.

11. Kwon KY, Myers JL, Swensen SJ, et al. Middle lobe syndrome: a clinicopathological study of 21 patients. *Hum Pathol.* 1995;26:302.

    This study reviewed the clinical and pathologic findings in 21 patients with MLS caused by nonneoplastic conditions. The most common findings were bronchiectasis and chronic bronchitis/bronchiolitis with lymphoid hyperplasia.

---

17. COMPLICATIONS AFTER PULMONARY RESECTION

David P. Kapelanski

Thorough preoperative evaluation and preparation for lung resection is the most effective way to minimize postoperative complications. Specific objectives include (1) assessment of the extent and consequences of parenchymal resection required for disease management; (2) determination of concurrent cardiac and pulmonary status; (3) recognition and amelioration of disorders, such as malnutrition and reactive airway disease, that might compromise postoperative ventilatory mechanics; and (4) reduction in tracheobronchitis by smoking cessation. Postoperative pain can reduce spontaneous ventilatory volume and interfere with effective coughing, thereby promoting retention of secretions. Consequently, prudent preoperative planning should include selecting an operative approach that minimizes disruption of chest wall mechanics whenever possible. Furthermore, because respiratory depression can limit postoperative narcotic administration, regional analgesic techniques should be considered. Recent experience with lung volume reduction surgery suggests that safe anatomic or wedge resection is often possible, even in higher risk patients with scrupulous preoperative preparation, meticulous intraoperative technique, careful anesthetic management, and exacting postoperative care. *It is important to emphasize that all physicians who care for patients after lung resection surgery should be aware of the common and unusual complications that can arise in this setting.*

Bleeding can occur during and after lung resection. During an operation, knowledge of variation in segmental pulmonary anatomy and avoidance of intemperate dissection in inflamed tissue provide the best prophylaxis against catastrophic hemorrhage that may not be manageable without sacrificing lung parenchyma. The risk of perioperative hemorrhage can be reduced further by circumspect introduction of pleural drains and pericostal sutures. Finally, meticulous inspection of the hemithorax before wound closure facilitates opportune management of previously unappreciated mediastinal or pleural bleeding points.

Postoperative pleural effusion is relatively common. After resection, the volume drained by pleural catheters is highly variable but is rarely more than 300 mL in the initial 24 hours, unless significant pulmonary inflammation is present at operation. Whenever pleural drainage exceeds a rate of 200 mL/hour for 2 or more hours or 100 mL/hour for 4 or more hours, reexploration should be considered. Clinical factors that should encourage a more aggressive approach to reoperation include the development of hemodynamic instability, radiographic evidence of retained intrapleural blood, or difficulty obtaining blood components that may be required either to sustain oxygen delivery or correct coagulation system defects.

Atelectasis is a common complication after thoracotomy. The frequency of postresectional atelectasis can be reduced by preoperative management of purulent tracheobronchitis and bronchospasm; several studies suggest that even short periods of tobacco abstinence can be beneficial. After operation, adequate analgesia is essential to facilitate maintenance of normal ventilatory volumes and effective secretion clearance. Properly coached incentive spirometry, intermittent positive pressure breathing, and encouragement of early ambulation are useful. If airway secretions are copious or cough ineffectual, mucolytics, chest physiotherapy, and careful nasotracheal aspiration can be instituted. Although lobar or segmental collapse may be evident after careful clinical examination of a patient with fever, tachypnea, or desaturation, radiographic diagnosis is important. When clinically significant, atelectasis is best treated by bronchoscopy, which permits rapid evacuation of secretions and early reexpansion. If a prolonged problem is anticipated, minitracheostomy may be useful.

Bronchial stump integrity after resection should be routinely tested under saline during sustained inflation to an airway pressure of 25 to 30 cm H_2O. Continuous air leaks should be repaired immediately. After partial lung resection, low-volume air leaks from residual parenchyma are common but can be minimized if caution is exercised during the development of intersegmental and interlobar planes. Reinforcement of parenchymal staple lines with glutaraldehyde fixed bovine pericardial strips or bovine collagen should be considered whenever undertaking resection in an abnormal lung. Major parenchymal air leaks identified at operation should be carefully repaired with absorbable suture; pedicled or free pleural flaps or bovine pericardium and collagen can be used to buttress the repair when the pulmonary parenchyma is diseased. Massive air leak occurring within the initial 24 hours of operation suggests a failure of surgical technique because of unrecognized injury to pulmonary parenchyma or airway dehiscence. Bronchoscopy and reoperation should be strongly considered to prevent the development of empyema or the need for prolonged pleural drainage. Most postoperative air leaks resolve within 96 hours of operation without adjunctive maneuvers, provided the residual lung fills the hemithorax. If a low-volume air leak persists beyond this time, the integrity of the drainage system should be confirmed. In the absence of a postresection space, increasing the magnitude of pleural suction has limited value and can perpetuate the leak. Partially withdrawing the pleural catheters may displace drainage apertures from raw parenchymal sites and allow fusion of these sites with adjacent tissue. Chemical sclerosis and autologous blood patches are both used with variable success in the management of low-volume leaks. If these relatively simple interventions fail and hospitalization is prolonged beyond 1 week for the sole purpose of managing an air leak, a Heimlich valve can be substituted for the water seal system, with further management on an outpatient basis.

The management of postresectional spaces depends on the extent of resection. A postresectional space after pneumonectomy is unavoidable; after lesser resections, the remaining parenchyma may only partially fill the hemithorax. In ordinary circumstances, the residual space will be obliterated or minimized with some combination of compensatory mediastinal shift, hemidiaphragmatic elevation, and narrowing of the intercostal spaces. These mechanisms can fail in the presence of pulmonary or visceral pleural restriction or if mediastinal mobility has been reduced by prior inflammatory disease or preoperative radiation therapy. Improperly positioned or managed pleural drains, postoperative atelectasis, and prolonged air leaks are all factors that further contribute to incomplete expansion of the residual parenchyma. Although most postresectional spaces are clinically innocuous, it is hazardous to assume that all will resolve in benign fashion. If a significant space is recognized as inevitable at the conclusion of a limited resection, myoplasty or osteoplastic or tailoring thoracoplasty merit consideration, particularly when operation is undertaken in the management of infectious disease. Pleural tents are more readily created, but their utility largely resides in their capacity to help seal parenchymal air leaks.

After operation, maneuvers to prevent or manage atelectasis are paramount. It is relatively simple to increase the magnitude of suction on pleural drains, although the response is unpredictable. Therapeutic pneumoperitoneum, which is used less frequently, can be useful, particularly in the presence of a persistent air leak. If the pleural drains are patent and an uninfected space remains after cessation of any postoperative air leak, suction should be discontinued. If the residual space is stable and the air leak does not recur after 24 hours on water seal drainage, the pleural tubes should be withdrawn. If the space enlarges or the air leak recurs, a brief additional trial of suction is generally warranted, if still within the initial 2 weeks of operation. Failure at that juncture warrants management by conversion to an open drainage system and secondary consideration of space reduction by myoplasty or thoracoplasty, especially if the volume of the residual space is large and the duration of open drainage likely to be unduly prolonged.

A bronchopleural fistula complicating pulmonary resection generally develops in the second week after operation and is usually heralded by fever, hemoptysis, and increased cough. Preoperative treatment of malnutrition and tracheobronchitis and careful intraoperative management of the bronchus during dissection and closure are essential to minimize the risk of fistula. A recurrence or delayed increase in the magnitude of postresectional air leak, the late development of subcutaneous emphysema, or the recurrence, enlargement, or new development of a postresectional space should each be assessed with this potential development in mind. The most pressing management goals are protecting the residual parenchyma from soilage and preserving adequate minute ventilation.

The first goal is met by promptly reestablishing closed pleural drainage; after pneumonectomy, the patient should be positioned, with the operated side dependent, until the pneumonectomy space has been drained. A balanced drainage system prevents excessive mediastinal shift and, thus, confers some advantage in the initial management of early postpneumonectomy bronchopleural fistula; if such is not readily available, a standard water seal system will ordinarily suffice. Suction should not be done in an unbalanced system if mediastinal stability is questionable. The resumption of pleural drainage can secondarily unmask a high-volume air leak, particularly in the setting of positive pressure ventilation; the consequent ventilation maldistribution can precipitate respiratory compromise. Under these circumstances, the most expediently available method to reestablish effective tidal ventilation should be used. After pneumonectomy, this generally dictates selective intubation of the remaining main stem bronchus; after lesser resections, insertion of a dual-lumen tube is preferable. Bronchoscopy is indicated whenever a bronchopleural fistula is suspected. Careful examination of the bronchial stump will generally confirm the diagnosis, although a smaller fistula can elude detection. If early reoperation to close the fistula is a consideration, the viability of the bronchial mucosa at potential sites of stump revision or more proximal resection should be verified. A fibrin glue patch, applied at the time of bronchoscopy, may seal small-caliber fistulas. Myoplastic closure is increasingly preferred for definitive management of a bronchopleural fistula.

The capacity of the patient to withstand additional parenchymal resection after lobectomy, segmental resection, or bronchoplasty must be determined, because debridement of the initial repair and reclosure may not always be possible. If the patient's medical condition is tenuous or the success of early repair is questionable, it is prudent to deliberately temporize and maintain closed drainage. A small proportion of fistulas will seal without further intervention. If, after stabilization, myoplastic repair is not considered to be an option, an Eloesser flap should be created.

Infection of the pleural space after pulmonary resection can be minimized by careful adherence to the principles of operative preparation, operative technique, and postoperative care described above. Although postpneumonectomy empyema can occur several months or years after operation, most are diagnosed during the second postoperative week. Diagnostic features include enlargement or development of new air-fluid levels in the postresectional space, accompanied by constitutional symptoms and signs of infection. Aspiration of the pleural fluid under ultrasound or radiographic guidance may be necessary if pleural drains are no longer present.

Reestablishing effective pleural drainage is the first therapeutic goal once the diagnosis of empyema has been verified. Closed irrigation of the empyema space with antibiotic solutions, coupled with systemic antibiotics, may sterilize the space and allow subsequent removal of the pleural catheters without further intervention. If this technique fails and the patient is judged a suitable candidate to withstand a major operative procedure, myoplastic obliteration of the space should be considered. An Eloesser flap is generally used in those instances in which medical circumstances preclude a more aggressive approach.

Lobar torsion can occur whenever a lung lobe is peripherally untethered. Operative division of the pulmonary ligament and completion of the anatomic fissures may permit unconstrained rotation of a retained lobe about the bronchovascular pedicle, with infarction the ultimate consequence. Careful examination of lobar orientation during tidal ventilation is required before chest closure. Unusual mobility of a remaining lobe should be restricted, either by fixation to adjoining mediastinal tissue or by peripheral attachment to an adjacent lobe. After operation, clinical and radiographic signs may not permit discrimination between torsion, atelectasis, or parenchymal hematoma. The diagnosis is readily confirmed by bronchoscopy. Immediate reoperation may allow salvage of the involved lobe. If recognition or operation is delayed, lobectomy is required.

Inadvertent obstruction of pulmonary venous return or interruption of both pulmonary and bronchial arterial circulation can cause lobar or segmental gangrene in the absence of torsion. Arterial insufficiency, although less common, is generally not recognized until infarction or gangrene has developed, whereas venous compromise may be recognized at operation. Immediate resection of the involved segments is imperative whenever the diagnosis of gangrene is established.

Cardiac herniation is a rare problem that can develop if the pericardium is breached during pneumonectomy. Herniation, which generally occurs shortly after the operation is concluded, is characterized by the precipitous development of systemic venous obstruction and cardiovascular collapse. Immediate reoperation is mandatory to reintroduce the heart into the pericardial sac and restore effective circulation. A generous pericardiectomy prevents cardiac entrapment after left but not right pneumonectomy; thus, right-sided defects are best managed by closure using autologous tissue or prosthetic material. If available tissue is inadequate and prosthetic material undesirable, the pericardial edges can be carefully sutured to the adjacent atrial and ventricular epicardium.

The postpneumonectomy syndrome is an infrequent problem caused by extreme mediastinal shift after right pneumonectomy or, in the presence of a right aortic arch, after left pneumonectomy. Malacia of the trachea or main stem bronchus as a result of compression between the aorta and pulmonary artery can cause dyspnea and recurring pulmonary infections. Interventions to eliminate the compression have been successful when malacic changes are not severe.

---

1. Ali MK, Mountain CF, Ewer MS, et al. Predicting loss of pulmonary function after pulmonary resection for bronchogenic carcinoma. *Chest.* 1980;77:337.

2. Olsen GN, Weiman DS, Bolton JW, et al. Submaximal invasive exercise testing and quantitative lung scanning in the evaluation for tolerance of lung resection. *Chest*. 1989;95:267.
3. Epstein SK, Faling LJ, Daly BD, et al. Predicting complications after pulmonary resection: preoperative exercise testing vs. a multifactorial cardiopulmonary risk index. *Chest*. 1993;104:694.
4. McKenna RJ Jr, Fischel RJ, Brenner M, et al. Combined operations for lung volume reduction surgery and lung cancer. *Chest*. 1996;110:885.
5. Korst RJ, Ginsberg RJ, Ailawadi M, et al. Lobectomy improves ventilatory function in selected patients with severe COPD. *Ann Thorac Surg*. 1998;66:898.
   Accurately assessing cardiopulmonary reserve and predicting tolerance for lung resection are an art tempered by a solid appreciation of physiology. The scientific underpinnings of the art and the limitations of the science are evident after careful reading of the preceding references.
6. Slinger PD. Anaesthesia for lung resection. *Can J Anaesth*. 1990;37:Sxv.
   Optimal perioperative care requires careful planning. The strategic considerations and one tactical approach are well described here.
7. Nagasaki F, Flehinger BJ, Martini N. Complications of surgery in the treatment of carcinoma of the lung. *Chest*. 1982;82:25.
8. Ginsberg RJ, Hill LD, Eagan RT, et al. Modern thirty-day operative mortality for surgical resections in lung cancer. *J Thorac Cardiovasc Surg*. 1983;86:654.
9. Keagy BA, Lores ME, Starek PJ, et al. Elective pulmonary lobectomy: factors associated with morbidity and operative mortality. *Ann Thorac Surg*. 1985;40:349.
   Three fairly large surveys detailing the risks inherent in pulmonary resection are described in references 7 to 9.
10. Peterffy A, Henze A. Hemorrhagic complications during pulmonary resection: a retrospective review of 1428 resections with 113 haemorrhagic episodes. *Scand J Thorac Cardiovasc Surg*. 1983;17:283.
    Most bleeding complications were associated with a failure in technique. The authors conclude that a purse-string suture is safer than a transfixion suture-ligature for control of major vessels.
11. Issa MM, Healy DM, Maghur HA, et al. Prophylactic minitracheotomy in lung resections: a randomized controlled study. *J Thorac Cardiovasc Surg*. 1991;101:895.
    Minitracheotomy provides a low-risk advantage when used in patients with marginal pulmonary reserve, excessive secretions, and ineffective cough. Routine use is not warranted.
12. Asamura H, Naruke T, Tsuchiya R, et al. Bronchopleural fistulas associated with lung cancer operations: univariate and multivariate analysis of risk factors, management, and outcome. *J Thorac Cardiovasc Surg*. 1992;104:1456.
13. Ginsberg RJ, Pearson FG, Cooper JD, et al. Closure of chronic postpneumonectomy bronchopleural fistula using the transsternal transpericardial approach. *Ann Thorac Surg*. 1989;47:231.
14. Pairolero PC, Arnold PG, Trastek VF, et al. Postpneumonectomy empyema: the role of intrathoracic muscle transposition. *J Thorac Cardiovasc Surg*. 1990;99:958.
    The management of postresectional empyema and bronchopleural fistula is a challenging and often futile endeavor. The preceding three articles provide a concise perspective. Fistula occurrence in the patient at high risk may be reduced by prophylactic muscle transposition. The latter two papers describe complementary approaches to reduce the postpneumonectomy space and control the fistula.
15. Larsson S, Lepore V, Dernevik L, et al. Torsion of a lung lobe: diagnosis and treatment. *J Thorac Cardiovasc Surg*. 1988;36:281.
    Early recognition and reoperation are essential in managing this preventable complication.
16. Grillo HC, Shepard JA, Mathisen DJ, et al. Postpneumonectomy syndrome: diagnosis, management, and results. *Ann Thorac Surg*. 1992;54:638, 650.
    The best single reference for management of this rare, delayed complication.

17. PetersRM, Toledo J, eds. *Current Topics in General Thoracic Surgery. Volume 2: Perioperative Care.* New York: Elsevier; 1992.
18. WaldhausenJA; Orringer MB, eds. *Complications in Cardiothoracic Surgery.* St. Louis: Mosby-Year Book; 1991.

Comprehensive and timely discussions of each of the topics discussed in this brief chapter. Essential resources for anyone managing patients with thoracic disease.

18. KEY PULMONARY SYMPTOMS: COUGH AND DYSPNEA

Thomas E. Lawrie and Michael S. Stulbarg

Cough and dyspnea are the key symptoms of pulmonary disease. Virtually all conditions involving the respiratory system can present with dyspnea, whereas cough occurs in a more limited spectrum. Understanding these symptoms is important for appropriate evaluation and management. In general, the diagnosis of dyspnea is easier than the diagnosis of cough.

Cough usually results from reflex stimulation by mucus, foreign material, stretch, or inflammation of irritant neuroreceptors located in the vocal cords, trachea, and airways. Similar receptors are present in the ear canal, nose, sinuses, pericardium, diaphragm, esophagus, and stomach, but their role is less clear. Afferent impulses travel to the brain by the trigeminal, glossopharyngeal, superior laryngeal, and vagus nerves; efferent signals are then transmitted to the glottis, intercostals, and abdominal muscles, culminating in (1) inspiration; (2) glottic closure; (3) diaphragmatic relaxation; and (4) active contraction of the expiratory muscles (intrapleural pressure usually rises to 100 to 200 mmHg). When the glottis opens suddenly, the large transpulmonary pressure gradient between the pleura and the airway results in explosive release of intrathoracic air (i.e., a cough). Expiratory volume is no greater than during a forced exhalation, but narrowing of the airway caused by the pressure gradient leads to a high linear velocity (close to the speed of sound) which is generally effective in dislodging mucus and foreign materials. Patients with airway obstruction produce normal intrathoracic pressures but generate lower linear velocities and a less effective cough because of airway narrowing.

Occasional cough caused by minor irritations (e.g., aspiration of oral secretions) is normal. Cough accompanying upper or lower viral respiratory tract infections may continue for 6 to 8 weeks; beyond that time, further evaluation may be warranted. Chronic cough is a nonspecific symptom of a heterogeneous group of diseases that can (1) alter mucus quantity or quality (e.g., chronic bronchitis, parenchymal infection, some tumors); (2) increase sensitivity of cough receptors (e.g., asthma, cigarette smoking); (3) inadequately protect against acid stimulation of the esophageal mucosa (e.g., esophageal reflux) or cause actual aspiration of food or oral secretions (e.g., gastric reflux, neurologic dysfunction); (4) stimulate cough receptors directly (e.g., foreign body, tumor, thyroiditis, or thyromegaly) or indirectly (e.g., interstitial lung disease, pulmonary edema); or (5) affect psychological health. Cough can cause severe complications, including sleep disruption, rib fractures, emesis, stress incontinence, syncope, and social isolation.

Dyspnea is the clinical term for the discomfort associated with effort in breathing (e.g., bronchospasm) or the urge to breathe (e.g., hypoxemia, hypercapnia). It is a visceral sensation somewhat analogous to hunger or nausea and results from neural activity within the part of the cerebral cortex responsible for sensory perception. Dyspnea arises from stimuli that have different neurophysiologic pathways (e.g., exercise, breathholding, hypoxemia), but all have in common stimulation of the respiratory center. The greater the respiratory center stimulation (e.g., with hypoxia plus acidosis, pulmonary hypertension, pulmonary infiltrates), the greater the dyspnea. At the same time, anything that weakens respiratory muscles (e.g., thyrotoxicosis, myopathy) or puts them at mechanical disadvantage (e.g., hyperinflation, pleural effusion) will increase dyspnea. Other factors can affect the perception of dyspnea (e.g., belief about its significance, emotional state, airway inflammation, distraction). Dyspnea can be considered part of the warning system for humans to know when they are at risk of receiving inadequate ventilation. Dyspnea may be normal (e.g., with exercise), but patients with a variety of diseases experience it at lower than normal levels of physical activity.

The cause of cough or dyspnea is often apparent after a careful history, physical examination, and chest radiograph. Some data from the history are key (e.g., smoking history or occupational exposures), whereas others (e.g., timing, frequency, aggravating factors, and presence of sputum) have been shown not to be as helpful as previously thought. However, information about prior or current responses to empiric treatment (e.g., antibiotics, corticosteroids) can be especially helpful. Cough that follows an upper respiratory illness may be considered normal for up to 2 months and is probably caused by transient bronchial hyperreactivity or injury to airway receptors. Hyperreactivity persisting beyond 2 months may indicate asthma. Symptoms caused by occult asthma can be triggered by nonspecific irritants, such as cold air, fumes, or smoke, as well as by specific allergens. Nocturnal cough or dyspnea is frequently caused by asthma, esophageal reflux, or congestive heart failure. A personal or family history of allergies increases the probability that unexplained symptoms may be caused by asthma. Although chronic cough occurs in up to 75% of cigarette smokers, a changing pattern of cough or sputum production in this population should prompt evaluation for occult malignancy. Some patients cannot distinguish true *chest cough* from *throat clearing*. Frequent throat clearing, rhinorrhea, sinus congestion, or a feeling of drainage in the back of the throat suggests a diagnosis of postnasal drip or sinusitis. Cough caused by chronic bronchitis may be indistinguishable from that of bronchiectasis, although classically the latter is associated with more sputum production. Bronchiectasis can be quiescent for years until reactivated by a viral infection. Bronchiectasis may become evident in midlife because of chronic infection by *Mycobacterium avium* complex, particularly in women. Cough associated with blood-streaked sputum requires consideration of endobronchial malignancy, although it is usually caused by airway infection. Dyspnea from chronic lung or heart disease usually increases with exertion and improves with rest. Obesity increases ventilatory demands and, therefore, dyspnea for any activity. Cachexia of any cause can weaken respiratory muscles and increase dyspnea. Dyspnea or cough independent of activity or exposure should raise the possibility of psychogenic causation.

A thorough physical examination can provide clues to the etiology of cough and dyspnea. The patient's appearance may suggest a diagnosis (e.g., obesity, cachexia, central cyanosis, and use of accessory muscles). A nasal quality to the voice may suggest sinus disease. Hoarseness or inspiratory stridor suggests laryngotracheal disease. The sound of the cough can be helpful: (1) a *musical* cough suggests asthma, (2) a *wet* cough suggests airway infection, and (3) a *brassy* cough suggests tracheal narrowing. Upper airway examination should include a search for (1) hairs or impacted cerumen impinging on the tympanic membrane; (2) nasal secretions, bogginess, or polyps (rhinitis); (3) oropharyngeal cobblestoning or mucopurulent secretions (postnasal drip); and (4) tenderness over the maxillary sinuses (sinusitis). Examination of the neck may reveal unexpected masses or an enlarged thyroid pressing on the trachea. Auscultation may reveal wheezing, rhonchi, or rales, which are suggestive of chronic obstructive pulmonary disease, interstitial lung disease, or heart failure. Unilateral wheezing on forced inspiration or expiration may be caused by a partially obstructing endobronchial lesion (e.g., tumor, foreign body, mucus plug). A negative chest examination does not exclude primary lung disease. Signs of occult cardiac disease include jugular venous distention, gallops, and murmurs.

Diagnosis of either cough or dyspnea often requires supplemental laboratory and radiologic tests. The persistence and severity of the symptom will determine the extent of testing needed. Simple laboratory screening may uncover anemia, renal failure, or eosinophilia, each of which will lead to a different diagnostic pathway. Elevation of the sedimentation rate is nonspecific but may lead to a diagnosis of collagen vascular disease (e.g., giant cell arteritis), malignancy, or chronic infection (e.g., sinusitis).

The pulmonary function laboratory can be very useful in making a diagnosis. Spirometry can reveal airflow limitation or a reduction in vital capacity. More complete pulmonary function tests with measurement of lung volumes and diffusing capacity may suggest restrictive or pulmonary vascular diseases. Bronchoprovocation testing with histamine or methacholine can uncover occult asthma, but such testing should not be performed within 2 months of a viral syndrome because hyperreactivity is considered a normal consequence during that period. Cardiopulmonary exercise testing with measurements of arterial blood and expired gases may uncover exercise-induced hypoxemia, cardiac ischemia or arrhythmias, and ventilatory limitations to exercise.

Imaging studies beyond the chest radiograph may also be important. Sinus computed tomography (CT) scans are far more sensitive than sinus x-ray studies for the diagnosis of sinusitis, which can be found even in the absence of signs or symptoms. CT scanning of the chest is useful for the diagnosis of occult tumors, infiltrates, or adenopathy. High-resolution chest CT scanning has become the standard radiologic means of identifying occult emphysema, bronchiectasis, interstitial lung disease (including infection), and even pulmonary emboli. High resolution CT has essentially replaced gallium scanning in the search for occult parenchymal lung disease (e.g., pneumocystosis). The diagnosis of esophageal reflux can be elusive and requires esophagoscopy with biopsy or overnight pH monitoring, the latter of which has proven to be both highly sensitive and highly specific. Occult heart failure can present with dyspnea, cough, or both; diagnosis may require evaluation of ventricular function with echocardiography or even cardiac catheterization. Ultimately, bronchoscopy should be performed to exclude an endobronchial process (e.g., tumor, foreign body, broncholith, and stenosis) in any patient with a persistent cough. Bronchoscopy or ear, nose, and throat evaluation may reveal paradoxical vocal cord motion, which usually is not recognized unless it is included in the differential diagnosis. The diagnosis of psychogenic cough or dyspnea is one of exclusion and should only be considered when a clear impact on emotional status of the symptom is seen or after all other diagnoses have been excluded. A small group of patients with chronic cough or dyspnea cannot be diagnosed. In such patients, reassurance and surveillance for development of disease are important.

The treatment of cough or dyspnea is most effective when directed to a specific condition, but clinicians often prescribe empiric therapy first before subjecting a patient to an expensive and complex diagnostic algorithm. The severity and persistence of symptoms will determine when a more aggressive workup is warranted. A trial of antihistamine-decongestants, bronchodilators, inhaled corticosteroids, antireflux therapy, or other medications may be appropriate for both diagnosis and treatment, and specific algorithms have been proposed. Antihistamines and decongestants can be helpful, especially in the patient with chronic rhinorrhea or nasal stuffiness, but vasoconstrictor solutions should be avoided as they can lead to rebound rhinitis. Topical nasal steroids are sometimes effective in the treatment of postnasal drip (chronic rhinitis or sinusitis), even in the absence of a history of allergy or of laboratory evidence of eosinophilia. Oral leukotriene antagonists and nasal or inhaled cromolyn or nedocromil may be helpful, particularly if allergy is playing a role. Oral antibiotics are indicated if cough is associated with purulent sputum; prolonged or cyclic treatment may be necessary for sinusitis or bronchiectasis. Empiric trials of oral corticosteroids are often given because of the severity of the symptom. When a clear-cut clinical response occurs, it is not unreasonable to continue therapy, but the dosage should be reduced as much as possible. Partial response should lead to the search for multiple causes, which may need to be treated in a stepwise manner to achieve an adequate clinical response.

Nonspecific recommendations for cough treatment include hydration, steam inhalation, expectorants (e.g., guaifenesin), lozenges, and mucolytic drugs, but their benefits have not been scientifically established. Attempts at cough suppression with dextromethorphan or opiates (e.g., codeine) are not dangerous as long as side effects (e.g., sedation, constipation) are considered and a search for the underlying cause continues. In the occasional patient with persistent cough, oral benzonatate perles or nebulized lidocaine (e.g., 5 mL of 4% solution) sometimes provides substantial relief. As diagnosis of dyspnea is generally easier than diagnosis of persistent cough, non-specific recommendations are required less frequently. Strategies for dyspnea control can include supplemental oxygen, education (e.g., optimal use of medications, avoidance of triggers), distraction, social support, breathing control techniques (e.g., pursed lips breathing), or an exercise program. Education and exercise are generally best administered within a comprehensive pulmonary rehabilitation program, if available. Such programs have been shown to produce significant improvements in dyspnea and exercise tolerance in patients with chronic lung diseases.

Because intractable cough or dyspnea can be debilitating, narcotics should be used compassionately, as for severe pain, with appropriate attention to tachyphylaxis, dependence, and side effects.

Cough

1. Buist AS, Sexton GJ, Nagy JM, et al. The effect of smoking cessation and modification on lung function. *Am Rev Respir Dis*. 1976;114:115.

   Evidence that even after many years of smoking, cessation of smoking will dramatically reduce cough and sputum production.

2. Corrao WM, Braman SS, Irwin RS. Chronic cough as the sole presenting manifestation of bronchial asthma. *N Engl J Med*. 1979;300:633.

   Classic description of the cough variant of asthma, established by demonstration of bronchial hyperreactivity and response to bronchodilators in the absence of the usual stigmata of asthma (e.g., wheezing, airflow limitation).

3. Irwin RS, Curley FJ, French CL. Chronic cough. The spectrum and frequency of causes, key components of the diagnostic evaluation, and outcome of specific therapy. *Am Rev Respir Dis*. 1990;141:640.

   The classic and enthusiastic presentation of the anatomic diagnostic protocol made famous by the lead author. A specific cause of cough was determined in 101 of 102 patients: one cause in 73%, two in 23%, and three in 3%. Postnasal drip syndrome was a cause 41% of the time, asthma 24%, gastroesophageal reflux 21%, chronic bronchitis 5%, and bronchiectasis 4%. Cough was often the sole presenting manifestation of asthma (28%) and reflux (43%). Of note, methacholine challenge was falsely positive 22% of the time, although our experience has not been as encouraging.

4. Sen RP, Walsh TE. Fiberoptic bronchoscopy for refractory cough. *Chest*. 1991; 99:33.

   Bronchoscopy provided a diagnosis in seven of 25 patients with chronic unexplained cough.

5. Weiss W, Seidman H, Boucot KR. The Philadelphia Pulmonary Neoplasm Research Project. Symptoms in occult lung cancer. *Chest*. 1978;73:57.

   Symptoms are seldom useful in the detection of lung cancer, but the appearance of changing expectoration and chronic cough in older male smokers should raise a suspicion of the disease.

6. Brightling CE, Ward R, Goh KL, et al. Eosinophilic bronchitis is an important cause of chronic cough. *Am J Respir Crit Care Med*. 1999;160:406.

   Eosinophilic bronchitis is an important, recently recognized cause of cough. It presents with chronic cough and sputum eosinophilia (>3%) without abnormal spirometry or bronchial hyperreactivity and responds to inhaled corticosteroids. In this study, eosinophilic bronchitis was the final diagnosis in 12 of 91 patients referred for unexplained cough. After treatment with inhaled budesonide (400 mcg twice daily), cough improved and sputum eosinophilia fell from 16.8 to 1.6%.

7. Luque CA, Vazquez Ortiz M. Treatment of ACE inhibitor-induced cough. *Pharmacotherapy*. 1999;19:804.

Angiotensin-converting enzyme (ACE) inhibitors continue to be important drugs for cardiovascular disease. This article reviews options when the drugs cannot be discontinued safely.

8. Palombini BC, Villanova CA, Araujo E, et al. A pathogenic triad in chronic cough: asthma, postnasal drip syndrome, and gastroesophageal reflux disease. *Chest.* 1999;116:279.

   Yet another group finds that some combination of asthma, gastroesophageal reflux, and postnasal drip explains most (i.e., here 93.6%) chronic coughs and suggests that this be known as the pathogenic triad for chronic cough.

9. Tam TW, Bentsi-Enchill A. The return of the 100-day cough: resurgence of pertussis in the 1990s. *Can Med Assoc J.* 1998;159:695.

10. Birkebaek NH, Kristiansen M, Seefeldt T, et al. *Bordetella pertussis* infection and chronic cough in adults. *Clin Infect Dis.* 1999;29:1239.

    Several recent articles, including these, have emphasized that approximately 20% of patients with persistent cough have culture or serologic evidence of B. pertussis infection. These infections usually respond to macrolide therapy.

11. Irwin RS. The diagnosis and treatment of cough. *N Engl J Med.* 2000;343:1715.

12. Irwin RS, Madison JM. The persistently troublesome cough. *Am J Resp Crit Care Med.* 2002;165:1469.

    Two excellent articles that are highly recommended reading. The first is a comprehensive approach to acute and chronic cough, with an algorithm for diagnosis and treatment. The second emphasizes a novel approach to the patient with chronic cough, particularly the one in whom a diagnostic and therapeutic workup has been unrevealing.

13. Irwin RS, Boulet LP, Cloutier MM, et al. Managing cough as a defense mechanism and as a symptom. A consensus panel report of the American College of Chest Physicians. *Chest.* 1998;114:133S–181S.

    Consensus panel report on the diagnosis and treatment of cough. Highly recommended.

14. Allen CJ, Anvari M. Preoperative symptom evaluation and esophageal acid infusion predict response to laparoscopic Nissen fundoplication in gastroesophageal reflux patients who present with cough. *Surg Endosc.* 2002;16:1037.

    This is one of numerous articles emphasizing the high correlation between esophageal reflux and cough. This study emphasizes that fundoplication can be dramatically helpful in people who have failed proton pump therapy, particularly if these patients experienced no change in cough symptoms with these agents. Additionally, a positive result on esophageal infusion of acid was strongly predictive of a greater improvement in cough after surgery.

15. Pratter MR, Bartter T, Akers S, et al. An algorithmic approach to chronic cough. *Ann Intern Med.* 1993;119:977.

    An excellent article outlining an algorithmic approach to cough, initially using antihistamine-decongestant combination therapy, which was beneficial in 39 of 45 patients and the only treatment needed in 16. Methacholine challenge had a negative predictive value of 100% and a positive predictive value of 74% for cough caused by asthma. Recurrence of cough at 3 months was common (18%).

16. Trochtenberg S. Nebulized lidocaine in the treatment of refractory cough [see comments]. *Chest.* 1994;105:1592.

    Convincing case report of prolonged treatment of refractory cough with nebulized lidocaine. Mild dysphonia was the only side effect.

Dyspnea

17. Zeppetella G. The palliation of dyspnea in terminal disease. *Am J Hosp Palliat Care.* 1998;15:322.

18. Markowitz AJ, Rabow M. Management of dyspnea in patients with far-advanced lung disease. *J Am Med Assn.* 2002;287:2261.

    Two excellent reviews of dyspnea management in the terminally ill.

19. National Emphysema Treatment Trial Research Group. A randomized trial comparing lung-volume-reduction surgery with medical therapy for severe emphysema. *N Engl J Med.* 2003;348:2059.

A large multicenter study funded by Medicare and the National Institutes of Health demonstrating that in select patients with severe emphysema, LVRS can significantly improve survival and quality of life.

20. Mahler D. Dyspnea. In: Lenfant C, ed. *Lung Biology in Health and Disease*. Vol. 111. New York, NY: Marcel Dekker; 1998.

    An excellent monograph on dyspnea. Well worthwhile for those seriously interested in the symptom.

21. Poole PJ, Veale AG, Black PN. The effect of sustained-release morphine on breathlessness and quality of life in severe chronic obstructive pulmonary disease. *Am J Respir Crit Care Med*. 1998;157:1877.

    Disappointing results from a trial of oral morphine for dyspnea in patients with severe dyspnea. Doses were high enough to cause side effects; thus, inadequate dosing was not the cause of lack of benefit. This does not exclude the appropriateness of morphine for treatment of dyspnea in the terminally ill.

22. Foral PA, Malesker MA, Huerta G, et al. Nebulized opioids use in COPD. *Chest*. 2004;125:691.

    A literature review evaluating the role of nebulized narcotics for dyspnea relief. Besides one study that demonstrated efficacious use in terminal patients, the authors found no solid evidence from placebo-controlled studies that this therapy was beneficial in COPD.

23. Ferrari K, Goti P, Misuri G, et al. Chronic exertional dyspnea and respiratory muscle function in patients with chronic obstructive pulmonary disease. *Lung*. 1997;175:311.

    Demonstrates that the level of chronic exertional dyspnea in chronic obstructive pulmonary disease increases as the ventilatory muscle derangement increases. Unfortunately, therapeutic interventions to improve ventilatory muscle function are limited.

24. O'Donnell DE, Bain DJ, Webb KA. Factors contributing to relief of exertional breathlessness during hyperoxia in chronic airflow limitation. *Am J Respir Crit Care Med*. 1997;155:530.

    Evidence is provided that oxygen relieves dyspnea in chronic obstructive pulmonary disease, by reducing both ventilatory demand and blood lactate.

25. Ries AL, Kaplan RM, Myers R, et al. Maintenance therapy after pulmonary rehabilitation in chronic lung disease: a randomized trial. *Am J Respir Crit Care Med*. 2003;167:880.

    A randomized trial demonstrating that the beneficial effects of pulmonary rehabilitation in reducing dyspnea and improving quality of life may be enhanced with intensive maintenance therapy up to 1 year after such programs. However, the benefits of such an intervention were not significantly different from those enjoyed by the control group at 2 years of follow-up. Nonetheless, pulmonary rehabilitation is considered a standard of care in treating patients with advanced lung disease.

26. Lynch DA. High-resolution CT of idiopathic interstitial pneumonias. *Radiol Clin North Am*. 2001;29:1153.

    Excellent review of the utility of high-resolution CT (HRCT) in interstitial lung disease, along with descriptions of typical findings.

27. Mahler DA, Franco MJ. Clinical applications of cardiopulmonary exercise testing. *J Cardiopulm Rehabil*. 1996;16:357.

    Nice review of the utility of cardiopulmonary exercise testing in the workup of dyspnea.

28. Carrieri-Kohlman V, Gormley JM, Douglas MK, et al. Exercise training decreases dyspnea and the distress and anxiety associated with it. Monitoring alone may be as effective as coaching. *Chest*. 1996;110:1526.

    Evidence that exercise training alone is a powerful treatment for dyspnea.

29. Dyspnea. Mechanisms, assessment, and management: a consensus statement. *Am J Respir Crit Care Med*. 1999;159:321.

    The best review article available on the subject of dyspnea per se. This consensus statement presents a physiologic approach to understanding the mechanisms of the symptom and a physiologic approach to its treatment.

19. THE LUNG IN PREGNANCY

Ann M. Romaker

Pregnancy is characterized by a series of dynamic physiologic changes that can have an impact on multiple organ system functions. It is associated with a variety of changes in pulmonary anatomy and physiology and, by itself, predisposes to several pulmonary disorders.

The anatomic alterations of pregnancy include increases in (1) the level of the diaphragm (3 to 4 cm); (2) the transverse diameter of the chest (2 cm); and (3) the subcostal angle (68 to 103°). These changes take place earlier than can be accounted for by the enlarging uterus. Additionally, capillary engorgement throughout the respiratory tract results in mucosal edema and hyperemia. Multiple biochemical alterations occur concomitantly; progesterone, estrogen, prostaglandin, corticosteroid, and cyclic nucleotide levels rise during the course of pregnancy. The multiple functional consequences of these alterations are not clear, but the increased progesterone is thought to be responsible for the hyperventilation observed during pregnancy. The absolute rise in free cortisol (two to three times baseline levels) can modify the course of some steroid-responsive respiratory diseases.

Pulmonary function tests reveal multiple deviations from the nonpregnant state. Lung volumes are altered: functional residual capacity (FRC) diminishes by 10 to 25% because of diaphragmatic elevation, which in turn is associated with an 8 to 40% fall in expiratory reserve volume and a 7 to 22% fall in residual volume. Vital capacity and total lung capacity are preserved, although at term a slight drop occurs in total lung capacity. Because the motion of the diaphragm and the inspiratory muscles is preserved, inspiratory capacity actually increases about 10% and tidal volume increases about 28%. Changes in flow rates have not been observed, although airways resistance appears to fall. In general, closing volume remains unchanged (individual variations are reported). A normal closing volume coupled with a low FRC may result in airway closure near or above FRC.

During pregnancy, minute ventilation rises significantly; this rise is accomplished mainly by an increase in tidal volume. Consequently, the resting carbon dioxide in alveolar gas ($Paco_2$) drops to 27 to 32 mmHg. The pH is usually maintained by an increased renal excretion of bicarbonate, with a fall in serum bicarbonate to 18 to 21 mEq/L. The decline in $Paco_2$ leads to a rise in partial pressure of oxygen in arterial blood (Pao_2). The alveolar to arterial oxygen gradient also rises, possibly related to airway closure at or near FRC.

Pregnancy also results in an increased value of the respiratory quotient, possibly related to an increased utilization of carbohydrate and an increased resting oxygen consumption paralleling an increase in body weight. No differences have been noted in the response to mild to moderate exercise in the pregnant versus the nonpregnant state. During sleep, no significant difference in arterial oxygen saturation is seen in pregnancy. Apneas and hypopneas, however, may appear or worsen in obese women during their pregnancies.

Approximately 60 to 70% of women complain of dyspnea during pregnancy, generally in the first or second trimester. Dyspnea usually improves near term, suggesting that mechanical factors are not responsible. Dyspnea appears to be related to the increased minute ventilation.

Pregnant women suffer from respiratory diseases more than their age-matched, nonpregnant counterparts. An increased mortality is associated with influenza and varicella infections and an increase in primary varicella pneumonias. Pregnant women do not have a higher risk for bacterial pneumonia than nonpregnant women. It should be stressed that pregnancy is not a contraindication to chest radiography if it is clinically indicated. Radiation exposure sustained during a standard chest film is 50 mrad to the chest and 0.0025 to 0.005 cGy to the gonads. The minimal dose related to adverse effects on the fetus is considered to be 0.01 to 0.05 Gy. Nevertheless, appropriate lead shielding should be provided.

Pregnancy exerts little effect on the natural history of tuberculosis. The indications for treatment and recommended primary drug regimens are unchanged. Although isoniazid and rifampin cross the placenta, extensive experience indicates that these agents are not teratogenic. In addition, adverse effects have not been demonstrated with ethambutol. Both streptomycin and ethionamide, however, have been associated with fetal abnormalities.

The course of asthma during pregnancy is unpredictable. If severe disease antedates pregnancy and the expected fall in immunoglobulin E concentrations during pregnancy do not occur, clinical deterioration can develop. In a review of 1,059 pregnancies, Turner et al. found 49% experienced no change in their disease during pregnancy, 29% improved, and 22% worsened. In general, the care of the pregnant patient does not differ from that of nonpregnant asthmatics. Extensive experience with methylxanthines and beta-agonist bronchodilators, as well as corticosteroids, has not demonstrated adverse outcomes during pregnancy. Data suggest that untreated asthma has a more deleterious effect on the outcome of pregnancy than the judicious use of these drugs.

Several reports have documented an improved or unchanged pulmonary status during pregnancy among women with sarcoidosis. In general, the chest radiograph remains normal throughout pregnancy if the disease had cleared before conception; if it was resolving before pregnancy, improvement continues. Patients with inactive interstitial fibrotic disease remain stable during pregnancy. Those with active interstitial inflammatory disease often manifest partial or even complete clearing on their chest radiograph films. Unfortunately, most of these patients subsequently experience an exacerbation of their disease within 3 to 6 months postpartum.

Several other lung conditions are associated with pregnancy. Rib fractures can occur during the last trimester. These fractures are most often preceded by a chronic cough and are the result of mechanical factors related to an increasing abdominal volume. The lower ribs are pushed upward into a more horizontal position by the abdomen and pulled out by the intercostal and oblique muscles, thereby exerting a great force in the opposite direction. An asynchronous pull caused by an acute burst of coughing probably results in the so-called *cough fracture*. The differential diagnosis of thoracic pain also should include pulmonary embolism, pneumothorax, and acute intervertebral disk disease.

The risk of thromboembolic disease appears to be primarily associated with the postpartum period rather than with pregnancy. Several large studies have reported a pregnancy-related incidence of deep venous thrombosis of 1.2% and of pulmonary embolism of 0.2 to 0.4%. Despite its infrequency, pulmonary embolism is second only to abortion as a cause of maternal death. Doppler ultrasonography and impedance plethysmography are most helpful in the first and second trimesters. However, an accurate diagnosis is important, given the potentially disastrous consequences of a missed diagnosis and because of the difficulties associated with therapy.

The diagnosis of deep venous thrombosis is difficult to make in pregnant women; tests can pose significant risk to the fetus (venography, radiolabeled fibrinogen) or fail to detect thrombosis in pelvic veins. D-dimer levels may be helpful diagnostic aids, although they can rise up to 50% during the last trimester. Warfarin (Coumadin) crosses the placenta, producing both fetal hemorrhage and congenital abnormalities. Heparin can be safely used up to and immediately after labor, because it does not cross the placenta. However, the risk of excessive bleeding remains a consideration. Although the efficacy of low-molecular-weight heparin during pregnancy has not been established, its use is widespread. Careful monitoring of factor Xa levels is required. Estimates of radiation exposure to the fetus for the various procedures available to diagnose deep venous thrombosis and pulmonary embolism are listed in Table 19-1.

Amniotic fluid embolism, which is peculiar to pregnancy, accounts for 4 to 10% of total maternal mortality. Because this condition carries a mortality risk higher than 80%, it demands prompt recognition. Death is often immediate, or it can occur within several hours of labor and delivery. Clinical features include respiratory distress syndrome, cardiovascular collapse, and disseminated intravascular coagulation.

Table 19-1. Estimates of amount of radiation absorbed by the fetus for different procedures

Procedure	Estimated fetal radiation (cGy)
Bilateral venography without abdominal shield	0.628
Unilateral venography without abdominal shield	0.314
Limited venography, abdomen shielded	<0.050
Pulmonary angiography via femoral route	0.405
Pulmonary angiography via brachial route	<0.050
Perfusion lung scan using ^{99m}Tc MAA	
3 mCi	0.018
1–2 mCi	0.006–0.012
Ventilation lung scan	
Using ^{133}Xe	0.004–0.019
Using ^{99m}Tc DTPA	0.007–0.035
Using ^{99m}Tc SC	0.001–0.005
Radioisotope venography	0.205
Radioactive fibrinogen uptake scanning	2.000
Chest radiography	<0.001

Adapted from Ginsberg JS, Hirsh J, Rainbow AJ, Coates G. Risks to the fetus of radiologic procedures used in the diagnosis of maternal venous thromboembolic disease. *Thromb Haemost.* 1989;61:189.

Predisposing factors include a tumultuous labor, the use of intrauterine stimulants, the presence of meconium in the amniotic fluid, advanced maternal age, multiparity, and intrauterine fetal death. Treatment is supportive, as no specific therapy yet exists.

The effects of scuba diving on pregnancy are unclear. As this sport increases in popularity, more and more physicians are consulted regarding its suitability for the pregnant woman (e.g., How dangerous is decompression sickness? What are the effects of the decompression chamber on the fetus and mother?). In a study of pregnant ewes, bubbles in the placenta were demonstrated at depths greater than 60 feet. In a more relevant but retrospective study of 208 female divers, no increased risk of abortion or fetal abnormalities was noted. It is currently suggested that women of child-bearing age limit their dive to 60 feet and to a duration of one half the limits of the US Navy decompression tables. Additionally, they should avoid strenuous dives, hypoventilation, and chilling.

Premature labor occurs in approximately 7 to 10% of deliveries. Systemic tocolysis of these patients has produced dramatic improvements in fetal survival but also has resulted in sometimes life-threatening maternal complications. Noncardiogenic pulmonary edema has been reported with most tocolytic agents, including magnesium sulfate, terbutaline, and ritodrine. The incidence is low, approximately 3%, and appears to be higher in the presence of coexisting maternal infection. Other risk factors include multiple gestations, hydramnios, hypertension, and the use of glucocorticoid steroids. Treatment involves cessation of tocolytic therapy, antibiotics, if clinically indicated, and aggressive support.

1. Alaily AB, Carroll KB. Pulmonary ventilation in pregnancy. *Br J Obstet Gynaecol.* 1978;85:518.

   A well-done study comparing pulmonary function testing results during pregnancy and postpartum.
2. Anonymous. Guidelines for diagnostic imaging during pregnancy. The American College of Obstetricians and Gynecologists. *Int J Gynaecol Obstet.* 1995; Dec;51:288–291.

3. Gee JB, Packer BS, Millen JE, et al. Pulmonary mechanics during pregnancy. *J Clin Invest.* 1967;46:945.
   An excellent study of compliance and resistance.
4. Brownell LG, West P, Kryger MH. Breathing during sleep in normal pregnant women. *Am Rev Respir Dis.* 1986;133:38.
   The only such investigation.
5. Clark SL. Amniotic fluid embolism. *Crit Care Obstet.* 1986;13:801.
   A concise review.
6. Esplin MS, Clark SL. Outpatient management of asthma during pregnancy. *Clin Obstet Gynecol.* 1998;3:555.
   A well-written review of the effects of asthma, on both mother and child, with treatment recommendations.
7. Even-Tov I, Yedwab GA, Persitz E, et al. Stress fractures of ribs in late pregnancy. *Int Surg.* 1979;64:86.
   An interesting and unusual problem succinctly presented.
8. Cugell DW, Frank NR, Gaensler EA, et al. Pulmonary function in pregnancy. I. Serial observations in normal women. *Am Rev Tuberc.* 1953;67:568.
9. Gaensler EA, Patton WE, Verstraeten JM, et al. Pulmonary function in pregnancy. III. Serial observations in patients with pulmonary insufficiency. *Am Rev Tuberc.* 1953;67:779.
   References 7 and 8 are classic studies.
10. Ginsberg JS, Hirsch J. Use of anticoagulants during pregnancy. *Chest.* 1989; 95:1575.
    These authors review all the available literature to make their recommendations.
11. Ginsberg JS, Hirsh J, Rainbow AJ, et al. Risks to the fetus of radiologic procedures used in the diagnosis of maternal venous thromboembolic disease. *Thromb Haemost.* 1989;61:189.
    An in-depth review of the risks to the fetus of various diagnostic procedures.
12. Hatjis CG, Swain M. Systemic tocolysis for premature labor is associated with an increased incidence of pulmonary edema in the presence of maternal infection. *Am J Obstet Gynecol.* 1988;159:723.
    A well-done study of predisposing factors.
13. Jacobs RF, Abernathy RS. Management of tuberculosis in pregnancy and the newborn. *Clin Perinatol.* 1988;15:305.
    Includes a discussion of tuberculosis mastitis and the evaluation and treatment of the neonate.
14. Knuttgen HG, Emerson K. Physiologic response to pregnancy at rest and during exercise. *J Appl Physiol.* 1974;36:549.
    An elegant study scrutinizing pulmonary function at rest and during both weight-bearing and non–weight-bearing exercise.
15. Mitler JM, ed. Pulmonary diseases in pregnancy. *Clin Obstet Gynecol.* 1996;39:3.
    A collection of articles reviewing common pulmonary problems in pregnancy.
16. Niederman MS. *Clinics in Chest Medicine.* Philadelphia, Pa: Saunders; 1992.
    A thorough compilation of the pathophysiology of pregnancy and its pulmonary consequences.
17. Newhall JF Jr. Scuba diving during pregnancy: a brief review. *Am J Obstet Gynecol.* 1981;140:893.
    Very little work is available on the subject, but this brief article is state of the art.
18. Snider D. Pregnancy and tuberculosis. *Chest.* 1984;86:10S.
    Current American Thoracic Society recommendations.
19. Weinberger SE, Weiss ST, Cohen WR, et al. Pregnancy and the lung. *Am Rev Respir Dis.* 1980;121:559.
    An outstanding state-of-the-art review.
20. Wolff F, Fischer JH. Aspects of the pathophysiology of maternal lung edema during tocolytic therapy. *J Perinat Med.* 1988;16:50.
    Actual Swan-Ganz data on the physiology of tocolytic therapy.

20. HYPERBARIC OXYGEN THERAPY

Paul Cianci

Hyperbaric oxygen (HBO) therapy is the intermittent administration of 100% oxygen at pressure greater than sea level. The technique can be implemented in a walk-in (multiplace) chamber, compressed to depth with air, in which the patient breathes 100% oxygen through a mask, head tent, or endotracheal tube. Alternatively, the patient can be treated in a monoplace (one-person) chamber pressurized with 100% oxygen. In either case, the arterial partial pressure of oxygen Po_2 will approach 1500 mmHg at a pressure equivalent of 33 feet of seawater.

During the 1930s, oxygen at pressure was proposed as a treatment for decompression sickness (*the bends*). In the early 1960s, Dutch investigators showed the efficacy of HBO in the treatment of gas gangrene and anemic states. Later in that decade, it became the standard therapy for US Navy diving casualties. Subsequent studies have shown the importance of oxygen in the treatment of problem wounds, enhancement of white blood cell (WBC) killing ability, preservation of compromised tissue, and angiogenesis. Some centers are using this modality in the treatment of acute thermal injury. The clinical indications for the use of HBO as an adjunct to traditional medical and surgical regimens continue to be expanded and refined.

The indications for HBO include gas embolism, carbon monoxide poisoning, crush injury, acute traumatic ischemia, decompression sickness, gas gangrene, clostridial myonecrosis, necrotizing anaerobic infections, osteomyelitis (refractory), osteoradionecrosis, hard- and soft-tissue radiation injury, compromised skin grafts and flaps, enhancement of healing in selected problem wounds, exceptional blood loss anemia, intracranial abscesses, and thermal burns. The mechanism of action of HBO relates to its ability to deliver substantial increases of oxygen to hypoxic peripheral tissue. Oxygen inhaled at pressure dissolves in plasma. At 3 atm, an arterial Po_2 of nearly 2200 may be achieved. Under these conditions, up to 6.9 volumes percent of oxygen can be forced into the plasma, a quantity sufficient to maintain life in the absence of hemoglobin. Exposure to oxygen at pressure causes a 20% reduction in blood flow, resulting in less diapedesis and bleeding in areas of capillary damage and a reduction of edema. The tenfold increase in oxygen content of plasma more than compensates for decreased arterial flow.

Tissue oxygen levels play a major role in the physiology of wound healing, WBC function, and blood flow. Abnormally low tissue Po_2 (5 to 15 mmHg) is often present in nonhealing tissue. This results in diminished WBC killing ability and decreased collagen synthesis by fibroblasts. Raising tissue oxygen tensions to 30 to 40 mmHg provides the milieu necessary to lay down a collagen matrix for support of capillary ingress into avascular or damaged areas. HBO can increase tissue oxygen tensions to levels sufficient for effective WBC killing of bacteria, fibroblast production of collagen, and stimulation of angiogenesis, possibly through increased production of vascular endothelial growth factor. Although treatments are usually 90 to 120 minutes once or twice daily, tissue O_2 levels remain above baseline values for some time after a treatment. This is especially true in ischemic tissue, which can act as an oxygen capacitance system. Of course, a necessary condition for oxygen transport using HBO is plasma flow to the area through an intact circulation.

HBO therapy is the treatment of choice for decompression sickness and arterial gas embolism caused by diving accidents or iatrogenically induced gas embolism (e.g., lung biopsy or invasive vascular procedures). Treatment in a recompression chamber is mandatory for these disorders. HBO compresses the gas bubbles, encourages counter-diffusion of bubbles, and hyperoxygenates compromised tissue.

Carbon monoxide (CO) poisoning results in noncompetitive binding of CO with hemoglobin and myoglobin and reversible binding to the cytochrome system. HBO reverses hypoxia, displaces CO from the heme proteins (hemoglobin, myoglobin, cytochrome system), prevents WBC adherence to endothelium, and reduces lipid peroxidation in the central nervous system. Candidates for therapy include those with mental aberration, cardiac ischemia, or a history of unconsciousness and coma, particularly if hypotension has been present. Treatment within 6 hours of exposure has yielded the best results. Prompt treatment reduces the long-term mental disability often associated with CO poisoning.

Gas gangrene is caused by necrotizing toxins released by pathologic clostridial organisms. Bacterial growth may be severely restricted by tissue oxygen levels of 70 mmHg; tensions of 250 mmHg halt alpha-toxin production. Organisms other than *Clostridia* also can cause necrotizing infections. These are generally synergistic combinations of bacteria with differing oxygen requirements. HBO can serve as a useful adjunct to definitive surgical and antibiotic treatment, often preventing the need for amputation or ablative surgery.

Crush injury involves severe trauma to bones, soft tissue, nerves, and vascular structures and often results in marginal oxygenation of peripheral tissue. In this setting, HBO should be initiated as soon as possible to enhance support of marginally viable tissue, leukocyte killing, and edema reduction. A reduction in surgery and improved salvage rates have been demonstrated, particularly in patients older than age 40.

In chronic refractory osteomyelitis, periodic elevation of bone O_2 levels from hypoxic to normal or above-normal levels promotes fibroblast division, collagen production, capillary angiogenesis, increased leukocyte killing, and osteoclast activity. HBO must be used as an adjunct to surgical debridement, wound care, and appropriate long-term antibiotic administration.

Radiation necrosis, soft-tissue radiation injury, and osteoradionecrosis share a common pathophysiology of obliterative endarteritis, secondary tissue ischemia, and hypoxia. Daily HBO can restore a functioning capillary bed and facilitate surgical intervention. Surgery in previously irradiated tissue is otherwise associated with a high incidence of potentially fatal complications. HBO also is indicated postoperatively to ensure adequate capillarity for healing.

Hyperbaric oxygen therapy is not usually necessary for normal skin flaps, grafts, or surgical wounds. However, it can be useful for preparing a granulating base for skin grafting where viability of a graft or flap is compromised or uncertain or when previous grafts have failed. Preoperative HBO therapy is effective in promoting capillary proliferation to prepare a site in poorly granulating wounds. In selected problem wounds (e.g., diabetic ulcers, chronic nonhealing wounds), HBO therapy can be used as an adjunct in a regimen of meticulous wound care, careful attention to nutritional status, metabolic control, and revascularization, when indicated.

Adjunctive HBO for thermal injury is controversial. Some burn centers experienced in its use have reported reductions in length of hospital stay, need for grafting, and mortality rates. HBO for this indication should be restricted to facilities associated with a burn center.

Recent data suggest that HBO may have a beneficial effect on ischemia reperfusion injury. This effect appears to be mediated by nitric oxide (NO), providing temporary but reversible blocking of the CD11/CD18 integrins and their binding with endothelial cellular adhesion molecules. High doses of oxygen appear to have a profound effect on this reaction, ameliorating many of the effects of reperfusion injury by increasing NO synthesis.

Risks involved in the use of HBO therapy are related to pressure changes and the toxic effects of oxygen. They include barotrauma to the ears or sinuses, pulmonary overpressure accidents with pneumothorax, and pulmonary toxicity. Trauma to the ears or sinuses can be averted with slow compression, the use of decongestants, and patient education. Occasionally, myringotomy is necessary. Pulmonary overpressure accidents are rare, occurring approximately once per 50,000 treatments, and can be avoided by careful pretreatment screening for pulmonary blebs, air trapping caused by bronchospasm or secretions, and preexisting pneumothorax, which may have occurred undetected after chest compression, central lines, ventilatory support, or other forms of trauma. An undetected pneumothorax at sea level can be converted to a tension pneumothorax on ascent as ambient pressure decreases. Relief requires immediate insertion of a chest tube, which will allow the hyperbaric treatment to continue if warranted.

Overdose of oxygen itself may have definite toxic effects, usually affecting the brain or lungs. Exposure to oxygen at depth can cause grand mal seizures, possibly related to interference with gamma-aminobutyric acid metabolism. Susceptibility varies widely. The risk of seizures increases as the plasma Po_2 rises. For this reason, oxygen treatments are limited to a maximum depth of 3 ATA (atmosphere absolute), or 66 feet of sea water, 20 m. Fever and certain medications can predispose to this complication, and careful attention to potential drug enhancement is mandatory. Fortunately, oxygen seizures are rare, occurring about once in every 10,000 to 12,000 treatments. They are self limited and treated by cessation of high-pressure oxygen therapy. HBO treatment can be reestablished after seizure activity has ceased, although patients who have seized should be checked for any underlying pathology.

Damage to lung tissue, manifested by a decrement in vital capacity and irritation to the large airways, is a predictable complication of oxygen exposure at depth. The mechanism is believed to be loss of surfactant and changes in the pulmonary macrophages. Because toxicity is related to the depth and duration of exposure, treatment protocols are designed to use the shallowest depth consistent with the desired results. In practice, pulmonary toxicity from currently used wound healing protocols is virtually unheard of. Additional minor side effects are a change in visual acuity that reverts to baseline within a few weeks to months after treatment. No evidence indicates that protocols presently used in the United States predispose to cataract formation.

Although not a complication of treatment, confinement anxiety can be a problem for patients being treated in hyperbaric chambers. Sedation and reassurance usually remedy the problem. However, a small percentage of patients cannot tolerate HBO treatment for this reason.

Although expensive, HBO is a cost-effective treatment for some disorders. For example, the ability to preserve a functional extremity can reduce the high cost of disability resulting from amputation. The shortened healing time for chronic wounds will reduce the cost of frequent, repeated surgical procedures. Most important, however, is the reduction in morbidity associated with acute and chronic tissue injury. Reversal of local ischemia with HBO appears to be a new and useful application of this treatment in selected cases.

1. Bennett PB, Elliott DH, eds. *The Physiology and Medicine of Diving*. 4th ed. London, England: Saunders & Company; 1993.
   A major reference textbook in the field of diving medicine.
2. *US Navy Diving Manual*. Washington, DC: Government Printing Office; 1995.
   The standard of therapy throughout the Armed Forces and a good part of the diving community.
3. Peirce EC. Cerebral gas embolism (arterial) with special reference to iatrogenic accidents. *HBO Review*. 1980;1:161.
   An excellent review of the pathophysiology and incidence of air embolism.
4. Strauss MB. Role of hyperbaric oxygen therapy in acute traumatic ischemias and crush injuries—an orthopedic perspective. *HBO Review*. 1981;2:87.
   A summary of the world's experiences, with extensive references.
5. Kindwall EP, Goldmann RW. *Hyperbaric Medicine Procedures* (rev.). Milwaukee, Wis: St. Luke's Medical Center; 1995.
   An excellent handbook guide for the use of HBO therapy; contains numerous, timely references.
6. Davis JC, Hunt TK, eds. *Hyperbaric Oxygen Therapy*. Bethesda, Md: Undersea and Hyperbaric Medical Society; 1977.
   This reference established state-of-the-art status of hyperbaric medicine in 1977 and serves as a basis for all further work.
7. Davis JC, Hunt TK, eds. *Problem Wounds—The Role of Oxygen*. New York, NY: Elsevier; 1988.

This comprehensive review of wound healing presents basic physiology on the role of oxygen in the normal sequence of wound closure and its application in the problem wound.

8. Kindwall EP, ed. *Hyperbaric Medicine Practice.* 2nd ed. Flagstaff, Ariz: Best Publishing; 1999.
   A state-of-the art reference, with heavy emphasis on physiology, basic mechanisms, and patient management; a must for the practicing hyperbarist.
9. *Hyperbaric Oxygen Therapy: A Committee Report* (rev.). Bethesda, Md: Undersea and Hyperbaric Medical Society; 2003.
   This comprehensive report explains the experimental and physiologic aspects of hyperbaric medicine, its clinical efficacy and cost effectiveness, methods for avoiding misuse of this clinical entity, and key references for all covered and investigational conditions.
10. Bakker DJ. *The Use of Hyperbaric Oxygen in the Treatment of Certain Infectious Diseases, Especially Gas Gangrene and Acute Dermal Gangrene.* Wageningen, Holland: Drukkerij Veenman BV; 1984.
    A comprehensive review of adjunctive HBO in the treatment of gas gangrene and necrotizing fasciitis. Written by an experienced surgeon.
11. Hart GB, Lamb RC, Strauss MB. Gas gangrene I, a collective review. *J Trauma.* 1983;23:991.
    The definitive review of the subject. Written by surgeons experienced in the application of HBO to this disorder.
12. Marx RE. Radiation injury to tissue. In: Kindwall EP, Whelan HT, eds. *Hyperbaric Medicine Practice.* 2nd ed. Flagstaff, Ariz: Best Publishing; 1999:665.
    State-of-the-art review of this subject by the leading expert in the field.
13. Marx RE, Johnson RP. Problem wounds in oral and maxillofacial surgery: the role of hyperbaric oxygen. In: Davis JC, Hunt TK, eds. *Problem Wounds—The Role of Oxygen.* New York, NY: Elsevier; 1988:65.
    A comprehensive review of the pathophysiology and treatment of osteoradionecrosis with HBO therapy.
14. Kindwall EP, Gottlieb LJ, Larson DL. Hyperbaric oxygen therapy in plastic surgery: a review article. *Plast Reconstr Surg.* 1991;88:898.
    An excellent review of the applications of HBO in the field of plastic and reconstructive surgery.
15. Niezgoda JA, Cianci P, Folden BW, et al. The effect of hyperbaric oxygen therapy on a burn wound model in human volunteers. *Plast Reconstr Surg.* 1997;99:1620.
    A randomized, controlled study with normoxic controls demonstrating a reduction in wound size, inflammation, and wound exudation in human volunteers.
16. Zamboni WA, Roth AC, Russell RC, et al. Morphologic analysis of the microcirculation during reperfusion of ischemic skeletal muscle and the effect of hyperbaric oxygen. *Plast Reconstr Surg.* 1993;91:1110.
    This work proposes that leukocyte venular endothelial adherence and microarteriolar vasoconstriction are important morphologic events leading to reperfusion injury of skeletal muscle. Also suggests that HBO treatment does not exacerbate reperfusion injury, but rather appears to protect the microcirculation by reducing venular leukocyte adherence and inhibiting progressive adjacent arteriolar vasoconstriction.
17. Thom SR. Leukocytes in carbon monoxide-mediated brain oxidative injury. *Toxicol Appl Pharmacol.* 1993;123:234.
    In this paper, oxidative brain injury after carbon monoxide was shown to occur in the following sequence: leukocyte sequestration in the microvasculature, B2 integrin-dependent adherence, protease-mediated conversion of endothelial xanthine dehydrogenase to xanthine oxidase, O_2 radical-dependent lipid peroxidation.
18. Thom SR. Functional inhibition of leukocyte B2 integrins by hyperbaric oxygen in carbon monoxide-mediated brain injury in rats. *Toxicol Appl Pharmacol.* 1993;123:248.
    It was shown that HBO (3.0 ATA O_2) inhibits CO-mediated brain injury caused by leukocyte adherence mediated by B2 integrins.

19. Bonomo SR, Davidson JD, Yu Y, et al. Hyperbaric oxygen as a signal transducer: upregulation of platelet derived growth factor-beta receptor in the presence of HBO2 and PDGF. *Undersea Hyperb Med.* 1998;25:211.

   Hyperbaric oxygen serves as the stimulus for the production of platelet-derived growth factor beta, which plays a major role in wound repair.

20. Siddiqui A, Davidson JD, Mustoe TA. Ischemic tissue oxygen capacitance after hyperbaric oxygen therapy: a new physiologic concept. *Plast Reconstr Surg.* 1997;99:148.

   Ischemic tissue may actually store oxygen.

21. American Diabetes Association. Consensus development conference on diabetic foot wound care, 7–8 April 1999, Boston, Mass. *Diabetes Care.* 1999;22:1354.

   Recognition by a consensus panel that HBO is useful in selected cases of diabetic foot infection, particularly when ischemia is a prominent feature.

22. Hehenberger K, et al. Dose-dependent hyperbaric oxygen stimulation of human fibroblast proliferation. *Wound Repair and Regeneration* 1997;5:147.

   The authors describe stimulation of fibroblast activity in human cell cultures in diabetic patients.

23. Cianci P. Hyperbaric therapy for radiation injury. In: Meyer JL, ed. *Radiation Injury—Advances in Management and Prevention.* Basel: Karger; 1999:98.

   A comprehensive review of the indications for HBO therapy in radiation damage to various tissues.

24. Cianci P, Hunt TK. Adjunctive hyperbaric oxygen therapy in treatment of diabetic foot wounds. In: Bowker JH, Pfeifer MA, eds. *The Diabetic Foot.* 6th ed. Philadelphia, Pa: Mosby; 2000.

   The definitive reference on diagnosis and therapy of diabetic foot problems. This chapter summarizes state-of-the art application of HBO therapy in the management of diabetic foot problems.

25. Lowenstein C, Synder S. Nitric oxide, a novel biologic messenger. *Cell.* 1992;70:705.

   A good reference for understanding the role of nitric oxide.

26. Leitch DR, Greenbaum LJ, Hallenbeck JM. Cerebral arterial air embolism I, II, III, IV. *Undersea Biomed Res.* 1984;11:221.

   This work suggests, in a carefully controlled animal study, that compression beyond 60 feet of sea water is of no benefit in the treatment of gas embolization.

27. Goldbaum LR, Ramirez RG, Absalon KB. What is the mechanism of carbon monoxide toxicity? *Aviat Space Environ Med.* 1975;46:1289.

   This study established that CO toxicity cannot be attributed solely to carboxyhemoglobin-mediated hypoxia.

28. Brown SD, Piantadosi CA. In vivo binding of carbon monoxide to cytochrome c oxidase in rat brain. *J Appl Physiol.* 1990;68:604.

   The authors demonstrate reversible binding of CO to cytochrome in the brain.

29. Thom SR. Carbon monoxide-mediated brain lipid peroxidation in the rat. *J Appl Physiol.* 1990;68:997.

   The author describes a rat model in which brain lipid peroxidation developed during the recovery phase of CO poisoning.

30. Thom SR. A delayed carbon monoxide-induced change in rat brain and its antagonism by hyperbaric oxygen. *Undersea Biomed Res.* 1987;14(suppl):40.

   The author suggests that lipid peroxidation, which has been postulated as a possible mechanism of damage in CO injury, is antagonized by HBO therapy.

31. Goulon M, et al. Intoxication oxycarbone et anoxie par inhalation de gay de charbon et d'hydrocarbures. *Annales de Medecine Interne (Paris)* 1969;120:335. (English translation in *Journal of Hyperbaric Med.* 1986;1:23).

   Prompt treatment (within 6 hours) improved survival and long-term outcome.

32. Thom SR, Taber RL, Mendiguren II, et al. Delayed neuropsychiatric sequelae after carbon monoxide poisoning: prevention by treatment with hyperbaric oxygen. *Ann Emerg Med.* 1995;25:474.

33. Weaver LK, Hopkins RO, Chan KJ, et al. Hyperbaric oxygen for acute carbon monoxide poisoning. *New Engl J Med.* 2002;347:1057–1067.

Randomized, controlled studies demonstrate the absence / reduction of neurologic sequelae in patients receiving HBO therapy versus significant incidence in untreated controls.

34. Nylander G, Lewis D, Nordstrom H, et al. Reduction of postischemic edema with hyperbaric oxygen. *Plast Reconstr Surg.* 1985;76:596.
    A seminal work on the use of HBO to reduce postischemic edema and myonecrosis with the preservation of adenosine triphosphate.

35. Shupak A, et al. Hyperbaric oxygenation in acute peripheral post-traumatic ischemia. *J Hyperbaric Med.* 1987;2:7.
    Documents Israeli experience in acute trauma.

36. Hollabaugh RS Jr, Dmochowski RR, Hickerson WL, et al. Fournier's gangrene: therapeutic impact of hyperbaric oxygen. *Plast Reconstr Surg.* 1998;101:94.
    A clinical paper showing decreased mortality and increased salvage when HBO is used as an adjunct to surgical treatment.

37. Bevers RFM, Bakker DJ, Kurth KH. Hyperbaric oxygen treatment for haemorrhagic radiation cystitis. *Lancet.* 1995;346:803.
    The authors describe experience in palliation and long-term outcomes in patients with radiation cystitis treated with HBO therapy.

38. Davis JC, Heckman JD, DeLee JC, et al. Chronic nonhematogenous osteomyelitis treated with adjuvant hyperbaric oxygen. *J Bone Joint Surg Am.* 1986;68A:1210.
    The authors report an 89% arrest of chronic osteomyelitis with disease-free periods of 2 to 10 years.

39. Mader JT, Brown GL, Guckian JC, et al. A mechanism for the amelioration by hyperbaric oxygen of experimental staphylococcal osteomyelitis in rabbits. *J Infect Dis.* 1980;142:915.
    Experimental work measuring tissue oxygen tensions in infected bone, enhancement of WBC killing ability, and amelioration of an experimentally induced chronic osteomyelitis in the rabbit tibia.

40. Calhoun JH, Mader JT, Shirtliff ME. The use of HBO in the treatment of osteomyelitis. In: Kindwall EP, Whelan HT, eds. *Hyperbaric Medicine Practice.* 2nd ed. Flagstaff, Ariz: Best Publishing; 1999:603.
    An excellent explanation of the rationale and indications for HBO therapy in a selected group of patients with osteomyelitis.

41. Faglia E, Favales F, Aldeghi A, et al. Adjunctive systemic hyperbaric oxygen therapy in treatment of severe prevalently ischemic diabetic foot ulcer. *Diabetes Care.* 1996;19:1338.
    This randomized, controlled study demonstrated the efficacy of HBO in preventing amputation in the ischemic diabetic foot.

42. Kalani M, Jorneskog G, Naderi N, et al. Hyperbaric oxygen (HBO) therapy in treatment of diabetic foot ulcers. Long-term follow-up. *J Diabetes Complications* 2002;16:153–158.
    Increase in healing and durable effect of hyperbaric-treated group.

43. Abidia A, et al. Hyperbaric oxygen therapy for diabetic leg ulcers—a double-blind randomized controlled trial. *Undersea Hyperb Med.* 2001;28(suppl):64.
    Randomized studies show faster healing in hyperbaric-treated group.

44. Cianci P, Hunt TK. Long-term results of aggressive management of diabetic foot ulcers suggest significant cost effectiveness. *Wound Repair Regen.* 1997;5:141.
    The authors demonstrate a 55-month durability of repair when an aggressive wound care program, including HBO, is used in difficult (grade 4 Wagner) diabetic foot infections.

45. Cianci P. Advances in the treatment of the diabetic foot: Is there a role for adjunctive hyperbaric oxygen therapy? *Wound Repair Regen.* 2004;12:2–10.
    Represents state of the art in 2004.

46. Niu AKC, et al. Burns treated with adjunctive hyperbaric oxygen therapy: a comparative study in humans. *J Hyperb Med.* 1987;2:75.
    The authors describe experience in nearly 300 patients treated with HBO, showing a statistically significant difference in survival in patients treated with HBO.

47. Cianci P, Lueders HW, Lee H, et al. Adjunctive hyperbaric oxygen therapy reduces length of hospitalization in thermal burns. *J Burn Care Rehabil.* 1989;10:432.
    Statistically significant reduction in length of hospital stay with adjunctive HBO therapy.
48. Cianci P, Williams C, Lueders H, et al. Adjunctive hyperbaric oxygen in the treatment of thermal burns. An economic analysis. *J Burn Care Rehabil.* 1990;11:140.
    Authors report cost-effective reduction in length of stay.
49. Cianci P, Sato R. Adjunctive hyperbaric oxygen therapy in the treatment of thermal burns: a review. *Burns.* 1994;20:5.
    Up-to-date, comprehensive, state-of-the-art review.
50. Gibson JJ, Angeles AP, Hunt TK. Increased oxygen tension potentiates angiogenesis. *Surg Forum.* 1997;48:696.
    Production of vascular endothelial growth factor increases with HBO, and it appears to be a dose-dependent mechanism.
51. Warren DC, Feehan P, Slade JB, et al. Chronic radiation proctitis treated with hyperbaric oxygen. *Undersea Hyperb Med.* 1997;24:181.
    A multicenter report showing benefit of HBO therapy in the treatment of radiation-induced proctitis.
52. Buras JA, Stahl GL, Svoboda KK, et al. Hyperbaric oxygen downregulates ICAM-1 expression induced by hypoxia and hypoglycemia: the role of NOS. *Am J Physiol.* 2000;278:C292.
    This paper shows the downregulation of intercellular adhesion molecule expression induced by hypoxia and hypoglycemia and the stimulation of eNOS by HBO.
53. Banick PD, Chen Q, Xu YA, et al. Nitric oxide inhibits neutrophil beta-2 integrin function by inhibiting membrane-associated cyclic GMP synthesis. *J Cell Physiol.* 1997;172:12.
    Enhancement of NO production inhibits beta-2 integrin function and appears to be regulated by cyclic GMP.
54. Schoenrock GJ, Cianci P. Treatment of radiation cystitis with hyperbaric oxygen. *Urology.* 1986;27:271.
    This report documents spontaneous healing of a bladder fistula with HBO.
55. Fisher AB. Reactive oxygen species and cell signaling with lung ischemia. *Undersea Hyperb Med.* 2004;31:97–103.
    This paper describes the cascade of events in endothelium and the effect of reactive oxygen species on cell-signaling activation of transcription factors and cell division. The author postulates the mechanism is an attempt at restoration of blood flow.
56. Thom SR. Effects of hyperoxia on neutrophil adhesion. *Undersea Hyperb Med.* 2004;31:123–131.
    Prevention of white cell adhesion to endothelium is modulated through an increase in NO flux.

21. LUNG IN IMMUNOCOMPROMISED HOST

Shazia M. Jamil

Patients who develop increased susceptibility to infection as a result of qualitative and quantitative defects in inflammatory and immunologic host defenses are considered "immunocompromised hosts" (IH). These defects are caused by a wide range of processes, including, but not limited to, primary congenital syndromes, cancer, retroviral infection, malnutrition, and drug therapy. Pulmonary complications in immunocompromised hosts are becoming more common, owing to increases in solid organ transplantation, hematopoietic stem cell transplantation (HSCT), and the use of more potent chemotherapeutic regimens in cancer. Lung involvement may be either infectious or noninfectious; however, infectious causes are reported in the majority of patients (50–75%) with complications. IH are more susceptible to pulmonary infection because of compromised (1) granulocyte number and function; (2) immune function (i.e., lymphocyte activity); (3) mechanical barriers to colonization and infection; and (4) exposure to pathogens. Infections carry a high risk of morbidity and mortality in IH, warranting a careful diagnostic and therapeutic approach.

Infections in IH can be bacterial, viral, fungal, parasitic, or mycobacterial. Bacterial pneumonia is the most common cause of focal pulmonary infiltrates in patients with the AIDS or leukemia (before, during, and after chemotherapy). *Pneumococcus* and *Haemophilus* are as common in IH as they are in the general population. In addition, encapsulated gram-positive cocci (e.g., *Staphylococcus aureus*) and the Enterobacteriaceae spp. (e.g., *Escherichia coli, Klebsiella,* and *Pseudomonas* spp.) are more prevalent among those with granulocytopenia ($<500/mm^3$) and hospitalized patients. Nosocomially acquired *Legionella* infection also has been reported in IH. *Rhodococcus equi,* an unusual bacterial pathogen in normal hosts, may cause pneumonia and lung abscesses in AIDS patients and in solid organ transplant recipients, especially after heart transplantation.

Fungal infections common in IH include both the filamentous fungi (e.g., *Aspergillus* spp. and the mucormycosis) and the dimorphic fungi (e.g., *Candida* spp., *Cryptococcus neoformans, Blastomycoses dermatitidis, Coccidioides immitis,* and *Histoplasma capsulatum*). Some other emerging fungi include *Ochroconis, Trichosporon, Fusarium,* and Zygomycetes. Neutropenia, phagocyte dysfunction, and corticosteroid use are the major risks for fungal infection. *Aspergillus* is the most common cause of fungal pneumonia in the IH; patients with HSCT are particularly prone to invasive aspergillosis. *Candida* spp. (e.g., *C. albicans*) are part of the normal flora within the gastrointestinal tract. Local overgrowth in the mouth (thrush), vagina, esophagus, and gut is frequent in patients with deficient granulocyte number or function or those receiving broad-spectrum antibiotics. *Candida* pneumonia is rare, with the exception of lung transplant recipients. Prophylactic fluconazole in the setting of marrow transplantation is associated with a decreased incidence of *C. albicans* infections, but a rise in more antifungal-resistant *Candida* spp. (e.g., *C. krausei* and *C. glabrata*). The fungus *Ochroconis gallopavum* is a dematiaceous hyphomycete that is an emerging opportunistic and possibly fatal fungal infection. Fungi of the genus *Ochroconis* produce characteristic darkly pigmented, septate hyphae or conidia. In humans, infection by this species occurs infrequently and almost exclusively in immunocompromised patients. *O. gallopavum* has been reported to involve the brain, lung, and spleen in IH. Although no definitive guidelines can be recommended for treatment, surgical excision in combination with amphotericin B has been used. Itraconazole or flucytosine are reasonable effective alternative agents if there is concern about the toxicity of amphotericin B. The optimal duration and dosage of these antifungal agents to treat this infection have not been determined.

Viruses, such as cytomegalovirus (CMV), herpes, varicella, respiratory syncytial virus, adenovirus, influenza virus, and parainfluenza virus, are of major concern because of high morbidity, mortality, and an increase in the chance of rejection in solid organ transplant recipients. The infection is either newly acquired or reactivation of a dormant process. CMV is the most common viral respiratory pathogen in non-HIV IH. The development of CMV infection is also closely related to the donor and recipient's prior CMV serostatus.

Pneumocystis carinii is an opportunistic infection that can cause fulminant and fatal pneumonia in AIDS patients and other IH. The incidence of *P. carinii* pneumonia is decreased in at-risk patients who use trimethoprim-sulfamethoxazole for prophylaxis. However cases still arise, especially in those with adjustments in immunosuppressives (e.g., tapering of corticosteroids), those noncompliant with prophylaxis, and in patients with lymphoid malignancies treated with fludarabine.

Mycobacterium tuberculosis (MTB) infections are particularly common in AIDS patients and recipients of solid organ transplantation (especially renal transplant recipients), compared with other IH. The infection is either newly acquired (in endemic areas) or a reactivation of a latent infection. MTB may involve the lung very early during HIV infection, whereas extrapulmonary or atypical manifestations are associated with more profound immunodeficiency, presenting with mycobacteremia and multidrug resistance in IH. In patients with relatively high CD4+ T cell counts, a typical pattern of pulmonary reactivation occurs with fever, cough, weight loss, night sweats, and a radiograph revealing cavitary apical upper lobe disease. Disseminated MTB infection is more common in patients with low CD4+ T cell counts and appears with diffuse bilateral reticulonodular infiltrates consistent with miliary spread, pleural effusions, and hilar and/or mediastinal adenopathy.

The nontuberculous mycobacteria (NTM) are seen more frequently in the AIDS population compared with non–AIDS-immunocompromised patients, and usually appear as disseminated disease. In contrast to MTB, these are seen with increasing frequency as a late complication in AIDS patients. *Mycobacterium avium-intracellulare* (MAC) and *Mycobacterium kansasii* are the two most common causes of NTM lung infection. Some other NTM include *M. fortuitum, M abscessus, M. chelonae, M. bovis, M xenopi*, and *M. marinum*. Chest radiographs in these patients may show hilar or mediastinal adenopathy, cavitation and/or pleural effusion.

Noninfectious etiologies involving lung in IH deserve special mention. These are difficult to diagnose and differentiate from infectious causes. Common examples are cardiogenic pulmonary edema, acute lung injury/acute respiratory distress syndrome (ALI/ARDS), transfusion-related acute lung injury (TRALI), diffuse alveolar hemorrhage (DAH), alveolar hemorrhage secondary to thrombocytopenia, lung involvement by the hematopoietic malignancies (such as leukemic lung infiltration) and solid organ metastasis, posttransplant lymphoproliferative disease (PTLD), drug-induced lung disease, engraftment syndrome, radiation toxicity, idiopathic pneumonia syndrome, and bronchiolitis obliterans organizing pneumonia. Large-volume fluid infusion, as with chemotherapy and transfusion or direct cardiotoxicity from chemotherapeutic agents (e.g., anthracyclines), leads to increase capillary hydrostatic pressure and, hence, pulmonary edema. On the other hand, sepsis, chemotherapeutic agents (such as interleukin-2 and cytarabine), and transfusion may cause lung injury by increasing capillary leak leading to noncardiogenic pulmonary edema (ALI/ARDS).

PTLD, DAH, idiopathic pneumonia syndrome, and engraftment syndrome are seen more commonly after HSCT. The majority of PTLD are of B cell origin and related to immunosuppressive regimen and infection with Epstein-Barr virus. DAH complicates about 2 to 14% of HSCT. To make the diagnosis, pulmonary infection must be ruled out as the etiology of the hemorrhage. In addition, alveolar hemorrhage related to thrombocytopenia, uremia, or endogenous anticoagulants occurs without lung injury and is a entity separate from DAH.

Idiopathic pneumonia syndrome (IPS) is a noninfectious, frequent, and often fatal complication of allogeneic bone marrow transplantation (BMT). This syndrome usually develops during 31 to 100 days post-BMT and must be distinguished from CMV pneumonitis. The pathogenesis has not been fully elucidated. However, several contributing factors have been proposed, including lung injury caused by reactive oxygen and nitrogen intermediates during preconditioning and development of graft-versus-host disease (GVHD). Engraftment syndrome occurs during neutrophil recovery after HSCT and is difficult to differentiate from ALI/ARDS and pulmonary edema.

The first approach to diagnosis is a thorough assessment of the clinical history, including infection risk, and a detailed physical examination. The history should clarify the exact time of the onset of symptoms and the progression and relationship of symptoms to the institution of immunosuppression or transplantation. Other relevant facts include previous and current use of chemotherapeutic agents and other medications, immunization history, place of birth and residence (to explore the possibility of exposure to endemic fungi or mycobacteria), and history of positive tuberculosis skin test and positive CMV serology.

Common clinical features include fever, dry or productive cough, hemoptysis, dyspnea, wheezing, chest pain with or without pleurisy, hypoxemia, tachycardia, hypotension, and respiratory failure. Unfortunately, none of these can specifically differentiate between infectious and noninfectious etiologies. Sputum production may be scant in patients with bacterial pneumonia due to granulocytopenia. A paucity of clinical symptoms may be seen in patients with *Aspergillus* infection, especially early in the course of disease. Viruses such as herpes and CMV may cause tracheobronchitis or bronchiolitis, and may present with wheezing alone.

Key factors in evaluating lung involvement in immunocompromised patient are the: (1) rapidity of onset; (2) severity of illness; (3) relationship with immunosuppression; (5) radiologic pattern; and (6) presence of extrapulmonary manifestations. Lung infections with the most explosive onsets tend to be bacterial in nature. However, herpes viruses and *P. carinii* pneumonia can also progress to respiratory failure in a matter of days. *Legionella* infection commonly follows a prodromal period of fever and constitutional symptoms. Insidious onset is frequently seen in infections from various fungi, *Nocardia,* and mycobacteria. Gradual onset of symptoms is also more common with noninfectious etiologies, such as leukemic infiltration and drug-related lung injury. Notable exceptions to this maxim are cardiogenic pulmonary edema, ALI/ARDS, and pulmonary hemorrhage.

The time after transplantation may help predict the most likely etiologies of infectious and noninfectious pulmonary complications. For example, bacterial and invasive fungal pneumonia usually presents within a month of these procedures, whereas the risk of developing most opportunistic infections and CMV is highest between 1 and 3 months. On the other hand, mycobacterium, *Nocardia,* and delayed CMV infections are more likely to occur after 3 months. Noninfectious etiologies such as DAH, ALI/ARDS, and cardiogenic pulmonary edema should be strongly considered when pulmonary manifestations appear shortly after the procedure or within the first month.

Chest radiographs may be entirely normal early in the course of and remain normal during viral infections that have a predilection for airways rather than pulmonary parenchyma. Radiographs are useful in differentiating diffuse, multifocal, and focal processes. A diffuse interstitial or alveolar filling process is highly suggestive of either an opportunistic infection or a noninfectious cause of lung injury. Although diffuse presentation is not typical of bacterial or filamentous fungal or *Candida* pneumonias, bacteria or fungi can complicate diffuse lung disease of other causes. Viruses in the herpes group, *P. carinii,* and dimorphic fungi (e.g., *Histoplasma, Coccidioides*) often result in diffuse pneumonias without pleural effusions. Drug-induced injury, ALI/ARDS, cardiogenic pulmonary edema, DAH, and pulmonary leukostasis are the usual noninfectious causes of diffuse involvement.

Focal findings include alveolar consolidation, cavitation, abscesses, and mass lesions. The most frequent cause of focal consolidation is bacterial pneumonia. Cavitation suggests a diagnosis of *S. aureus, Pseudomonas, Klebsiella, E. coli,* anaerobes, *Legionella, Nocardia, Mycobacterium* spp., or *Rhodococcus equi.* Multiple areas of bronchopneumonia with cavitation are often seen in herpes simplex virus (HSV) pneumonia secondary to aspiration of infected oral secretions. Mycobacterial infection appears as either a focal infiltrate or miliary process. Mass-like lesions (especially those with cavitation), which expand without constraint by lobar fissures and tissue plains, are suggestive of invasive filamentous fungi. Common noninfectious causes of focal infiltrate are local hemorrhage (which, in fact, may be caused by infections) and focal leukemic infiltrates.

Extrapulmonary manifestations, such as pleural effusions, cardiomegaly, extrapulmonary soft-tissue masses, and bony lesions, may point to specific causes. Endemic fungi, mycobacterium and *Nocardia* infections often involve extrapulmonary organs.

Initial laboratory investigation should include complete blood counts with manual differential, electrolytes, liver enzyme and function, blood urea nitrogen, serum creatinine, urinalysis, and a good-quality posteroanterior and lateral chest radiograph (if possible).

Microbiologic evaluation is crucial. Specimens from all sites (e.g., blood, urine, sputum, bronchoalveolar lavage [BAL], transbronchial biopsy [TBB], pleural fluid, needle aspirate from abscess, or suspicious skin lesion) should be examined on Gram's stain, acid-fast stain, and fungal stain, and sent for respective culture on appropriate medium. In patients with high suspicion of fungal, *P. carinii,* or *Nocardia* infection, methenamine silver, Wright–Giemsa, and modified acid-fast stains should also be included. Blood cultures should be obtained as early as possible. AIDS and solid organ transplant patients with insidious onset pneumonia or lung abscess should have mycolic acid staining of specimens if Gram's stain or culture signifies diphtheroids to rule out *R. equi* (usually a misdiagnosed pathogen). Unilateral pleural effusion should be sampled by thoracentesis. Rapid detection methods using monoclonal antibody techniques for *L. pneumophila* and *L. micdadei* may be useful. Rapid viral culture and fluorescent antibody stains for viruses such as herpes group and influenza should be considered.

Chest computerized tomography (CT) scan should be considered early in the course. A chest CT scan is more sensitive and more specific than a chest radiograph in detecting lung disease. Up to 50% of IH patients with lung disease on thin section CT may have a normal chest radiograph. CT also helps guide invasive procedures, such as sampling of a peripheral lung mass or drainage of pleural effusion. It can provide an anatomic map to guide the bronchoscopist in performing BAL or TBB and the surgeon in performing lung biopsy.

Early detection of a pulmonary process and early institution of specific therapy increases the likelihood of survival; therefore, diagnostic procedures to obtain secretions, washings, or even lung tissue should be performed as soon as possible. Fiberoptic bronchoscopy (FOB) is the procedure of choice for sampling areas of radiographic abnormality by telescoping (protected-specimen) brush, BAL, or TBB for diagnosis. Although the yield of culture in patients receiving antibiotics may be lower, a positive culture is highly suggestive of infection and may warrant immediate treatment. TBB adds significantly in detecting tissue-invasive fungi such as *Candida* and *Aspergillus,* or leukemic infiltration.

Percutaneous fine needle aspiration (FNA) is a useful technique for sampling peripheral lesions. A larger lung sample can be achieved at thoracotomy with an open lung biopsy or video-assisted thoracoscopic surgery (VATS). VATS potentially offers a less morbid approach with the same diagnostic yield and expense. Lung biopsy is indicated in (1) rapidly progressive severe pneumonia with insufficient time to wait for response from empiric therapy (or when empirical therapy is relatively contraindicated), and (2) persistent, undiagnosed lung disease, despite attempts at less invasive diagnostic procedures and empiric therapy. IH patients with rapidly deteriorating pulmonary status often are placed on empiric antibacterial and antifungal agents until the results of medical evaluation are completed. This is especially true when suspicion is high or risk factors for bacterial pneumonia and *Aspergillus* infection are present. Increasingly, immunosuppressed patients with respiratory failure are successfully managed with noninvasive mechanical ventilation in the hospital and ICU setting.

---

1. Schmitt J, Adam D. Pulmonary infiltrations in febrile patients with neutropenia. Risk factors and outcome under empirical antimicrobial therapy in a randomized multicenter study. *Cancer.* 1994;73:2296.

Reports on the high risk of fungal infection in patients with febrile neutropenia and pneumonia.

2. Chanock SJ, Pizzo PA. Infectious complications of patients undergoing therapy for acute leukemia: current status and future prospects. *Semin Oncol.* 1997;4:132.
   An excellent review of the topic.

3. Gerson SL, Talbot GH, Hurwitz S, et al. Prolonged granulocytopenia: the major risk factor for invasive pulmonary aspergillosis in patients with acute leukemia. *Ann Intern Med.* 1984;100:345.
   A classic study of risks for invasive aspergillosis.

4. Marr KA, Carter RA, Crippa F, et al. Epidemiology and outcome of mould infections in hematopoietic stem cell transplant recipients. *Clin Infect Dis.* 2002;34:909.
   Study showing an increase in fungal/Aspergillus infection in allogenic HSCT patients.

5. Kahn FW, Jones JM, England DM. The role of bronchoalveolar lavage in the diagnosis of invasive pulmonary aspergillosis. *Am J Clin Pathol.* 1986;86:518.
   Report showing that bronchoscopic yield for invasive aspergillosis is only approximately 50%.

6. Maertens J, Verhaegen J, Lagrou K, et al. Screening for circulating galactomannan as a noninvasive diagnostic tool for invasive aspergillosis in prolonged neutropenic patients and stem cell transplantation recipients: a prospective validation. *Blood.* 2001;97:1604.
   A promising report of enzyme-linked immunosorbent assay for detection of aspergillus infection.

7. Goodrich J. A comparison of cytomegalovirus and community respiratory viruses in immunocompromised patients. *Am J Med.* 1997;102:37.
   Excellent review of viral pathogens in immunocompromised host.

8. Singh N, Paterson DL. Mycobacterium tuberculosis infection in solid organ transplant recipients: impact and implications for management. *Clin Infect Dis.* 1998;27:1266.

9. Aronchick JM, Miller WT Jr. Disseminated nontuberculous mycobacterial infections in immunosuppressed patients. *Semin Roentgenol.* 1993;28:150–157.
   Comprehensive clinical/radiologic presentation of tuberculous and nontuberculous mycobacterial infection in the immunocompromised host.

10. Thomas CF, Limper AH. Pneumocystic pneumonia: clinical presentation and diagnosis in patients with and without acquired immune deficiency syndrome. *Semin Respir Infect.* 1998;13:289.
    Reviews P. carinii infection in various immunocompromised hosts.

11. Perez MGV, Vassal T, Kemmerly SA. Rhodococcus equi infection in transplant recipients: a case of mistaken identity and review of literature. *Transpl Infect Dis.* 2002;4:52.

12. Wang TK, Chiu W, Chim S, et al. Disseminated ochroconis gallopavum infection in a renal transplant recipient: the first reported case and a review of literature. *Clin Nephrol.* 2003;60:415

13. Boutati EI, Anaissie EJ. Fusarium, a significant emerging pathogen in patients with hematologic malignancy: ten years' experience at a cancer center and implications for management. *Blood.* 1997;90:999.
    References 11 to 13 review rare but important pathogens in immunocompromised hosts.

14. Shelhamer JH, Gill VJ, Quinn TC, et al. The laboratory evaluation of opportunistic infections. *Ann Intern Med.* 1996;124:585.
    An excellent review of diagnostic approaches to various opportunistic infections.

15. Saito H, Anaissie EJ, Morice RC, et al. Bronchoalveolar lavage in the diagnosis of pulmonary infiltrates in patients with acute leukemia. *Chest.* 1988;94:745.
    Contains a discussion of the relevance of detection of Candida in BAL.

16. Crawford SW. Noninfectious lung disease in the immunocompromised host. *Respiration.* 1999;66–385.
    Excellent detailed review of possible noninfectious etiologies of lung disease in IH.

17. Shorr AF, Susla GM, O'Grady NP. Pulmonary infiltrates in the non-HIV infected immunocompromised patient. *Chest.* 2004;125:260.
    Excellent review of etiologies, diagnostic strategies and outcomes of lung infiltrates in IH.
18. Rano A, Agusti C, Jimenez P, et al. Pulmonary infiltrates in non-HIV immunocompromised patients: a diagnostic approach using noninvasive and bronchoscopic procedures. *Thorax.* 2001: 56:379.
    Infectious etiologies were responsible for more than three fourths of pulmonary infiltrates in a prospective study of 200 immunocompromised patients.
19. Crawford SW, Hackman RC, Clark JG. Biopsy diagnosis and clinical outcome of focal pulmonary lesions after marrow transplantation. *Transplantation.* 1989;48:266.
    A study of sequential fine needle aspirates in patients with focal lung lesions.
20. Heussel CP, Kauczor HU, Heussel G, et al.. Early detection of pneumonia in febrile neutropenic patients: use of thin-section CT. *Am J Roentgenol.* 1997;169:1347.
    Reported increased sensitivity of CT scan in detecting lung lesions compared with chest radiograph.
21. White DA, Wong PW, Downey R. The utility of open lung biopsy in patients with hematological malignancies. *Am J Respir Crit Care Med.* 2000;161:723.
    High utility of this procedure prompting changes in therapy in about 57% of such patients.
22. Hilbert G, Gruson D, Vargas F, et al. Noninvasive ventilation in immunosuppressed patients with pulmonary infiltrates, fever, and acute respiratory failure. *N Engl J Med.* 2001;344:481.
    A randomized trial of IH with pulmonary infiltrates and early respiratory failure showed that patients managed with noninvasive ventilation had decreased mortality compared with those who received standard care (endotracheal intubation).
23. Yen KT, Lee AS, Krowka MJ, et al. Pulmonary complications in bone marrow transplantation: a practical approach to diagnosis and treatment. *Clin Chest Med.* 2004;25:189–120.
    In this article, the authors describe an algorithmic approach to the diagnosis and management of the infectious and noninfectious pulmonary complications in bone marrow transplant patients.

22. THE LUNG IN DRUG ABUSE

Tristan J. Huie, Robert J. Kruklitis, and Charles A. Read

The lungs are particularly vulnerable to medical complications in drug abuse because the most common routes of administration are inhalation and intravenous (IV) injection. Drug abuse may cause infectious and noninfectious lung disorders (Table 22-1). The epidemiology and typical presentation may facilitate timely diagnosis and appropriate treatment.

Illicit drug users are susceptible to numerous infections that arise because the host's immune defenses are suppressed or bypassed. The increased prevalence of HIV infection among drug abusers leads to many infectious and noninfectious complications, such as pneumocystis pneumonia, bacterial pneumonia, tuberculosis and Kaposi sarcoma (see Chapter 47). In addition to the immune suppression that occurs with HIV infection, the drug user's immune system may be suppressed by the direct effects of the drug itself. Recent studies in cocaine and marijuana users demonstrate impaired function of alveolar macrophages. Alveolar macrophages exposed to marijuana smoke have reduced phagocytosis, bacterial cell killing, and fungicidal activity. Marijuana

Table 22-1. Pulmonary complications of illicit substance abuse

Infectious
—Aspiration pneumonia
—Septic emboli
—Bacterial pneumonia
—Acute bronchitis
—Tuberculosis
—Fungal pneumonia
Noninfectious
—Vascular complications
—Noncardiogenic pulmonary edema
—Pulmonary hemorrhage
—Pulmonary hypertension
—Interstitial complications
—Talc granulomas
—Pulmonary fibrosis
—Airway complications
—Bronchospasm/asthma
—Chronic bronchitis
—Bullous disease
—Bronchiectasis
—BOOP (bronchiolitis obliterans with organizing pneumonia)
—Pleural complications
—Pneumothorax/pneumomediastinum
—Pleural effusions/empyema
—Respiratory failure
—Carcinogenesis

exposure results in decreased expression of proinflammatory cytokines, such as tumor necrosis factor (TNF)-α and interleukin (IL)-6. T cell proliferation is shifted from T helper 1 (Th1) cells that are responsible for cell-mediated immunity to T helper 2 (Th2) cells that mediate allergy and atopy. This shift may cause an increased risk of infection and malignancy in marijuana users. Macrophages exposed to crack cocaine are less able to kill bacteria or tumor cells, possibly because of decreased production of reactive oxidant species. Marijuana and cocaine smoking also harm the lungs' primary defenses by replacing ciliated epithelium with nonciliated mucus-secreting cells or metaplastic squamous epithelium. These findings help explain the enhanced susceptibility to infections observed in drug addicts.

Aspiration into the lower respiratory tract commonly occurs after the use of many illicit drugs. Heroin overdose is complicated by pneumonia in up to half of cases. Overdose depresses the state of consciousness and diminishes gag and cough reflexes; consequently, the risk for aspiration of oropharyngeal or gastric contents and pneumonia increases. The initial inflammatory response can result in significant alveolar edema. Patients are seen with fever, tachypnea, and hypoxia. Radiographs may be normal or may show localized or bilateral diffuse infiltrates, depending on the volume of aspiration and the severity of resulting inflammation. Treatment is generally supportive. The use of antibiotics is controversial, but if they are used, they should be directed primarily against the oropharyngeal flora.

Septic pulmonary emboli are common in injection drug users and may occur in up to one quarter of hospitalized drug addicts with pulmonary complaints. Emboli originate from endocarditis, typically of the tricuspid valve, or from thrombophlebitis at the injection site. Presenting symptoms typically include pleuritic chest pain, hemoptysis, and fever. Physical examination in the case of thrombophlebitis reveals erythema, induration, and warmth at the injection site. A palpable cord may be present. In contrast, tricuspid valve endocarditis is often difficult to detect on examination. Tricuspid murmurs are usually soft, and the peripheral stigmata of endocarditis are not present with right-sided lesions. Typical radiographic manifestations include diffuse infiltrates or peripheral nodules, which may cavitate. Sequentially appearing nodules suggest endocarditis. Pleural effusions may occur; hilar and mediastinal lymphadenopathy is rarely seen. Blood cultures are usually positive. *Staphylococcus aureus* causes 80% of cases; gram-negative bacteria and *Candida* are rarer causes. Complications include abscess, empyema, and bronchopleural fistula. Appropriate antimicrobial therapy should be continued for 4 to 6 weeks and is typically effective if compliance is achieved.

Community-acquired pneumonia is recognized with increased frequency in drug abusers. Drug abusers have a tenfold increased risk of pneumococcal pneumonia compared with nonusers. The presentation, course of illness, and response to treatment are similar in drug-using and nonusing populations. The usual community-acquired organisms are most common in drug users; however, aspiration is often associated with anaerobes, and intravenous drug use is associated with gram-negative bacilli and *S. aureus*. In addition, drug use increases risk of methicillin-resistant *S. aureus* infection.

Acute bronchitis develops at an increased frequency in marijuana users. This increased incidence partially may result from the respiratory irritants in marijuana smoke. Although not well studied, other inhaled drugs may also predispose to acute bronchitis. The treatment of acute bronchitis in drug abusers is similar to that in nonabusers.

Pulmonary tuberculosis develops more frequently in drug abusers and appears to be related to lower socioeconomic status and the decreased immunity and higher rate of reactivation in this population. Clinically and radiographically, tuberculosis in drug abusers is indistinguishable from that of nonusers and should be treated with the standard multidrug antimycobacterial regimen. However, directly observed therapy is advisable in drug addicts to ensure compliance and avoid development of resistance.

Fungal pulmonary infections have been linked to illicit drug use. Invasive aspergillosis has been reported in immunocompromised patients who smoked marijuana contaminated with the fungus. Cases have been described in patients with advanced HIV, chronic granulomatous disease, after bone marrow transplant, and in patients with lung cancer treated with chemotherapy. Aspergillus-laden marijuana has been implicated in allergic bronchopulmonary aspergillosis. Lobar candidal pneumonia and systemic candidiasis resulting in the adult respiratory distress syndrome (ARDS) have been reported in heroin users. The likely source of candidal infection in this population is the lemon used to acidify the heroin fix. Although these severe fungal infections are rare, drug abusers have a high prevalence of serum precipitins against these fungi, suggesting widespread fungal contamination of illicit drugs. Treatment should focus on standard aggressive antifungal therapy.

Illicit substance abuse is also responsible for numerous noninfectious lung disorders that may occur within the pulmonary vasculature, interstitium, airways, or pleura.

Noncardiogenic pulmonary edema is perhaps the most frequent fatal complication of illicit drug abuse. A large number of drugs, including narcotics, cocaine, amphetamines, sedatives, tranquilizers, and hydrocarbons, can acutely produce pulmonary edema. Heroin is a particularly common offender. In one large series, 18% of those with heroin-induced pulmonary edema died. Pulmonary edema has been documented in both the first-time user and the experienced addict; it can occur immediately or up to 24 hours after use. Patients typically are stuporous or comatose, with fever, cyanosis, and crackles. Constricted pupils suggest opiate-induced disease. Chest films classically demonstrate fluffy, bilateral alveolar infiltrates without cardiomegaly. The pathophysiology appears to differ depending on the drug involved, but increased permeability is suggested by studies that demonstrate equivalent protein concentrations in the alveolar fluid and serum. Treatment is generally supportive with supplemental oxygen and mechanical ventilation as needed. Naloxone should be considered in opiate-induced edema to reverse respiratory depression. Typically the edema resolves within 24 to 72 hours, but it can take several weeks until the lung volumes, compliance, and diffusing capacity normalize.

Crack lung is an acute lung injury syndrome that includes fever, cough, chest pain, wheezing, and hypoxia. Chest radiographs show diffuse alveolar infiltrates.

Eosinophilia is usually present in both peripheral blood and bronchoalveolar lavage. Crack lung can develop immediately or up to 48 hours after smoking crack cocaine. Increased neutrophil activation and IL-8 expression may cause the lung injury from cocaine smoking. The infiltrates resolve spontaneously with supportive treatment. Corticosteroid therapy has been used with mixed success, and there is no convincing evidence to support the routine use of steroids.

Pulmonary hemorrhage has been well described in crack cocaine smokers. Volatile hydrocarbons and heroin have also been associated with at least subclinical pulmonary vascular hemorrhage. The amount of pulmonary hemorrhage may be massive or barely detectable. Massive hemoptysis has been associated with pulmonary infarction after cocaine use. Crack users more commonly experience trace hemoptysis; many report black or blood-tinged sputum after crack use. One third of cocaine smokers have hemosiderin-laden macrophages in their lungs at autopsy, pointing to occult episodes of bleeding. It has been postulated that pulmonary hemorrhage occurs from either the intense vasoconstriction caused by cocaine or the direct alveolar injury. Chest radiographs are usually normal. Treatment depends on the extent of hemoptysis, but is mainly supportive. Bronchoscopy is indicated with significant hemoptysis to locate the site of the bleeding and direct further interventions.

Pulmonary hypertension can develop in patients who inject aqueous suspensions of medications intended for oral use only. Addicts often prepare and inject suspensions of tablets containing insoluble filler components such as talc or cellulose. The most frequently crushed and injected tablets include amphetamines, methylphenidate (Ritalin), methadone, and propoxyphene. Heroin and other drugs may be diluted with insoluble adulterants such as starch or inadvertently contaminated with the cotton used to filter the liquid drug. Repeated embolization of these particles results in thrombosis, fibrosis, and ultimately pulmonary vessel occlusion. Progressive loss of pulmonary microcirculation leads to pulmonary hypertension and, if untreated, to cor pulmonale. Treatment options are limited; the most important step is cessation of IV drug use.

Interstitial lung disease, in the form of pulmonary fibrosis and granulomatosis, can also result from the embolization of insoluble particles. Embolized foreign bodies cause endothelial injury in the pulmonary vasculature. Initially a focal inflammatory process develops that leads to damage of the arterial walls. Transvascular migration of the insoluble particles occurs next with the formation of perivascular and interstitial granulomas. *Talcosis* develops after long-term, chronic injection of pills that contain magnesium silicate (i.e., talc). Patients complain of insidious progressive dyspnea, mild cough, and, occasionally, wheezing. Fundoscopic examination often reveals glistening white spots around the macula. Chest radiography is normal in 50% of cases or may have diffuse reticulo-nodular infiltrates most prominent at the lung bases. Lower lung emphysema is common in patients who inject Ritalin. Patients with talcosis classically have a decreased diffusion capacity and an obstructive pattern on pulmonary function testing; however, a restrictive pattern may also be seen. Definitive diagnosis requires that either a transbronchial or open lung biopsy demonstrate foreign body granulomas containing birefringent talc or other foreign particle. Anecdotal evidence suggests that steroids may be of mild benefit in some patients. A series of six patients, however, showed that all developed severe respiratory insufficiency during long-term follow-up regardless of steroid use, and three died of respiratory failure.

Thermal injury can occur from smoking crack cocaine because of the extremely high temperatures of inhaled chemicals or secondary to ignition of the highly volatile ether residue used in processing the free-base form of cocaine. *Thermal epiglottitis* has been described in a small series of drug abusers who presented with acute epiglottitis. Treatment is supportive with corticosteroids to reduce swelling and airway compromise. Repeated thermal injury to the trachea can lead to *tracheal stenosis*, which has been described in crack cocaine use. Such patients will have wheezing, which may be irreversible, and occasionally with stridor. Severe tracheal stenosis may require a mechanical correction, including tracheostomy placement.

Bronchospasm can occur after the use of a variety of inhaled drugs, with crack cocaine and heroin being the most frequent offenders. The drugs themselves, or their adulterants, result in inflammation of the respiratory epithelium and can result in the direct release of histamine. Bronchospasm is most threatening in patients with poorly controlled asthma prior to drug use. Several case studies have reported that asthma deaths are associated with substance abuse in up to 30% of cases. Treatment involves avoiding the precipitating drug and using standard bronchodilators and inhaled steroids as necessary.

Chronic bronchitis and impaired gas exchange occur with the repeated use of marijuana. Marijuana causes bronchodilation and was once evaluated as a possible therapy for asthma. Bronchodilation results from tetrahydrocannabinol (THC) binding to a cannabinoid receptor that is independent of antimuscarinic or beta-agonistic activity. Unfortunately, these bronchodilatory effects are only transient, and the other combustion byproducts tend to worsen asthma. The chronic use of marijuana causes increased cough, sputum production, and wheezing similar to chronic bronchitis.

Bullous lung disease occurs occasionally in IV drug users—up to 2% in one large retrospective study. It is associated with methylphenidate injection and with marijuana use. Bullous disease, predominately located in the upper lobes, occurs much earlier than expected from cigarette smoking alone. The pathophysiology of bullae formation is uncertain, but is speculated to result from the coalescence of microbullae, which are formed indirectly from either emboli or foreign body granulomas. Barotrauma also appears to play a role. Patients present with obstructive symptoms similar to those of patients with moderate to severe emphysema. Obstructive lung disease can also result from damage to the medium and small airways.

Bronchiectasis has been reported in drug users after one or more episodes of noncardiogenic pulmonary edema. Aspiration, hypoxia, and direct irritant effects may all contribute to the development of bronchiectasis. *Bronchiolitis obliterans with organizing pneumonia* (BOOP) has been associated with cocaine in several case reports. Typically these patients improve with steroids, but several cases of ARDS and death have occurred. The best available long-term therapy for bronchiectasis and bronchiolitis obliterans is cessation of drug use. Continued exposure generally leads to progression of the disease.

A *pneumothorax* or *pneumomediastinum* can result from the use of either intravenous or inhaled drugs. As sites for peripheral access are exhausted, IV drug abusers often attempt to access the subclavian or internal jugular veins. A "pocket shot" is an injection lateral to the sternocleidomastoid muscle immediately above the clavicle; pneumothorax, pneumomediastinum, pseudoaneurysm formation, and paralysis of the vocal cords because of recurrent laryngeal nerve trauma have been reported. Pneumomediastinum and pneumothorax can also occur with inhalation drug use. This occurs because of weakening of the alveolar walls and from an increased pressure gradient across the alveolar membrane. An increased gradient occurs during "shotgunning," as one person forcibly exhales smoke into another person's mouth, and during a Valsalva maneuver performed after inhalation to increase absorption of the inhaled drug. There have been case reports of pneumothorax and pneumomediastinum after ecstasy use with prolonged dancing.

Respiratory failure, through suppression of the respiratory drive, occurs with many different drug classes. Narcotics and sedatives suppress ventilation; their use may result in carbon dioxide retention, decreased consciousness, respiratory failure, and death. Treatment should be individualized and may include naloxone to antagonize opiates and reverse respiratory depression or, in some cases, flumazenil to antagonize benzodiazepines. Mechanical ventilation may be required. Abuse of volatile inhalants, common among adolescents, may lead to asphyxiation from suppressed respiratory drive and physical displacement of oxygen by the inhalant. The increased abuse of ketamine and gamma hydroxybutyrate has shown that they can also cause respiratory failure.

Lung cancer occurs with increased frequency in tobacco smokers. The link between various illicit drugs and cancer has been difficult to prove because of the frequent concurrent use of tobacco in drug users and difficulty in enrolling drug users in prospective studies. Indirect evidence suggests that cancers and precancerous changes occur with increased frequency in marijuana and cocaine users. Histologic and molecular alterations that are linked to carcinogenesis have been identified in the bronchial epithelium of marijuana and cocaine smokers. Surrogate endpoint markers, such as increased epidermal growth factor receptor, occur with increased frequency in cell lines that develop lung cancers. Epidemiologic evidence also supports a link between drug use and cancer. Marijuana use has been reported at an increased frequency in patients who develop early head and neck and lung cancers. Although not well studied, other illicit substances may have similar carcinogenic effects.

The effects of illicit drug use on the lungs are diverse and most commonly follow smoking or intravenous injection. Many infectious and noninfectious complications may arise acutely or chronically. Patterns of drug abuse frequently change as different drugs gain popularity. Thus, the clinician must maintain a high suspicion for drug use and must remain informed of current drug use trends to provide optimal care for drug users.

1. Heffner JE, Harley RA, Schabel SI. Pulmonary reactions from illicit substance abuse. *Clin Chest Med.* 1990;11:151.
   A comprehensive review that divides subject material by both drug type and common complications.
2. Hind CRK. Pulmonary complications of intravenous drug misuse. I: Epidemiology and non-infective complications. *Thorax.* 1990;45:891.
3. Hind CRK. Pulmonary complications of intravenous drug misuse. II: Infective and HIV related complications. *Thorax.* 1990;45:957.
   References 3 and 4 provide an excellent review of the subject.
4. Wolff AJ, O'Donnell AE. Pulmonary effects of illicit drug use. *Clin Chest Med.* 2004;25:203–216.
   An excellent, detailed review of the literature.
5. Tashkin DP. Airway effects of marijuana, cocaine, and other inhaled illicit agents. *Curr Opin Pulm Med.* 2001;7:43–61.
   An excellent review of the pathophysiology and consequences of inhaled drugs.
6. Cruz R, Davis M, O'Neil H, et al. Pulmonary manifestations of inhaled street drugs. *Heart Lung.* 1998;27:297.
   A review article providing a historical prospective of street drugs, along with their common clinical sequelae.
7. Joseph WL, Fletcher HS, Giordano JM, et al. Pulmonary and cardiovascular implications of drug addiction. *Ann Thorac Surg.* 1973;15:263.
   A good general reference.
8. Haim DY, Lippmann ML, Goldberg SK, et al. The pulmonary complications of crack cocaine. A comprehensive review. *Chest.* 1995;107:233.
   A thorough review of the pulmonary manifestations of cocaine use.
9. Thadani PV. NIDA conference report on cardiopulmonary complications of crack cocaine use. *Chest.* 1996;110:1072.
   Summarizes the pulmonary and cardiac complications of crack cocaine use.
10. Saba GP II, James AE Jr, Johnson BA, et al. Pulmonary complications of narcotic abuse. *Am J Roentgenol Radium Ther Nucl Med.* 1974;122:733.
    Reviews the radiographic appearances of the various complications that result from narcotic abuse.
11. O'Donnell AE, Pappas LS. Pulmonary complications of intravenous drug abuse. Experience at an inner-city hospital. *Chest.* 1988;94:251.
12. O'Donnell AE, Selig J, Aravamuthan M, et al. Pulmonary complications associated with illicit drug use. An update. *Chest.* 1995;108:460.
    References 10 and 11 catalog the experiences of a pulmonary consult service with an inner city drug-abusing patient population.
13. Jaffe RB, Koschmann EB. Septic pulmonary emboli. *Radiology.* 1970;96:527.
    Compilation of the radiographic manifestations of septic pulmonary emboli in 17 patients.
14. Reichman LB, Felton CP, Edsall JR. Drug dependence, a possible new risk factor for tuberculosis disease. *Arch Intern Med.* 1979;139:337.
    Demonstrates that drug dependence is a risk factor for the development of active tuberculosis.

15. Baldwin GC, Tashkin DP, Buckley DM, et al. Marijuana and cocaine impair alveolar macrophage function and cytokine production. *Am J Respir Crit Care Med.* 1997;156:1606.

    Demonstrates impairment of cytokine function from the alveolar macrophages in users of marijuana or cocaine.

16. Hamadeh R, Ardehali A, Locksley RM, et al. Fatal aspergillosis associated with smoking contaminated marijuana, in a marrow transplant recipient. *Chest.* 1988;94:432.

    Contaminated marijuana caused invasive aspergillosis in an immunosuppressed host.

17. Llamas R, Hart DR, Schneider NS. Allergic bronchopulmonary aspergillosis associated with smoking moldy marijuana. *Chest.* 1978;73:871.

    Case report that associates allergic bronchopulmonary aspergillosis with smoking Aspergillus-laden marijuana.

18. Steinberg AD, Karliner JS. The clinical spectrum of heroin pulmonary edema. *Arch Intern Med.* 1968;122:122.

    A series of 16 patients that emphasizes the variability in the presentation of heroin-induced noncardiogenic pulmonary edema.

19. Duberstein JL, Kaufman DM. A clinical study of an epidemic of heroin intoxication and heroin-induced pulmonary edema. *Am J Med.* 1971;51:704.

    A series of 149 cases of heroin intoxication and its complications.

20. Murray RJ, Albin RJ, Mergner W, et al. Diffuse alveolar hemorrhage temporally related to cocaine smoking. *Chest.* 1988;93:427.

    A case report linking cocaine inhalation with life-threatening hemoptysis.

21. Waller BF, Brownlee WJ, Roberts WC. Self-induced pulmonary granulomatosis. A consequence of intravenous injection of drugs intended for oral use. *Chest.* 1980;78:90.

    An instructive case report that reviews the pathophysiology of pulmonary hypertension and pulmonary granulomatosis.

22. Ward S, Heyneman LE, Reittner P, et al. Talcosis associated with IV abuse of oral medications: CT findings. *Am J Roentgenol.* 2000;174:789–93.

    This report describes the CT findings of 12 patients with talcosis.

23. Douglas FG, Kafilmout KJ, Patt NL. Foreign particle embolism in drug addicts: respiratory pathophysiology. *Ann Intern Med.* 1971;75:865.

    A series of cases outlining the sequelae of foreign body granulomas.

24. Tashkin DP, Kleerup EC, Koyal SN, et al. Acute effects of inhaled and IV cocaine on airway dynamics. *Chest.* 1996;110:904.

    Demonstrates a decrease in airway conductance after the use of inhaled cocaine.

25. Goldstein DS, Karpel JP, Appel D, et al. Bullous pulmonary damage in users of intravenous drugs. *Chest.* 1986;89:266.

    A retrospective study linking bullous pulmonary disease to use of illicit drugs.

26. Corbridge T, Cygan J, Greenberger P. Substance abuse and acute asthma. *Intensive Care Med.* 2000;26:347–349.

    An overview of several recent studies, including two medical examiner studies, that evaluates the role of substance abuse in fatal asthma.

27. Mayo-Smith MF, Spinale J. Thermal epiglottitis in adults: a new complication of illicit drug use. *J Emerg Med.* 1997;15:483–485.

    Reports four cases of acute epiglottitis caused by thermal injury after crack or marijuana use.

28. Banner AS, Rodriguez J, Sunderrajan EV, et al. Bronchiectasis: a cause of pulmonary symptoms in heroin addicts. *Respiration.* 1979;37:232.

    A series of seven case reports linking the development of bronchiectasis to heroin use.

29. Lewis JW Jr, Groux N, Elliott JP Jr, et al. Complications of attempted central venous injections performed by drug abusers. *Chest.* 1980;78:613.

    A series of case reports that document the various complications related to IV drug injected into the central venous system.

30. Seaman ME. Barotrauma related to inhalational drug abuse. *J Emerg Med.* 1990;8:141.

Reports of inhaled drug use resulting in pneumothorax and pneumomediastinum.

31. Barsky SH, Roth MD, Kleerup EC, et al. Histopathologic and molecular alterations in bronchial epithelium in habitual smokers of marijuana, cocaine and/or tobacco. *J Natl Cancer Inst.* 1998;90:1198.

Marijuana and cocaine smokers have alterations at the histologic and molecular levels consistent with carcinogenesis.

32. Yuan M, Kiertscher SM, Cheng Q, et al. Delta 9-tetrahydrocannabinol regulates Th1/Th2 cytokine balance in activated human T cells. *J Neuroimmunol.* 2002;133:124–131.

THC was shown to alter T cell proliferation and decrease T cell immunity.

23. TOBACCO CONTROL

David M. Burns

Cigarette smoking causes lung cancer, oral cancer, laryngeal cancer, esophageal cancer, kidney cancer, bladder cancer, pancreatic cancer, leukemia, cervical cancer, stomach cancer, abdominal aortic aneurysm, atherosclerotic peripheral vascular disease, cerebrovascular disease, coronary heart disease, and chronic obstructive pulmonary disease. The use of oral contraceptives increases the risk of vascular disease in women who smoke, and there are higher fetal and maternal complications of pregnancy if women smoke during the last 6 months of pregnancy. In addition, there is sufficient evidence to suggest that smoking causes cataracts, hip fractures, low bone density, peptic ulcer disease, and adverse surgical outcomes resulting from poor wound healing and respiratory complications in women (or in both men and women).

The major goals of tobacco control interventions are prevention of tobacco initiation and cessation of tobacco use. Prevention of smoking initiation is an important public health goal in itself, but near-term reduction in disease rates can only be achieved by cessation, which is also the only means by which current cigarette smokers can reduce their risk of disease. Prevention of initiation among adolescents contributes little to reduction in disease rates until 30 years or more after the point at which they would have started to smoke.

Tobacco control is intended to influence individual tobacco use, but tobacco control interventions may be focused on the individual smoker (e.g., pharmacologic treatment) or the environment (e.g., restrictions on where smoking is allowed). Since the 1960s, tobacco control strategies have gradually transitioned from being focused exclusively on the individual smoker toward an understanding of the role of the environment in promoting and enhancing cessation. Efforts to educate the smoker and clinic-based cessation assistance have been supplemented by efforts to change community norms, increase the cost of cigarettes, restrict where smoking is allowed, and provide societal-based persistent and inescapable messages to quit coupled with support for cessation. The current belief is that an effective program is a multilayered approach that offers a menu of options for cessation assistance supported by changes in social norms, restrictions on smoking behavior, and increased psychological and financial cost of tobacco use.

Changes in public policies on tobacco can affect large numbers of individuals at minimal cost, and they are currently felt to be the most powerful tools in altering smoking behavior. Increases in the price of cigarettes have repeatedly been linked to a reduction in total and per capita cigarette consumption; most studies have shown a relatively consistent effect of a 4% decline in consumption for each 10% increase in price. More limited data are available for cessation, but it appears that an increase in the cost of cigarettes can also influence both short-term cessation attempts and long-term cessation success.

There has been a dramatic increase in the fraction of the working population protected by total bans on smoking in the workplace, from 3% in 1986 to 70% in 2001. Multiple workplace observations have demonstrated that instituting a change in workplace smoking restrictions is accompanied by an increase in cessation attempts and a reduction in number of cigarettes smoked per day. Once restrictions on smoking in the workplace have been successfully implemented, they continue to reduce the number of cigarettes smoked per day and increase the success rate of smokers attempting to quit.

The healthcare system has long been recognized as a logical and potentially productive means of reaching smokers with a cessation message and increasing the chances of successful cessations. Approximately 70% of smokers see a physician each year, offering the potential to reach large numbers of smokers with advice to quit. The fraction of patients who report receiving cessation advice in the last year by their physician remains too low, but it has been increasing over time and now exceeds 50% of all smokers. The US Food and Drug Administration has approved a variety of pharmacologic approaches to smoking cessation over the last 2 decades, including nicotine replacement therapy with gum, patches, nasal and oral inhalers; clonidine; and bupropion. The nicotine patch and gum have been approved for over-the-counter sale since 1996.

Multiple controlled clinical trials have demonstrated that both physician advice and pharmacologic treatment have substantial effects on long-term successful smoking cessation. In their offices, physicians should record a patient's smoking history, motivate the smoker to quit, negotiate a quit date, follow up the quit attempt, and notify the smoker about additional cessation assistance. When physicians provide this type of intervention, they can double the rate of long-term successful cessation in their patients. In addition, physician encouragement can also double the likelihood that a patient will participate in more structured cessation assistance, such as a smoking clinic. Once these interventions move beyond the controlled investigational setting, with the careful attention to detail of the intervention protocol, and are used in isolation without the structure and support provided by a clinical trial, it is likely that they have less impact on the smoker.

The gap between the effect achieved in clinical trials and population-based data defines the potential that can be achieved if these strategies are delivered in a more comprehensive, organized manner and integrated with other available cessation resources. If physician advice can achieve the effectiveness demonstrated in clinical trials, it could result in as many as 750,000 additional quits among the 35 million smokers who visit physicians each year. If the success rate of pharmacologic interventions matched that in clinical trials, as many as 500,000 additional quits could be achieved each year; and an even greater number could be expected if more smokers who are trying to quit could be persuaded to use pharmacologic aids.

Improving the effectiveness of these interventions requires focusing resources on enhancing the capacity of other tobacco control structures to support pharmacologic- and physician-based interventions. This can be accomplished by reducing barriers to access (particularly cost) of cessation aids and linking them with other existing tobacco control interventions. For example, linking physician advice with telephone hotline counseling, providing information at community events on how to use over-the-counter medications effectively, and encouraging healthcare systems to view cessation as a population-based intervention in messages delivered by various media rather than coming exclusively from physicians could enhance effectiveness. To obtain maximal benefit, we need to integrate tobacco control interventions into healthcare delivery systems, link them to community cessation resources, and create an environment that encourages access. When this is done, dramatic improvements in population-based rates of cessation are possible.

There is concern that successful cessation by more than half those who have ever smoked has left behind a residual population of smokers who have more difficulty quitting and are more resistant to tobacco control interventions. Despite this compelling logic, there is little evidence that current smokers are quitting at lower rates or that tax increases and other tobacco control efforts are losing their influence on smoking behavior.

Two common components of most comprehensive tobacco control programs are mass media and self-help materials. They share the ability to reach large numbers of individuals at relatively low cost. However, they also share the misconception that they are autonomous interventions whereby cessation goals are achieved simply by delivering self-help materials or exposing the smoker to the media message. It is clear that both of these tobacco control channels are just that: channels. They are methods by which other tobacco control interventions can be facilitated, reinforced, and publicized and by which agendas can be set; however, in isolation, without integration into a more comprehensive approach, they have little effect.

Changing the environment in which the smoker lives and smokes to provide persistent and inescapable messages to quit while giving support for cessation has been a goal of most comprehensive tobacco control approaches, but accomplishing this goal has been problematic. Comprehensive statewide programs in California and Massachusetts have reduced smoking behaviors and disease risks, and are models for programs in other states. Unfortunately, downturns in tax revenue and political pressures have dramatically reduced or eliminated the funding for state tobacco control efforts and are likely to minimize their future impact.

Considerable data support the effectiveness of telephone counseling services in promoting long-term successful cessation. Several newer approaches to individualized counseling have recently been developed that can provide assistance to the general population of smokers. Computer-based interactive software can tailor the intervention and counseling provided to the individual smoker. The possibility of providing this kind of customized intervention over the Internet, in public locations where smokers have access, on home computers, or in hand-held devices could overcome some of the traditional resistance of smokers to the more intensive, but more effective, smoking cessation interventions.

Community and local activities are the foundations of comprehensive tobacco control programs. However, because they are so broad-based, it is difficult to independently quantify them as interventions and to demonstrate their association with individual or population-based cessation activity and success. Nevertheless, the fact that we have limited tools to measure community interventions accurately does not necessarily mean that community programs have a limited effect.

Current models of smoking behavior postulate that smokers cycle through stages during which they are disinterested in cessation, contemplate quitting, make a quit attempt, and are either successful or relapse back to smoking. Smoking relapse can be followed by a period of disinterest in cessation or the smoker may think about making an additional cessation attempt. Individual components of a comprehensive tobacco control program may affect the process of cessation at different stages. For example, public information campaigns can help smokers think about the need to quit, physician advice may trigger a cessation attempt, and working in a smoke-free environment may facilitate cessation once the attempt is made. Public information about the risks of smoking, negative images of the smoker, and physician warnings about risks can all convince a smoker to attempt to quit. In addition, the desire to set a good example for children and concern about being dependent on smoking are reasons smokers give for wanting to quit. Acute illness can also trigger cessation activity.

The forces influencing smoking cessation attempts may be different from those that lead to longer term successful cessation. For example, older smokers are less likely to report making a cessation attempt in the last 12 months, but they are more likely to quit successfully for 3 or more months based on that attempt. This observation suggests that efforts to promote cessation among older smokers can yield important benefits even in the face of their lower rates of attempts.

---

1. Agency for Health Care Policy and Research. *Smoking Cessation: Clinical Practice Guideline*. Rockville, Md: US Department of Public Health and Human Services, Public Health Service, Agency for Health Care Policy and Research; 2000.

A comprehensive review of what has been proved to be effective with interventions in the clinical practice setting, based on comprehensive meta-analyses of existing literature and best judgment of experts.

2. Brownson RC, Eriksen MP, Davis RM, et al. Environmental tobacco smoke: health effects and policies to reduce exposure. *Annu Rev Public Health.* 1997;18: 163.

    A good review of the health effects of environmental tobacco smoke exposure and the effects of implementing a smoke-free workplace on reducing the number of cigarettes smoked per day and increasing smoking cessation.

3. Centers for Disease Control and Prevention. *Best practices for comprehensive tobacco control programs—August 1999.* Atlanta, Ga: Department of Health and Human Services, Centers for Disease Control and Prevention, National Center for Chronic Disease Prevention and Health Promotion, Office on Smoking and Health; August 1999.

    Recommendations for content and budgets of comprehensive state tobacco control campaigns.

4. Centers for Disease Control and Prevention. Cigarette smoking among adults— United States, 2002. *MMWR.* 2004;53:427.

    Recent data on the prevalence of smoking in the United States from the National Health interview survey.

5. Curry SJ, Grothaus LC, McAfee T, et al. Use and cost effectiveness of smoking-cessation services under four insurance plans in a health maintenance organization. *N Engl J Med.* 1998;339:673.

    Describes the effectiveness of a comprehensive healthcare, systems-based smoking cessation program, which increased successful cessation by 2.4-fold and demonstrated the importance of removing financial barriers to accessing cessation assistance on increasing participation in cessation assistance programs.

6. Johnston LD, O' Malley PM, Bachman JG, et al. *Monitoring the Future: National Survey Results on Drug Use, 1975–2003. Vol I. Secondary School Students* (NIH Publication No. 04-5507). Bethesda, Md: National Institute on Drug Abuse; 2004. http://monitoringthefuture.org/

    Demonstrates the recent national trends of declining adolescent initiation of cigarette smoking in the context of other adolescent drug use.

7. Jorenby DE, Leischow SJ, Nides MA, et al. A controlled trial of sustained release bupropion, a nicotine patch, or both for smoking cessation. *N Engl J Med.* 1999;340:685.

    A clinical trial demonstrating the clinical utility of bupropion and nicotine patches in treating nicotine dependence, with a suggestion that the two therapies used together may be even more effective than when they are used independently.

8. National Cancer Institute. Cigar smoking in the United States: health effects and trends. Burns D, Cummings KM, Hoffman D, eds. Smoking and Tobacco Control Monograph No. 9. USDHHS NIH NCI, 1998.

    A comprehensive review of cigar smoking and its disease consequences, recent changes in cigar smoking behavior, and the chemical composition of cigar smoke.

9. National Cancer Institute. Those who continue to smoke: is achieving abstinence harder and do we need to change our interventions? Smoking and Tobacco Control Monograph No. 15. USDHHS, NIH, NCI, NIH Pub. No. 03-5370, 2003. http://cancercontrol.cancer.gov/tcrb/monographs/15/index.html

    A review of the trends in cessation demonstrating that existing tobacco control efforts continue to work and that the residual smoking population continues to be influenced by them.

10. National Cancer Institute. Risks associated with smoking cigarettes with low machine-measured yields of tar and nicotine. Smoking and Tobacco Control Monograph, No. 13 USDHHS, PHS, NIH, NCI, 2001. http://cancercontrol.cancer.gov/tcrb/monographs/13/

    A review of existing evidence, which reaches the conclusion that the changes in cigarette design over the past 50 years have not reduced the disease risks of smoking.

11. Prochaska JO, DiClemente CC. Stages and processes of self-change in smoking: toward an integrative model of change. *J Consult Clin Psychol.* 1991;59:295.
    A classic article demonstrating the repetitive cycling of smokers through stages of smoking behavior, which sequentially reflect (1) disinterest in cessation, (2) interest in cessation, (3) cessation attempts, and (4) success or failure.
12. Schroeder SA. Tobacco control in the wake of the 1998 master settlement agreement. *N Engl J Med.* 2004;350:293–301.
    A thoughtful review of the current challenges in tobacco control.
13. US Department of Health and Human Services. *Reducing Tobacco Use: A Report of the Surgeon General.* Atlanta, Ga: US Department of Health and Human Services, Public Health Service, Centers for Disease Control and Prevention, National Center for Chronic Disease Prevention and Health Promotion, Office on Smoking and Health, 2000 http://www.cdc.gov/tobacco/sgr/sgr_2000/index.htm.
    A careful review of the current evidence for major tobacco control interventions.
14. US Department of Health and Human Services. *The Health Consequences of Smoking: A Report of the Surgeon General.* Atlanta, Ga: US Department of Health and Human Services, Public Health Service, Centers for Disease Control and Prevention, National Center for Chronic Disease Prevention and Health Promotion, Office on Smoking and Health,2004 http://www.cdc.gov/tobacco/sgr/sgr_2004/index.htm.
    An encyclopedic description of the disease consequences of smoking and the evidence supporting a causal relationship with smoking.
15. US Department of Health and Human Services. *The Health Consequences of Involuntary Exposure to Tobacco Smoke.* Atlanta: US Department of Health and Human Services, Public Health Service, Centers for Disease Control and Prevention, National Center for Chronic Disease Prevention and Health Promotion, Office on Smoking and Health, (in preparation, 2006).
    Extensively documented review of the disease consequences of environmental tobacco smoke exposure.

Web Sites
CDC web site for state-specific tobacco control information
http://www.cdc.gov/tobacco/statehi/statehi.htm
Department of Agriculture web site for tobacco consumption data
http://www.ers.usda.gov/publications/so/view.asp?f=specialty/tbs-bb/
Agency for Health Care Policy Research web site for clinical practice guidelines
http://text.nlm.nih.gov/ftrs/tocview
National Cancer Institute Smoking and Tobacco Control monograph series
http://www.naccho.org/LINK185.cfm

24. TERRORISM: DISASTER MEDICINE FROM THE PULMONOLOGIST'S PERSPECTIVE

Dennis Amundson, Asha Devereaux, and John Parrish

A comprehensive approach to disaster medicine requires a blend of Emergency and Public Health Medicine principles. Planning for disasters is oriented to low probability-high impact occurrences. Most disasters result from natural events and produce injuries familiar to acute care physicians. However, acts of terrorism involving chemical, biological, and nuclear agents present unique situations beyond the practical experience of most healthcare providers. Because of the nature of these injuries, pulmonologists will likely play a prominent role in managing these patients.

CHEMICAL EXPOSURE

After intentional chemical exposure, patients most frequently present with manifestations of toxic inhalation of common industrial agents, such as chlorine and organophosphate products or products of combustion. Chemical substances can be classified as inhalational toxins that primarily affect the lungs or neurotoxic agents that primarily involve the central nervous system. If appropriate hazardous materials (HAZMAT) assessment is available, prompt identification of the agent will allow the clinician to prepare specific antidotes and treatment supplies before the patient's arrival.

Inhalational Toxins

Inhalational toxins may be classified as (1) direct respiratory irritants and (2) airway vesicants. Chemical asphyxiants such as carbon monoxide, hydrogen cyanide, and hydrogen sulfide may produce significant morbidity, but do not cause pulmonary injury.

Direct Respiratory Irritants (Chlorine, Phosgene)

Chlorine is a highly reactive greenish yellow gas that is 2.5 times as dense as air. It is used in the production of chemicals, bleaching and plastics processing, and in a variety of recreational and household settings (e.g., swimming pools, cleaning solutions). Previously it was thought that chlorine reacted with tissue water to form hydrochloric acid and oxygen radicals and caused significant mucosal irritation. However, hydrochloric acid is much less toxic than chlorine, and recent animal studies demonstrate that chlorine directly damages the respiratory system via oxidative injury of epithelial proteins. Severe or prolonged exposures can result in ulcerative tracheobronchitis, diffuse alveolar damage with hyaline membrane formation, and pulmonary edema.

Phosgene and diphosgene have both been used in chemical warfare. These agents are poorly soluble in water and, thus, have a delayed onset of action (30 minutes to 8 hours). Initial exposure produces a burning sensation of the mucus membranes of the eyes, nose, throat, and upper respiratory tract. More severe exposures can result in cough, wheezing, stridor, dyspnea, hypotension, and noncardiogenic pulmonary edema. Development of acute lung injury after exposure to phosgene carries a poor prognosis.

Treatment of respiratory irritant exposure is supportive with bronchodilators and local care. The use of steroids has been advocated, but is of unproven benefit.

Vesicants (Mustards)

The mustard compounds are a family of similar agents that have had significant use on the battlefield, either alone or in combination with other chemical and biological agents. The most common agent is sulfur mustard, which has a simple structure and is easily produced with ingredients typically used to manufacture plastics. Mustards are oily, light yellow-brown, fat-soluble substances that are heavier than water and become liquids at room temperature. Mustard vapor, which smells like garlic, is heavier than air and concentrates in low-lying areas. Because of its low volatility, mustard can persist in an environment for up to 5 days. Liquid mustard is rapidly absorbed and hydrolyzed in extracellular fluid. Within 2 minutes of exposure, mustard can irreversibly alkylate cellular DNA, resulting in necrotic cell death. Also, within minutes target organs irreversibly bind the chemical agent, making delayed elimination difficult, if not impossible. Skin, eye, airway, bone marrow, gastrointestinal, and nervous system findings predominate. The clinical effects of mustard toxicity typically begin 2 to 48 hours after exposure. More severe exposures are heralded by earlier onset of signs and symptoms. Typical manifestations include skin blistering, eye, and airway symptoms resulting from direct irritant effects. Incapacitating respiratory tract injury can occur at vapor exposures significantly lower than those that cause skin blistering. A sore throat or productive cough that begins within 4 hours of exposure implies lower respiratory tract involvement and should prompt immediate airway evaluation and intervention. Sloughing and ulceration of the trachea and bronchi can lead to obstruction. Pseudomembrane formation may cause necrotic obstruction that can complicate airway management. Mortality soon after exposure is most often related to pulmonary complications. Later mortality is usually due to bone marrow suppression and septic complications of lung injury and superficial skin lesions.

The initial approach to mustard gas contact is to minimize further exposure. Primary preventive techniques with barriers, such as protective clothing and lotions, may provide limited protection. Effective and early decontamination maneuvers (within 5 minutes) can remove residual agents on the skin. In contrast to treatment of thermal burns, care of chemical dermal wounds should include addressing large blisters or bullae with frequent irrigation and application of topical antibiotics. Because of the superficial nature of chemical burns compared with heat-related burns, skin grafting is seldom needed and initial fluid requirements are not as great. Pain management includes the judicious use of oral or systemic narcotics. Topical mydriatics, lubricating ocular gels, and local anesthetics can help relieve irritant ocular pain and later scarring. Humidified air and cough suppressants help soothe inhalational injury. Bronchodilator therapy is the mainstay of treatment. Airway control should be considered if dysphonia, cough, or respiratory distress occurs soon after exposure. The role of corticosteroids is controversial; however, they may be useful in severe cases. Antibiotics should be reserved for confirmed cases of infectious pneumonia. Sulfur-containing drugs should be avoided because they may potentiate the cellular injury caused by sulfur mustard exposure. In some animal studies, pretreatment or treatment within 20 minutes of exposure with N-acetylcysteine (Mucomyst, Mucosil-20) eliminated some of the organ damage. Some experts recommend post-exposure treatment with intravenous sodium thiosulfate (500 mg/kg per day) for 48 hours, followed by 10 days of oral N-acetylcysteine and vitamin C. Although sulfates are contraindicated with mustard exposure, preparations that act as sulfur donors have minimized systemic effects and elevated the lethal dose in research animals. Persons who have been exposed to mustard are at significant risk for long-term effects, particularly lung and upper airway cancers. Persons with respiratory exposure may experience asthma or syndromes similar to chronic obstructive pulmonary disease.

Neurotoxic Agents

In the 1930s, German scientists developed toxic "nerve agents" in industrial organophosphate factories. The four major compounds are tabun, sarin, soman, and VX. These agents inhibit the ability of acetylcholinesterase to hydrolyze acetylcholine. The accumulation of acetylcholine produces excess stimulation of nicotinic and muscarinic receptors.

The attachment of the nerve agent to the enzyme becomes permanent through a process called "aging" when acetylcholinesterase cleaves a portion of the bound nerve agent to produce a stable bond. The time required for aging varies, ranging from 2 minutes for soman to hours for other nerve agents. If administered prior to aging, several compounds can remove the nerve agent from the enzyme. The most important group of such compounds is the oximes. Nerve agents are liquids that may constitute both a liquid hazard and a vapor hazard during dispersal. All the agents except VX are volatile at room temperature. The vapors, which are heavier than air, are concentrated in low-lying areas. All nerve agents rapidly penetrate clothing, skin, and mucous membranes. They may be absorbed by inhalation, ingestion, or dermal contact. Symptoms depend on the route of exposure and dose. After dermal contact, symptoms may be delayed for up to 18 hours; however, after inhalation, symptoms occur within seconds to minutes.

The clinical manifestations of nerve agent toxicity reflect the hyperstimulation of muscarinic and nicotinic receptors in the nervous system. Muscarinic effects include rhinorrhea, pinpoint pupils, blurred vision, hypersecretion by glands (e.g., salivary, lacrimal, sweat, respiratory), bronchospasm, nausea, vomiting, diarrhea, bradycardia, abdominal pain, and bowel and bladder incontinence. Nicotinic effects include skeletal muscle twitching, cramping, weakness, tachycardia, and hypertension. Mild exposure results in rhinorrhea, pinpoint pupils, bronchospasm, increased secretions, and dyspnea. More severe exposures cause muscle fasciculations, nausea, vomiting, diarrhea, unconsciousness, seizures, paralysis, apnea, and death. Patients who survive exposure to nerve agents may experience fatigue, irritability, and memory impairment for weeks after recovery from the short-term effects.

The management of patients begins with a careful assessment of airway, breathing, and circulation. Victims should be separated from the source of exposure and rapidly decontaminated. Clothing should be removed, eyes flushed with water for 5 to 10 minutes, and skin washed with soap and water. Antidotes for nerve agent poisoning are atropine sulfate and pralidoxime chloride (2-PAM Protopam Chloride). The initial dose of atropine is 2 to 6 mg intramuscularly (IM), depending on the severity of exposure, followed by 2 mg IM every 5 to 10 minutes until secretions and dyspnea or airway obstruction are minimized. As an oxime, 2-PAM acts as an acetylcholinesterase reactivator that binds the nerve agent and removes it from the enzyme. The initial dose is 600 to 1,800 mg IM, depending on the severity of exposure. Diazepam (Valium) can be used as an adjunct to control seizures.

In the case of exposure to a chemical agent or "dirty" bomb radiation, the critical care physician should not assume that the patient has been adequately decontaminated. It is likely that many casualties will either arrive directly at area hospitals or be transported with only partial decontamination owing to the presence of an agent in traumatic wounds. Prompt removal of clothing will significantly reduce further systemic absorption and has been shown to be approximately 90% effective in decontamination when performed at the site of exposure. Providing medical care to a contaminated patient will tax even the most practiced clinician. Personal protective equipment (PPE) such as gas masks, respirators, and thick overgarments lead to heat stress within 30 minutes and make adequate communication with the patient and staff nearly impossible. Manual dexterity is also compromised. It should be noted that chemical agents traverse latex gloves readily and double gloves should be changed every 20 minutes. Wash the patient with lukewarm water and mild soap rather than hypochlorite bleach solution because bleach can potentiate further chemical injury. Eyes, mucus membranes, and wounds should be irrigated for at least 2 minutes with normal saline. In late 2003, the Food and Drug Administration (FDA) cleared, for limited use, a reactive skin decontamination lotion (RSDL): a broad-spectrum, viscous liquid decontamination solution that can neutralize chemical warfare agents and T-2 fungal toxin in the skin. This lotion, created by the Defense R&D of Canada, leaves a nontoxic residue, which then washes off safely with water.

Biologic Agents
The biologic agents that concern pulmonary physicians include "biologic toxins" (Ricin and botulinum), "infecting zoonoses" (anthrax, plague, tularemia), and communicable viruses (smallpox, viral encephalitides). The agents that pose the most likely threat include: anthrax, smallpox, plague, and Ricin. Recently, anthrax and Ricin have been intentionally released; smallpox and plague present a substantial communicable risk to the population.

Anthrax
Anthrax is caused by the spore-forming *Bacillus anthracis*. Historically it is a disease of skin contamination (Woolsorter's disease). Recently it has been used as an aerosolized bioweapon. To produce respiratory infection, 3,000 to 5,000 airborne spores (3 to 5 microns in size) must be inhaled and transported to hilar and mediastinal lymph nodes. Rapid transition to the bacillary form leads to massive toxin production. Acute disease initially resembles a severe influenza-like illness, followed by rapid progression to sepsis, shock, multiorgan failure, and death. Hemorrhagic transformation occurs in mediastinal lymph nodes. Inhalational anthrax has a high fatality rate (50 to 70%). Diagnosis requires clinical suspicion and assessment for mediastinal widening in a severely ill patients. Treatment is predicated on the early use of effective antibiotics (usually a combination of ciprofloxacin, rifampin, and/or clindamycin), complete pleural drainage, and meticulous intensive care unit (ICU) care. A vaccine against the bacterial toxin has been developed and is an integral part of the epidemiologic approach to an anthrax event. Prolonged chemoprophylaxis with ciprofloxacin or doxycycline, with or without vaccine, has been used in potentially exposed patients.

Plague

Plague is caused by *Yersinia pestis,* a gram-negative coccobacillary organism. It holds a historic place in pandemic human diseases. A rodent zoonosis, plague occurs naturally in endemic areas and is usually acquired by direct exposure to infected animals. There are three forms: (1) bubonic (lymphadenitis); (2) septicemic (usually from hematogenous spread); and (3) pneumonic (the greatest threat as a biowarfare agent). Pneumonic plague produces a severe, overwhelming pneumonia with hemoptysis and, usually, mediastinal and hilar lymphadenopathy. Shock and death occur within 2 to 6 days with mortality approaching 60%. Treatment is with IM streptomycin or gentamycin (IV/IM). Alternative agents include doxycycline, ciprofloxacin or chloramphenicol. Antibiotics must be administered early to improve survival. Persons with possible exposure should receive chemoprophylaxis with oral doxycycline or ciprofloxacin. No plague vaccine is currently available.

Smallpox

Smallpox is caused by the *Variola* virus and is responsible for an historical infection that was believed to be eradicated in 1980. It is likely that it still exists in bioweapons arsenals in many countries. Smallpox is extremely contagious and clinical disease carries a 30% mortality rate. A rash/fever syndrome occurs after a prolonged incubation period. The rash is similar to chickenpox and any severe case of "chickenpox" should be suspect for smallpox. Respiratory symptoms can occur owing to mucosal lesions or secondary infection. Currently, there is no effective treatment for acute infections. The public health approach is predicated on prevention and control by isolation, cohorting, and ring vaccination strategies. An antiretroviral agent, cidofovir, shows promise and is being tested for therapy.

Ricin

Ricin is a biologic toxin consisting of a protein extracted from the seed of the castor bean plant. It is easy to produce and highly toxic. Exposure to the freeze-dried powder can occur through inhalation, ingestion, or injection. Ricin causes ribosomal inactivation in cells to produce necrotic cell death. Inhaled Ricin causes rapidly progressive, severe respiratory failure with pulmonary edema within 3 hours and is frequently fatal. There is no antidote, although a vaccine is under development.

Ionizing Radiation Exposure

Ionizing radiation exposure arising from accidents or acts of terrorism has the potential for creating catastrophic mass casualties. Significant exposure to ionizing radiation may result from a single point source (e.g., radiation dispersal device [RDD], or "dirty bomb"]), accident or sabotage in a nuclear power plant, or detonation of a nuclear weapon. The potential use of an RDD, a device that combines conventional explosives and radioactive material, is of significant concern, given the widespread availability of these materials in industry, research, and healthcare within our society. The effects following exposure can be predicted from the type and duration of exposure. An individual's radiation dose can be estimated by determining the time to onset and severity of prodromal symptoms (nausea and vomiting), the decline in absolute lymphocyte count over the first 48 hours, and the appearance of chromosome aberrations in peripheral blood lymphocytes. Exposure can be in the form of local irradiation, whole body irradiation, external contamination, internal contamination, or a combination. Frequently the adverse effects of radiation exposure are seen in association with traumatic injuries. Regardless of the scenario, the principles of decontamination and treatment of casualties arising from radiation events remain the same.

The management of radiation exposure initially should consist of actions to: (1) minimize exposure time, (2) increase distance from the source, and (3) maximize shielding. Decontamination efforts should be initiated in the field. All uninjured but externally contaminated individuals can be decontaminated without medical interventions. Simply removing clothing and washing the skin with soap and warm water is effective in removing more than 99% of external contamination. Injured contaminated patients pose unique problems for the healthcare facility. Treatment of life-threatening injuries always takes precedence over decontamination (i.e., pay attention to the ABCs first). All casualties with non–life-threatening injuries should be decontaminated before treatment. Internal contamination can result from wounds, ingestion, or inhalation of radioactive material. Wounds can be decontaminated by irrigation and removal of foreign material. Debridement should be limited to devitalized tissue. Gastrointestinal decontamination may include the use of cathartics or chelating agents. Whole-lung lavage can potentially remove as much as 50% of the radioactivity after inhalation of significant amounts of material. This reduction in radioactivity is accomplished primarily through the removal of alveolar macrophages, which have engulfed contaminated particles in the alveoli and alveolar ducts.

Acute Radiation Syndrome

Acute radiation syndrome (ARS) may develop after systemic irradiation. Generally, ARS results from acute whole-body doses above 1 Gray (Gy). With exposures exceeding 10 Gy, survival is unlikely and treatment should be limited to comfort care. The syndrome progresses through four distinct phases: prodromal, latent, manifest illness, and recovery/death. After exposure, prodromal symptoms may develop within hours, but also may develop as late as 6 days after exposure. Prodromal symptoms classically consist of nausea, vomiting, and diarrhea. The duration to onset of these symptoms depends upon the dose received. Rapid onset of prodromal symptoms suggests shorter latency and predicts a more severe acute illness. After the prodromal phase, symptoms may remit for hours to days suggesting recovery, but this transient latent phase is followed by the manifest illness phase. This stage may last for weeks and is characterized by profound immunosuppression. The time course and severity of ARS depends upon the degree of exposure. A person exposed to a supralethal dose of radiation may experience all phases within hours before death. At lower doses, ARS may consist predominantly of a hematopoietic syndrome. With increasing exposure, gastrointestinal and cerebrovascular syndromes will be seen. After significant exposure, interstitial radiation pneumonitis can develop, which can progress to fibrosis.

The management of patients exposed to ionizing radiation consists of prompt decontamination and treatment of injuries, followed by a radiologic survey to determine the dose, assess prodromal symptoms, and collect samples for biodosimetry. Patients can then be triaged based on the estimated dose received and the presence or absence of other injuries. Surgery for traumatic injuries, if indicated, should be performed within 36 hours of exposure. Further surgery should be delayed for 6 weeks to allow recovery of immune function and normalization of wound healing. Depending upon the severity of the hematopoietic syndrome, treatment with cytokines, transfusions, or stem-cell transplantation may be indicated. Supportive care may include administration of antibiotics, antiemetics, antidiarrheal medications, fluids, electrolytes, and analgesics. Critical care should be provided for patients who develop multiorgan failure days to weeks after exposure, as their dose received is likely to have been less than 10 Gy. Patients who experience multiorgan failure within hours of exposure (>10 Gy) should receive expectant care.

1. Borak J, Sidell FR. Agents of chemical warfare: sulfur mustard. *Ann Emerg Med.* 1992;21:303–308.
   One of the first reviews and often-cited complete works on chemical and biologic agents.
2. Burgess J. Hospital evacuations due to hazardous materials incidents. *Am J Emerg Med.* 1999;17:16.
3. Chilcott R, Jenner J, Hotchkiss SA, et al. Evaluation of barrier creams against sulphur mustard. I. In vitro studies using human skin. *Skin Pharmacol Appl Skin Physiol.* 2002;15:225–235.
   Scientific study of differing creams as protection from mustard.

4. Cooper G, Ryan J, Galbraith K. The surgical management in war of penetrating wounds contaminated with chemical warfare agents. *J R Army Med Corps*. 1994;140:113–118.
5. Devereaux A, Amundson DE, Parrish JS, et al. Vesicants and nerve agents in chemical warfare. *Postgrad Med*. 2002;112:90–96.
   Review of chemicals used in military warfare and the clinical approach to management.
6. Feldman KA, Russel EE, Lathrop SL. An outbreak of primary pneumonic tularemia on Martha's Vineyard. *N Engl J Med*. 2001;345:1601–1606.
7. Kadivar H, Adams SC. Treatment of chemical and biological warfare injuries: insight derived from the 1984 Iraqi attack on Majnoon Island. *Mil Med*. 1991;156:171–177.
8. Kales S, Christiani DC. Acute chemical emergencies. *N Engl J Med*. 2004;19:350:800–808.
9. Lazarus A, Deveraux AV. Potential agents of chemical warfare. *Postgrad Med*. 2002;112:133–140.
10. Leiken KB, McFee RB, Walter FG, et al. *A Primer for Nuclear Terrorism*. Vol 49. St. Louis, Mo: Mosby, Inc; 479–516.
11. *Management of Terrorist Events Involving Radioactive Material*. NCRP Publication No. 138. Bethesda, Md: National Council on Radiation Protection and Measurements; 2001:54–73.
12. Martin J, Campbell HR, Iijima H, et al. Chlorine-induced injury to the airways in mice. *Am J Respir Crit Care Med*. 2003;168:568–574.
    Discussion of the pathophysiologic mechanism of chlorine injury.
13. Maynard RM, Tetley TD. Bioterrorism: the lung attack. *Thorax*. 2004;59:188–189.
14. *Medical Management of Radiological Casualties Handbook*. 2nd ed. Bethesda, Md: Armed Forces Radiology Research Institute; 2003.
15. Mettler FA, Voelz GL. *Major radiation exposure—what to expect and how to respond*. *N Engl J Med*. 2002;346:20.
16. Ricks RC, Berger ME, O'Hara F, eds. *The Medical Basis for Radiation-Accident-Preparedness. The Clinical Care of Victims*. New York, NY: Parthenon; 2002.
17. Rorison D, McPherson SJ. Acute toxic inhalations. *Environ Emerg*. 1992;10:409–435.
18. Safarinejad M, Moosavi SA, Montazeri B. Ocular injuries caused by mustard gas: diagnosis, treatment, and medical defense. *Mil Med*. 2001;166:67–70.
19. Sidell F, Borak J. Chemical warfare agents: II. Nerve agents. *Ann Emerg Med*. 1992;21:865–871.
20. Smith W, Dunn MA. Medical defense against blistering chemical warfare agents. *Arch Dermatol*. 1991;127:1207–1203.
21. Swartz MN. Recognition and management of anthrax: an update. *N Engl J Med*. 2001;345:1621–1626.
22. *The Medical Management of Chemical Casualties Handbook*. 3rd ed. USAMRICD. Bethesda, Md: Office of the Army Surgeon General; 2000.
23. Waselenko JK, MacVittie TJ, Blakely WF, et al. Medical management of the acute radiation syndrome: recommendations of the Strategic National Stockpile Radiation Working Group. *Ann Intern Med*. 2004;140:1037–1051.
    Excellent resource that provides specific guidance for the triage and management of radiation casualties. (91 ref)
24. Yu C, Burklow TR, Madsen JM. Vesicant agents and children. *Pediatr Ann*. 2003;32:254–257.

Useful Web Sites

United States Army Office of the Surgeon General. This site offers detailed military-relevant information on chemical and nerve agents. *http://sis.nlm.nih.gov/Tox/ChemWar.html*

REAC/TS Radiation Emergency Assistance: Center/Training site. Provides support to the US Department of Energy, WHO, and the International Atomic Energy Agency in the medical management of radiation accidents. Web site contains information for management of radiation emergencies and guidance for initial hospital medical management.*www.orau.gov/reacts*

Armed Forces Radiobiology Research Institute web site. Multiple references available at this web site for download including (1) *Medical Management of Radiological Casualties Handbook,* (2) *Pocket Guide for Responders to Ionizing Radiation Terrorism,* and (3) *Textbook of Military Medicine: Consequences of Nuclear Warfare. www.afrri.usuhs.mil*

Center for Disease Control and Prevention web site for Emergency Preparedness and Response. Excellent web site geared toward both natural disasters and acts of terrorism. *www.bt.cdc.gov*

American College of Radiology. Provides access to the handbook *Disaster Preparedness for Radiology Professionals. www.acr.org*

III. PULMONARY INFECTION

25. PNEUMONIA: GENERAL CONSIDERATIONS

Gordon L. Yung

Pneumonia is a term used to describe infections of the lower respiratory tract. The causative agent can be bacterial, viral, fungal, or even parasitic. In the United States, pneumonia is the sixth leading cause of death with an incidence of approximately 4 to 10 million cases each year. The term pneumonia is sometimes used interchangeably with the word pneumonitis, which describes the nonspecific state of inflammation of the lungs. Less commonly, the cause of pneumonia/pneumonitis may be unknown (idiopathic), or the result of noninfectious agents such as chemicals, stomach contents, radiation, or an autoimmune disease.

Microbial agents can be introduced into the lungs by several routes: aspiration of oropharyngeal secretions, inhalation, hematogenous spread via the pulmonary or bronchial circulation, and direct spread from surrounding structures. In many cases, breakdown in normal body defenses is responsible for infection. The interplay between body defense and microbial inoculation, including the size and virulence of the inoculum, ultimately determines the occurrence and severity of pneumonia. A thorough understanding of these factors is important in the diagnosis and management of patients with pneumonia.

Upper airway colonization of organisms and subsequent aspiration may be the most common mechanism in the pathogenesis of pneumonia. The pattern of colonization depends on the location and the patient's underlying health. Some bacteria, such as *Streptococcus pneumoniae* and *Haemophilus influenzae,* can transiently colonize healthy individuals. Mixed anaerobic flora are often found in those with poor dental hygiene. *Staphylococcus aureus* and *Pseudomonas* species can be isolated in upper airways of hospitalized patients. Some 45% of healthy adults experience microaspiration at night, but normal body defenses like cough and mucociliary clearance usually prevent bacterial colonization from progressing to infection. These defenses are compromised in patients who are intubated, debilitated, or who have altered consciousness. *Legionella* species, mycobacteria, endemic fungi, *Mycoplasma pneumoniae, Chlamydia pneumoniae,* and most viral infections are examples of pneumonia resulting from direct inhalation of organisms. Direct inhalation of airborne droplets partially accounts for the geographic and seasonal clustering of cases caused by these organisms. Hematogenous or embolic causes of pneumonia are uncommon, and usually originate from infected heart valves or thrombophlebitis. In these cases, the pulmonary circulation acts as a sieve for venous blood, with microorganisms lodging in the small vessels of the lungs to become the source of infection. Because bacteria are released in clusters from the source, they are likely to reach multiple parts of the pulmonary circulation simultaneously. Hematogenous pneumonias are, therefore, often multifocal and affect the peripheral regions of the lungs.

Patients with pneumonia resulting from infection typically present with the acute onset of cough, sputum production, fever, dyspnea, and, sometimes, pleuritic chest pain and hemoptysis. However, pneumonia resulting from noninfectious etiologies, such as malignancy, pulmonary hemorrhage, and drugs, can also occur with similar symptoms. Certain clinical and radiographic features may suggest specific organisms as the cause of pneumonia. These are discussed in subsequent chapters. In practice, however, these features are often nonspecific, and empirical treatment is usually necessary until a definitive diagnosis is made.

The initial antibiotic choice should be guided by Gram's stain results. This requires the demonstration of a satisfactory sputum sample (defined >25 polymorphonuclear leukocytes and <10 epithelial cells in each low power field) and the presence of a predominant organism (>8–10 organisms per high power field), particularly if the same bacteria is found within white blood cells. The presence of inflammatory cells without identifiable organisms should alert physicians to noninfectious causes of pneumonitis, as well as "atypical" pathogens, such as viruses, *M. pneumoniae, Legionella* species, and *Chlamydia* species. A more definitive identification of organisms and their sensitivity to antibiotics is often necessary if patients do not respond to initial treatment. For nonintubated patients, expectorated sputum is usually obtained, although its clinical utility has been debated for many years. This method is noninvasive, but the yield is decreased if antibiotics are given prior to sample collection. In addition, conventional culture techniques of sputum samples will not detect the "atypical" organisms. Finally, up to 30% of patients with pneumonia have a nonproductive cough. Although induced sputum is often obtained, its role has only been validated in pneumonia caused by tuberculosis or *Pneumocytes carinii*. For intubated patients, a negative Gram's stain and culture of an endotracheal aspiration sampled prior to antibiotic administration may be helpful to rule out pneumonia. Interpretation of a positive endotracheal aspirate is, however, more difficult because of frequent contamination of specimens derived from the endotracheal tube and upper airways in intubated patients.

Despite extensive laboratory testing, a causative organism can only be identified in about 50% of all pneumonia cases. Many patients, particularly those hospitalized and on ventilator support, may also have conditions that mimic pneumonia (e.g., atelectasis, pulmonary embolism, pulmonary hemorrhage, and vasculitis). Invasive tests are therefore used in selective cases to improve diagnostic yield.

Flexible bronchoscopy is probably the most common invasive procedure used to diagnose pneumonia. It is particularly useful in patients unable to produce a satisfactory sputum sample. It allows direct sampling of distal airway secretions from selective bronchial segments that correspond to the changes on chest radiographs. Samples are obtained either by simple washing of a bronchial segment or by bronchial alveolar lavage (BAL). Because of potential contamination while passing through upper airways, a protected brush specimen (PBS) is sometimes obtained. In most bacterial pneumonia, flexible bronchoscopy does not appear to provide any significant advantage over the noninvasive techniques in making a definitive bacterial identification. Some investigators believe that semiquantitative culture by bronchoscopy, defined as PBS $>10^3$ or BAL $>10^4$ or 10^5 colony forming units/mL, may improve the diagnostic yield. One meta-analysis showed a sensitivity and specificity of 91% and 95% for PBS, and 86 to 100% and 100% for BAL, respectively. These results may be affected by prior antibiotic administration, operator skill, and laboratory support. At this time, routine use of PBS or BAL is not recommended. However, bronchoscopy appears to have a role in identifying infection in several conditions: *P. carinii* in patients with AIDS, cytomegalovirus in posttransplant patients, and tuberculosis when there is a strong clinical suspicion despite negative expectorated sputum. In addition, bronchoscopy allows sampling for opportunistic organisms in immunocompromised patients, as well as direct visualization of airways, when bronchial obstruction is suspected. Transbronchial biopsy provides tissue evidence of invasion by microorganisms such as *Aspergillus* species, and its role appears to be limited to cases in which a differentiation between colonization and invasive disease is required. It has also been used to diagnose noninfectious causes of pneumonitis.

Other invasive techniques have been used to bypass the upper airways. Percutaneous transthoracic lung aspiration, with or without the use of fluoroscopy, uses a small-bore needle to aspirate approximately 0.5 to 2 mL of lung tissue sample. The technique appears to increase the diagnostic yield of pneumonia when combined with blood culture results, but suffers similar problems in patients who receive prior antibiotics. It is useful in cases in which mass-like lesions are present and, because contamination is less likely, it provides valuable information in cases in which multiple organisms are involved. Transtracheal aspiration was used extensively in the 1970s, primarily for the diagnosis of anaerobic infections, and in immunocompromised patients. Because of side effects and lack of expertise, its use has largely been replaced by flexible bronchoscopy. Finally, open lung biopsy, by minithoracotomy or thoracoscopy, can provide adequate tissue for histologic examination but the risks and discomfort of the procedure limit its clinical usefulness. It is only used in cases of unresolved "pneumonia," in which a noninfectious cause or an atypical organism is suspected.

In the last few years, many practice guidelines have been developed to provide a systematic approach to managing community-acquired pneumonia. Specific guidelines may concentrate on different aspects of pneumonia management, reflecting local patterns of practices. In the United States, excellent guidelines have been developed by the American Thoracic Society and the Infectious Diseases Society of America. A new joint guideline by these two societies is expected to be published in 2004. These recent guidelines focus on the identification of risk factors leading to poor outcome (often used to determine need of hospitalizations), preventive measures such as immunizations, and discharge criteria. Two questions should be asked in the initial evaluation of pneumonia: (1) Is the pneumonia community-acquired or hospital acquired? (2) What are the risk factors that may predict unusual pathogens and poor outcome?

Community-acquired pneumonia is twice as common in the winter season, and people at the extremes of age (younger than age 5 and older than age 65) are at increased risks. *S. pneumoniae* is the most common causative agent and is responsible for about 50% of all cases. Other common causes include *M. pneumoniae, C. pneumoniae,* and *H. influenzae;* and patients with comorbid conditions or who are older than age 65 are also at risk of pneumonia from *Legionella* species, *S. aureus,* and gram-negative organisms. Risk factors for increased mortality have been identified and they are used to assist physicians in deciding whether a patient should be hospitalized for treatment: age older than 65, comorbidity (e.g., diabetes mellitus, renal or congestive heart failure), altered mental status, tachycardia (>125 beats/min), tachypnea (>30/min), high fever (>38.3–40°C), hypotension (systolic blood pressure <90 mmHg), hypoxia (SaO_2 <90% or PaO_2 <60 mmHg), multilobar involvement on chest radiograph, and identification of "high-risk" pathogens such as gram-negative organisms and *S. aureus.*

Outpatient management of community-acquired pneumonia usually includes a chest radiograph and complete blood count. The role of routine sputum and blood cultures is controversial. The typical initial treatment for community-acquired pneumonia is either an extended macrolide (clarithromycin or azithromycin), or an extended spectrum fluoroquinolone (levofloxacin, moxifloxacin, or gatifloxacin). Increasingly, physicians are reluctant to use narrow spectrum antibiotics such as erythromycin or sulfamethoxazole/trimethoprim because of changes in antibiotic resistance patterns. The choice of treatment may also be influenced by local antibiotic resistance patterns, different antibiotic side effects, and spectrum of activities such as need of anaerobic coverage.

Inpatient management of community-acquired pneumonia should include sputum Gram's stain and culture, and blood culture. For hospitalized patients, initial therapy for community-acquired pneumonia usually includes a cephalosporin (such as ceftriaxone or cefuroxime) plus an extended macrolide, or an extended spectrum fluoroquinolone alone. The fluoroquinolones have subtle differences in side effects and antibacterial activities that may have significant therapeutic implications. Antibiotic treatment should be given as soon as possible, as mortality can increase even after a short delay (i.e., more than 8 hours) in receiving appropriate antibiotics.

Hospital-acquired pneumonia, also termed *nosocomial pneumonia,* is the second most common infection in hospitalized patients and the most common infection in the intensive care unit. Intubated patients are 6 to 21 times more likely to develop pneumonia, and the incidence increases with the duration of intubation and poor infection control practices. In the first 5 days of hospitalizations, *H. influenzae, S. pneumoniae,* and *S. aureus* are often isolated. Common causative organisms after the initial period of hospitalization include *P. aeruginosa, S. aureus,* anaerobic microbes, *Acinetobacter* species and other gram-negative enteric bacilli. Unlike the case in community-acquired pneumonia, mixed flora and resistant organisms also are commonly isolated in hospital-acquired pneumonia, with important therapeutic implications. Initial therapy depends on factors such as the length of hospital stay, severity of pneumonia, risk of aspiration, and other comorbidities. The respective roles of directed therapy and empiric therapy are the subject of much controversy. Details of management of hospital-acquired pneumonia are covered by a subsequent chapter.

Identification of factors that may encourage development of pneumonia is extremely important in the initial management. Patients with AIDS or who are immunosuppressed from chemotherapy or post-organ/bone marrow transplantation have increased risk of developing pneumonia from a wide variety of bacteria, viruses, fungi, and even parasites. Encapsulated organisms such as *S. pneumoniae, H. influenzae,* and *Neisseria meningitidis* commonly cause pneumonia in patients with hypogammaglobulinemia or after splenectomy. In addition, neutropenic patients are more prone to infection by gram-negative bacilli and *Aspergillus* species. Anaerobic infections should also be considered in patients with aspiration risks, whereas patients with recent influenza infection are at risk of developing *S. aureus* and pneumococcal pneumonia. Recognition of these associations would help physicians tailor their initial management of these patients.

Because of the high incidence of pneumonia by some organisms in immunocompromised patients, prophylactic therapy is being used increasingly, with promising results. Typical examples are the use of trimethoprim/sulfamethoxazole to prevent *P. carinii* pneumonia in patients with HIV disease, and ganciclovir in cytomegalovirus-mismatch transplant recipients.

In summary, patients presenting with clinical features of pneumonia should be separated into different categories, according to their presentation and comorbidities. Subsequent evaluation and treatment depend on the severity and progression of disease. It is important for physicians to differentiate pneumonia from noninfective causes of pneumonitis. Identification of individual patient's risk factors for different types of pneumonia will allow the appropriate use of diagnostic tools and early administration of treatment.

1. Barlett JG, Breiman RF, Mandell LA, et al. Community-acquired pneumonia in adults: guidelines for management. *Clin Infect Dis.* 1998;26:811–838.
   Up-to-date guidelines from the Infectious Diseases Society of America, developed by experts in infectious diseases. Provides a rational approach to community-acquired pneumonia.
2. Hospital-acquired pneumonia in adults: diagnosis, assessment of severity, initial antimicrobial therapy, and preventive strategies. A consensus statement of American Thoracic Society. *Am J Respir Crit Care Med.* 1995;153:1711–1725.
   A detailed and systematic approach to hospital-acquired pneumonia. Prepared by a panel of experts in pulmonary medicine and infectious diseases.
3. Marrie TJ. Community-acquired pneumonia: epidemiology, etiology, treatment. *Infect Dis North Am.* 1998;12:723–740.
   The article provides a good overview of community-acquired pneumonia, with in-depth discussion of management of the condition.
4. Torres A, El-Ebiary M. Invasive diagnostic techniques for pneumonia: protected specimen brush, bronchoalveolar lavage, and lung biopsy methods. *Infect Dis North Am.* 1998;12:701–721.
   A comprehensive review of the role, technique, and complications of different invasive diagnostic tools for pneumonia.
5. Scott JAG, Hall AJ. The value and complications of percutaneous transthoracic lung aspiration for the etiologic diagnosis of community-acquired pneumonia. *Chest.* 1999;116:1716–1732.
   A recent review of historic background, as well as the utility and complications of percutaneous transthoracic aspiration.
6. Fine MJ, Auble TE, Yealy DM, et al. A prediction rule to identify low-risk patients with community-acquired pneumonia. *N Engl J Med.* 1997;336:243–250.
   From data of 14,199 adult patients hospitalized for pneumonia, the authors described a predictive rule that assigned points to different clinical, radiographic, and laboratory abnormalities, to predict adverse outcomes.
7. Fang GD, Fine M, Orloff J, et al. New and emerging etiologies for community-acquired pneumonia with implication for therapy: a prospective multicenter study of 359 cases. *Medicine.* 1990;69:307–316.

Chlamydia pneumoniae *and* Legionella *spp. were noted in 13% of cases, whereas the etiology of pneumonia was not found in 32.9% of cases. The majority of patients had either chronic obstructive pulmonary diseases, malignancy, or were immuno-compromised.*

8. Reed WW, Byrd GS, Gates RH, et al. Sputum Gram's stain in community-acquired pneumococcal pneumonia: a meta-analysis. *West J Med.* 1996;165:197–204.

   A meta-analysis of 12 articles that found a wide range in sensitivity and specificity of sputum Gram's stain, with the results subjected to errors in interpretation.

9. Cassiere HA, Fein AM. Duration and route of antibiotic therapy in community-acquired pneumonia: switch and step-down therapy. *Semin Respir Infect.* 1998;13:36–42.

   A practical approach to identifying low risk patients to allow switching antibiotics from intravenous to oral preparations.

10. Louthan FB, Meduri GU. Differential diagnosis of fever and pulmonary densities in mechanically ventilated patients. *Semin Respir Infect.* 1996;11:77–95.

    A review of differential diagnosis of conditions that mimics pneumonia. Multiple conditions may coexist in patients presenting with fever and changes on chest radiograph.

11. Fagon JY, Chastre J, Domart Y, et al. Nosocomial pneumonia in patients receiving continuous mechanical ventilation: prospective analysis of 52 episodes with use of a protected specimen brush and quantitative culture techniques. *Am Rev Respir Dis.* 1989;139:877–884.

    Using PBS through flexible bronchoscopy, the authors found that the risk of pneumonia in intubated patients increased with duration of mechanical ventilation, age, and underlying illness. P. aeruginosa *and* S. aureus *were the commonest organisms isolated.*

12. Chastre J, Fagon JY, Bornet Lecso M, et al. Evaluation of bronchoscopic techniques for the diagnosis of nosocomial pneumonia. *Am J Respir Crit Care Med.* 1995;152:231–240.

    PBS and BAL were reliable in identifying microorganisms, both qualitatively and quantitatively, in ventilated patients, when compared with postmortem lung examinations.

13. Sternberg RI, Baughman RP, Dohn MN, et al. Utility of bronchoalveolar lavage in assessing pneumonia in immunosuppressed renal transplant recipients. *Am J Med.* 1993;95:358–364.

    Results of BAL in this group of patients with pneumonia significantly affected the type of antibiotics used.

14. Bartlett JG, Dowell SF, Mandell LA, et al. Practice guidelines for the management of community-acquired pneumonia in adults. *Clin Infect Dis.* 2000;31:347–382.

15. Guidelines for the management of adults with community-acquired pneumonia—diagnosis, assessment of severity, antimicrobial therapy, and prevention. The official statement of the American Thoracic Society. *Am J Respir Crit Care Med.* 2001;163:1730–1754.

16. Mandell LA, Barlett JG, Dowell SF, et al. Update of practice guidelines for the management of community-acquired pneumonia in immunocompetent adults. *Clin Infect Dis.* 2003;37:1405–1433.

26. PNEUMOCOCCAL PNEUMONIA

Julian P. Lichter

Pneumococcal pneumonia is the most common infection leading to hospitalization in the United States. It occurs in all age groups and is responsible for 500,000 cases of pneumonia and approximately 40,000 deaths annually. Pneumococcal pneumonia accounts for more than 50% of community-acquired pneumonias and 10% of nosocomial pneumonias. A resurgence of outbreaks of pneumococcal pneumonia has occurred, especially in chronic care facilities where the strains are increasingly resistant to antibiotics. Although pneumococcal pneumonia can occur in any season, it is more common in winter and early spring.

The pneumococcus frequently inhabits the nasopharynx of normal individuals. The probability and severity of infection are influenced by host factors and by the biologic properties of the bacterium itself. Patients who are most susceptible to pneumococcal infection include those with (1) disorders of swallowing and impairment of airway clearance mechanisms and mucociliary defenses, such as advanced age, seizure and other neurologic disorders, chronic bronchitis, bronchiectasis); (2) alveolar fluid accumulation, such as congestive heart failure, burns, acute respiratory distress syndrome; and (3) impaired phagocytosis and compromised humoral immunity, such as surgical or functional asplenia (e.g., sickle cell anemia), hypogammaglobulinemia, diabetes, AIDS, multiple myeloma, lymphoma, cirrhosis. Such individuals are also susceptible to protracted or complicated pneumonias. Viral upper respiratory illness also seems to predispose patients to subsequent pneumococcal pneumonia. Viral disruption of respiratory epithelium increases expression of receptors for pneumococcal attachment and, thus, predisposes the patient to pneumococcal invasion.

Of the more than 82 strains of pneumococci, only a few commonly cause pneumonia. The pathogenicity and virulence of particular strains are related to properties of the outer capsules and cell walls, as well as surface and cytoplasmic regulatory mechanisms. They may be identified in the laboratory by a characteristic capsular swelling (quellung reaction) when incubated with specific antibody. Current evidence suggests that the pneumococcal capsule protects the organism from phagocytosis and enhances its pathogenicity. Recent studies suggest that the development of type-specific, anti-capsular antibody correlates with the resolution of fever and recovery in untreated patients.

Pneumococci are aerosolized from the nasopharynx to the alveolus, then pass from alveolus to alveolus through the pores of Cohn, resulting in a mostly lobar distribution of consolidation. They invade alveolar type II cells, a process initiated through binding of bacterial surface choline to the receptor for platelet-activating factor (up-regulated on the alveolar cell surface, presumably by viral infection). Pathologically the consolidated lung evolves through well-described stages of alveolar engorgement followed by red hepatization and, after a few days, grey hepatization with alveoli packed with leukocytes. There is, however, little tissue destruction, and resolution occurs with minimal organization or permanent scarring. Dying pneumococci produce a potent cytotoxin, pneumolysin, which binds to cholesterol on the host's cell membranes, forming pores and killing the cells. Pneumolysin also promotes intra-alveolar bacterial replication, penetration from alveoli to interstitium, and dissemination into the bloodstream. Approximately 25% of cases of pneumococcal pneumonia have associated bacteremia.

The clinical manifestations of classic pneumococcal pneumonia include high fever (100% in one series, although high fever may be absent in the elderly or in uremic patients), productive cough (98%), pleuritic chest pain (70%), and the abrupt onset of shaking chills (7%). The sputum is blood streaked or rusty (75%). Pleuritic pain may radiate into the abdomen, masquerading as an acute abdomen. The individual characteristically appears acutely ill and tachypneic, with signs of consolidation apparent on chest examination. A pleural rub is occasionally present. Herpes labialis is a relatively common finding. The chest roentgenogram usually reveals a lobar, alveolar-filling process, frequently with an ipsilateral pleural effusion. The roentgenographic presentations, however, are diverse and include a patchy bronchopneumonia, adult respiratory distress syndrome, and an interstitial appearance when in an emphysematous lobe.

As with other bacterial pneumonias, the methods and criteria for establishing a diagnosis are controversial. Gram's stain of expectorated sputum typically reveals numerous polymorphonuclear granulocytes and lancet-shaped gram-positive diplococci. However, the predominant organism may not be obvious on some specimens because of heavy smear contamination with oropharyngeal flora. Sputum Gram's stain and culture also can be misleading in patients who have received prior antibiotics and in patients with chronic obstructive pulmonary disease. Isolation of the organism in the sputum is not sensitive for the presence of infection; in fact, only 45% of patients with pneumonia and blood cultures positive for pneumococci grow the organism on sputum culture. For this reason, many culture-negative cases of pneumonia may be caused by the pneumococcus. Isolation of the organism from blood, pleural fluid, or other involved closed tissue space (e.g., joint, cerebrospinal fluid, pericardium) may be required for a firm diagnosis. A rapid urinary antigen test (Binax NOW) is available to detect pneumococcal pneumonia earlier in its course. Sensitivity is 60 to 70% but higher for bacteremic patients, whereas specificity is close to 100%.

Much of our understanding of the natural history of pneumococcal pneumonia comes from experience during the preantibiotic era, when three clinical patterns were observed: (1) a 5- to 10-day course characterized by high fevers with defervescence and recovery occurring either gradually (lysis) or dramatically (crisis); (2) a protracted or recrudescent febrile course indicative of complications such as empyema, meningitis, endocarditis, and pericarditis; or (3) rapid respiratory deterioration and death. An initial leukocytosis exceeding 20,000 correlated with a good prognosis, whereas a normal or low leukocyte count implied a grave prognosis. An abrupt fall in leukocyte count often preceded resolution by crisis, but persistent leukocytosis frequently was a harbinger of complications such as empyema.

Although antibiotics have improved survival, pneumococcal pneumonia remains a serious disease. In the preantibiotic era, the overall mortality rate was 25 to 35%. In bacteremic patients, it exceeded 80%. Antibiotics have reduced the mortality rate to 5% and 20%, respectively. Nevertheless, the mortality in bacteremic patients infected with type 3 pneumococcus currently remains at 51%. Of patients who die despite antibiotic therapy, 35% die within the first 24 hours of antibiotic treatment, underscoring the fulminant course this disease can pursue. Mortality in those who require mechanical ventilation remains high. Advanced age, inability to mount a fever and nosocomially acquired pneumococcal pneumonia are the greatest risk factors for respiratory failure or death.

Penicillin G continues to be the drug of choice for sensitive pneumococcal pneumonia. It is effective either orally or intramuscularly in moderately to severely ill patients but should be administered intravenously in the critically ill and in those with empyema or extrapulmonary foci of infection. Therapy of uncomplicated pneumonia should be continued for at least 3 to 5 days after defervescence. Although monotherapy with a single effective antibiotic for pneumococcal pneumonia is standard, a recent study has shown a significant survival benefit for dual effective therapy in patients with bacteremic pneumococcal pneumonia.

It is becoming more common to find pneumococci that have become resistant to penicillin, probably through alteration of cellular penicillin-binding proteins. Approximately 5 to 10% of pneumococcal strains in the United States show an intermediate resistance, indicated by a mean inhibitory concentration of 0.1 to 1.0 μg/mL. In some areas (e.g., Alaska), as many as 20 to 25% of the strains demonstrate such resistance. In this setting, increasing the penicillin dose to 12 to 18 million units per day may be effective, as would administration of cefotaxime, ceftriaxone, imipenem, or one of the newer fluoroquinolones once sensitivities have been confirmed. Highly resistant pneumococcal isolates (types 6, 9, 14, 19, and 23), with a mean inhibitory concentration of at least 2 μg/mL, are common in Spain (44%), Hungary (>50%), and South Africa, and have been encountered in the United States as well. A recent multicenter study in the United States of 368 children with pneumococcal pneumonia determined that 10% were resistant to penicillin, 13% had intermediate resistance to penicillin, and 7.5% were resistant to ceftriaxone. A recent international multicenter study of 638 cases of community-acquired pneumococcal pneumonia identified multidrug resistance in 22%, and the overall mortality rate was 14.5%. Multiresistant strains (resistant to penicillin, trimethoprim-sulfamethoxazole, chloramphenicol, tetracycline, macrolides, and even second- and third-generation cephalosporins) have been isolated in the United States. Resistance to levofloxin has now been reported as well. Vancomycin, newer fluoroquinolones, or an alternative agent based on in vitro sensitivities should be used for strains with high-level penicillin resistance or resistance to multiple antibiotics. Drug-resistant infections have been observed in certain institutional settings, particularly daycare centers, hospitals, and nursing homes. Interestingly, recent studies seem to indicate that antibiotic resistance to the pneumococcus is not necessarily associated with increased morbidity or mortality in patients with pneumococcal pneumonia.

The response to antibiotic therapy is usually apparent. In one large study (358 patients), 71% of patients were afebrile within 5 days of therapy. A protracted febrile course may indicate antibiotic resistance but also can occur in individuals who are elderly, anemic, or alcoholic, and in those whose disease is characterized by bacteremia, multilobar involvement, or leukopenia. Survival in patients with bacteremic community-acquired pneumococcal pneumonia is much improved when the patient receives, within 24 hours of hospitalization, empiric antibiotics that have in vitro activity against the isolated strain. A slow clinical response is frequently associated with delayed radiographic resolution. In one series of bacteremic patients, only 13% had complete roentgenographic clearing within 2 weeks. Of the others, 61% cleared by 6 weeks, 78% cleared by 10 weeks, and 100% cleared by 18 weeks. Conversely, the chest roentgenogram can appear worse or unchanged, despite clinical improvement with antibiotics. Thus, slow radiographic resolutions do not indicate treatment failure in the face of clinical response.

Complications of pneumococcal pneumonia include necrotizing pneumonia, lung abscess, meningitis, endocarditis, septic arthritis, and pleural disease. Pleural complications are common, and most patients have pleuritic chest pain. A pleural friction rub has been reported in 17% of cases. Pleural effusions can be detected in nearly 60% of patients if repetitive lateral decubitus chest radiographs are obtained. Although the effusions usually are sterile (parapneumonic) exudates, the incidence of empyema is approximately 15%. Diagnostic thoracentesis is mandatory for all large effusions occurring with pneumococcal pneumonia. A pleural fluid pH less than 7.2 suggests that a complicated parapneumonic effusion or frank empyema is present and that chest tube drainage is indicated. Conservative treatment with antibiotics is usually successful if the pH is greater than 7.3. Both parapneumonic effusions and empyemas can accumulate during antibiotic therapy. Generally, the patient with empyema usually appears ill, with a persistent or recrudescent fever and leukocytosis. The degree of pleural disease correlates well with the extent of the initial pneumonia. Early therapy decreases the incidence of empyema.

Pneumococcal vaccines are an important weapon against the pneumococcus, especially in view of the increasing prevalence of multiple antibiotic-resistant strains. For adults, the vaccine has evolved since 1983 to include 23 purified capsular polysaccharide antigens (the 23-valent vaccine) chosen to represent 90% of the serotypes that cause invasive disease in the United States. Pneumococcal infections have the highest mortality rate of any vaccine-preventable disease; about half these deaths are felt to be preventable by the polysaccharide vaccine. Many trials have shown failure to protect against nonbacteremic community-acquired pneumonia, as well as those at the highest risk for pneumococcal pneumonia. There is a paucity of evidence to show that the polysaccharide vaccine protects against pneumococcal pneumonia in patients who are HIV positive, whereas antiretroviral cocktails are highly protective. In one large recent Swedish study, the vaccine was shown to be effective in lowering hospitalization and mortality by 50% in individuals older than age 65. There is also consistent evidence that the polysaccharide vaccine significantly reduces the risk of pneumococcal bacteremia. A serotype prevalence study based on the Centers for Disease Control's pneumococcal surveillance system demonstrated a 57% overall protective effect of this vaccine against invasive disease. The reduction in pneumococcal bacteremia is felt to be reason enough to administer the vaccine. Pneumococcal vaccine can be administered concurrently with other vaccines. The antibody levels to most vaccine antigens remain elevated for at least 5 years in healthy adults. Vaccination is recommended for all persons older than age 65; those with chronic medical illnesses; patients who are immunosuppressed, especially by asplenia; and patients in chronic-care facilities. Routine revaccination of immunocompetent persons is not recommended. A single repeat vaccination is recommended for persons older than age 2 who are at highest risk for serious pneumococcal infection, provided that 5 years have elapsed since the first dose.

In February 2000, a promising new vaccine formulation was approved by the Food and Drug Administration (FDA) for use in children younger than age 2—the protein conjugate heptavalent vaccine. This vaccine links the capsular polysaccharide of seven serotypes to a protein carrier, thereby making it immunogenic in children younger than age 2. Recent studies have shown high efficacy (80–100%) against invasive disease in children, modest efficacy against noninvasive vaccine type pneumococcal otitis media, and reduction in the carriage and transmission of nasopharyngeal pneumococcus including antibiotic-resistant isolates. One year after the licensing of the conjugate vaccine, a dramatic reduction in invasive disease was documented in children; also noted over this period was a reduction in disease rates for adults coupled with a reduction in penicillin-resistant pneumococcus. This suggests that vaccinating children with the conjugate vaccine is of decided benefit to adults as well. Nine- and 11-valent conjugate vaccines are currently in development.

1. Austrian R, Gold J. Pneumococcal bacteremia with special reference to bacteremic pneumococcal pneumonia. *Ann Intern Med.* 1964;60:759.
   A classic paper describing the natural history of pneumococcal pneumonia and the benefits (and limitations) of antibiotic therapy.
2. Austrian R. Pneumococcal pneumonia: diagnostic, epidemiologic, therapeutic, and prophylactic considerations. *Chest.* 1986;90:738.
   A general update from the previous paper.
3. Barret-Connor E. The nonvalue of sputum culture in the diagnosis of pneumococcal pneumonia. *Am Rev Respir Dis.* 1971;103:845.
   The isolation of pneumococci from sputum may be both difficult and misleading.
4. Bartlett JG, Mundy LM. Community-acquired pneumonia. *N Engl J Med.* 1995;333:24:1618.
   Pneumonia is the sixth leading cause of death in the United States. Prevention of influenza and pneumococcal pneumonia by vaccination should be assigned a high priority.
5. Davies D, Hodgson G, Whitby L. A study of pneumococcal pneumonia. *Lancet.* 1935;1:791.
   A clinical description of this disease in the preantibiotic era.
6. Waterer GW, Somes GW, Wunderink RG. Monotherapy may be suboptimal for severe bacteremic pneumococcal pneumonia. *Arch Intern Med.* 2001;161:1837–1842.
   Dual effective therapy reduces mortality compared with single effective therapy in bacteremic pneumococcal pneumonia.
7. Moroney JF, Fiore AE, Harrison LH, et al. Clinical outcomes of bacteremic pneumococcal pneumonia in the era of antibiotic resistance. *Clin Infect Dis.* 2001;33:797–805.
   Antimicrobial resistance in cases of invasive pneumococcal pneumonia appears to have no impact on mortality or need for ICU. Potential reasons discussed.

8. Doern GV. Antimicrobial resistance with *Streptococcus pneumoniae:* much ado about nothing? *Semin Respir Infect.* 2001;16:177–185.

   In vitro antibiotic resistance to S. pneumoniae *does not necessarily translate into diminished effectiveness in vivo.*

9. Aspa J, Rajas O, Rodriguez de Castro F, et al. Drug-resistant pneumococcal pneumonia: clinical relevance and related factors. *Clin Infect Dis.* 2004;38:787–798.

   Multicenter study of 638 cases of pneumococcal pneumonia in which high incidence of antibiotic resistance did not increase morbidity. Complications were, in fact, more common in penicillin-sensitive patients.

10. Marcos MA, Jimenez de Anta MT, et al. Rapid urinary antigen test for diagnosis of pneumococcal community-acquired pneumonia in adults. *Eur Respir J.* 2003;21:209–214.

    The Binax NOW urinary antigen test is sensitive and specific for detecting pneumococcal pneumonia.

11. Lujan M, Gallego M, Fontanals D, et al. Prospective observational study of bacteremic pneumococcal pneumonia: Effect of discordant therapy on mortality. *Crit Care Med.* 2004;32:625–631.

    Survival is improved if an antibiotic with in vitro activity against the isolated strain is administered within 24 hours.

12. Anderson KB, Tan JS, File TM Jr, et al. Emergence of levofloxacin-resistant pneumococci in immunocompromised adults after therapy for community-acquired pneumonia. *Clin Infect Dis.* 2003;37:376–381.

    Levofloxacin resistance is more likely in immunosuppressed patients after a recent prior course of levofloxacin.

13. Tan TQ, Mason EO Jr, Wald ER, et al. Clinical characteristics of children with complicated pneumonia caused by Streptococcus pneumonia. *Pediatrics.* 2002;110(pt 1):1–6.

    Multicenter study of 368 children hospitalized with pneumococcal pneumonia showed that the increasing frequency of complicated pneumonia in children is not related to antibiotic-resistant isolates.

14. O'Brien KL, Santosham M. Potential impact of conjugate pneumococcal vaccines on pediatric pneumococcal diseases. *A J Epidemiol* 2004;159:634–644.

    Up-to-date review of the effectiveness of the new conjugated vaccine.

15. Jackson LA, Neuzil KM, Yu O, et al. Effectiveness of pneumococcal polysaccharide vaccine in older adults. *N Engl J Med.* 2003;348:1747–1755.

    The vaccine is effective for prevention of bacteremia but not pneumococcal pneumonia in older adults.

16. Pierce AB, Hoy JF. Is the recommendation for pneumococcal vaccination of HIV patients evidence based? *J Clin Virol.* 2001;22:255–261.

    Pneumococcal vaccination in HIV patients is much less effective than taking antiretroviral medications to reduce incidence of pneumococcal disease.

17. Davidson M, Schraer CD, Parkinson AJ, et al. Invasive pneumococcal disease in an Alaska native population, 1980 through 1986. *JAMA.* 1989;261:715.

    Reports on a high incidence of disease and high case-fatality rates.

18. Drew WL. Value of sputum culture in diagnosis of pneumococcal pneumonia . *J Clin Microbiol.* 1977;6:62.

    Positive sputum cultures were obtained in 94% of bacteremic pneumococcal pneumonias. Poor culture yields may result from suboptimal technique.

19. Fine MJ, Smith MA, Carson CA, et al. Efficacy of pneumococcal vaccination in adults. A meta-analysis. *Arch Intern Med.* 1994;154:2666.

    Vaccine appears efficacious in reducing bacteremic pneumococcal pneumonia in low-risk adults, but does not protect against pneumonia (all causes), bronchitis, or mortality from pneumonia or pneumococcal infection.

20. Janoff EN, Breiman RF, Daley CL, et al. Pneumococcal disease during HIV infection. Epidemiologic, clinical, and immunologic perspectives. *Ann Intern Med.* 1992;117:314.

    Streptococcus pneumoniae is the leading cause of invasive bacterial respiratory disease in patients with HIV infection. Prompt diagnosis and treatment are associated with favorable outcome.

21. Jay SJ, Johanson W, Pierce A. The radiographic resolution of *Streptococcus pneumoniae* pneumonia. *N Engl J Med*. 1975;293:798.
    A good study in bacteremic patients.
22. Ort S, Ryan JL, Barden G, et al. Pneumococcal pneumonia in hospitalized patients: clinical and radiologic presentations. *JAMA*. 1983;249:214.
    Atypical presentations are common.
23. Marfin AA, Sporrer J, Moore PS, et al. Risk factors for adverse outcome in persons with pneumococcal pneumonia. *Chest*. 1995;107:2.
    Risk factors identified at hospital admission can predict the outcome in persons with pneumococcal pneumonia and bacteremia.
24. Nuorti JP, Butler JC, Crutcher JM, et al. An outbreak of multidrug-resistant pneumococcal pneumonia and bacteremia among unvaccinated nursing home residents. *N Engl J Med*. 1998;338:1861.
    The first report in the United States of an epidemic outbreak of multidrug-resistant pneumococcal pneumonia in unvaccinated nursing home residents.
25. Pallares R. Risk factors and response to antibiotic therapy in adults with bacteremic pneumonia caused by penicillin-resistant pneumococci. *N Engl J Med*. 1987;317:18.
    Addresses an infrequent but important problem.
26. Spika JS, Facklam RR, Plikaytis BD, et al. Antimicrobial resistance of *Streptococcus pneumoniae* in the United States, 1979–1987. *J Infect Dis*. 1991;163:1273.
    Antimicrobial resistance among pneumococcal isolates remained at low levels in the United States through 1987. Resistance was more likely in the southwestern United States.
27. Taryle DA, Sahn SA. The incidence and clinical correlates of parapneumonic effusions in pneumococcal pneumonia. *Chest*. 1978;74:170.
    Effusions are common when looked for carefully. Their presence correlates with duration of symptoms before admission, bacteremia, and prolonged fever after therapy.
28. Tilghman R, Finland M. Clinical significance of bacteremia in pneumococcic pneumonia. *Arch Intern Med*. 1937;59:602.
    A classic review of 1,586 cases.
29. Tuomanen EI, Austrian R, Masure HRN. Pathogenesis of pneumococcal infection. *N Engl J Med*. 1995;332:1280.
    A review of some of the molecular details of the pathogenesis of pneumococcal infection in relation to the current understanding of the genesis of the clinical symptoms and signs.
30. Update on adult immunization: recommendations of the Immunization Practices Advisory Committee (ACIP). *MMWR*. 1991;40:42.
    Recommends pneumococcal vaccine every 6 years for high risk individuals. Also outlines vaccine indications and data on vaccine efficacy.
31. Van Vetre T. Pneumococcal pneumonia treated with antibiotics: the prognostic significance of certain clinical findings. *N Engl J Med*. 1954;251:1048.
    Prognostic correlates in 358 cases.
32. Williams JH Jr., Moser KM. Pneumococcal vaccine and patients with chronic lung disease. *Ann Intern Med*. 1986;104:106.
    The need for and utility of vaccination are not established in this group of patients.

27. STAPHYLOCOCCAL AND STREPTOCOCCAL PNEUMONIAS

Thomas E. Lawrie

Streptococci and staphylococci are human pathogens responsible for a wide spectrum of infections, including community-acquired and nosocomial pneumonias. The emergence of penicillin-resistant strains of *Streptococcus pneumoniae* and methicillin-resistant strains of *Staphylococcus aureus* has had a significant impact over the last decade on our approach to infection caused by these organisms.

Streptococci are spherical gram-positive bacteria that grow in pairs or chains. The bacteria are classified according to (1) the pattern of hemolysis demonstrated when the organism is cultured on blood agar (alpha refers to partial hemolysis, beta refers to complete hemolysis, and gamma refers to nonhemolytic strains); (2) antigenic composition (Lancefield group); (3) colony morphology; and (4) other biochemical reactions and genetic analyses.

S. pneumoniae, or pneumococcus, is an alpha hemolytic streptococcus that typically appears as diplococci on Gram's stain. It is the pathogen most commonly isolated in hospitalized patients with community-acquired pneumonia (CAP), accounting for 9 to 55% of isolates. In addition, pneumococcal pneumonia is responsible for 11 to 37% of patients with CAP requiring admission to intensive care units, and 6 to 26% of nursing home-acquired pneumonia. Risk factors for pneumococcal infections include immunosuppression (HIV infection, transplant recipients); immune deficiencies; aspiration (alcoholism, stroke, and seizure); sickle cell anemia; diabetic ketoacidosis congestive heart failure; chronic obstructive lung disease; and crowding (jail, military, and nursing home).

Clinically, patients are seen with sudden onset of rigors, fever, pleuritic chest pain, and cough productive of rust-colored sputum. However, the presentation also can be more subtle and associated with predominantly nonspecific symptoms (e.g., malaise, coryza, and gastrointestinal symptoms). The diagnosis is confirmed by Gram's stain and culture of sputum; however, diagnosis can be difficult because the culture of pneumococci may simply reflect colonization of the upper airway. In addition, many patients have received antibiotics before sputum collection for culture and, therefore, may be culture negative. Other diagnostic tools, such as blood cultures, bronchoscopically derived tracheal cultures, and serum pneumolysin antibodies may be useful. Radiographic patterns vary from lobar consolidation (usually unilobar, but occasionally two or more lobes are involved) to patchy diffuse opacities. Pleural effusions and empyema may be present; cavitation is rare. Overall mortality for hospitalized patients ranges from 7 to 36% and is influenced by age, comorbid illness, the presence of bacteremia, and the development of complications (e.g., respiratory failure, meningitis, empyema, or other organ failure).

Pneumococcal isolates with minimum inhibitory concentrations (MIC) below 0.1 mcg/mL are classified as penicillin susceptible. Penicillin is the treatment of choice for patients with sensitive organisms. Amoxicillin is recommended by the Infectious Disease Society of America as appropriate outpatient oral treatment for pneumococcal pneumonia caused by penicillin-sensitive pneumococci. Alternative agents for penicillin-allergic patients include macrolides, clindamycin, or one of the newer fluoroquinolones. Hospitalized patients should be treated with intravenous penicillin or ceftriaxone.

Pneumococci that are relatively resistant to penicillin have intermediate susceptibility to penicillin with an MIC of 0.1 to 1.0 mcg/mL. Isolates that are highly resistant have MICs greater than 2.0 mcg/mL. Penicillin-resistant *S. pneumoniae* was first reported in 1967 in New Guinea natives, followed in 1977 by a report of a multidrug-resistant strain. Currently, resistant strains are found throughout the world and have developed resistance to several classes of antibiotic, including trimethoprim-sulfamethoxazole, tetracycline, erythromycin, chloramphenicol, and quinolones. The recent increase in isolates resistant to penicillin is alarming. In the United States as of June 1999, approximately 25 to 35% of all isolates were intermediately resistant or resistant to penicillin. Rates are substantially higher in European countries, with the notable exceptions of Germany and the Netherlands, where accepted prescribing standards significantly limit antibiotic usage. Extremes of age (<18 months and the elderly), recent β-lactam use, overcrowding, malignancy, and HIV positivity are risk factors for nonsusceptible strains. Because the development of relative resistance to penicillin involves lower affinity of penicillin-binding proteins to β-lactams, cephalosporin sensitivity can also be affected. Nevertheless, cefotaxime and ceftriaxone are effective treatments for most pulmonary infections caused by pneumococci that are relatively resistant to penicillin, but strains resistant to these cephalosporins have been reported. A 10-year prospective study conducted in Barcelona of 504 patients with severe pneumococcal pneumonia revealed no significant difference in mortality rate between infections caused by penicillin-susceptible and relatively resistant strains when adjusted for other factors. The authors concluded that high-dose intravenous penicillin G may be effective for strains with intermediate susceptibility, and that ceftriaxone or cefotaxime is effective for penicillin-resistant strains with MICs for cephalosporins that are less than 2.0 mcg/mL.

For multidrug-resistant pneumococci with MICs greater than 2.0 mcg/mL for cephalosporins, alternative agents such as vancomycin, clindamycin, imipenem, meropenem, or fluoroquinolones should be considered. For invasive disease, especially meningitis, recommendation is to add vancomycin to cefotaxime or ceftriaxone for initial therapy. Fluoroquinolones concentrate in respiratory tissue and may be useful in treating infections caused by pneumococci that are relatively resistant to penicillin, and their use has been shown to be effective. Quinapristine/dalfopristin or linezolid are other potentially appropriate choices, but their use is tempered by limited experience with these agents. Patients should begin to improve within 24 to 48 hours, and recommended duration of therapy is 7 to 14 days.

Preventing pneumococcal infection is clearly an important goal in reducing morbidity and mortality. The 23 capsular antigen vaccine has been shown to be cost effective and efficacious, although highly underutilized. It induces an antibody response within 1 week and remains active for 5 years in healthy adults. These 23 antigens represent 85 to 90% of the serotypes responsible for invasive pneumococcal infections based on surveillance data from the CDC. The CDC recommends vaccination for all persons aged 65 or older, patients with functional or anatomic asplenia, and patients who are immunocompromised (e.g., HIV infection, hematologic malignancy, chronic renal failure or nephrotic syndrome, immunosuppressive therapy, or organ transplant recipient). According to the Advisory Committee for Immunization Practices (ACIP), revaccination is indicated for those older than age 65 who were given the vaccine more than 5 years previously and were less than age 65 at initial vaccination, for those with the highest risk for pneumococcal disease, and for those at increased risk for rapid antibody decline.

Other streptococci can also cause serious lung infections, albeit less commonly than pneumococcus. *Streptococcus pyogenes* (β-hemolytic, Lancefield group A) causes pyogenic infections such as pharyngitis, cellulitis, necrotizing fasciitis, arthritis, sepsis, toxic shock-like syndrome, and scarlet fever. *S. pyogenes* can result in severe necrotizing pneumonia and even empyema, especially in the postinfluenza or postmeasles setting, and has been responsible for cluster outbreaks in military recruits and nursing home residents. *S. agalactiae* (β-hemolytic, group B) is a common cause of neonatal infections such as sepsis, meningitis, and pneumonia. Group B, C, G, and *S. viridans* are uncommon causes of pneumonia in adults.

Staphylococci are gram-positive bacteria that appear as clusters on Gram's stain. They are normal inhabitants of skin and mucous membranes, including the upper respiratory tract. The species that cause disease in humans are classified as coagulase-positive (*S. aureus*) or coagulase-negative (*S. epidermidis*, *S. saprophyticus*, and *S. hemolyticus*). *S. epidermidis* infection is almost always acquired in the hospital and coagulase-negative staphylococci are the major cause of catheter-related bacteremia. *S. epidermidis* can cause endocarditis, especially of prosthetic valves. *S. aureus* can cause severe pyogenic infections, including pneumonia, lung abscess, empyema, tracheitis, skin and soft tissue infections, endophthalmitis, osteomyelitis, septic arthritis, catheter-related bacteremia, and toxic-shock syndrome. *S. aureus* is isolated in approximately 3% of patients with community-acquired pneumonia, 15 to 20% of patients with nosocomial pneumonia, and up to 30% of those patients with nursing home-acquired pneumonia. Patients may initially describe symptoms of an upper respiratory tract illness. This is occasionally followed by a transient improvement with subsequent rapid progression to fevers, chills, cough, and chest pain. Risk factors for *S. aureus* pneumonia include diabetes, alcoholism, cystic fibrosis, bronchiectasis, and postinfluenza bacterial pneumonia. Presentation is characterized by high fever, productive cough with purulent sputum, and pleuritic chest pain. Radiologically, several patterns are seen (consolidation, diffuse or patchy infiltrates) and, classically, *S. aureus* pneumonia is known to cavitate. Diagnosis is made by culture and Gram's stain of sputum.

Staphylococci first developed resistance to penicillin in 1942 and later to the semisynthetic penicillins (e.g., methicillin) in 1961. Risk factors for acquiring methicillin-resistant *S. aureus* from the community include intravenous drug use, serious underlying illness, previous antibiotic therapy, and previous hospitalization. For strains sensitive to the semisynthetic penicillins, oxacillin, nafcillin, or first generation cephalosporins (e.g., cefazolin) should be used. Vancomycin should be used for penicillin-allergic patients (although it is less effective than penicillin derivatives) and for methicillin-resistant *S. aureus* infections. Therapy for staphylococcal pneumonia, especially for abscesses or other deep-seated infections, may require 4 to 6 weeks of antibiotics. Staphylococcal empyemas need to be drained by chest tube in addition to antibiotics for cure. Prevention remains a major emphasis for controlling staphylococcal infections. Strict handwashing and careful attention to infection control measures are of utmost importance in limiting the rate of nosocomial transmission.

1. Mandell GL, ed. *Principles and Practice of Infectious Diseases.* 5th ed. Philadelphia, Pa: Churchill Livingstone; 2000.

   Basic resource for streptococci and staphylococci microbiology, disease, and treatment.

2. Sarosi GA, ed. The pneumococcus. *Semin Respir Infect.* 1999;14:197.

3. Sanders CV. Pneumococcal disease: a symposium in honor of Robert Austrian, MD—a summary. *Am J Med.* 1999;107:86S.

   Two excellent reviews of pneumococcal pathophysiology, disease, and treatment.

4. File TM. Community-acquired pneumonia. *Lancet.* 2003;362:1991.

5. Halm EA, Teirstein AS. Management of community-acquired pneumonia. *N Engl J Med.* 2002;347:2039.

   Two excellent and comprehensive reviews of community-acquired pneumonia, with emphasis on diagnosis and empiric management.

6. Bartlett JG, Dowell SF, Mandell LA, et al. Practice guidelines for the management of community acquired pneumonia in adults. *Clin Infect Dis.* 2000;31:347.

7. Mandell LA, Bartlett JG, Dowell SF, et al. Update of practice guidelines for the management of community acquired pneumonia in immunocompetent adults. *Clin Infect Dis.* 2003;37:1405.

   Consensus statement of the Infectious Disease Society of America, with recent update.

8. Kaplan SL, Mason EO. Management of infections due to antibiotic-resistant *Streptococcus pneumonia. Clin Microbiol Rev.* 1998;11:628.

   Basic guidelines for treatment of antibiotic-resistant pneumococcal infections, including meningitis, bacteremia, and pneumonia.

9. Richards MJ, Edwards JR, Culver DH. Nosocomial infections in medical intensive care units in the United States. National Nosocomial Infections Surveillance System. *Crit Care Med.* 1999;27:887.

   Epidemiologic survey of nosocomial infections in critically ill patients.

10. Hansman D, Bullen MM. A resistant pneumococcus. *Lancet.* 1967;ii:267.

    The first report of pneumococcal resistance.

11. Appelbaum PC. World-wide development of antibiotic resistance in pneumococci. *Eur J Clin Microbiol Infect Dis*. 1987;6:367.
12. Geographic variation in penicillin resistance in *Streptococcus pneumonia*— selected sites, United States. *MMWR*. 1997;48:656.
    These two references review the global and US epidemiology of pneumococcal antibiotic resistance.
13. Pallares R, Linares J, Vadillo M, et al. Resistance to penicillin and cephalosporin and mortality from severe pneumococcal pneumonia in Barcelona, Spain. *N Engl J Med*. 1995;333:474.
    This study showed no difference in mortality rate between patients with penicillin-sensitive and penicillin-resistant pneumococcal pneumonia.
14. Leggiadro RJ. The clinical impact of resistance in the management of pneumococcal disease. *Infect Dis Clin North Am*. 1997;11:867.
15. Klugman KP. Pneumococcal resistance to antibiotics. *Clin Microbiol Rev*. 1990;3:171.
    A concise review of options for penicillin-resistant pneumonia.
16. Butler JC. Polysaccharide pneumococcal vaccine efficacy: an evaluation of current recommendations. *JAMA*. 1993;270:1826.
    A review with indications for use of the pneumococcal vaccine.
17. Centers for Disease Control and Prevention. Prevention of pneumococcal disease: recommendation of the Advisory Committee on Immunization Practices (ACIP). *MMWR*. 1997;46:1.
18. Centers for Disease Control and Prevention. Pneumococcal and influenza vaccination levels among adults aged equal to or greater than 65. *MMWR*. 1997;46:913.
    Recommendations for immunization and infection control measures.
19. Kalima P, Riordan T. Necrotizing pneumonia associated with group A streptococcal bacteremia. *Eur J Clin Microbiol Infect Dis*. 1998;17:296.
    A case report of severe necrotizing pneumonia with complicating bronchopleural fistula formation.
20. Maranan MC. Antimicrobial resistance in staphylococci. Epidemiology, molecular mechanisms, and clinical relevance. *Infect Dis Clin North Am*. 1997;11:813.
    Reports on mechanisms for resistance.

28. *HAEMOPHILUS INFLUENZAE* INFECTIONS

Dennis E. Amundson and Frank T. Grassi

Haemophilus influenzae are small, pleomorphic, nonmotile gram-negative rods that occur in both encapsulated and nonencapsulated forms. The encapsulated forms (types a–f), and particularly *H. influenzae* type B (Hib), have increased virulence and are associated with invasive disease (e.g., meningitis, bacteremia, epiglottitis, pneumonia, and septic arthritis), primarily in children younger than age 5. In contrast, the genetically diverse unencapsulated (nontypeable) strains of *H. influenzae* commonly cause community-acquired pneumonia in adults, sinusitis in children and adults, otitis media in children, and bronchitis in patients with chronic lung disease. All strains of *H. influenzae* are fastidious, tend to be overgrown by other bacteria in culture, and require special growth factors (X, hemin and V, nicotinamide adenine dinucleotide) to grow aerobically. These factors can be supplied with chocolate or supplemented agars. The capsular forms are identified and differentiated from the nontypeable *H. influenzae* strains by a variety of serotyping methodologies (e.g., latex particle slide agglutination, countercurrent immunoelectrophoresis). Although relatively accurate, these assays can misidentify a nontypeable *H. influenzae* as encapsulated *H. influenzae*.

A dramatic shift has occurred in the epidemiology of *H. influenzae* infections in developed countries since the early 1990s, because of the universal implementation of Hib vaccines in infancy. *H. influenzae* type B was the cause of more than 90% of all invasive *H. influenzae* infections, with an estimated incidence of 1 of every 200 children; Hib-related disease is now uncommon in developed countries. Concurrently, there has been increasing global recognition of the importance of nontypeable *H. influenzae* strains as causative agents for respiratory tract infections and, less commonly, for invasive disease.

Humans are the only known hosts for *H. influenzae*. The organisms, predominately the nontypeable strains, colonize the nasopharynx throughout life, beginning in infancy. They can be cultured from 25 to 80% of asymptomatic individuals, depending on the population sampled. Higher rates and more prolonged duration of carriage are observed in those with underlying lung disease (e.g., cystic fibrosis, chronic obstructive pulmonary disease [COPD]) as well as in those with relative immunosuppression (e.g, alcoholism, diabetes). Colonization can be a very dynamic process, with coinfection and strain turnover within days to weeks. Unlike the nontypeable strains, *H. influenzae* type B and other encapsulated strains colonize only a few percent of healthy individuals. The rate of carriage of Hib has substantially declined in countries using the Hib vaccine.

Bacterial transmission occurs through respiratory droplets or contact with secretions and fomites. Increased transmission occurs in closed settings, such as households, child day care centers, and nursing homes. *H. influenzae*, primarily nontypeable strains, cause approximately 20% of all otitis media infections in children and 20 to 25% of all sinus infections in adults. In addition, nontypeable *H. influenzae* strains are second only to *Streptococcus pneumoniae* as the causative agents in community-acquired pneumonia (12–28% of cases) and are the most common cause of exacerbations of COPD and bronchiectasis. Infection with *H. influenzae* in bronchiectasis is particularly interesting in that the eradication of one strain of the bacteria is quickly followed by reacquisition of another. Additionally, the degree of bacterial load in bronchiectasis is associated with evidence of inflammatory infiltration of the airways and increased airway injury. Risk factors for *H. influenzae* pneumonia include (1) antecedent viral respiratory tract infection (especially influenza A); (2) chronic lung disease (e.g., COPD or bronchiectasis); (3) systemic diseases associated with immunosuppression (e.g., diabetes or cancer); (4) environmental exposures (e.g., exposure to smoke); and in some cases, (5) strain-specific virulence factors.

The pathogenesis of disease is very different between encapsulated and unencapsulated strains. The encapsulated strains are better able to survive in the bloodstream because the polysaccharide capsules confer virulence, as in the case of the polyribosylribitol phosphate moieties of *H. influenzae* type B. Hib invades the nasopharyngeal vascular space; the ensuing bacteremia can result in sepsis, meningitis, epiglottitis, and other deep-seated infections. Other encapsulated serotypes (especially a and f) can cause invasive disease, especially in the immunocompromised population and in a small minority of immunocompetent individuals.

Pathogenesis of disease for the unencapsulated strains is by contiguous spread from a colonized nasopharynx, resulting in localized upper and lower respiratory tract infections. Studies have shown that the oligoliposaccharide of *H. influenzae* plays a major role in microbe adherence and colonization. Unencapsulated strains of *H. influenzae* historically rarely caused tissue invasion. Recent reports from developing countries suggest they are becoming more prevalent as causes of both invasive disease and pneumonia in healthy children and adults.

Nontypeable *H. influenzae* are common causes of pneumonia in adults and resemble other pneumonias in clinical presentation. Radiographically, multilobar involvement often occurs with patchy or lobar distribution of infiltrates. As with other bacterial pneumonias, bacteremia, parapneumonic effusions, and empyema can occur. Blood cultures and culture of other accessible specimens (e.g., parapneumonic pleural effusion) should be done, although the yield from blood cultures for nontypeable strains is low. Gram's stain and culture of tracheobronchial secretions can be difficult to interpret, given the frequent colonization of the respiratory tract by *H. influenzae*. The diagnosis is supported if a predominance of gram-negative bacilli and polymorphonuclear leukocytes are seen in a Gram's stain of expectorated sputum (or transtracheal or bronchoscopic specimens). H. influenzae, however, may not be evident as the cause of pneumonia, by either Gram's stain or culture. More invasive sampling (e.g., protected bronchial brush catheterization or needle aspiration of lung tissue) can increase the likelihood of a definitive diagnosis. These procedures, however, are not usually necessary in stable, immunocompetent individuals presenting with community-acquired pneumonia. Rather, most patients are treated with empiric antibiotic therapy that covers the more common causes of community-acquired pneumonia.

Nontypeable H. influenzae is also a common cause of acute bacterial exacerbation of COPD and bronchiectasis. Recently, colonization with H. influenzae in "stable" COPD patients has been shown to increase total symptoms during an exacerbation and to prolong the recovery of peak flow after the exacerbation. Additionally, bacteria isolated from patients with COPD subjected to molecular typing demonstrate that the acquisition of a new strain of H. influenzae is associated with a significantly increased risk of exacerbation. The clinical signs of an exacerbation can be subtle: low-grade fever; mild, increased shortness of breath; or a change in tracheobronchial secretions. Because of the ubiquity of the organism and the limitations of sputum Gram's stain and culture (described above), empiric antibiotic therapy for COPD exacerbation should include coverage of nontypeable H. influenzae.

Acute epiglottis, as with the other clinical syndromes primarily associated with Hib, is declining in incidence; however, it is a presentation that requires prompt recognition and management to circumvent progression to lethal airway obstruction. Acute epiglottitis is more common in children, but it can also affect adults with serious clinical implications. It should be suspected in the setting of a severe sore throat and painful swallowing. In later stages, the voice is often muffled and stridor is evident with rapid progression to severe upper airway obstruction. The epiglottis is bright red and edematous when visualized by indirect laryngoscopy; it is seen as an enlarged structure compromising the air column on lateral roentgenograms of the neck. In expert hands, laryngoscopic evaluation can be performed with relative safety and is diagnostically helpful. Establishing a patent airway is essential until the edema and inflammation subside. Although tracheostomy will bypass the obstruction, management of the airway by endotracheal intubation is increasingly used such that tracheostomy is not usually required. Importantly, as manipulation of swollen laryngeal tissues by attempts at visualization or intubation can result in more edema and obstruction, the provisions and expertise for tracheostomy should be immediately available. Management also includes appropriate antibiotics and may include systemic steroids, although the benefit of the latter has not been definitely established.

Serious infections with H. influenzae should be treated with parenteral antibiotics. Appropriate options include (1) selected second-generation cephalosporins (e.g., cefuroxime); (2) third-generation cephalosporins (e.g., ceftriaxone, cefotaxime); (3) fluoroquinolones (e.g., levo-, gati-, moxifloxacin); (4) monolactams (e.g., aztreonam); (5) extended-spectrum penicillins (e.g., piperacillin); and (6) imipenem-cilastatin. Less serious infections, including otitis media, sinusitis, bronchitis, and community-acquired pneumonia, may be treated with oral agents. A major consideration in selection of an oral agent is the occurrence of β-lactamase-producing H. influenzae strains, which were first reported in the 1970s. Both encapsulated and nontypeable strains can produce β-lactamase. Most recent national estimates suggest that approximately 20–35% of all isolates produce β-lactamase. Thus, ampicillin or amoxicillin is only appropriate when the particular isolate has been shown to be sensitive. Reasonable options for either empiric oral therapy or therapy with a documented β-lactamase-producing strain include (1) trimethoprim-sulfamethoxazole (although resistance is as high as 20% in some areas); (2) cefuroxime axetil; (3) amoxicillin-clavulanate; (4) doxycycline; (4) azithromycin; and (5) fluoroquinolones. Erythromycin, first-generation cephalosporins, clindamycin, and tetracycline have poor activity against H. influenzae and should not be prescribed empirically.

Currently, a number of licensed Hib conjugate vaccines incorporate capsular polysaccharide into protein carriers and are highly immunogenic, even in infancy. The Hib vaccines have been shown to be protective for invasive disease and to reduce carriage of Hib, contributing to *herd immunity*. No cross-protection with other capsular strains or nontypeable *H. influenzae* strains exists. Since the addition of these vaccines in routine infant immunization schedules, follow-up surveillance has demonstrated significant reductions in the overall incidence of Hib infections and the near elimination of invasive Hib infection (without concomitant increases in the prevalence of other encapsulated *H. influenzae* infections). Research is ongoing to develop vaccines to prevent infections caused by nontypeable *H. influenzae;* however, the heterogeneity of the surface molecules of the various strains has made attempts challenging thus far. An oral monobacterial vaccine has shown some promise in small studies in reducing the frequency and severity of recurrent bronchitis exacerbations in adults, and a nasal vaccine used in mice was able to protect against middle ear and pulmonary infections. However, further work needs to be done.

In summary, *H. influenzae* is an important respiratory tract pathogen with a changing epidemiology and resistance pattern noted over the last decade. Encapsulated forms, predominately Hib, and nontypeable strains are both pathogenic, with different mechanisms of disease pathogenesis and outcomes, however. The introduction of Hib immunization in infancy has sharply reduced the incidence of Hib infections, which were predominately invasive infections of childhood. Nonencapsulated forms, which are common colonizers of the respiratory tract, primarily cause mucosal disease. Additionally, they are responsible for a significant proportion of otitis media in children, sinusitis and community-acquired pneumonia in adults, and lower respiratory tract infection in patients with chronic lung disease. Approximately 20–35% of both encapsulated and nontypeable strains produce β-lactamase; thus, empiric antibiotic therapy strategies should include agents with β-lactamase resistance. Research is in progress to develop an effective vaccine for nontypeable *H. influenzae*.

1. Lipsitch M. Bacterial vaccines and serotype replacement: lessons from *Haemophilus influenzae* and prospects for *Streptococcus pneumoniae*. *Emerg Infect Dis*. 1999;5:336.
2. Acar JF. Resistance patterns of *Haemophilus influenzae*. *J Chemother*. 1999;11(suppl):44.
3. Thornsberry C, Ogilvie P, Kahn J, et al., and the Laboratory Investigator Group. Surveillance of antimicrobial resistance in *Streptococcus pneumoniae*, *Haemophilus influenzae*, and *Moraxella catarrhalis* in the United States in 1996–1997 respiratory season. *Diagn Microbiol Infect Dis*. 1997;29:249.
4. Takala AK, Eskola J, van Alphen L, et al. Spectrum of invasive *Haemophilus influenzae* type B disease in adults. *Arch Intern Med*. 1990;150:2573.
5. Booy R, Kroll JS. Is *Haemophilus influenzae* finished? *J Antimicrob Chemother*. 1997;40:149.
6. Nizet V, Colina KF, Almquist JR, et al. A virulent nonencapsulated *Haemophilus influenzae*. *J Infect Dis*. 1996;173:180.
7. Klein JO. Role of nontypeable *Haemophilus influenzae* in pediatric respiratory tract infections. *Pediatr Infect Dis J*. 1997;16:S5.
8. Shann F. *Haemophilus influenzae* pneumonia: type b or non-type b? *Lancet*. 1999;354:1488.
9. St. Geme JW. Insights in the mechanism of respiratory tract colonization by nontypeable *Haemophilus influenzae*. *Pediatr Infect Dis J*. 1997;16:931.
10. Murphy TF. Respiratory infections caused by non-typeable *H. influenzae*. *Curr Opin Infect Dis*. 2003;16:129.
11. Barker AF. Bronchiectasis. *N Engl J Med*. 2002;346:1383.
12. Gilsdorf JR. Antigenic diversity and gene polymorphisms in *Haemophilus influenzae*. *Infect Immun*. 1998;66:5053.
13. Quinones CA, Memon MA, Sarosi GA. Bacteremic *Hemophilus influenzae* pneumonia in the adult. *Semin Respir Infect*. 1989;4:12.
14. Levin DC, Schwarz MI, Matthay RA, et al. Bacteremic *Hemophilus influenzae* pneumonia in adults: a report of 24 cases and a review of the literature. *Am J Med*. 1977;62:219.

15. Patel IS, Seemungal TA, Wilks M, et al. Relationship between bacterial coloniza-
    tion and the frequency, character, and severity of COPD exacerbations. *Thorax.*
    2002;57:759.
16. Sethi S, Evans N, Brydon JB, et al. New strains of bacteria and exacerbations of
    chronic obstructive pulmonary disease. *N Engl J Med.* 2002;347:465.
17. Kurono Y, Shimanmura K, Mogi G. Inhibition of nasopharyngeal colonization
    of *Hemophilus influenzae* by oral immunization. *Ann Otol Rhinol Laryngol.*
    1992;157:11.
18. Ryan M, Hunt M, Snowberger T. A changing pattern of epiglottis. *Clin Pediatr*
    (Phila). 1992;31:532.
19. Quintiliani R, Hymans PJ. The association of bacteremic *Haemophilus influenzae*
    pneumonia in adults with typeable strains. *Am J Med.* 1971;50:781.
20. Wallace RJ Jr, Musher DM, Martin RR. *Hemophilus influenzae* pneumonia in
    adults. *Am J Med.* 1978;64:87.
21. Fainstein V, Berkey P, Elting L, et al. *Haemophilus* species bacteremia in patients
    with cancer: a 13-year experience. *Arch Intern Med.* 1989;149:1341–1345.
22. Gleckman R, DeVita J, Hibert D, et al. Sputum gram stain assessment in
    community-acquired bacteremic pneumonia. *J Clin Microbiol.* 1988;26:846.
23. Hershey CO, Panaro V. Round pneumonia in adults. *Arch Intern Med.*
    1988;148:1155.
24. MayoSmith MF, Hirsch PJ, Wodzinski SF, et al. Acute epiglottitis in adults: an
    eight-year experience in the state of Rhode Island. *N Engl J Med.* 1986;314:1133.
25. Baker AS, Roland DE. Adult supraglottitis (epiglottitis). *N Engl J Med.*
    1986;314:1185. Editorial.
26. Shih L, Hawkins DB, Stanley RB Jr. Acute epiglottitis in adults: a review of
    48 cases. *Ann Otol Rhinol Laryngol.* 1988;97:527.
27. Doern GV, Brown SD. Antimicrobial susceptibility among community-acquired
    respiratory tract pathogens in the USA: data from PROTEKT US 2000–2001.
    J Infect. 2004;48:56.
28. Foxwell AR, Cripps AW, Dear KB. *Haemophilus influenzae* oral whole cell vaccina-
    tion for preventing acute exacerbations of chronic bronchitis. *Cochrane Database
    Syst Rev.* 2003;(3):CD001958.
29. Bertot GM, Becker PD, Guzman CA, et al. Intranasal vaccination with recom-
    binant P6 protein and adamantylamide dipeptide as mucosal adjuvant con-
    fers efficient protection against otitis media and lung infection by nontypeable
    Haemophilus influenzae. J Infect Dis. 2004;189:1304.

29. *KLEBSIELLA* PNEUMONIA

Bao Q. Luu

Klebsiella pneumonia is often described as the classic community-acquired gram-
negative bacillary pneumonia (Friedlander's pneumonia). Medical textbooks continue
to list *Klebsiella* as an important cause of community-acquired pneumonia; however,
recent epidemiologic studies demonstrate that the incidence of community-acquired
Klebsiella pneumonia is declining in the United States. In fact, it is estimated that
K. pneumoniae is responsible for less than 1% of cases of community-acquired pneumonias requiring hospitalization. On the other hand, *K. pneumoniae* has now emerged
as an important cause of hospital-acquired pneumonia.

Klebsiella species are lactose-fermenting gram-negative bacteria belonging to the
Enterobacteriaceae family. *K. pneumoniae* has a very large polysaccharide capsule with antiphagocytic property, which contributes to its virulence. Encapsulated

K. pneumoniae strains have a mucoid appearance in culture plates, and Gram's stain demonstrates bipolar gram positivity, as seen in other enteric organisms. *K. pneumoniae* may be suspected on Gram's stain if there are clear zones around apparently gram-negative bacteria.

Nasopharyngeal carrier rates among normal hosts range from 1 to 6%. The carrier rate increases in the hospital environment in direct proportion to the length of stay and appears to be associated with the use of antibiotics. In hospitalized patients, the pharyngeal carrier rate has been reported to be as high as 19%.

K. pneumoniae also colonizes the pharynx of ambulatory alcoholics in rates as high as 30%. Undoubtedly, this accounts for the common observation that community-acquired *Klebsiella* pneumonia occurs more frequently in alcoholics than in normal hosts. However, other debilitating conditions, such as diabetes mellitus and chronic pulmonary disease, and immunocompromised status resulting from hematologic malignancy, cytotoxic chemotherapy and steroids, and neutropenia also predispose to infection and disease. Aspiration is likely the precipitating event in both community- and hospital-acquired *Klebsiella* pneumonia.

The classic presentation of community-acquired *Klebsiella* pneumonia is the acute onset of prostration, pleuritic chest pain, dyspnea, high fever, and productive cough in a debilitated host. The sputum is classically described as looking like "currant jelly," a term used to describe the thick, bloody-appearing (but heme negative) and mucoid-viscid sputum. Physical examination discloses tachypnea and signs of lung consolidation. The posterior segment of the right upper lobe and superior segment of the right lower lobe are the most often affected areas of the lungs, consistent with aspiration as the mechanism for infection. Patients may present with sepsis and septic shock, and blood cultures are positive in approximately 25% of the cases. Leukocyte counts can be high, normal or low. Neutropenia indicates a poorer prognosis. Respiratory distress or failure requiring endotracheal intubation and mechanical ventilation upon presentation is common. Lung abscess, cavitation, and pulmonary gangrene may complicate the course of illness. Pulmonary gangrene is described as a large cavity containing fragments of necrotic lung. Pleural effusion and empyema also are common and, after a recovery, unclosed cavities, residual fibrosis, and reduced lung volumes are often detected.

The presentation of hospital-acquired *Klebsiella* pneumonia generally is less dramatic than that seen in community-acquired pneumonia. Depending on the patient's underlying illness and ability to respond immunologically, localizing symptoms, physical findings, and radiographic appearances may be less apparent or less specific. Outbreaks of hospital-acquired *Klebsiella* pneumonia with sepsis in intensive care units have been reported.

Klebsiella species may also cause "chronic" pneumonia. This is thought to occur occasionally when a patient recovers from the acute phase of pneumonia but passes into a chronic phase of disease characterized by cavitation and scarring resembling that of tuberculosis.

On chest radiograph, *Klebsiella* pneumonia has been described classically as a lobar consolidation with a "bulging" or "bowed" fissure sign more commonly affecting the upper lobes and on the right more often than the left. Pathologically, the "bulging" fissure sign is thought to result from the necrotizing pneumonia seen more often with *Klebsiella* pneumonia than pneumococcal pneumonia. Destruction of parenchyma within larger areas of consolidative lung is thought to lead to the loss of elastic recoil, and thus the "bulging" fissure sign. Subsequent investigation has revealed that the "bulging" fissure sign is not specific to *Klebsiella* pneumonia and has been reported in *Haemophilus influenza* and *Streptococcus pneumoniae* pneumonia as well.

A prospective study of the radiographic appearance of bacteremic *Klebsiella* pneumonia in 15 patients showed bilateral involvement just as often as unilateral involvement. Moreover, diffuse patchy infiltrates occur just as often as discrete infiltrates. Pleural effusion was seen in 10 of the 15 patients studied. None of the cases showed evidence of the "bulging" fissure sign. It is thought that these changes in the radiographic appearance of *Klebsiella* pneumonia reflect the changes seen in the patient population in terms of their underlying diseases (more immunocompromised host) as well as the shift of *Klebsiella* pneumonia from being mostly a community-acquired pneumonia to that of a hospital-acquired one.

The mortality rate for *Klebsiella* pneumonia remains high (25–50%), especially among alcoholics and other immunocompromised hosts. Empyema and abscess are common. Other unusual complications include arthritis, meningitis, and pericarditis.

Like other members of the Enterobacteriaceae family, *Klebsiella* species have acquired the extended-spectrum beta-lactamase (ESBL) genes through plasmids transmission. In vitro, ESBL-producing organisms are susceptible to combination therapy with beta-lactam/beta-lactamase inhibitors, third- and fourth-generation cephalosporins, aminoglycosides, and quinolones. In severe infection, however, treatment with carbapenem has been shown to be associated with a lower mortality rate.

1. Korvick JA, Hackett AK, Yu VL, et al. *Klebsiella* pneumonia in the modern era: clinicoradiographic correlations. *South Med J*. 1991;84:200.

   A prospective study of 15 patients with bacteremic Klebsiella *pneumonia demonstrating the changes in clinical presentation and radiographic findings of this disease from the classic gram-negative community-acquired pneumonia described by Friedlander to that of a predominantly hospital-acquired one affecting more immunocompromised hosts.*

2. Yinnon AM, Butnaru A, Raveh D, et al. *Klebsiella* bacteremia: community versus nosocomial infection. *Q J Med*. 1996;89:933.

   The incidence of bacteremic hospital-acquired Klebsiella *pneumonia was 25% compared with 7% in community-acquired pneumonia in this study done in Israel.* Klebsiella *bacteremia was associated with high mortality rates: 42% in hospital-acquired disease compared with 22% for community acquired. This study also showed a high incidence of extended-spectrum beta–lactamase-containing strains.*

3. Schmidt AJ, Stark P. Radiographic findings in Klebsiella (Friedlander's) pneumonia: the bulging fissure sign. *Semin Respir Infect*. 1998;13:80.

   A succinct discussion on the changes in the classic presentation of Friedlander's *pneumonia to the current more hospital-acquired* Klebsiella *pneumonia. This article provides the historic perspective and discusses the nonspecificity of the bulging fissure sign.*

4. Podschun R, Ullmann U. *Klebsiella* spp. As nosocomial pathogens: epidemiology, taxonomy, typing methods, and pathogenicity factors. *Clin Microbiol Rev*. 1998; 11:589.

   A review of the microbiology of Klebsiella *species.*

5. Ko WC, Paterson DL, Sagnimeni AJ, et al. Community-acquired Klebsiella *pneumoniae* bacteremia: global differences in clinical patterns. *Emerg Infect Dis*. 2002; 8:160.

   A worldwide collaborative study showing that community-acquired Klebsiella *pneumoniae bacteremia is decreasing in incidence in the United States, Argentina, Europe, and Australia, with no cases reported in association with alcoholism. In South Africa and Taiwan, the incidence remains high and the association with alcoholism persists.*

6. Paterson DL, Ko WC, Von Gottberg A, et al. Antibiotic therapy for *Klebsiella pneumoniae* bacteremia: implications of production of extended-spectrum beta-lactamases. *Clin Infect Dis*. 2004;39:31.

   A multinational study showing that the prevalence of extended-spectrum beta-lactamase approaches 50% in some countries. This study shows that the mortality rate is lower when treatment of severe ESBL Klebsiella *pneumoniae bacteremia is initiated with at least one carbapenem.*

7. Hoban DJ, Biedenbach DJ, Mutnick AH, et al. Pathogen of occurrence and susceptibility patterns associated with pneumonia in hospitalized patients in North America: results of the SENTRY Antimicrobial Surveillance Study (2000). *Diagn Microbiol Infect Dis*. 2003;45:279.

*Among patients hospitalized with pneumonia in North America, Klebsiella spp.
were isolated 7.5% of the time. Extended-spectrum beta-lactamases were detected at
a rate of 5.4% among Klebsiella spp. They remain 100% susceptible to carbapenem
(imipenem and meropenem).*

30. OTHER GRAM-NEGATIVE PNEUMONIAS: PSEUDOMONAS AERUGINOSA, ESCHERICHIA COLI, PROTEUS, SERRATIA, ENTEROBACTER, ACINETOBACTER

James H. Williams, Jr.

BACKGROUND AND ETIOLOGY

The gram-negative bacilli (GNB) *Pseudomonas aeruginosa*, *Escherichia coli*, and organisms of the *Proteus*, *Serratia*, *Enterobacter*, and *Acinetobacter* species are most commonly associated with nosocomial, or hospital-acquired pneumonia (HAP). GNB are associated with less than 20% of pneumonias among ambulatory patients, with *Klebsiella* species being common. However, these GNB are more commonly recovered from the airways of debilitated, institutionalized patients with pneumonia and are associated with half the deaths from bacterial pneumonia in this population. They represent the majority of bacteria demonstrated among acutely ill patients diagnosed with pneumonia after being admitted to the hospital.

Predisposing factors for GNB pneumonia vary with the population at risk. In the community, chronic bronchitis, bronchiectasis, alcoholism, diabetes, altered mental status, and neutropenia appear to be the major risk factors for GNB pneumonia. In the hospital, GNB pneumonia most often occurs with prolonged intubation, including tracheostomy, and labeled ventilator-associated pneumonia (VAP). Additional risk factors include a prolonged hospital stay, particularly those requiring an intensive care unit (ICU), recent thoracic or abdominal surgery, advanced age, and severe underlying illness. Relative deficiencies in some micronutrients during acute and chronic illness are associated with increased risk, potentially reflecting altered host responses. More frankly immunocompromised hosts are at particular risk for adverse outcomes from these infections.

Although contaminated respiratory equipment has caused occasional outbreaks, particularly due to *Serratia* and *Pseudomonas* species, these outbreaks are uncommon with use of disposable equipment and aseptic techniques. Medical staffs are believed to facilitate colonization of patients with potentially resistant organisms by careless hygiene (which can be diminished by careful cleansing of hands) and other commonly shared contact sites (e.g., stethoscopes, doors handles, bed controls, etc.). Some GNB pneumonias result from bacteremia introduced by bladder catheters, intravenous catheters, as well as from infections in the abdomen or elsewhere. However, GNB causing HAP are most commonly delivered to the lungs via the upper airways.

Colonization of the upper airway by GNB generally precedes pneumonia associated with these organisms, including the pharynx and nasal sinuses. Reflux of gastric contents into the posterior pharynx is enhanced in the supine position and by large gastric volume. Nasal tubes increase retention of secretions in the nasal sinuses that drain into the posterior pharynx. Selection of GNB is encouraged in a hospital by a number of additional factors commonly encountered in the ICU, particularly antibiotic selection pressure and increased adherence of GNB to the airway epithelium and retained secretions of seriously ill patients. Suppression of gastric acidity selectively promotes GNB proliferation in the stomach, but the role of this emergence in the development of GNB HAP/VAP is unclear and simply reflects pharyngeal colonization in many. Nasogastric tubes used for medications and feeding may enhance risk of aspiration, and passage of feeding tubes beyond the stomach only inconsistently and incompletely reduces this risk.

Access of nasopharyngeal flora to the lower airways is facilitated by a number of factors inherent to ICU patients, particularly intubated patients. Translaryngeal intubation mechanically holds open the epiglottis and vocal cords. Although cuffed endotracheal tubes diminish the rate with which large volumes can enter the lower airways, the reservoir of secretions above the cuff continue to ooze down around the balloon, which is kept at low pressure to avoid tracheal necrosis. Efforts to diminish the size of this subglottic pool of secretions with specially designed endotracheal tubes has been associated with some promising, but variable, results, perhaps reflecting their tenacious character and limited accessibility. Bacteria adherent to the endotracheal tube provide an additional nidus for infection.

The normal reflex clearance of airway secretions is attenuated by many factors as well. Endotracheal and tracheostomy tubes create a smaller lumen through which to expectorate and become a nidus for adherence of secretions and bacteria. The effort and effectiveness of expectoration is also inhibited by central nervous system (CNS) depression (narcotics, sedatives, metabolic instability, CNS lesions), local reflex depression (topical anesthetic, learned tolerance of foreign nasotracheal or nasogastric tubes), and pain (particularly chest and abdominal surgery). Mucociliary activity can be decreased (alcohol, chronic inflammation, metabolic disorders), and phagocytic activity can be impaired (immunocompromised patients, alcohol, overwhelmed reserves).

Tracheostomy has advantages for patients requiring prolonged intubation, including stabilization of airway access, patient comfort, and less physical interruption of airway closure during swallowing. However, tracheostomy also delays re-establishment of normal airway architecture during patient recovery. After weaning from ventilator support, clearance of secretions is still inhibited by diminished ability to generate a high positive pressure and by physical obstruction of the tube. Airway protection during swallowing also is impaired by limiting the positive airway pressure normally generated in this process, and potentially by hindering tracheal lift for epiglottis closure, and applying pressure to the upper esophagus through the membranous posterior tracheal surface. These factors, along with the underlying problems of these patients, lead to a high incidence of recurrent pneumonia, often with GNB.

COMMON CLINICAL PRESENTATIONS

The clinical features of GNB infections are intertwined with the underlying diseases with which they are usually associated. The classic descriptions of GNB pneumonias focus on community-acquired cases, uncomplicated by adult respiratory distress syndrome (ARDS), heart failure, and fluid imbalance, and therefore incompletely represent the spectrum of nosocomial GNB pneumonias. Regardless, they provide useful comparisons of pathologic responses in otherwise relatively fit individuals. However, it is important to remember that immunocompromised patients may exhibit relatively few signs or symptoms, and conversely, that underlying acute or chronic lung injury may present with similar symptoms and signs, making diagnosis challenging.

P. aeruginosa frequently colonizes the skin or mucosa of patients, as well as the hospital environment (soap, liquid media, and hospital staff). It can colonize or infect tracheostomy sites, burns, wounds, and the urinary tract, and mucoid strains often emerge in the airways of patients with cystic fibrosis. Pneumonia, usually acquired via the airway, is predominantly located in dependent lung zones, whereas hematogenous infections may lead to more widespread distribution. Pathologically there is severe focal necrosis, with nodular infarcts and vessel wall necrosis leading to hemorrhage and formation of small cavities. Purulent pleural effusion is often found at autopsy. Clinically, patients usually appear toxic, presenting with chills, fever, and dyspnea; sputum often is copious and can be blood tinged. Pleuritic chest pain is less common. Ecthyma gangrenosum is an uncommon cutaneous maculopapular eruption representing infection and necrosis in vessel walls, which may present as hemorrhagic bullae, ulcers, or nodular lesions; although classically linked to bacteremia with these organisms, it can be seen with other infections. Radiographically, consolidation in dependent areas is most commonly seen, and less consistently recognized are abscesses varying in size from 2 to 11 cm. Small effusions may be present. Hematogenous pneumonias are more typically bilateral, with patchy infiltrates or nodular shadows.

E. coli pneumonia may follow aspiration or hematogenous dissemination from urinary tract or gastrointestinal infections. Pathologically, a diffuse, hemorrhagic pneumonia is often present, but abscess formation is less common. Clinically, patients generally appear toxic, with fever, dyspnea, productive cough, and, more often, pleuritic chest pain. Classically, one may see a relative bradycardia for the degree of temperature elevation and a paucity of signs of the parenchymal consolidation. The chest roentgenogram usually demonstrates a patchy bronchopneumonia, often in lower lobes. Pleural effusion may be present.

Proteus species less commonly cause respiratory tract infection, and is frequently associated with an altered state of consciousness, potentially leading to aspiration. Pathologically, the pneumonia is hemorrhagic and associated with small abscesses. Clinically, the patients usually appear less toxic, although chills, fever, dyspnea, productive cough, and pleuritic chest pain may be present. The chest roentgenogram demonstrates dense infiltrates, more often in the dependent segments of the upper lobes and superior segment of the lower lobes, and volume contraction may be seen. Pleural effusion is less common.

Serratia species also occasionally cause pneumonia. Clustered cases have been linked in the past to contaminated respiratory equipment. Pathologically, a diffuse bronchopneumonia can occur with small (2–3 mm) abscesses. Patients typically are toxic, with fever, chills, and productive cough. Pseudohemoptysis, the production of sputum tainted with a red pigment produced by some strains, is uncommon. The chest radiograph generally demonstrates a diffuse, patchy, bronchopneumonia similar to *Pseudomonas* pneumonia, although abscess formation is less common. Pleural effusion and empyema may occur.

Enterobacter pneumonia is less well characterized than the other GNB pneumonias. In one small series, symptoms included fever, dyspnea, and cough productive of yellow sputum, although pleuritic pain was uncommon. Chest radiographs most often demonstrate bilateral bronchopneumonia, but abscesses and empyema formation are uncommon. The emergence of drug-resistant strains has increased the frequency and seriousness of infection from these organisms.

Acinetobacter species have more recently emerged as a multidrug-resistant organism associated with HAP/VAP, in response to the prolific use of broad-spectrum antibiotics. Colonization of hospitalized patients with these organisms is being observed with increasing frequency. The presence of multidrug-resistant *Acinetobacter* species in airway cultures of febrile intubated patients with pulmonary infiltrates presents diagnostic and therapeutic dilemmas. The chest roentgenogram may demonstrate multilobar infiltrates, occasionally with signs of necrosis (cavitation) or effusion.

DIAGNOSIS

The diagnosis of gram-negative pneumonia by examination of airway secretions is problematic because of the frequency with which GNB colonize the airways of patients at risk, many of whom may have infiltrates on chest films for other reasons. Demonstrating numerous GNB and neutrophils on smears of airway secretions provides presumptive evidence, particularly with intracellular organisms providing evidence of a host response, but still may reflect bronchitis rather than pneumonia. Attempting to bypass the upper airway via bronchoscopic brushing or lavage samples ignores the fact that the upper airways are traversed in the process, contaminating the sampling channel with suctioning to maintain visualization. The fewer organisms sometimes recovered with these techniques may simply reflect a smaller or diluted sample. Therefore, these presumptive diagnoses are more firmly supported by positive cultures from blood or pleural fluid. However, while routine use in this setting is debated, bronchoscopy can provide important access to samples in patients who cannot provide adequate lower airway samples, and sometimes demonstrates organisms not reported in cultures of upper airway samples laden with other bacteria. Occasionally, if the patient is deteriorating while undergoing treatment, demonstration of tissue infection via lung biopsy may be warranted.

TREATMENT

The decision of when and how to treat HAP/VAP is particularly difficult, knowing the issues causing diagnostic uncertainty will similarly complicate recognition of a response and that initiation of antibiotic therapy immediately adds selection pressure for emergence of drug-resistant organisms. However, the high mortality associated with HAP/VAP with GNB is worsened by a delay in the start of antibiotics to which the organism is sensitive. This argues *for* aggressive, broad-spectrum empiric coverage initially, particularly among those who are critically ill, and *against* limited coverage while waiting for cultures.

The initial drug or drugs chosen should be based on current resistance patterns in the hospital and organisms likely to be present based on the patient's presentation and risk profile. For example, *Pseudomonas* is more likely among patients with VAP and those previously receiving antibiotics, particularly those with recurrent respiratory tract infections associated with bronchiectasis. To limit antibiotic selection pressure, current opinion favors a "de-escalation" strategy, starting with relatively broad coverage, particularly with critically ill patients, and then narrowing subsequent coverage based on the results of cultures. However, subsequent de-escalation is often difficult when a patient is clinically improving, given the uncertain sensitivity of cultures, especially among patients with limited ability to tolerate deterioration. Another approach that has been suggested is to rotate routinely every few months the classes of drugs selected to shift the emerging resistance patterns. Underlying these antibiotic use strategies/guidelines is a desire to save classes of drugs for use with subsequent infections in the individual and the institution and to reduce the emergence of multidrug resistance profiles, although evidence of outcome benefit from specific approaches remains limited.

Two parenteral antibiotics directed at *Pseudomonas* species have been commonly used when these species are suspected or demonstrated, because drug resistance often emerges with these organisms. Traditional use of a semisynthetic penicillin (piperacillin) and aminoglycoside has in many centers been modified, often replacing the aminoglycoside with a less toxic alternative, such as very high doses of fluoroquinolones (ciprofloxacin, possibly levofloxacin), particularly among older, sicker patients who are at increased risk of ototoxicity and nephrotoxicity from aminoglycosides. A number of drugs can be used in substitution for piperacillin, including a β-lactamase inhibitor combination (piperacillin-tazobactam), which enhances efficacy against many other organisms but requires a higher dose for *Pseudomonas* than for other organisms. Additional alternatives include some third- and fourth-generation cephalosporins, monobactams (aztreonam) and thienamycin-derived carbapenems (imipenem, less CNS-toxic meropenem, less pseudomonas-effective ertapenem). However, emergence of multidrug-resistant strains, notoriously among *Acinetobacter baumannii,* force consideration of agents uncommonly considered in recent years, including tetracyclines and more toxic drugs, such as colistin and polymyxin B.

A single broad-spectrum drug has been successful in the initial treatment of patients with HAP pending results of cultures, unless there is concern for resistant organisms, including some GNB or *Staphylococcus* species. However, because adequacy of initial therapy improves survival in HAP/VAP, the patient's potential tolerance for worsening if cultures prove the single drug inadequate must be considered. A growing list of orally active agents effective against GNB has facilitated outpatient management of persons with less severe pneumonia. Options include very high-dose quinolones (ciprofloxacin, levofloxacin), second- and fourth-generation cephalosporins, and β-lactam inhibitor combinations (e.g., amoxicillin plus clavulanate), only some of which treat *Pseudomonas* (e.g. piperacillin plus tazobactam), as well as carbapenems (e.g. imipenem, meropenem). Specific choice(s) should take into account institutional sensitivity patterns.

Prior exposure to a class of antibiotics increases the probability of resistance progressively, which argues for use of a different drug class with each new event. However, this must be weighed against the risk of broadening antibiotic selection pressure in the individual patient, if recurrent infection is likely, which may be shared with others as well. As such, the potential tolerance of the individual for a delay in appropriately targeted therapy should be considered in making the best decision for the patient, both short term and long term.

Delivery of antibiotics to infected regions of the lungs is inherently complicated by hypoxic vasoconstriction, and accumulated secretions may further diminish local concentrations. Bacteriocidal activity increases with higher local concentrations of aminoglycoside and quinolones, whereas activity of beta-lactam drugs is not similarly enhanced by raising local concentrations above the bacteriocidal level. Therefore, although drug penetration is always an issue, it carries additional significance with quinolones and aminoglycosides. Quinolones enjoy good tissue penetration and (some) good tolerance at higher systemic doses. However, aminoglycosides penetrate tissues more poorly, and toxicity precludes systemic administration of higher doses. Airway instillation of aminoglycosides as an adjuvant to intravenous therapy more rapidly clears GNB from secretions, but direct instillation of less-than-usual systemic doses of aminoglycoside has little impact on the overall course of VAP, when added to systemic administration. In contrast, repeated nebulization of very high doses of tobramycin (300 mg bid) alone has improved long-term outcomes among patients with cystic fibrosis and suppresses symptoms among patients with other types of bronchiectasis. The role of nebulizing high-dose aminoglycosides as an adjunct to systemic therapy in HAP/VAP with GNB has not yet been well characterized. Aerosolization of other classes of antibiotics with systemic toxicity is also of interest, but data are not sufficient for specific recommendations.

The potential role of passive immunotherapy for treatment or prevention of GNB infections continues to be investigated. However, results from clinical trials have overall been variable and generally disappointing. Therefore, new isolated reports should be reviewed with caution, particularly where the intervention is potentially toxic and/or costly. Examples of failed, logical approaches include efforts to suppress potentially excessive host responses and, conversely, to enhance apparently weak responses. Unfortunately, these interventions may dysregulate overall host response sufficiently to result in ineffective, or even harmful, overall effects. Commercially available agents include immunosuppressants (corticosteroids, tumor necrosis factor [TNF] antagonists, etc.) and immunostimulants (granulocyte colony-stimulating factor [G-CSF], granulocyte-macrophage colony-stimulating factor [GM-CSF], interferons, etc.). Although the value of these agents in most patients is unclear, severe neutropenia (neutrophils $<500/mm^3$) is associated with very high risk and should usually be treated (for example with G-CSF, GM-CSF). Immunoglobulin supplements (IVIG) should be administered to patients with severe deficiencies, but a role in others with HAP/VAP with GNB is not established.

PROGNOSIS

Unfortunately, the mortality rate associated with GNB pneumonia remains high, ranging from 20 to 90%. Mortality is largely determined by the severity of the underlying illness. Although bacteremia with GNB is not necessarily associated with higher mortality, neutropenic patients with *P. aeruginosa* pneumonia and bacteremia have a mortality exceeding 80%. Supportive measures directed at the underlying illnesses, improving multiorgan dysfunction, and reducing risk factors for development of pneumonia, are likely important for overall outcome.

PREVENTION

A persistently high mortality rate from GNB pneumonia continues to stimulate interest in preventative therapy. Unfortunately, the need for intubation and antibiotics for apparent infections, as well as the underlying serious illnesses of these patients, significantly limit the impact of prevention efforts. Nevertheless, risk factors may be modified in some patients.

Avoidance of prolonged intubation can diminish HAP/VAP. Noninvasive (mask) ventilation (NIV) applied initially to patients with respiratory insufficiency may reduce HAP/VAP and associated mortality among patients with respiratory insufficiency, including those with neutropenia. However, the role of NIV after extubation for respiratory failure is more complex. NIV may be helpful when applied routinely at the time of extubation of marginal patients, perhaps diminishing fatigue leading to respiratory failure, but it appears potentially harmful when used to delay reintubation of patients with signs of respiratory failure after extubation.

If intubation is required, an oral rather than nasal route is recommended to avoid obstructing sinuses and, if feasible, with a dorsal lumen above the cuff for continuous or intermittent suction to reduce secretions in the subglottic space. At the time of extubation, careful attention to clearing these secretions is recommended to avoid large volume aspiration. One practical approach, which this author suggests, is as follows. (1) Temporarily increase positive pressure in the trachea (increase positive end expiratory pressure [PEEP], return to AC with larger volumes) just before and during a very slow deflation of the balloon, capturing the few secretions that fall into the trachea with an endotracheal suction catheter. (2) Then rapidly clear the larger volume of secretions thrown up into the posterior pharynx with an oral suction device. (3) Lastly, pull the endotracheal tube out while continuing suctioning with the catheter extended through the endotracheal tube.

Among patients with a tracheostomy who no longer require ventilatory support but still need access for suctioning, deflation of the balloon and application of a one-way value (e.g., Passey valve) not only facilitates speech, but also can reduce aspiration during swallowing. These valves permit inhalation via the tracheostomy tube and are generally more easily removed than locking tracheostomy tube caps when access is needed urgently. Among those who continue to require ventilator support, clearance of condensate in ventilator tubing is recommended, but frequent replacement of the tubing itself has little impact in patients who remain connected to the ventilator. Careful cleansing of hands and other contact surfaces is too often forgotten when moving from patient to patient.

Among high-risk patients, elevation of the head of the bed 30 to 45° to avoid gastric reflux appears important, as does limiting gastric residua, but protracted efforts to advance feeding tubes beyond the stomach are more costly, can delay onset of feedings, and have demonstrated benefit less consistently. The role of sucralfate for gastric protection without alkalization is not clear; sucralfate must be delivered directly to an acidic stomach to have an effect, is less effective for treatment of ulcers than acid inhibitors, and has inconsistently been demonstrated to reduce HAP/VAP with GNB. Prophylactic administration of antibiotics intratracheally, intravenously, or by oral paste to achieve selective gut decontamination can reduce colonization with organisms susceptible to the agents, but resistant strains appear and mortality has been inconsistently improved.

The potential value of augmenting immune responses in high-risk patients continues to be explored both for prevention and treatment, including active immunization of high-risk individuals and passive enhancement of host responses in established infections. Dietary supplements to restore micronutrient deficiencies (e.g., selenium, zinc) may enhance host immunity and epithelial repair, and may reduce risk of infection, although existing data regarding many selective nutrients remain inconsistent and insufficient for specific recommendations.

Continued research in this area holds the promise of reducing the unacceptably high mortality rate caused by infection with GNB, but large randomized, controlled clinical trials are needed before recommending routine use of specific interventions. Because the role of the GNB recovered from the airways in these patients is often unclear, valued endpoints for such studies should include reduced mortality, shortened stays, and reduced costs, and not simply an impact on recovery of the organisms that crudely define GNB pneumonia.

Recent General Reviews

1. Richards MJ, Edwards JR, Culver DH, et al. Nosocomial infections in medical intensive care units in the United States. National Nosocomial Infections Surveillance System. *Crit Care Med.* 1999;27:887.
   Incidence and character of nosocomial pneumonia.
2. Tablan OC, Anderson LJ, Besser R, et al. Guidelines for preventing health-care–associated pneumonia, 2003. Recommendations of CDC and the Healthcare Infection Control Practices Advisory Committee. *MMWR.* 2004;53:1–36.

More recent review, listing 433 references, with specific recommendations that were carefully considered and generally not overstated.

3. Kollef MH. The prevention of ventilator-associated pneumonia. *N Engl J Med.* 1999;340:627.
   A good review of prevention efforts circa 1999.
4. Mandell LA, Campbell GD. Nosocomial pneumonia guidelines. An international perspective. *Chest.* 1998;113:188–193S.
   Critical review of previous guidelines.
5. Bernstein JM, Campbell GD Jr. Emerging resistance and therapeutic options. *Chest.* 1999;115:1S.
6. Collard HR, Saint S, Matthay MA. Prevention of ventilator-associated pneumonia: an evidence-based systematic review. *Ann Intern Med.* 2003;138:494–502.
   Review in support of head elevation in most, and sucralfate, subglottic aspiration, and oscillating beds in some patients to prevent VAP.
7. Fiel S. Guidelines and critical pathways for severe hospital-acquired pneumonia. *Chest.* 2001;119:412–418S.
   Review of prior 1995 ATS recommendations.
8. Montejo JC, Zarazaga A, Lopez-Martinez J, et al. Immunonutrition in the intensive care unit. A systematic review and consensus statement. *Clinical Nutr.* 2003;22:221–233.
   Reviews nutritional value in the ICU, concluding data are inconsistent, but supporting consideration of supplements that may support immune function.
9. Marik PE, Zaloga GP. Gastric versus post-pyloric feeding: a systematic review. *Crit Care.* 2003;7:46–51.
   Pneumonia not significantly reduced by passing feeding tube past pylorus, but delays initiation of feeding.

Recent Relevant Studies
10. El-Solh AA, Pietrantoni C, Bhat A, et al. Microbiology of severe aspiration pneumonia in institutionalized elderly. *Am J Respir Crit Care Med.* 2003;167:1650–1654.
11. El-Solh AA, Aquilina AT, Dhillon RS, et al. Impact of invasive strategy on management of antimicrobial treatment failure in institutionalized older people with severe pneumonia. *Am J Respir Crit Care Med.* 2002;166:1038–1043.
    While sampling adjusted therapy, there was no impact on mortality.
12. Esteban A, Frutos-Vivar F, Ferguson ND, et al. Noninvasive positive-pressure ventilation for respiratory failure after extubation. *N Engl J Med.* 2004;350:2452–2460.
    Multicenter trial of delaying reintubation with trial of NIV: outcome worse, including greater ICU mortality with NIV.
13. Ferrer M, Esquinas A, Arancibia F, et al. Noninvasive ventilation during persistent weaning failure: a randomized, controlled trial. *Am J Respir Crit Care Med.* 2003;168:70–76.
    Routine application of NIV immediately after extubation trials of selected patients with marginal weaning parameters, having failed 2-hour T-piece trials on 3 consecutive days, but who were cooperative and lacked excessive secretions, had better outcomes, including survival.
14. Antonelli M, Conti G, Rocco M, et al. A comparison of noninvasive positive-pressure ventilation and conventional mechanical ventilation in patients with acute respiratory failure. *N Engl J Med.* 1998;339:429.
    Earlier study that demonstrated decreased mortality with early application of NIV in patients at risk of intubation, tending to reduce nosocomial pneumonia.
15. Ioanas M, Cavalcanti M, Ferrer M, et al. Hospital-acquired pneumonia: coverage and treatment adequacy of current guidelines. *Eur Respir J.* 2003;22:876–882.
    ATS 1996 guidelines adequately described GNB pneumonia, but antibiotic recommendations were inadequate, reflecting resistant strains. Therefore, antibiotic use should not bezealously restricted to those listed in available guidelines, as antibiotic selection pressure willcontinually shift the target.

16. Chastre J, Wolff M, Fagon JY, et al. Comparison of 8 vs 15 days of antibiotic therapy for ventilator-associated pneumonia in adults: a randomized trial. *JAMA*. 2003;290:2888–2898.

   Seeking to reduce antibiotic selection pressure time, the shorter course unfortunately diminished efficacy for clearing nonfermenting, gram-negative organisms.

17. Gruson D, Hilbert G, Vargas F, et al. Strategy of antibiotic rotation: long-term effect on incidence and susceptibilities of gram-negative bacilli responsible for ventilator-associated pneumonia. *Crit Care Med*. 2003;21:1908–1914.

   Unfortunate swing of late outcome data that eroded initially published enthusiasm for the approach.

18. Hamer DH. Treatment of nosocomial pneumonia and tracheobronchitis caused by multi-drug resistant Pseudomonas aeruginosa with aerosolized colistin. *Am J Respir Crit Care Med*. 2000;162:328–330.

   Three patients treated by nebulization of systemically toxic drug.

19. de Jonge E, Schultz MJ, Spanjaard L, et al. Effects of selective decontamination of digestive tract on mortality and acquisition of resistant bacteria in intensive care: a randomized, controlled trial. *Lancet*. 2003;362:1011–1016.

   A complex approach renews hope for a role of selective gut decontamination in reducing colonization with GNB, without increased resistance.

20. Berger MM, Spertini F, Shenkin A, et al. Trace element supplementation modulates pulmonary infection rates after major burns: a double-blind, placebo-controlled trial. *Am J Clin Nutr*. 1998;68:365.

   Selenium, zinc, and copper supplement reduces pulmonary infections in burn patients.

21. Girodon F, Galan P, Monget AL, et al. Impact of trace elements and vitamin supplementation on immunity and infections in institutionalized elderly patients: a randomized controlled trial. MIN. VIT. AOX. geriatric network. *Arch Intern Med*. 1999;159:748.

   Selenium plus zinc supplement enhances influenza vaccine titers and tends to reduce respiratory infections.

22. Conejero R, Bonet A, Grau T, et al. Effect of a glutamine-enriched enteral diet on intestinal permeability and infectious morbidity at 28 days in critically ill patients with systemic inflammatory response syndrome: a randomized, single-blind, prospective, multicenter study. *Nutrition*. 2002;18:716.

   HAP declined; additional supportive studies needed.

23. Holzapfel L, Chastang C, Demingeon G, et al. A randomized study assessing the systematic search for maxillary sinusitis in nasotracheally mechanically ventilated patients. Influence of nosocomial maxillary sinusitis on the occurrence of ventilator-associated pneumonia. *Am J Respir Crit Care Med*. 1999;159:695.

   Suggests early recognition and treatment of sinusitis reduces the incidence of nosocomial pneumonia in intubated patients.

Historically Important References

24. Reyes MP. The aerobic gram-negative bacillary pneumonias. *Med Clin North Am*. 1980;64:363.

   A readable review with many classic references.

25. Unger JD, Rose HD, Unger GF. Gram-negative pneumonia. *Radiology*. 1973; 107:283.

   Discusses classic radiologic features.

26. Dorff GJ, Rytel MW, Scanlon G. Etiologies and characteristic features of pneumonia in a municipal hospital. *Am J Med Sci*. 1973;266:349.

   A study of 178 cases of pneumonia before the initiation of antibiotics.

27. Polednak AP. Postmortem bacteriology and pneumonia in a mentally retarded population. *Am J Clin Pathol*. 1977;67:190.

   Postmortem diagnosis that was most accurate!

28. Valdivieso M, Gil-Extremera B, Bodey GP. Gram-negative bacillary pneumonia in the compromised host. *Medicine* (Baltimore). 1977;55:214.

   A classic, large study of patients receiving tumor chemotherapy, with good discussions.

29. Zornoza J, Goldman AM, Bodey GP. Radiologic features of gram-negative pneumonias in the neutropenic patient. *AJR*. 1976;127:989.
30. Andrews CP, Coalson JJ, Johanson WG. Diagnosis of nosocomial bacterial pneumonia in acute, diffuse lung injury. *Chest*. 1981;80:254.
    Gram-negative bacterial pneumonia is difficult to diagnose in adult respiratory distress syndrome.
31. Rose HD, Heckman MG, Unger JD. *Pseudomonas aeruginosa* pneumonia in adults. *Am Rev Respir Dis*. 1973;107:416.
    A classic description.
32. Fuchshuber PR, et al. *Ecthyma gangrenosum* secondary to *E. coli* sepsis. *Infect Med*. 1998;15:798.
    The finding discussed is seen in infections other than Pseudomonas. *This is a well-written case report of it in* E. coli *sepsis, with an illustrative description and thoroughly referenced list of the associated infectious agents.*
33. Jonas M, Cunha BA. Bacteremic *Escherichia coli* pneumonia. *Arch Intern Med*. 1982;142:2157.
    A good study and review.
34. Tillotson JR, Lerner MA. Characteristics of pneumonias caused by *Bacillus proteus*. *Ann Intern Med*. 1968;68:287.
    A classic study of outpatients.
35. Yu VL. *Serratia marcescens*: historical perspective and clinical review. *N Engl J Med*. 1979;300:887.
36. Hurley EJ, Viroslav J, Gray WR, et al. Pharyngeal aspiration in normal adults and patients with depressed consciousness. *Am J Med*. 1978;64:564.
    Aspiration is common, even in normals.
37. Torres A, Serra-Batlles J, Ros E, et al. Pulmonary aspiration of gastric contents in patients receiving mechanical ventilation: the effect of body position. *Ann Intern Med*. 1992;116:540.
    Emphasizes the importance of elevating the head of the bed after intubation, because the endotracheal tube only reduces acute aspiration volumes, not aspiration per se.
38. Mann HJ, Canafax DM, Cipolle RJ, et al. Increased dosage requirements of tobramycin and gentamicin for treating *Pseudomonas pneumonia* in patients with cystic fibrosis. *Pediatr Pulmonol*. 1985;1:238.
    Higher aminoglycoside doses were required to maintain levels in cystic fibrosis patients.
39. Johanson WG Jr, Seidenfeld JJ, Gomez P Jr, et al. Bacteriologic diagnosis of nosocomial pneumonia following prolonged mechanical ventilation. *Am Rev Respir Dis*. 1988;137:259.
    An important animal (baboon) study, suggesting bronchoalveolar lavage is more sensitive and correlates better with burden than protected brush and needle aspirates, although it is not more specific.
40. Brown RB, Kruse JA, Counts GW, et al. Double-blind study of endobronchial tobramycin in the treatment of gram-negative bacterial pneumonia. *Antimicrob Agents Chemother*. 1990;34:269.
    Added to intravenous therapy, aminoglycoside instillation accelerates bacterial clearance without a significant impact on overall hospital course.
41. Intravenous Immunoglobulin Collaborative Study Group. Prophylactic intravenous administration of standard immune globulin as compared to core-lipopolysaccharide immune globulin in patients at high risk of postsurgical infection. *N Engl J Med*. 1992;327:234.
    Nonimmune globulin inhibited GNB infections more effectively than specific immune globulin.
42. Hospital-acquired pneumonia in adults: diagnosis, assessment of severity, initial antimicrobial therapy, and preventive strategies. A consensus statement, American Thoracic Society, November 1995. *Am J Respir Crit Care Med*. 1996;153:1711–1725.

31. ANAEROBIC PULMONARY INFECTIONS

David M. Shaw and Jayne E. Chu

Anaerobic infection is relatively common in the lung and pleural space. Anaerobic bacteria, which have been isolated in 85 to 93% of lung abscesses and in 29 to 76% of empyemas, are a major cause of both community-acquired and hospital-acquired pneumonias. However, the role of anaerobic pathogens in pulmonary infections is often overlooked because of the difficulty in isolating and culturing these organisms. Blood cultures are positive in less than 3% of anaerobic pulmonary infections. Anaerobic bacteria are part of the normal oropharyngeal flora. Expectorated sputum and bronchoscopy aspirates are, therefore, often contaminated by oropharyngeal flora. Transtracheal aspirates, transthoracic aspirates, and quantitative protected brush specimens, all of which avoid contamination from the upper airway, are difficult to obtain and maintain under the anaerobic conditions necessary for culture. (An empyema sample, however, can be collected by thoracentesis anaerobically.) Because of the limitations of culture techniques, most anaerobic infections are diagnosed presumptively, based on the clinical presentation.

Anaerobic pulmonary infection is caused by aspiration of oral secretions, direct extension from continuous foci such as subphrenic abscesses, or by hematogenous spread. More than 70% of cases are caused by aspiration. Aspiration is commonly associated with states of impaired consciousness, such as alcoholism, cerebrovascular disease, drug overdose, general anesthesia, head trauma, or seizure disorder. Other predisposing conditions include neuromuscular disease, esophageal dysmotility, intestinal obstruction, use of nasogastric or orogastric tubes, periodontal disease, gingivitis, bronchial obstruction, and smoking (which compromises the activity of respiratory cilia). The most common sites of infection are the dependent portions of the lung: if aspiration occurs in the recumbent position, the posterior segments of the upper lobes and superior segments of the lower lobes are generally involved; if aspiration occurs in the upright position, the basal segments of the lower lobes are involved. When infection develops in other pulmonary segments, an underlying process other than aspiration (e.g., bronchial obstruction or metastatic infection) should be suspected.

The most common bacteria causing anaerobic infections resemble flora found in the gingival crevice, with *Fusobacterium nucleatum*, *Peptostreptococcus* species, and *Prevotella melaninogenicus* being the predominant organisms. *Bacteroides fragilis* is a notable exception. It is isolated in 7 to 21% of anaerobic infections and is not commonly present in the oropharyngeal cavity. Unlike aerobic pneumonias, most anaerobic infections are polymicrobial, with an average of three organisms per infection. In approximately half of anaerobic infections, only anaerobic bacteria are recovered. The remaining half have aerobic bacteria concurrently present, although no specific clinical characteristics distinguish between exclusively anaerobic infections and those caused by anaerobic–aerobic mixtures. Aerobic bacteria associated with anaerobic infections include *Klebsiella* species, *Staphylococcus aureus*, *Streptococcus* species, and *Haemophilus influenzae*. Hospital-acquired aspiration pneumonia is more likely caused by mixed aerobic–anaerobic infections in which the aerobic component is often gram-negative rods.

Because the bacteriology of most anaerobic pneumonias is similar, the degree of virulence depends on the host factors and the size of the inoculum. Although aspirating small amounts of mouth contents is relatively common, infection usually does not occur, owing to the less virulent nature of anaerobic bacteria in general. However, aspiration can lead to pneumonia if either large amounts of oropharyngeal secretions are aspirated or chronic infections in the gingivodental crevice increase the concentration of anaerobic bacteria in the mouth. Anaerobic pneumonias also can occur when focal areas of the lung are subject to tissue necrosis or stasis of secretions from conditions such as pulmonary infarction, bronchial obstruction (resulting from a foreign body or neoplasm), or bronchiectasis. Underlying conditions that compromise host defense (e.g., malnutrition, diabetes mellitus, steroids, and cytotoxic agents) are also risk factors for anaerobic lung infection.

The clinical course of anaerobic pulmonary infections is progressive, and the natural history of uncontrolled disease can be divided into several distinct stages: (1) pneumonitis, (2) necrotizing pneumonia, (3) abscess formation, and (4) empyema. Pneumonitis mimics common bacterial aerobic pneumonia with an acute presentation of fever, cough, pleuritic chest pain, and patchy infiltrates seen on chest radiograph. The only distinguishing clinical features of acute anaerobic infection are putrid sputum and the absence of rigors, though neither occurs frequently enough to reliably differentiate between an anaerobic and aerobic infection. An underlying predisposing condition may also be found in most patients. If the anaerobic infection is treated promptly, the pneumonitis resolves without residual lesions. Necrotizing pneumonia can develop after 7 to 16 days if the anaerobic pneumonitis is untreated or unchecked by normal host defenses. Necrotizing pneumonia commonly has a more subacute presentation, with patients often having symptoms for more than a week before presentation. Signs and symptoms include fever, pleuritic chest pain, putrid sputum, and multiple microabscesses (<1 cm in diameter as seen on chest radiograph). The response to treatment at this stage of infection is slow, and pulmonary complications are frequent. Large lung abscesses can form if the microabscesses enlarge and coalesce. Lung abscesses often represent an indolent stage of the infection, which can mimic tuberculous infection or lung cancer. Patients usually present, after several weeks, with fever, anorexia, weight loss, anemia, pleuritic chest pain, putrid sputum, clubbing, and thick-walled cavitary lesions (>1 cm as seen on chest radiograph). If the infection remains uncontrolled, the next stage often is empyema formation caused by necrosis extending to involve the pleura. A bronchopleural fistula can occur if the necrosis communicates with the airways.

Treatment of anaerobic pulmonary infections is usually empiric because of the difficulty in obtaining valid cultures. Special techniques are required for transport and processing of specimens, and extended periods are required to isolate anaerobic organisms in culture. Even when appropriate specimens are collected and rigorous culturing techniques are used, most laboratories do not perform in vitro sensitivity testing on anaerobes. Most importantly, most infections involve three to five microbial species and the pathogenic potential of each one may be uncertain. The National Committee for Clinical Laboratory Standards does not recommend routine sensitivity testing of anaerobic bacteria; empiric treatment of anaerobic pulmonary infections is usually effective without it.

The three most commonly recommended antibiotic regimens for anaerobic pulmonary infections are penicillin, clindamycin, and the combination of metronidazole plus penicillin. In the 1960s, nearly all anaerobic pulmonary infections were treated with penicillin, and treatment failures were few. Although penicillin has proved to be an effective treatment for anaerobic pulmonary infections, in vitro sensitivity testing demonstrates that 15 to 25% of patients have strains that are resistant to penicillin because of the production of β-lactamases. Resistance is most commonly found in *Prevotella* and *Fusobacterium* spp. Clindamycin, however, is effective against β-lactamase–producing pathogens. One large prospective study comparing antibiotic regimens for the treatment of anaerobic lung abscesses found a statistically significant difference favoring clindamycin over penicillin in terms of number of treatment failures, number of relapses, mean duration of fever, and mean duration of putrid sputum. However, penicillin is still the drug of choice for some clinicians because of its low cost and because clinical failures with penicillin remain rare. A recent trial also has demonstrated that amoxicillin-clavulanic acid is an effective regimen. Another antibiotic for the treatment of anaerobic infections is metronidazole, which has bactericidal activity against virtually all anaerobes and good penetration into abscess cavities (and through the blood–brain barrier). However, treatment of anaerobic lung infections with metronidazole alone has been associated with an unacceptably high proportion of treatment failures, possibly because of its poor activity against coexisting aerobic and microaerophilic streptococci. Thus, metronidazole is a viable treatment option for anaerobic infections only when used in combination with penicillin.

The treatment duration necessary for an anaerobic lung infection must be individualized, because the rate of response to therapy can vary. Patients with uncomplicated pneumonitis usually show signs of resolution within the first few days of treatment, whereas those with necrotizing pneumonia and abscesses may take weeks to improve. The response to treatment of patients with empyema may be extensively delayed and fevers can recur and persist if the empyema is not completely drained. Parenteral antibiotics are usually given initially; oral medications can be substituted once fever and other signs of toxicity have subsided. Oral (outpatient) therapy usually continues for 6 to 12 weeks. Chest radiographs are obtained at intervals of 2 to 4 weeks. Treatment should continue until radiographs demonstrate complete resolution of parenchymal opacities or show only stable, residual scars.

Antibiotics are the mainstay of treatment for anaerobic lung infections. Although empyema almost always requires surgical drainage, lung abscesses usually resolve with antibiotics alone; drainage can even be hazardous because of risk of bacteria spillage into other pulmonary segments. Fiberoptic bronchoscopy is indicated to rule out bronchial occlusion as a cause of lung abscess when occlusion is suspected, either on clinical grounds or because the abscess fails to resolve within a reasonable time. Surgical intervention may be required in 10 to 12% of lung abscesses and is indicated under the following circumstances: (1) rapid enlargement of the abscess despite antibiotics; (2) life-threatening hemorrhage caused by erosion into a major blood vessel; (3) bronchial obstruction with poor drainage; (4) symptomatic bronchiectasis; or (5) associated lung cancer. Some patients with urgent needs for abscess drainage may, however, have prohibitive operative risks. A suggested approach in such cases is percutaneous drainage of pulmonary abscesses, which has been successful in some severely septic and debilitated patients.

The mortality rate for untreated anaerobic pulmonary infections is 30 to 35%; it is reduced to 5 to 10% with antibiotics and other appropriate therapy. Inadequate or delayed effective therapy may allow the progressive destruction of parenchymal tissue, resulting in bronchiectasis, pulmonary fibrosis, chronic empyema, persistent bronchopleural or pleurocutaneous fistula, and recurrent pulmonary infection. In addition, the infection can disseminate to distant sites, particularly to the brain. Conditions associated with poor prognosis include large abscess cavity size, necrotizing pneumonia, prolonged symptoms lasting more than 8 weeks, advanced age, bronchial obstruction, and comorbid diseases. However, with prompt diagnosis and effective treatment, the prognosis for anaerobic pulmonary infections generally has been favorable.

1. Bartlett JG, Finegold SM. Anaerobic infections of the lung and pleural space. *Am Rev Respir Dis.* 1974;110:56.

   A classic review of anaerobic pulmonary infections.
2. Beerens H, Tahon-Castel M. *Infections Humaines a Bacteries Anaerobies Nontoxigenes.* Brussels, Belgium: Presses Academiques Europeenes; 1965:91.

   Transthoracic needle aspiration was used to characterize the flora of lung abscesses, and anaerobes were recovered in 22 of 26 patients.
3. Brook I, Finegold SM. Bacteriology and therapy of lung abscess in children. *J Pediatr.* 1979;94:10.

   Bacteriologic data and clinical findings of pediatric patients with lung abscesses found Peptococcus *species,* Peptostreptococcus *species,* Bacteroides melaninogenicus, *and* Bacteroides fragilis *to be the most frequent isolates.*
4. Fernandez-Sabe N, Carratala J, Dorca J, et al. Efficacy and safety of sequential amoxicillin-clavulanate in the treatment of anaerobic lung infections. *Eur J Clin Microbiol Infect Dis.* 2003;22:185–187.

   Forty patients with lung abscess or necrotizing pneumonia were treated successfully with I.V. and then oral amoxicillin-clavulanic acid without treatment failure or adverse reaction.

5. Gudiol F, Manresa F, Pallares R, et al. Clindamycin vs penicillin for anaerobic lung infections: high rate of penicillin failures associated with penicillin-resistant *Bacteroides melaninogenicus*. *Arch Intern Med*. 1990;150: 2525.
   Anaerobes were isolated in 37 of 41 patients with lung abscesses using transthoracic needle aspiration.
6. Bartlett JG, Gorbach SL, Thadepalli H, et al. Bacteriology of empyema. *Lancet*. 1974;1:338.
   Anaerobic bacteria were isolated in 76% of 83 cases of empyema.
7. Lemmer J, Botham MJ, Orringer MB. Modern management of adult thoracic empyema. *J Thorac Cardiovasc Surg*. 1985;90:849.
   Shift in bacteriology of empyemas, with a decrease in pneumococcal empyemas to 5 to 10% and an increase in anaerobic empyemas to 25 to 40%.
8. Ries K, Levison ME, Kaye D. Transtracheal aspiration in pulmonary infection. *Arch Intern Med*. 1974;133:453.
   Transtracheal aspiration in 134 patients with suspected bronchopulmonary infection revealed anaerobic organisms in 33%.
9. Pollock HM, Hawkins EL, Bonner JR, et al. Diagnosis of bacterial pulmonary infections with quantitative protected catheter cultures obtained during bronchoscopy. *J Clin Microbiol*. 1983;17:255.
   Protected fiberoptic bronchoscopy brush specimens from 172 patients revealed anaerobic organisms in 22% of cases of infection.
10. Bartlett JG, O'Keefe P, Tally FP, et al. Bacteriology of hospital-acquired pneumonia. *Arch Intern Med*. 1986;146:868.
   Anaerobic bacteria were the predominant isolate in 35% of 159 patients with hospital-acquired pneumonia.
11. Bartlett JG. Anaerobic bacterial infections of the lung. *Chest*. 1987;91:901.
   An excellent review of anaerobic pulmonary infections.
12. Bartlett JG, Finegold SM. Anaerobic pleuropulmonary infections. *Medicine*. 1972;51:413.
   A comprehensive review of anaerobic pleuropulmonary infections.
13. Lorber B, Swenson RM. Bacteriology of aspiration pneumonia. A prospective study of community- and hospital-acquired cases. *Ann Intern Med*. 1974;81: 329.
   Anaerobic bacteria were isolated in 21 of 24 patients with community-acquired infections and 8 of 23 of those with hospital-acquired aspiration pneumonias.
14. Brook I, Finegold SM. Bacteriology of aspiration pneumonia in children. *Pediatrics*. 1980;65:1115.
   Aspiration pneumonia in children commonly involved anaerobic gram-positive cocci, Bacteroides melaninogenicus, and Fusobacterium.
15. Cesar L, Gonzalez C, Calia FM. Bacteriologic flora of aspiration-induced pulmonary infections. *Arch Intern Med*. 1975;135:711.
   Anaerobes isolated in 100% of patients who were aspiration susceptible, usually with multiple species isolated.
16. Bartlett JG, Gorbach SL, Finegold SM. The bacteriology of aspiration pneumonia. *Am J Med*. 1974;56:202.
   Anaerobic bacteria were the most common isolates in aspiration pneumonia, but aerobes concomitantly presented in half of infections.
17. Socransky SS. Microbiology of periodontal disease—present status and future considerations. *J Periodontol*. 1977;48:497.
   Anaerobes originate in and around gingival crevices and achieve high concentrations with periodontal infections.
18. Bartlett JG. Anaerobic bacterial pneumonias. *Am Rev Respir Dis*. 1979; 119:19.
   Clinical features of 46 patients with anaerobic bacterial pneumonitis were compared with patients with pneumococcal pneumonia. Patients were comparable in age, fever, leukocyte count, and radiographic abnormalities. Differences included putrid sputum in two patients, lack of chills, tendency to develop abscess, and underlying neoplasms in patients with anaerobic infections.

19. Drugs for anaerobic infections. *Med Lett Drugs Ther*. 1984;26:87.
    Recommended regimens for treatment of anaerobic pulmonary infections: penicillin, clindamycin, or metronidazole plus penicillin.
20. Weiss W. Oral antibiotic therapy of acute primary lung abscess: comparison of penicillin G and tetracycline. *Curr Ther Res*. 1970;12:154.
    Forty patients with lung abscesses were treated with penicillin G, and all but three responded. The three failures were treated successfully with tetracycline.
21. Kirby BD, George WL, Sutter VL, et al. Gram-negative anaerobic bacilli: their role in infection and patterns of susceptibility to antimicrobial agents. I. Little-known *Bacteroides* species. *Rev Infect Dis*. 1980;2:914.
    Some Bacteroides species were resistant to β-lactam antibiotics because of the production of β-lactamases.
22. Levison ME, Mangura CT, Lorber B, et al. Clindamycin compared with penicillin for the treatment of anaerobic lung abscess. *Ann Intern Med*. 1983;98:466.
    Clindamycin was superior to penicillin in the treatment of pulmonary abscesses, with a shorter febrile period and with fewer days of fetid sputum, treatment failures, and relapses.
23. Tally FP, Sutter VL, Finegold SM. Treatment of anaerobic infections with metronidazole. *Antimicrob Agents Chemother*. 1975;7:672.
    Ten patients with anaerobic infections treated with metronidazole: six patients were cured; three initially responded but subsequently required change to another drug and one did not respond.
24. Perlino CA. Metronidazole vs. clindamycin treatment of anaerobic pulmonary infection. Failure of metronidazole therapy. *Arch Intern Med*. 1981;141:1424.
    Metronidazole is less effective than clindamycin for the treatment of anaerobic pulmonary infections.
25. Sanders CV, Hanna BJ, Lewis AC. Metronidazole in the treatment of anaerobic infections. *Am Rev Respir Dis*. 1979;120:337.
    Thirteen patients with anaerobic pleuropulmonary infections treated with metronidazole: five were cured and five did not respond; the effect could not be assessed in the remaining three patients.
26. Weiss W. Cavity behavior in acute, primary, nonspecific lung abscess. *Am Rev Respir Dis*. 1973;108:1273.
    The courses of 71 acute, primary lung abscesses treated with antibiotics were followed over a 10-year period.
27. Sosenko A, Glassroth J. Fiberoptic bronchoscopy in the evaluation of lung abscesses. *Chest*. 1985;87:489.
    Recommends fiberoptic bronchoscopy evaluation in patients whose lung abscesses are likely related to underlying bronchogenic carcinoma. Does not recommend routine bronchoscopy in all patients with abscess.
28. Harber P, Terry PB. Fatal lung abscesses: review of 11 years' experience. *South Med J*. 1981;74:281.
    A review of the outcome of 440 patients with lung abscess revealed that advanced age and concomitant disease were associated with a higher risk of death.
29. Hagan JL, Hardy JD. Lung abscess revisited. A survey of 184 cases. *Ann Surg*. 1983;197:755.
    A survey of 184 patients with lung abscess.
30. Pohlson EC, McNamara JJ, Char C, et al. Lung abscess: a changing pattern of the disease. *Am J Surg*. 1985;150:97.
    A survey of 89 patients treated for lung abscess. Twenty three patients underwent surgical therapy when cancer was suspected or they failed to improve with medical management.
31. Weissberg D. Percutaneous drainage of lung abscess. *J Thorac Cardiovasc Surg*. 1984;87:308.
    Seven patients with lung abscess and severe sepsis were treated successfully with percutaneous drainage.
32. Snow N, Lucas A, Horrigan TP. Utility of pneumonotomy in the treatment of cavitary lung disease. *Chest*. 1985;87:731.

Three patients underwent percutaneous drainage for cavitary pulmonary lesions instead of resection because of high operative risks.

33. Bartlett JG, Gorbach SL, Tally FP, et al. Bacteriology and treatment of primary lung abscess. Am Rev Respir Dis. 1974;109:510.

Bacteriologic data in 26 cases of lung abscesses indicated Fusobacterium nucleatum, Bacteroides melaninogenicus, *and anaerobic gram-positive cocci to be the principal isolates.*

---

32. EMPYEMA

Carl A. Riddick

Pulmonary infection is frequently complicated by the development of pleural inflammation and infection; both are associated with increased morbidity and mortality. Parapneumonic effusions are typically classified as uncomplicated or complicated. Uncomplicated effusions resolve with antibiotic therapy alone; complicated effusions require drainage to effect a cure. Empyema is defined as the presence of pus in the pleural space. Pulmonary parenchymal infection is the most common cause of empyema. Postsurgical, posttraumatic and iatrogenic etiologies are now encountered with increasing frequency. Less common causes include bacteremic seeding of the pleural space, septic emboli from distant sites of infection, esophageal perforation, and direct extension from perithoracic sites of infection (e.g., subphrenic abscess). The bacteriology of empyema has shifted over the years and *Streptococcus pneumoniae* is no longer the most commonly isolated organism in most published series. *Staphylococcus aureus*, gram-negative enteric organisms and anaerobes are now increasingly isolated. Anaerobic organisms are responsible for 11 to 76% of reported cases depending on the reported series and the meticulousness of the search for these organisms. Many cases are polymicrobial. The incidence of opportunistic and unusual organisms has also increased, coincident with the increasing numbers of patients seen with underlying immunodeficiency.

Untreated parapneumonic effusions can progress through three phases of variable duration. The initial response to an underlying parenchymal focus of infection is the exudation of sterile fluid across the visceral pleura into the pleural space. This fluid is thin, free flowing and characterized by a low white blood cell count and normal pH and glucose concentration. This so-called *exudative phase* can last from hours to days. During the next (fibrinopurulent) phase, neutrophils accumulate in the fluid in response to the invasion and multiplication of microorganisms. During this phase, pleural fluid increases in volume and pH and glucose concentration fall. A rise in lactic dehydrogenase (LDH) is caused by cellular metabolism and lysis. The pleural fluid subsequently thickens, fibrin is deposited on both pleural surfaces and loculation and the formation of a limiting membrane (i.e., the pleural peel) are initiated. After a variable interval ranging from days to weeks, the organization stage begins, characterized by migration and increased activity of, fibroblasts in the developing membrane and the subsequent formation of an inelastic pleural peel. Untreated, empyema and uncomplicated pleural effusions rarely resolve. The latter can spontaneously rupture into lung parenchyma (bronchopleural fistula) or through the chest wall (empyema necessitatis). The inflammatory response is largely orchestrated by the release of soluble mediators of inflammation from both resident and recruited inflammatory cells, including the mesothelial cells lining the pleural surfaces.

Empyema should be considered whenever pneumonia is diagnosed and a pleural effusion is detected. The clinical presentation is nonspecific and is frequently conditioned by host factors, including associated disease processes, the immune status of the host and coincidental medical therapy. Fever, cough, dyspnea, pleuritic chest pain, and leukocytosis are common but not always present. Empyema can also present as an indolent process with malaise, low-grade fever, weight loss, and anorexia. Patients with post-pneumonectomy empyema can develop postoperative fever, expectorate large quantities of purulent sputum, and develop purulent drainage from the thoracotomy wound. Contralateral mediastinal shift can occur. Debilitated patients and those on corticosteroid and other immunosuppressive therapy can be afebrile and the peripheral blood leukocyte count may not be elevated. Empyema should always be suspected when patients with pneumonia fail to respond to seemingly appropriate antibiotic therapy. Delays in diagnosis and therapy are common.

The chest radiographs of patients with pneumonia should be carefully inspected for the presence of pleural fluid. If pleural effusion is noted or suspected, decubitus views should be obtained to confirm its presence, estimate the volume of fluid, assess for loculation and further assess the underlying parenchyma. Larger effusions and those present in non-dependent locations on plain radiographs may not require decubitus imaging. Radiographic findings are not specific for the different causative organism(s), but can have prognostic value. Fluid that is not free flowing on decubitus views or is present in fixed or nondependent locations suggests loculation. An air–fluid level is associated with empyema caused by a gas-forming organism, bronchopleural fistula or lung abscess abutting the pleural space.

Ultrasound and CT are increasingly used as a substitute or an adjunct to decubitus radiographs. Ultrasound has several applications, including the evaluation of the pleural fluid for loculation, localization of fluid for thoracentesis and guidance for the placement of thoracostomy tubes. However, ultrasound cannot image through bone or aerated lung which limits its effectiveness in localizing small fluid loculations within fissures, near the mediastinum and in paramediastinal locations. It is also not useful for evaluating the status of the underlying lung and airways. Contrast-enhanced chest computed tomography (CT) scanning is superior to both plain chest radiography and ultrasonography in defining the empyema space and assessing adequacy of drainage. Pleural thickening and the attenuation of subpleural fat are frequently noted but their presence or absence does not obviate the need for diagnostic thoracentesis. CT is useful for differentiating lung abscess from empyema with bronchopleural fistula. CT also can detect other conditions that may impact management decisions (e.g., lung masses, foreign bodies and bronchopleural fistulas).

Diagnostic thoracentesis is nearly always required for patients with parapneumonic effusions, as clinical parameters alone do not allow the clinician to reliably differentiate effusions requiring drainage from those likely to resolve with antibiotic therapy alone. However, if the pleural fluid layers to less than 1 cm on decubitus view or is less than 1 cm thick on ultrasound imaging, pleural fluid aspiration is usually not necessary. When thoracentesis is performed, the fluid should be collected carefully and visually inspected. The gross appearance of the aspirated fluid in pleural space infections ranges from thin and nonpurulent to thick and putrid. The latter is associated with anaerobic infection and is virtually diagnostic. Pleural fluid analysis should include determination of pH, differential leukocyte count and appropriate stains and cultures. If pH is not available, the glucose concentration should be measured. In the setting of a free-flowing parapneumonic effusion, a carefully obtained pH (collected anaerobically in a heparinized syringe and quickly placed on ice) or glucose concentration is commonly used to determine therapy. A small, free-flowing pleural effusion with a pH greater than 7.3 is usually associated with a positive response to antibiotic therapy alone, whereas a fluid pH less than 7.2 or a glucose level less than 60 suggest the need for drainage. Patients having free-flowing effusions with a pH between 7.2 and 7.3 can be started on antibiotic therapy alone and monitored. A repeat thoracentesis in 12 to 24 hours and clinical parameters can then be used to further guide therapy. An increasing volume of fluid, continued signs and symptoms suggestive of ongoing pleural sepsis and falling pH and glucose suggest the need for drainage.

The use of biochemical parameters should augment, not replace, clinical judgment regarding the treatment of parapneumonic effusions. The threshold for consideration of tube drainage needs to be individualized according to the patient's estimated risk for complicated effusion, empyema, and the likelihood of poor outcome. Pleural fluid

Gram's stains and cultures are not infrequently negative, especially in the setting of prior antibiotic therapy. In addition, pleural fluid in loculated effusions may not be homogeneous; i.e., fluid sampled from one locule may have unremarkable biochemical parameters and stain negative, whereas fluid in other locules may have features that suggest the need for drainage. Finally, pleural fluid biochemical parameters do not carry the same prognostic significance in the setting of other processes known to produce effusions with a low pH, in particular, rheumatoid pleuritis, tuberculous pleurisy and malignancy.

Antibiotic therapy and complete pleural space drainage are the mainstays of initial therapy for pleural empyema. The initial choice of antibiotics should be based on the clinical presentation, patient characteristics and risk factors, whether the infection was contracted in the community or in a hospital and the results of microbial stains and cultures of specimens of the fluid and from other sites. Anaerobes are commonly present in empyemas and empiric antibiotic regimens should usually include therapy directed against them. Keeping these facts in mind, several drug regimens may be effective, including (1) modified penicillin/beta-lactamase inhibitors; (2) clindamycin plus a third-generation cephalosporin (or aztreonam); and (3) penicillin, metronidazole, and a third-generation cephalosporin. For nosocomial or other suspected gram-negative empyemas, a fluoroquinolone, a third-generation cephalosporin or a broad-spectrum penicillin/β-lactamase inhibitor combination should be considered. A carbapenem can be used as *monotherapy*. Although most antibiotics adequately penetrate into the infected pleural space, aminoglycosides penetrate less well and can be inactivated by the acidic milieu of an empyema. They are, therefore, not appropriate as monotherapy. As with any infection, antibiotic therapy should be conditioned on the local susceptibilities of the commonly encountered organisms and adjusted once culture and sensitivity results are available. Therapy duration depends on the clinical circumstances; however, as in other necrotizing intrathoracic infections, antibiotic therapy should be continued until clinical and radiographic evidence of resolution of infection is seen.

Prompt and adequate drainage is indicated for (1) large or loculated effusion and one associated with thickened parietal pleura; (2) an effusion with a positive pleural fluid Gram's stain or culture; (3) one with frank pus on thoracentesis; (4) and, in the case of a parapneumonic effusion, one with a pleural fluid pH less than 7.2. (A possible exception is empyema associated with pneumococcal infection for which some experts recommend antibiotic therapy alone.) For free-flowing or uniloculate effusions, closed thoracostomy tube drainage is usually adequate. A large bore (28 to 36 Fr) chest tube should be placed in the dependent portion of the pleural space by one experienced in this procedure. After placement, adequacy of drainage should be confirmed by appropriate imaging studies, usually posteroanterior and lateral chest radiography. Image-guided drainage with fibrinolytic therapy, video-assisted thoracoscopic surgery and thoracotomy are all acceptable approaches. Fibrinolytic therapy with urokinase, streptokinase and, more recently, tissue plasminogen activator, has been used with success and a time-limited trial of this therapy may be considered before proceeding to surgery. Urokinase may avoid the risk of allergic reactions observed with streptokinase and may be less prone to antibody mediated deactivation.

Video-assisted thoracoscopic surgery is considered an appropriate intervention as either the initial approach or for those patients who fail to respond to image-guided drainage and fibrinolytic therapy. It has the advantage of allowing direct visualization of the pleural space, lysis of adhesions and optimal placement of chest tubes. If a pleural peel is present at thoracoscopy, the decision can be made to proceed directly to standard thoracotomy and pleural decortication. Minithoracotomy with digital lysis of adhesions and thoracostomy tube placement is another commonly used technique. For the most complex pleural space infections or after the development of a pleural peel, one may proceed directly to standard thoracotomy and decortication. This approach may shorten hospitalization and the duration of chest tube drainage and can usually be performed with reasonable safety, even when the duration of empyema is unknown. For patients too debilitated to undergo decortication, open drainage, with or without an Eloesser flap, can be an effective alternative, albeit one that is frequently associated with prolonged hospitalization. Surgical repair using a muscle or omental flap may be necessary for a bronchopleural fistula-associated empyema unresponsive to aggressive tube drainage, or for an empyema complicating a pulmonary resection. Thoracoplasty can also be considered in these settings.

1. Medical Section of the National Tuberculosis Association of the American Thoracic Society. Management of nontuberculous empyema: a statement of the Subcommittee on Surgery. *Am Rev Respir Dis.* 1962;85:935.
   This statement outlines the pathologic stages of empyema.
2. Light RW, et al. Parapneumonic effusions. *Am J Med.* 1980;69:507.
   Patients with parapneumonic effusions can be separated into those requiring drainage and those who do not on the basis of pleural fluid pH, glucose, and LDH.
3. Heffner JE, et al. Pleural fluid chemical analysis in parapneumonic effusions. A meta-analysis. *Am J Respir Care Med.* 1995;151:1700.
   A meta-analysis of studies examining the application of pleural fluid biochemical analysis to management decisions regarding treatment of parapneumonic effusions. They suggest that pleural fluid pH has the highest diagnostic accuracy when receiver operating characteristic techniques are used. Specific decision thresholds for instituting pleural drainage are presented.
4. Himelman RB, Callen PW. The prognostic value of loculations in parapneumonic pleural effusions. *Chest.* 1986;90:852.
   Ultrasound and CT scanning are more sensitive than plain chest radiographs in detecting pleural fluid loculations. Loculations have diagnostic and prognostic significance.
5. Light RW, Rodriguez RM. Management of parapneumonic effusions. *Clin Chest Med.* 1998;19:373.
   As part of their review of parapneumonic pleural effusions, the authors present a classification and treatment scheme.
6. Hughes CE, Van Scoy RE. Antibiotic therapy of pleural empyema. *Semin Respir Infect.* 1991;6:94.
   Initial empiric antibiotic regimens for empyema are offered.
7. Heffner JE. Infection of the pleural space. *Clin Chest Med.* 1999;20:607.
   An excellent, well-referenced review on the evaluation and management of pleural space infections.
8. Davies CW, Gleeson FV, Davies RJ. BTS guidelines for the management of pleural infection. *Thorax* 2003;58 Suppl 2:ii18.
   The British Thoracic Society's Pleural Diseases Group, Standards of Care Committee's clinical practice guideline on the management of parapneumonic effusion.
9. Colice GL, Curtis A, Deslauriers J, et al, for the American College of Chest Physicians Parapneumonic Effusions Panel. Medical and Surgical Treatment of Parapneumonic Effusions—An Evidence-Based Guideline. *Chest.* 2000;118:1158.
   A clinical practice guideline on the medical and surgical treatment of PPE from the Health and Sciences Policy Committee (HSP) of the American College of Chest Physicians.
10. Moulton JS. Image-guided management of complicated pleural fluid collections. *Radiologic Clinics of North America.* 2000;38:345.
    This article reviews image-guided thoracostomy drainage and intra-cavity fibrinolytic therapy.
11. Bouros D, et al. Intrapleural urokinase versus normal saline in the treatment of complicated parapneumonic effusions and empyema. *Am J Respir Crit Care Med.* 1999;159:37.
    A small randomized clinical trial showing that, as adjunctive treatment to thoracostomy tube drainage, intrapleural urokinase was superior to saline in the treatment of multiloculated pleural space infections.
12. Roberts JR. Minimally invasive surgery in the treatment of empyema: intraoperative decision making. *Ann Thorac Surg.* 2003;76:225.
    Examines the role of minimally invasive thoracic surgery in the treatment of empyema.

13. Waller DA. Thoracoscopy in management of postpneumonic pleural infections. *Curr Opin Pulm Med.* 2002;8:323.

   The author reviews recent studies and outcomes regarding the use of thoracoscopic intervention in the management of pleural space infection. While acknowledging its apparent utility he concludes that there are insufficient data to support its routine use.

---

33. ATYPICAL PNEUMONIAS: *MYCOPLASMA,* CHLAMYDOPHILA (CHLAMYDIA), Q FEVER, AND *LEGIONELLA*

Philip A. LoBue

Historically, the term *atypical pneumonia* was applied to pulmonary infections that differed clinically and radiographically from classic bacterial lobar pneumonia. Subsequently, a variety of causative organisms were identified as causes of pneumonia, including *Mycoplasma pneumoniae, Chlamydophila* (formerly *Chlamydia*) *psittaci* (psittacosis or ornithosis), *Chlamydophila* (formerly *Chlamydia*) *pneumoniae* (formerly *C. psittaci,* strain TWAR), *Coxiella burnetii* (Q fever), *Legionella* species, and various viruses. These agents cause pneumonia very commonly, accounting for about one fourth of all community-acquired pneumonias. Although illnesses caused by these organisms differ in their epidemiology and natural history, they are all thought to be transmitted via particle or droplet inhalation.

   M. pneumoniae accounts for 10 to 30% of pneumonias in ambulatory patients, depending on whether an outbreak is in progress. Although generally a disease of healthy children and young adults, *M. pneumoniae* also causes pneumonia in elderly patients, who are more likely to require hospitalization. *M. pneumoniae* has an incubation period averaging 14 to 21 days. The infection is usually endemic, but outbreaks do occur, especially in the fall and winter months, and appear to have a periodicity of 2 to 4 weeks. The rate of infection is greatest in areas of close personal contact (e.g., military bases, fraternity houses, households). *M. pneumoniae* infection is most commonly manifested as tracheobronchitis (75–80%) and relatively few infected persons develop frank pneumonia (3–6%). In addition to respiratory illness, *M. pneumoniae* can cause myringitis and a pharyngitis that is clinically indistinguishable from streptococcal pharyngitis. Other extrapulmonary manifestations have been described. The best known is cold agglutinin-induced hemolysis, which results from immunoglobulin M (IgM) antibodies that cross-react with the I antigen of red blood cells. Raynaud's syndrome, peripheral gangrene, and disseminated intravascular coagulation also can occur in this setting. Other complications include hepatitis, erythema multiforme, the syndrome of inappropriate antidiuretic hormone, migratory polyarthritis, pericarditis, myocarditis, and neurologic abnormalities, such as aseptic meningitis, meningoencephalitis, transverse myelitis, and Guillain-Barré syndrome. The overall mortality rate is 0.1%, which is largely attributed to neurologic and cardiac involvement. Overall, only 2% of patients with *M. pneumoniae* require hospitalization.

   The bacterial genus *Chlamydophila* contains three species: *C. trachomatis, C. psittaci,* and *C. pneumoniae. C. trachomatis* causes conjunctivitis and pneumonia in newborn infants but has not been implicated as a cause of adult respiratory disease.

   C. psittaci is primarily an avian pathogen but it also causes infection in humans (psittacosis) after contaminated droppings from diseased birds are inhaled. Parrots and parakeets (psittacine birds) are the most common sources of human infection, but domestic (chickens, ducks, and turkeys) and urban (pigeons) fowl also have been described as a source of infection. Psittacosis occurs sporadically but frequently is seen in association with avian outbreaks. It is a serious occupational hazard in poultry-processing plants, with turkeys being the most commonly involved bird in the United States and ducks in Europe. After the organism gains access to the upper respiratory tract, it spreads hematogenously to the lungs and to the reticuloendothelial system. The incubation period is 7 to 21 days. Human-to-human transmission is unusual, although infection of healthcare workers by patients has been described. Because human-to-human transmission is very rare, routine respiratory isolation of hospitalized patients is not recommended.

The clinical spectrum of psittacosis is variable and includes (1) a flulike illness (the majority); (2) pneumonia that, although generally mild, can be a severe multilobar consolidative process characterized by splenomegaly and relative bradycardia; and (3) a fulminant toxic syndrome with multiorgan failure. Common extrapulmonary manifestations include severe headache, photophobia, myalgias, arthralgias, nausea and vomiting, lymphadenopathy, hepatosplenomegaly, and epistaxis. Less commonly, endocarditis, myocarditis, disseminated intravascular coagulation, and thyroiditis are seen. Dermatologic manifestations include erythema nodosum, erythema marginatum, and a pink, roselike, macular rash (Horder's spots). High, spiking fevers (100–105°F), shaking chills, severe headache, and stupor characterize severe psittacosis, with renal failure and jaundice signifying fulminant infection. Poor prognostic signs include increased age, confusion, leukopenia, severe hypoxemia, and renal and multilobar pulmonary involvement. The mortality rate was 20% in the preantibiotic era and now is about 1% with appropriate treatment.

C. pneumoniae is currently recognized as a cause of respiratory illness. Initially it was believed to be a strain of *C. psittaci;* later, it was demonstrated to be a separate species. In contrast to *C. psittaci,* no animal vector (other than humans) has been discovered. Transmission is likely from person to person through respiratory secretions. Serologic evidence indicates that infection is common throughout the world. Five to 15% of community-acquired pneumonia is attributed to this organism, although serologic tests used to make such estimates have suffered from poor specificity. Dual infections in combination with *Streptococcus pneumoniae* or *M. pneumoniae* have been reported. Illness caused by *C. pneumoniae* is clinically similar to that caused by *Mycoplasma* species. Often the patient has a brief prodrome of headache and myalgias and then high fever and shaking chills. Cough is almost always present, associated with pharyngitis in up to 50% of patients. Other clinical manifestations include sinusitis and delirium. Extrapulmonary signs and symptoms are less common than with *M. pneumoniae.* In addition to causing pneumonia, *C. pneumoniae* has been identified as an etiology of acute exacerbations of chronic obstructive pulmonary disease.

C. burnetii, the etiologic agent of Q fever, is an obligate intracellular parasite with a large natural reservoir that includes rodents, cattle, sheep, and goats. In nature, a tick vector maintains the disease. Humans acquire the disease through contact with infected milk, feces, urine, or placentas of farm animals. The disease is virtually nonexistent in urban areas but can be spread in a rural community by contaminated dust, hay, and clothing. Human-to-human spread, although theoretically possible, has never been documented. The incubation period averages 2 to 3 weeks. Outbreaks have been reported in stockyard and meat packinghouse employees, dairy workers, animal hair processors, and medical school employees (in research facilities using contaminated sheep placentas). Many cases of Q fever appear to be flulike with high fever, cough, headache, and myalgias. Significant pulmonary symptoms occur in up to 50% of patients. Other more severe extrapulmonary disorders include endocarditis with a predilection for the aortic valve, myocarditis, and pericarditis. Endocarditis can occur in up to 11% of infected patients and can appear months or years after the initial infection. Q fever pneumonia is usually a self-limited illness with a mortality rate of less than 1%.

Legionnaires' disease (also known as legionellosis) is an acute pneumonic illness caused by gram-negative bacterial organisms of the genus *Legionella.* At present, approximately 49 species of *Legionella* are known. Most cases of Legionnaires' disease are caused by *L. pneumophila,* serogroups 1 to 15 (80% are *L. pneumophila* serogroup 1), but other *Legionella* species are known to cause similar human disease. *Legionella* organisms are mainly intracellular parasites, distinguished by their very weak gram-negative staining and fastidious growth requirements in culture. The organisms are found in water sources, such as cooling towers, evaporative condensers, humidifiers, and nebulizers, as well as potable water systems. Superheating and hyperchlorination can eradicate the organism. *Legionella* is often an opportunistic pathogen. Smokers, the elderly, and patients with immunosuppression and other chronic illnesses are at increased risk for infection, although some cases do occur in previously healthy individuals. It is not unusual for patients with *L. pneumophila* infection to be severely ill, as manifested by a high fever, rigors, and significant hypoxemia. Failure to institute appropriate therapy rapidly in these cases is likely to result in a poor outcome, especially in older individuals. The greater severity of illness seen with *Legionella*, frequently requiring hospitalization and intensive care, distinguishes it from the other atypical pneumonias. For this and other reasons, classifying atypical pneumonias as a single entity can be misleading. In rare cases, Legionnaires' disease can be complicated by endocarditis, pericarditis, pancreatitis, skin abscesses, and rhabdomyolysis. Pontiac fever, an acute, febrile, self-limited, flulike illness, is a distinct nonpneumonic syndrome resulting from *Legionella* infection.

Although important differences in severity and outcome exist, the clinical manifestations of Q fever, psittacosis, *M. pneumoniae* infection, Legionnaires' disease, and *C. pneumoniae* infection can be similar and nonspecific. An appropriate medical history should be obtained, including history of contact with other ill persons and environmental exposures. Initial complaints can include coryza, pharyngitis, fever, headache, malaise, and, occasionally, chills. A bradycardia relative to high fever can occur with significant illness. Cough is usually present and may be nonproductive or associated with small amounts of mucoid sputum. Dyspnea is a prominent feature only when pneumonia is extensive. Pleuritic chest pain is rare, except in Q fever. Gastrointestinal symptoms, especially diarrhea, are a prominent finding in 20 to 40% of patients with Legionnaires' disease.

In all these entities, the physical findings are often less impressive than would be predicted from the chest radiograph. Rales are usually present over involved areas, but findings of frank consolidation are uncommon. However, no diagnostic features on the chest radiograph reliably distinguish these infections from each other or from typical (e.g., pneumococcal) pneumonias; infiltrates can be unilateral, bilateral, patchy, or dense.

Routine laboratory tests also are nonspecific. Leukocytosis, which may be present or absent in most atypical pneumonias, is more common in Legionnaires' disease. Proteinuria may accompany high fever. In *M. pneumoniae* infection, serologic abnormalities may appear, including the presence of rheumatoid factor, false-positive serologic tests for syphilis, and cold agglutinins (>50%). Occasionally, the latter occurs in titers high enough to cause hemolysis. However, a rise in cold agglutinins is not specific for *M. pneumoniae* disease and can be seen in up to 25% of viral pneumonias. *Chlamydophila* infections and Q fever do not share this proclivity for nonspecific antigenic stimulation. Legionnaires' disease is often associated with elevated liver enzymes, especially LDH levels greater than 700 U/mL, and hyponatremia (Na <130). In one study of community-acquired pneumonia, the combination of high fever (>39°C), hyponatremia (Na <130), high LDH (>700 U/mL), and central nervous system abnormalities was found to be predictive for the diagnosis of Legionnaires' disease.

A hallmark of all these pneumonic illnesses is the absence of bacterial pathogens on Gram's stain and routine culture of clinical samples. Although specialized cultures and antigen, polymerase chain reaction (PCR), and serologic tests for atypical organisms exist, their use is not routinely recommended for all pneumonia patients. These tests should be used for hospitalized patients, particularly those requiring intensive care, or when a definitive diagnosis could assist with investigation of an outbreak or other public health intervention.

Culture of atypical organisms is difficult. *Chlamydophila* organisms and *C. burnetii* are known causes of laboratory-acquired infection and, for this reason, are handled only in special laboratories. Isolation of *Chlamydophila* species requires specialized tissue culture techniques and 4 to 5 days for detection of growth. *Mycoplasma* organisms can be handled safely in most laboratories, but their growth requires specialized cell-free media, and 2 to 3 weeks of growth are necessary for detection.

The culture of *Legionella* species requires special culture media but can be performed in many laboratories. Other techniques are most often used for establishing a diagnosis. A fourfold or greater rise in complement-fixing antibodies between acute and convalescent sera assays run simultaneously is considered definitively diagnostic for *Mycoplasma*, *Chlamydophila*, *C. burnetii*, and *Legionella*. PCR assays exist for *Mycoplasma*, *Chlamydophila*, and *Legionella* organisms, but no United States Food and Drug Administration (FDA)-approved commercial test kits exist, and such tests are available only through research and reference laboratories. Direct immunofluorescence can rapidly detect *Legionella* in sputum or lung tissue, although the sensitivity of this test is less than desirable (<75%). The *Legionella* urine antigen test is more reliable and can be positive for weeks after acute illness. The test only detects serogroup 1, although this is the most common cause of *Legionella* disease. Testing for *Legionella* using the urine antigen test and culture is recommended for all patients with community-acquired pneumonia requiring intensive care.

As with all pneumonias, a decision to treat must be made before laboratory confirmation of a specific diagnosis is made. Single empiric antibiotic options for outpatient therapy that will cover atypical pathogens include (1) macrolides (clarithromycin or azithromycin); (2) fluoroquinolones (e.g., levofloxacin, moxifloxacin, or gatifloxacin); or (3) tetracyclines (tetracycline or doxycycline). All three antibiotic classes are equally efficacious for treating *M. pneumoniae* and *C. pneumoniae*; however, tetracyclines are generally preferred for the treatment of psittacosis and are clearly the first choice in *C. burnetii* infections. For patients with documented psittacosis or Q fever, 14 days of a tetracycline antibiotic is recommended. In hospitalized patients, empiric therapy should include coverage of pneumococcus in addition to atypical organisms. For a confirmed diagnosis of *Legionella*, macrolides are considered the drugs of choice; azithromycin is recommended for hospitalized patients because it can be given intravenously. Alternatives are levofloxacin, moxifloxacin, or gatifloxacin, which are also available as intravenous preparations. Some suggest adding rifampin for patients who are severely ill with Legionnaires' disease. The Infectious Diseases Society of America has developed useful guidelines for empiric treatment of these and other community-acquired pneumonia (see Reference 25).

After the patient has improved sufficiently, oral medication can be substituted and continued for a total of 2 weeks. Macrolides and fluoroquinolones are preferred for *Legionella*, with tetracyclines available as second-line agents. In all but the most severe cases, complete healing of atypical pneumonia is the rule. Radiographic resolution can be slow but is usually complete by 6 to 8 weeks. Significant pulmonary tissue necrosis is rare in *Mycoplasma* disease, but it sometimes occurs in fulminant cases of Q fever and psittacosis.

Several of the atypical pneumonias have important public health implications. Therefore, individual cases of Legionnaires' disease and psittacosis and outbreaks of *M. pneumoniae* should be reported to the local health department. Prompt reporting may prevent additional cases of disease.

---

1. Smith G, Hosker H. Diagnosing and treating atypical pneumonia. *Practitioner.* 2001;245:736.
   Concise review of diagnosis and treatment of atypical pneumonias.
2. Hindiyeh M, Carroll KC. Laboratory diagnosis of atypical pneumonia. *Semin Respir Infect.* 2000;15:101.
   Detailed review of various laboratory tests for diagnosing Mycoplasma, Chlamydia, Q fever, and Legionella.
3. File TM, Tan JS, Plouffe JF. The role of atypical pathogens: *Mycoplasma pneumoniae*, *Chlamydia pneumoniae*, and *Legionella pneumophila* in respiratory infection. *Infect Dis Clin North Am.* 1998;12:562.
   An excellent review of lower respiratory infections caused by these pathogens.
4. Casey KR. Atypical pneumonia and environmental factors: where have you been and what have you done? *Clin Chest Med.* 1991;12:285.

Underscores the importance of obtaining a thorough occupational, environmental, travel, and social history in patients with atypical pneumonias. Clues obtained from the history are crucial in trying to identify a specific cause of acute pneumonitis, whether it be infectious or noninfectious.

5. Daxboeck F, Krause R, Wenisch C. Laboratory diagnosis of *Mycoplasma pneumoniae* infection. *Clin Microbiol Infect.* 2003;9:263.

   Reviews culture, serology, antigen detection, and PCR techniques used to diagnosis Mycoplasma pneumoniae.

6. Hammerschlag MR. Mycoplasma pneumoniae infections. *Curr Opin Infect Dis.* 2001;14:181.

   Overview of epidemiology, diagnosis, and treatment of Mycoplasma pneumoniae.

7. Watkins-Riedel T, Stanek G, Daxboeck F. Comparison of SeroMP IgA with four other commercial assays for serodiagnosis of Mycoplasma pneumoniae pneumonia. *Diagn Microbiol Infect Dis.* 2001;40:21.

   In this study, five Mycoplasma *serodiagnostic assays were compared. Sensitivity ranged from 87 to 100%. The IgA enzyme-linked immunosorbent assay (ELISA) had the best sensitivity and had a specificity of 96%.*

8. Reittner P, Muller NL, Heyneman L, et al. Mycoplasma pneumoniae pneumonia: radiographic and high-resolution CT features in 28 patients. *AJR Am J Roentgenol.* 2000;174:37.

   High-resolution computed tomographic (CT) findings of M. pneumoniae *pneumonia include centrilobular nodules, unilateral or bilateral consolidation in a lobular distribution, and thickening of the peribronchovascular and interlobular interstitium. The lobular distribution, centrilobular involvement, and interstitial abnormalities are often difficult to recognize on plain radiography.*

9. Kirchner JT. Psittacosis: is contact with birds causing your patient's pneumonia? *Postgrad Med.* 1997;102:181.

   Description of pathophysiology, clinical features, diagnosis, treatment, and prevention of psittacosis.

10. Wainwright AP, Beaumont AC, Kox WJ. Psittacosis: diagnosis and management of severe pneumonia and multi organ failure. *Intensive Care Med.* 1987;13:419.

    A report of two cases of psittacosis in which the patients developed respiratory failure, septic shock, and renal and hepatic impairment. Both patients recovered after treatment with tetracyclines.

11. Gregory DW, Scaffner W. Psittacosis. *Semin Respir Infect.* 1997;12:7.

    A concise review of the presentation and management of psittacosis.

12. Grimes JE. Zoonoses acquired from pet birds. *Vet Clin North Am Small Anim Pract.* 1987;17:209.

    An appropriate chapter from a volume devoted to zoonoses.

13. Monno R, De Vito D, Losito G, et al. Chlamydia pneumoniae in community-acquired pneumonia: seven years of experience. *J Infect.* 2002;45:135.

    Of 311 patients with community-acquired pneumonia, 39 (12.5%) met with diagnostic criteria of acute C. pneumoniae infection. Four had coinfection with other organisms. Incidence was greater in the winter and early spring. Macrolides and levofloxacin were effective for treatment.

14. Lieberman D, Ben-Yaakov M, Lazarovich Z, et al. Chlamydia pneumoniae infection in acute exacerbations of chronic obstructive pulmonary disease: analysis of 250 hospitalizations. *Eur J Clin Microbiol Infect Dis.* 2001;20:698.

    Among 250 patients hospitalized for acute exacerbations of chronic obstructive pulmonary disease, 73 (33%) met serologic criteria for the diagnosis of C. pneumoniae infection.

15. File TM Jr, Plouffe JF Jr, Breiman RF, et al. Clinical characteristics of Chlamydia pneumoniae infection as the sole cause of community-acquired pneumonia. *Clin Infect Dis.* 1999;29:426–428.

    Description of clinical characteristics of C. pneumoniae based on 26 patients diagnosed with community-acquired pneumonia caused by the organism.

16. Kleemola M, Saikku P, Visakorpi R, et al. Epidemics of pneumonia caused by TWAR, a new *Chlamydia* organism, in military trainees in Finland. *J Infect Dis.* 1988;157:230.

Retrospective serologic evidence of four TWAR epidemics from 1957–1985. Clinical data and antibody responses documented.

17. Sampere M, Font B, Font J, et al. Q fever in adults: review of 66 clinical cases. *Eur J Clin Microbiol Infect Dis*. 2003;22:108.

    The most common clinical presentation was pneumonia (56%); eight patients had hypoxia and five developed respiratory failure. Over 70% of patients received empiric treatment with macrolides (the intent being to cover for the organisms that most frequently cause atypical pneumonia in the region; the patients were recognized to have Q fever at a later time). Nevertheless outcomes were favorable, although the authors acknowledge that use of macrolides in Q fever is controversial, and tetracyclines are the drugs of choice.

18. Marrie TJ. Q fever pneumonia. *Curr Opin Infect Dis*. 2004;17:137.

    A brief, current review of this disease.

19. Scola BL. Current laboratory diagnosis of Q fever. *Semin Pediatr Infect Dis*. 2002;13:257.

    Reviews use of PCR, culture, and serology in the diagnosis of Q fever.

20. Gikas A, Kofteridis D, Bouros D, et al. Q fever pneumonia: appearance on chest radiographs. *Radiology*. 1999;210:339.

    In 85 patients with Q fever pneumonia, the most common abnormalities were segmental (62%) and lobar (18%) opacities. Most abnormalities were unilateral and located in the upper lobes.

21. Gacouin A, Le Tulzo Y, Lavoue S, et al. Severe pneumonia due to Legionella pneumophila: prognostic factors, impact of delayed appropriate antimicrobial therapy. *Intensive Care Med*. 2002;28:686.

    This study examined patients with severe Legionella pneumonia admitted to an ICU. Delays in admission to the ICU and the need for intubation were associated with increased mortality. Starting a fluoroquinolone within 8 hours of ICU admission significantly reduced mortality.

22. Oren I, Zuckerman T, Avivi I, et al. Nosocomial outbreak of *Legionella* pneumophila serogroup 3 pneumonia in a bone marrow transplant unit: evaluation, treatment and control. *Bone Marrow Transplant*. 2002;30:175.

    Contamination of the water supply in a bone marrow transplant unit resulted in four cases of Legionella pneumonia. After decontamination of the water and ciprofloxacin prophylaxis for the other patients in the unit, no additional Legionella cases were detected.

23. Lindsay DSJ, Abraham WH, Findlay W, et al. Laboratory diagnosis of Legionnaires' disease due to *Legionella* pneumophila serogroup 1: comparison of phenotypic and genotypic methods. *J Med Microbiol*. 2004;53:183.

    Both the urine antigen test and PCR were found to be sensitive and specific for the diagnosis of legionnaires' disease.

24. Franzin L, Dal Conte I, Cabodi D, et al. Culture proven *Legionella* pneumophila pneumonia in an HIV-infected patient: case report and review. *J Infect*. 2004;45:199.

    In a human immunodeficiency virus (HIV)-infected patient, the diagnosis was first made by culture that was positive 3 days after collection. Urine antigen was initially negative but did become positive 20 days later.

25. Bartlett JG, Dowell SF, Mandell LA, et al. Practice guidelines for the management of community-acquired pneumonia in adults. *Clin Infect Dis*. 2000;31:347–382.

    Comprehensive guidelines for the management of community-acquired pneumonia from the Infectious Diseases Society of America.

26. American Veterinary Medical Association. Compendium of measures to control *Chlamydophila psittaci* (formerly *Chlamydia psittaci*) infection among humans (psittacosis) and pet birds, 2004. Available at *http://www.avma.org/pubhlth/psittacosis.asp*.

    Describes measures indicated to control psittacosis as recommended by the American Veterinary Medical Association.

34. VIRAL PNEUMONIA

Bao Q. Luu

Viral pneumonia in the immunocompetent adult remains a diagnostic and clinical challenge. In a recent study of 338 immunocompetent patients admitted with community-acquired pneumonia, a virus was found to be the sole causative agent in 31 patients and a coinfecting agent in another 30. In general, most viral respiratory tract infections appear similarly; therefore, a specific diagnosis depends more on epidemiologic, serologic, and immunohistochemical data. Recent advances in cellular and molecular biologic techniques may rapidly identify viral antigens and nucleic acids.

Influenza viruses remain the most common cause of respiratory tract viral infections. They are enveloped single-stranded RNA viruses belonging to the Orthomyxoviridae family. There are three types of influenza viruses, but only type A and B are human pathogens. On the surface of influenza A and B are spikelike projections of glycoproteins that possess hemagglutinin (H) or neuraminidase (N) activity. Hemagglutinin is necessary for binding to and penetrating the host cellular membrane. Neuraminidase aids in the release and spread of replicated viral particles. The complete nomenclature of a strain of influenza virus includes the viral type (A or B), the geographic location of discovery, the strain number, the year, and the H and N numbers (e.g., the A/Sydney/5/97/H3/N2 strain). Most of the host immune response is directed against hemagglutinin. Minor mutations can lead to small antigenic changes in the hemagglutinin glycoprotein and are characterized as an *antigenic drift*. Reassortments between strains can result in major changes in the hemagglutinin protein and are characterized as an *antigenic shift*. The effect of *antigenic drift* on a population is usually minor. In contrast, *antigenic shift* may result in a devastating pandemic because of the lack of immunity to the new antigen.

Influenza infections occur in annual epidemics and in sporadic cases. Outbreaks occur in the winter in temperate zones; in tropical zones, seasonal association is less clear. In the setting of a confirmed influenza outbreak, 63 to 71% of patients were found to have influenza if they were acutely ill with fever ($>37.8°C$) and reported at least two other symptoms, such as headache, myalgia, cough, or sore throat. Shortness of breath has been reported as a very useful indicator of pneumonia complicating influenza. Influenza pneumonia is more common in patients with congestive heart failure and other chronic illnesses, such as chronic obstructive pulmonary disease (COPD), renal disease, diabetes, and immunosuppression.

The laboratory may be enormously helpful in diagnosing influenza infection. The gold standard technique is viral culture in cell cultures or in embryonated hen eggs followed by hemagglutination inhibition testing. Serologic diagnosis requires the demonstration of a fourfold increase in influenza-specific antibody titer in convalescent sera as compared with acute sera. Recently, rapid diagnostic techniques, such as enzyme immunoassays and direct immunofluorescence assays, have become available. These tests use nasal or pharyngeal cells obtained by brushing or washing (a process that takes approximately 15 minutes) and have excellent sensitivity and specificity that range from 65 to 96% and 90 to 99%, respectively. Polymerase chain reaction (PCR)-based testing to detect low quantities of viral RNA is now available, but this technique is costly to perform and not routinely used.

Chest radiographs in influenza pneumonia usually demonstrate patchy, bilateral infiltrates. Segmental or subsegmental infiltrates also can occur. Most often, infiltrates are self limited and resolve within 3 weeks. Occasionally, patients develop diffuse pneumonia, hypoxemia, and acute respiratory distress syndrome.

Superinfection or mixed infection with bacteria such as *Streptococcus pneumoniae, Staphylococcus aureus,* and *Haemophilus influenza* can occur and is a significant factor in producing high mortality rates associated with epidemics. Recrudescence of fever and a productive cough with purulent sputum are important clinical signs of superinfection. The clinical presentation is similar to that of a community-acquired bacterial pneumonia. The clinical course is determined in part by the specific bacterial pneumonia. Complications such as abscess formation (especially with *S. aureus*), sepsis, empyema, and toxic shock syndrome have been reported.

Neurologic sequelae of influenza, including Guillain-Barré syndrome, seizure, and transverse myelopathy, have been reported. Severe myositis with elevated serum creatinine and phosphokinase levels also has been noted. Unusual complications include myoglobinuria, Reye's syndrome, thrombocytopenia, renal failure, myocarditis, and disseminated intravascular coagulopathy.

Treatment of influenza should be considered in patients who present within 48 hours of onset of typical symptoms, including fever and cough, in the setting of known influenza activity in the community. The use of a rapid diagnostic test is not necessary prior to initiation of antiviral therapy in typical cases of febrile influenza during the epidemic period; however, it may permit physicians to withhold antibiotics with some degree of confidence. There are currently four drugs available to treat influenza in the Unites States. Amantadine and rimantadine are related antiviral drugs with similar mechanisms of action and are only effective against influenza A. These drugs act by blocking an ion channel formed by the M2 protein that spans the viral membrane. Both are effective in preventing influenza A infection and illness. Beneficial effects are reported in clinical studies if treatment is started during the first days of illness. Side effects are more prominent from amantadine than from rimantadine and may target the central nervous system, manifesting as anxiety, depression, lightheadedness, difficulty concentrating, and insomnia. Rarely, hallucination and seizures can occur. Newer treatments for influenza include zanamivir and oseltamivir. Both are neuraminidase inhibitors and are effective against influenza A and B. Zanamivir is available in inhalational form and oseltamivir in oral form. Side effects are generally less problematic than those seen with amantadine and rimantadine. However, zanamivir is known to cause bronchospasm and reduction in airflow, limiting its use in patients with severe obstructive lung disease. Oseltamivir can cause gastrointestinal side effects, such as nausea and vomiting; however, generally it is well tolerated. Although these medications have been shown to be effective in both prophylaxis and treatment of influenza illness, their specific efficacy in the treatment of influenza pneumonia has not been studied. A potential benefit of treatment is reduction in transmission rates, particularly among household contacts.

Vaccination remains the most important preventive measure against the annual epidemic of influenza. The current vaccines are inactivated viruses containing two influenza A subtypes and influenza B. The annual selection of the subtypes to include in the vaccine is based on the occurrence of the latest "drift" virus that is causing outbreaks of influenza somewhere in the world. The recommendations for annual influenza vaccination are developed by the Advisory Committee on Immunization Practices of the Centers for Disease Control and Prevention (CDC) and include several groups. The first are people at high risk for a complication of influenza: persons age 50 or older; residents of long-term care facilities; adults and children with chronic pulmonary and cardiovascular diseases, chronic metabolic diseases, renal dysfunction, hemoglobinopathy, or immunosuppression (including human immunodeficiency virus infection). Other groups include (1) women in their second or third trimester of pregnancy during the influenza season; (2) children on long-term aspirin therapy (a risk factor for Reye's syndrome); and (3) individuals who may transmit influenza to those at high risk (such as healthcare personnel, employees of long-term care facilities, household members, and home care providers). For unvaccinated people at high risk of complication, or unvaccinated persons caring for people at high risk and those living in households with people at high risk, oseltamivir at 75 mg per day for the duration of peak influenza activity in the community should also be considered.

Adenovirus is a nonenveloped, double-stranded DNA virus that causes a particularly aggressive form of pneumonia in neonates, triggering necrotizing bronchiolitis and alveolitis. In adults, it may cause a pneumonia with a similar presentation to "atypical" pneumonia, particularly in large, closely quartered populations, such as military recruits. In the general population, adenovirus rarely causes pneumonia but is a common cause of pharyngitis, tracheobronchitis, and conjunctivitis. Treatment is supportive with analgesic and cough suppressants. Effective, enteric-coated live vaccines have been developed for military recruits, but they are not used in other settings.

Respiratory syncytial virus (RSV) is the leading cause of respiratory tract infection in infants and young children. It is responsible for 25% of hospital admissions for pneumonia and 75% of bronchiolitis in children younger than age 6 months. In adults, it typically causes an influenza-like illness with cough, coryza, and pharyngitis, and can lead to exacerbations of chronic lung disease (e.g., COPD and asthma). In the elderly, it causes a viral bronchopneumonia that can be complicated by secondary bacterial pneumonia, as with influenza. Serologic diagnosis is possible but less reliable in children younger than age 4 months. Cultures for direct diagnosis can be obtained from respiratory secretions, nasopharyngeal washing, or throat swabs. Immunofluorescence techniques are frequently used and allow for a reliable and more rapid detection in nasal scrapings or washings. Aerosolized ribavirin improves the clinical course and has been associated with a reduction in viral titers and improvement in blood gas abnormalities. Systemic corticosteroids have also been given to those who suffer the most severe involvement.

Parainfluenza viruses, responsible for up to 20% of respiratory infections (croup, rhinitis, pharyngitis, laryngitis, and bronchitis) that occur in children, are found infrequently in immunocompetent adults. In adults, the disease can be completely asymptomatic or may present as a common upper respiratory tract infection with rhinitis and pharyngitis. Fever is unusual, as is progression to pneumonia. However, parainfluenza infection is often a cause of exacerbation of chronic lung diseases (e.g., COPD and asthma).

Varicella-zoster virus (VZV) causes varicella, a highly contagious childhood exanthem with variable systemic symptoms. Reactivation of latent VZV in adults results in herpes zoster. In normal children, it is rarely associated with respiratory manifestation. In adults, viral pneumonia is a major complication of varicella. When pneumonia occurs, it generally appears within the first 4 to 5 days after the onset of the rash. Symptoms include cough, fever, dyspnea, hemoptysis, and pleuritic chest pain (from herpetic vesicles on the pleural surface). Respiratory failure is fairly common. Radiographically, varicella pneumonia has a diffuse nodular (1–10 mm) pattern radiating from the hila, which may resolve into military calcified densities. Intravenous acyclovir is the treatment of choice and should be started early. Preventive oral acyclovir in adults who have varicella may be prudent, especially in elderly patients, pregnant women, or patients with chronic pulmonary diseases. Zoster immune globulin is recommended to reduce the severity of illness in immunocompromised patients exposed to varicella. Resolution generally coincides with clearing of the cutaneous vesiculopapular rash. The mortality rate is 10 to 15%.

Measles *(rubeola)* is another highly contagious systemic viral illness of childhood that can cause serious pneumonias in susceptible adults. Pulmonary infection is a common complication in older children and young adults, some with acute respiratory failure. In the United States, pneumonia is the cause of 60% of measles-related deaths in children. Measles pneumonia can cause hilar lymphadenopathy and pleural effusions, in addition to reticulonodular parenchymal infiltrates. Secondary bacterial pneumonia also can occur. Treatment is supportive, and antibiotics are for secondary bacterial pneumonia. No consistent data are available on the effects of corticosteroids.

Hantavirus Pulmonary Syndrome (HPS) can result from several hantaviruses, such as the Sin Nombre virus (SNV). The deer mouse *(Peromyscus maniculatus)* is the primary reservoir of the hantavirus that causes HPS in the United States; however, other rodents such as cotton and rice rats and the white-footed mouse also have been known as rodent carriers of hantaviruses. HPS is transmitted to humans through aerosolization of infected rodents' urine, droppings, and saliva. Clinically the syndrome should be suspected in any previously healthy individuals with the appropriate exposure risk, who develop a febrile prodrome lasting 3 to 5 days followed by a rapidly deteriorating pneumonia with bilateral patchy opacities resembling acute respiratory distress syndrome (ARDS). In addition to the fever, early symptoms include myalgia, headache, nonproductive cough, nausea, vomiting, and other gastrointestinal symptoms. Signs that reduce the likelihood of this diagnosis include rashes, conjunctival or other hemorrhages, throat or conjunctival erythema, petechiae, and peripheral or periorbital edema. Patients with HPS develop rapid respiratory failure from non-cardiogenic pulmonary edema caused by massive pulmonary capillary leaks. Serous respiratory secretions high in protein and lactate dehydrogenase are found. Routine laboratory findings are nonspecific, but certain findings make HPS more likely. The combination of atypical lymphocytes (circulating immunoblasts), a significant bandemia, and thrombocytopenia in the setting of pulmonary edema is strongly suggestive of a hantavirus infection. Other findings include a fall in serum albumin and a rise in hematocrit as the patient is becoming hemoconcentrated with a fluid shift from the systemic circulation into the lungs. Disseminated intravascular coagulopathy occurs in the most severe cases. Renal insufficiency and rhabdomyolysis and elevated liver enzymes have been reported. The diagnosis can be made by a positive serologic test, evidence of antigen in tissue by immunohistochemistry, or the presence of amplifiable viral RNA sequences in the blood or tissue of a patient with compatible history and clinical syndrome. An enzyme-linked immunosorbent assay using specific viral antigens from SNV to detect immunoglobulin M (IgM) antibodies to SNV is now available. Acute and convalescent sera with a fourfold rise in IgG can be considered diagnostic for hantaviral disease. Also in use is a rapid immunoblot strip assay (RIBA). Immunohistochemistry of formalin-fixed tissues with specific monoclonal and polyclonal antibodies can be used to detect hantavirus antigens. In addition, reverse transcriptase-PCR (RT-PCR) can be used to detect hantaviral RNA in fresh frozen lung tissue, blood clots, or nucleated blood cells. However, this method is prone to cross-contamination and should be considered an experimental technique.

HPS patients often progress rapidly to respiratory failure and septic shock and require intubation and mechanical ventilation. A unique feature of shock from HPS is a much more profound myocardial depressant effect than generally observed in septic shock. Moreover, cardiac output does not improve after a fluid challenge, as might be expected. Fluid management should be conservative, given the potential for massive pulmonary capillary leaks. Inotropic support and vasopressors are often needed. Early transfer to centers capable of hemodynamics monitoring and management has been recommended. Intravenous ribavirin has not been shown to be effective in a placebo-controlled trial despite its effects on a related disease caused by another hantavirus. The mortality rate of HPS has been reported to be as high as 76%.

Severe acute respiratory syndrome (SARS) is a viral respiratory illness caused by the SARS-associated corona virus (SARS-CoV). SARS was first reported in Asia in February 2003. Outbreaks have been reported in North America, South America, and Europe. The CDC divides the clinical criteria of the diagnosis of SARS into early illness, mild-to-moderate respiratory illness, and severe respiratory illness. Early illness is defined as the presence of two or more of the following: fever, chills, rigors, myalgia, headache, diarrhea, sore throat, or rhinorrhea. Mild-to-moderate respiratory illness requires temperature greater than 38°C and one or more clinical findings of respiratory illness (e.g., cough, shortness of breath, or hypoxia). Severe respiratory illness is defined as a mild-to-moderate illness plus one or more of the following: radiographic evidence of pneumonia, ARDS, and autopsy findings consistent with pneumonia or ARDS without an identifiable cause. Given these extremely broad case definitions, the CDC has published a clinical guide on the identification and evaluation of possible SARS-CoV disease among persons presenting with community-acquired illness. This document stresses that early clinical recognition of SARS-CoV disease relies on a combination of clinical and epidemiologic features. The vast majority of patients with SARS-CoV illness have pneumonia severe enough to require hospitalization and have a clear history of exposure either to a SARS patient(s) or to a setting in which SARS-CoV transmission is occurring (e.g., in the laboratory with live SARS-CoV). The clinician should be suspicious of SARS in an appropriate clinical setting and obtain a travel history for the patient and household contacts. Laboratory tests, although helpful, do not reliably detect infection early in the illness.

Based on the clusters of cases in Hong Kong and Canada, SARS-CoV is spread from person to person and can be acquired from face-to-face contact suggesting droplet spread—similar to varicella-zoster virus. Transmission to healthcare workers has been a common feature of outbreaks. The incubation period for SARS is usually 2 to 7 days prior to the onset of symptoms (typically fever). The World Health Organization

(WHO) and the CDC have recommended home isolation and monitoring for the development of symptoms for at least 10 days after possible exposure.

Laboratory findings may include normal or slightly elevated white blood cell counts with lymphopenia. Leukopenia and thrombocytopenia may be present as the respiratory phase peaks. Other findings include elevated serum aminotransferases and creatinine kinase. Elevated lactate dehydrogenase is associated with poor prognosis. Renal function is usually normal. Chest radiographs often show bilateral interstitial opacities; however, areas of focal consolidation have also been described. Computed tomographic (CT) scanning can reveal parenchymal abnormalities not seen on chest radiographs.

SARS is a two-stage illness beginning with a prodrome of fever associated with nonspecific symptoms such as malaise, headache, and myalgia. Diarrhea can occur. However, rash and neurologic symptoms have not been described. In the second phase, typically beginning within 3 to 7 days of the fever, respiratory illness predominates. A nonproductive cough and dyspnea are typically described. This may be followed by progression to respiratory failure requiring intubation and mechanical ventilation.

The diagnosis of SARS (in the United States) currently requires clinical criteria fitting the case definition in the appropriate epidemiologic context and positive serologic test(s) to SARS-CoV or the detection of SARS-CoV RNA by RT-PCR validated by the CDC. Currently, there is no specific treatment recommended for SARS except for meticulous supportive care. Multiple antiviral agents have been used, but the efficacy of these drugs has not been established.

Infection control clearly decreased the number of cases during outbreaks in Singapore and Hong Kong. Hospitalized patients should be isolated in negative pressure rooms and healthcare workers and visitors should be wearing N-95 masks, gowns, gloves, and protective eyewear to prevent inhalation of respiratory droplets and guard against contact transmission. Suspected cases of SARS in the community should be house quarantine for a full 10 days after the resolution of fever and other symptoms.

1. de Roux A, Marcos MA, Garcia E, et al. Viral community-acquired pneumonia in nonimmunocompromised adults. *Chest.* 2004;125:1343.

   Viruses were the only cause for community acquired pneumonia in 9% of the patients in this study. In addition, viral serology was positive in another 9% of patients with other bacterial causes for pneumonia, suggesting coinfection or superinfection.

2. Couch RB. Prevention and treatment of influenza. *New Engl J Med.* 2000; 343:1778.

   Review article discussing the current recommendation for vaccination chemoprophylaxis and treatment of influenza.

3. Monto AS, Gravenstein S, Elliott M, et al. Clinical signs and symptoms predicting influenza infection. *Arch Intern Med.* 2000;160:3243.

   A study of clinical features of influenza. A cough with a fever has a positive predictive value of 79% for influenza.

4. Oliveira EC, Marik PE, Colice G. Influenza pneumonia: a descriptive study. *Chest.* 2001;119:1717.

   Implementation of rapid diagnostic tests for influenza increases the recognized number of hospital admissions for pneumonia caused by influenza. The study recognizes that influenza pneumonia occurs in both immunocompromised and healthy patients and has a high mortality rate. Staphylococcus aureus was a common bacterial superinfection in this study. Oseltamivir and rimantadine were used in treating patients, but their effectiveness remains to be determined.

5. Oliveira EC, Lee B, Colice GL. Influenza in the intensive care unit. *Jour Intensive Care Med.* 2003;18:80.

   A review of the current concepts, recent advances, and management strategies in influenza-associated pneumonia with discussion of pertinent issues in the intensive care unit.

6. Gerberding JL, Morgan JG, Shepard JA, et al. Case9–2004: An 18-year-old man with respiratory symptoms and shock. *New Engl J Med*. 2004;350:1236.

   A case presentation of an 18-year-old man with influenza and myopericarditis with refractory cardiogenic shock, rhabdomyolysis, and renal failure. This case illustrates the potential lethality of influenza.

7. Treanor JJ, Hayden FG, Vrooman PS, et al. Efficacy and safety of the oral neuraminidase inhibitor oseltamivir in treating acute influenza, a randomized controlled trial. *JAMA*. 2000;283:1016.

   Treatment of acute influenza with oseltamivir reduces the duration and severity of the illness and may decrease the incidence of secondary complication. Pneumonia was not specifically studied.

8. Smith D, Letendre S. Viral pneumonia as a serious complication of etanercept therapy. *Ann Intern Med*. 2002;136:174.

   A case report of parainfluenza pneumonia in a patient taking etanercept for rheumatoid arthritis.

9. Harger JH, Ernest JM, Thurnau GR, et al. Risk factors and outcome of varicella-zoster virus pneumonia in pregnant women. *J Infect Dis*. 2002;185:422.

   This is a descriptive study of pregnant women with VZV pneumonia. Risk factors for pneumonia in this population were found to be smoking and having 100 or more skin lesions.

10. Triebwasser JH, Harris RE, Bryant RE, et al. Varicella pneumonia in adults. *Medicine*. 1967;46:409.

    A classic review.

11. Duchin JS, Koster FT, Peters CJ, et al. Hantavirus pulmonary syndrome: a clinical description of 17 patients with a newly recognized disease. *N Engl J Med*. 1994;330:949.

    This now-classic paper describes the first cluster of deaths from HPS in the Four Corners region of the United States.

12. http://www.cdc.gov/ncidod/diseases/hanta/hps/index.htm

    An excellent website maintained by the CDC for public information on the hantavirus pulmonary syndrome. Last accessed October 17, 2004.

13. Peiris JSM, Yuen KY, Osterhaus AD, et al. The severe acute respiratory syndrome. *New Engl J Med*. 2003;349:2431.

    A review of SARS.

14. http://www.cdc.gov/ncidod/sars/index.htm

    An excellent website maintained by the CDC for public information on SARS. Last accessed October 17, 2004.

35. TUBERCULOSIS: EPIDEMIOLOGY, DIAGNOSIS, AND TREATMENT OF LATENT INFECTION

Philip A. LoBue

Tuberculosis is a pulmonary and systemic disease caused by *Mycobacterium tuberculosis*. It is spread from person to person by airborne transmission of droplet nuclei 1 to 5 μm in diameter. Several factors determine the probability of transmission: (1) infectiousness of the source patient—a positive sputum smear for acid-fast bacilli or a cavity on chest radiograph being strongly associated with infectiousness; (2) host susceptibility of the contact; (3) duration of exposure of the contact to the source patient; and (4) the environment in which the exposure takes place: a small, poorly ventilated space providing the highest risk. Even among household contacts of active tuberculosis patients, the risk of infection is surprisingly low; the United States

Public Health Service (USPHS) reported an approximate 28% incidence of infection in household contacts. In addition, animal and human studies have demonstrated that tuberculosis transmission may dramatically decrease within days to weeks of instituting effective treatment.

Despite this relatively low transmission rate, tuberculosis remains a major global public health problem. Approximately one third of the world's population is infected with tuberculosis, and 2 million people die of the disease each year. The human immunodeficiency virus (HIV) epidemic has dramatically altered tuberculosis epidemiology and is driving much of the global epidemic, especially in Africa. Approximately 13% of worldwide HIV deaths are tuberculosis related. The current epidemic has been accompanied by a rise in multidrug-resistant tuberculosis cases (defined as resistance to at least isoniazid and rifampin).

In the United States, there had been a steady 4 to 7% annual decline in the case rate until 1984. Between 1985 and 1992, however, the annual incidence of tuberculosis increased by 20%. This increase was concentrated in young (predominantly aged 25 to 44), urban (especially New York, New Jersey, and California), racial and ethnic minority populations. Tuberculosis was also found to be prevalent among the homeless, injection and noninjection drug users, and inmates of correctional facilities. In many of these groups, the rise in tuberculosis was linked to high rates of HIV infection. A second epidemiologic trend emerged with increased immigration to the United States of persons from countries where tuberculosis is prevalent (especially Latin America, South and Southeast Asia, Africa, and Eastern Europe). Before 1986, foreign-born persons accounted for 22% of tuberculosis cases. By 1997, this number had increased to 39% and in 2003, it reached 53%. In some locations, this phenomenon is even more pronounced. In California, for example, nearly 70% of tuberculosis cases occur in persons born outside the United States. Because of extensive national, state, and local control efforts, the annual incidence of tuberculosis has been on the decline again since 1992, falling 44% between 1992 and 2003. Despite this welcome decline, the associations of this disease with conditions such as HIV infection, homelessness, injection drug use, and foreign birth remain. Of perhaps even greater concern, the decrease in reported cases in 2003 was the smallest since 1992, and 19 states, including California, Texas, and New York (three of the highest-morbidity states) reported increases in case numbers.

The tuberculin skin test (TST) is a major tool for investigating tuberculosis infection. It can be used diagnostically in the individual patient and epidemiologically in the general population. The TST (Mantoux method) is performed by the intracutaneous injection of a standardized, stabilized dose of 5 TU of purified protein derivative (PPD). The extent of induration is measured 48 to 72 hours later. Multiple puncture techniques (e.g., tine test) are not recommended. The interpretation of the TST is based on an individual's epidemiologic risk factors for tuberculosis infection. The 2000 American Thoracic Society (ATS)/American Thoracic Society (ATS) guidelines for interpretation of TST results are as follows: (a) 5-mm induration is considered positive for (i) individuals with HIV infection or other comparable immunosuppression (equivalent to receiving 15 mg or greater of prednisone for 1 month or more), (ii) close contacts to an active tuberculosis case, or (iii) patients with a chest radiograph suggestive of prior tuberculosis (e.g., fibronodular) disease (also termed inactive disease); (b) 10-mm induration is considered positive for (i) recent immigrants (within the last 5 years) from high-incidence countries, (ii) injection drug users, (iii) residents and employees of high-risk congregate facilities, such as nursing homes, homeless shelters, or prisons, (iv) mycobacterial laboratory personnel, (v) persons with underlying medical conditions, such as diabetes, silicosis, end-stage renal disease, certain malignancies, and low body weight (loss of at least 10% of ideal body weight), or (vi) children younger than age 4 and infants, children, or adolescents exposed to adults at high risk; and (c) 15-mm induration is considered positive for all others.

A positive TST result is considered to indicate the presence of infection with *M. tuberculosis*. In the United States, it is recommended that persons who test positive receive treatment for latent tuberculosis to prevent progression to disease. Thus an intent to test for latent tuberculosis should indicate an intent to treat for latent tuberculosis when found. Consequently, testing should be reserved for persons at high risk for latent infection or at high risk to progress to disease based on their epidemiologic profile.

In a number of situations, the TST is neither sensitive nor specific for tuberculosis infection. A positive TST result is a manifestation of type IV delayed hypersensitivity. Certain biologic conditions, such as viral illnesses (including HIV infection), malignancies, other debilitating illness (including advanced active tuberculosis) and certain medications will suppress the type IV response and T-lymphocyte function. In addition, proper application of the TST requires careful attention to technique and interpretation. Tuberculin skin testing should be performed by well-trained, experienced operators. False-positive test findings can occur for a number of reasons, including cross-reactions caused by nontuberculous (atypical) mycobacterial infection.

In 2001, a new test, the QuantiFeron-TB test (QFT), was approved by the Food and Drug Administration for the diagnosis of latent tuberculosis infection. This test, which measures γ-interferon response to PPD in whole blood, has been found to have good agreement with the TST in a number of populations that have been studied. Currently, its use is recommended for testing in persons at increased risk for tuberculosis infection, such as recent immigrants and residents of congregate facilities; persons who by history are at low risk for tuberculosis infection but whose future activity may place them at high risk such as healthcare workers; and persons at low risk for tuberculosis infection for whom tuberculosis infection screening is required, such as occurs with workplace or school screening. There are inadequate data at present to recommend its use in the evaluation of children, close contacts of tuberculosis patients, and persons suspected of having active tuberculosis. Ongoing studies, however, are likely to provide evidence to extend the QFT's use to such groups in the near future.

Two methods have been used for tuberculosis prevention: bacille Calmette-Guérin (BCG) vaccination and isoniazid therapy for latent infection. BCG is a live, attenuated bacterial vaccine that has been evaluated extensively. The World Health Organization recommends administering BCG once at birth in endemic countries. Except for occasional local reactions, its toxicity is minimal. In controlled trials, the efficacy of case reduction has varied from 0 to 80%. In most trials, the incidence of miliary and meningeal tuberculosis in children has been greatly reduced. Variations in the efficacy of case reduction have been explained by differences in vaccine potency. A large trial conducted in India using a very potent BCG vaccine failed to show a protective effect against tuberculosis in adults, however, suggesting that vaccine potency is not the only factor determining efficacy. BCG is best used in the noninfected (TST-negative) population. The vaccine generally converts an individual's TST to positive, at least in the short term; however, the TST response has been somewhat variable with different vaccines and in different individuals and it correlates poorly with vaccine effectiveness. BCG may, therefore, limit the diagnostic value of the TST in certain circumstances. BCG has not been used in the United States because of the low incidence of tuberculosis. It has been most useful in areas of the world where the case rate and new infection rate remain high.

The principal preventive tool in the United States has been treatment of latent infection with isoniazid. In the 1950s, when isoniazid became available as an inexpensive, bactericidal, and relatively nontoxic drug for the treatment of active tuberculosis disease, controlled trials were instituted to determine its efficacy for the treatment of latent infection. In more than 70,000 patients, the USPHS and others consistently demonstrated a 60 to 70% case reduction rate attributable to isoniazid therapy. Follow-up for as long as 15 years confirmed the long-term protection isoniazid provides against progression to disease.

Concern regarding toxicity, especially hepatotoxicity, and the need for adherence to a prolonged course of therapy have limited isoniazid therapy's effectiveness as a public health intervention. Older studies revealed that isoniazid-associated liver injury occurred in about 1% of patients, and deaths secondary to isoniazid-induced liver injury were reported. More recently, however, public health clinics in Seattle and San Diego reported incidences of hepatotoxicity of 0.1 and 0.3%, respectively, among more than 14,000 patients treated. There were no deaths reported and only one hospitalization. Despite the low incidence of liver injury, completion rates for 6 months of therapy were below 65% in both reports.

ATS and CDC recommend that all persons with latent tuberculosis infection receive treatment. Clinical monitoring, on a monthly basis at minimum, is recommended for all patients receiving isoniazid. Routine transaminase monitoring should be reserved for individuals at particular risk for hepatotoxicity, including those who are pregnant or in the immediate postpartum period (first 3 months) or those with HIV infection, a history of liver disease, a history of excess alcohol use, or other risks for liver disease. The preferred duration of isoniazid therapy is 9 months for all groups of patients, including those with HIV infection, those with a chest radiograph suggestive of prior tuberculosis disease (inactive tuberculosis), and children. Six months of treatment is considered an acceptable alternative for immunocompetent adults without evidence of prior tuberculosis on chest radiograph, but this shorter duration is felt to be less effective based on existing data.

Initial studies done in HIV-infected patients suggested that the combination of daily rifampin and pyrazinamide for 2 months was equally efficacious and safe for the treatment of latent tuberculosis when compared with 6 or 12 months of isoniazid. Subsequently, as this regimen came in to general use, multiple hospitalizations and deaths resulting from hepatotoxicity associated with this regimen were reported. ATS and CDC now recommend that the combination of rifampin and pyrazinamide should generally not be offered to persons with latent tuberculosis infection for either HIV-negative or HIV-infected persons.

For contacts exposed to isoniazid-resistant, rifampin-susceptible tuberculosis patients, rifampin (4 months duration) can be used. It is important to note that rifampin and a closely related medication, rifabutin, interact with protease inhibitors and nonnucleoside reverse transcriptase inhibitors used to treat HIV. Consultation with an expert familiar with both HIV and tuberculosis treatment is recommended in this situation. For multidrug-resistant tuberculosis exposures, some have suggested the use of pyrazinamide and ethambutol or pyrazinamide in combination with a fluoroquinolone. Data on the efficacy of these regimens are not available, however.

1. McDermott LJ, Glassroth J. Tuberculosis. Part I: natural history and epidemiology. *Dis Mon.* 1997;43:113.
   A comprehensive review of tuberculosis epidemiology.
2. Mehta JB, Dutt AK. Tuberculosis. Part I: public health issues of tuberculosis. *Dis Mon.* 1997;43:156.
   Reviews issues of tuberculosis transmission, screening (including skin testing), and prevention (including isoniazid therapy).
3. World Health Organization. Global tuberculosis control. Geneva: World Health Organization; 2004.
   WHO annual report on global TBcontrol. It includes data on case notifications and treatment outcomes from all national TBcontrol programs that have reported to WHO.
4. Centers for Disease Control and Prevention. Trends in tuberculosis—United States, 1998–2003. *MMWR.* 2004;53:209.
   Analysis of national tuberculosis surveillance data from 1998–2003. Notes continued decline of tuberculosis cases into 2003, but an increase in cases from 2002 to 2003 in 19 states, including California, Texas, and New York.
5. Centers for Disease Control and Prevention. Trends in tuberculosis morbidity—United States, 1992–2002. *MMWR.* 2003;52:217.
   Documents decline in tuberculosis cases in the United States over the past decade with increasing proportion of tuberculosis cases occurring in immigrants.
6. Weis SE, Moonan PK, Pogoda JM, et al. Tuberculosis in the foreign-born population of Tarrant county, Texas by immigration status. *Am J Respir Crit Care Med.* 2001;164:953.

Study of tuberculosis among immigrants in a high-morbidity county in a United States–Mexico border state.

7. American Thoracic Society and Centers for Disease Control and Prevention. Targeted tuberculin testing and treatment of latent tuberculosis infection. *Am J Respir Crit Care Med.* 2000;161:s1.
   Comprehensive guidelines for tuberculin skin testing and treatment of latent tuberculosis. These guidelines included the use of rifampin and pyrazinamide as a recommended treatment regimen. However, after multiple reports of severe liver injury associated with this combination, an amendment was published recommending that this regimen not be used for treatment of latent tuberculosis.

8. Jasmer R, Nahid P, Hopwell P. Clinical practice. Latent tuberculosis infection. *N Engl J Med.* 2002;347:1860.
   Review of current practices and recommendations surrounding latent tuberculosis diagnosis and treatment.

9. Chee CB, Soh CH, Boudville IC, et al. Interpretation of the tuberculin skin test in Mycobacterium bovis BCG-vaccinated Singaporean schoolchildren. *Am J Respir Crit Care Med.* 2001;164:958.
   Relatively recent article that examines the effect of BCG vaccination on TST results.

10. Mazurek GH, LoBue PA, Daley CL, et al. Comparison of a whole-blood interferon gamma assay with tuberculin skin testing for detecting latent Mycobacterium tuberculosis infection. *JAMA.* 2001;286:1740.
    Multicenter study of more than 1,200 adults comparing TST to QFT. Overall agreement between tests was 83%.

11. Mazurek GH, Villarino ME. Guidelines for using the QuantiFERON-TB test for diagnosing latent Mycobacterium tuberculosis infection. *MMWR.* 2003;52(RR-2):15.
    Guideline for use of QFT published by the CDC.

12. Ferebee S. Controlled chemoprophylaxis trials in tuberculosis: a general review. *Adv Tuberc Res.* 1969;17:29.
    The classic review by the Unites States Public Health Service that summarizes controlled chemoprophylaxis trials in more than 70,000 patients. A consistent 60 to 70% reduction in case rate was found. Isoniazid was effective for 10 to 15 years.

13. Nolan CM, Goldberg SV, Buskin SE. Hepatotoxicity associated with isoniazid preventive therapy: a 7-year survey from a public health tuberculosis clinic. *JAMA.* 1999;281:1014.
    During a 7-year period in Seattle, only 11 of 11,141 patients starting isoniazid had significant liver injury develop. There were no deaths and only one hospitalization.

14. LoBue PA, Moser KS. Use of isoniazid for latent tuberculosis infection in a public health clinic. *Am J Respir Crit Care Med.* 2003;168:443.
    In findings similar to the Seattle study, patients treated with isoniazid had a very low rate of hepatotoxicity (0.3 %, no deaths or hospitalizations), but also had a modest treatment completion rate (64%).

15. Centers for Disease Control and Prevention. Update: adverse event data and revised American Thoracic Society/CDC recommendations against the use of rifampin and pyrazinamide for treatment of latent tuberculosis infection—United States, 2003. *MMWR.* 2003;52:735.
    Of 7,737 patients reported to have started rifampin and pyrazinamide for treatment of latent tuberculosis, 204 discontinued using the regimen because of transaminase concentrations greater than five times the upper limit of normal. Forty-eight patients had severe liver injury, defined as death or hospitalization resulting from the medication. This regimen is no longer recommended for the treatment of latent tuberculosis.

16. Polesky A, Farber HW, Gottlien DJ, et al. Rifampin preventive therapy for tuberculosis in Boston's homeless. *Am J Respir Crit Care Med.* 1996;154:1473.
    Rifampin is shown to be safe and effective for prevention of tuberculosis reactivation and appears to be the drug of choice if infection with isoniazid-resistant tuberculosis is likely.

17. Centers for Disease Control and Prevention. Updated guidelines for the use of rifamycins for the treatment of tuberculosis among HIV-infected patients taking protease inhibitors or nonnucleoside reverse transcriptase inhibitors. *MMWR.* 2004;53:37.

   Latest update from the Centers for Disease Control and Prevention on management of drug interactions resulting from concurrent use of rifamycins and HIV therapy.

36. TUBERCULOSIS: CLINICAL MANIFESTATIONS AND DIAGNOSIS OF DISEASE

Philip A. LoBue

Tuberculosis has a wide array of clinical manifestations, both pulmonary and extrapulmonary. Inhaled droplet nuclei of *Mycobacterium tuberculosis* initially lodge in the middle or lower lung zones where regional ventilation is greatest, resulting in a local inflammatory reaction with spread to regional lymph nodes and subsequent hematogenous dissemination. Distant organs, especially the kidneys, bone, central nervous system, as well as the lung apices, are seeded, but overt clinical disease of these areas does not usually ensue. A low-grade fever and symptoms of an upper respiratory illness also may be present. The chest radiograph may show a small area of pneumonitis and often hilar and paratracheal lymphadenopathy. Prominent hilar adenopathy is frequent in children; it is found less commonly in adults.

This initial infection, termed *primary tuberculosis,* resolves spontaneously in most individuals. Healed lesions appear on chest radiograph as calcified parenchymal nodules and are often associated with calcified hilar lymph nodes. In a small percentage of individuals, the initial infection progresses and can manifest as (1) rupture of subpleural infectious foci into the pleural space, resulting in tuberculous pleuritis; (2) extensive caseous pneumonia; (3) enlargement of tuberculous lymph nodes, causing bronchial obstruction (collapse–consolidation lesion); (4) rupture of a tuberculous focus into a bronchus, leading to extensive endobronchial spread throughout one or both lungs; or (5) rupture of a tuberculous focus into a pulmonary blood vessel with hematogenous spread leading to acute disseminated disease.

Tuberculosis can reactivate months to years after containment of the primary infection. The factors causing reactivation lesions are poorly understood. Certain conditions increase the likelihood of progression of latent tuberculosis infection to disease, including malnutrition, alcoholism, poorly controlled diabetes mellitus, silicosis, immunosuppression (by disease processes or drugs), the postpartum period, gastrectomy, chronic hemodialysis, and jejunoileal bypass surgery. In most patients, however, no predisposing factor can be identified.

Radiographically, reactivation or postprimary pulmonary tuberculosis usually presents as an infiltrate in the apical and posterior segments of the upper lobes. The patient can be entirely asymptomatic or have nonspecific symptoms of chronic respiratory infection (e.g., fever, weight loss, productive cough, and hemoptysis). The chest radiograph may reveal a somewhat nondescript fibronodular or fluffy alveolar filling process in the upper lung fields but frequently shows cavity formation, fibrosis with volume loss, or both. The process occasionally heals spontaneously but more frequently progresses locally in the absence of drug therapy.

Advanced disease can be associated with rupture of a hypertrophied pulmonary artery (Rasmussen's aneurysm) into a cavity, resulting in massive hemoptysis, although this is exceedingly uncommon in the era of effective therapy. Rapid progression of pulmonary disease with severe ventilation–perfusion disturbances presenting as the adult respiratory distress syndrome is also seen in rare instances. New hematogenous dissemination and extrapulmonary disease may follow pulmonary reactivation.

Routine laboratory studies in pulmonary tuberculosis are nonspecific. Hematologic studies often reveal a mild anemia, leukopenia, or a monocytosis, but more profound pancytopenia or leukocytosis has been reported. Hyponatremia, usually attributable to the syndrome of inappropriate antidiuretic hormone production, occurs in more than 10% of patients with pulmonary tuberculosis. Addison's disease is a very rare cause of hyponatremia in patients with tuberculosis.

The definitive diagnosis of pulmonary tuberculosis depends on obtaining a positive culture from infected secretions or tissue. If cultures are negative or obtaining a culture is not possible, a presumptive diagnosis can be made from clinical inference and therapeutic trial. The tuberculin skin test (TST) provides information as to whether a tuberculous infection is present but does not distinguish between disease and latent infection. False-negative TST results are common in immunosuppressed patients (advanced tuberculosis, itself, being sufficiently immunosuppressive). A typical chest radiograph is helpful but nonspecific: a variety of nontuberculous processes can have a similar appearance. Spontaneous or aerosol-induced sputum sampling (at least three specimens) is the initial method of choice for bacteriologic assessment. Initially, the specimens are stained by the Ziehl-Neelsen's or fluorescent techniques for acid-fast bacilli (AFB). When sputum analyses are unrevealing, bronchoscopy with lavage, brushings, transbronchial biopsy, or needle aspiration may be considered. Bronchoscopic sampling can enhance both the speed and likelihood of making a diagnosis for an individual patient. Recent systematic studies have not found bronchoscopy to provide an aggregate diagnostic yield superior to aerosol-induced sputum sampling, however. All sputum, lavage, and tissue specimens should be cultured for mycobacteria. Cultures are essential, because (1) smears alone will miss up to 50% of active tuberculosis cases, (2) mycobacteria other than *M. tuberculosis* can produce positive smears, and (3) cultures are necessary for drug susceptibility testing. Special culture media are required, and the laboratory should have proficiency in mycobacterial techniques.

One of the major limitations of mycobacterial culture in the past was that 6 to 8 weeks were required to obtain results. Newer laboratory diagnostic techniques significantly reduced culture times. Using the BACTEC™ system, a rapid radiometric culture technique, mycobacterial growth can be detected in as few as 5 to 8 days, although on average it takes 2 to 3 weeks. Deoxyribonucleic acid (DNA) probe technology can provide a very rapid (within hours) method of differentiating *M. tuberculosis* complex from nontuberculous mycobacteria in growing cultures. This technique has proved to be highly specific and sensitive.

The newest laboratory tools for the diagnosis of tuberculosis are nucleic acid amplification (NAA) tests performed on direct specimens (i.e., without the need for a growing culture). Two commercially available NAA tests have been approved by the Food and Drug Administration (FDA) for use on AFB smear-positive respiratory specimens: the polymerase chain reaction and transcription-mediated amplification. NAA tests can be performed in 6 to 8 hours. The combination of a positive AFB smear and positive NAA test is essentially diagnostic of active tuberculosis. A negative NAA test in the face of a positive AFB smear suggests that the patient has infection with nontuberculous mycobacteria. NAA tests are also approximately 25% more sensitive than the AFB smear and can be of use when the smear is negative and the clinical suspicion for tuberculosis remains moderate or high. Transcription-mediated amplification has also been FDA approved for use on AFB smear-negative specimens. There is less experience with the use of NAA tests for nonrespiratory specimens. Several studies suggest they can be useful for the diagnosis of extrapulmonary tuberculosis, especially for meningitis. The finding of a positive NAA test does not obviate the need for cultures, as NAA tests do not give any information about drug susceptibilities.

Extrapulmonary tuberculosis can occur with or without concurrent active pulmonary tuberculosis. Most frequently, the pathogenesis is that of recrudescence of a previously quiescent hematogenous lesion. However, upper airway and laryngeal disease, lymphatic tuberculosis, and pleural or pericardial tuberculosis commonly arise by extension from contiguous structures. Gastrointestinal tuberculosis can follow ingestion of expectorated infectious sputum or of unpasteurized dairy products from cattle infected with *Mycobacterium bovis* (a rare cause of human tuberculosis).

Large airway (endobronchial) and laryngeal tuberculosis can be present with a normal chest radiograph but is usually associated with extensive cavitary pulmonary disease. Hoarseness is a common presenting symptom. Classically, laryngeal tuberculosis has been considered extremely infectious; however, it may be that the often-associated extensive pulmonary disease, rather than the laryngeal disease per se, is responsible for the increased contagiousness.

Pleural tuberculosis usually presents as a unilateral, exudative, predominantly lymphocytic, pleural effusion often associated with ipsilateral pulmonary tuberculosis. Symptomatic improvement frequently occurs spontaneously. With thoracentesis and pleural biopsy, the diagnosis can be made in 80 to 90% of cases. High levels of adenosine deaminase and interferon-γ in the pleural fluid have been associated with pleural tuberculosis in numerous studies, and these tests should be considered if available. Younger patients with an idiopathic pleural effusion and a positive TST reaction are often treated for pleural tuberculosis solely on clinical grounds. However, multiple closed pleural biopsies or thoracoscopic or surgical exploration should be strongly considered when resolution is not prompt.

Pericardial tuberculosis can present with clinical features of tamponade or chronic constrictive pericarditis. Pericardial involvement should be considered in all tuberculosis patients with cardiomegaly, unexplained heart failure, or arrhythmias. A calcified pericardium on chest radiograph strongly suggests the diagnosis. Echocardiography may demonstrate the presence of pericardial fluid; however, pericardiocentesis and possibly pericardiectomy are necessary to confirm the diagnosis. Cultures of pericardial fluid are positive in only 50% of cases.

Miliary tuberculosis refers to widespread dissemination of *M. tuberculosis* from a previously established focus. It is seen more commonly in primary tuberculosis or in association with immunosuppression (HIV, organ transplantation, tumor necrosis factor α antagonists). Sputum AFB smears and cultures are positive in 30 to 60% of patients. Extrapulmonary sources of culture material (e.g., liver biopsy, bone marrow biopsy, and urine) should be obtained if the diagnosis is being considered, and sputum AFB smears are negative.

Tuberculous meningitis usually results from acute hematogenous spread and is present in up to 33% of cases of miliary disease. Rarely, it can result from breakdown in a silent granuloma or residua from remote hematogenous dissemination and, in children, by direct spread from a tuberculous otitis. Meningitis can present insidiously with lethargy, confusion, and headache. The cerebrospinal fluid (CSF) often shows a lymphocytic pleocytosis, a glucose level less than 20 mg/dL, and a significantly elevated protein level. The CSF smear is positive in only 10 to 20% of cases, whereas cultures are positive in 45 to 70%. Pathologically, an occlusive cranial arteritis can lead to infarction, cranial nerve palsies, and hydrocephalus.

Genitourinary tuberculosis classically presents as painless hematuria and sterile pyuria, but dysuria and secondary bacterial infection are not infrequent. Of all tuberculosis patients, 5 to 7% may have positive urine cultures for *M. tuberculosis*, despite the absence of urinary symptoms and normal urinalyses. The renal parenchyma, caliceal system, ureters, bladder, and reproductive organs all can be affected. If renal tuberculosis is suspected, early-morning urine cultures, an intravenous pyelogram, renal ultrasound, or cystoscopy may be indicated.

Bone and joint tuberculosis can be difficult to diagnose in the early stages of disease. Pain and joint swelling can occur, and there may be paraosseus (cold) abscesses and sinus tract formation. The weight-bearing bones and joints are most commonly affected, especially the spine (Pott's disease), hips, and knees. Early diagnosis by joint aspiration or biopsy is essential to prevent significant disability and to avoid the need for surgery.

Tuberculosis in HIV-infected patients often presents differently than it does in immunocompetent patients. Atypical features of tuberculosis found in HIV patients include (1) higher frequency of negative TSTs (61% vs. 10%); (2) higher frequency of extrapulmonary sites (60% vs. 28%); (3) higher frequency of diffuse or miliary infiltrates (60 vs. 32%); (4) higher frequency of hilar adenopathy (20% vs. <5%); (5) higher frequency of normal chest radiographs with pulmonary involvement (15% vs. <1%); (6) lower frequency of focal infiltrates (35% vs. 68%); and (7) lower frequency of cavities (18% vs. 67%). Atypical clinical and radiographic features of TB in HIV patients are more likely to be seen in those patients with lower CD4 counts, especially below 200. Patients infected with HIV are much more likely to develop rapidly progressive, sometimes fatal disease.

1. LoBue PA, Perry S, Catanzaro A. Diagnosis of tuberculosis. In: Reichman LB, Hershfield ES, eds. *Tuberculosis: A Comprehensive International Approach*. New York, NY: Marcel Dekker, 2000;341–375.
   A general review of the approach to the diagnosis of pulmonary and extrapulmonary tuberculosis.
2. Schluger NW, Rom WN. Current approaches to the diagnosis of active pulmonary tuberculosis. *Am J Respir Crit Care Med*. 1994;149:264.
   A review of both older and newer diagnostic techniques.
3. Havlir DV, Barnes PF. Tuberculosis in patients with human immunodeficiency virus infection. *N Engl J Med*. 1999;340:367.
   Reviews the clinical presentations of tuberculosis in HIV-positive patients, the diagnostic approach including use of NAA testing, and treatment.
4. McAdams HP, Erasmus JE, Winter JA. Radiologic manifestations of pulmonary tuberculosis. *Radiol Clin North Am*. 1995;33:655.
   Reviews chest radiographic findings in pulmonary tuberculosis.
5. Leung AN, Muller NL, Pineda PR, et al. Primary tuberculosis in childhood: radiographic manifestations. *Radiology*. 1992;182:87.
   Chest radiographic abnormalities in primary tuberculosis include infiltrates, atelectasis, and intrathoracic adenopathy often in the lower lobes, findings that are different from the classic abnormalities seen in reactivation tuberculosis, such as upper lobe predominance and cavitation.
6. Jones BE, Young SM, Antoniskis D. Relationship of the manifestations of tuberculosis to CD4 cell counts in patients with human immunodeficiency virus. *Am Rev Respir Dis*. 1993;148:1292.
   Extrapulmonary tuberculosis and atypical chest radiographic abnormalities are associated with lower CD4 counts in patients with HIV.
7. Catanzaro A, Perry S, Clarridge JE, et al. The role of clinical suspicion in evaluating a new diagnostic test for active tuberculosis: results of a multicenter prospective trial. *JAMA*. 2000;283:639.
   Multicenter study of the use of an NAA test for the diagnosis of pulmonary tuberculosis. The NAA test was found to be more sensitive and specific than the acid-fast bacillus smear. Determination of clinical suspicion of tuberculosis was helpful in targeting areas of the clinical spectrum in which NAA tests can make an important contribution.
8. Hiraki A, Aoe K, Eda R, et al. Comparison of six biological markers for the diagnosis of tuberculous pleuritis. *Chest*. 2004;125:987.
   Pleural fluid levels of six biologic markers, including adenosine deaminase and interferon-γ, were measured in 55 patients with pleural effusions. Interferon-γ was the most accurate marker of tuberculous pleuritis.
9. Conde MB, Soares SL, Mello FC, et al. Comparison of sputum induction with fiberoptic bronchoscopy in the diagnosis of tuberculosis: experience at an acquired

immune deficiency syndrome reference center in Rio de Janeiro, Brazil. *Am J Respir Crit Care Med.* 2000;162:2238.

   Aerosol-induced sputum sampling and bronchoscopy were found to have similar diagnostic yields in HIV-positive patients.

10. Lee KC, Tami TA, Lalwani AK, et al. Contemporary management of cervical tuberculosis. *Laryngoscope.* 1992;102:60.

    An algorithm-based approach to diagnosis and management of tuberculous lymphadenitis. Fine needle aspirates (FNA) are recommended as initial diagnostic tools, reserving excisional biopsy for cases where FNA is nondiagnostic.

11. Ogawa S, Smith MA, Brennessel DJ, et al. Tuberculous meningitis in an urban medical center. *Medicine.* 1987;66:317.

    Describes clinical and laboratory presentation and outcome of tuberculous meningitis.

12. Fowler NO, Manitsas GT. Infectious pericarditis. *Prog Cardiovasc Dis.* 1973;16:323.

    Of 19 cases of tuberculous pericarditis, only 32% had associated pulmonary parenchymal infiltrate on chest roentgenograph; 58% had pleural effusion.

13. Gorse GJ, Pais MJ, Kusske JA, et al. Tuberculous spondylitis: a report of six cases and a review of the literature. *Medicine.* 1983;62:178.

    Reviews diagnosis and management of spinal tuberculosis.

14. Berney S, Goldstein M, Bishko F. Clinical and diagnostic features of tuberculous arthritis. *Am J Med.* 1972;53:36.

    Underlying disease was present in 50%. Six patients had previous joint trauma; 19 of 20 had an abnormal synovial biopsy showing granulomatous changes.

15. Christensen WI. Genitourinary tuberculosis: a review of 102 cases. *Medicine.* 1974;53:377.

    A review of urinary tract and genital tuberculosis.

16. Shakil AO, Korula J, Kanel GC, et al. Diagnostic features of tuberculous peritonitis in the absence and presence of chronic liver disease: a case control study. *Am J Med.* 1996;100:179.

    Characteristics of ascitic fluid in patients with tuberculous peritonitis can vary, depending on whether the patient has significant underlying liver disease.

17. Abrams JS, Holden WD. Tuberculosis of the gastrointestinal tract. *Arch Surg.* 1964;89:282.

    The ileocecal area is most commonly affected. The differential diagnosis from Crohn's disease can be difficult.

18. Maartens G, Willcox PA, Benatar SR. Miliary tuberculosis: rapid diagnosis, hematologic abnormalities, and outcome in 109 treated adults. *Am J Med.* 1989;89:291.

    Transbronchial lung biopsy, bone marrow biopsy, and liver biopsy are the best diagnostic tests and should be considered if sputum samples are nondiagnostic.

19. Christie JD, Callihan DR. The laboratory diagnosis of mycobacterial diseases. *Clin Lab Med.* 1995;15:279.

    An excellent review of current smear and culture techniques.

37. TUBERCULOSIS: TREATMENT OF DISEASE

Philip A. LoBue

Although the principles of effective antituberculous chemotherapy are reasonably straightforward, even well-trained physicians may treat tuberculosis patients inappropriately. This likely reflects the relatively limited experience many physicians have had with this disease. As a consequence, local health departments have assumed a greater role in the management of patients with tuberculosis. Whether care is being managed primarily by a private physician or the health department, the medical provider has two major responsibilities: (1) prescribe a treatment regimen with appropriate drugs, dosages, and duration, and (2) ensure adherence to the regimen until the treatment is complete. When non–health department providers assume a primary patient management role, they should work in partnership with the health department to ensure these responsibilities are met.

Drugs used to treat tuberculosis can be divided into first- and second-line agents. The first-line (i.e., most effective and least toxic) drugs consist of isoniazid, rifampin, pyrazinamide, and ethambutol. Isoniazid and rifampin are very effective bactericidal drugs. Isoniazid's major adverse reactions include hepatitis and neuritis. The major adverse effects of rifampin are hepatotoxicity and hypersensitivity reactions. Some evidence suggests that the combination of rifampin and isoniazid can be associated with a greater incidence of liver injury than with either drug alone. Hypersensitivity reactions, including a flulike syndrome, thrombocytopenia, and, rarely, acute renal failure, have been reported, usually occurring with intermittent rifampin therapy. Rifampin increases hepatic metabolism of some drugs, causing important drug interactions. Oral contraceptives can be ineffective at normal doses because their hepatic metabolism is increased. In addition, rifampin can induce methadone withdrawal. Pyrazinamide is used for the first 2 months in many treatment regimens. Its principal side effects are hepatotoxicity and hyperuricemia, with the latter rarely leading to gout or renal failure. Ethambutol is a bacteriostatic agent that has been in general use for over 3 decades. A dose of 25 mg/kg daily is used for 2 to 3 months and then decreased to 15 mg/kg. Retrobulbar optic neuritis has occasionally complicated therapy with doses in excess of 20 mg/kg for prolonged periods, but is almost never seen when using 15 mg/kg.

Second-line medications are generally reserved for therapy of drug-resistant disease or for patients intolerant of first-line medications. Fluoroquinolones are among the latest additions to the antituberculous array of drugs. They are generally well tolerated and several have good in vitro activity against *Mycobacterium tuberculosis*. Levofloxacin is the first choice of medications in this class because it has in vitro activity superior to other older fluoroquinolones and a good safety profile with long-term use. The newer fluoroquinolones, moxifloxacin and gatifloxacin, have better *in vitro* activity, but there is less clinical experience with their use for tuberculosis treatment. Rare gastrointestinal side effects, such as nausea and bloating, and neurologic side effects, including dizziness, insomnia, tremulousness, and headache, may occur with fluoroquinolones. Several aminoglycoside antibiotics are of proven efficacy in the therapy of tuberculosis. Unfortunately, they all require intramuscular or intravenous administration and have a high incidence of serious side effects. Streptomycin, the first drug available for tuberculosis therapy, is still used occasionally; however, its value is limited by dose-related renal and eighth cranial nerve toxicities and an increasing incidence of drug resistance. Other aminoglycosides, such as capreomycin, kanamycin, and amikacin have similar toxicities and may be slightly less effective. Para-aminosalicylic acid (PAS), ethionamide, and cycloserine are oral preparations that are usually used only in multidrug-resistant (MDR) tuberculosis. PAS and ethionamide can cause severe gastrointestinal distress, whereas cycloserine is associated with personality changes, depression, frank psychoses, and, in high doses, seizures.

Since the first antituberculous medications were developed in the late 1940s, the treatment of tuberculosis has changed considerably. Although clinical investigations are ongoing and individual patients or situations can require tailored regimens, the combination of isoniazid, rifampin, and pyrazinamide is currently the mainstay of treatment for patients with susceptible organisms. Other drugs, however, especially ethambutol and the fluoroquinolones, have important roles in certain contexts.

For patients with isoniazid- and rifampin-susceptible pulmonary tuberculosis standard treatment is divided into an initial phase of 2 months (8 weeks) followed by a continuation phase of 4 months (18 weeks). Because of the relatively high rate of isoniazid resistance found in adults, their initial-phase treatment should consist of isoniazid, rifampin, pyrazinamide, and ethambutol for 2 months. For children, ethambutol usually is not needed, unless there is particular concern for isoniazid resistance or the child has a clinical pattern usually seen in adults (i.e., upper lobe infiltration, cavity formation). Once susceptibility results become available, ethambutol may be discontinued (or omitted if drug susceptibility results are known before treatment is started) if the organism is susceptible to isoniazid and rifampin. If pyrazinamide cannot be included in the initial phase of treatment, or if the isolate is resistant to pyrazinamide alone, the initial phase should consist of isoniazid, rifampin, and ethambutol (at least until drug susceptibility results are known; see above) given daily for 2 months. Situations where pyrazinamide may be withheld include severe liver disease, gout, and pregnancy. The initial phase may be given daily throughout, daily for 2 weeks and then twice weekly for 6 weeks, or three times weekly throughout. Twice-weekly therapy is never recommended for human immunodeficiency virus (HIV)-infected patients with CD4 counts less than 100 in the initial or continuation phase of tuberculosis treatment (see below).

The standard continuation-phase therapy for tuberculosis susceptible to isoniazid and rifampin consists of isoniazid and rifampin. Treatment may be given daily, two times weekly (except if HIV-infected and CD4 count below 100), or three times weekly. For HIV-seronegative patients with noncavitary pulmonary tuberculosis and negative sputum smear results at the completion of 2 months of treatment, an alternative continuation phase treatment is isoniazid and rifapentine (a long-acting analog of rifampin) given once weekly. The duration of the continuation phase is 4 months (6 months total treatment) for most patients with drug-susceptible tuberculosis. However, patients who did not have pyrazinamide included in their initial phase should have their continuation phase extended to 7 months (9 months total treatment). In addition, a recent clinical trial involving more than 1000 patients demonstrated that patients with positive sputum cultures after 2 months of therapy and cavities on chest radiograph were more likely to fail treatment or relapse. Therefore, such patients should also have their continuation phase extended to 7 months, as should patients being treated with once-weekly isoniazid and rifapentine with positive sputum cultures after 2 months of treatment, regardless of chest radiographic findings.

Since the 1990s, use of directly observed therapy (DOT) by local health departments has become a major tool in tuberculosis control. With DOT, some or all doses of medication are taken in the presence of a nurse or other ancillary healthcare worker. This can be done by having the patient come to the clinic or by sending an outreach worker to the patient's home. Use of DOT minimizes the risk of treatment failure and acquired drug resistance due to nonadherence. DOT is considered a core management strategy for patients with tuberculosis. It is considered mandatory when using intermittent (i.e., other than daily) therapy. Because DOT is resource intensive, some health departments may not have the resources to provide it to all patients. Priority for DOT is usually given to children, individuals with drug-resistant disease, and those who are likely to be nonadherent (e.g., intravenous drug users, those with psychiatric disorders, the homeless).

Completion of treatment is defined not just by the duration of therapy, but by the number of doses taken. For example, a patient receiving daily standard treatment for drug-susceptible disease should take 56 doses (over 8 weeks) of medication in the initial phase and 126 doses (over 18 weeks) in the continuation phase. This should be kept in mind when deciding when to discontinue therapy.

To monitor response to therapy, sputum cultures should be collected every month until cultures are negative for 2 consecutive months. Since more than 90% of patients have negative sputum cultures after 3 months of treatment, any individual with a positive sputum culture at this point should be carefully evaluated to try to identify the etiology of this delayed response to therapy. A patient with a positive sputum culture after 4 months of treatment is considered a treatment failure. Possible reasons for treatment failure include nonadherence and medication malabsorption. In addition to addressing the reasons for treatment failure, repeat susceptibility testing should be performed to assess for acquired drug resistance. If the treatment regimen is going to be modified, at least three new drugs to which the patient's organism would be expected to be susceptible should be added. A cardinal rule of tuberculosis therapy is that a single drug should never be added to a failing regimen.

Patients infected with organisms that are resistant to isoniazid, rifampin, or both, require modifications in their drug regimens. For tuberculosis that is isoniazid resistant (but rifampin susceptible), the recommended regimen is daily rifampin, ethambutol, and pyrazinamide for 6 months. A fluoroquinolone may be added to strengthen this regimen in patients with extensive disease. For tuberculosis resistant to rifampin (but isoniazid susceptible), the recommended therapy is isoniazid, ethambutol, and a fluoroquinolone for 12 to 18 months with pyrazinamide added for the first 2 months. Tuberculosis that is resistant to at least isoniazid and rifampin is termed *MDR*. Treatment of MDR tuberculosis is often complex and should be done with the consultation of a tuberculosis expert. MDR tuberculosis should be treated with four to six medications to which the organism is susceptible. Therapy should continue for 18 to 24 months (24 months is strongly recommended if there is also resistance to ethambutol or pyrazinamide). Surgical resection of heavily diseased areas of the lung is sometimes used as an adjunctive therapy for MDR tuberculosis and should be considered in suitable candidates.

Chemotherapy for extrapulmonary tuberculosis does not differ in principle from that for pulmonary tuberculosis. Duration of therapy is the same as for pulmonary disease, with the exceptions of (1) meningitis, for which 9 to 12 months of treatment is recommended and (2) bone and joint disease, for which some experts recommend extending treatment to 9 months. Corticosteroids should be used routinely in the treatment of central nervous system tuberculosis including meningitis and pericarditis but are not recommended as an adjunct for treatment of other forms of tuberculosis.

Tuberculosis treatment of HIV-infected patients is similar to that of HIV-negative patients, although there are several differences. The combination of once-weekly isoniazid and rifapentine should never be used in HIV-infected individuals, as this has resulted in high rates of treatment failure and relapse associated with acquired rifampin resistance. Biweekly therapy should not be used in HIV-infected patients with CD4 counts below 100 for the same reason. Rifampin should not be used in patients in conjunction with most protease inhibitors (ritonavir is an exception) or nonnucleoside reverse transcriptase inhibitors (NNRTI) (efavirenz is an exception). For this reason, consideration should be given to substituting rifabutin (a comparably effective rifamycin) for rifampin. Rifabutin can be used with most protease inhibitors (saquinavir is an exception) and most NNRTIs (delavirdine is an exception) if appropriate dosage adjustments are made. Because of the complex drug interactions between many antiretroviral medications and rifamycins, it is strongly recommended that tuberculosis treatment of patients on such drugs be carried out in consultation with a clinical HIV expert.

Temporary exacerbation of tuberculosis symptoms and lesions can occur in patients with HIV who are taking antiretroviral therapy. This phenomenon, known as the paradoxical reaction, has been attributed to recovery of the delayed hypersensitivity response in these patients and increased exposure to tuberculosis antigens after the initiation of bactericidal antituberculous therapy. In general, modifications of tuberculosis therapy and antiretroviral therapy are not necessary, and a short course of corticosteroids may ameliorate symptoms associated with this reaction if it is severe.

Tuberculosis in children is treated similarly to adult disease. In the past, concern was expressed about the use of ethambutol in very young children because of the difficulty in screening for retrobulbar neuritis. More recent data, however, suggest that ethambutol is safe in this population.

Isoniazid, ethambutol, and rifampin have been used successfully and safely in pregnancy. Pyrazinamide has not been shown to be teratogenic, but there is insufficient experience with this drug in pregnancy to assure its safety; its use during pregnancy is not generally recommended. Streptomycin causes eighth cranial nerve damage to the fetus and should not be used. All other second-line drugs, with the possible exception of PAS, either have known teratogenic effects or are lacking sufficient safety data to endorse their use in pregnancy.

Adverse drug reactions can occur at any time during treatment. Often difficult to diagnose, they can be confused with manifestations of tuberculosis or other concurrent illnesses. Sometimes drug reactions are relatively mild so that stopping therapy is not warranted. Specific reactions can be handled by discontinuing the suspect drug. Often drugs have overlapping toxicity and reactions are nonspecific (e.g., fever, rash, jaundice). In such cases, all drugs should be stopped for a brief period (e.g., 1 week) and then reintroduced singly, the least likely offender first. Some clinicians reinitiate drugs at low doses, whereas others resume full-dose therapy. If a reaction appears a second time, then another drug may need to be substituted. (One drug can be added to a successful regimen as long as the entire regimen is adequate.)

All patients being treated for tuberculosis should be counseled and tested for HIV infection. Patients with risk factors for hepatitis B or C should be tested for these viruses. Baseline serum transaminase, bilirubin, alkaline phosphatase, and creatinine levels and a platelet count should be measured for all adults. Visual acuity and color testing should be performed for all patients receiving ethambutol. Routine follow-up measurements of liver or renal function or platelet count are not necessary unless there were abnormalities at baseline or there are clinical indications for additional blood tests. Patients who have stable abnormalities of hepatic or renal function at initial testing should have repeat measurements early in the course of treatment, then less frequently to ensure that there is no deterioration. At minimum, patients receiving ethambutol should be questioned regarding visual disturbances at monthly intervals; however, formal monthly repeat testing of visual acuity and color vision is often done routinely and is strongly recommended for individuals receiving more than 15 mg/kg or for those taking the medication for more than 2 months. Monitoring tests for individual second-line drugs can be found in the American Thoracic Society/Centers for Disease Control and Prevention/Infectious Diseases Society of America 2003 Treatment of Tuberculosis statement.

Surgery is rarely necessary except in selected cases of MDR tuberculosis and for complications of tuberculosis such as (1) emergency treatment of massive hemoptysis, (2) therapy of bronchopleural fistulas, (3) drainage of true (purulent) tuberculous empyemas (*not free flowing, nonpurulent effusions, which are much more common*), or (4) relief of mechanical problems in skeletal tuberculosis, such as spinal stabilization procedures in selected individuals with Pott's disease.

1. American Thoracic Society, Centers for Disease Control and Prevention, Infectious Diseases Society of America. Treatment of tuberculosis. *MMWR*. 2003; 52(RR-11):1.

   National guidelines for the treatment of active tuberculosis. Also gives background information on various tuberculosis medications and guidelines for special situations, such as children, pregnancy, and drug resistance.
2. The Tuberculosis Trials Consortium. Rifapentine and isoniazid once a week versus rifampicin and isoniazid twice a week for treatment of drug-susceptible pulmonary tuberculosis in HIV-negative patients: a randomized clinical trial. *Lancet*. 2002;360:528.

Randomized clinical trial involving more than 1000 patients. Important findings included: (1) isoniazid and rifapentine once weekly could be used successfully in the continuation phase in selected low-risk patients and (2) patients with positive cultures after 2 months of treatment and a cavity on chest radiograph were at higher risk for treatment failure or relapse regardless of treatment regimen.

3. Combs DL, O'Brien RJ, Geiter LJ. USPHS Tuberculosis Short Course Chemotherapy Trial 21: effectiveness, toxicity, and acceptability. The report of final results. *Ann Intern Med.* 1990;112:397.

   A 6-month regimen, beginning with isoniazid, rifampin, and pyrazinamide for 2 months, followed by isoniazid and rifampin for 4 months, is similar in effectiveness and toxicity to the 9-month regimen.

4. Chan ED, Laurel V, Strand MJ, et al. Treatment and outcome analysis of 205 patients with multidrug-resistant tuberculosis. *Am J Respir Crit Care Med.* 2004; 169:1103–1109. (Epub ahead of print as doi:10.1164/rccm.200308-1159OC.)

   Compared to a prior cohort of MDR patients, this group had more favorable initial treatment responses and long-term outcomes. Use of fluoroquinolones and adjunctive surgery was associated with improved clinical and microbiologic outcomes.

5. Telzak EE, Sepkowitz K, Alpert P, et al. Multidrug-resistant tuberculosis in patients without HIV infection. *N Engl J Med.* 1995;333:907.

   Report of 26 HIV-negative patients treated for MDR tuberculosis in New York City. Twenty-four (96%) had a response to therapy and only 4 of 23 treated with second-line drugs required discontinuation of therapy.

6. Centers for Disease Control and Prevention. Prevention and treatment of tuberculosis among patients infected with human immunodeficiency virus: principles of therapy and revised recommendations. *MMWR.* 1998;47:1.

   CDC guidelines for tuberculosis treatment in HIV-positive patients. Reviews recent trials of tuberculosis treatment in HIV, drug interactions between tuberculosis medications and antiretrovirals, and the paradoxical reaction. More recent updates are available at the CDC's website (www.cdc.gov).

7. Havlir DV, Barnes PF. Tuberculosis in patients with human immunodeficiency virus infection. *N Engl J Med.* 1999;340:367.

   An excellent recent review of all aspects of tuberculosis in patients infected with HIV.

8. Chaisson RE, Clermont HC, Holt EA, et al. Six-month supervised intermittent tuberculosis therapy in Haitian patients with and without HIV infection. *Am J Respir Crit Care Med.* 1996;154:1034.

   Six-month intermittent therapy was efficacious for the treatment of tuberculosis in patients infected with HIV.

9. Narita M, Ashkin D, Hollender ES, et al. Paradoxical worsening of tuberculosis following antiretroviral therapy in patients with AIDS. *Am J Respir Crit Care Med.* 1998;158:157.

   Describes the paradoxical reaction which can occur in patients being treated for HIV and tuberculosis.

10. Weis SE, Slocum PC, Blais FX, et al. The effect of directly observed therapy on the rates of drug resistance and relapse in tuberculosis. *N Engl J Med.* 1994;330:1179.

    Use of DOT results in decreased rates of relapse, acquired drug resistance, and primary drug resistance in the community.

11. Moore RD, Chaulk PC, Griffiths R, et al. Cost-effectiveness of directly observed versus self-administered therapy for tuberculosis. *Am J Respir Crit Care Med.* 1996;154:1013.

    DOT is more cost effective than self-administered therapy.

12. Trebucq A. Should ethambutol be recommended for routine treatment of tuberculosis in children? A review of the literature. *Int J Tuberc Lung Dis.* 1997;1:12.

    Ethambutol can be used safely in children younger than age 5.

13. Yee D, Valiquette C, Pelletier M, et al. Incidence of serious side effects from first-line antituberculosis drugs among patients treated for active tuberculosis. *Am J Respir Crit Care Med.* 2003;167:1472.

Among 430 patients, the incidence of all major adverse effects was 1.48 per 100 person-months of exposure. The incidence of pyrazinamide-induced hepatotoxicity and rash during treatment for active TB was substantially higher than with the other first-line anti-TB drugs, and higher than previously recognized.

14. Patel AM, McKeon J. Avoidance and management of adverse reactions to antituberculous drugs. *Drug Saf.* 1995;12:1

   Comprehensive review of adverse effects of medications used to treat tuberculosis, including sections on prevention, monitoring, and management.

---

38. MYCOBACTERIAL INFECTION DUE TO MYCOBACTERIA OTHER THAN TUBERCULOSIS (MOTT)

Jana Cooke and Antonio Catanzaro

Nontuberculous mycobacterial (NTM) infections encompass a variety of acid-fast bacilli that are biologically distinct from *Mycobacterium tuberculosis, Mycobacterium leprae,* and *Mycobacterium bovis.* They had long been considered saprophytes or culture contaminants. More recently, however, they have been recognized as significant human pathogens, with the potential to cause disease in virtually any organ in the body, particularly in immunosuppressed patients or anatomically disrupted sites. Although the rates of tuberculosis are declining in many industrialized countries, the prevalence of disease caused by these environmental opportunistic mycobacteria appears to be increasing.

The distribution of NTM is worldwide, although there appear to be important regional predominances of certain species. For example, *Mycobacterium kansasii* is most commonly found in urban inhabitants of some midwestern and southernmost states. Mycobacterium avium-intracellulare (MAI) complex, also known as MAC, is more common in rural inhabitants of the southeastern states. Unlike the *M. tuberculosis* complex, NTM are widely dispersed in the environment and commonly isolated from soil, drinking water, rivers, hospital instruments (i.e., bronchoscopes), and dairy products, specifically raw milk. There have been increasing reports of nosocomial infections resulting from NTM, specifically MAC, presumably due in part to reduced hot water temperatures in hospitals. Unlike tuberculosis, there is no person-to-person transmission.

Diagnosis of disease caused by NTM is difficult, as the organisms are commonly isolated from environmental sources, and therefore, most isolates are in fact contaminants. Further complicating the diagnosis is the fact that these organisms are frequently isolated from the sputum of patients with chronic lung disease. Skin testing with homologous antigens contributes little to the diagnosis of NTM disease and suffers many shortcomings, such as cross-reactivity, frequent inapparent infection, and lack of availability of antigens. The American Thoracic Society published an official statement outlining diagnostic criteria for NTM pulmonary disease in 1997. To make a diagnosis of NTM, these guidelines require a compatible clinical presentation and the recovery of large numbers of organisms, as indicated by a positive smear as well as a positive culture, repeated isolates from sputum or bronchial wash of a given species, a compatible roentgenographic picture, and the exclusion of other potential etiologic agents. These criteria essentially put the burden of proof on the clinician who wants to treat and are based on experience with common and well-described respiratory pathogens, such as MAC. There is little experience or published series with many of the other NTM to know if these criteria also are applicable. *M. kansasii* is a notable exception. It is considered to be the most virulent NTM pathogen, and most experts consider a single isolate to be all that is needed to make a diagnosis in the proper clinical context.

Several recent advances enable laboratories to detect and identify mycobacteria more rapidly and accurately. The use of liquid-based culture media such as BACTEC (Becton Dickinson, Sparks, Md.) has greatly reduced the time in which results are available; many NTM can now be recovered in days rather than weeks. The increased use of liquid culture probably is also a factor in the increase in isolation of some of these organisms. Chemiluminescent DNA probes (such as AccuProbe; GeneProbe Inc., San Diego, Calif.) are now being used to identify some of the most common species of NTM, including MAC and *M. kansasii*. These probes are reported to be nearly 100% sensitive and specific and have become the most commonly used method of rapid mycobacterial identification. Although not yet commercially available, two other new methods include polymerase restriction endonuclease analysis (PRA) and deoxyribonucleic acid (DNA) sequence analysis.

Pulmonary infection with NTM is most often caused by MAC. Two main types of presentation are currently recognized in HIV-negative patients with pulmonary disease caused by MAC. The first is an apical fibrocavitary disease, often multistrain, seen mostly in men in their late 40s and early 50s who have a history of heavy cigarette use and, often, alcohol abuse. The second is a bilateral or isolated right middle lobe/lingular nodular and interstitial/nodular disease with a much slower progression over a 5- to 10-year period. This type of manifestation is predominantly seen in nonsmoking elderly females and is usually owing to one strain. A variation on the second type of presentation is the combination of bronchiectasis, small nodules, and focal mass-like opacities, the so-called "Lady Windermere syndrome," which was first described in 1992. In addition to its occurrence in the above-mentioned at-risk patient populations, pulmonary disease due to MAC is increasingly being recognized as a pathogen in patients with cystic fibrosis. One potentially important discovery is the presence of CFTR mutation (the gene responsible for cystic fibrosis) in patients without cystic fibrosis who have a diagnosis of bronchiectasis, pulmonary NTM, or both.

MAC infection in HIV-positive patients differs somewhat from how it presents in those who are immunocompetent, as it tends to manifest as disseminated disease. Pulmonary disease due to MAC has been reported to occur in fewer than 5% of cases of dissemination and can occur without evidence of dissemination. As with immunocompetent individuals, pulmonary disease due to MAC in the HIV-positive patient has a variety of presentations, including nodules, infiltrates, cavities, and lymphadenopathy. Overall, the incidence of disseminated MAC has dramatically decreased over the past decade owing to the introduction of highly active antiretroviral therapy (HAART).

The initiation of this potent therapy has introduced a new clinical entity, called *immune reconstitution syndrome*. It is thought to be caused by the recovery of pathogen-specific immune responses to infections that are already present but not clinically detectable. It typically presents with a fever, leukocytosis, and lymphadenitis but can have symptoms related to any site where the infection has remained previously quiescent. The symptoms are fairly mild, occur within the first few weeks of the initiation of therapy, and usually resolve with continued HAART. Of note, it can occur each time the patient is challenged with HAART.

The diagnosis of MAC pulmonary infection remains difficult and complicated. The American Thoracic Society (ATS) guidelines, which are applicable to both HIV-negative and -positive patients, recommend an integrated approach of clinical presentation, radiographic findings, and laboratory data. A single positive sputum culture is insufficient to make a diagnosis. However, if the organism is isolated from a transbronchial or lung biopsy or from a bronchial wash, a single positive culture is adequate. According to these guidelines, three separate sputum specimens should produce at least two positive cultures, with the third being smear-positive, or three positive cultures, regardless of smear results. It should be noted that these guidelines remain controversial and debates regarding the diagnosis of MAC are ongoing. Furthermore, making a diagnosis does not necessarily imply that treatment should be initiated.

M. kansasii is the second most common NTM to cause pulmonary disease and in some regions, it has become the most common. Of all the NTM, *M. kansasii* most closely parallels the clinical course of *M. tuberculosis,* with up to 90% of HIV-negative patients presenting with cavitary infiltrates. Risk factors for developing pulmonary disease by *M. kansasii* include pneumoconiosis, chronic obstructive pulmonary disease, previous mycobacterial disease, malignancy, and alcoholism. This NTM primarily affects middle aged white men. *M. kansasii* also produces pulmonary disease in HIV-infected patients who usually have the same symptoms as immunocompetent patients. Radiographically, interstitial infiltrates and hilar adenopathy are more commonly seen with HIV-infected patients than cavitations. *M. kansasii* can also appear as disseminated disease, particularly in severely immunocompromised patients, such as those with advanced AIDS and those who have undergone organ transplantation. As stated above, in the appropriate clinical setting, a single culture-positive specimen for *M. kansasii* is sufficient to make a diagnosis and initiate therapy as this NTM is considered to be the most virulent.

Rarely, pulmonary infections may be caused by some of the rapidly growing nontuberculous mycobacteria (RGM) such as *Mycobacterium abscessus, Mycobacterium fortuitum,* and *Mycobacterium chelonei*. In general, constitutional symptoms are less severe and the course more indolent than in classic tuberculosis. Pulmonary infection with these NTM is more prevalent among white, female nonsmokers who are at least age 60. Approximately 40% of these patients have an underlying medical condition such as previously treated mycobacterial lung disease. In general, these RGM are very difficult to treat.

Well-documented infections involving bone, joints, urinary tract, skin, soft tissues, lymph nodes, liver, kidney, and meninges have been reported with a variety of NTM. Widely disseminated disease may occur, especially in immunosuppressed individuals and those with hematologic abnormalities.

Lymphadenitis due to NTM is found almost exclusively in children. The causative organism is usually MAC but may be *M. kansasii*. Lymphadenitis due to *Mycobacterium scrofulaceum* has diminished greatly in frequency in recent years. Infection presumably results from an inapparent breach of the tonsillar mucosa. Patients most frequently present with asymptomatic, unilateral, anterior cervical adenopathy. Less commonly, other nodes may be involved, and in advanced cases, draining sinuses and fistulae may appear. The chest radiograph is often clear.

Swimming pool granuloma (*Mycobacterium marinum*) is a superficial cutaneous ulceration that usually presents on the extremities. Healing generally occurs spontaneously, although complete resolution may take 3 to 4 months. However, treatment may be needed in selected cases, particularly when resolution is indolent. In contrast, *Mycobacterium ulcerans* may produce extensive tissue necrosis (*Buruli* or Bairnsdale ulcer) requiring surgical debridement and skin grafting. Subcutaneous abscesses due to *M. fortuitum* may result from inoculation with contaminated surgical implements.

The approach to management of pulmonary disease due to nontuberculous mycobacteria depends primarily on the causative species. It is important to stress that, as no documentation of communicability exists, the standard measures for reducing communicability used in patients with *M. tuberculosis* are not necessary. In fact health departments do not typically tabulate these cases.

The optimal treatment of previously untreated pulmonary disease due to MAC is not known. Many experts recommend a four-drug regimen that includes a macrolide (clarithromycin or azithromycin), rifampin, ethambutol, plus inhaled amikacin for the first 2 to 3 months. Bronchial hygiene is an important, often overlooked adjunctive therapy for those patients with preexisting lung disease; there is no role for rotating antibiotics, however. A recent study found that the efficacy of thrice weekly treatment was comparable to daily therapy—good news for patients who have trouble tolerating the side effects of the various medications. Routine drug susceptibility testing is not recommended as the organism shows in vitro resistance to most antituberculous drugs. However, in vitro sensitivities should be obtained for those patients who are failing therapy or experiencing a relapse after prior treatment. After 6 months of triple drug treatment, up to 92% of patients without preexisting lung disease have sputum conversion compared with 62 to 74% of patients with underlying preexisting pulmonary disease. Patients who have no pulmonary disease and who have MAC sporadically recovered may not require treatment. Sputum should be sampled monthly to document negative conversion, and blood tests should be monitored routinely while on treatment as the potential for drug toxicity is high.

The optimal length of drug treatment for pulmonary disease due to MAC also has not yet been established. Some advocate therapy for 12 months after sputum conversion. One study using 12 months of negative sputum cultures as an endpoint observed no relapses with a mean follow-up period of 18 months. Of note, early relapses were observed if 10 months of culture negativity was used as a therapy endpoint. Others recommend 24 months of therapy although the extended treatment benefits have not been clearly proven. In addition, some advocate stopping therapy all together for those patients who have difficulty tolerating the medications or who do not show clear improvement after 6 months or more of treatment. In general, patients on a macrolide-containing regimen should show clinical improvement in 3 to 6 months. When anatomically feasible, early surgical intervention (under chemotherapeutic coverage) is indicated. Bacteriologic conversion rates varying from 40 to 90% have been achieved with such combined medical and surgical therapy.

Patients with AIDS and disseminated MAC should be treated with the aforementioned four-drug therapy. However, the drugs used to treat MAC are associated with frequent adverse effects in this population. For example, rifampin increases the hepatic metabolism of protease inhibitors. Some argue that the toxicity of these drugs in AIDS patients is prohibitive and that the goal in treating disseminated MAC should be to improve the immune function of the patient.

In patients without immune function recovery, treatment of MAC should be life-long. Optimal duration of treatment for those patients whose immune system responds to HAART is not known. Finally, the United States Public Health Service/Infectious Diseases Society of America (USPHS/IDSA) recommends that all patients who have CD4 counts less than 50 cells/mm^3 receive prophylaxis for disseminated MAC. The most commonly used regimen is clarithromycin given twice daily or azithromycin given once weekly. Both agents have been proven to reduce the incidence of MAC bacteremia.

M. kansasii responds well to chemotherapy. In vitro susceptibility studies do not necessarily correlate with in vivo drug efficacy. The initial regimen should include isoniazid, ethambutol, and most importantly, rifampin. Rarely, regimens including four or five drugs may be necessary to achieve a bacteriologic cure. Medication should be continued for 18 months, and many experts feel that successful treatment requires the documentation of negative sputum cultures for at least 1 year. More than 90% success has been achieved with drug therapy alone. Adjunctive surgery is rarely indicated, except in well-localized disease that has responded poorly to adequate chemotherapy.

Strict guidelines regarding the less common pathogens are not possible because of the relative lack of available information. Treatment of RGM is difficult, however, as they are resistant to most antituberculous drugs. Chemotherapeutic regimens similar to those for MAC have yielded only limited success. Clarithromycin, amikacin, doxycycline, cefoxitin, imipenem, levofloxacin, and trimethoprim-sulfamethoxazole may show in vitro sensitivity and can be clinically useful. Because of the difficult nature of treating these NTMs, it is recommended that broad sensitivity studies be obtained. In general, 3 to 5 drugs are needed for an extended duration. Surgical resection, if feasible, should also be considered.

---

1. American Thoracic Society. Diagnosis and treatment of disease caused by nontuberculous mycobacteria. *Am J Respir Crit Care Med.* 1997;156:S1–S25.

   This official statement covers diagnostic criteria that work best with MAC, M. abscessus, *and* M. kansasii. *Disease should be suspected if any of the following criteria are met: If three sputum/bronchial wash results are available from the previous 12 months: two or three positive cultures with negative acid-fast bacilli smear results. If only one bronchial wash is available: positive culture with a* positive acid-fast bacilli smear or moderate to heavy growth on solid media. Lab features for NTM include staining and culture, species identification, and susceptibility testing. Treatment of NTM can include the following: isoniazid, rifampin, ethambutol, clarithromycin, azithromycin, rifabutin, and streptomycin.

2. French AL, Benator DA, Gordin FM. Nontuberculous mycobacterial infections. Med Clin North Am. 1997;81:361–379.

An excellent review article covering MAC, M. kansasii, and other nontuberculous mycobacteria, with special emphasis on involvement with AIDS.

3. Tanaka E, Kimotot T, Tsuyuguchi K, et al. Effect of clarithromycin regimen for Mycobacterium avium complex pulmonary disease. Am J Respir Crit Care Med. 1999;160:866–872.

The authors examined the efficacy of a four-drug regimen for MAC that contained clarithromycin. They found that the regimen benefited newly treated patients, but problems remained for retreated patients, such as adverse side effects and low sputum conversion rates.

4. Rosenzweig DY, Schlueter DP. Spectrum of clinical disease in pulmonary infection with Mycobacterium avium-intracellulare. Rev Infect Dis. 1981;3:1046.

Cases usually occur in middle-aged men with underlying lung diseases, but variations in age, sex, presentation, and severity of disease are wide.

5. Corpe RF. Surgical management of pulmonary disease due to Mycobacterium avium-intracellulare. Rev Infect Dis. 1981;3:1064.

Of 131 patients with pulmonary infections due to MAC, 124 had excisional surgery plus chemotherapy; and 7 had definitive thoracoplasties.

6. Reich JM, Johnson RE. Mycobacterium avium complex pulmonary disease. Am Rev Respir Dis. 1991;143:1381.

The experience with pulmonary disease caused by MAC was examined during a 12-year period in a nonreferral setting.

7. Reich JM, Johnson RE. Mycobacterium avium complex pulmonary disease presenting as an isolated lingular or middle lobe pattern: the Lady Windermere syndrome. Chest. 1992;101:1605.

Pulmonary disease due to MAC radiographically resembles that due to tuberculosis. It preferentially affects elderly white men with predisposing pulmonary disorders.

8. Swensen SJ, Hartman TE, Williams DE. Computed tomographic diagnosis of Mycobacterium avium-intracellulare complex in patients with bronchiectasis. Chest. 1994;105:49.

Of 24 patients with multiple pulmonary nodules, 19 had lung nodules and bronchiectasis in the same lobe. Of 15 patients with lung nodules, 8 (53%) had cultures positive for MAC, as did 2 of the 48 (4%) patients with no computed tomographic evidence of lung nodules.

9. Prince DS, Peterson DD, Steiner RM, et al. Infection with Mycobacterium avium complex in patients without predisposing conditions. N Engl J Med. 1989;321:863.

The authors describe 21 patients (mean age, 66 years) with MAC infection without the usual predisposing factors, representing 18% of the 119 patients surveyed.

10. Gribetz AR, Damsker B, Bottone EJ, et al. Solitary pulmonary nodules due to nontuberculous mycobacterial infection. Am J Med. 1981;70:39.

Of 20 specimens in which acid-fast bacilli were seen and that roentgenographically were solitary pulmonary nodules, 12 (60%) were due to infection with MAC. In five granulomas, acid-fast bacilli were seen but failed to grow on culture. In one instance each, M. tuberculosis, M. fortuitum, and M. gordonae grew on culture.

11. Mitchison DA, Ellard GA, Grosset J. New antibacterial drugs for the treatment of mycobacterial disease in man. Br Med Bull. 1988;44:757.

A nice review of the mechanism of action of drugs used to treat tuberculosis or infection due to MAC.

12. Hornick DB, Dayton CS, Bedell GN, et al. Nontuberculous mycobacterial lung disease: Substantiation of a less aggressive approach. Chest. 1988;93:550.

Eighteen MAC patients were treated with three or four antituberculosis agents, resulting in sputum conversion and clinical improvement in 12 (67%). When

M. kansasii was identified as the etiologic agent, all patients were treated with four or fewer antituberculosis agents, and 14 of 16 patients (88%) achieved sputum conversion and clinical improvement.

13. O'Brien RJ, Geiter LJ, Snider DE, Jr. The epidemiology of nontuberculous mycobacterial diseases in the United States: Results from a national survey. Am Rev Respir Dis. 1987;135:1007.

The data suggested a changing epidemiologic picture of nontuberculous mycobacterial disease due perhaps to the decreased incidence of tuberculosis, the increased prevalence of chronic lung disease, and increased culturing of diagnostic specimens, as well as possibly a change in the ecology of these organisms.

14. Woods GL, Washington JA. Mycobacteria other than Mycobacterium tuberculosis: review of microbiologic and clinical aspects. Rev Infect Dis. 1987;9: 275.

The epidemiologic, pathologic, and clinical features of the individual nontuberculous mycobacteria species are discussed.

15. Davidson PT. The diagnosis and management of disease caused by M. avium complex, M. kansasii, and other mycobacteria. Clin Chest Med. 1989;10:431.

A scheme to categorize patients with MAC according to the nature of their disease, together with subsequent management strategies, is presented.

16. Kahana LM, Spino M. Ciprofloxacin in patients with mycobacterial infections: experience in 15 patients. DICP. 1991;25:919.

This article presents treatment results of 11 patients with tuberculosis and 4 with nontuberculous mycobacterial infections who were treated with combinations of ciprofloxacin and 1 or 2 other antituberculosis agents.

17. Kotloff RM. Infection caused by nontuberculous mycobacteria: clinical aspects. Semin Roentgenol. 1993;28:131.

A discussion of the differential diagnosis of nontuberculous mycobacterial disease from the perspective of a radiologist.

18. MacDonell KB, Glassroth J. Mycobacterium avium complex and other nontuberculous mycobacteria in patients with HIV infection. Semin Respir Infect. 1989; 4:123.

Initiation of drug therapy for MAC may decrease the severity of disease symptoms in some HIV-infected patients.

19. Novick RJ, Moreno-Cabral CE, Stinson EB, et al. Nontuberculous mycobacterial infections in heart transplant recipients: a seventeen-year experience. J Heart Transplant. 1990;9:357.

Nontuberculous mycobacterial infections occur late after heart transplantation; drug treatment is usually successful (although difficult), and long-term survival is not adversely affected if the infection is successfully controlled.

20. Stover DE, White DA, Romano PA, et al. Diagnosis of pulmonary disease in acquired immune deficiency syndrome (AIDS): role of bronchoscopy and bronchoalveolar lavage. Am Rev Respir Dis. 1984;130:659.

The effectiveness of fiberoptic bronchoscopy with the addition of bronchoalveolar lavage was evaluated in 72 patients with AIDS and parenchymal pulmonary disease.

21. Nightingale SD, Cameron DW, Gordin FM, et al. Two controlled trials of rifabutin prophylaxis against Mycobacterium avium complex infection in AIDS. N Engl J Med. 1993;329:828.

MAC infection eventually develops in most patients with AIDS. Two randomized, double-blind, multicenter trials of daily prophylactic treatment with either rifabutin (300 mg) or placebo were conducted.

22. Nightingale SD, Byrd LT, Southern PM, et al. Incidence of Mycobacterium avium-intracellulare complex bacteremia in human immunodeficiency virus-positive patients. J Infect Dis. 1992;165:1082.

The product-limit incidence of MAC bacteremia in 1006 HIV-positive patients followed at one institution over a 3-year period from the day of AIDS diagnosis with monthly lysis centrifugation blood cultures was 21% +/− 2% SE at 1 year and 43% +/− 3% at 2 years.

23. Huebner RE, Schein MF, Cauthen GM, et al. Evaluation of the clinical usefulness of mycobacterial skin test antigens in adults with pulmonary mycobacterioses. *Am Rev Respir Dis.* 1992;145:1160.

    This report provides an update on the potential of these antigens. Unfortunately, these antigens are no longer available.

24. O'Brien RJ. The epidemiology of nontuberculous mycobacterial disease. *Clin Chest Med.* 1989;10:407.

    The most common forms of disease are chronic pulmonary disease resembling tuberculosis, benign cervical adenopathy in children, skin and soft tissue infection, and disseminated disease in immunocompromised persons.

25. Good RC, Snider DE, Jr. Isolation of nontuberculous mycobacteria in the United States, 1980. *J Infect Dis.* 1982;146:829.

    A survey of results from 48 state laboratories gives the incidence of isolation and pathology associated with those isolations. Incidence data for MAC and M. kansasii are presented.

26. Kirschner RA, Jr., Parker BC, Falkinham JO. Epidemiology of infection by nontuberculous mycobacteria. *Am Rev Respir Dis.* 1992;145:271.

    M. avium, M. intracellulare, and M. scrofulaceum in acid, brown-water swamps of the southeastern United States and their association with environmental variables.

27. von Reyn CF, Maslow JN, Barber TW, et al. Persistent colonisation of potable water as a source of Mycobacterium avium infection in AIDS. *Lancet.* 1994;343:1137.

    As part of a prospective epidemiologic study, the investigators isolated multiple colonies of MAC from patients with AIDS and from potable water to which they had been exposed.

28. Catanzaro A, Daley CL. Clinics in chest medicine: Lung disease due to nontuberculous mycobacterial infections. September 2002.

    An excellent, thorough review of this topic including epidemiology, pathogenesis, diagnosis, and treatment.

29. Heifets L. Mycobacterial infections caused by nontuberculous mycobacteria. *Semin Respir Crit Care Med.* 2004;25:283–295.

    A relatively concise review on the topic of NTM with excellent references and a focus on pulmonary disease.

30. Phillips MS, von Reyn, CF. Nosocomial infections due to nontuberculous mycobacteria. *Clin Infect Dis.* 2001;33:1363–1374.

    A review of the spectrum of potential nosocomial infections due to NTM.

31. Griffith DE, Brown-Elliott BA, Wallace RJ. Diagnosing nontuberculous mycobacterial lung disease. A process in evolution. *Infect Dis Clin North Am.* 2002;16:235–239.

    A discussion of the ongoing controversies in diagnosing NTM pulmonary disease.

32. Chemlal K, Portaels F. Molecular diagnosis of nontuberculous mycobacteria. *Curr Opin Infect Dis.* 2003;16:77–83.

    A review of the various molecular diagnostic tools available to diagnose NTM.

33. Brown-Elliott BA, Griffith DE, Wallace RJ. Diagnosis of nontuberculous mycobacterial infections. *Clin Lab Med.* 2002;22:911–925.

    This article reviews the methods of laboratory diagnosis of NTM.

39. COCCIDIOIDOMYCOSIS

Antonio Catanzaro

Coccidioidomycosis is the infection caused by *Coccidioides*. In addition to *Coccidioides immitis,* a second species, *Coccidioides posadii,* recently has been identified. The two organisms are genetically distinct and geographically separated, but there are no known differences between the two species, either in terms of the immune response or clinical disease. Coccidioides is a dimorphic fungus that grows in the soil in endemic areas, including the lower Sonoran life zone (southern California, Arizona, Nevada, New Mexico, and Texas), an in northern Mexico and parts of South America. It proliferates in the mycelial form during the rainy season and forms arthrospores when the climate becomes hot and dry. Coccidioidomycosis outbreaks can follow natural disasters such as earthquakes, which can vigorously disturb soil and cause the release of coccidioidomycosis arthrospores.

The primary coccidioidal infection is asymptomatic in 60% of individuals; the remainder experience variable degrees of fever, chills, malaise, cough, dyspnea, chest pain, arthralgias, pharyngitis, and rash. Skin manifestations are common in primary infection, occurring in approximately 5% of men and 25% of women. A fine erythematous maculopapular exanthem, toxic cutaneous erythema, is said to be very common but is an extremely evanescent, early event. San Joaquin Valley Fever represents a characteristic symptom complex of primary coccidioidomycosis and classically includes erythema nodosum (with or without erythema multiforme), arthralgias, malaise, and fever. The chest roentgenogram is often abnormal, even in asymptomatic individuals, and infiltrates are observed in 80% of patients requiring hospitalization. The infiltrates vary widely in size, location, character, and duration. Hilar adenopathy occurs in 20% of cases and does not influence the prognosis unless it is persistent and accompanied by rising serologic titers. Pleural effusion is detected roentgenographically in less than 10% of symptomatic individuals; in most patients, the effusion is small (<1 L).

In general, physical findings in primary coccidioidomycosis are nonspecific and consistent with those of a "flu" syndrome. Signs of pulmonary parenchymal consolidation may be present and often are very localized and transient; pleural rubs are unusual. The risk of dissemination is increased in patients with depressed cell-mediated immune (CMI) responses. Certain individuals appear predisposed to severe, prolonged, or disseminated infections. These include, in order of decreasing risk, immunocompromised individuals, most notably those with AIDS; patients taking immunosuppressive drugs, particularly prednisone; individuals of black, Filipino, or American Indian extraction; and, possibly, those in the last trimester of pregnancy. Pregnancy has long been considered a risk factor, but its importance is unclear. Age older than 55 carries a greater risk of continuing illness even after 1 year of treatment.

Coccidioidomycosis is considered persistent or progressive when symptoms or signs of pulmonary involvement are present or increasing beyond 6 to 8 weeks. Manifestations of persistent pulmonary coccidioidomycosis may include acute progressive pneumonia that is usually symptomatic; chronic progressive pneumonia; pulmonary nodule or nodules; and pulmonary cavities that may hemorrhage, rupture into the pleural space, or undergo spontaneous closure. Coccidioidomas represent isolated residua of active pulmonary disease, and organisms have been cultured from lesions that remained unchanged for decades. Cavities may be thin walled and often represent the initial roentgenographic manifestation of infection. The thin-walled cavities have a tendency to expand, presumably owing to a check-valve mechanism at their bronchial communication. Most coccidioidal cavities are clinically silent, but hemorrhage, rupture leading to bronchopleural fistulas, and secondary bacterial infection may occur. Empyema may result and be either bacterial or fungal in etiology. In persistent pulmonary coccidioidomycosis, serologic evidence of activity (e.g., elevated complement fixation [CF] titers may be absent but, when present, should raise the possibility of intrapulmonary dissemination. A few individuals develop progressive pulmonary disease or disseminated infection.

A worse prognosis and an increased risk of dissemination may be indicated by the findings of (1) elevated CF titers, (2) pulmonary infiltrates or hilar or paratracheal adenopathy that persists more than 6 weeks, and (3) significant weight loss. Disseminated coccidioidomycosis occurs infrequently, usually in individuals with impaired CMI. CMI may be depressed by an obvious cause such as systemic illness (e.g., AIDS, Hodgkin's disease) or certain pharmacologic agents (e.g., steroids or cytotoxic agents), but usually such depression is of obscure cause. Typical miliary lesions occur in 4% of cases. The most frequent sites of dissemination are the skin, bones, soft tissues, and meninges; however, single- or multiple-mass lesions or abscesses may occur in any organ. Cutaneous fistula formation from deep-seated lesions is common. Arsura et al. found that patients with facial lesions due to coccidioidomycosis had a greater chance of developing meningitis than patients who had lesions on the body only. This association may allow for earlier detection and treatment of coccidioidomycosis meningitis. Meningitis is the most ominous form of dissemination because of the anatomic disruption that ensues, and because of the difficulty in getting drugs to the site of infection. If dissemination has occurred or is suspected, a careful evaluation of its extent should be undertaken, including analysis of the cerebrospinal fluid for CF titer. Cerebrospinal fluid may be negative in 25% of cases on an initial examination. If clinical suspicion is high, a spinal tap should be repeated in 1 or 2 weeks. Bone scans are very useful in the search for subclinical sites of dissemination.

Coccidioidomycosis was often diagnosed by appropriate interpretation of the skin test and serology. Unfortunately the skin test reagent has been unavailable for a number of years, but it may be reintroduced. Fortunately serology is widely available. The precipitin tests become positive early in the course of infection (1–3 weeks), whereas CF and immunodiffusion tests are more delayed in their conversion to positive. The latex agglutination test is problematic. It detects both immunoglobulin G and M (IgG, IgM) antibodies; unfortunately, it is positive in up to 10% of normals and negative in 30% of confirmed cases of coccidioidomycosis. For these reasons, it is usually necessary to confirm the results of latex agglutination. The CF and immunodiffusion tests are important, because titers tend to correlate with the extent of infection and are useful with respect to prognosis and management. CF titers are greater than 1:32 or 1:64 in 90% of disseminated disease; however, a high titer is not always present in disseminated disease. That notwithstanding, a high titer by itself is not sufficient evidence to diagnose dissemination. The coccidioidal CF test may give some reaction in other fungal infections, most notably in patients with histoplasmosis. CF tests using spherulin antigen are even more nonspecific. The immunodiffusion test is ideally suited to demonstrate antigenic cross-reactivity. A new enzyme-linked immunosorbent assay (ELISA) for coccidioidal antigens has become available. This test has very good sensitivity and is technically much easier to automate and more widely available than the older tests. At this point in time, it may be best to confirm positive ELISA test results with one of the other serologic tests described above. This is particularly the case for following the patient, as it is sometimes difficult to correlate the results of this test with benchmarks established for complement fixation antibody levels.

Treatment considerations are largely influenced by the specifics of the case, such as the extent of disease, the immune response and risk factors such as age, gender, and ethnicity. It is necessary to establish the extent of disease, particularly involvement of the central nervous system or bones, as well as the immune response of the host to the infection in terms of cell-mediated immunity and antibody response. These steps will allow a better estimation of the prognosis, as well as establish a baseline that is necessary to monitor treatment.

Amphotericin B was the first antifungal that showed efficacy in the treatment of coccidioidomycosis and for many years was the drug of choice for this and many other fungal infections. Amphotericin B is not absorbed orally, tissue distribution is poor, and it is highly toxic. For these reasons it is not considered the drug of choice in many situations.

Many experts now consider the triazoles, fluconazole and itraconazole, to be first line drugs to treat coccidioidomycosis. They have been demonstrated to be efficacious in open trials. Each should be started at 400 mg/day. Fluconazole can be given intravenously or at higher doses as needed. Fluconazole or itraconazole at a dose of 200 to 400 mg/day is effective in more than half the cases. Itraconazole is more toxic, particularly at higher doses, and interacts with many drugs. Itraconazole is not available in a parenteral formulation and has unacceptable toxicities at dosages of more than 600 mg/day. Further, itraconazole is much better absorbed from the liquid formulation than the tablet and is preferred in difficult cases, particularly when the bones are involved. Fluconazole is less toxic and can be given at much higher doses in those cases that do not respond to conventional doses. In refractory cases, as much as 2 g/day can be given without toxicity. In these cases, the dose can be lowered when control of the disease is established. Treatment with a 200 or 400 mg/day dose of fluconazole is well tolerated and fairly effective for the treatment of chronic coccidioidomycosis. However, alopecia is a side effect associated with higher doses (400 mg/day) or fluconazole given for 2 months or longer. Alopecia is usually reversed when therapy is stopped. Although ketoconazole is active against coccidioides, the safety margin is small and at the effective dose, 200 to 600 mg/day, it may cause gastrointestinal irritation, hepatitis, and adrenal and testicular dysfunction. The triazoles, fluconazole and itraconazole, are more active and less toxic than ketoconazole. Relapse is a risk when treatment with any azole is completed. Relapses are seen in 50% of cases treated with ketoconazole and 25 to 30% of patients treated with fluconazole or itraconazole. Oldfield et al. confirmed a long-held clinical suspicion that negative skin tests and a titer of $\geq 1:256$ were associated with increased risk of coccidioidomycosis relapse.

With the advent of the azoles, amphotericin B has been moved to a niche drug. Reduction in kidney function is a nearly universal side effect of this drug. This complication can be highly problematic, particularly in diabetic patients. Liposomal formulations of amphotericin are clearly less nephrotoxic. In addition they alter the distribution of the drug, which can be a distinct advantage. Amphotericin B or its liposomal formulations are very useful, but only for special situations, for example, patients who are pregnant, those who are critically ill, and those who have failed therapy with azoles.

Coccidioidal meningitis is usually treated with fluconazole. Although the best study reported the results of treatment with 400 mg/day, most clinicians start at 800 to 1000 mg/day. Either fluconazole or itraconazole can be used to treat meningitis. However, when the drug is stopped, meningitis is likely to recur. Occasionally meningitis continues even with azole treatment. In these cases amphotericin must be used. Amphotericin B is probably best considered as second-line therapy for meningitis. It does not cross the blood-brain barrier in concentrations needed to treat coccidioidal meningitis, so it must be administered intrathecally. Lumbar injections are easiest to deliver amphotericin to the cerebrospinal fluid (CSF), but almost always result in chemical arachnoiditis. Cisternal injections may reduce the incidence of chemical arachnoiditis, but must be performed by a specially trained practitioner. An intraventricular catheter with an Ommaya reservoir circumvents some problems, but if outflow of fluid from the ventricles becomes obstructed, the drug may not get to the site of the infection.

In general, coccidioidomycosis is not a surgical disease. However, surgery is critical in several situations, specifically in establishing the diagnosis in difficult cases, for draining pus, in treating certain problems, such as life-threatening hemoptysis, or as an adjunct to medical treatment of tenosynovitis.

Control and prevention of coccidioidomycosis can be improved by early diagnosis, through careful clinical evaluation (including a thorough travel history) and specific testing, as well as individualized case management, including a multidisciplinary approach. Further progress is possible through scientific research efforts and intelligent institutional policies. The Valley Fever Vaccine Project has funded several investigators to develop candidate vaccine molecules. They have started testing their most promising agents in primates and have plans to follow quickly with human trials.

---

1. Koehler AP, Cheng AF, Chu KC, et al. Successful treatment of disseminated coccidioidomycosis with amphotericin B lipid complex. *J Infect.* 1998;36:113–115.

   This article discusses a case of coccidioidomycosis contracted while the patient traveled to an endemic area. It notes that the patient did not respond favorably to typical antifungal treatments but responded well to amphotericin B lipid complex.

2. Arsura EL, Kilgore WB, Caldwell JW, et al. Association between facial cutaneous coccidioidomycosis and meningitis. *West J Med.* 1998;169:13–16.

   Through a retrospective review, the authors determined that patients are more likely to develop meningitis if they have facial lesions than those with lesions on the body only.

3. Oldfield EC, Bone WD, Martin CR, et al. Prediction of relapse after treatment of coccidioidomycosis. *Clin Infect Dis.* 1997;25:1205–1210.

   The authors report on their findings of a retrospective cohort study designed to determine factors associated with relapse after successful treatment of coccidioidomycosis.

4. Einstein HE, Johnson RH. Coccidioidomycosis: new aspects of epidemiology and therapy. *Clin Infect Dis.* 1993;16:349.

   A good summary of the extent of the epidemic of coccidioidomycosis in 1992 to 1994 and some of the clinical experiences arising from the epidemic confirming many presumed risk factors for poor outcomes.

5. Richardson HB, Jr., Anderson JA, McKay BM. Acute pulmonary coccidioidomycosis in children. *J Pediatr.* 1967;70:376.

   Excellent description of coccidioidomycosis in the pediatric population.

6. Greendyke WH, Resnick DL, Harvey WC. The varied roentgen manifestations of primary coccidioidomycosis. *Am J Roentgenol Rad Ther Nucl Med.* 1970;109:491.

   Categorizes roentgenographic abnormalities. The article states that 46% demonstrated segmental pneumonias, 27% had minimal infiltrates, and 19% each had hilar lymphadenopathy or pleural effusions.

7. Bronnimann DA, Adam RD, Galgiani JN, et al. Coccidioidomycosis in the acquired immunodeficiency syndrome. *Ann Intern Med.* 1987;106:372.

   Of seven patients with coccidioidomycosis and AIDS, six had diffuse nodular pulmonary infiltrates as well as many extrapulmonary sites. Six patients had temporary responses to amphotericin B taken alone and in combination with ketoconazole, but all died within 14 months of the diagnosis of coccidioidomycosis.

8. Catanzaro A. Pulmonary mycoses in pregnant women. *Chest.* 1984;86:145.

   Pregnancy has long been regarded as a major risk factor in the successful localization of coccidioidomycosis. A careful review of the literature suggests that the disastrous courses described are more a reflection of race and patterns of healthcare than strictly consequences of pregnancy on the host defense system. Pregnancy may shift the balance slightly in favor of the fungus, primarily because of the stimulatory effect of progesterone and beta estradiol on the growth of C. immitis.

9. Wack EE, Ampel NM, Galgiani JN, et al. Coccidioidomycosis during pregnancy: an analysis of ten cases among 47,120 pregnancies. *Chest.* 1988;94:376.

   The argument about the extent to which pregnancy is a risk factor for disseminated coccidioidomycosis continues. This paper says, "Yes, it is."

10. Wallace JM, Catanzaro A, Moser KM, et al. Flexible fiberoptic bronchoscopy for diagnosing pulmonary coccidioidomycosis. *Am Rev Respir Dis.* 1981;123:286.

    Flexible fiberoptic bronchoscopy (FFB) is an excellent tool for obtaining specimens for culture of C. immitis.

11. Raab SS, Silverman JF, Zimmerman KG. Fine-needle aspiration biopsy of pulmonary coccidioidomycosis: spectrum of cytologic findings in 73 patients. *Am J Clin Pathol.* 1993;99:582.

This report describes the spectrum of cytologic findings in 73 patients who were diagnosed with pulmonary coccidioidomycosis by fine-needle aspiration (FNA) biopsy.

12. Hyde L. Coccidioidal pulmonary cavitation. *Dis Chest.* 1968;54:273.

    With nonsurgical therapy, 25% of the cavities (211 cases) closed spontaneously; with surgery, 18% developed new cavities during the postoperative period and 30% had postoperative bronchopleural fistula.

13. Bouza E, Dreyer JS, Hewitt WL, et al. Coccidioidal meningitis: an analysis of thirty-one cases and review of the literature. *Medicine* (Baltimore). 1981;60:139.

    Clinical and laboratory features of 31 patients with coccidioidal meningitis are presented. Many had long-term follow-up.

14. Wrobel CJ, Meyer S, Johnson RH, et al. MR findings in acute and chronic coccidioidomycosis meningitis. *Am J Neuroradiol.* 1992;13:1241.

    Magnetic resonance (MR) findings in acute and chronic coccidioidomycosis meningitis were found to show hydrocephalus and intense enhancement of the cervical subarachnoid space, basilar, sylvian, and interhemispheric cisterns on postcontrast MR scans. In addition, focal parenchymal signal abnormalities suggesting ischemia or infarction were common.

15. Williams PL, Johnson R, Pappagianis D, et al. Vasculitic and encephalitic complications associated with Coccidioides immitis infection of the central nervous system in humans: Report of 100 cases and review. *Clin Infect Dis.* 1992;14:673.

    Six cases of apparent and four cases of histopathologically confirmed vasculitis of the central nervous system are presented. Vasculitic complications included changes in mental status, as well as stroke-like findings of aphasia, hemianopsia, and hemiparesis. Seven patients died.

16. Vincent T, Galgiani JN, Huppert M, et al. The natural history of coccidioidal meningitis: VA-Armed Forces cooperative studies, 1955–1958. *Clin Infect Dis.* 1993;16:247.

    This new analysis of old cases of meningitis shows rather surprising cerebrospinal fluid findings in a review of the clinical course of 699 patients who had coccidioidomycosis before the advent of effective antifungal therapy.

17. Pappagianis D, Zimmer BL. Serology of coccidioidomycosis. *Clin Microbiol Rev.* 1990;3:247.

    A very nice updating of the use of serology in the diagnosis of this disease.

18. Como JA, Dismukes WE. Oral azole drugs as systemic antifungal therapy. *N Engl J Med.* 1994;330:263.

    A very nice general review of the antifungal agents available and their indications for certain mycoses.

19. Graybill JR, Stevens DA, Galgiani JN, et al. Itraconazole treatment of coccidioidomycosis. NAIAD Mycoses Study Group. *Am J Med.* 1990;89:282.

    Fifty-one patients with nonmeningeal coccidioidomycosis were considered for treatment with itraconazole. Itraconazole was taken orally in dosages of 100 to 400 mg/day for periods up to 39 months. Of these patients, 12 had osteoarticular disease, 23 had chronic pulmonary disease, and 14 had skin or soft tissue disease. Of the 44 patients no longer receiving therapy, 25 (57%) achieved remission.

20. Ampel NM. Coccidioidomycosis among persons with human immunodeficiency virus infection in the era of highly active antiretroviral therapy (HAART). *Semin Respir Infect.* 2001;16:257–262.

    Coccidioidomycosis remains an important opportunistic infection among individuals infected with human immunodeficiency virus (HIV) who live in the coccidioidal endemic area. There are several manifestations of coccidioidomycosis during HIV infection, but pulmonary disease, either diffuse or focal, is the most common. The most important factor associated with the risk for developing clinically active coccidioidomycosis is a CD4 peripheral blood lymphocyte count of less than $250/\mu L$.

21. Ampel NM, Mosley DG, England B, et al. Coccidioidomycosis in Arizona: increase in incidence from 1990 to 1995. *Clin Infect Dis.* 1998;27:1528–1530.

    The number of cases (incidence) of coccidioidomycosis reported to the Arizona Department of Health Services increased from 255 (7.0 per 100,000 population) *in 1990 to 623 (14.9 per 100,000 population) in 1995 (P < .001). Cases in persons aged 65 or older and men were reported more frequently (for both, P < .001). These data demonstrate that coccidioidomycosis is a growing health problem in Arizona.*

22. Arsura EL, Bellinghausen PL, Kilgore WB, et al. Septic shock in coccidioidomycosis. *Crit Care Med.* 1998;26:62–65.

Eight patients were diagnosed with septic shock from infection with C. immitis from September 1991 to December 1993. Septic shock was diagnosed using criteria formulated by the American College of Chest Physicians Consensus Conference / Society of Critical Care Medicine. Septic shock that follows infection with C. immitis is an ominous yet underrecognized condition. Hemodynamic parameters and cytokine concentrations were not significantly different from values seen in gram-negative septic shock. Clinical clues to the diagnosis include duration of illness and conspicuous pulmonary involvement. Patient outcome in this series was poor, but may improve with increased recognition of septic shock in infections from C. immitis.

23. Bergstrom L, Yocum DE, Ampel NM, et al. Increased risk of coccidioidomycosis in patients treated with tumor necrosis factor alpha antagonists. *Arthritis Rheum.* 2004;50:1959–1966.

Thirteen cases of documented coccidioidomycosis were associated with TNF alpha antagonist therapy. Twelve cases were associated with the use of infliximab and 1 case with etanercept. Among the cohort of patients from a single medical center, 7 of the 247 patients receiving infliximab and 4 of the 738 patients receiving other therapies developed symptomatic coccidioidomycosis (relative risk 5.23, 95% confidence interval 1.54–17.71; P <0.01). Patients with inflammatory arthritis who are undergoing treatment with infliximab appear to be at higher risk for developing symptomatic coccidioidomycosis as compared with those not receiving infliximab.

24. Catanzaro A, Galgiani JN, Levine BE, et al. Fluconazole in the treatment of chronic pulmonary and nonmeningeal disseminated coccidioidomycosis. NIAID Mycoses Study Group. *Am J Med.* 1995;98:249–256.

Of 78 patients enrolled, 22 had soft-tissue, 42 had chronic pulmonary, and 14 had skeletal coccidioidomycosis. Forty-nine had at least one concomitant disease, seven of whom had HIV infection. Patients were given oral fluconazole 200 mg/day. Nonresponders were increased to 400 mg/day. Treatment courses were long: a mean of 323 +/− 230 days at 200 mg and 433 +/− 178 days at 400 mg. Among 75 evaluable patients, a satisfactory response was observed in 12 (86%) of the 14 patients with skeletal, 22 (55%) of the 40 patients with chronic pulmonary, and 16 (76%) of the 21 patients with soft-tissue disease. Five patients (7%) required modification of treatment due to toxicity. Forty-one patients who responded were followed up off-drug. Fifteen (37%) of them experienced reactivation of infection. Fluconazole 200 or 400 mg/day is well tolerated and a moderately effective treatment for chronic pulmonary or nonmeningeal disseminated coccidioidomycosis. The relapse rate after therapy is high. Treatment trials with higher doses appear warranted. The relative efficacy of fluconazole versus other azoles or amphotericin B remains unknown.

25. Dewsnup DH, Galgiani JN, Graybill JR, et al. Is it ever safe to stop azole therapy for Coccidioides immitis meningitis? *Ann Intern Med.* 1996;124:305–310.

Fourteen of 18 patients with coccidioidal meningitis (78% [95% CI, 52% to 94%]) had relapse with disseminated disease after discontinuation of therapy, for a total of 1 nonmeningeal and 15 meningeal relapses to date. Relapse occurred both soon and late (range, 0.5 to 30 months) after therapy was discontinued. Relapse had serious consequences in some patients; three died.

26. Galgiani JN, Catanzaro A, Cloud GA, et al. Comparison of oral fluconazole and itraconazole for progressive, nonmeningeal coccidioidomycosis. A randomized, double-blind trial. Mycoses Study Group. *Ann Intern Med.* 2000;133:676–686.

One hundred ninety-eight patients with chronic pulmonary, soft tissue, or skeletal coccidioidal infections were studied. Oral fluconazole, 400 mg/day, or itraconazole, 200 mg twice daily was given. Overall, 50% of patients (47 of 94) and 63% of patients (61 of 97) responded to 8 months of treatment with fluconazole and itraconazole, respectively (difference, 13 percentage points [95% CI, −2 to 28 percentage points]; P = .08). Patients with skeletal infections responded twice as frequently to itraconazole as to fluconazole. By 12 months, 57% of patients had responded to fluconazole and 72% had responded to itraconazole (difference, 15 percentage points [CI, 0.003 to 30 percentage points]; P = .05). Soft tissue disease was associated with increased likelihood of response, as in previous studies. Relapse rates after discontinuation of therapy did not differ significantly between groups (28% after fluconazole treatment and 18% after itraconazole treatment). Both drugs were well tolerated.

27. Galgiani JN, Ampel NM, Catanzaro A, et al. Practice guideline for the treatment of coccidioidomycosis. Infectious Diseases Society of America. *Clin Infect Dis.* 2000;30:658–661.

    Management of patients diagnosed with coccidioidomycosis involves defining the extent of infection and assessing host factors that predispose to disease severity. Patients with relatively localized acute pulmonary infections and no risk factors for complications often require only periodic reassessment to demonstrate resolution of their self-limited process. On the other hand, patients with extensive spread of infection or at high risk of complications because of immunosuppression or other preexisting factors require a variety of treatment strategies that may include antifungal therapy, surgical debridement, or both. Amphotericin B is often selected for treatment of patients with respiratory failure due to C. immitis or rapidly progressive coccidioidal infections. With other more chronic manifestations of coccidioidomycosis, treatment with fluconazole, itraconazole, or ketoconazole is common. Duration of therapy often ranges from many months to years, and, for some patients, chronic suppressive therapy is needed to prevent relapses.

28. Kushwaha VP, Shaw BA, Gerardi JA, et al. Musculoskeletal coccidioidomycosis. A review of 25 cases. *Clin Orthop.* 1996;(332):190–199.

    Twenty-five patients with musculoskeletal coccidioidomycosis are described. There were 36 lesions among the 25 patients, 8 located in the spine, with the remainder distributed throughout the body. Seventeen patients had a delay in diagnosis of more than 1 month. Eight patients had an elevated white blood cell count, and 10 had an elevated sedimentation rate. Only seven of the patients had an overt pneumonia before the musculoskeletal presentation. Twenty-four patients underwent formal irrigation and debridement and 22 had at least one course of amphotericin B. The average follow-up after the initiation of treatment was 3.5 years, ranging from 2 to 10 years. Seven patients had recurrent lesions that required further surgical intervention, four of whom had a delay in diagnosis of more than 1 month. There were three deaths. All surviving patients were free of disease at final follow-up.

29. Martins TB, Jaskowski TD, Mouritsen CL, et al. Comparison of commercially available enzyme immunoassay with traditional serological tests for detection of antibodies to Coccidioides immitis. *J Clin Microbiol.* 1995;33:940–943.

    A newly released commercially available ELISA was evaluated for its ability to detect IgM and IgG antibodies against the tube precipitin and CF antigens of C. immitis. The ELISA was compared with more traditional diagnostic assays, CF, latex agglutination (LA), and immunodiffusion (ID). When the IgM-specific portion of the ELISA was compared with LA, there was an agreement of 81.8%, a specificity of 75.0%, and a sensitivity of 84.6%. For the determination of the presence of IgG antibodies, the results of the IgG-specific part of the ELISA were compared with the combined results of ID and CF. After resolution of discrepant results, there was an agreement of 95.6%, a specificity of 98.3%, and a sensitivity of 92.6%. When the results of the IgG- and IgM-specific portions of the ELISA combined were compared with the results of the three traditional assays (CF, LA, and ID), there was an agreement of 96.7%, a specificity of 98.5%, and a sensitivity of 94.8%. The ELISA proved to be a reliable assay for the detection of antibodies against the tube precipitin and CF antigens and did not suffer from the objectivity required to interpret the results of the traditional assays and anticomplement interference associated with the traditional assays.

30. Schneider E, Hajjeh RA, Spiegel RA, et al. A coccidioidomycosis outbreak following the Northridge, Calif, earthquake. *JAMA.* 1997;277:904–908.

   In Ventura County, between January 24 and March 15, 1994, 203 outbreak-associated coccidioidomycosis cases, including 3 fatalities, were identified (attack rate [AR], 30 cases per 100,000 population). The majority of cases (56%) and the highest AR (114 per 100,000 population) occurred in the town of Simi Valley, a community located at the base of a mountain range that experienced numerous landslides associated with the earthquake. Disease onset for cases peaked 2 weeks after the earthquake. The AR was 2.8 times greater for persons age 40 and older than for younger persons (relative risk, 2.8; 95% confidence interval [CI], 2.1–3.7; P < .001). Environmental data indicated that large dust clouds, generated by land-slides after the earthquake and strong aftershocks in the Santa Susana Mountains north of Simi Valley, were dispersed into nearby valleys by northeast winds. Simi Valley case-control study data indicated that physically being in a dust cloud (odds ratio, 3.0; 95% CI, 1.6–5.4; P <.001) and time spent in a dust cloud (P <.001) significantly increased the risk for being diagnosed with acute coccidioidomycosis.

40. HISTOPLASMOSIS

Mehran Mandegar

The term *histoplasmosis* refers to any one of a variety of disorders resulting from infection with the dimorphic fungus *Histoplasma capsulatum*. Histoplasmosis and its causative agent are found worldwide, and it is the most prevalent endemic mycosis in the United States and in certain areas of Latin America. Up to 50 million people in the United States have been infected by *H. capsulatum* and up to 500,000 new infections occur each year, although the number of persons in whom infection causes disease is much less.

In the United States, most cases occur within the Ohio and Mississippi River valleys. Infection with *H. capsulatum* by inhalation is ubiquitous in those areas. This particular endemic distribution pattern is thought to be enabled by local conditions favorable to the fungus, such as humidity, moderate climate, and soil components. *H. capsulatum* lives as a mycelium in nitrogen-rich soil, especially near bird droppings and in starling roosts or chicken houses. Bats may carry the fungus enterically, making bat guano particularly infested with *H. capsulatum*. Bird and bat excrement accelerates the sporulation of this organism and enhances its localized growth in soil in what is referred to as *microfoci*.

Activities that disturb the soil cause aerosolization of the spores and mycelial fragments. The air currents carry these elements for miles, exposing individuals who are generally unaware of the exposure. Only the mycelia generate spores (microconidia). Spores are small enough to be aerosolized and to reach the alveoli, if inhaled. At the host's body temperature, the microconidia grow into the yeast form. After an in-effective neutrophil response, alveolar macrophages phagocytize the yeast but they are unable to kill the fungi. Infected macrophages serve to disseminate the infection hematogenously via regional lymph nodes.

The severity of infection due to inhalation of the spores or mycelial fragments varies, depending on the intensity of the exposure, presence of underlying lung disease, and the immunity of the host. In the normal host, histoplasmosis is usually asymptomatic. Some patients suffer an influenza-like syndrome 1 to 2 weeks after infection, which in women can be accompanied by erythema nodosum. Others may develop acute pulmonary histoplasmosis, a self-limited pneumonia-like condition that can be localized or diffuse. It is generally characterized by consolidation and hilar lymphadenopathy.

Typical symptoms of this form of histoplasmosis are fever, chills, headache, myalgia, anorexia, cough, and pleuritic chest pain, which are seen in 85 to 100% of cases. Physical findings are generally nonspecific and may include fever, pulmonary crackles, or pleural friction rubs. Recovery generally occurs within 2 weeks. Treatment is not indicated in the typical patient with acute pulmonary histoplasmosis because the illness is usually self limited and associated with minimal morbidity. Therapy may be helpful in symptomatic patients whose conditions have not improved during the first month of infection. Treatment with itraconazole, 200 mg once daily for 6 to 12 weeks, is often recommended in such cases. Illnesses lasting longer than 3 weeks may portend progressive dissemination.

A notable exception may occur in individuals who acutely inhale a large inoculum. They may develop severe, potentially fatal, diffuse pulmonary inflammation that can be followed by progressively disseminated disease. A massive inhalation inoculum can occur if fungal deposits are stirred up and inhaled in an enclosed space (such as can happen if a spelunker disturbs a large bat lair). The resulting disease resembles acute respiratory distress syndrome (ARDS) in both presentation and severity.

Hematogenous dissemination probably occurs in all infected individuals during the first 2 weeks of infection and before specific immunity has developed. It is generally self limited, however, and in the majority of cases, the development of calcified granulomas in the liver, spleen, or both is the only remnant of the disease. *Progressive* disseminated histoplasmosis is defined as pulmonary and extrapulmonary disease caused by histoplasmosis, characterized by interstitial pneumonitis and involvement of the spleen, liver, bone marrow, lymph nodes, gastrointestinal tract, adrenal glands, meningeal vessels, or heart valves, particularly the aortic valves. Although dissemination itself is usually clinically silent, the most common symptoms are fever and weight loss, whereas the most common physical findings are hepatomegaly or splenomegaly.

In immunocompetent hosts, T-lymphocytes develop a specific cell-mediated immunity within 2 weeks post exposure and *arm* macrophages to eradicate the fungus throughout the body, whereas in the absence of intact cell-mediated immune response, progressive dissemination occurs inside macrophages. In areas where the yeast collections are too large, they are not killed but are contained within a fibrotic granuloma, which eventually calcifies. Granulomata in the liver and spleen containing *H. capsulatum* may later be discovered incidentally at biopsy or autopsy. Indeed, the high frequency of pulmonary and splenic calcifications in residents of endemic areas is evidence of the ubiquitous nature of this infection.

An enormous inflammatory reaction to the dissemination of histoplasma can cause acute respiratory insufficiency and hypoxemia about 2 weeks after exposure. Shock, hepatic and renal failure, and coagulopathy may complicate severe cases. Chest radiographs demonstrate scattered infiltrates and hilar adenopathy. Patients with more severe manifestations may require ventilatory supportive therapy. About 5 to 20% of cases present with CNS involvement, such as chronic meningitis or focal brain lesions, rarely involving the spinal cord. Mortality without treatment is 80% but can be reduced to less than 25% with antifungal therapy. The treatment of choice is amphotericin B, being effective in 68 to 92% of immunocompetent patients. A dose of 0.7 mg/kg per day (or one of the lipid preparations at a dose of 3 mg/kg per day for patients with renal impairment) should be used for a total recommended course of 35 mg/kg over 2 to 4 months, followed by maintenance therapy for a minimum of 6 months to life. Additionally, corticosteroids may be helpful in taming the inflammatory response that may contribute to the pathogenesis of the respiratory compromise. Prednisone at a dosage of 60 mg daily for 2 weeks may be helpful. In patients with disseminated histoplasmosis and those with AIDS, life-long maintenance therapy is needed to prevent relapse. Therapy is not considered curative for patients with AIDS. Life-long suppression therapy can be provided by itraconazole, 200 mg daily.

A variety of conditions can predispose individuals to progressive disseminated histoplasmosis. These include extremes of age; AIDS; idiopathic CD4 lymphocytopenia or other immunosuppressive disorders; immunosuppressive medications, such as steroids and methotrexate, AIDS-blocking therapies (infliximab, etanercept); and other immunosuppressants. Furthermore, progressive disseminated histoplasmosis has been recognized recently as an opportunistic infection in patients with rheumatoid arthritis or Crohn's disease treated with TNF-alpha blocking agents, and in chronic diseases such as diabetes, hepatic insufficiency, and chronic renal failure. Progressive disseminated histoplasmosis in solid organ transplant recipients is well known and may result from exogenous infection by inhalation of spores or reactivation of quiescent disease from both the donor and recipient of the transplanted organ. The presence of underlying lung disease, such as centrilobular emphysema, predisposes one to progressive pulmonary infection. Depending on the degree of immune insufficiency, the course can run from severe sepsis to chronic consumption. An acute form occurs in infants and severely immunosuppressed adults, which can lead to death within weeks if untreated. In other cases, a deteriorating course can run for several months or even years. Smears and cultures of the involved sites usually provide the diagnosis.

Histoplasma capsulatum can also colonize the distorted architecture of an emphysematous lung, causing chronic pulmonary histoplasmosis. Infected cavities can enlarge and worsen gas exchange in the already compromised lungs. In addition, periodic spillage of the fungi can cause recurrent pneumonia and eventual fibrosis in dependent lung parenchyma. The clinical and radiographic findings resemble that of reactivation tuberculosis. Although the appearance can simulate cavitary tuberculosis, the sputum culture will grow *H. capsulatum* in one third to one half of cases. Without treatment, the illness is progressive, causing loss of pulmonary function in most patients and death in up to half. All patients with chronic pulmonary histoplasmosis require treatment. Itraconazole, 200 mg once or twice daily for 12 to 24 months, is the treatment of choice for chronic pulmonary histoplasmosis and is effective in 75 to 85% of cases, but its use is complicated by high relapse rates. Amphotericin B has been shown effective in 59 to 100% of cases. A dose of 50 mg daily, or about 0.7 mg/kg per day, is recommended for patients who require hospitalization because of ventilatory insufficiency or general debilitation and those unable to take itraconazole or who have failed to respond to at least 12 weeks of itraconazole therapy. A total dose of 35 mg/kg should be given over 2 to 4 months to complete the course of therapy, if tolerated. In most patients, however, treatment can be changed to itraconazole once the fungal burden is reduced. Fluconazole, 200 to 400 mg daily, is less effective than amphotericin B or itraconazole, yielding a mere 64% response rate. Higher doses of up to 400 to 800 mg daily have been suggested for use in patients who cannot take itraconazole or are unable to achieve detectable blood concentrations with itraconazole. Ketoconazole is generally less well tolerated, and its use is discouraged due to its toxicity. Because of a high relapse rate among patients with chronic pulmonary histoplasmosis, some authors recommend at least 12 months of therapy. If the patient's lung function will allow surgery, resection of the infected cavity is generally curative.

Unusual inflammatory or fibrotic responses to histoplasmosis may present with a variety of acute and chronic manifestations, such as rheumatologic syndromes and pericarditis, during the first year after exposure. Chronic mediastinal inflammation or fibrosis (fibrosing or sclerosing mediastinitis), broncholithiasis, and enlarging parenchymal granulomas occur later. In the mediastinum, enlarging caseous lymph nodes can mat together to form a large mass inside a common capsule. The resulting mediastinal granuloma is most commonly found in the right peritracheal area; it can enlarge up to 10 cm, causing extrinsic compression of nearby structures (e.g., the esophagus). Symptomatic mediastinal granuloma can be cured by surgical resection, although some authors recommend a trial of oral antifungal agents first.

Sclerosing mediastinitis is the most extreme example of immunologic overreaction, in which a small amount of *H. capsulatum* antigen stimulates severe fibrosis. The reaction is so intense that fibroblasts from inside adjacent vital structures are recruited and fuse the mediastinal contents into a rock-hard mass. Constriction of the esophagus, pulmonary arteries, pulmonary veins, pericardium, and even the bronchi may ensue. Corticosteroids are of equivocal benefit. Reports of live organisms in surgical specimens from these patients prompt some optimistic clinicians to treat fibrosing mediastinitis with antifungal agents. Although surgical resection is not possible, heroic surgical procedures have been performed to bypass obstructed blood vessels.

Should the granulomatous response to *H. capsulatum* antigen be vigorous in the lung parenchyma, 1- to 2-cm nodules called *histoplasmomas* can form.

The histoplasmoma can enlarge at a rate of 2 mm/year, but poses no danger and does not require treatment. It can be mistaken for a lung cancer, however, and prompt unnecessary resection. The presence of a small central calcification with concentric calcified laminations may identify this lesion on chest radiograph.

Although there is no evidence to support a more severe course of histoplasmosis during pregnancy or that dissemination occurs to the fetus, histoplasmosis during pregnancy poses a special challenge to the clinician. Azole-class antifungal agents cause potential teratogenic complications to the fetus and should not be used in pregnant women. Amphotericin B, however, is considered to be generally safe during pregnancy and is the treatment of choice. The safety of the lipid preparations of amphotericin B during pregnancy is unknown.

Fungal blood cultures are positive in 50 to 70% of progressive disseminated histoplasmosis and should be performed in all cases. Bone marrow aspiration or biopsy for fungal stains and culture should be considered in patients with negative tests for antigen, especially if they are anemic, leukopenic, or thrombocytopenic. Bone marrow cultures are positive in more than 75% of cases. In patients with diffuse interstitial or miliary pulmonary infiltrates, *H. capsulatum* may be recovered from sputum, alveolar lavage specimens, or lung tissue in up to 70% of cases.

The diagnosis of histoplasmosis is best made by culture of the affected sites; however, the yield of culture is variable among different manifestations of the disease. Two specific tests that are readily available for rapid diagnosis of disseminated histoplasmosis are antigen determination and fungal stain of tissues. Histoplasma polysaccharide antigen (HPA) can be rapidly detected in the urine of 90% and serum of 70% of cases of progressive disseminated histoplasmosis. Histoplasma urinary antigen is now the most commonly performed test for detection of histoplasmosis. Tests for antigen in urine and serum should be performed in all patients with suspected disseminated histoplasmosis. Antigen concentrations in urine or serum fall with effective therapy and rise by at least 2 units in 90% of patients at the time of relapse. This provides a useful tool for monitoring therapy. Urine and serum specimens should be tested at 3- to 6-month intervals during maintenance therapy to ensure effectiveness of the treatment. Failure of antigen concentrations to fall after at least 3 months of therapy suggests that treatment may not be effective. Tissue biopsy of the affected organs can lead to the diagnosis by demonstrating the presence of the organism by hematoxylin and eosin or methenamine sliver staining.

A variety of nonspecific laboratory abnormalities may also give clues as to the sites of involvement in disseminated histoplasmosis. For example, anemia, leukopenia, and thrombocytopenia suggest bone marrow infection; hepatic enzyme and bilirubin elevations signal hepatic involvement; and significant elevation of the serum lactate dehydrogenase has been useful in the diagnosis of disseminated histoplasmosis in patients with AIDS. The fungi can be seen within macrophages on Wright's or silver stain, but care must be taken to distinguish them from other intracellular pathogens.

Antibodies to histoplasmin appear in the serum 2 to 3 weeks after exposure and can be detected by complement fixation in 85% of cases. Because of the prevalence of positive reactions in endemic areas, presumptive evidence of infection requires a dilution titer of greater than 1:32 or an acute fourfold rise in titer. Unfortunately, titers this high are seen in only about half of active infections. Immunodiffusion or counterimmunoelectrophoresis detects antibodies against two *Histoplasma* antigens, *m* and *h*. Antibodies to m are found in most histoplasmosis patients but can also be induced by remote asymptomatic exposure or even skin testing. Finding both m and h antibodies is specific for histoplasmosis but much less sensitive than other serologic tests. Skin testing is generally considered not useful and is no longer done. Another consideration is that skin testing can cause false-positive results on serologic tests.

The T cell deficit in patients with AIDS makes them particularly vulnerable to infection from *Histoplasma* organisms. Progressive disseminated histoplasmosis has been found in up to 5% of patients with AIDS living in endemic areas and even in a few who had relocated from endemic areas years ago. Progressive dissemination can occur either from reactivation of latent infection or from new exposure. Although fever is present in nearly all patients, respiratory complaints and chest radiograph changes are found in only half. Of patients with AIDS, 12% with histoplasmosis present with a sepsis syndrome. The enormous fungal load frequently results in positive smears and cultures of blood, respiratory secretions, urine, and bone marrow. However, up to 15% of these patients can have negative smears and cultures despite multiple sampling. Furthermore, standard antibody testing in this population is more frequently negative. A more reliable test in this population is the detection of HPA in body fluids. In AIDS patients with progressive disseminated histoplasmosis, HPA can be rapidly detected in urine (97% of cases), blood (83%), and cerebrospinal fluid (66%).

1. Bullock WE. Interactions between human phagocytic cells and *Histoplasma capsulatum*. *Arch Med Res*. 1993;24:219.
2. Eissenberg LG, Goldman WE. Histoplasma variation and adaptive strategies for parasitism: new perspectives on histoplasmosis. *Clin Microbiol Rev*. 1991;4:411.
3. Goodwin RA, Des Prez RM. Histoplasmosis. *Am Rev Respir Dis*. 1978;117:929.
4. Wheat LJ, Slama TG, Eitzen HE, et al. Large urban outbreak of histoplasmosis: clinical features. *Ann Intern Med*. 1981;94:331.
5. Leggiadro RJ, Luedtke GS, Convey A, et al. Prevalence of histoplasmosis in a midsouthern population. *South Med J*. 1991;84:1360.
6. Williams B, Fojtasek M, Connolly-Stringfield P, et al. Diagnosis of histoplasmosis by antigen detection during an outbreak in Indianapolis, Ind. *Arch Pathol Lab Med*. 1994;118:1205.
7. Hay RJ. Histoplasmosis. *Semin Dermatol*. 1993;12:310.
8. Connell JV, Muhm JR. Radiographic manifestations of pulmonary histoplasmosis: a 10-year review. *Radiology*. 1976;121:281.
9. Sobel JD. Practice guidelines for the treatment of fungal infections. *Clin Infect Dis*. 2000;30:652.
10. Goodwin RA Jr, Owens FT, Snell JD, et al. Chronic pulmonary histoplasmosis. *Medicine* (Baltimore). 1976;55:413.
11. Wheat J. Histoplasmosis: recognition and treatment. *Clin Infect Dis*. 1994;19 (suppl 1):S19.
12. Dunn EJ, Ulicny KS Jr, Wright CB, et al. Surgical implications of sclerosing mediastinitis. *Chest*. 1990;97:338.
13. Sarosi GA, Voth DW, Dahl BA, et al. Disseminated histoplasmosis: results of long-term follow-up. *Ann Intern Med*. 1971;75:511.
14. Mathisen DJ, Grillo HC. Clinical manifestation of mediastinal fibrosis and histoplasmosis. *Ann Thorac Surg*. 1992;54:105.
15. Zajtchuk R, Strevey TE, Heydorn WH, et al. Mediastinal histoplasmosis: surgical considerations. *J Thorac Cardiovasc Surg*. 1973;66:300.
16. Cordasco EM Jr, Ahmad M, Mehta A, et al. The effects of steroid therapy on pulmonary hypertension secondary to fibrosing mediastinitis. *Cleve Clin J Med*. 1991;57:647.
17. Kaufman L. Laboratory methods for the diagnosis and confirmation of systemic mycoses. *Clin Infect Dis*. 1992;14:s23.
18. Penn RL, Lambert RS, George RB. Invasive fungal infections: the use of serologic test in diagnosis and management. *Arch Intern Med*. 1983;143:1215.
19. Kappe R, Seeliger HPR. Serodiagnosis of deep seated fungal infections. *Curr Top Med Mycol*. 1993;5:247.
20. Parker JD, Sarosi GA, Doto IL, et al. Treatment of chronic pulmonary histoplasmosis. *N Engl J Med*. 1970;283:225.
21. Edwards PQ, Parker CE. Nationwide histoplasmin sensitivity and histoplasmal infection.
22. Jordan MM, Chawla J, Owens MW, et al. Significance of false-positive serologic tests for histoplasmosis and blastomycosis in an endemic area. *Am Rev Respir Dis*. 1990;141:1487.
23. Johnson P, Sarosi G. Current therapy of major fungal diseases of the lung. *Infect Dis Clin North Am*. 1991;5:6351.

24. National Institute of Allergy and Infectious Diseases Mycosis Study Group. Treatment of blastomycosis and histoplasmosis with ketoconazole: results of a prospective randomized clinical trial. *Ann Intern Med.* 1985;103:861.
25. National Institute of Allergy and Infectious Diseases Mycosis Study Group. Itraconazole therapy for blastomycosis and histoplasmosis. *Am J Med.* 1992;93:489.
26. Wheat LJ, Connolly-Stringfield PA, Baker RL, et al. Disseminated histoplasmosis in the acquired immune deficiency syndrome: clinical findings, diagnosis and treatment, and review of the literature. *Medicine* (Baltimore). 1990;69:361.
27. Wheat LJ, Connolly-Stringfield P, Blair R, et al. Histoplasmosis relapse in patients with AIDS: detection using *Histoplasma capsulatum* variety capsulatum antigen levels. *Ann Intern Med.* 1991;115:936.
28. Conces DJ Jr, Stockberger SM, Tarver RD, et al. Disseminated histoplasmosis in AIDS: findings on chest radiographs. *AJR.* 1993;160:15.
29. Wheat J. Histoplasmosis in the acquired immunodeficiency syndrome. *Curr Top Med Mycol.* 1996;7:7.
30. Ankobiah WA, Vaidya K, Powell S, et al. Disseminated histoplasmosis in AIDS: clinicopathologic features in seven patients from a non-endemic area. *NY State J Med.* 1990;90:234.
31. Wheat LJ, Connolly-Stringfield P, Williams B, et al. Diagnosis of histoplasmosis in patients with the acquired immunodeficiency syndrome by detection of *Histoplasma capsulatum* polysaccharide antigen in bronchoalveolar lavage fluid. *Am Rev Respir Dis.* 1992;145:1421.
32. Wheat LJ, Connolly-Stringfield P, Blair R, et al. Effect of successful treatment with amphotericin B on *Histoplasma capsulatum* variety capsulatum polysaccharide antigen levels in patients with AIDS and histoplasmosis. *Am J Med.* 1992;92:153.
33. Drew RH. Pharmacotherapy of disseminated histoplasmosis in patients with AIDS. *Ann Pharmacother.* 1993;27:1510.
34. Wheat J, Hafner R, Wulfsohn M, et al. Prevention of relapse of histoplasmosis with itraconazole in patients with the acquired immunodeficiency syndrome. *Ann Intern Med.* 1993;118:610.
35. Hostetler JS, Denning DW, Stevens DA. U.S. experience with itraconazole in *Aspergillus*, *Cryptococcus*, and *Histoplasma* infections in the immunocompromised host. *Chemotherapy.* 1992;38(suppl 1):12.
36. Negroni R, Taborda A, Robies AM, et al. Itraconazole in the treatment of histoplasmosis associated with AIDS. *Mycoses.* 1992;35:281.
37. McKinsey DS, Kauffman CA, Pappas PG, et al. Fluconazole therapy for histoplasmosis. The National Institute of Allergy and Infectious Diseases Mycoses Study Group. *Clin Infect Dis.* 1996;23:996.
38. Wheat J, MaWhinney S, Hafner R, et al. Treatment of histoplasmosis with fluconazole in patients with acquired immunodeficiency syndrome. National Institute of Allergy and Infectious Diseases Acquired Immunodeficiency Syndrome Clinical Trials Group and Mycoses Study Group. *Am J Med.* 1997;103:223.
39. Norris S, Wheat J, McKinsey D, et al. Prevention of relapse of histoplasmosis with fluconazole in patients with the acquired immunodeficiency syndrome. *Am J Med.* 1994;96:504.
40. Wheat J, Hafner R, Korzun AH, et al. Itraconazole treatment of disseminated histoplasmosis in patients with the acquired immunodeficiency syndrome. AIDS Clinical Trial Group. *Am J Med.* 1995;98:336.
41. Hecht FM, Wheat J, Korzun AH, et al. Itraconazole maintenance treatment for histoplasmosis in AIDS: a prospective, multicenter trial. *J Acquir Immune Defic Syndr Hum Retrovirol.* 1997;16:100.
42. Reddy PA, Gorelick DF, Brasher CA, et al. Progressive disseminated histoplasmosis as seen in adults. *Am J Med.* 1970;48:629.
43. Sathapatayavongs B, Batteiger BE, Wheat LJ, et al. Clinical and laboratory features of disseminated histoplasmosis during two large urban outbreaks. *Medicine* (Baltimore). 1983;62:263.
44. McKinsey DS, Spiegel RA, Hutwagner L, et al. Prospective study of histoplasmosis in patients infected with human immunodeficiency virus: incidence, risk factors, and pathophysiology. *Clin Infect Dis.* 1997;24:1195.

41. BLASTOMYCOSIS

David Wayne Dockweiler

Blastomycosis is a relatively uncommon disease caused by the dimorphic fungus *Blastomyces dermatitidis*. After inhalation of fungal spores by the host, the organism may give rise to a spectrum of clinical syndromes ranging from an acute, self-limited, flu-like illness to rapidly progressive, widely disseminated, fatal disease. *B. dermatitidis* grows in mycelial form when cultured at 25°C and as a single budding yeast with a characteristically thick refractive cell wall at 37°C. The primary reservoir for human infection by is soil that is moist and rich in organic debris.

The vast majority of cases have been described in North America in endemic areas that include the southeastern and south-central United States and the region around the Great Lakes; thus, the disease also has been known as North American blastomycosis. With the demonstration of cases in Europe, Africa, South America, and the Middle East, this term is clearly not appropriate.

Blastomycosis most often is a disease of young to middle-aged men, although cases have been described in both sexes and in ages ranging from newborn to the elderly. A significant number of patients have a history of outdoor activities, especially hunting. Interestingly, canine blastomycosis, a condition similar to human disease, is more commonly seen in animals that are used in hunting, pointing to exposure of both humans and animals from a common outdoor source. Blastomycosis is not considered an opportunistic infection, per se, and has not been identified in immunocompromised patients to the same degree as other fungal pathogens, such as histoplasmosis or cryptococcosis; however, cases have occurred in patients with renal transplants, chronic steroid use and AIDS. Not surprisingly, disseminated disease and an increased incidence of central nervous system (CNS) involvement are seen in such individuals.

Primary infection with *B. dermatitidis* almost always results from inhalation of fungal spores. Far less commonly, the disease is sexually transmitted through prostatic secretions or spread by maternal–fetal transmission. A laboratory accident associated with percutaneous inoculation has resulted in disease. Person-to-person transmission by aerosol has never been documented.

After deposition of the spores in the alveoli, an inflammatory response is initiated that consists of polymorphonuclear leukocytes, monocytes, and alveolar macrophages. Granuloma formation follows in most cases. Several clinical courses may ensue, depending on factors such as host resistance and the inhaled dose. First, there may be spontaneous resolution of mild or clinically silent pulmonary involvement that, in a presumably small number of cases, may disseminate. Second, there may be the development of acute pneumonitis with nonspecific symptoms, such as fever, cough, purulent sputum, chills, myalgias, pleuritic chest pain, and occasionally erythema nodosum. Third, patients may present with a severe progressive pulmonary process leading to hypoxemia, respiratory failure, and prostration. Fourth, the infection may present as a chronic pulmonary infiltrate, easily confused with other fungal diseases or tuberculosis. Patients with this chronic form of blastomycosis often present with a long history of constitutional complaints, such as malaise, weight loss, chronic cough, fever, and blood-tinged sputum. Significant hemoptysis is rare. Dissemination is said to take place in up to 70% of patients with chronic pulmonary blastomycosis, and multiple organ involvement is the rule. Lastly, there may be disseminated disease, which may occur with the previously mentioned patterns of pulmonary involvement or in isolation, representing reactivation of the disease long after the primary focus of infection has resolved.

Although disseminated blastomycosis may present anywhere, the skin, as the organism's name suggests, is by far the most commonly involved organ. The skin lesions typically begin as small subcutaneous nodules or pustules that may grow rapidly and ulcerate to form large verrucose ulcers with heaped-up edges. Although skin lesions may occur at any site, the face and trunk are favored. Bony lesions, typically osteolytic, are next in frequency. Areas commonly involved include the bones of the extremities, vertebral bodies, skull, ribs, and pelvis. Overlying soft tissue may be involved, joint spaces may be infected by direct extension, and vertebral body disease may give rise to paraspinous abscesses. The male genital tract (epididymis, testes, prostate) has been estimated to be involved in about 10% of patients with disseminated disease. Infected prostatic secretions have been documented and presumably explain sexual transmission of the disease. Less often, laryngeal involvement is seen and may be difficult to distinguish grossly from carcinoma. Adrenal involvement with adrenal insufficiency has been reported. Meningeal blastomycosis is rare in immunocompetent hosts but occurs more frequently in patients with AIDS.

Roentgenographic findings are variable and correlate only moderately well with the clinical presentation. In patients with acute disease, the chest radiograph and computed tomogram (CT) are more likely to demonstrate pneumonic, consolidative, nodular, or interstitial infiltrates that are segmental or nonsegmental. Multiple lobes may be involved, though upper lobe involvement appears to be more common. Despite the relatively common occurrence of pleurisy, pleural effusions are unusual. Cavitary changes have been reported in up to 10% of cases. Chronic forms of blastomycosis are somewhat more likely to present as central mass lesions and may closely mimic bronchogenic carcinoma. Hilar and mediastinal adenopathy appear to be infrequent, even on CT examination. Lymph node calcification, common in histoplasmosis, is rare in blastomycosis.

Standard laboratory studies are nonspecific. Hematologic abnormalities (e.g., anemia, leukocytosis) are variable and rarely significant. Serum chemistries are usually normal. Skin testing for blastomycosis is not useful. Serologic tests are available, but they are too nonspecific and insensitive to be helpful clinically.

Definitive diagnosis of the disease requires the demonstration of the fungus in the tissues, either microscopically or by culture. *B. dermatitidis* is often found in sputum smears (potassium hydroxide [KOH] or Papanicolaou), bronchoscopy washings, pleural fluid, urine (especially after prostate massage), or tissue biopsy specimens. The organism is best demonstrated with methenamine silver or para-aminosalicylic acid (PAS) stains. Culture of the organism from all the above sources has a very high diagnostic yield, but growth requires up to 5 weeks, a delay that is problematic in the acutely ill patient. Once cultured, the yeast form of the fungus is relatively easy to identify microscopically. Because tissue colonization with blastomycosis does not occur, finding the organism provides a definitive diagnosis.

The decision regarding which patients with blastomycosis to treat is not without some controversy. Although most experts agree that the majority of cases of blastomycosis are usually self limited, treatment is now recommended for all cases of both acute and chronic pulmonary blastomycosis.

Itraconazole, an oral antifungal triazole, is the drug of choice in the treatment of nonmeningeal, non–life-threatening forms of blastomycosis. Early studies have found response rates of >90%, results as good or better than with ketoconazole, with significantly less toxicity. Furthermore, itraconazole has been shown to be effective in treating ketoconazole-treatment failures. Like the other oral azoles, itraconazole is fungistatic and does not cross the blood-brain barrier; therefore, its use should be limited to treating immunocompetent individuals with nonmeningeal, non–life-threatening disease. A dosage of 200 mg/day for 6 months is recommended, unless progression of disease occurs, in which case the dosage should be increased to 400 mg/day. Itraconazole is recommended as maintenance therapy for patients with AIDS and disseminated blastomycosis who have already had an initial course of amphotericin B.

Ketoconazole was the first oral azole shown to be effective, though less so than itraconazole, in cases of both disseminated and pulmonary disease. Treatment failures and relapses have also been documented.

A third oral antifungal, fluconazole, does not appear to be as effective as itraconazole, based on the need for higher drug doses to achieve nearly comparable results. The higher incidence of side effects and higher cost of the drug make it a second- or third-line treatment choice for blastomycosis. However, because of its greater penetration into the CNS, fluconazole may be useful in patients with meningeal blastomycosis after initial treatment with amphotericin.

Amphotericin B remains the drug of choice for severe life-threatening infections, meningeal disease, pregnant patients, AIDS patients with blastomycosis, and oral antifungal treatment failures. The clinical response to treatment is usually excellent, although side effects can be troublesome. When given in a cumulative dose of 1.5 to 2.5 g, the incidence of relapse in the immunocompetent patient is probably less than 5%.

---

1. Bradsher RW, Chapman SW, Pappas PG. Blastomycosis. *Infect Dis Clin North Am.* 2003;17:21–40.
   Excellent, comprehensive review of the subject.
2. Brown LR, Swensen SJ, Van Scoy RE, et al. Roentgenologic features of pulmonary blastomycosis. *Mayo Clin Proc.* 1991;66:29.
   In 35 cases of pulmonary blastomycosis, consolidation (26%) and mass lesion (31%) were the most common findings. Hilar adenopathy, pleural effusion, and calcification were uncommon.
3. Kauffman CA, Hajjeh R, Chapman SW. Practice guidelines for the management of patients with blastomycosis. Infectious Disease Society of America. *Clin Infect Dis.* 2000;30:679–683.
   Recent treatment guidelines.
4. Farber ER, Leahy MS, Meadows TR. Endometrial blastomycosis acquired by sexual contact. *Obstet Gynecol.* 1968;32:195.
   First well-documented case of sexually transmitted blastomycosis.
5. Hebert CA, King JW, George RB. Late dissemination of pulmonary blastomycosis during ketoconazole therapy. *Chest.* 1989;95:240.
   Despite apparent good compliance and adequate dosage, the patient described suffered relapse with dissemination after 5 months of therapy.
6. Dismukes WE, and the NIAID Mycoses Study Group. Itraconazole therapy for blastomycosis and histoplasmosis. *Am J Med.* 1992;93:489.
   Itraconazole was found to be highly effective for nonmeningeal, non–life-threatening blastomycosis, with minimal drug toxicity.
7. Klein BS, Vergeront JM, Weeks RJ, et al. Isolation of Blastomyces dermatitidis in soil associated with a large outbreak of blastomycosis in Wisconsin. *N Engl J Med.* 1986;314:529.
   First convincing demonstration of soil as the reservoir for the organism.
8. Kravitz GR, Davies SF, Eckman MR, et al. Chronic blastomycotic meningitis. *Am J Med.* 1981;71:501.
   All three cases presented as a chronic meningitis and obstructive hydrocephalus developed. Cerebrospinal fluid cultures from lumbar taps were not diagnostic, but ventricular taps were.
9. Jordan MM, Chawla J, Owens MW, et al. Significance of false-positive serologic tests for histoplasmosis and blastomycosis in an endemic area. *Am Rev Respir Dis.* 1990;141:1487.
   False-positive fungal serologies were found to be of no use in suggesting a specific category of disease other than a pulmonary mycosis.
10. Martynowicz MA, Prakash UBS. Pulmonary blastomycosis: an appraisal of diagnostic techniques. *Chest.* 2002;121:768–773.
    Noninvasive specimens were positive on culture in 86%, compared with a 92% yield from specimens obtained by bronchoscopy.
11. Pappas PG. Blastomycosis in the immunocompromised patient. *Semin Respir Infect.* 1997;12:343–351.
    Clinical disease in this patient population is much more likely to disseminate and involve multiple organs, especially the central nervous system.
12. Pappas PG, Bradsher RW, Kauffman CA, et al. Treatment of blastomycosis with higher doses of fluconazole. The National Institute of Allergy and Infectious Diseases Mycoses Study Group. *Clin Infect Dis.* 1997;25:200–205.

Fluconazole is found to be nearly as effective as itraconazole when given at higher doses (400–800 mg/day).
13. Patel RG, Patel B, Petrini MF, et al. Clinical presentation, radiographic findings, and diagnostic methods of pulmonary blastomycosis: a review of 100 consecutive cases. *South Med J.* 1999;92:289–295.
    Clinical presentation was found to correlate with findings on chest radiograph in about 60 to 70% of cases. Diagnosis was made in most cases with sputum examination, culture, or cytology.
14. Vasquez JE, Mehta JB, Agrawal R, et al. Blastomycosis in northeast Tennessee. *Chest.* 1998;114:436–443.
    A quadrupling of the incidence rate of blastomycosis in northeast Tennessee during the last 18 years was found to coincide with major new construction in that region.
15. Watts EA, Gard PD, Tuthill SW. First reported case of intrauterine transmission of blastomycosis. *Pediatr Infect Dis.* 1983;2:308.
    A case of maternal-to-fetal transmission of blastomycosis is described.
16. Winer-Muram HT, Beals DH, Cole FH. Blastomycosis of the lung: CT features. *Radiology.* 1992;182:829.
    CT scans of 16 patients with blastomycosis found a low incidence of pleural effusion and hilar and mediastinal adenopathy.

---

42. *ASPERGILLUS* LUNG DISEASE

Judd W. Landsberg

Aspergillus species are responsible for a diverse spectrum of human pulmonary diseases, ranging from hypersensitivity reactions to necrotizing angioinvasive infection. Overall, the incidence of *Aspergillus* lung disease is on the rise, largely as a result of increased numbers of immunosuppressed patients. Worldwide, *Aspergillus* is the most common cause of invasive mold infection. Although host immune status influences disease susceptibility (e.g., allergic reaction with atopy vs. invasive aspergillosis with neutropenia), the notion that invasive disease is seen exclusively in neutropenic recipients is incorrect. Only 31% of patients with invasive pulmonary aspergillosis (IPA) are neutropenic when diagnosed. Increasingly, IPA has been recognized as complicating systemic glucocorticoid therapy for chronic lung disease in otherwise immunocompetent patients.

There are more than 200 species of *Aspergillus*, but *Aspergillus fumigatus* is responsible for more than 90% of human disease; the remainder is mostly caused by *Aspergillus flavus* (5–10%), *Aspergillus terreus* (2–5%) or *Aspergillus niger* (1–2%). *Aspergillus* is ubiquitous and found worldwide in organic debris and soil. It commonly contaminates sputum and laboratory specimens exposed to unfiltered air. *Aspergillus* can be isolated from sputum in 1 to 6% of healthy individuals; higher rates of asymptomatic colonization are found in cigarette smokers and patients with chronic lung disease or HIV infection.

In the environment, the fungi produce small spores that, when inhaled, may result in hypersensitivity, saprophytic colonization, or invasive disease. Person-to-person transmission has not been reported, but clustered minioutbreaks of aspergillosis in immunocompromised patients have been reported from environmental exposure.

Aspergillus can cause at least seven distinct pulmonary syndromes, depending on host susceptibility: (1) immunoglobulin E (IgE)-mediated asthma; (2) hypersensitivity pneumonitis (HP); (3) allergic bronchopulmonary aspergillosis (ABPA); (4) aspergilloma; (5) chronic invasive pulmonary aspergillosis (CIA); (6) acute IPA; and

(7) tracheobronchial aspergillosis. Although each syndrome has a unique pathogenesis, there is significant overlap between these syndromes in individual patients (e.g., saprophytic colonization of bronchiectatic airways in patients with ABPA or angioinvasion after high-dose glucocorticoids in patients with chronic aspergillosis).

IgE-Mediated Asthma

Patients with extrinsic IgE-mediated asthma attributable to environmental *Aspergillus* antigens must be differentiated from those with asthma and ABPA. Immediate skin test reactivity to *A. fumigatus* is present in up to 25% of patients in asthma clinics. The absence of *Aspergillus*-specific IgE-Af and IgG-Af antibodies argues against ABPA. As in all allergies, avoidance of antigen and anti-inflammatory therapy is primary.

Hypersensitivity Pneumonitis

Inhalation of organic matter contaminated with *Aspergillus* species has been associated with HP. *Aspergillus* antigens are associated with Malt-worker's lung, paper mill worker's lung, and more recently a cluster of HP cases in plaster workers exposed to *Aspergillus*-contaminated esparto fibers (see Chapter 85).

Allergic Bronchopulmonary Aspergillosis

ABPA refers to a clinical syndrome occurring most commonly in atopic patients with long-standing reactive airway disease. It is characterized by episodic chest radiograph infiltrates, IgE elevations, and poorly controlled asthma. The peak incidence is in the fourth to fifth decades. The clinical course is characterized by a cough productive of golden-brown sputum plugs (containing *Aspergillus* hyphae), hemoptysis, intermittent fever, chest pain, and recurrent pneumonias. Often there is a discrepancy between significant chest radiograph consolidation and muted clinical findings. During disease flares, serum IgE levels are typically elevated >1000 ng/mL. Exacerbations may be clinically silent, requiring vigilant chest radiograph and serum IgE surveillance.

Radiographic findings include fleeting upper lobe infiltrates, branching homogeneous (gloved finger) shadows of mucoid impaction, and tramline and ring shadows indicative of thickened bronchial walls. Computed tomographic (CT) scans may identify central bronchiectasis that characteristically terminates abruptly, leaving distal airways uninvolved. Recurrent episodes can lead to bronchiectasis and, ultimately, severe mixed restrictive–obstructive lung disease and respiratory failure. ABPA is classified by the presence or absence of bronchiectasis and clinically staged according to disease activity. Treatment now focuses on both control of inflammation and organism eradication.

The essential features required for the diagnosis of ABPA are (1) bronchospasm, (2) immediate cutaneous reactivity to *A. fumigatus* and, in patients not on systemic glucocorticoids (3) total serum (IgE) >1000 ng/mL, (4) precipitating antibodies to *A. fumigatus,* and (5) elevated serum IgE-Af and IgG-Af specific to *A. fumigatus*. Common, but not required features include (6) episodic chest radiograph infiltrates and (7) peripheral eosinophilia. During flares, sputum stains may be positive for fungal elements and cultures positive for *Aspergillus*. In the absence of cystic fibrosis, central bronchiectasis suggests ABPA. The differential diagnosis of ABPA includes IgE-mediated asthma, pulmonary infiltration with eosinophilia syndromes, helminthic lung disease, and other types of hypersensitivity pneumonitis.

Clinically, patients with ABPA can be divided into five stages: (I) acute, (II) remission, (III) exacerbation, (IV) corticosteroid-dependent asthma, and (V) fibrotic. Stage I (acute) describes patients who initially present with classic ABPA. Stage II (remission) is defined as no recurrence for at least 6 months after corticosteroid therapy is discontinued. Remissions can be permanent, but relapses have occurred as long as 7 years after initial remission. Stage III (exacerbation) may be clinically asymptomatic, consisting of only asymptomatic infiltrate or an increase in IgE levels (doubling is generally accepted as the criterion for exacerbation, but tenfold increases are common). Stage IV (corticosteroid-dependent asthma) is diagnosed when steroids cannot be discontinued without exacerbation. Infiltrates may or may not recur, and IgE is only variably elevated. Occasionally the diagnosis of ABPA will be made at stage IV during evaluation of a patient with long-standing steroid-dependent asthma. In this situation serology is less useful. The presence of proximal bronchiectasis on chest CT scan is very suggestive, as are previous chest radiographs revealing fleeting upper lobe infiltrates. Stage V (fibrotic) refers to patients with ABPA who develop mixed obstructive–restrictive lung disease with pulmonary fibrosis, often complicated by hypoxia, cor pulmonale, bacterial superinfection, and respiratory failure.

Treatment of ABPA should produce rapid improvement with resolution of infiltrates by 4 weeks, improved asthma, reduced sputum with clearing of *Aspergillus*, decreased peripheral blood eosinophilia, and decreased total serum IgE (by at least 35% in 6 weeks). Standard treatment for stages I (acute) and III (exacerbation) is prednisone 40 mg (about 0.5 mg/kg) daily for at least 2 weeks, followed by every other day dosing for 2 months. Prednisone can then be tapered rapidly and stopped unless infiltrates, clinical symptoms, or a rise in total serum IgE recur.

A randomized clinical trial of itraconazole for patients with stage IV ABPA showed a 46% response rate with no significant adverse events. Another randomized trial demonstrated that itraconazole (400 mg/day) over 16 weeks resulted in fewer exacerbations requiring oral glucocorticoid therapy, reduced eosinophilic airway inflammation, and reduced IgE levels in patients with stage II (remission). Anecdotal evidence suggests itraconazole also may be used as a steroid-sparing agent for stage V (fibrotic) disease. The role of itraconazole and newer azoles in the treatment of stage I and III disease remains to be defined.

Because repeated exacerbations of ABPA lead to progressive bronchiectasis and, ultimately, end-stage lung disease, periodic chest imaging and IgE serology are warranted despite apparent clinical stability. With adequate management, the prognosis for ABPA is good and long remissions are often achieved.

Aspergilloma (mycetoma or fungus) refers to a mass of fungal mycelia, inflammatory cells, and tissue debris, typically occurring in a preexisting, poorly draining lung cavity. Cavities occur most commonly in association with tuberculosis (TB), emphysematous bullae, endemic fungal infection, *Pneumocystis carinii* (PCP) infection (in HIV disease), sarcoidosis, bronchiectasis, and bronchial cysts.

An aspergilloma may be discovered on routine chest imaging in asymptomatic individuals or may be associated with recurrent mild hemoptysis in 45 to 85%. Most aspergillomas remain stable and 10% regress spontaneously. However, aspergillomas may progress to locally invasive infection, complicated by parenchymal necrosis, vessel invasion, and massive hemoptysis resulting from bronchial vessel involvement. Immunosuppression increases the risk of invasive disease. Clinical signs of invasive disease include radiographic progression, massive hemoptysis, and increasing *Aspergillus*-specific IgG titers.

Patients with aspergilloma complicating obstructive lung disease may experience varying degrees of chronic cough and increased dyspnea. Fever, weight loss, and constitutional signs are less common and should prompt a search for another explanation, such as TB, *Mycobacterium avium-intracellulare* complex (MAC), bacterial infection, or neoplasm. Typically, imaging reveals an upper lobe cavity with an intraluminal irregularity. Fluoroscopy may demonstrate mobility of the shadow with positional changes. Sputum culture for *Aspergillus* may be negative in 50% of cases. Serum IgG *Aspergillus*-specific antibodies are present in >90% but may be falsely negative in patients on high-dose corticosteroids, or in patients infected with non-*A. fumigatus* species. *Aspergillus* skin testing is uniformly negative in patients with aspergilloma. Lesions tend to be solitary, but bilateral disease is reported in 5 to 10%.

Asymptomatic patients with stable chest radiographs require no therapy. Systemic antifungal agents (I.V. amphotericin B and oral itraconazole) have been ineffective, probably reflecting poor intracavitary penetration. Bronchial artery embolization is an appropriate initial step in the management of massive, life-threatening, hemoptysis, though recurrent bleeding from collateral blood vessels is very common. Although surgical resection of the cavity provides definitive treatment, mortality and morbidity can be very high (7 to 23%) in the presence of coexisting lung disease. In a recent study of 87 younger patients without significant underlying lung disease, reported mortality was 1.5% with morbidity of 18%. In general, surgery should be reserved for massive hemoptysis in patients with adequate pulmonary reserve. Although parenchymal progression and increased hemoptysis may represent concomitant bacterial infection, the clinician must also consider chronic invasive aspergillosis, in which case antifungal therapy is warranted.

CIA, also known as semi-invasive aspergillosis or chronic necrotizing aspergillosis, describes an indolent clinical syndrome occurring in patients with underlying lung disease and often mild degrees of immunosuppression in which saprophytic colonization of abnormal parenchyma progresses to local invasion. Chronic invasive aspergillosis typically occurs in middle-aged and elderly patients with chronic obstructive pulmonary disease (COPD), prior granulomatous disease (both mycobacterial and fungal), cystic fibrosis, and other diseases involving parenchymal distortion. Alternatively, parenchymal consolidation and necrosis can occur de novo, often mimicking necrotic tumor or tuberculosis. Patients may be immunocompetent but typically have varying degrees of mild immunosuppression secondary to diabetes mellitus, low-dose oral glucocorticoid therapy, alcoholism, poor nutrition, or connective tissue disease. Typically, patients complain of dry cough with recurrent small hemoptysis, often with increased wheezing and dyspnea in those with obstructive lung disease. Weight loss and low-grade fever are less common and should prompt consideration of mycobacterial disease or bacterial superinfection. Imaging classically reveals an infiltrative process, often with adjacent pleural thickening, in the upper lobes or superior segments of the lower lobes. Nearly 50% of the time consolidation occurs in areas surrounding an aspergilloma. Given the presence of underlying lung disease, old imaging studies are essential to look for subtle changes surrounding preexisting areas of parenchymal distortion or aspergilloma.

Biopsy is the diagnostic gold standard. However, given the poor yield from transbronchial biopsy and complications associated with thoracoscopic or open-lung biopsy in patients with severe underlying lung disease, diagnosis is usually made on clinical grounds. Diagnostic criteria include: (1) compatible clinical and radiographic features; (2) isolation of Aspergillus species in sputum or bronchoalveolar lavage fluid (if cultures are negative but suspicion is high, the presence of IgG-specific Aspergillus antibodies can further suggest the diagnosis); and (3) exclusion of other conditions with similar presentations (e.g., active tuberculosis, atypical mycobacterial infection, and chronic cavitary histoplasmosis or coccidioidomycosis), often through combined bronchoalveolar lavage (BAL), skin testing, and serology results.

Given the invasive nature of the disease and the often unmodifiable immune status of the host, antifungal therapy is warranted. Clinical data are lacking, but voriconazole has replaced amphotericin as first-line therapy for invasive and chronic invasive aspergillosis. Itraconazole has emerged as an effective oral agent, either alone for mild to moderate disease, or after a course of intravenous therapy for severe CIA. Duration of therapy ranges from 6 months to chronic suppressive therapy for patients with substantial immunosuppression. Surgical resection remains an option for the rare young patient with focal disease and good pulmonary reserve. The long-term prognosis for patients with CIA has not been well studied, but 2-year survival is reported to be 70%, with the majority of deaths attributed to underlying lung disease or comorbidities, rather then Aspergillus infection.

The incidence of acute IPA has increased in the last several decades from 6 to 11% owing to more at-risk patients. Although the majority of IPA occurs in patients with underlying hematologic malignancies (28%) or allogeneic hematopoietic stem cell transplants (HSCT) (25%), up to 9% of cases occur in patients with chronic lung disease and only modest immunosuppression. Solid organ transplant (9%), AIDS (8%), autologous HSCT (6%), and other immune deficiencies (6%) account for the rest. Up to 2% of cases are reported in patients with no underlying disease; therefore the diagnosis of IPA should be considered in immunocompetent patients if clinical suspicion is high. The majority of invasive infections involve rapidly progressive, multifocal, necrotizing bronchopneumonia that, if untreated, lead to vascular invasion, dissemination, and death. Reported mortality rates vary and may be as high as 90% or as low as 16%, depending on the speed of diagnosis, aggressiveness of therapy, and host immune system recovery. CT scan and BAL are the mainstays of diagnosis. Therapy is often started empirically based on clinical and radiographic features. Voriconazole has replaced amphotericin B as first line therapy for IPA, demonstrating improved survival and less toxicity. In addition a new class of antifungals, the echinocandins, may provide a better tolerated alternative salvage therapy to lipid amphotericin preparations.

Invasive aspergillosis has become a leading cause of death in allogeneic HSCT recipients, in addition to being the most common cause of community-acquired pneumonia in those with graft-versus-host disease (GVHD). The epidemiology of IPA after allogeneic HSCT shows a bimodal peak, with an early onset at 2 weeks and a late onset at 3.5 months. The clinical presentation of IPA is variable. Early in the disease, up to 30% of neutropenic patients may be asymptomatic. Initial symptoms include fever, dry cough, pleurisy, and, occasionally, hemoptysis. If untreated, the disease will progress rapidly. Physical examination is nonspecific but may reveal a pleural rub. Differential diagnosis includes pneumonia from other opportunistic pathogens in immunocompromised hosts (e.g., other fungi, *Nocardia*, viruses, *Pneumocystis*, bacteria), as well as pulmonary involvement by an underlying neoplasm or pneumonitis owing to the toxicity from radiation or chemotherapy.

A definitive diagnosis of invasive pulmonary aspergillosis requires lung biopsy, demonstrating septate hyphae with acute-angle branching in tissue (best seen with silver stain), and simultaneous growth of the organism in culture. Unfortunately, both transbronchial biopsy and sputum culture have a high false-negative rate. Thoracoscopic or open lung biopsy may delay diagnosis and carry significant bleeding risk in the thrombocytopenic patient. For most patients at high risk for IPA, a less invasive diagnosis can be made by combining clinical, radiographic, and microbiologic or BAL results.

CT is a significant tool in the early diagnosis of invasive pulmonary aspergillosis. Common CT findings include multiple peripheral nodules (1 to 3 cm, typically at the pleural surface), and consolidation with wedge-shaped infarcts. Less common are multiple tiny (<1 cm) nodules scattered throughout the lung. Other less common findings include tracheobronchial thickening, pleural invasion, and hilar or mediastinal masses. The halo sign, a circumferential low attenuation ground-glass opacity surrounding a nodule (resulting from hemorrhage) occurs in 95% of patients at the time of diagnosis but is present in only 19% at 2 weeks. Conversely, the air crescent sign (necrosis of the nodule after neutrophils and inflammation return) is absent at diagnosis but present 63% after 2 weeks. Serial CT imaging should not be used to assess early response to therapy. Despite response, the volume of lesions typically increases fourfold from the first week and then remains stable between days 7 and 14.

Growing *Aspergillus* in sputum or BAL has a positive predictive value of 80 to 90% in high-risk patients. Additionally, identifying branching hyphae on BAL cytology defines invasion in the right clinical setting. Traditional *Aspergillus* serology (i.e., specific IgG-Af and IgE-Af) are often falsely negative in the immunosuppressed, but new serodiagnostic techniques that detect circulating fungal DNA and fungal cell-wall components such as β-glucan are under development. A commercial sandwich enzyme-linked immunosorbent assay (ELISA) *Aspergillus* antigen detection kit (Platelia) has recently been approved by the Food and Drug Administration (FDA) for use in cancer patients but, at present, sensitivity is low (30%), and testing requires serial measurements over 2 to 3 days.

Voriconazole has replaced amphotericin B as first-line therapy for invasive pulmonary aspergillosis. Herbrecht et al. found that after 12 weeks of therapy, patients treated with voriconazole had improved survival (71% vs. 58%) and fewer severe side effects compared with amphotericin B. The echinocandins, fungistatic peptides that inhibit the synthesis of fungal cell wall glucan, have been approved for second-line or salvage therapy and may be superior to lipid preparations of amphotericin B. Caspofungin is dosed 70 mg intravenously daily × 1 (load) followed by 50 mg intravenously per day.

The optimal duration of therapy is unknown and must be weighed against the extent of infection, degree and rate of immune reconstitution, and degree of radiographic resolution. Practice guidelines suggest induction therapy with intravenous medication should be continued until the infection stabilizes, followed by oral maintenance therapy until complete resolution of radiographic findings or immune reconstitution occurs. The role of surgical resection remains controversial. Patient's most likely to benefit from surgery are those with focal residual disease, often threatening a great vessel, and those who will be significantly immunosuppressed again in the future. The role of granulocyte colony-stimulating factor (GCSF), interferon-γ, (IFN-γ), and other immune-based therapies are currently under investigation.

Tracheobronchial Aspergillosis

Beyond mucoid impaction seen in ABPA, *Aspergillus* causes a range of invasive tracheobronchial diseases in the immunosuppressed. Tracheobronchial aspergillosis represents a unique presentation of invasive pulmonary aspergillosis in which large airway mucosal invasion leads to thick, adherent, nodular plaques that cause endobronchial narrowing, obstruction, and significant distal plugging. The manifestations of tracheobronchial aspergillosis vary from obstructing tracheobronchitis to ulcerative tracheobronchitis, to an extensive pseudomembranous tracheobronchitis. Symptoms include cough, dyspnea, fixed wheeze, and radiographic evidence of atelectasis. Diagnosis is made by bronchoscopy with biopsy and culture. If the condition is not promptly diagnosed and treated, respiratory failure may result from airway obstruction, progression to frank invasive pulmonary aspergillosis, or, rarely, perforation of the trachea or bronchi.

Beyond the obvious risk factors of hematologic malignancy and HIV infection, cases of fulminant tracheobronchitis have been reported in patients with only modest immunosuppression. Individuals with HIV infection and lung transplant recipients have a predilection for tracheobronchial aspergillosis.

In the 6 months after lung transplant, the bronchial anastomosis (BA) is uniquely vulnerable to saprophytic *Aspergillus* colonization and subsequent invasion, given its poor perfusion. The reported incidence of posttransplant *Aspergillus* colonization is approximately 30%, with isolated tracheobronchial aspergillosis occurring 5 to 25% of the time. The median time of diagnosis is 35 days posttransplant. Prognosis is good with a more than 80% response rate to combined antifungal therapy and bronchoscopic debridement. Mortality ranges from 1 to 5%. Residual airway complications after BA *Aspergillus* infection occur about 20% of the time consisting mainly of bronchial stenosis and less frequently bronchomalacia. Routine, posttransplant surveillance bronchoscopy is recommended. Treatment consists of antifungal therapy for invasive aspergillosis and bronchoscopic debridement.

1. Baron O, Guillaume B, Moreau P, et al. Aggressive surgical management in localized pulmonary mycotic and nonmycotic infections for neutropenic patients with acute leukemia: report of eighteen cases. *J Thorac Cardiovasc Surg.* 1998;115:63.
   Eighteen patients with hematologic diseases diagnosed as localized invasive pulmonary aspergillosis were treated with aggressive surgical resection. No perioperative deaths or complications occurred. Sixty-six percent of patients were alive after a mean follow-up of 29.1 months. No statistically significant difference was found between the invasive and the noninvasive pulmonary aspergillosis groups.
2. Binder RE, Faling LJ, Pugatch RD, et al. Chronic necrotizing pulmonary aspergillosis: a discrete clinical entity. *Medicine* (Baltimore). 1982;61:109–124.
   Original description of chronic necrotizing pulmonary aspergillosis as a clinical entity.
3. Buchheidt D, Weiss A, Reiter S, et al. Pseudomembranous tracheobronchial aspergillosis: a rare manifestation of invasive aspergillosis in a non-neutropenic patient with Hodgkin's disease. *Mycoses.* 2003;46:51–55.
   Case report of pseudomembranous tracheobronchial aspergillosis occurring in a patient with recurrent Hodgkin's disease.
4. Cornet M, Mallat H, Somme D, et al. Fulminant invasive pulmonary aspergillosis in immunocompetent patients—a two-case report. *Clin Microbiol Infect.* 2003;9:1224–1227.
   Report describing two cases of fulminant invasive pulmonary aspergillosis in immunocompetent patients with chronic lung disease treated with a short course of systemic corticosteroids.

5. Davies SF, Sarosi GA. Fungal pulmonary complications. *Clin Chest Med.* 1996;17: 725.

   An excellent general review.

6. Herbrecht R, Denning DW, Patterson TF, et al. Voriconazole versus amphotericin B for primary therapy of invasive aspergillosis. *N Engl J Med.* 2002;347:408–415.

   Prospective randomized trial of 277 patients with invasive aspergillosis, 144 in the voriconazole group and 133 in the amphotericin B group. The survival rate at 12 weeks was 70.8% in the voriconazole group compared with 57.9% in the amphotericin B group, changing the standard of care for invasive pulmonary aspergillosis to voriconazole.

7. Husain S, Kwak EJ, Obman A, et al. Prospective assessment of Platelia Aspergillus galactomannan antigen for the diagnosis of invasive aspergillosis in lung transplant recipients. *Am J Transplant.* 2004;4:796–802.

   Prospective clinical trial investigating the utility of the Platelia Aspergillus galactomannan antigen test for the early diagnosis of invasive aspergillosis, in 70 lung transplant recipients. Although the specificity of the test was 95%, the sensitivity was only 30%.

8. Kahn FW, Jones JM, England DM. The role of bronchoalveolar lavage in the diagnosis of invasive pulmonary aspergillosis. *Am J Clin Pathol.* 1986;86: 518.

   Demonstrated was 97% specificity, but only 53% sensitivity, of bronchoalveolar lavage in patients suspected of having invasive aspergillosis pneumonia.

9. Marr KA, Patterson T, Denning D. Aspergillosis. Pathogenesis, clinical manifestations, and therapy. *Infect Dis Clin North Am.* 2002;16:875–894.

   Thorough, up-to-date review.

10. McCarthy DS, Pepys J. Pulmonary aspergilloma: clinical immunology. *Clin Allergy.* 1973;3:57.

    Serology findings in patients with aspergilloma.

11. McCarthy DS, Simon G, Hargreave FD. The radiological appearances in allergic bronchopulmonary aspergillosis. *Clin Radiol.* 1970;21:366.

    A classic description.

12. Mehrad B, Paciocco G, Martinez FJ, et al. Spectrum of Aspergillus infection in lung transplant recipients: case series and review of the literature. *Chest.* 2001;119:169–175.

    Retrospective review of 133 transplantations demonstrating airway colonization, isolated tracheobronchitis, and invasive pneumonia due to Aspergillus species occurred in 29%, 5%, and 8%, respectively.

13. Mennink-Kersten MA, Donnelly JP, Verweij PE. Detection of circulating galactomannan for the diagnosis and management of invasive aspergillosis. *Lancet Infect Dis.* 2004;4:349–357.

    Review reporting that in all studies thus far the specificity of the galactomannan assay was greater than 85%; however, the sensitivity of the assay varied considerably between 29 and 100%. Reasons for variable performance are discussed in detail.

14. Moreno-Ancillo A, Dominguez-Noche C, Carmen Gil-Adrados A, et al. Familial presentation of occupational hypersensitivity pneumonitis caused by aspergillus-contaminated esparto dust. *Allergol Immunopathol.* 2003;31:294–296.

    Case report of a cluster of HP cases in plaster workers exposed to Aspergillus-contaminated esparto fibers.

15. Munoz P, Alcala L, Sanchez Conde M, et al. The isolation of Aspergillus fumigatus from respiratory tract specimens in heart transplant recipients is highly predictive of invasive aspergillosis. *Transplantation.* 2003;75:326–329.

    Study demonstrating that the isolation of Aspergillus from the respiratory tract of heart transplant recipients is highly predictive of invasive aspergillosis.

16. Nunley DR, Gal AA, Vega JD, et al. Saprophytic fungal infections and complications involving the bronchial anastomosis following human lung transplantation. *Chest.* 2002;122:1185–1191.

    Review of 61 lung transplant recipients who underwent surveillance bronchoscopy demonstrating saprophytic fungal infection of the bronchial anastomosis

(80% Aspergillus, 20% Candida) in 24.6%. Infection was associated with bronchial stenosis nearly 20% of the time.

17. Patterson R, Greenberger PA, Halwig JM, et al. Allergic bronchopulmonary aspergillosis: natural history and classification of early disease by serologic and roentgenographic studies. Arch Intern Med. 1986;146:916.

   A classification system for allergic bronchopulmonary aspergillosis, including specific recommendations regarding treatment and disease parameters to be monitored.

18. Rello J, Esandi ME, Mariscal D, et al. Invasive pulmonary aspergillosis in patients with chronic obstructive pulmonary disease: report of eight cases. Clin Infect Dis. 1998;26:1473.

   A seminal description of hospital-acquired disease.

19. Robinson LA, Reed EC, Galbraith TA, et al. Pulmonary resection for invasive Aspergillus infections in immunocompromised patients. J Thorac Cardiovasc Surg. 1995;109:1182.

   In immunocompromised patients with hematologic diseases or liver transplantation with invasive pulmonary aspergillosis, early pulmonary resection should be strongly considered when the characteristic clinical and radiographic pictures appear.

20. Rosenberg M, Patterson R, Roberts M, et al. The assessment of immunologic and clinical changes occurring during corticosteroid therapy for allergic bronchopulmonary aspergillosis. Am J Med. 1978;64:599.

   Serum IgE levels, both specific and nonspecific for Aspergillus, are elevated in individuals with ABPA and mirror disease activity. Elevated IgE levels generally precede clinical exacerbations and fall toward normal in response to steroid therapy.

21. Safirstein BH, D'Souza MF, Simon G, et al. Five-year follow-up of allergic bronchopulmonary aspergillosis. Am Rev Respir Dis. 1973;108:450.

   Oral corticosteroids may be important in prevention of long-term sequelae.

22. Salez F, Brichet A, Desurmont S, et al. Effects of itraconazole therapy in allergic bronchopulmonary aspergillosis. Chest. 1999;116:1665.

   An interesting report on the efficacy of itraconazole in long-standing ABPA in reducing steroid requirements and improving lung function.

23. Stevens DA, Schwartz HJ, Lee JY, et al. A randomized trial of itraconazole in allergic bronchopulmonary aspergillosis. N Engl J Med. 2000;342:756–762.

   Randomized, double-blind, placebo-controlled trial of 16 weeks of itraconazole treatment in 28 patients with ABPA and corticosteroid-dependent allergic asthma, demonstrating a 46% response rate with no significant adverse events. A response was defined as a reduction of at least 50% in corticosteroid dose, a decrease of at least 25% in serum IgE concentration, and one of the following: an improvement of at least 25% in exercise tolerance or pulmonary function tests or resolution or absence of pulmonary infiltrates.

24. Stevens DA. Practice guidelines for diseases caused by Aspergillus. Infect Diseases Society of America. Clin Infect Dis. 2000;30:696–709.

   Diagnosis and treatment recommendations.

25. Wark PA, Hensley MJ, Saltos N, Boyle MJ, et al. Antiinflammatory effect of itraconazole in stable allergic bronchopulmonary aspergillosis: a randomized controlled trial. J Allergy Clin Immunol. 2003;111:952–957.

   A randomized, double-blind, placebo-controlled trial of itraconazole in 29 stable subjects with ABPA showing reduced eosinophilic airway inflammation, systemic immune activation, and exacerbations requiring glucocorticoid therapy.

43. NOCARDIOSIS

John Verrilli and Antonio Catanzaro

Nocardia is a genus of gram-positive, partially acid-fast bacteria, in the family Mycobacteriaceae. These Actinomycetes are responsible for a wide spectrum of suppurative and granulomatous disease in humans with both normal and abnormal immune systems. The bacteria was first described in 1888 by Edward Nocard, who isolated it from cattle, but the first documentation of human infection came later in 1890. *Nocardia* was previously misclassified as a fungus because of its mycelial development with true branching filaments; however, it was reclassified as a bacterium because of its lack of chitin or cellulose within its cell wall and other biochemical properties.

The current incidence of nocardiosis is not known, but probably 500 to 1,000 new cases are recognized each year in the United States. It is diagnosed with increasing frequency, possibly because of improved diagnostic methods, higher levels of suspicion, and an increasing number of immunocompromised patients. Recently, new species have been identified by gene sequencing (e.g., *Nocardia africana*, *Nocardia paucivorans*, and *Nocardia veterana*). Infection occurs primarily in men (90%). The reason for this is unclear but may relate to hormonal differences. The male predominance is not as apparent in patients with malignancies or organ transplant.

Nocardia is a soil saprophyte, and infection is acquired from inhalation of airborne mycelial fragments and spores or by direct inoculation. Human-to-human transmission has not been reported. Although clusters of hospitalized patients in close proximity having the same strain of *Nocardia* have been reported, it is not known whether this represents nosocomial infection or a common environmental source.

Infections in humans typically involve the lungs, but skin, soft tissue, ocular and disseminated disease, including the brain or visceral organs, also occur. *Nocardia brasiliensis* is usually responsible for direct inoculations to the skin and lymphangitic spread. Acute *Nocardia* infections produce large numbers of small abscesses with sinus tracts, a cellular infiltrate of lymphocytes, giant and foam cells, and extensive fibrosis.

Nocardiosis is usually an opportunistic infection. At least half of all cases are associated with one of the following: malignancy, chronic granulomatous diseases, systemic immunosuppression, such as in AIDS, organ transplantation, alcoholism, systemic lupus erythematosus, diabetes mellitus, or corticosteroid use. Other predisposing factors to infection include pulmonary parenchymal pathology, such as chronic obstructive pulmonary disease, bronchiectasis, and pulmonary fibrosis.

In cases in which no systemic immunosuppression is present, infection is usually confined to the lungs and can be acute, subacute, or a chronic suppurative infection with periods of remission and exacerbation. The most common symptoms are cough, purulent sputum (occasionally bloody), chest pain, weight loss, high fever, chills, and night sweats.

Acute infection can appear as an isolated lung abscess or a bronchopneumonia that may lead to a lung abscess. Consolidation and large irregular nodules are common and may be cavitary. Nodules, masses, and interstitial patterns also occur. Pleural involvement is seen in approximately 25% of cases, ranging from simple, uncomplicated effusion to empyema. Lymph nodes can be enlarged. Spread to other parts of the lung or chest wall rarely happens; however, sinus tracts and perforation of the chest wall can occur.

Chronic infection can appear as small abscesses or chronic fibronodular disease. Such lesions may be confined to a small portion of the lungs or scattered throughout the lungs, mimicking miliary tuberculosis. Airway colonization is possible, and a few well-documented cases have been described in which the organism was repeatedly isolated from the sputum in the absence of disease. Nocardia also can invade preexisting pulmonary cavities, forming a fungus ball.

Extrapulmonary presentations may include primary cutaneous inoculation with lymphangitic spread or hematogenous dissemination after a pulmonary or oropharyngeal infection. Hematogenous spread is usually to the central nervous system, causing meningitis or multiple brain abscesses. Rare cases of widespread dissemination have been reported, usually in individuals with diseases known to interfere with cell-mediated immunity.

Most clinicians feel that the isolation of *Nocardia* organisms from sputum, tissue, or other body fluids represents prima facie evidence for nocardiosis. In identifying *Nocardia* organisms, multiple clinical specimens should be submitted to the laboratory for Gram's stain and culture. Because the organism can be difficult to detect, identification is more likely if the specimen comes from pus from a fistula or abscess (if possible). Skin testing is unreliable and serologic tests are neither reliable nor available commercially. Polymerase chain reaction (PCR) testing has been used to classify isolates but is not used in the clinical setting. Isolation of *Nocardia* organisms from a gastric washing is of no significance, because they can be present in food.

The organism can be identified on Gram's stain, with a typical appearance of delicate, gram-positive, irregularly staining, beaded, branching filaments. These filaments can fragment easily however, into nondescript, coccobacillary forms. The organism is partially acid-fast and must be identified under oil immersion because of the extremely fine nocardial filaments (0.5–1.0 μm in diameter). It does not stain on hematoxylin-eosin and will be missed unless special tissue stains are performed. Expectorated sputum may or may not yield positive smears or cultures in established pulmonary infection, and various invasive procedures, including bronchoscopic biopsy, percutaneous lung aspiration, and open lung biopsy, have a very high yield. Although *Nocardia* has been reported to form sulfur granules, the diagnosis is best established by identification of the organisms themselves.

Successful treatment of nocardiosis includes the use of appropriate antibiotics and, if necessary, surgical drainage. Sulfa-containing antibiotics have been the mainstay of treatment since the 1940s and are active against the two most common organisms, *Nocardia asteroides* and *N. brasiliensis*. Trimethoprim along with sulfamethoxazole (TMP-SMX) has shown a synergistic effect and is still the initial treatment for nocardiosis infection as it is well absorbed and distributed in most bodily tissues. TMP-SMX is usually well tolerated; however, adverse effects do occur, including nausea, vomiting, anorexia, and diarrhea; more serious side effects include myelotoxicity. Several potential alternative treatments have been used, such as minocycline, the newer macrolides, amikacin, imipenem, linezolid, third-generation cephalosporins such as ceftriaxone and cefotaxime, fluoroquinolones, and amoxicillin-clavulanate. Species identification and susceptibility testing are useful in choosing a successful alternative treatment. Combination therapy with a sulfa-containing agent and one of the alternative agents has been recommended for serious, systemic disease. The duration of therapy is uncertain, but 6 to 12 months is usually recommended to prevent dissemination or recurrence. Immunosuppressed patients should be treated for a minimum of 12 months with the possibility of an ongoing suppressive regimen.

1. Lerner PI. Nocardiosis. *Clin Infect Dis*. 1996;22:891.
   Excellent summary of recent studies. Discusses the whole spectrum of disease in this review.
2. Smilack JD. Trimethoprim-sulfamethoxazole. *Mayo Clin Proc*. 1999;74:730.
   Thorough review of TMP-SMX, including its mechanism of action, antimicrobial activity, pharmacologic properties and dosage, toxicity, and side effects.
3. Menendez R, Cordero PJ, Santos M, et al. Pulmonary infection with Nocardia species: a report of 10 cases and review. *Eur Respir J*. 1997;10:1542.
   Reviews the clinical features and prognostic factors of 10 cases of pulmonary infection by Nocardia species.
4. Palmer SM Jr, Kanj SS, Davis RD, et al. A case of disseminated infection with Nocardia brasiliensis in a lung transplant recipient. *Transplantation*. 1997;63:1189.

A discussion of a patient's course with the unusual presentation of N. brasiliensis *after lung transplant.*

5. Yoon HK, Im JG, Ahn JM, et al. Pulmonary nocardiosis: CT findings. *J Comput Assist Tomogr.* 1995;19:52.

   Discusses the computed tomographic (CT) results of five immunocompromised patients and recommends that nocardiosis should be included in the differential diagnosis with certain findings.

6. Boiron P, Provost F, Chevrier G, et al. Review of nocardial infections in France 1987 to 1990. *Eur J Clin Microbiol Infect Dis.* 1992;11:709.

7. Bross JE, Gordon G. Nocardial meningitis: case reports and review. *Rev Infect Dis.* 1991;13:160.

8. Feigin DS. Nocardiosis of the lung: chest radiographic findings in 21 cases. *Radiology.* 1986;159:9.

9. Heffner JE. Pleuropulmonary manifestations of actinomycosis and nocardiosis. *Semin Respir Infect.* 1988;3:352.

10. Kramer MR, Uttamchandani RB. The radiographic appearance of pulmonary nocardiosis associated with AIDS. *Chest.* 1990;98:382.

11. Schulman LL, Epson Y. Nocardia pneumonitis and the adult respiratory distress syndrome. *Am J Med Sci.* 1987;293:315.

    References 6 to 11 discuss the clinical and radiographic presentations of nocardiosis.

12. Chapman SW, Wilson JP. Nocardiosis in transplant recipients. *Semin Respir Infect.* 1990;5:74.

13. Haramati LB, Schulman LL, Austin JH. Lung nodules and masses after cardiac transplantation. *Radiology.* 1993;188:491.

14. Javaly K, Horowitz HW, Wormser GP. Nocardiosis in patients with immunodeficiency virus infection. *Medicine* (Baltimore). 1992:71:128.

15. Kim J, Minamoto GY, Grieco ME. Nocardial infection as a complication of AIDS: report of six cases and review. *Rev Infect Dis.* 1991;13:624.

16. Perschak H, Gubler J, Speich R, et al. Pulmonary nocardiosis concurrent with Pneumocystis carinii pneumonia in two patients undergoing immunosuppressive therapy. *J Infect.* 1991;23:183.

17. Raby N, Forties G, Williams R. Nocardia infection in patients with liver transplants or chronic liver disease: radiologic findings. *Radiology.* 1990;174:713.

18. Wilson JP, Turner HR, Kirchner KA, et al. Nocardial infections in renal transplant recipients. *Medicine* (Baltimore). 1989;68:38.

19. Husain S, McCurry K, Dauber J, et al. Nocardia infection in lung transplant recipients. *J Heart Lung Transplant.* 2002;21:354–359.

20. Peraira JR, Segovia J, Fuentes R, et al. Pulmonary nocardiosis in heart transplant recipients: treatment and outcome. *Transplant Proc.* 2003;35:2006–2008.

    References 12 to 20 review the influence of comorbid conditions, particularly those involving immunosuppression on the occurrence of nocardial infection.

21. Angeles AM, Sugar AM. Rapid diagnosis of nocardiosis with an enzyme immunoassay. *J Infect Dis.* 1987;155:292.

22. de Vivo F, Pond GD, Rhenman B, et al. Transtracheal aspiration and fine needle aspiration biopsy for the diagnosis of pulmonary infection in heart transplant patients. *J Thorac Cardiovasc Surg.* 1988;96:696.

23. Rodriguez JL, Barrio JL, Pitchenik AE. Pulmonary nocardiosis in the acquired immunodeficiency syndrome: diagnosis with bronchoalveolar lavage and treatment with non-sulphur containing drugs. *Chest.* 1986;90:912.

    References 21 to 23 review the approach to the diagnosis of nocardiosis.

24. Garlando F, Bodmer T, Lee C, et al. Successful treatment of disseminated nocardiosis complicated by cerebral abscess with ceftriaxone and amikacin: Case report. *Clin Infect Dis.* 1992;15:1039.

25. Overkamp D, Waldmann B, Lins T, et al. Successful treatment of brain abscess caused by Nocardia in an immunocompromised patient after failure of cotrimoxazole. *Infection.* 1992;20:365.

26. Yew WW, Wong PC, Kwan SY, et al. Two cases of Nocardia asteroides sternotomy infection treated with ofloxacin and a review of other active antimicrobial agents. *J Infect.* 1991;23:297.

　　References 24 to 26 review the therapeutic approaches to nocardial infection.

27. Lerner PI. Nocardia species. In: Mandell GL, Bennett JE, Dolin R, eds. *Principles and Practice of Infectious Diseases.* 4ᵗʰ ed. New York, NY: Churchill Livingston; 1995:2273–2280.

　　Discusses the epidemiology, classification, pathology, diagnosis, and treatment of Nocardia infections.

28. Mari B, Monton C, Mariscal D, et al. Pulmonary nocardiosis: clinical experience in ten cases. *Respiration.* 2001;68:382–388.

29. Hui CH, Au VW, Rowland K, et al. Pulmonary nocardiosis re-visited: experience of 35 patients at diagnosis. *Respir Med.* 2003;97:709–717.

30. Matulionyte R, Rohner P, Uckay I, et al. Secular trends of nocardia infection over 15 years in a tertiary care hospital. *J Clin Pathol.* 2004;57:807–812.

　　References 28 to 30 discuss the incidence, predisposing factors, diagnosis, treatment, and systems involved with Nocardia infection.

31. Saubolle MA, Sussland D. Nocardiosis: review of clinical and laboratory experience. *J Clin Microbiol.* 2003;41:4497–4501.

32. Burgert SJ. Nocardiosis: a clinical review. *Infect Dis Clin Pract.* 1999;8:27–32.

33. Corti ME, Villafane Fioti MF. Nocardiosis: a review. *Int J Infect Dis.* 2003;7:243–250.

　　References 31 to 33 are recent review articles that discuss the challenges of diagnosis and treatment of Nocardia infection.

34. Kiska DL, Hicks K, Pettit DJ. Identification of medically relevant Nocardia species with an abbreviated battery of tests. *J Clin Microbiol.* 2002;40:1346–1351.

　　Proposes an algorithm for rapid species identification and for directed therapy in nocardial infections.

44. CRYPTOCOCCOSIS AND ACTINOMYCOSIS

Jana Cooke and Antonio Catanzaro

Cryptococcus neoformans is a unimorphic fungus that produces a granulomatous disease in humans known as *cryptococcosis*. The organism occurs as a single-budding yeast and has a thick polysaccharide capsule that is responsible for its characteristic visualization by India ink. The major environmental reservoir appears to be avian, primarily pigeons, and therefore cryptococcosis tends to be an urban disease.

C. neoformans enters the body through the respiratory tract with at least four potential outcomes: clearance of the organism, acute infection with or without dissemination, chronic infection, or development of latent infection. In immunocompetent individuals, two thirds of infections are confined to the lungs. Cryptococcal infection in the lung may lead to (1) subpleural fibrotic nodules, usually less than 1 cm in diameter; (2) "torulomas" or larger granulomatous lesions up to 6 cm or more in diameter, which are often gelatinous and may undergo central necrosis and cavitation; (3) the poorly defined mass or "infiltrative mass"; and (4) miliary dissemination to both lungs resulting in diffuse edema, necrosis, and hemorrhagic exudate filling the alveoli and airways.

Most cryptococcal infections are associated with conditions that compromise cell-mediated immunity, including advanced HIV infection, lymphoproliferative disorders, corticosteroid therapy, solid organ transplantation, rheumatologic disorders, and sarcoidosis. The use of tumor necrosis factor-α (TNF-α) antagonists has recently been associated with the development of disseminated cryptococcosis.

The epidemiology of cryptococcosis has changed over the past 10 years with the introduction of more effective antiretroviral treatment, specifically HAART (highly active antiretroviral therapy) and the widespread use of oral fluconazole for oropharyngeal candidiasis. Surveillance data document the decreasing incidence of cryptococcosis among individuals with AIDS in the United States during the 1990s. Those individuals with AIDS who did develop cryptococcosis in the late 1990s were shown to have limited access to routine HIV medical care. The expensive nature of HAART and poor access to medical care in less developed countries, such as those in Africa and Asia, have resulted in an increased prevalence of AIDS and with it, cryptococcosis.

The prevalence of infection is thought to be high despite the overall low incidence of disease in non–HIV-infected individuals. Serologic studies of children indicate that seroconversion occurs in early childhood, with the majority of individuals converting before the age of 10. Data support the theory that, like *Mycobacterium tuberculosis*, a significant proportion of cryptococcosis results from reactivation of latent infection. There is no evidence of human-to-human transmission.

The clinical manifestations of pulmonary infection vary considerably. There is speculation that asymptomatic pulmonary infection occurs frequently, as nearly all adults have serum antibody to *C. neoformans*. However, the lack of a reliable epidemiologic tool (e.g., skin test) makes this difficult to prove. Symptoms may be acute or subacute and include cough, sputum (rarely bloody), shortness of breath, chest discomfort, malaise, and low-grade fever. Pulmonary infection is often asymptomatic in the normal host, whereas the majority of immunocompromised hosts develop constitutional symptoms and can present with a rapidly progressing pneumonia and even adult respiratory distress syndrome (ARDS).

The risk of dissemination is greatest in individuals with those underlying diseases that depress cell-mediated immunity. The central nervous system is the most common site of dissemination, and immunosuppressed patients may present with a meningeal rather than a pulmonary syndrome. In patients with AIDS, the risk of developing cryptococcosis is inversely related to the CD4 lymphocyte count, with the risk rapidly rising once the CD4 count drops below $100/\mu$L.

Roentgenographic abnormalities vary from well-defined, noncalcified, single, or multiple nodules that resemble bronchogenic carcinoma to ill-defined masslike infiltrates. These may cavitate (10–15%) and become secondarily infected with other fungi or, rarely, with tuberculosis. Hilar adenopathy and pleural effusions can also occur. In the immunosuppressed individual, alveolar and interstitial infiltrates are more common. Some patients develop a "primary complex," consisting of a pulmonary lesion and hilar node involvement, as seen with tuberculosis, further supporting the theory of latent infection.

The diagnosis of *C. neoformans* infection depends on demonstration of the organism in body fluids or tissue. Positive cultures may be difficult to obtain from sputum, cerebrospinal fluid, or blood, although it will grow on most routine mycologic or bacteriologic media. *C. neoformans* antigens (CRAG) can be identified using the latex agglutination test, which has a specificity and sensitivity of more than 90%. This test is the primary tool used for both diagnosis and following the response to treatment. A positive test at titers of greater than or equal to 1:4 in a biologic fluid strongly suggests infection. If the infection is limited to the lung, the serum CRAG may be negative, although the bronchoalveolar lavage CRAG may be positive. Some believe that a positive serum CRAG implies dissemination, which should prompt an examination of the individual's cerebral spinal fluid to rule out simultaneous central nervous system (CNS) infection with or without symptoms. Others believe that a positive serum CRAG in an immunocompetent patient with isolated pulmonary disease reflects those individuals who may be at increased risk of more severe disease or for dissemination. Further evaluation of this aspect of the serum CRAG is warranted to define more clearly the nature of this relationship.

Fortunately, the increase in cases of cryptococcal infection in the 1980s came when several new treatments became available. A recent executive summary from the National Institute of Allergy and Infectious Diseases (NIAID) Mycoses Study Group outlines treatment guidelines with graded recommendations. Treatment for HIV-infected patients with isolated cryptococcal pneumonia remains clear, and all such patients should be treated because of the high risk of dissemination. Patients who are mildly to moderately symptomatic should be treated with fluconazole 200 to 400 mg/day for life. Itraconazole remains an acceptable alternative at 400 mg/day for life. Starting with the combination of fluconazole 400 mg/day plus flucytosine 150 mg/kg per day for a minimum of 10 weeks is one treatment option, although the toxicity with this regimen limits its utility. For more severe disease, amphotericin B, 0.3 mg/kg per day should be instituted until symptoms are controlled, at which time fluconazole may be substituted. Experience with liposomal amphotericin preparations remains limited but AmBisone 4 mg/kg may be substituted for amphotericin B. Maintenance therapy with fluconazole is highly effective in preventing recurrence.

Immunocompromised patients with isolated pulmonary cryptococcosis should be treated as if they have CNS disease with amphotericin B 0.3 mg/kg per day and 5-flucytosine 150 mg/kg per day administered every 6 hours for 2 weeks followed by fluconazole 400 mg/day for a minimum of 10 weeks. Significant predictors of mortality include age older than 60, underlying hematologic malignancy, and organ failure. Immunocompetent patients with mild to moderate symptoms may be treated with fluconazole 200 to 400 mg/day for 6 to 12 months. Itraconazole is an effective alternative, 200 to 400 mg/day for 6 to 12 months. Amphotericin B may also be used at the onset of disease, particularly if the disease is severe or progressing or for patients who do not respond to azoles, at 0.4 to 0.7 mg/kg per day for a total dose of 1,000 to 2,000 mg.

Treatment of non–HIV-infected, immunocompetent patients is not as clear. The debate continues regarding treatment of the asymptomatic immunocompetent patient with positive sputum cultures, as in a number of case series and retrospective reviews, patients have done well without therapy. These patients, however, can be treated with fluconazole, 200 to 400 mg/day for 3 to 6 months. Long-term chronic suppression with fluconazole should be reserved for those patients with ongoing immunosuppression and persistent disease.

Voriconazole and caspofungin are two relatively new antifungals. Both are highly active against *C. neoformans* in vitro. There is little experience with voriconazole's in vivo activity against *C. neoformans* and caspofungin has little activity against the yeast in animal models. Albaconazole, a new azole, is currently under investigation and to date, has been shown to have potent in vitro activity against *C. neoformans* with some signs of fungicidal activity in rabbit models.

Actinomyces israelii, the organism causing human actinomycosis, is a gram-positive, usually non-acid-fast anaerobic organism that is often considered with fungi because of its morphology; however, its responsiveness to antibiotics and its cell-wall composition establish it as a true bacterium. It is a normal inhabitant of the oropharynx, gastrointestinal tract, and female genital tract in humans. Men develop infection more often than women, and there is no occupational or environmental predisposition. In humans, the organism may cause disease in the mandibulofacial area, intestinal tract, and lung, in decreasing frequency. There is no person-to-person transmission, and it usually occurs in immunocompetent individuals. Pulmonary infection is thought to be caused by aspiration of organisms residing around carious teeth. The incidence appears to be greatest between ages 11 and 20, and 35 and 50, corresponding to the time when infection is most common in tonsils and teeth.

Thoracic actinomycosis can involve the lung parenchyma, pleura, mediastinum, or chest wall. There are several possible routes of infection, including aspiration of oropharyngeal secretions or gastric contents, direct extension of cervicofacial infection, transdiaphragmatic or retroperitoneal spread from the abdomen or, rarely, hematogenous dissemination. Pathologically, infection results in a chronic granulomatous infiltrate, often with abscess formation. The organism is usually obvious on hematoxylin-eosin stain, forming a mass of filamentous hyphae staining densely with hematoxylin.

Clinically, pulmonary actinomycosis may present with cough, often productive of purulent or blood-tinged sputum, chest pain, weight loss, and fever, mimicking that of tuberculosis or malignancy. Chest-wall swelling may occur, although cutaneous abscesses or frank bronchocutaneous fistulas rarely develop. Pleural extension with resultant empyema is a frequent complication of primary pulmonary actinomycosis; rarely, secondary bacterial infection may complicate empyema.

Examination may reveal rales, digital clubbing, and signs of consolidation or pleural effusion. Roentgenographically, actinomycosis may appear acutely with a diffuse alveolar-filling process typical of any other acute bacterial pneumonia. Alternatively, chronic infection may appear as a large mass, resembling bronchogenic carcinoma. This mass may extend across fissures or into the pleural space or chest wall, creating a soft-tissue mass or causing rib destruction. Extensive pulmonary fibrosis has been noted in a few patients with chronic infection. Extrapulmonary extension to the pericardium, mediastinum, pulmonary arteries, and beneath the diaphragm are recognized complications to pulmonary infection. Hematogenous dissemination is rare.

The diagnosis of actinomycosis is based on demonstration of the organisms in tissue or pleural fluid, although this remains a difficult task. Advancements in both tissue sampling and radiographic techniques have improved our diagnostic abilities. In a retrospective review, a ringlike peripheral rim enhancement was seen on contrast computed tomography (CT) in 77% of patients with histopathologically proven thoracic actinomycosis. The presence of sulfur granules (white or yellow, 1-mm to 2-mm clumps of mycelia) in sputum or in drainage from a sinus tract is highly suggestive of the diagnosis; however, cultural confirmation is required.

Penicillin in large doses and for long duration is the treatment of choice. Administration should be intravenous for the first 4 to 6 weeks, followed by oral administration for 6 to 12 months. Other effective alternatives are tetracycline, chloramphenicol, erythromycin, and clindamycin. One case report documents the successful use of a third-generation cephalosporin. There is also a small series of patients who were successfully treated with imipenem–cilastatin. A shorter duration of penicillin therapy was recently used successfully in two patients with esophageal and cervicofacial actinomycosis. To date, however, there are little data to support an abbreviated course in patients with thoracic disease. Suppurative lesions (empyema) should be excised or drained, or both. Surgical debridement of soft-tissue lesions is believed by some to be of critical importance. Appropriate therapy yields an approximate 80% recovery rate.

Cryptococcosis References

1. Saag MS, Graybill RJ, Larsen RA, et al. Practice guidelines for the management of cryptococcal disease. *Clin Infect Dis*. 2000;30:710.

   The National Institute of Allergy and Infectious Disease (NIAID) Mycoses Study Group's guidelines for the management of cryptococcal disease.

2. Yamaguchi H, Ikemoto H, Watanabe K, et al. Fluconazole monotherapy for cryptococcosis in non-AIDS patients. *Eur J Clin Microbiol Infect Dis*. 1996;15:787.

   Monotherapy with fluconazole 200 to 400 mg/day was used to treat 44 non–HIV-infected patients with cryptococcosis, with a clinical response rate of 89%.

3. Perfect JR, Casadevall A. Cryptococcosis. *Infect Dis Clin North Am*. 2002;16:837–874.

   An excellent thorough review of cryptococcosis.

4. Saag MS, Cloud GA, Graybill JR, et al. A comparison of itraconazole versus fluconazole as maintenance therapy for AIDS-associated cryptococcal meningitis. National Institute of Allergy and Infectious Diseases Mycoses Study Group [see comments]. *Clin Infect Dis*. 1999;28:291–296.

   Saag et al. sought to determine the equivalency of itraconazole versus fluconazole through a randomized, double-blind, controlled clinical trial and found that these drugs for maintenance treatment for cryptococcal meningitis were not equivalent.

5. Nightingale SD. Initial therapy for acquired immunodeficiency syndrome-associated cryptococcosis with fluconazole. *Arch Intern Med*. 1995;155:538–540.

   Nightingale performed a retrospective review of 30 AIDS patients who acquired cryptococcosis to determine whether fluconazole used as initial therapy was successful.

6. Joly V, Geoffray C, Reynes J, et al. Amphotericin B in a lipid emulsion for the treatment of cryptococcal meningitis in AIDS patients. *J Antimicrob Chemother*. 1996;38:117–126.

Joly et al. discuss the results of this phase II trial assessing two dosages of deoxycholate-amphotericin B mixed with Intralipid (ILd-AmB).

7. Dromer F, Mathoulin S, Dupont B, et al. Comparison of the efficacy of amphotericin B and fluconazole in the treatment of cryptococcosis in human immunodeficiency virus-negative patients: retrospective analysis of 83 cases. French Cryptococcosis Study Group. *Clin Infect Dis.* 1996;22(suppl 2):S154–160.

This retrospective study found fluconazole to be as effective as amphotericin B for this population.

8. Yu FC, Perng WC, Wu CP, et al. Adult respiratory distress syndrome caused by pulmonary cryptococcosis in an immunocompetent host: a case report. *Zhonghua Yi Xue Za Zhi (Taipei).* 1993;52:120.

The development of ARDS can be associated with a variety of clinical disorders. Pulmonary cryptococcosis has been reported with increasing frequency. Here a rare case of pulmonary cryptococcosis is reported in an immunocompetent host who developed ARDS. The clinical course, radiologic patterns, methods of diagnosis, and treatment are reviewed.

9. Flickinger FW, Sathyanarayana, White JE, et al. Cryptococcal pneumonia occurring as an infiltrative mass simulating carcinoma in an immunocompetent host: plain film, CT, and MRI findings. *South Med J.* 1993;86:450.

Radiographic findings of pulmonary cryptococcosis are variable and include single and multiple masslike infiltrates, nodules, and segmental infiltrates. The authors have compared MRI, CT, and plain film radiographic findings in a case of cryptococcal pneumonia occurring as a mass simulating carcinoma in an immunocompetent individual.

10. Carter EA, Henderson DW, McBride J, et al. Case report: complete lung collapse—an unusual presentation of cryptococcosis. *Clin Radiol.* 1992;46:292.

Cryptococcosis presenting as an intrabronchial mass is not a recognized cause of complete lung collapse. This case illustrates this extremely rare manifestation, which mimicked primary pulmonary carcinoma clinically, radiologically, and bronchoscopically.

11. Ziomek S, Weinstein W, Margulies M, et al. Primary pulmonary cryptococcosis presenting as a superior sulcus tumor. *Ann Thorac Surg.* 1992;53:892.

After resection of a superior sulcus tumor, primary pulmonary cryptococcosis was diagnosed. Management is presented along with a review of the literature.

12. Mitchell DH, Sorrell TC. Pancoast's syndrome due to pulmonary infection with Cryptococcus neoformans variety gattii. *Clin Infect Dis.* 1992;14:1142.

A case of right lung mass and Pancoast's syndrome due to locally invasive C. neoformans variety gattii in a normal host. Lobectomy followed by therapy with amphotericin B and flucytosine was curative.

13. Conces DJ Jr, Vix VA., Tarver RD. Pleural cryptococcosis. *J Thorac Imaging.* 1990;5:84.

Pleural infection by C. neoformans is uncommon and, when present, typically occurs in the immunocompromised host. The authors report two renal transplant patients who developed pleural cryptococcosis.

14. Zeluff BJ. Fungal pneumonia in transplant recipients. *Semin Respir Infect.* 1990;5:80.

Fungal pneumonia is an infrequent but devastating complication of solid organ transplantation. Some fungi, such as C. neoformans, Candida, and Mucor, are associated with concomitant diabetes mellitus. The level of immunosuppressive therapy is also a major predisposing factor. For some fungi, such as Coccidioides immitis and C. neoformans, serologic tests may assist in diagnosis. For Aspergillus, Candida, and Mucor, culture evidence is not sufficient to determine pulmonary involvement, as these fungi may be nonpathogenic saprophytes. Histopathologic proof is required. Amphotericin B exhibits synergistic nephrotoxicity with cyclosporine, and ketoconazole competes with cyclosporine for hepatic metabolism in an unpredictable manner that may result in increased cyclosporine toxicity.

15. Chechani V, Kamholz SL. Pulmonary manifestations of disseminated cryptococcosis in patients with AIDS. *Chest.* 1990;98:1060.

Forty-eight patients with disseminated cryptococcosis and AIDS were retrospectively studied. Symptoms and roentgenographic manifestations were diverse. Interstitial infiltrates predicted the presence of another opportunistic lung infection besides cryptococcosis in five patients. Endobronchial abnormalities were identified in four patients at bronchoscopy. Bronchoalveolar lavage (9 of 9) and pleural fluid (3 of 3) cultures were sensitive tests for detection of pulmonary involvement with C. neoformans.

16. Sider L, Westcott MA. Pulmonary manifestations of cryptococcosis in patients with AIDS: CT features. *J Thorac Imaging.* 1994;9:78.

    The CT scans and chest radiographs of 10 patients with AIDS and proven pulmonary cryptococcal infections were reviewed. In seven (70%), CT demonstrated pulmonary opacities that ranged in appearance from a perihilar interstitial pattern to dense alveolar consolidation. Pulmonary nodules were identified in three patients (30%) by CT but were identifiable on the chest radiograph in only one. The chest radiograph suggested hilar adenopathy in three, although CT confirmed hilar adenopathy in only one patient. In one patient, a small pleural effusion, not appreciated on the chest radiograph, was detected by CT.

17. Baughman RP, Rhodes JC, Dohn MN, et al. Detection of cryptococcal antigen in bronchoalveolar lavage fluid: a prospective study of diagnostic utility. *Am Rev Respir Dis.* 1992;145:1226.

    A prospective study in 220 immunocompromised patients (188 with HIV infection, 32 with other causes of immunosuppression) undergoing BAL for fever and pulmonary symptoms led to the eventual diagnosis of cryptococcal pneumonia in 8 patients. All eight patients had a cryptococcal antigen titer greater than or equal to 1:8. There were four patients without cryptococcal pneumonia who had cryptococcal antigen titers of 1:8; none had higher titers. For a cryptococcal antigen titer of 1:8 or higher, there was 100% sensitivity, 98% specificity, a positive predictive value of 67%, and a negative predictive value of 100%. The measurement of cryptococcal antigen in the bronchoalveolar lavage can be a rapid, simple way to make a diagnosis of cryptococcal pneumonia in immunosuppressed patients with pneumonia.

18. Lee LN, Yang PC, Kuo SH, et al. Diagnosis of pulmonary cryptococcosis by ultrasound guided percutaneous aspiration. *Thorax.* 1993;48:75.

    In this study, 608 patients who had ultrasound-guided lung aspirations were reviewed retrospectively, and 9 aspirates documenting pulmonary cryptococcosis were collected. Five patients also underwent bronchoscopy and biopsy. The diagnostic yield with needle aspiration was higher than that of bronchoscopy.

19. Patz EF Jr, Goodman PC. Pulmonary cryptococcosis. *J Thorac Imaging.* 1992;7:51.

    The most common finding is a poorly marginated nodule or mass. Lobar or segmental parenchymal opacities and, less commonly, a diffuse scattered nodular or reticulonodular pattern have also been observed. Associated adenopathy, pleural effusions, and cavitation are uncommon, but when present, occur chiefly in immunocompromised patients.

20. Powderly WG, Saag MS, Cloud GA, et al. A controlled trial of fluconazole or amphotericin B to prevent relapse of cryptococcal meningitis in patients with the acquired immunodeficiency syndrome. The NIAID AIDS Clinical Trials Group and Mycoses Study Group. *N Engl J Med.* 1992;326:793.

    A multicenter, randomized trial that compared fluconazole (200 mg/day P.O.) with a ~~phot~~ericin B (1 mg/kg of body weight per week I.V.) in patients with AIDS who h~~a~~~~ c~~ompleted primary therapy for cryptococcal meningitis with amphotericin B (≤15 mg/kg) is presented. After a median follow-up of 286 days, 14 of 78 receiving amphotericin B (18%) and 2 of 111 assigned to fluconazole (2%) had relapses of symptomatic cryptococcal disease (P < .001 by Fisher's exact test). Serious drug-related toxicity was more frequent in the amphotericin B group (P = .02), as were bacterial infections (P = .004) and bacteremia (P = .002). Fluconazole taken by mouth is superior to weekly intravenous therapy with amphotericin B to prevent relapse after primary treatment with amphotericin B.

21. Coker RJ, Viviani M, Gazzard BG, et al. Treatment of cryptococcosis with liposomal amphotericin B (AmBisome) in 23 patients with AIDS. *AIDS.* 1993;7:829.

A *phase II, multicenter, European, noncomparative, open study to assess the use of AmBisome in 23 patients (26 enrollments) with cryptococcosis. The drug was well tolerated with little renal, hepatic, or hematologic toxicity. Eighteen of 23 (78%) patients responded clinically. Nineteen patients had cryptococcal meningitis. Sterilization of spinal fluid was achieved in 12; 14 (74%) responded clinically.*

22. Garcia-Hermoso D, Janbon G, Dromer F. Epidemiological evidence for dormant cryptococcus neoformans infection. *J Clin Microbiol.* 1999;37:3204.

A genetic analysis of isolates from nine African expatriates diagnosed with cryptococcosis while living in France a median of 110 months and without contact with an African environment for as long as 13 years. These isolates were significantly different than those isolates recovered from 17 European patients and were more similar to those isolates known to be from Africa.

23. Pappas PG, Perfect JR, Cloud GA, et al. Cryptococcosis in human immunodeficiency virus-negative patients in the era of effective azole therapy. *Clin Infect Dis.* 2001;33:690.

A case study of HIV-negative patients with cryptococcosis that further highlights the demographics, therapies, and prognostic factors associated with this disease.

Actinomycosis References

1. Cheon JE, Im JG, Kim MY, et al. Thoracic actinomycosis: CT findings. *Radiology.* 1998;209:229–233.

   Discusses CT findings of 22 immunocompetent patients from a retrospective review.

2. Hsu WH, Chiang CD, Chen CY, et al. Ultrasound-guided fine needle aspiration biopsy in the diagnosis of chronic pulmonary infection. *Respiration.* 1997;64:319–325.

   After studying 14 patients with abnormal chest x-rays, the authors found that ultrasound-guided fine needle aspiration biopsy was useful for pinpointing the diagnosis of chronic pulmonary infections.

3. Hamed KA. Successful Treatment of primary Actinomyces viscosus endocarditis with third-generation cephalosporins. *Clin Infect Dis.* 1998;26:211–212.

   A case review of a patient with endocarditis caused by Actinomyces species who was allergic to penicillin and treated successfully with third-generation cephalosporins.

4. Yew WW, Wong PC, Lee J, et al. Report of eight cases of pulmonary actinomycosis and their treatment with imipenem-cilastatin. *Monaldi Arch Chest Dis.* 1999;54:126–129.

   A prospective study of eight patients explored the efficacy of treatment with imipenem–cilastatin. The study showed that this treatment alternative strategy shows promise.

5. Brown JR. Human actinomycosis: a study of 181 subjects. *Hum Pathol.* 1973;4:319.

   Concise clinical review. Thoracic (lung or chest wall) involvement was present in 24%.

6. Frank P, Strickland B. Pulmonary actinomycosis. *Br. J. Radiol.* 1974;47:373.

   Most frequent alternative diagnosis is bronchogenic carcinoma. There is often a history of oral trauma, loss of consciousness, epileptic episodes, or dental caries.

7. Newsom BD, Hardy JD. Pulmonary fungal infection: Survey of 159 cases with surgical implications. *J Thorac Cardiovasc Surg.* 1982;83:218.

   One hundred fifty-nine cases of pulmonary fungal disease treated at the Hospital of the University of Mississippi are presented. This clinical review describes the presentation of the various fungal infections as well as the results of treatment regimens used at that hospital.

8. Smith R, Heaton CL. Actinomycosis presenting as Wegener's granulomatosis. *JAMA.* 1978;240:247.

   Sulfur granules were absent in biopsied lesions. Ultimate diagnosis confirmed by an aerobic growth in thioglycolate broth.

9. Merdler C, Greif J, Burke M, et al. Primary actinomycotic empyema. *South Med J.* 1983;76:411.

The clinical findings of this entity are described, along with a response to treatment with cefazolin and pleural drainage.
10. Smego RA, Foglia G. Actinomycosis. *Clin Infect Dis.* 1998;26:1255.
   An excellent concise review of the spectrum of disease, diagnosis, and treatment.
11. Sudhakar SS, Ross JJ. Short-term treatment of actinomycosis: two cases and a review. *Clin Infect Dis.* 2004;38:444.
   Two case reports of successful shorter durations of treatment for esophageal and cervicofacial actinomycosis.

45. NEMATODE AND TREMATODE DISEASES OF THE LUNG

Gregory A. Ruff and Richard T. Mahon

Helminthic (worm-related) pulmonary infections are caused by nematodes (roundworms) or trematodes (flat worms). Both types of parasites are metazoan worms, a group that also includes cestodes (segmented worms). Helminthic infection is ubiquitous in nature; however, human helminthic lung disease is relatively infrequent in North America. The diagnosis is usually considered in travelers returning from endemic regions. The parasites reach the lungs by hematogenous spread or direct migration, and disease is caused by the parasites themselves or by the host's immune response to helminthic antigens. Pulmonary manifestations vary from asymptomatic to catastrophic. The pathologic nematodes include *Ascaris*, hookworm species, *Strongyloides*, and *Filaria*.

Ascaris lumbricoides is among the most common intestinal nematodes in the world. Though found predominately in the tropics, it also infects up to 4 million people living in the southern United States, especially in rural areas. Humans are infected by ingestion of contaminated soil or food that contains the *Ascaris* egg, which then hatches in the gastrointestinal tract. The larvae subsequently migrate through the venous system to the right ventricle and to the lungs, where they enter the alveoli and ascend the tracheobronchial tree.

Pulmonary disease results from a hypersensitivity response to migrating larvae. The manifestations are usually limited to transient pulmonary infiltrates and peripheral eosinophilia. A few patients develop the stigmata of Löffler's syndrome (mild fever, cough, dyspnea, wheezing, sternal pain, and mild hemoptysis associated with migratory pulmonary infiltrates and peripheral eosinophilia). This typically occurs 1 to 2 weeks after egg ingestion. Secondary bacterial pneumonia is common, and mechanical airway obstruction has been described in the presence of a high worm burden.

Eosinophilia and elevated serum immunoglobulin E (IgE) levels are common. Chest radiographs may show patchy consolidation or diffuse military infiltrates. Sputum is rich in eosinophils and in crystallized protein from fragmented eosinophils (Charcot-Leyden crystals). Eggs are rarely found in the sputum but may be recovered from gastric aspirates. The diagnosis can be made by demonstration of *Ascaris* eggs in the stool within 3 months of a self-limited eosinophilic pneumonitis. Serum serologies are available, but their use is mainly as a research tool in endemic areas.

The hookworms, *Ancylostoma duodenale* and *Necator americanus,* infect humans through direct penetration of skin by larvae found in moist contaminated soil. The geographic distribution is worldwide and includes the southeastern Unites States *(N. americanus).* As with *Ascaris,* the hookworm larvae migrate to the lung through the venous system and can produce a self-limited Löffler's syndrome (see above) before they inhabit the small intestine. Also similar to ascariasis, the stool examination may not be positive for up to 2 months after the pulmonary symptoms develop. Symptoms are usually self limited and treatment for pulmonary complaints is generally not necessary, but inhaled bronchodilators may provide symptomatic relief. Eradication of the parasite can be achieved with mebendazole (100 mg two times a day for 3 days or a 500-mg single dose).

Strongyloides stercoralis is endemic in tropical and subtropical areas and in the southeastern United States. A relatively unique feature of S. stercoralis is its ability to complete its lifecycle entirely within the human, potentially leading to a substantial worm burden. Although the acute and chronic stages generally produce only mild symptoms in normal hosts, in immunocompromised conditions (AIDS, steroids, and malignancy), it can be devastating. Strongyloides migrate hematogenously to the lungs after the larvae penetrate the skin. From here, they ascend the tracheobronchial tree and are swallowed. In the duodenum, they mature and produce larvae, some of which can penetrate the colonic mucosa or perianal skin, resulting in autoinfection.

The initial skin penetration by S. stercoralis may lead to local inflammation, edema, and a serpiginous erythematous track that rarely comes to medical attention. The gastrointestinal manifestations include duodenitis, abdominal pain, and malabsorption that can be seen with high worm burdens. The pulmonary manifestations in the immunocompetent patient include cough, wheezing, and a recurrent pneumonitis. Peripheral blood eosinophilia is not necessarily present. Asthma induced by chronic strongyloides will paradoxically worsen with corticosteroid administration.

In the immunocompromised host (e.g., those using corticosteroids), the colonic penetration of filariform larvae occurs unchecked and can widely disseminate to lungs, liver, the central nervous system, and other organs. This so-called *hyperinfection syndrome* carries an extremely high mortality (>90%). The pulmonary manifestations at this stage include adult respiratory distress syndrome (ARDS) or secondary bacterial infections caused by enteric gram-negative bacilli translocating with the worms. Interestingly, the hyperinfection syndrome is uncommon in individuals infected with HIV in endemic areas. Also curious is the observation that cyclosporine in transplant patients may have a theoretical protective effect from this syndrome.

The diagnosis of *Strongyloides* infection rests on finding larvae by stool examination or a duodenal string test; however, these tests lack adequate sensitivity. Enzyme-linked immunosorbent assays (ELISA) are about 90% sensitive and have a negative predictive value of 95% in some populations. In hyperinfection syndrome, strongyloides has been diagnosed by examination of sputum or cerebral spinal fluid. Thiabendazole (25 mg/kg twice a day for 2 days) or ivermectin (200 μg/kg per day for 2 days) are treatment options. The relapse rate with thiabendazole is significant.

Infection by members of the *Filaria* superfamily (filariasis) can be asymptomatic but can also cause acute or chronic tropical pulmonary eosinophilia (TPE). TPE is a relatively uncommon manifestation of human filarial disease (mostly seen with *Wuchereria bancrofti* and *Brugia malayi*). It is most common in India, Southeast Asia, and Sri Lanka, and is more prevalent in men. TPE is considered to be a hypersensitivity reaction to filarial antigen. In the acute phase, TPE causes paroxysmal nonproductive cough and wheeze, which are typically worse at night. Physical examination may reveal hepatomegaly and generalized lymphadenopathy. Laboratory evaluation typically reveals significant peripheral eosinophilia, elevated IgE, and eosinophilic alveolar exudates. Filarial antibodies are usually present, but microfilariae are not seen. The chest radiograph shows fluffy reticulonodular shadows in the mid and lower lung zones; a miliary pattern also has been described. Up to 20% of patients may have normal radiographs. Some patients develop chronic TPE, manifested by a restrictive fibrotic pulmonary process without peripheral or alveolar eosinophilia.

Most patients with acute TPE respond to diethylcarbamazine (6 mg/kg for 21 days), but relapse (or reinfection) and chronically unresponsive disease are well described. Other treatment options included thiabendazole and ivermectin. Concurrent corticosteroids may be useful. The clinical response to therapy is poor in chronic disease.

Dirofilaria immitis (dog heartworm) can be transmitted to the human by a mosquito vector and has been reported increasingly in the United States. In dogs and cats, the larvae develop into sexually mature worms that travel to the right ventricle. In the human host, larvae cannot mature and subsequently die but are passively transported to the lung through the venous system, where they may cause thrombosis, infarction, and a granulomatous reaction. The infection generally manifests itself as an asymptomatic pulmonary nodule but can present with cough, chest pain, and hemoptysis. Because of its radiographic similarities to lung cancer, *D. immitis* manifested as a pulmonary nodule is often diagnosed by surgical resection.

Toxocariasis (visceral larvae migrans) is caused by human infection with a dog or cat ascarid. Endemic to North America, England, and Mexico, *Toxocara canis* and *Toxocara cutis* eggs are ingested from contaminated soil and food. As is the case with dog heartworm, the human is an imperfect host and maturation of the larvae cannot occur. The eggs hatch in the gut and the larvae migrate through host tissue, including the lungs. This migration causes an inflammatory granulomatous response that is considered the source of the clinical manifestations of the disease. Serum and bronchoalveolar lavage (BAL) show increased IgE, as well as an increased eosinophil count. Pulmonary involvement is present in 20 to 80% of cases. Severity of symptoms is related to the worm burden. Visceral larva migrans is generally asymptomatic but can have a fulminant course with central nervous system involvement, acute pneumonia, or severe asthma.

Infection is most common in children (especially those with pica) and can be associated with cough, wheezing, and pulmonary infiltrates. Peripheral eosinophilia is significant and hepatosplenomegaly may be present. A definitive diagnosis depends on the demonstration of larvae in tissue; however, ELISA (using antitoxocara antibodies) and specific larva-related IgE tests are useful. Examination of stool for eggs is useless, as the ascarid cannot reproduce in the human host.

Generally, the disease is self-limited and treatment is generally not indicated; however, diethylcarbazine or thiabendazole is recommended if drug treatment is necessary. The use of corticosteroids in severe cases has been associated anecdotally with clinical improvement.

Two types of trematodes (flat worms or flukes) can cause human infection: Schistosoma and Paragonimus. Schistosomiasis is caused by a digenetic parasitic trematode that infects an estimated 200 million people worldwide. Several species can cause human disease: (1) *Schistosoma japonicum,* found in Japan, China, and the Philippines; (2) *Schistosoma mansoni,* found in Africa, Arabia, and South America; (3) *Schistosoma haematobium* found in Africa and the Middle East; and (4) *Schistosoma intercalatum,* found in western Africa. Infection occurs through contact with fresh water that contains infective cercariae released from snails, which are intermediate hosts. The cercariae penetrate the intact skin of the definitive mammalian host and undergo transformation into migrating larvae. Mature adults localize in mesenteric (*S. mansoni* and *S. japonicum*) or bladder vesicle venules (*S. haematobium*) after passing through the lungs and liver. Mature adults produce eggs that are excreted in the urine and stool, completing the lifecycle. Eggs are also carried in the venous system to the pulmonary vascular beds.

Pulmonary manifestations of schistosomiasis occur in acute and chronic forms. Acute pulmonary schistosomiasis occurs in nonendemic patients, typically manifests 3 to 8 weeks after schistosome penetration, and is characterized by shortness of breath, wheezing, and dry cough. Symptoms may be temporally related to a well-described febrile illness (Katayama fever), but respiratory complaints persist after resolution of fever. Eosinophilia (30–40% of total leukocytes) with leukocytosis, elevated IgE and abnormal liver function tests are common. Radiographic abnormalities (ill-defined nodules, increased interstitial markings, hilar prominence) may be absent or may only appear after antischistosomal therapy is instituted. It is thought that these manifestations are immunologically related and are seen after release of schistosomal antigens. Transbronchial biopsy and BAL may only show eosinophils. The sensitivity of stool and urine for detecting ova is low because of sporadic passage of eggs and the low fluke burden. Serologies may be helpful, but at present, are only available at research centers.

Chronic pulmonary schistosomiasis is a syndrome of endemic individuals consisting of chest pain, dyspnea, fatigue, and cough. Cor pulmonale and right-sided congestive heart failure may be present. The syndrome results from an inflammatory reaction to eggs in the circulatory system, which lodge in the distal pulmonary vasculature and cause granulomatous inflammation. Serologies are not helpful, nor are transbronchial biopsies, because of the sporadic nature of the pathology. Lesions are typically fibrotic and thus respond poorly to therapy. However, because of the relative safety of praziquantel, a course of therapy may be warranted.

Paragonimiasis is a disease with a widespread geographic range that is caused by the trematode *Paragonimus*. The best known species (also having the widest distribution) is *Paragonimus westermani*, which is prevalent in Asia, India, Latin America, and Africa. Humans become definitive hosts by consuming uncooked crustaceans that harbor the larvae of this lung fluke. Infection may also result from eating undercooked pork that carries the larvae. Once ingested, the larvae penetrate into the peritoneal cavity and migrate through the diaphragm and pleura into the lung. Here, they mature and produce eggs that are either expectorated or swallowed. Unlike most other helminths, pulmonary involvement is essential in this fluke's development. Early infection can cause pleuritic chest pain with unilateral small to massive eosinophilic pleural effusions. Fleeting infiltrates and pulmonary hemorrhage may also be seen.

Once in the lungs, the larvae become encysted and eggs are produced. Clinically, this stage of infection can last for several years and carry few symptoms. Rupture of the cysts will cause blood-streaked sputum containing parasite eggs, necrotic tissue, and Charcot-Leyden crystals. Radiographically, small cavitary nodules, ring shadows, and masslike lesions may be present in addition to unilateral, eosinophilic, exudative pleural effusions. A peripheral eosinophilia is generally present in the acute setting, although the total leukocyte count may be normal. Eosinophilia is more common in patients who complain of pleurisy and less common with parenchymal disease. In the absence of eosinophilia, the clinical picture may be confused with tuberculosis, fungal infection, or cancer.

The diagnosis is established by demonstrating parasite eggs in sputum, feces, pleural fluid, or tissue. A single sputum examination has a sensitivity of 30 to 45%, and the yield is increased with multiple collections. BAL samples have a sensitivity of 60 to 70%. Stool examination is generally less sensitive than sputum or pleural fluid analysis. ELISA and immunoblotting assay techniques can help make the diagnosis also. An intradermal test is available but used only in highly endemic areas and in research studies. The first-line therapy is with praziquantel (25 mg/kg three times a day for 3 days) with cure rates approaching 100%.

In summary, pulmonary helminthic infections may present with a broad array of signs and symptoms. A high index of suspicion should be maintained in patients with a pertinent travel history, underlying immune deficiency, or both. Diagnosis and therapy should be tailored to the specific infective agent. The Centers for Disease Control and Prevention (CDC) maintains a Web site at *www.cdc.gov/travel/diseases.htm,* which provides helpful information for travelers and physicians.

1. Drugs for parasitic infections. *Med Lett Drugs Ther.* 1998;40:1–12.
   An overview of available antiparasitic drugs with side effects, dosing schedules, and availability.
2. Allen JN, Davis WB. Eosinophilic lung diseases. *Am J Respir Crit Care Med.* 1994;150:1423–1438.
   Excellent overview of PIE (pulmonary infiltrates and eosinophilia) syndromes to include helminthic diseases.
3. Flieder DB, Moran CA. Pulmonary dirofilariasis: a clinicopathologic study of 41 lesions in 39 patients. *Hum Pathol.* 1999;30:251–256.
   Good clinical and pathologic information on dirofilariasis with excellent photomicrographs and description of lifecycle.
4. Kagawa FT. Pulmonary paragonimiasis. *Semin Respir Infect.* 1997;12:149–158.
   Broad overview of paragonimiasis with epidemiologic, pathophysiologic, diagnostic, and therapeutic information for this lung fluke.
5. Morris W, Knauer CM. Cardiopulmonary manifestations of schistosomiasis. *Semin Respir Infect.* 1997;12:159–170.
   Well-written description of pulmonary manifestations of schistosomiasis. This entire text has valuable information on a variety of helminthic infections.

6. Ong RK, Doyle RL. Tropical pulmonary eosinophilia. *Chest.* 1998;11:1673.
   A good review of this uncommon cause of eosinophilia and pulmonary infiltrates with information on how to obtain recommended antifilarial medications.
7. Ryan ET, Kain KC. Health advice and immunizations for travelers. *N Engl J Med.* 2000;342:1716–1725.
   A nice resource for both patients and providers. Information on recommended immunizations, preventative therapy, and endemic diseases.
8. Sarinas PS, Chitkara RK. Ascariasis and hookworm. *Semin Respir Infect.* 1997; 12:130–137.
   This series has comprehensive information on nematode infections.
9. Schwartz E. Pulmonary schistosomiasis. *Clin Chest Med.* 2002;23:433–443.
   This Clinics on tropical lung diseases has many valuable sections including this one on schistosomiasis. Reviews the lifecycle and epidemiology as well as diagnosis and therapy.
10. Shah MK. Human pulmonary dirofilariasis: review of the literature. *South Med J.* 1999;92:276–279.
    Comprehensive look at pulmonary manifestations of Dirofilaria.
11. Siddiqui AA, Berk SL. Diagnosis of Strongyloides stercoralis infection. *Clin Infect Dis.* 2001;33:1040–1047.
    Current opinion and review of the different testing entities for diagnosis of this blood fluke.
12. Udwadia FE. Tropical eosinophilia: a review. *Respir Med.* 1993;87:17.
    A classic description of this pulmonary helminthic disease.
13. Velez ID, Ortega JE, Velasquez LE. Paragonimiasis: a view from Columbia. *Clin Chest Med.* 2002;23;421–431, ix–x.
    Up-to-date review of paragonimiasis including some atypical presentations.
14. Zaha O, Hirata T, Kinjo F. Strongyloidiasis: progress in diagnosis and treatment. *Intern Med.* 2000;39:695–700.
    Includes information on therapeutic interventions, as well as a review of common and specialized tests for diagnosis of strongyloides.

46. AMEBIASIS AND ECHINOCOCCAL DISEASES OF THE LUNG

William L. Ring

Amebiasis is caused by the protozoan *Entamoeba histolytica* and is most common in tropical and subtropical regions. In the United States, infection is observed most commonly in (1) travelers and immigrants exposed in endemic areas; (2) patients in mental health institutions; (3) HIV-positive patients; and (4) sexually active male homosexuals. The organism is usually confined to the colon, producing either no symptoms or amebic dysentery. The disease is usually contracted by ingestion of food or water contaminated by feces or by fecal–oral contact.

Rarely, mature organisms (trophozoites) penetrate the bowel wall and migrate to the liver by the hepatic veins, where an abscess may form. This invasive form of amebiasis is three to ten times more common in men, is associated with alcohol abuse, and is more common in individuals who are malnourished or immunosuppressed. Most patients with invasive disease present with several weeks of right upper quadrant abdominal pain and fevers. By the time a hepatic abscess forms, no dysenteric symptoms are present in up to two thirds of patients and most patients do not have parasites detectable in their stool.

Thoracic involvement occurs in 13 to 35% of patients with hepatic amebiasis. The usual route of pleuropulmonary infection is by extension from a hepatic or subdiaphragmatic abscess. Less commonly, direct parasitic migration occurs into the thorax. In addition, hematogenous spread to the lung rarely occurs by hemorrhoidal veins or lymphatics. All modes of spread can result in empyema or lung abscess. Pleuropulmonary disease can also occur without actual parasitic invasion in the form of lower lobe infiltrates and exudative effusions; the mechanism for this is not clear, but it is presumably a response to subdiaphragmatic infection.

Amebic pleuropulmonary disease is 10 to 15 times more common in men than women, with a peak incidence between ages 20 and 40. Patients usually have a history of amebic dysentery and may complain of right upper quadrant pain, weight loss, and cough. Rarely, the cough is productive of thick, dark *chocolate sauce* or *anchovy paste* sputum or even bile (biliptysis), indicating hepatobronchial and bronchobiliary fistulas, respectively. Fever and signs of empyema or consolidation may also be present. Chest roentgenogram typically reveals a right-sided effusion or right lower lobe lung abscess. In addition, areas of consolidation may be seen in the right lower lobe, middle lobe, or both. The right diaphragm may be elevated and have decreased motility. In cases involving the left lobe of the liver, changes can occur in the left lung field. Computerized tomography will show the liver abscess. Magnetic resonance imaging can directly visualize the secondary diaphragmatic rupture. Thoracentesis usually reveals a sterile exudate; however, organisms are rarely present.

Routine laboratory examination may show a mild leukocytosis and eosinophilia. Cysts are rarely found in the sputum or the pleural fluid; however, when present, they confirm the diagnosis. A serum hemagglutination test for antibodies to amebae is positive in up to 95% of invasive infections, and will remain positive for years after the infection. Commercial polymerase chain reaction (PCR) assays for amebae are now available and may become the "gold standard" for diagnosis.

In the appropriate clinical picture, it is reasonable to initiate therapy. Metronidazole (750 mg tid) orally for 10 days followed by a luminal agent such as iodoquinol (650 mg tid for 20 days), paromomycin (25–35 mg/kg per day in three divided doses for 7 days), or diloxanide furoate (500 mg tid for 10 days) is generally recommended for extraintestinal amebiasis. Failure to respond to treatment should call into question the diagnosis or suggest the possibility of a secondary bacterial infection. The rare patient with invasive amebiasis who does not respond to this regimen should be treated with chloroquine and percutaneous drainage of the liver abscess and any pleural fluid. Surgery is rarely indicated.

Echinococcosis or hydatid disease is caused by the postlarval metacestode stage of the tapeworm *Echinococcus*. Humans are an intermediate host for this parasite. After ingestion of contaminated food, water, or soil, the oncosphere migrates through the portal circulation, whereby it is ultimately deposited within an organ. Once in an organ, cellular differentiation occurs, resulting in the development of a cyst. The mature cyst consists of an inner germinal layer, the endocyst; an outer chitinous layer, the exocyst; and a peripheral fibrous layer caused by host reaction, the pericyst.

Four species of *Echinococcus* cause human disease. *Echinococcus granulosus* is the most common because of its wide distribution and its high prevalence in sheep; it involves the lung 60% of the time and often has a protracted and relatively benign course. *Echinococcus granulosus* causes cystic echinococcosis, the classic hydatid disease, with often large, unilocular cysts. *Echinococcus multilocularis* is less common. It is primarily a liver disease with occasional involvement of the lung and typically has an aggressive, malignant course. *E. multilocularis* causes alveolar echinococcosis, with somewhat smaller, multilocular cysts, which at pathology appear to have an alveolar appearance. *Echinococcus vogeli* and *Echinococcus oligarthus* are restricted to parts of Central and South America and only rarely cause human disease. They cause polycystic echinococcosis.

E. granulosus is endemic in sheep-raising regions of the Mediterranean, Russia, Australia, and parts of South America and Africa. In North America, it has been reported in both Canada and the United States, particularly in the Mississippi River Valley and Alaska. Dogs and other carnivores serve as the definitive hosts, whereas humans, sheep, and cattle are intermediate hosts.

Pulmonary hydatid cysts are typically 1 to 10 cm in diameter, but can grow much larger. The cysts usually grow at a rate of 1 cm per year in diameter, but growth rates of up to 5 cm per year have been reported. The cysts are usually located in the lower lobes and are twice as frequent on the right. When multiple (20–30%), they are most often unilateral (80%). A cyst can rupture into the bronchial tree, in which case the fluid is replaced with air, or into the pleural space. Pulmonary cysts often (10–60%) coexist with hepatic cysts. Clinically, most patients are asymptomatic. Hydatid cysts are discovered most frequently on routine chest radiographs. Cough, hemoptysis, and chest pain occur uncommonly. Mediastinal cysts can erode into adjacent structures, causing bone pain, hemorrhage, or airflow obstruction. Uncommonly, rupture of a cyst, either spontaneously or during surgery, can result in an acute hypersensitivity reaction. Roentgenographically, the cyst(s) appears as a dense, well-circumscribed oval or spherical mass that can reach enormous dimensions and fill an entire hemithorax. Debris within the fluid of the cyst, which is called *hydatid sand*, has typical characteristics. If bronchial communication has occurred, air between the pericyst and exocyst can produce the appearance of a thin layer around the cyst—the meniscus or moon skin sign. Air penetrating the interior of the cyst may outline the inner surface of the exocyst, producing parallel arches of air—Cumbo's sign. As air fills the space, the endocyst and the exocyst may detach, showing an irregular air fluid layer with the collapsed membranes floating on the fluid surface; this is known as the water lily, lotus on water, or camelot sign. Calcification of the cyst is rare. Eosinophilia, usually not prominent, is found in less than 50% of patients. A skin test (Casoni) for delayed hypersensitivity to cyst material is generally positive but does not correlate with disease activity.

A number of sensitive, serologic tests are available, but they are of limited clinical value because of poor specificity. Fiberoptic bronchoscopy may reveal whitish–yellow gelatinous material in the bronchi. Conclusive diagnosis can be made if components of the hydatid cysts, including possibly scolexes or degenerated hooklets, are identified in bronchoalveolar lavage fluid, pleural fluid, or sputum. Although some risk is seen to percutaneous aspiration of a cyst, some studies have suggested that this can be done safely. Traditionally, the treatment of choice has been surgical resection. Some studies have suggested that medical treatment alone with a benzimidazole (albendazole or mebendazole) can be a safe, initial strategy.

E. multilocularis is endemic in an area extending from the White Sea to the Bering Straits, including the former Soviet Union, the European alpine countries, southern and central Canada, northeastern United States, Alaska, Japan, and China. The red fox, Arctic foxes, coyotes, and wolves are the definitive hosts, and certain wild rodents are intermediate hosts. The infection originates from larval penetration through the duodenal wall and transit through the portal vein. Most are trapped in the hepatic sinusoids, but some larvae pass through and are subsequently trapped in the alveolar capillaries. Cysts can form in the liver, the lung, or in both organs. Progressive larval invasion to contiguous regions, as well as occasional metastases to distant sites, leads to massive tissue destruction. When the lung is involved by direct invasion from the diseased liver, typically only the right lower lung field is abnormal, often appearing roentgenographically as an abscess. With hematogenous spread, multiple small cysts can form diffusely in the lung. Typically, pulmonary symptoms are overshadowed by hepatic dysfunction.

Serologic testing, particularly the Em2-enzyme-linked immunosorbent assay (ELISA), is both sensitive and specific and useful to both assist in the diagnosis of the disease and monitor for recurrence. Alveolar echinococcosis is uniformly fatal if not treated. Surgical resection remains the treatment of choice. In cases with limited disease, radical resection can lead to cure. Prolonged drug therapy with mebendazole or albendazole has a significant impact on disease progression.

1. Haque R, Huston CD. Current concepts: amebiasis. *N Engl J Med.* 2003;348:16.
   A concise, overall review of amebiasis.
2. Shamsuzzaman SM, Hashiguchi Y. Thoracic amebiasis. *Clin Chest Med.* 2002;23: 479.
   A detailed, overall review of thoracic amebiasis.

3. Tanyuksel M, Petri WA. Laboratory diagnosis of amebiasis. *Clin Microbiol Rev.* 2003;16:713.

   An overview of amebiasis with a detail discussion of diagnostic strategies, including the potential use of PCR.

4. Stephen SJ, Uragoda CG. Pleuro-pulmonary amoebiasis: a review of 40 cases. *Br J Dis Chest.* 1970;64:96.

   A classic review from Ceylon of pleuropulmonary amebiasis.

5. Cameron EW. The treatment of pleuropulmonary amebiasis with metronidazole. *Chest.* 1978;73:647.

   Describes the management of 140 cases classified by chest radiographic findings; revises the indications for surgical intervention in view of the efficacy of metronidazole.

6. Landay MJ, Setiawan H, Hirsch G, et al. Hepatic and thoracic amebiasis. *AJR Am J Roentgenol.* 1980;135:449.

   Reviews sonographic and radiographic findings in 27 cases of hepatic amebiasis; half had nonspecific findings on chest radiographs, including elevated right hemidiaphragm, basilar infiltrates, and pleural effusions.

7. Huch Boni RA, Peter J, Marincek B. Amebic abscess of the liver manifested as "hemoptysis": US, CT, and MRI findings. *Abdom Imaging.* 1995;20:214.

   A case report of the use of magnetic resonance imaging in diagnosing a bronchohepatic fistula in a patient with amebiasis.

8. Deshmukh H, Prasad S, Patankar T, et al. Percutaneous management of a bronchobiliary fistula complicating ruptured amebic liver abscess. *Am J Gastroenterol.* 1999;94:289.

   A recent case report of external biliary diversion as part of the treatment of a bronchobiliary fistula.

9. McManus DP, Zhang W, Li J, et al. Echinococcis. *Lancet.* 2003;362:1295.

   A concise review of this disease.

10. Eckert J, Deplazes P. Biological, epidemiological, and clinical aspects of echinococcosis, a zoonosis of increasing concern. *Clin Microbiol Rev.* 2004;17:107.

    An extensive, detailed review of echinococcosis.

11. Bottstein B, Reichen J. Hydatid lung disease (echinococcosis/hydatidosis). *Clin Chest Med.* 2002;23:397.

    A detailed review of pulmonary echinococcosis.

12. Amir-Jahed AK, Fardin R, Farzad A, et al. Clinical echinococcosis. *Ann Surg.* 1975; 182:541.

    A retrospective study of 221 patients in Iran with hydatid disease, who were treated before benzimidazoles were available.

13. Sarsam A. Surgery of pulmonary hydatid cysts: review of 155 cases. *J Thorac Cardiovasc Surg.* 1971;62:663.

    A review of the various surgical approaches to treating cystic echinococcosis.

14. Lewal DB. Hydatid disease: biology, pathology, imaging and classification. *Clin Radiol.* 1998;53:863.

    A review of the radiology of hydatid disease, including the nomenclature and sequelae of ruptured cysts.

15. Oztek I, Baloglu H, Demirel D, et al. Cytologic diagnosis of complicated pulmonary unilocular cystic hydatidosis: a study of 131 cases. *Acta Cytol.* 1997;41: 1159.

    Reports on the cytology of E. granulosus *pulmonary cysts.*

16. Mawhorter S, Temeck B, Chang R, et al. Nonsurgical therapy for pulmonary hydatid cyst disease. *Chest.* 1997;112:1432.

    One of a number of case reports in the literature on safely performing percutaneous drainage of pulmonary cysts caused by E. granulosus.

17. Franchi C, Di Vico B, Teggi A. Long-term evaluation of patients with hydatidosis treated with benzimidazole carbamates. *Clin Infect Dis.* 1999;29:304.

    A prospective study of 448 patients with 929 E. granulosus *hydatid cysts (195 cysts in the lung), treated with mebendazole or albendazole and followed up for up to 15 years; 74% responded to treatment, but 25% of those relapsed; however, more than 90% of the relapsed cases responded to additional medical treatment.*

18. Keshmiri M, Baharvahdat H, Fattahi SH, et al. Albendazole versus placebo in treatment of echinococcosis. *Trans R Soc Trop Med Hyg.* 2001;95:190.

   This study compared 400 mg of albendazole twice daily in three cycles of 6 weeks, with 2 weeks between cycles, versus placebo, for the treatment of E. granulosus *pulmonary cysts and found a significant improvement in the treatment group. The authors concluded that patients with uncomplicated hydatid disease should be given a trial of albendazole before surgery is considered.*

19. Senyuz OF, Yesildag E, Celayir S. Albendazole therapy in the treatment of hydatid liver disease. *Surg Today.* 2001;31:487.

   One of a number of small studies suggesting that albendazole may be incorporated in the treatment of E. multilocularis *cystic disease.*

47. PULMONARY INFECTIONS AND COMPLICATIONS IN HIV INFECTED PATIENTS

Denis Jones

Patients infected with HIV are predisposed to a variety of infectious, inflammatory, and neoplastic pulmonary diseases. Over the past decade, significant changes in the spectrum of HIV-related pulmonary complications have been observed after the introduction of highly active antiretroviral therapy (HAART) (i.e., combination of protease inhibitors taken with reverse transcriptase inhibitors) and the widespread use of effective prophylaxis against opportunistic infection. Moreover, changes in population characteristics and risk factors for HIV infection have evolved; AIDS is observed increasingly in women, children, and intravenous drug abusers (IVDAs). Homosexual and bisexual men now represent a decreasing percentage of cases. The most prevalent opportunistic infection in patients infected with HIV is *Pneumocystis carinii* pneumonia (PCP), although the incidence has declined in recent years. Person-to-person airborne transmission is the most likely mode of new infection; however, respiratory isolation of PCP-infected patients is not currently recommended. The risk of infection with PCP in HIV-infected patients increases sharply once the CD4 count drops below 200 cells/mm or there is a history of oropharyngeal candidiasis. In addition, the annual risk of recurrence after an episode of PCP is greater than 60%. For these reasons, all HIV-infected patients with CD4 counts less than 200 or with a prior history of PCP should receive chemoprophylaxis. Primary or secondary prophylaxis can be discontinued in patients who have a response to HAART vigorous enough to raise the CD4 count to more than 200 for a period of 3 months. However, prophylaxis should be reinstituted if the CD4 cell count drops to less than 200. Drugs recommended for the prophylaxis are listed in Table 47-1.

The presentation of PCP is usually insidious with a nonproductive cough, dyspnea, and fever developing over 2 to 3 weeks. This is in contrast to the abrupt onset of symptoms observed in cancer patients. The physical examination is dominated by tachypnea and tachycardia; auscultatory findings are generally minimal or absent. The presence of physical findings on lung examination should raise the possibility of an alternative diagnosis. Symptoms may be mild and permit outpatient management with oral therapy; however, severe hypoxemia mandates hospital admission and intravenous therapy.

Laboratory abnormalities often are nonspecific, revealing lymphopenia and anemia. Serum lactate dehydrogenase is almost always elevated, likely reflecting lung inflammation rather than a specific marker for PCP. The chest radiograph is abnormal in 80 to 90% of cases and typically displays bilateral perihilar interstitial infiltrates that

Table 47-1. Medications for PCP prophylaxis

Drug	Dose	Comments
Trimethoprim-sulfamethoxazole (TMP-SMX)	1 double-strength tablet daily or 1 single-strength tablet daily or 1 double-strength tablet 3×/week	Most effective and most widely recommended Short-term intolerance is common and prophylaxis can frequently be continued.
Pentamidine	300 mg monthly	Given by inhalation
Dapsone	100 mg daily	Ensure patient does not have G6PD deficiency
Atovaquone	1500 mg daily	Give with meals to improve absorption

can progress to diffuse and homogenous opacities. Less common radiographic findings include solitary or multiple nodules, upper lobe infiltrates in patients receiving inhaled pentamidine, pneumatoceles, and pneumothorax. Although the chest radiograph may be normal in 5 to 10% of patients, high-resolution computed tomography (HRCT) may reveal extensive ground-glass attenuation or cystic lesions. An HRCT with normal findings essentially rules out the diagnosis of PCP. Pleural effusions and thoracic lymphadenopathy are suggestive of another diagnosis (e.g., Kaposi's sarcoma or mycobacterial disease).

The arterial PO_2 is abnormal in most cases and is a key prognostic indicator; patients presenting with near-normal oxygenation generally survive. An abnormal carbon monoxide diffusing capacity, oxygen desaturation during exercise, and an abnormal gallium lung scan are sensitive but nonspecific for PCP infection.

Because the organism cannot be cultured, microscopic examination of an appropriate specimen is required to make the diagnosis. Patients with AIDS and PCP have significantly more organisms in their lungs than do PCP patients without AIDS. Based on this higher organism burden, induced sputum has a diagnostic yield of 50 to 90% and should be the initial diagnostic procedure if PCP is suspected. If induced sputum is either negative or not available, bronchoalveolar lavage (BAL) fluid obtained by fiberoptic bronchoscopy should be examined (90–95% sensitivity). Transbronchial or open lung biopsy is seldom needed. However, with an atypical presentation (e.g., focal disease), other diseases become more likely and transbronchial biopsy should be considered. The clinician should be aware that cysts can persist for weeks to months after successful treatment, so a positive result on repeat testing does not necessarily indicate relapse.

Trophic forms of *Pneumocystis* can be detected with modified Papanicolaou or Wright-Giemsa stain. Cysts can be stained with Gomori methenamine silver, toluidine blue O, or calcofluor white. Immunohistochemical stains detect both the trophic forms and cysts and have higher sensitivity and specificity in induced sputum samples than conventional tinctorial stains. However, BAL fluid usually contains such a high density of organisms that immunohistochemistry is unnecessary.

Nucleic acid amplification using polymerase chain reaction (PCR) with respiratory specimens has greater sensitivity and specificity for the diagnosis of PCP than conventional staining. In patients with a positive PCR but a negative smear, treatment is recommended if the patient is immunosuppressed. PCR testing of serum samples has not yet been shown to be useful.

Those with mild cases of PCP can be treated as outpatients with close follow-up; however, hospitalization is usually indicated when the alveolar-arterial oxygen gradient ($P_{[A-a]}O_2$) is greater than 35 mmHg or the chest radiograph is clearly abnormal.

Trimethoprim-sulfamethoxazole is the preferred form of therapy. In moderate to severe disease, parenteral therapy for 3 weeks is preferred. Drugs used in the treatment of PCP are listed in Table 47-2.

Administration of adjunctive corticosteroids is indicated in patients with a PaO_2 < 70 mmHg or $P_{(A-a)}O_2$ >35 mmHg. A recommended treatment regimen is prednisone given orally at a dose of 40 mg twice daily for 5 days, then 40 mg daily on days 6 through 11, and then 20 mg daily on days 12 through 21.

With the widespread use of sulfa drugs for prophylaxis and treatment of PCP, there is growing concern about mutations in the dihydropteroate synthase (DHPS) gene of *P. carinii*. Some investigators have reported a correlation between prior sulfa prophylaxis and the occurrence of this mutation; however, at this time the clinical significance of this mutation is poorly understood.

Pneumothoraces in the setting of PCP can lead to prolonged air leaks and long-term morbidity. Conservative management is associated with high failure rates and prolonged hospitalization. Needle drainage, tube thoracostomy, Heimlich valve drainage, pleurodesis, pleurectomy, video-assisted thoracoscopic surgery, and thoracotomy may be needed. The reported success rates of tube thoracostomy in the evacuation of pneumothorax are variable. Heimlich valve drainage has been shown to facilitate earlier discharge from acute care facilities. Surgery is needed if tube thoracostomy does not resolve the pneumothorax. The reported recurrence rates of spontaneous pneumothorax in AIDS are high (11–60%), with pneumothorax in PCP being an independent predictor of mortality.

The introduction of HAART in patients successfully treated for PCP led to the description of a new phenomenon: "the immune reconstitution syndrome." This syndrome, first described in patients with tuberculosis, is now being increasingly reported in patients with PCP who develop a pneumonic syndrome after PCP treatment and subsequent HAART initiation. During this illness, no pathogens are identified on bronchoscopy, and the BAL CD4/CD8 ratio is much higher than in the initial illness. This suggests that an influx of CD4 cells may be responsible. This syndrome may be severe enough to cause respiratory failure requiring mechanical ventilation.

Bacterial pneumonia remains a common complication of HIV infection. *Streptococcus pneumonia* and *Haemophilus influenzae* are the most common causes of community-acquired pneumonia (CAP). "Atypical" organisms are found in approximately 3% of cases, usually with another organism. Nosocomial organisms are usually associated with advanced disease, recent hospitalization, and prior antibiotic exposure. Although the clinical presentation of CAP is similar in HIV-infected and non–HIV–infected patients, bacteremia occurs more frequently in the presence of HIV, and the incidence and severity increases with worsening immunodeficiency. In HIV-infected patients, the yield from routine sputum cultures in the diagnosis of CAP equals that of other, more invasive diagnostic procedures. Treatment of bacterial pneumonia in patients infected with HIV is no different than in immunocompetent patients, although mortality may be higher. Although pneumococcal vaccination is recommended for HIV-infected patients, there is still debate about its efficacy in these patients.

Mycobacterium tuberculosis (see Chapters 35–37) is a serious threat to patients with HIV. Patients with HIV infection and a positive tuberculin skin test have an 8 to 10% risk per year of developing clinical tuberculosis (TB). For this reason, tuberculin skin testing and appropriate TB prophylaxis are essential in the care of those with HIV infection. In this patient group, 5-mm induration should be considered to represent a positive tuberculin skin test and justify prophylaxis with isoniazid (INH) monotherapy or, alternatively, one of several short-course multidrug combinations with comparable efficacy but a higher incidence of adverse effects. However, recent studies suggest that, in HIV-infected patients, INH monotherapy may provide only temporary protection from TB activation and that combination regimens that include rifampicin may provide longer lasting protection.

TB can occur as a primary infection, or as reactivation of a prior infection, and tends to present earlier in the course of HIV-related disease than most other infectious complications. Chest radiographic findings depend on the degree of immunosuppression.

Table 47-2. Medications used in the treatment of PCP

Medication	Dose	Route	Common adverse reactions	Comments
Trimethoprim-sulfamethoxazole (TMP-SMX)	15–20 mg/kg of the trimethoprim component	Oral or intravenous	Rash, fever, transaminase elevations, pancytopenia and hyperkalemia	First choice of therapy
Pentamidine	4 mg/kg daily	Intravenous	Nephrotoxicity, pancreatitis, leukopenia, arrhythmias and dysglycemia	Switching to pentamidine after failure of TMP-SMX does not improve prognosis
Primaquine plus clindamycin	30 mg daily + 600 mg three times a day	Oral	Abdominal pain, anemia, fever, and hemolysis	Screen for G6PD deficiency
Atovaquone	750 mg twice daily	Oral	Abdominal pain, nausea, anemia, and neutropenia	Should take with meals

Typical infiltrates are most common among patients with normal or mildly diminished CD4 cell counts. With advancing HIV infection, cavitation becomes rare, and nonapical or diffuse infiltrates predominate. The approach to the diagnosis and treatment of TB in the HIV-infected patient is similar to that in patients without AIDS. There is, however, some concern that shorter regimens (24 weeks) may be associated with a higher rate of recurrence or relapse in patients infected with HIV.

In patients in whom HAART is initiated during the treatment of tuberculosis, temporary worsening of TB signs and symptoms is thought to be secondary to immune reconstitution. This phenomenon, also known as the paradoxical response, is seen in as many as 30% of patients. Thorough evaluation to rule out other etiologies is necessary before this diagnosis can be made. In many patients, no change in therapy is required. However, a short course of corticosteroids may be required for those in whom the inflammatory response is exaggerated. This syndrome usually occurs within the first 45 days after initiation of HAART. For this reason, some authorities do not start HAART during the first 2 months of TB therapy.

Although infection resulting from *Mycobacterium avium complex* is common in advanced HIV disease (and is commonly cultured from pulmonary secretions), it is a rare cause of pulmonary signs and symptoms. On the other hand, *Mycobacterium kansasii, Mycobacterium xenopi,* and *Mycobacterium gordonae* can all cause pulmonary disease. Both antimycobacterial therapy and surgical resection have been described in the treatment of *M. xenopi.*

Fungal pneumonia is well described in advanced HIV disease. Commonly reported organisms are *Cryptococcus neoformans, Histoplasma capsulatum, Coccidioides immitis,* and *Blastomycosis dermatitidis.* Disseminated infection is often part of the clinical presentation, and the radiographic findings are extremely varied.

The presentation of aspergillosis (see Chapter 42) in the HIV-infected host is varied. In HIV-infected patients with pulmonary mycetoma, the clinical course differs in several ways from that seen in the immunocompetent host. HIV-infected patients are less likely to have hemoptysis but have a greater risk of disease progression. Invasive aspergillosis is associated with an extremely high mortality rate. However, combination therapy with antiretroviral and antifungal therapy has been reported to improve the outcome in these patients.

Although rarely reported, bronchiolitis obliterans organizing pneumonia (BOOP) should be considered in the differential diagnosis of bilateral patchy infiltrates in a patient with AIDS. The clinical presentation is nonspecific, with fever, cough, dyspnea, and night sweats reported most commonly. The diagnosis can be made with open or thoracoscopic lung biopsy and the response to corticosteroids is generally good. The recommended dose and duration of therapy is the same as that used in the immunocompetent host.

Kaposi's sarcoma (KS) is the most common HIV-related malignancy involving the lungs and occurs almost exclusively in homosexual or bisexual men. Mucocutaneous manifestations are seen in the majority of patients with pulmonary disease. Fever and dyspnea are the most common symptoms at presentation, and the chest radiograph may show patchy perihilar infiltrates with or without pleural effusions. Although lymphadenopathy may be seen, bulky disease suggests an alternative diagnosis. The visualization of characteristic reddish, flat, or raised endobronchial lesions is usually diagnostic. Biopsy of these lesions is usually not performed owing to the risk of bleeding and poor diagnostic yield from the small amount of tissue obtained.

In the absence of endobronchial disease, open lung biopsy may be necessary for diagnosis. Before the introduction of HAART, KS carried a very poor prognosis, with median survival for responders to chemotherapy of less than 12 months. The administration of HAART to patients receiving chemotherapy significantly improves survival.

Bronchogenic carcinoma occurs more frequently in HIV-infected patients in the post-HAART era. Unfortunately, the outcome remains poor despite HAART. HIV-infected patients are also at risk of developing B cell lymphoma, in which pulmonary involvement is common.

HIV-related pulmonary hypertension is a complication of HIV infection that has become recognized with increasing frequency over the past few years. Recently, an association between infection with human herpes virus (HHV)-8 and pulmonary hypertension was described. Although these patients carry a poor prognosis, there is some evidence to suggest that the introduction of HAART may be of benefit in the management of this disease.

1. Anonymous. 2002 USPHS/IDSA Guidelines for the Prevention of Opportunistic Infections in Persons Infected with Human Immunodeficiency Virus. U.S. Public Health Service and Infectious Diseases Society of America. *MMWR.* 2002;51:1.
   Comprehensive, up-to-date, evidence-based recommendations for prophylaxis of HIV-related infections.
2. Barry SM, Lipman MC, Deery AR, et al. Immune reconstitution pneumonitis following Pneumocystis carinii pneumonia in HIV-infected subjects. *HIV Med.* 2002;3:207–211.
   Indolent infection with P. carinii *may lead to inflammatory pneumonitis after the institution of HAART.*
3. Bower M, Powles T, Nelson M, et al. HIV-related lung cancer in the era of highly active antiretroviral therapy. *AIDS.* 2003;17:371–375.
   A description of the incidence of lung cancer in HIV-infected patients during the HAART era.
4. Bozzette SA, Sattler FR, Chiu J, et al. A controlled trial of early adjunctive treatment with cortico-steroids for Pneumocystis carinii pneumonia in the acquired immunodeficiency syndrome. California Collaborative Treatment Group. *N Engl J Med.* 1990;323:1451.
   In 251 patients, early adjunctive steroids reduced the risk of oxygenation failure from 30 to 14% and of death from 23 to 11%.
5. Cool CD, Rai PR, Yeager ME, et al. Expression of human herpesvirus 8 in pulmonary hypertension. *N Engl J Med.* 2003;349:1113–1122.
6. Cordero E, Pachon J, Rivero A, et al. Usefulness of sputum culture for diagnosis of bacterial pneumonia in HIV-infected patients. *Eur J Clin Microbiol Infect Dis.* 2002;21:362–367.
   Routine sputum cultures have a diagnostic yield comparable to other standard, more invasive diagnostic methods.
7. DeLorenzo LJ, Huang CT, Maguire GP, et al. Roentgenographic patterns of Pneumocystis carinii pneumonia in 104 patients with AIDS. *Chest.* 1987;91:323.
   Bilateral interstitial infiltrates occurred in 75%, but alveolar infiltrates (25%), cysts (7%), unilateral infiltrates (5%), and other atypical features were not rare.
8. Greenberg AK, Knapp J, Rom WN, et al. Clinical presentation of pulmonary mycetoma in HIV-infected patients. *Chest.* 2002;122:886–892.
   Presentation and outcome of aspergillosis in HIV-infected patients.
9. Gordin FM, Simon GL, Wofsy CB, et al. Adverse reactions to trimethoprim-sulfamethoxazole in patients with the acquired immunodeficiency syndrome. *Ann Intern Med.* 1984;100:495.
   Adverse reactions, including rash, fever, neutropenia, and transaminase elevation, occurred in 29 of 35 patients (79%) and was dose limiting in 19 (54%).
10. Huang L, Hecht FM, Stansell JD, et al. Suspected Pneumocystis carinii pneumonia with a negative induced sputum examination: is early bronchoscopy useful? *Am J Respir Crit Care Med.* 1995;151:1866.
    Large series of patients with suspected PCP and negative induced sputum in a center where the yield of induced sputum is more than 90%. Even so, bronchoscopy had a high yield for PCP and other pathogens.
11. Huang L, Schnapp LM, Gruden JF, et al. Presentation of AIDS-related pulmonary Kaposi's sarcoma diagnosed by bronchoscopy. *Am J Respir Crit Care Med.* 1996;153:1385.
    The largest case series published. Chest radiograph and serum lactate dehydrogenase, not clinical presentation, distinguished those with and without concomitant infection.
12. Johnson JL, Okwera A, Hom DL, et al. Duration of efficacy of treatment of latent tuberculosis infection in HIV-infected adults. *AIDS.* 2001;33:1762–1769.

Six months of isoniazid for latent tuberculosis infection is initially protective but efficacy is lost within a year of therapy.

13. Kagawa FT, Kirsch CM, Yenokida GG, et al. Serum lactate dehydrogenase activity in patients with AIDS and Pneumocystis carinii pneumonia. *Chest.* 1988;94:1031.
    Findings in all 30 patients were abnormal.

14. Khater FJ, Moorman JP, Myers JW, et al. Bronchiolitis obliterans organizing pneumonia as a manifestation of AIDS: case report and literature review. *J Infect.* 2004;49:159–164.
    Description of presentation, diagnosis, and treatment of BOOP in the HIV-infected patient.

15. Kovacs JA, Ng VL, Masur H, et al. Diagnosis of Pneumocystis carinii pneumonia: improved detection in sputum with use of monoclonal antibodies. *N Engl J Med.* 1988;318:589.
    Immunofluorescent staining was 92% sensitive, compared with 80% for the best tinctorial stain, toluidine blue O.

16. Kovacs JA, Gill VJ, Meshnick S, et al. New insights into transmission, diagnosis and drug treatment of Pneumocystis carinii pneumonia. *JAMA.* 2001;286:2450–2460.
    Gene mutations provide evidence for person-to-person transmission of P. carinii.

17. Koval CE, Gigliotti F, Nevins D, et al. Immune reconstitution syndrome after successful treatment of Pneumocystis carinii pneumonia in a man with human immunodeficiency virus type 1 infection. *Clin Infect Dis.* 2002;35:491–493.
    Pneumonitis following improvement in immune function.

18. Leoung GS, Feigal DW Jr, Montgomery AB, et al. Aerosolized pentamidine for prophylaxis against Pneumocystis carinii pneumonia: the San Francisco community prophylaxis trial. *N Engl J Med.* 1990;323:769.
    Aerosolized pentamidine was 50 to 75% effective.

19. Lopez-Palomo C, Martin-Zamorano M, Benitez E, et al. Pneumonia in HIV-infected patients in the HAART era: Incidence, risk, and impact of the pneumococcal vaccination. *Med Virol.* 2004;72:517–524.
    Evaluates the efficacy of pneumococcal vaccination in HIV-infected patients.

20. Magnenat JL, Nicod LP, Auckenthaler R, et al. Mode of presentation and diagnosis of bacterial pneumonia in human immunodeficiency virus-infected patients. *Am Rev Respir Dis.* 1991;144:917.
    Half of patients taken to bronchoscopy for undiagnosed HIV-related pneumonia had an atypical presentation of bacterial infection.

21. Masur H, Ognibene FP, Yarchoan R, et al. CD4 counts as predictors of opportunistic pneumonias in human immunodeficiency virus (HIV) infection. *Ann Intern Med.* 1989;111:223.
    CD4 counts obtained within 60 days were less than 200 in 46 of 49 episodes and less than 250 in 48 of 49 episodes. Patients with higher counts had other diseases.

22. Metersky ML, Colt HG, Olson LK, et al. AIDS-related spontaneous pneumothorax: risk factors and treatment. *Chest.* 1995;108:946.
    A large case series with multivariate analysis. Pneumatoceles and prophylactic aerosolized pentamidine predicted risk of pneumothorax. Surgical and chemical pleurodesis prevented recurrence.

23. Miller RF, Foley NM, Kessel D, et al. Community-acquired lobar pneumonia in patients with HIV infection and AIDS. *Thorax.* 1994;49:367.
    In order, the most common pathogens were S. pneumoniae, S. aureus, P. carinii, H. influenzae, and P. aeruginosa.

24. Narita M, Ashkin D, Hollender ES, et al. Paradoxical worsening of tuberculosis following antiretroviral therapy in patients with AIDS. *Am J Respir Crit Care Med.* 1998;158:157.
    Combination retroviral therapy initiated during treatment for TB induced temporary worsening of signs and symptoms in one third of patients, although usually not severe enough to warrant discontinuation of therapy. The phenomenon was associated with the return of a positive purified protein derivative (PPD) skin test and likely represented enhanced immune response to infection with TB.

25. Sattler FR, et al. Comparison of trimetrexate with leucovorin versus trimethoprim-sulfamethoxazole for moderate-severe episodes of Pneumocystis carinii pneumonia in patients with AIDS. *J Infect Dis*. 1994;170:165.

Trimethoprim-sulfamethoxazole therapy was superior to trimetrexate with leucovorin for patients presenting withP(A-a)o$_2$ greater than 30 mmHg, although trimetrexate was better tolerated.

26. Schneider MM, Hoepelman AI, Eeftinck Schattenkerk JK, et al. A controlled trial of aerosolized pentamidine or trimethoprim-sulfamethoxazole as primary prophylaxis against Pneumocystis carinii pneumonia in patients with human immunodeficiency virus infection. *N Engl J Med*. 1992;327:1836.

Of patients on monthly aerosolized pentamidine and patients on once or twice daily trimethoprim-sulfamethoxazole, 11% and 0, respectively, developed first-episode Pneumocystis *pneumonia.*

27. Selwyn PA, Pumerantz AS, Durante A, et al. Clinical predictors of Pneumocystis carinii pneumonia, bacterial pneumonia and tuberculosis in HIV-infected patients. *AIDS*. 1998;12:885.

At admission, simple clinical variables differentiate TB, PCP, and bacterial pneumonia.

28. Shafer RW, Kim DS, Weiss JP, et al. Extrapulmonary tuberculosis in patients with human immunodeficiency virus infection. *Medicine (Baltimore)*. 1991;70:384.

Diagnosis was often delayed because of decreased PPD reactivity and usually negative sputum smears (despite 90% of sputum eventually growing Mycobacterium tuberculosis*). Aspirates of lymph nodes, bone marrow, and the liver had the highest immediate yield.*

29. Staikowsky F, Lafon B, Guidet B, et al. Mechanical ventilation for Pneumocystis carinii pneumonia in patients with the acquired immunodeficiency syndrome: is the prognosis really improved? *Chest*. 1993;104:756.

Mortality rate was 50% if respiratory failure developed within 5 days of initial medical therapy and 95% if it developed after 5 days.

30. Toma E, Fournier S, Dumont M, et al. Clindamycin/primaquine versus trimethoprim-sulfamethoxazole as primary therapy for Pneumocystis carinii pneumonia in AIDS: a randomized, double-blind pilot trial. *Clin Infect Dis*. 1993;17:178.

Combination clindamycin-primaquine with trimethoprim-sulfamethoxazole as primary treatment for mild to moderately severe PCP. Efficacy of both regimens was equal, with no significant difference in toxicity, survival, or rate of relapse.

31. Thomas CF, Limper AH. Pneumocystis pneumonia. *N Engl J Med*. 350;2487–2498.

Comprehensive review of Pneumocystis *pneumonia, clinical presentation, diagnosis, treatment and biology of the disease.*

32. Visconti E, Ortona E, Mencarini P, et al. Mutations in dihydropteroate synthase gene of Pneumocystis carinii in HIV patients with Pneumocystis carinii pneumonia. *Int J Antimicrob Agents*. 2001;18:547–551.

Genetic mutations in P. carinii *occur as a result of selective pressure from sulfa therapy. Such mutations may not translate into worse outcome or nonresponse to therapy.*

33. Weverling GJ, Mocroft A, Ledergerber B, et al. Discontinuation of Pneumocystis carinii pneumonia prophylaxis after start of highly active antiretroviral therapy in HIV-1 infection. *Lancet*. 1999;353:1293.

During 247 person-years of follow-up after discontinuation of prophylaxis at median CD4 count of 270, no cases of PCP developed. Almost all had been receiving primary prophylaxis.

34. White DA, Stover DE. Pulmonary complication of HIV infection. *Clin Chest Med*. 1996;17:621.

A review of essentially all major clinical issues relating to HIV-related lung disease. Some of the chapters: P. carinii; *Mycobacterial complications of HIV infection; Approach to the patient with pulmonary disease.*

35. Woldehanna S, Volmink J. Treatment of latent tuberculosis infection in HIV infected persons. *Cochrane Database Syst Rev*. 2004;CD000171.

Review of the treatment of latent tuberculosis infection.

36. Wolff AJ, O'Donnell AE. HIV-related pulmonary infections: a review of the recent literature. *Curr Opin Pulm Med.* 2003;9:210–214.

   The authors review some of the more recent literature pertaining to HIV-related pulmonary infections.

37. Zuper JP, Calmy A, Evison JM, et al. Pulmonary arterial hypertension related to HIV infection: improved hemodynamics and survival associated with antiretroviral therapy. *Clin Infect Dis.* 2004;38:1178–1185.

   Antiretroviral therapy improved survival in HIV-infected patients with pulmonary hypertension.

48. HOSPITAL-ACQUIRED PNEUMONIA

Kim M. Kerr

Hospital-acquired pneumonia (HAP) is defined as pneumonia occurring 48 hours or later after hospital admission. The definition excludes pulmonary infection that may be incubating at the time of admission. Pneumonia is the second most common hospital-acquired infection, carrying the highest mortality rate of all nosocomial diseases. Between 5 and 10 cases of HAP occur per 1000 hospital admissions, but the incidence is 6 to 20 times higher in patients receiving mechanical ventilation. In patients who are mechanically ventilated, the development of pneumonia (ventilator-associated pneumonia, [VAP]) is associated with significant morbidity and higher mortality and substantially increases the cost of patient care.

In the immunocompetent host, HAP can be divided into early-onset and late-onset infections. Early pneumonia occurs during the first 4 days of hospitalization and is often caused by community-acquired pathogens such as *Streptococcus pneumoniae*, methicillin-sensitive *Staphylococcus aureus*, and *Haemophilus influenzae*. Specific risk factors can alter likely pathogens. For instance, if a patient has a witnessed aspiration, anaerobes, enteric gram-negative bacilli, and *S. aureus* should be considered. Recent thoracoabdominal surgery or the presence of an obstructing foreign body are additional risk factors for anaerobic pneumonias. Patients with coma, head injury, recent influenza, recent intravenous drug use, diabetes mellitus, or chronic renal failure are at increased risk for *S. aureus* pneumonias. Corticosteroids predispose patients to pneumonias from fungi, *Pseudomonas aeruginosa*, and, in some regions of the country, *Legionella* species.

Late-onset HAP, occurring 4 days or more after admission, is more commonly caused by *Enterobacter* species, *S. aureus*, *P. aeruginosa*, or *Acinetobacter* species. Resistant organisms such as methicillin-resistant *S. aureus* (MRSA), *P. aeruginosa*, and *Acinetobacter baumannii* tend to emerge after prolonged mechanical ventilation (>7 days), prior antibiotic use, and the use of broad-spectrum antibiotics (third-generation cephalosporins, fluoroquinolone, or imipenem).

Understanding the pathogenesis of HAP may help in developing mechanisms of prevention. In the normal nonsmoking host, the upper respiratory tract is colonized with aerobic and anaerobic bacteria, whereas the respiratory tract below the vocal cords is sterile. Changes in host defenses can lead to inoculation of the lower respiratory tract with potentially pathogenic bacteria. Colonization and potentially fatal infection can follow inoculation.

Although pathogens can gain access to the lung by inhalation, hematogenous seeding, and contiguous spread, aspiration is the major route of bacterial access in patients with and without endotracheal tubes. Organisms such as *P. aeruginosa* can be inoculated directly into the endotracheal tube of intubated patients, whereas *Enterobacteriaceae* usually colonize the oropharynx before the trachea.

Mechanical ventilation almost always requires the presence of an artificial airway (endotracheal tube or tracheostomy tube). However, the presence of such an airway reduces the effectiveness of the cough reflex, compromises mucociliary clearance, can cause direct injury to the tracheal epithelial surface, and provides a direct pathway for pathogens from the intensive care unit (ICU) environment to the lower respiratory tract. A biofilm of bacteria-laden accretions on the luminal surface of the endotracheal tube can also contribute to the development of VAP if accretions dislodge into distal airways. Novel solutions to the biofilm problem include the development of less-adhesive polymers to prevent accumulation of infected material in the lumen of the tube or coating the tube with antimicrobial agents. Aspiration around the cuff of the endotracheal tube is another mechanism by which bacteria can access the lower respiratory tract. To reduce the amount of secretions pooling on top of the endotracheal tube cuff, a specific endotracheal tube (HI-LO EVAC tube, Mallinckrodt, St. Louis, Mo.) was designed with a separate lumen that allows removal of secretions from the subglottic space above the tube. Randomized trials have shown a reduction in the incidence of VAP with the use of this technique. Problems with the use of this device are the additional cost and the need to have these endotracheal tubes available when patients undergo tracheal intubation (emergency room, operating room, ICU, wards). Noninvasive ventilation has been shown to reduce the need for endotracheal intubation and decrease the likelihood of HAP and should be considered in appropriate patients.

Nasogastric feeding tubes (NGT) have been implicated as a risk factor for pneumonia, presumably because NGT increase the incidence of gastroesophageal reflux and aspiration. The supine head position also has been linked to an increased incidence of aspiration and bacterial colonization of the lower airways in ventilated patients and is a risk factor for the development of VAP. Clinical data suggest that the simple maneuver of elevating the head of the bed, especially for patients with feeding tubes, may be a safe and inexpensive means of lowering the incidence of VAP.

The role of gastric colonization in facilitating VAP is controversial and has generated multiple clinical trials yielding conflicting data. Central to the controversy is the relationship between VAP, gastric colonization, and stress ulcer prophylaxis. The acidic environment of the gastric lumen prevents bacterial growth under normal physiologic circumstances. However, gastric acidity can be reduced by critical illness, by advanced age, and by administration of antacids or H_2 antagonists. The cytoprotective agent, sucralfate, has been claimed to prevent stress ulcers without altering gastric acidity. There have been 7 meta analyses of more than 20 randomized, controlled clinical trials trying to address the issue of the effect of stress ulcer prophylaxis on the development of VAP. Four studies reported a significant decrease in VAP with the use of sucralfate versus H_2 antagonists, and three studies showed a nonsignificant trend toward a reduction in VAP with the use of sucralfate. Given its relatively low cost and safe pharmacologic profile, sucralfate is an appealing way of providing stress-related upper gastrointestinal (GI) bleeding prophylaxis. However, sucralfate is not as effective as H_2 antagonists in preventing upper GI bleeding and one must weigh the benefit of the potential decreased risk of VAP against the potential decreased protection against GI bleeding. At present, there are no data on proton pump inhibitors for stress ulcer prophylaxis and the risk of VAP. In summary, the optimal agent that minimizes the risk of both stress ulcers and VAP has yet to be determined.

Although the role of gastric colonization in VAP is uncertain, convincing evidence indicates that colonization of the oropharynx often precedes colonization of the trachea and subsequent development of VAP. Selective decontamination of the digestive tract (SDD) is a strategy designed to prevent oropharyngeal and gastric colonization with aerobic gram-negative bacilli and *Candida* species without altering the anaerobic flora of the gut. Some proposed regimens use a combination of nonabsorbable antibiotics applied as a paste to the oropharynx or given through the NGT, whereas others also include a short course of a systemic antibiotic, such as intravenous cefotaxime. Some clinical trials have demonstrated a decrease in the rates of lower respiratory tract infections with SDD; others, however, have found no difference in the incidence of VAP. Because of concerns about the emergence of antibiotic-resistant organisms with these regimens, the routine use of SDD to prevent VAP is not recommended at present.

The diagnosis of HAP, and in particular VAP, has been the subject of numerous studies and heated debates. It is generally accepted that relying solely on clinical criteria (e.g., fever, leukocytosis, purulent tracheal secretions, and a new or progressive infiltrate on chest radiographs) often can be misleading. What has yet to be agreed on is the role of blind and bronchoscopically guided culture techniques in the diagnosis of VAP. At issue for all microbiologic techniques are (1) the accuracy and reproducibility of the collection methods used, (2) the appropriate bacteriologic thresholds to define pneumonia, (3) the costs and risks associated with each procedure, and (4) the effect of the techniques on overall clinical outcomes. One problem in assessing the various diagnostic maneuvers is that no true gold standard for accuracy exists with which to compare diagnostic techniques, such as quantitative tracheal aspirates, quantitative bronchoalveolar lavage (BAL), or protected brush specimens. Even when open lung biopsy has been performed, significant interobserver variability has been noted between pathologists when making the diagnosis of pneumonia based on histologic criteria.

Because of the significant questions regarding the sensitivity, specificity, and reproducibility of invasive diagnostic techniques for the diagnosis of HAP, a conservative approach seems warranted. When nosocomial pneumonia is suspected, a sputum or tracheal aspirate specimen should be obtained for Gram's stain and culture. The Gram's stain allows for the evaluation of the quality of the respiratory sample. Finding more than 10 squamous epithelial cells per low-powered field in an expectorated sputum specimen suggests oropharyngeal contamination; culture results will likely be unreliable. In addition, if the sample demonstrates fewer than 10 neutrophils per low-powered field, a diagnosis other than pneumonia should be suspected. However, the absence of neutrophils does not conclusively exclude an infectious process, because factors such as sampling errors and leukopenia can make this finding misleading. In the intubated patient, contamination of oropharyngeal specimens is less of a concern, but colonization of the endotracheal tube lumen itself can confound the interpretation of microbiologic studies. Cultures of tracheal aspirates are very sensitive for detecting the organism responsible for the pneumonia, but they are not very specific. Differentiating organisms that are colonizers from true pathogens is extremely difficult. Semiquantitative cultures can provide information regarding the relative number of pathogens in the specimen, but will not necessarily distinguish between colonizing and infecting bacteria. In addition, semiquantitative cultures are not available at all institutions, and many patients who develop HAP are already receiving antibiotics that may alter the results of this technique. Blood cultures should be obtained in the evaluation of suspected HAP, as should pleural fluid analysis in patients with pleural effusion. Isolation of organisms from these normally sterile fluids is diagnostic.

Treatment of nosocomial pneumonia should be initiated promptly and not await the results of microbiologic tests. Early use of appropriate antibiotic therapy, before obtaining culture results, appears to have the greatest likelihood of improving patient outcome. The American Thoracic Society published recommendations that, along with local (hospital/ICU) resistance patterns, may help in selecting appropriate antibiotics for empiric treatment of HAP. Consideration of previous antibiotics the patient may have received is also necessary when selecting empiric coverage for HAP. Inadequate initial empiric antibiotic therapy most frequently results from omission of treatment for MRSA or gram-negative bacteria (*P. aeruginosa, Acinetobacter* species, *Klebsiella pneumoniae,* and *Enterobacter* species) with resistance to previously used antibiotics and is associated with a high mortality.

Of particular relevance to the choice of empiric antibiotic regimens for HAP are (1) the presence or absence of underlying medical conditions; (2) the time during the hospital course that the patient developed HAP (early <4 days, or late >4 days); and (3) the presence of specific risk factors for infection with particular organisms. Previously healthy patients who develop early-onset HAP can usually be treated with a second-generation cephalosporin, a nonpseudomonal third-generation cephalosporin, or a combination β-lactam/β-lactamase inhibitor. Those who develop late-onset HAP, are critically ill, or have recently been on antibiotics should receive broader antibiotic coverage to include resistant and virulent organisms such as *P. aeruginosa, Acineto-bacter* and *Enterobacter* species, and MRSA. Empiric therapy in these circumstances commonly includes two synergistic antipseudomonal agents as well as vancomycin. Hospital-acquired *Pseudomonas* infections almost always occur in patients who have previously received antibiotics, so reuse of the same class of antibiotics should be avoided in selecting initial empiric therapy. The spectrum of antibiotic coverage frequently can be narrowed 2 to 3 days into the treatment course, based on culture and sensitivity results and on the patient's response. Tailoring of antibiotic treatment as soon as possible is important to minimize the development of resistant organisms and to avoid the cost and adverse effects of unnecessary medications. Treatment of specific organisms is addressed elsewhere in this book. The duration of therapy is usually 7 to 21 days, based on the severity of illness, the infecting pathogen, and the rapidity of clinical response.

1. Hospital-acquired pneumonia in adults: diagnosis, assessment of severity, initial antimicrobial therapy, and preventive strategies. A consensus statement, American Thoracic Society, November, 1995. *Am J Respir Crit Care Med.* 1996;153:1711.
   Guidelines for the initial antimicrobial therapy in hospital-acquired pneumonia. Supported by 110 references.
2. Bonten MJ, Gaillard CA, de Leeuw PW, et al. Role of colonization of the upper intestinal tract in the pathogenesis of ventilator-associated pneumonia. *Clin Infect Dis.* 1997;24:309.
   A critical assessment and comparison of 9 studies analyzing the sequence of bacterial colonization leading to respiratory tract colonization / VAP and 13 studies comparing the effects of sucralfate or acid-reducing agents on the incidence of VAP. The conclusion is that the results do not support that the gastropulmonary route of colonization is important in the pathogenesis of VAP and that sucralfate does not provide a preventive effect with respect to VAP.
3. Carter AB, Hornick DB. Therapy for ventilator-associated pneumonia. *Clin Chest Med.* 1999;20:681.
   A concise review of the microbiology of ventilator-associated pneumonia, empiric therapy, and modifications necessary in empiric therapy when the cause of VAP is identified. Other issues covered include antimicrobial resistance, tissue penetration, and pharmacodynamics.
4. Chastre J, Fagon J. Ventilator-associated pneumonia. *Am J Respir Crit Care Med.* 2002;165:867–903.
   An extensive review of the literature published between 1980 and 2001 on the epidemiology, diagnosis, and treatment of VAP.
5. Chastre J, Wolff M, Fagon J, et al. Comparison of 8 vs 15 days of antibiotic therapy for ventilator-associated pneumonia in adults. *JAMA.* 2003;290:2588–2598.
   Four hundred and one patients with VAP were randomized to 8 or 15 days of antibiotics. There was no difference in mortality, recurrent infection, duration of mechanical ventilation, or length of ICU stay between the two groups. Those with VAP caused by nonfermenting gram-negative bacilli who were treated with 8 days had a higher pulmonary infection recurrence than those who received 15 days of antibiotics.
6. Collard HR, Saint S, Matthay M. Prevention of ventilator-associated pneumonia: an evidence-based systematic review. *Ann Intern Med.* 2003;138:494–501.
   A systematic review of the literature published between 1966 and 2001 addressing methods of prevention of VAP.
7. Corley DE, Kirtland SH, Winterbauer RH, et al. Reproducibility of the histologic diagnosis of pneumonia among a panel of four pathologists: analysis of the gold standard. *Chest.* 1997;112:458.
   This study challenges histology as a gold standard in the diagnosis of VAP. Recognition of histologic pneumonia varies among pathologists.
8. Fagon JY, Maillet JM, Novara A. Hospital-acquired pneumonia: methicillin resistance and intensive care unit admission. *Am J Med.* 1998;104:17S.

A review of the importance of S. aureus as a pathogen in HAP and risk factors for the acquisition of MRSA.

9. Gallego M, Rello J. Diagnostic testing for ventilator-associated pneumonia. *Clin Chest Med.* 1999;20:671.
   Reviews the interpretation of the various diagnostic tests used in the evaluation of patients with suspected VAP.

10. Gerbeaux P, Ledoray V, Boussuges A, et al. Diagnosis of nosocomial pneumonia in mechanically ventilated patients. *Am J Respir Crit Care Med.* 1998;157:76.
    Results using BAL are reasonably reproducible in the absence of pneumonia, but in the presence of pneumonia, BAL is not repeatable.

11. Ibrahim EH, Tracy L, Hill C, et al. The occurrence of ventilator-associated pneumonia in a community hospital: risk factors and clinical outcomes. *Chest.* 2001; 120:555–561.
    Prospective study of a medical and a surgical ICU in a community hospital. VAP developed in 15% of the 880 mechanically ventilated patients. Logistic regression analysis demonstrated that tracheostomy, multiple central venous lines, reintubation, and the use of antacids were independently associated with the development of VAP.

12. Iregui M, Ward S, Sherman G, et al. Clinical importance of delays in the initiation of appropriate antibiotic treatment for ventilator-associated pneumonia. *Chest.* 2002;122:262–268.
    Delay in appropriate antibiotic treatment in occurred in 30.8% patients with VAP and was associated with a higher mortality (odds ratio [OR] 7.68). The most common reason for the delay in appropriate therapy was a delay in writing the antibiotic orders.

13. Kirtland SH, Corley DE,Winterbauer RH, et al. The diagnosis of ventilator-associated pneumonia: a comparison of histologic, microbiologic, and clinical criteria. *Chest.* 1997;112:445.
    No combination of clinical criteria correlated with the presence or absence of histologic pneumonia. Quantitative cultures (protected specimen brushing [PSB], BAL) did not accurately separate the histologic pneumonia and nonpneumonia groups. Tracheal aspirate had a sensitivity of 87% in recognizing bacterial species simultaneously present in lung parenchyma.

14. Kollef MH. Epidemiology and risk factors for nosocomial pneumonia: emphasis on prevention. *Clin Chest Med.* 1999;20:653.
    An excellent overview of the epidemiology and pathophysiology of HAP and a review of the recent literature on prevention of VAP.

15. Kollef MH, Ward S. The influence of mini-BAL cultures on patient outcomes: implications for the antibiotic management of ventilator-associated pneumonia. *Chest.* 1998;113:412.
    Selection of appropriate initial antibiotic therapy improves the mortality rate in patients with suspected VAP. The most common organisms not appropriately covered with initial therapy were gram-negative bacteria resistant to a prescribed third-generation cephalosporin.

16. Luna CM, Vujacich P, Niederman MS, et al. Impact of BAL data on the therapy and outcome of ventilator-associated pneumonia. *Chest.* 1997;111:676.
    Delay of adequate therapy until bronchoscopy is performed or until BAL results are known results in increased mortality in patients with suspected VAP.

17. Rello J, Olendorf D, Oster G, et al. Epidemiology and outcomes of ventilator-associated pneumonia in a large US database. *Chest.* 2002;122:2115–2121.
    US study with 842 VAP patients and 2,243. control subjects. The incidence of VAP was 9.3%; the mean interval between intubation and development of VAP was 3.3 ± 6.6 days. VAP resulted in an increase in ICU/hospital stay, duration of mechanical ventilation, and hospital charges.

18. Rello J, Torres A, Ricart M, et al. Ventilator-associated pneumonia by Staphylococcus aureus: comparison of methicillin-resistant and methicillin-sensitive episodes. *Am J Respir Crit Care Med.* 1994;150:1545.
    Risk factors for developing methicillin-resistant S. aureus ventilator-associated pneumonia (MRSA VAP) include previous antibiotic therapy, therapy with steroids,

mechanical ventilation more than 6 days, age older than 25 years, and preceding chronic obstructive pulmonary disease. MRSA VAP had a greater bacteremic rate and a worse outcome than MSSA VAP.

19. Tablan OC, Anderson LJ, Besser R, et al. Guidelines for preventing health-care-associated pneumonia, 2003: recommendations of CDC and the Health Care Infection Control Practices Advisory Committee. *MMWR Recomm Rep.* 2004;53:1–36.

    Extensive, detailed review of the most recent Centers for Disease Control and Prevention (CDC) guidelines for the prevention of pneumonia in acute-care hospitals and other healthcare settings.

20. Trouillet JL, Chastre J, Vuagnat A, et al. Ventilator-associated pneumonia caused by potentially drug-resistant bacteria. *Am J Respir Crit Care Med.* 1998;157:531.

    Using logistic regression analysis, three variables were identified as risk factors for the development of VAP with potentially drug-resistant bacteria: mechanical ventilation more than 7 days, prior antibiotic use, and prior use of broad-spectrum antibiotics.

IV. AIRWAYS DISEASE

49. ASTHMA: CLINICAL PRESENTATION AND DIAGNOSIS

Timothy D. Bigby

Asthma is characterized clinically by reversible airway obstruction in association with symptoms of dyspnea, cough, and sputum production. Asthma is defined in pathophysiologic terms by emphasizing the physiologic finding of airway hyperresponsiveness and the pathologic finding of airway inflammation.

Asthma is a common disorder worldwide. The World Health Organization recently stated that approximately 300 million people have asthma. Asthma is not distributed equally throughout the world; industrialized, Western countries have a higher incidence. In the United States, asthma afflicts 17 to 18 million people, including 5 million children. Asthma is the most common chronic disease of children. It is more common in urban than rural populations, and the incidence is higher among minority populations. Careful epidemiologic studies indicate that most asthma begins in early childhood, although it can develop at any age. At least one half of children who develop asthma will have remission as adults, but adult-onset asthma rarely abates. The prevalence, severity, and mortality rate associated with asthma have visibly increased over the last 40 years. The explanation is unclear, but urban living conditions, exposure to oxidant pollutants, passive smoking, and even current therapies have been implicated. More recent concerns have been raised about relationships to the modernization of western culture, including a decreased incidence of common childhood infectious diseases, widespread antibiotic use, declining physical fitness in children, and rising incidence of obesity beginning in childhood.

The hallmark of airway pathology in asthma is mixed inflammatory cell infiltration; eosinophils are the most striking feature, but these infiltrates also include large numbers of less easily recognized mast cells, neutrophils, lymphocytes, and macrophages. The inflammatory changes are also associated with denudation of airway epithelium and mucous gland hypertrophy. Long-standing asthma can be associated with subepithelial fibrosis and smooth muscle hypertrophy. Currently, substantial interest is seen in this remodeling of the airway, its long-term consequences, and potential treatments.

The etiology of asthma remains enigmatic. It does not appear to be a single disease, but a syndrome. An older hypothesis suggested that so-called *intrinsic asthma* (i.e., asthma in individuals without identifiable triggers) might be neurally mediated. However, a distinct abnormality of the sympathetic, parasympathetic, or peptidergic nervous systems has not been found in common for asthmatics. Mutations of the β_2 adrenergic receptor have now been described, but these mutations may be more important in dictating response to treatment. Substantial data support an allergic pathogenesis mediated predominantly by both inhaled and systemic antigens. Allergy appears to play a central role in sustained wheezing in early childhood that can be characterized clinically as asthma. Cytokines released by Th2 lymphocytes are increasingly recognized as important in allergic and, possibly, all asthma. Pivotal cytokines include interleukins 13, 4, 5, and 9. The regulation of the adaptive immune response and its interface with the innate immune response appear to play key roles in the pathogenesis of allergic asthma. This is an intense focus of investigation. This interface has been suggested to play a role in the increase in asthma prevalence. An attempt to link the increase in asthma in the industrialized world to improved healthcare and decreased childhood infections has been termed the *hygiene hypothesis*. If hygiene does play a role in the development of asthma, it may do so through the interface between the innate and adaptive immune response.

Multiple studies have demonstrated that airway inflammation precedes the development of hyperresponsiveness. In some models, hyperresponsiveness does not develop if this inflammatory cell influx is blocked. Most investigators now believe that, despite multiple triggers for the inflammatory cell influx, airway inflammation is the common pathway by which airway hyperresponsiveness is induced. These inflammatory cells also appear to be the source of mediators that induce acute bronchoconstriction, mucus hypersecretion, airway edema, and further inflammatory cell influx. However, the inflammatory milieu is complex, and a single inflammatory cell or inflammatory mediator is unlikely to explain all the clinical features of asthma. Although a genetic component of asthma clearly exists, it is not explained by a single gene, but instead is a complex genetic disorder. Asthma appears to be polygenic and the phenotypic expression of involved genes is significantly influenced by environmental factors. A variety of candidate genes in asthma are currently under investigation. Some large screens in inbred populations have revealed linkages to genes that would not have been predicted based on current knowledge of asthma pathogenesis. Thus, moving from phenotype to genotype or so-called *forward genetics* is likely to be a source of new insights into the pathogenesis of asthma.

Intermittent reversible airway obstruction, hyperresponsiveness, and inflammation characterize the asthma phenotype. The clinical hallmarks are well known: episodic wheezing with dyspnea, cough, and sputum production. Between acute episodes, symptoms improve or can fully remit. These symptoms can vary from mild to severe, with profound limitation of activity and symptoms at rest. Patients often do not notice symptoms of obstruction until their acute exacerbation is of moderate to severe intensity. A detailed history of factors that precipitate acute symptoms is critical in subsequent management.

The 1997 National Asthma Education and Prevention Program, Expert Panel Report II, provides a relatively simple classification of chronic asthma that has direct implications for treatment. This report stratifies severity of disease into *steps* of severity that can be used to determine appropriate therapy (a *step-care* approach). These guidelines have been well received by pulmonary and allergy clinicians. The stratification includes mild intermittent (step 1), mild persistent (step 2), moderate persistent (step 3), and severe persistent disease (step 4) (Table 49-1). Patients with mild intermittent asthma have only occasional symptoms (two or fewer times per week), normal pulmonary function, modest variability in peak expiratory flow (PEF), and use intermittent inhaled β_2 agonists no more than twice per week. Patients with mild persistent asthma have symptoms more than twice per week but less than once per day, normal pulmonary function between exacerbations, and more significant variability in PEF with exacerbations. Patients with moderate persistent asthma have daily symptoms that interfere with activity, require daily use of a β_2 agonist for quick relief, and have abnormal baseline pulmonary function with more severe variability of PEF. Patients with severe, persistent asthma have continuous symptoms that significantly impair their activities, limited physical activity, frequent exacerbations, and more abnormal baseline pulmonary function with more dramatic variability of PEF.

Historical details, such as age of onset, frequency and severity of episodes, requirements for medications, hospitalizations, and prior need for mechanical ventilation, are important to document. Daily fluctuations in symptoms also are important. Some patients have predominantly nocturnal symptoms, which can be associated with uncontrolled reflux esophagitis, sinusitis, or pharyngeal dysfunction. Daily fluctuations also can be precipitated by exertion or exposure to a variety of environmental agents, including cold, dry air, oxidant pollutants, tobacco smoke, perfumes, dust, or provocative agents in the workplace. Symptoms that increase throughout the work day or work week and tend to improve with days off from work suggest the possibility of occupational asthma. A history of allergy, atopy, eczema, allergic rhinitis, or nasal polyps may be elicited. Medication allergies or symptoms associated with the use of nonsteroidal anti-inflammatory drugs (NSAIDs) also can be associated with asthma. The syndrome of sensitivity to NSAIDs, nasal polyps, and asthma has been termed *triad asthma* or Samter's syndrome. Patients with asthma should be instructed to avoid these drugs and those with sensitivity to them should be advised to strictly avoid them.

Cough occasionally is the only symptom of asthma; in the evaluation of chronic cough, asthma should be included in the differential diagnosis. The cough associated with asthma can be dry, but it is often productive of thick, tenacious sputum that may contain mucous plugs. The sputum may become purulent as symptoms worsen. This may represent secondary bacterial infection but more often is caused by inflammatory

Table 49-1. Classification of Asthma Severity

	Symptoms	Nighttime Symptoms	Lung Function
Step 4 Severe Persistent	• Continual symptoms • Limited physical activity • Frequent exacerbations	Frequent	• $FEV_1/PEF \leq 60\%$ predicted • PEF variability >30%
Step 3 Moderate Persistent	• Daily symptoms • Daily use of inhaled short-acting β_2-agonist • Exacerbations ≥ 2 times a week; may last days	>1 time a week	• FEV_1/PEF >60%–<80% predicted • PEF variability >30%
Step 2 Mild Persistent	• Symptoms >twice a week but <once a day • Exacerbations may affect activity	>twice a month	• $FEV_1/PEF \geq 80\%$ predicted • PEF variability 20–30%
Step 1 Mild Intermittent	• Symptoms $\leq$twice per week • Asymptomatic and normal PEF between exacerbations • Exacerbations brief (from a few hours to a few days); intensity may vary	$\leq$twice per month	• $FEV_1/PEF \geq 80\%$ predicted • PEF variability <20%

Adapted from the National Asthma Education and Prevention Program, Expert Report II, 1997.

cell infiltration without viral or bacterial superinfection. This purulent sputum most often contains numerous eosinophils.

Physical findings in asthma correlate poorly with more objective measures of airway obstruction, such as pulmonary function tests. Nevertheless, the findings are clinically useful. In an asymptomatic asthmatic patient, physical findings may be absent; however, wheezing may be elicited by forced expiration. Mild bronchospasm, in general, is associated with wheezing only during expiration. With greater degrees of obstruction, wheezing is heard in both the inspiratory and expiratory phases, with prolongation of the expiratory phase. With profound obstruction, wheezes may be heard only during the inspiratory phase or may even be absent with profoundly diminished air movement. When wheezing is correlated with other physical examination findings, a more reliable assessment can be made of the severity of obstruction. Normally the inspiratory-to-expiratory ratio is less than 1:2, but this ratio increases in a graded fashion to 1:3 or more with increasing degrees of airway obstruction. With severe obstruction, the intensity of breath sounds diminishes. Patients also begin to use accessory muscles of respiration with moderate to severe acute bronchospasm and may have active rather than passive expiration. With significant obstruction, evidence also may be seen of hyperinflation with low diaphragms and an increased anteroposterior diameter. The degree of obstruction correlates crudely with pulsus paradoxus. A pulsus greater than 10 mmHg is abnormal, and greater than 20 mmHg suggests profound obstruction. However, this measure should not substitute for direct measures of the degree of obstruction by PEF measurements or measurement of forced expiratory volume in 1 second (FEV_1). With severely labored respirations, the patient can become diaphoretic, anxious, and unable to speak in full sentences. A respiratory rate greater than 30 breaths per minute and a heart rate of 120 beats per minute suggest severe bronchospasm. Agitation, confusion, somnolence, and cyanosis are foreboding findings and suggest impending respiratory failure. Unilateral loss of breath sounds can be consistent with mucous plugging and secondary atelectasis, but these findings also must raise the possibility of pneumothorax.

The clinical laboratory examination of asthmatics is often of limited value. Peripheral blood eosinophilia is frequently present but rarely exceeds 25%. Serum IgE is often elevated in asthmatics, and in allergic asthmatics specific antibodies can be detected. Very high serum IgE should raise the question of allergic bronchopulmonary aspergillosis. Likewise, examination of sputum or nasal mucus can often reveal the presence of increased numbers of eosinophils. None of these laboratory tests is specific for asthma or significantly alters management in most patients.

During bronchospasm, spirometry reveals obstruction with a decrease in FEV_1 and decreased midexpiratory flows. The FEV_1 to forced vital capacity (FVC) ratio also is reduced. With more severe obstruction, hyperinflation is evident, with an increased residual volume and functional residual capacity more than total lung capacity. The flow-volume loop reveals evidence of obstruction with diminished flows and caving inward of the expiratory limb. One of the hallmarks of asthma is partial or complete reversal of airway obstruction after the administration of a bronchodilator. This response also can be used to gauge the adequacy of treatment. However, the lack of response to a one-time dose of a bronchodilator does not preclude a reversible component to the patient's obstruction. Moreover, it is now recognized that asthma is associated with a progressive decline in lung function over years; presumably, this decline is caused by fixed airway obstruction associated with airway remodeling. The diffusing capacity of the lung for carbon monoxide is often increased in asthmatics who do not smoke. The exact mechanism of this increase is unknown, but it is thought to represent an increase in pulmonary capillary blood volume associated with obstruction. Peak expiratory flow measurements, which are inexpensive, simple measurements that patients can assess and interpret, are also reduced during bronchospasm.

Bronchial challenge testing can establish the presence of airway hyperresponsiveness. Nonspecific bronchial hyperresponsiveness is demonstrated by exaggerated bronchoconstriction to inhaled histamine or methacholine. Nonspecific bronchial challenge is most useful in the evaluation of cough or to establish the diagnosis of asthma when the history is compatible, but physical examination and pulmonary function evidence of obstruction are lacking. However, bronchial challenge can be hazardous and should not be performed when significant airway obstruction is present. Bronchial challenge with specific provocative agents has utility in selected cases. The most commonly used specific bronchial challenges are exercise or cold air. Specific airway challenges with other agents (e.g., antigen) should only be performed in specialized centers having experience with these procedures.

Assessment of arterial blood gases usually is not necessary in the management of mild to moderate asthma. However, pulse oximetry may be of value during moderately severe exacerbations, and arterial blood gas assessment may be indicated during severe exacerbations. Hypoxemia is a frequent finding in this setting, and the arterial Pco_2 is usually decreased. During prolonged and severe episodes of airway obstruction, the patient can develop respiratory muscle fatigue, and the Pco_2 may normalize or become elevated. A normal or elevated Pco_2 during a severe exacerbation is an ominous sign, suggesting impending respiratory failure.

In the setting of chronic asthma and in the absence of another underlying condition, chest radiographic findings are usually normal. During an exacerbation, chest radiographs are not required unless fever, sputum production, chest pain, leukocytosis, or physical evidence of barotrauma are present. Hyperinflation of the lung can be present during severe exacerbations.

The diagnosis of asthma is made principally on clinical grounds; laboratory data are used in a supplementary or confirmatory fashion. A history of episodic wheezing in a nonsmoking patient, with findings of wheezing on physical examination, is strongly suggestive of asthma. Other causes of wheezing should be excluded. The diagnosis is confirmed with spirometry, which demonstrates obstruction (a FEV_1 of 80% of predicted or less with a reduced FEV_1:FVC ratio) that normalizes or significantly improves with use of a bronchodilator. If spirometry is normal, it should be repeated after a forced expiratory maneuver, which usually induces a fall in FEV_1 in asthmatics. If spirometry still remains normal, bronchial challenge testing should be considered. Alternatively, the patient can be followed over time with serial spirograms (or PEF monitoring) to demonstrate variable obstruction.

Not all patients who wheeze have asthma. Additional diagnoses should be sought in both acute and chronic settings. Upper airway obstruction, tracheomalacia, and tracheal or bronchial masses can all masquerade as asthma. These disorders are usually distinguished by the presence of stridor or focal wheezing on physical examination with flow limitation on a flow-volume loop. Laryngeal (vocal cord) dysfunction can be clinically indistinguishable from asthma. This disorder is caused by inappropriate apposition of the vocal cords during the respiratory cycle, which can be successfully treated by speech therapy. Laryngeal dysfunctions are often misdiagnosed and, when severe, can be treated with systemic corticosteroids for presumed severe asthma. Flow-volume loops demonstrate normal or near-normal expiratory flow with a flow-limited inspiratory limb. Vocal cord dysfunction is confirmed by direct laryngoscopy.

Patients with chronic fixed airway obstruction (e.g., emphysema or chronic bronchitis) can have acute wheezing episodes, most often associated with exacerbations of their disease. These patients often have airway hyperresponsiveness that is enhanced during their exacerbation. Previously, these patients have been labeled as having *asthmatic bronchitis*. A history of smoking, poor response to aggressive bronchodilator therapy, and spirometric findings of obstruction that do not reverse over time differentiate them from asthmatics. Acute bronchitis can also be associated with the development of airway hyperresponsiveness, most commonly after a viral respiratory tract infection. Most patients have transient symptoms that resolve spontaneously, but a small subgroup may develop sustained clinical asthma. Similarly, other respiratory tract infections are associated with wheezing, and some patients may develop sustained asthma. Left ventricular failure, pulmonary embolus, hypersensitivity pneumonitis, sarcoidosis, lymphangiomyomatosis, and pulmonary helminth infections should also be considered. Eosinophilic vasculitis (Churg-Strauss syndrome) can also masquerade as asthma, with the symptoms or signs of vasculitis masked by the use of corticosteroids.

1. Boushey HA, Holtzman MJ, Sheller JR, State of the art: bronchial hyperreactivity. *Am Rev Respir Dis.* 1980;121:389.
   A classic article that is still one of the best reviews of our understanding of the physiology and pathophysiology of airway hyperresponsiveness.
2. Chan-Yeung M, Malo JL, Tarlo SM, et al. Proceedings of the first Jack Pepys Occupational Asthma Symposium. *Am J Respir Crit Care Med.* 2003;167:450–471.
   An authoritative review of and guideline on occupational asthma written by one of the best-recognized clinical experts.
3. Chilmonczyk BA, Salmun LM, Megathlin KN, et al. Association between exposure to environmental tobacco smoke and exacerbation of asthma in children. *N Engl J Med.* 1993;328:1665.
   This provocative study further expands our knowledge of the dangers of passive smoking. It clearly demonstrates that exacerbations of asthma can be precipitated by second hand smoke in children.
4. Christopher KL, Wood RP 2nd, Eckert RC, et al. Vocal-cord dysfunction presenting as asthma. *N Engl J Med.* 1983;308:1566.
   The initial description of a fascinating clinical entity. Vocal cord dysfunction is important to differentiate from asthma.
5. Cookson W. Genetics and genomics of asthma and allergic diseases. *Immunol Rev.* 2002;190:195–206.

A review of current data regarding the genetics of asthma, genome-wide screening, and candidate genes.

6. Corrao WM, Braman SS, Irwin RS. Chronic cough as the sole presenting manifestation of bronchial asthma. *N Engl J Med.* 1979;300:633.
    A classic article demonstrating that asthma can present as cough only, and that the cough can improve with bronchodilators.

7. Gergen PJ, Weiss KB. The increasing problem of asthma in the United States. *Am Rev Respir Dis.* 1992;146:823.
    An important editorial summarizing the argument that asthma mortality, morbidity, and prevalence are increasing in the United States. This is a call to focus effort on understanding these presumed changes.

8. Gern JE, Busse WW. Relationship of viral infections to wheezing illnesses and asthma. *Nat Rev Immunol.* 2002;2:132–138.
    A comprehensive and authoritative review of the role of viral infections and asthma.

9. Gern JE. Viral respiratory infection and the link to asthma. *Pediatr Infect Dis J.* 2004;23(1 suppl):S78–86.
    An update summary of the above article reviewing data in support of the role of viral infection in the pathogenesis of asthma.

10. Gold DR. Environmental tobacco smoke, indoor allergens, and childhood asthma. *Environ Health Perspect.* 2000;108(suppl 4):643–651.
    A careful review of the hazards of environmental tobacco smoke and its role in asthma.

11. Goldman J, Muers M. Vocal cord dysfunction and wheezing. *Thorax.* 1991;46:401.
    An early report of vocal cord dysfunction and some of its physiologic effects.

12. Martin RJ, Banks-Schlegel S. Chronobiology of asthma. *Am J Respir Crit Care Med.* 1998;158:1002.
    An authoritative review of asthma and its chronobiology, with a particular focus on nocturnal asthma.

13. Lange P, Parner J, Vestbo J, et al. A 15-year follow-up study of ventilatory function in adults with asthma. *N Engl J Med.* 1998;339:1194.
    An important study demonstrating that asthmatics lose lung function at an accelerated rate when compared with nonasthmatics, and that this loss is further accelerated by smoking. This article signaled the importance of focusing on chronic structural changes in the airways of asthmatics (airway remodeling) and the role that they might play in the loss of lung function.

14. Lette J, Cerino M, Laverdiere M, et al. Severe bronchospasm followed by respiratory arrest during thallium-dipyridamole imaging. *Chest.* 1989;95:1345.
    An interesting case report that raises two important issues: (1) intravenous dipyridamole may precipitate life-threatening bronchospasm; and (2) adenosine, in this case released by dipyridamole, may play a role in bronchospasm and, perhaps, asthma.

15. Martinez FD. Development of wheezing disorders and asthma in preschool children. *Pediatrics.* 2002;109(s suppl):362–367.
    An interesting and provocative review regarding the pathogenesis of asthma and the critical role of early childhood events. Written by a leader in the field.

16. McFadden ER, Kiser R, DeGroot WJ. Acute bronchial asthma: relations between clinical and physiologic manifestations. *N Engl J Med.* 1973;288:221.
    A classic article that documents the discordance between clinical manifestations of asthma and objective physiologic measurements of its severity. Also demonstrates the lag between improvement in clinical symptoms and improvement in pulmonary function tests during the treatment of acute exacerbations.

17. National Heart, Lung, and Blood Institute National Asthma Education Program Expert Panel Report 2: *Guidelines for the Diagnosis and Management of Asthma.* NIH publication No. 97-4051, 1997.

This landmark document attempts to educate American physicians regarding the management of asthma to improve the care of these patients and provide more uniform care. Comprehensive, detailed discussion of diagnostic and management issues. Exhaustively referenced. Familiarity with its contents is essential. Also available online at www.nhlbi.nih.gov.

18. National Heart, Lung, and Blood Institute National Asthma Education Program Expert Panel Report: *Guidelines for the Diagnosis and Management of Asthma— Update on Selected Topics 2002.* NIH publication No 02-5074, 2003.
    The follow-up of the 1997 report based on an exhaustive review of the interim literature. Also available online at www.nhlbi.nih.gov.
19. Samter M, Beers RF. Intolerance to aspirin: clinical studies and considerations of its pathogenesis. *Ann Intern Med.* 1968;68:975.
    The classic article describes the clinical syndrome of aspirin sensitivity, nasal polyposis, and asthma.
20. Sears MR, Greene JM, Willan AR, et al. A longitudinal, population-based, cohort study of childhood asthma followed to adulthood. *N Engl J Med.* 2003;349:1414–1422.
    This provides a stronger link between childhood and adult asthma and identifies factors that are associated with persistence of disease. This study provides insights that suggest that environmental interventions may have an impact on the prevalence and severity of asthma.
21. Snashall PD, Chung KF. State of the art: airway obstruction and bronchial hyperresponsiveness in left ventricular failure and mitral stenosis. *Am Rev Respir Dis.* 1991;144:945.
    An exhaustive review of mechanisms by which increased left-sided filling pressures of the heart might lead to airway obstruction and bronchial hyperresponsiveness.
22. Szczeklik A, Stevenson DD. Aspirin-induced asthma: advances in pathogenesis, diagnosis, and management. *J Allergy Clin Immunol.* 2003;111:913–921; quiz 922.
    Updated review of the clinical syndrome of aspirin hypersensitivity from well-recognized experts on this topic. Pathogenesis, clinical features, and desensitizing therapy are reviewed.
23. Umetsu DT, McIntire JJ, Akbari O, et al. Asthma: an epidemic of dysregulated immunity. *Nat Immunol.* 2002;3:715–720.
    An authoritative review of data supporting a critical role for T cells in the pathogenesis of asthma and our emerging understanding of allergic asthma.
24. Weiss KB, Sullivan SD. The health economics of asthma and rhinitis. I. Assessing the economic impact. *J Allergy Clin Immunol.* 2001;107:3–8.
    Updates the sobering details of the economic impact of asthma in the United States and breaks the numbers down into costs for inpatient and outpatient care.
25. Weiss KB, Wagener DK. Changing patterns of asthma mortality: identifying target populations at high risk. *JAMA.* 1990;264:1683.
    A classic article that documents the observed increase in asthma mortality during the 1980s. The increase is not explained by changes in disease coding or improved disease recognition.
26. Wills-Karp M, Santeliz J, Karp CL. The germless theory of allergic disease: revisiting the hygiene hypothesis. *Nat Rev Immunol.* 2001;1:69–75.
    A careful discussion of and challenge to the so-called hygiene hypothesis of asthma.
27. Wills-Karp M, Ewart SL. Time to draw breath: asthma-susceptibility genes are identified. *Nat Rev Genet.* 2004;5:376–387.
    State-of-the-art review of our current understanding of the genetics of asthma.
28. Young S, Le Souef PN, Geelhoed GC, et al. The influence of a family history of asthma and parental smoking on airway responsiveness in early infancy. *N Engl J Med.* 1991;324:1168.
    Early data regarding the impact of passive smoking on health. This study is especially concerning in that it suggests that exposure to tobacco smoke early in life plays a role in the pathogenesis of childhood asthma.

29. Yunginger JW, Reed CE, O'Connell EJ, et al. A community-based study of the epidemiology of asthma. *Am Rev Respir Dis.* 1992;146:888.

   A landmark epidemiologic study that carefully demonstrates that asthma appears to begin in early childhood, and that an alarming increase in incidence has occurred in a 20-year period from 1964 to 1983 in Rochester, Minnesota.

---

50. ASTHMA: MANAGEMENT

Shazia M. Jamil and Timothy D. Bigby

In 1997, the classification of asthma severity was modified to include the categories of (1) mild intermittent, (2) mild persistent, (3) moderate persistent, and (4) severe persistent asthma. These categories are based on the frequency of daytime and nocturnal asthma symptoms, as well as lung function. New medications in the last decade have included leukotriene modifiers (including cysteinyl leukotriene receptor antagonists and 5-lipoxygenase inhibitors), longer acting β_2-agonists, more potent inhaled corticosteroids, nedocromil, and omalizumab (a recombinant humanized monoclonal anti-IgE antibody). The primary goal of asthma therapy is to maintain a normal or near-normal lifestyle by (1) regular and personal monitoring of disease activity, (2) preventing chronic and recurrent symptoms, (3) controlling factors contributing to severity, (4) maintaining optimal pulmonary function, (5) ensuring appropriate pharmacotherapy, and (6) providing patient education.

Patient education is the most important nonpharmacologic intervention. A comprehensive understanding of asthma and its treatment allows the patient to participate actively in the care program, recognize potential problems, obtain early treatment, and avoid exacerbations that might lead to hospitalization. The correct use of metered-dose inhalers (MDIs) and the value of "spacers" (simple devices that connect to MDIs and improve the efficiency of aerosol delivery to the distal lung) should be emphasized. Inexpensive and portable peak flow meters may be of great value for patients with moderate to severe persistent asthma. Daily monitoring of peak expiratory flow (PEF) provides a simple, quantitative, and reproducible index of airflow obstruction and can detect early changes in airway function and disease status. Spirometry is indicated at baseline and after stabilization to document a patient's personal best function and should be repeated every 1 to 2 years to assess airway function. Optimal asthma management is best facilitated by a written action plan describing the steps a patient should take based on symptoms and PEF.

Successful long-term management of asthma can be challenging. Inhaled allergens, occupational precipitants, and irritants should be identified and exposure reduced. The patient should be asked about exposure to pets, house-dust mites, cockroaches, indoor molds, and outdoor allergens. Patients with an allergic component should avoid, or at least reduce, exposure to specific allergens. Patients with persistent asthma with an inconclusive allergic history may undergo skin testing. If a clear relationship between an allergen and symptoms is detected, immunotherapy may be considered if allergen avoidance and conventional pharmacotherapy fail to control symptoms. All asthmatics should abstain from smoking and avoid exposure to second-hand smoke. Patients with severe persistent asthma, nasal polyps, or a history of sensitivity to aspirin or other nonsteroidal anti-inflammatory drugs should obviously avoid these agents, as fatal exacerbations have occurred. However, subclinical sensitivity to these agents is more common, suggesting that asthmatics should avoid these agents whenever possible. Patients should also avoid nonselective β-blockers, including topical ophthalmologic preparations, as these agents may surreptitiously cause exacerbations. Patients with persistent asthma should receive yearly influenza vaccine.

Pneumococcal vaccine is no longer recommended routinely for asthmatics. Careful evaluation and treatment of concomitant conditions (e.g., chronic rhinitis, chronic sinusitis, vocal cord dysfunction, and gastroesophageal reflux disease) may alleviate particularly difficult-to-control asthmatic symptoms.

Asthma medications are classified as *quick-relief* (rescue) and *long-term* (control) medications. Quick-relief medications, taken to promptly reverse airflow obstruction and relieve symptoms, include short-acting β_2-agonists, anticholinergics, and systemic corticosteroids (the earliest effect of corticosteroids is the upregulation of β_2-receptors within 8 hours). Long-term medications, taken daily to maintain control of persistent asthma, include corticosteroids, leukotriene modifiers, long-acting β_2-agonists, theophylline, nedocromil, and cromolyn.

The mainstay of pharmacologic therapy for mild intermittent asthma is inhaled, short-acting β_2-agonists, as needed for symptoms without the use of daily, long-term control medication. Patients whose asthma is not adequately controlled with this medication alone are considered to have persistent disease. Mild persistent asthma is defined, in part, as asthma requiring inhaled β_2-agonists more than twice per week for relief of symptoms (*National Asthma Education and Prevention Program Guidelines [NAEPP], 1997*). Patients with persistent disease require long-term control medication in addition to a short-acting β_2-agonist as-needed. Inflammation plays a key role in asthma and medications with anti-inflammatory properties are most effective for long-term control.

For patients with mild persistent asthma, the control agent of choice is low-dose inhaled corticosteroids (equivalent to 8–10 puffs of beclomethasone per day). Cromolyn or leukotriene modifiers are regarded as alternative treatment. High-dose inhaled corticosteroids (equivalent to 16–20 puffs of beclomethasone per day) have not proved to be superior to the low-dose regimen. This is particularly important in light of recent data suggesting that inhaled corticosteroids may have clinically relevant long-term side effects. The use of a spacer device, followed by rinsing the mouth after inhalation, decreases local side effects and systemic absorption. A dose-dependent reduction in bone mineral content probably occurs with long-term inhaled corticosteroids. For this reason, physicians should consider calcium and vitamin D supplementation for older postmenopausal women. For patients who cannot or will not take inhaled corticosteroids, alternatives can include leukotriene modifiers, cromolyn, or theophylline. These agents are less effective than inhaled corticosteroids as first-line control therapy except in specific circumstances (see below). Long acting β_2-agonists should not be considered as a substitute for inhaled corticosteroids, because of a report suggesting increased mortality in patients using long-acting β_2-agonists in the absence of inhaled corticosteroids.

New recommendations for treatment of patients with moderate persistent asthma are daily low-dose inhaled corticosteroids in combination with long-acting inhaled β_2-agonists. This is based on scientific evidence from research studies in moderate asthmatic children older than age 12 and adults that indicate these patients benefit most from combination controller therapy. This approach is superior to increasing the dose of inhaled corticosteroid. Alternatively, medium-dose inhaled corticosteroids can be used as monotherapy, but this approach is clinically inferior (*NAEPP, 2002*). For patients with recurring severe exacerbations requiring oral prednisone, emergency department visits or hospitalizations, increasing the dose of inhaled corticosteroids to medium-dose range along with use of long-acting inhaled β_2-agonists is one strategy for management and probably the most economical. However, current data favor additional add-on therapies as more effective than increasing corticosteroids in this setting. Alternative therapy for patients intolerant of long acting inhaled β_2-agonists include addition of either a leukotriene modifier or theophylline to medium-dose inhaled corticosteroids. Nedocromil or long-acting oral β_2-agonists are not recommended alternatives to increasing the dose of inhaled corticosteroids. Daily use of a long-acting β_2-agonist is generally well tolerated but should not exceed 84 mcg (salmeterol; two puffs twice a day) and should not be used on an as-needed basis for acute symptoms. There is no evidence that anticholinergics provide added benefit to β_2-agonists in long-term asthma control therapy, although they may be moderately effective for a subset of asthmatics.

Patients with severe, persistent asthma typically have symptoms and altered pulmonary function that are not adequately controlled with low- to medium-dose inhaled corticosteroids along with other long-term control therapies. These patients are characterized by having continuous daily asthma symptoms despite therapy. Treatment recommendations (*NAEPP, 2002*) include high-dose inhaled corticosteroids and long-acting inhaled β_2-agonists, and, if needed, oral corticosteroids. The recommended dose of oral corticosteroid is 1 mg/kg per day, generally not to exceed 60 mg per day. Because of serious long-term consequences of chronic systemic corticosteroids, every attempt should be made to improve the management of these patients with environmental control and attempts to taper systemic corticosteroids to the lowest dose possible. Patients receiving chronic oral corticosteroids should be treated no more frequently than once per day, except in rare circumstances; alternate-day therapy is preferred whenever possible. They should also be monitored closely for adverse medication effects. All patients in this category should be referred to an asthma specialist. Occasionally, patients with severe persistent asthma may not be adequately controlled despite daily systemic corticosteroids. After careful re-evaluation and maximal adjustment of medications, these patients may be considered for cytotoxic or immunosuppressive therapy. This should only be considered by a specialist who is experienced in the use of such medications. Omalizumab, an anti-IgE antibody, is directed at human IgE and inhibits binding of IgE to mast cells without provoking mast cell activation. Clinical data from randomized controlled trials have shown that the addition of omalizumab to standard asthma therapy reduces asthma exacerbations and decreases inhaled corticosteroid and rescue medication use. However, at this time, the positioning of this therapy in step care and its specific indications have not been determined.

Written self-management plans, especially for patients with moderate or severe persistent asthma with good fundamental understanding of their disease, are useful both for chronic management and during acute exacerbations. The usual initial plan during an exacerbation is to increase the dose and shorten the interval of short-acting inhaled β_2-agonists. Ipratropium bromide used with a short-acting β_2-agonist may provide additional bronchodilation. Purulent sputum with fever requires early medical attention and evaluation for possible concomitant pneumonia. However, purulent secretions are common during exacerbations and often are due to inflammatory influx into the airways unassociated with infection. Antibiotics are not recommended for the treatment of acute asthma exacerbations, except as needed for comorbid or exacerbating infectious conditions, such as bacterial pneumonia or suspected bacterial sinusitis. When symptoms do not remit with more aggressive use of inhaled β_2-agonists, early intervention with systemic corticosteroids is pivotal and should always precipitate contact with a physician. A typical schedule would begin with 40 to 60 mg/day of prednisone, tapered over 10 to 14 days. The dosage can be tapered rapidly and discontinued if the total course is less than 14 days. However, patients with more severe or more frequent exacerbations or those with prior use of corticosteroids may require more gradual tapering to avoid treatment failure and readmission. When the dose of oral corticosteroid has been reduced to approximately 20 mg/day of prednisone, or equivalent, reinstitution of inhaled corticosteroids is appropriate. Usually, inhaled corticosteroids are discontinued during acute exacerbations because of the tendency for some of these preparations to exacerbate bronchospasm through irritant effects. This is most common for inhaled corticosteroids supplied as a suspension rather than a solution. This issue has been re-evaluated in recent years; some inhaled corticosteroids can provide therapeutic benefit during exacerbations. The physiologic abnormalities associated with exacerbation may persist well after symptomatic improvement and, therefore, intensive therapy and close follow-up should be continued for an extended period after resolution of symptoms.

Status asthmaticus is life-threatening asthma characterized by sustained, severe airway obstruction refractory to treatment. These patients should always seek emergent medical care. Initial treatment should include oxygen, higher and more frequent doses of inhaled β_2-agonists, and early institution of systemic corticosteroids because of the delay in the observed clinical response (i.e., 6–8 hours). Small volume nebulizers, MDIs, and continuous administration by a nebulizer are all effective methods for delivering β_2-agonists; however, numerous studies indicate that an MDI with a spacer is both as effective and more cost-effective than a nebulizer. Spacers are particularly important when an MDI is used for adults who are unable to coordinate their inspiratory effort with activation of the MDI. β-Agonists have been administered by the subcutaneous route in the past; however, this results in greater toxicity and has no greater benefit over the aerosol route. A commonly used corticosteroid is methylprednisolone in a dose of approximately 60 mg every 6 hours. These high doses are not benign; potential complications include hypokalemia, hyperglycemia, acute central nervous symptom alterations, hypertension, and peripheral edema. Use of parenteral theophylline in this setting is controversial; many studies have shown no added bronchodilator effect and substantial increases in toxicity. The value of magnesium sulfate in the treatment of status asthmaticus has not been studied rigorously. Available studies suggest that it can provide some modest, transient improvement in lung function as a temporizing measure in the acute setting, but it cannot be used repeatedly.

During severe exacerbations, respiratory failure can develop despite maximal therapy. Hypercapnia alone does not necessitate intubation and can be effectively managed in some cases with noninvasive mechanical ventilation by face mask. The goal is to allow time to optimize pharmacologic management. The presence of peak flows (<150 L/min), pulsus paradoxus (>20 mmHg), thoracoabdominal paradox, hypoxemia despite oxygen therapy, or an increasing $PaCO_2$ signal the potential for progression to respiratory failure requiring intubation and mechanical ventilation.

For patients requiring intubation and mechanical ventilation, hydration should be used to attenuate hypotension that is frequently observed after the institution of positive pressure ventilation. Sodium thiopental, etomidate, narcotics, ketamine, and benzodiazepines have all been used safely for sedation or anesthesia at the time of intubation in the acute asthmatic patient. Paralysis may be required to intubate the patient safely and can be accomplished with succinylcholine; however, acidemic patients should be monitored carefully because of the potential for hyperkalemia. Concomitant use of nondepolarizing, neuromuscular blocking agents with systemic corticosteroids has been associated with myopathy and severe peripheral muscle weakness; thus, they should be used with caution.

Once the patient is intubated, careful attention to tidal volumes, peak flows, and inspiration to expiration ratios is necessary to minimize barotrauma and dynamic hyperinflation, which are significant risks in this setting. Sedation with opioids, benzodiazepines, or propofol is required to facilitate ventilator synchrony. To minimize intrinsic positive end-expiratory pressure ($PEEP_i$), the time available for expiration should be maximized by increasing the inspiratory flow rate and reducing the respiratory frequency. It also may be necessary to reduce the tidal volume to increase expiratory time. In turn, permissive hypercapnia in some patients may help to avoid dramatically elevated airway pressures. Intravenous bicarbonate can be used with permissive hypercapnia to partially compensate for the resulting respiratory acidosis, but it must be used judiciously to maintain arterial pH greater than 7.20. Often higher doses of inhaled β_2-agonists and ipratropium bromide are required through in-line MDI treatments at more frequent intervals because of the severe bronchospasm and the decreased efficiency of aerosol delivery through the ventilator circuit. Intravenous theophylline is of questionable benefit and can be risky; if used, theophylline drug levels should be monitored closely. Monitoring of peak-to-plateau airway pressure gradients and auto-PEEP may help in assessing the severity of bronchospasm and response to therapy. These patients should receive an extended course of oral corticosteroids (at least 4–6 weeks) and should not be tapered below 20 mg/day until seen by a physician, preferably an asthma specialist, in follow-up.

Some specific circumstances warrant special considerations in asthma. Exercise-induced asthma is common, especially in young asthmatics. Symptoms are often controlled by use of short-acting, inhaled β_2-agonists before exercise. For more persistent symptoms, regularly scheduled long-acting β_2-agonists, leukotriene modifier, or chromone should be considered. Persistent nocturnal symptoms despite inhaled corticosteroids require addition of long-term control therapy with long-acting β_2-agonists, leukotriene modifiers, or theophylline. Patients with aspirin-sensitive asthma usually have moderate to severe symptoms that can be difficult to control.

Leukotrienes are thought to play a particularly important role; thus, leukotriene modifiers should be strongly considered in these patients.

Asthma is the most common potentially serious medical condition complicating pregnancy. Uncontrolled asthma during pregnancy can produce complications in both the mother and the fetus. A recent report by the Working Group on Asthma and Pregnancy found that undertreatment, principally attributable to unfounded fears of fetal effects of medication, is the major problem in asthma management during pregnancy. The greatest experience in the pregnant patient is with inhaled β_2-agonists and theophylline; however, corticosteroids, cromolyn, and anticholinergics have all been used safely. Thus, asthma should be treated as aggressively in pregnant as in nonpregnant women. A recent large study of pregnant women has raised concern about use of oral corticosteroids and theophylline. In this population, an increased risk of preterm delivery has been observed. Special emphasis should also be placed on nonpharmacologic measures to avoid asthma triggers. Asthma care should include monitoring of fetal growth, maternal symptoms, and maternal lung function. All pregnant asthmatics should be tested with spirometry; the single best index of severity is the forced expiratory volume in 1 second (FEV_1), which is not significantly altered by pregnancy. Patients with moderate or severe asthma should be monitored with twice-daily measurements of peak expiratory flow rate and should report the values to the physician at each prenatal visit. After the first trimester, patients should receive influenza vaccine.

The basic management of asthma during pregnancy is very similar to that in nonpregnant patients and is based on asthma severity classification. If the patient's asthma is more than mild intermittent, anti-inflammatory therapy is recommended. Cromolyn sodium is a reasonable first choice; however, if inhaled corticosteroids are used, beclomethasone is preferred. The immediate goals of therapy of severe asthma exacerbation in pregnancy are to correct hypoxemia, alleviate bronchospasm, avoid maternal exhaustion or respiratory failure, and prevent fetal morbidity and mortality. The management of acute exacerbation includes oxygen to maintain a minimum Pao_2 (>60 mmHg; oxygen saturation >95%), inhaled β_2-agonists, and a short course of systemic corticosteroids. During labor and delivery, patients who have required long-term systemic corticosteroids should be given hydrocortisone because of the risk of maternal adrenal suppression.

Asthmatics are at risk for respiratory complications during and after surgery, including acute bronchospasm triggered by intubation and hypoxemia. Therefore, patients with asthma should be evaluated before surgery, including a review of symptoms and medications, measurement of pulmonary function, and attempts made to optimize lung function. A short course of corticosteroids may be necessary. It is recommended that patients who have received systemic corticosteroids for more than 2 weeks during the past 6 months be given hydrocortisone (100 mg every 8 hours) intravenously on the day of surgery, with a rapid reduction of the dose within 24 hours after surgery.

All patients with severe persistent asthma, and possibly those with moderate persistent asthma, as well as those who have had a life-threatening asthma exacerbation, should be referred to an asthma specialist.

1. Abramson MJ, Puy RM, Weiner JM. Is allergen immunotherapy effective in asthma? A meta-analysis of randomized controlled trials. *Am J Respir Crit Care Med.* 1995;151:969.

   A meta-analysis of 20 randomized, placebo-controlled studies, confirming the effectiveness of immunotherapy in asthma.

2. Aubier M. Pharmacologic strategies for treating respiratory failure. *Chest.* 1990; 97:98S.

   A review of respiratory muscle function and dysfunction in respiratory failure and the effects of pharmacologic agents on respiratory muscle function.

3. Barnes PJ, Pederson S, Busse WW. Efficacy and safety of inhaled corticosteroids: new developments. *Am J Respir Crit Care Med.* 1998;157:S1.

A comprehensive review by leading investigators in the field, with new information about inhaled corticosteroids in regard to molecular mechanism, effects on asthmatic inflammation, systemic activity, safety, and clinical efficacy.

4. Blaiss MS. Managing asthma during pregnancy. The whys and hows of aggressive control. *Postgrad Med.* 2004;115:55–58, 61–64.

   A current, informed, and practical update of asthma management in the clinical setting of pregnancy.

5. Bracken MB, Triche EW, Belanger K, et al. Asthma symptoms, severity, and drug therapy: a prospective study of effects on 2205 pregnancies. *Obstet Gynecol.* 2003;102:739–752.

   This study prospectively examined whether asthma therapy influenced preterm delivery, intrauterine growth restriction, or birthweight in a large group of pregnant women.

6. Calhoun WJ. Summary of clinical trials with zafirlukast. *Am J Respir Crit Care Med.* 1998;157:S238.

   A review of clinical trials with zafirlukast, which concludes that zafirlukast reduced asthma symptoms, decreased as-needed β_2-agonist use, and improved pulmonary function.

7. Clark NM, Evans D, Mellins RB. Pulmonary perspective: patient use of peak flow monitoring. *Am Rev Respir Dis.* 1992;145:722.

   A "pulmonary perspective," reviewing the role of patient peak flow monitoring in the management of asthma.

8. Clark SL, Esplin MS. Outpatient management of asthma during pregnancy. *Clin Obstet Gynecol.* 1998;41:555.

   This article discusses the effect of asthma on pregnancy and outlines an aggressive approach to outpatient treatment designed to reduce or eliminate the increased risks of asthma during pregnancy.

9. Cohen NH, Eigen H, Shaughnessy TE. Status asthmaticus. *Crit Care Clin.* 1997;13:459.

   An extensive review of the pathophysiology, pharmacology, and clinical management options of status asthmaticus in adults and children. A total of 93 references.

10. Doerschug KC, Peterson MW, Dayton CS, et al. Asthma guidelines. An assessment of physician understanding and practice. *Am J Respir Crit Care Med.* 1999;159:1735.

    Results of a multiple-choice test of asthma knowledge based on 1997 National Heart, Lung, and Blood Institute guidelines in 108 physicians in an academic institution. Regardless of their level of training, physicians tended to score low when asked to classify the severity of chronic lung disease. The most common errors were not recognizing daily symptoms as mild persistent asthma, failure to recognize daily β_2-agonists as poorly controlling asthma, and failure to use objective disease monitoring, such as spirometry, as often as suggested by the guidelines.

11. Drazen JM, Israel E, O'Brian PM. Treatment of asthma with drugs modifying the leukotriene pathway. *N Engl J Med.* 1999;340:197.

    An excellent article that reviews the biochemistry of the cysteinyl leukotrienes and leukotriene modifiers, with special emphasis on the role of these drugs in chronic stable asthma.

12. Dutoit J, Salome CM, Woolcock AJ. Inhaled corticosteroids reduce the severity of bronchial hyperresponsiveness in asthma but oral theophylline does not. *Am Rev Respir Dis.* 1987;136:1174.

    A double-blind, crossover study demonstrating that 3 to 4 weeks of inhaled beclomethasone dipropionate (800 μg/day) reduces bronchial hyperresponsiveness. This effect was maintained through 10 weeks of therapy. On discontinuation of beclomethasone, the benefit was lost. Theophylline did not improve bronchial hyperresponsiveness.

13. Fanta CH, Rossing TH, McFadden Jr.ER. Emergency room treatment of asthma. *Am J Med.* 1982;72:416.

    In this study, 102 acutely ill asthmatics were randomized to inhaled β_2-agonist, inhaled β_2-agonist with intravenous aminophylline, or inhaled β_2-agonist with *oral theophylline. Theophylline or aminophylline was not better than β₂-agonist alone.*

14. Fanta CH, Rossing TH, McFadden Jr.ER.Glucocorticoids in acute asthma: a critical controlled trial. *Am J Med.* 1983;74:845.

    Documents a beneficial effect of intravenous hydrocortisone in patients who had not responded to 8 hours of intensive bronchodilator therapy. Based on plasma cortisol levels; no dose response to or optimal dose of corticosteroids could be determined. A several-hour delay was seen before the beneficial effects were manifest.

15. Jain S, Hanania NA, Guntupalli KK. Ventilation of patients with asthma and obstructive lung disease. *Crit Care Clin.* 1998;14:685.

    An extensive review that details the indications for mechanical ventilation in patients with acute severe asthma. Outlines important ventilator strategies to avoid complications, emphasizing the role of controlled hypoventilation with permissive hypercapnia.

16. Juniper EF, Kline PA, Vanzieleghem MA, et al. Effect of long-term treatment with an inhaled corticosteroid (budesonide) on airway hyperresponsiveness and clinical asthma in non-steroid-dependent asthmatics. *Am Rev Respir Dis.* 1990;142:832.

    This study extends previous work examining the effects of inhaled corticosteroids on airway hyperresponsiveness. In 32 patients treated for 1 year with budesonide, the authors found significant improvement in hyperresponsiveness and, in some cases, resolution. An associated significant clinical improvement in asthma occurred.

17. Lam A, Newhouse MT. Management of asthma and chronic airflow limitation. Are methylxanthines obsolete? *Chest.* 1990;98:44.

    Reviews literature, both pro and con, regarding the use of methylxanthines in asthma and chronic obstructive pulmonary disease. Concludes that methylxanthines add little to the acute or chronic management of asthma. They should be considered third-line or fourth-line therapy. Theophylline is recommended only if objective benefit can be demonstrated.

18. Lemanske RF, Busse WW. Asthma. *JAMA.* 1997;278:1855.

    A review article emphasizing the role of allergens, irritant exposure, and exercise on short-term and long-term management of asthma and the importance of correctly classifying patients based on disease severity.

19. Lin RY, Pesola GR, Bakalchuk L, et al. Superiority of ipratropium plus albuterol over albuterol alone in the emergency department management of adult asthma: a randomized clinical trial. *Ann Emerg Med.* 1998;31:208.

    A randomized, double-blind, placebo-controlled trial demonstrating that treatment with albuterol plus ipratropium bromide compared with albuterol alone provides a greater increase in peak expiratory flow rate and decreased hospital admission rate in patients with acute asthma.

20. Littenberg B, Gluck EH. A controlled trial of methylprednisolone in the emergency treatment of acute asthma. *N Engl J Med.* 1986;314:150.

    This controlled trial administered methylprednisolone, in addition to other standard therapies, to 97 asthmatics with acute exacerbations on arrival at the emergency department. The corticosteroid-treated group was found to require hospitalization less frequently.

21. Luskin AT. An overview of the recommendations of the working group on asthma and pregnancy. *J Allergy Clin Immunol.* 1999;103:S350.

    The working group was established by the National Asthma Education and Prevention Program to address issues surrounding asthma management during pregnancy. This article reviews the guidelines set up by the group and attempts to ensure the safety of mothers and their fetuses by emphasizing the importance of accurate diagnosis and appropriate management of asthma during pregnancy.

22. Mountain RD, Sahn SA. Clinical features and outcome in patients with acute asthma presenting with hypercapnia. *Am Rev Respir Dis.* 1988;138:535.

    A retrospective study identifying 61 episodes of hypercapnia at presentation of an acute exacerbation of asthma. Data refute the older notion that patients with a normal or elevated Pco_2 at presentation require intubation.

23. National Heart, Lung, and Blood Institute National Asthma Education and Prevention Program (NAEPP) Expert Panel Report 2. *Guidelines for the Diagnosis and Management of Asthma.* NIH publication No. 97-4051, 1997.

   This landmark document contains information to educate American physicians regarding the management of asthma to improve their ability to provide more uniform care. Comprehensive, detailed discussion of diagnostic and management issues. Exhaustively referenced. Familiarity with its contents is essential. This second report, in our opinion, is a vast improvement compared with the first.

24. National Heart, Lung, and Blood Institute National Asthma Education and Prevention Program (NAEPP) Expert Panel Report. *Guidelines for the Diagnosis and Management of Asthma—Update on Selected Topics 2002.* NIH publication No. 97-4051, 2002.

   The NAEPP keeps clinical practice guidelines up to date by identifying selected topics on asthma that warrant intensive review based on the level of research activity reflected in the published literature or the level of concern in clinical practice. This report provides an update to 1997 NAEPP guidelines in asthma management.

25. Naureckas ET, Solway J. Clinical practice. Mild asthma. *N Engl J Med.* 2001;345: 1257–1262.

   An authoritative review of the comprehensive management of asthma.

26. Roy SR, Milgrom H. *Management of the acute exacerbation of asthma. J Asthma.* 2003;40:593–604.

   This article reviews in depth the management of asthma exacerbation.

27. Sears MR, Taylor DR, Print CG, et al. Regular inhaled β-agonist treatment in bronchial asthma. *Lancet.* 1990;336:1391.

   A provocative, small study comparing regular and intermittent use of inhaled fenoterol in the management of asthma. Although concerns exist about the number of subjects and the quantitation of the data, patients using fenoterol regularly did worse than those treated intermittently. This study has been used to implicate β-agonists in rising asthma morbidity.

28. Storms W. Allergens in the pathogenesis of asthma: potential role of anti-immunoglobulin E therapy. *Am J Respir Med.* 2002;1:361–368.

   This article reviews the role of allergy in triggering asthma symptoms and the mechanism of IgE-mediated allergic reactions. It further reviews clinical data from randomized trials on omalizumab.

29. Weiner C. Ventilatory management of respiratory failure in asthma. *JAMA.* 1993;269:2128.

   A case report followed by an excellent discussion. The article emphasizes that by understanding the pathophysiology and consequences of auto-PEEP, mechanical ventilation of patients with severe airway obstruction can be accomplished with minimal risk of complication.

30. Wilding P, Clark M, Thompson Coon J, et al. Effect of long-term treatment with salmeterol on asthma control: a double blind, randomized crossover study. *BMJ.* 1997;314:1441.

   Double-blind, randomized, crossover study demonstrating that the addition of salmeterol to inhaled corticosteroid in patients with mild or moderate asthma is associated with a reduction in inhaled steroid use and improved lung function and symptom control.

31. Wilson SR, Scamagas P, German DF, et al. A controlled trial of two forms of self-management education for adults with asthma. *Am J Med.* 1993;94:564.

   Clear evidence that self-management programs can improve patient understanding and lead to improved compliance and decreased symptoms.

32. Woodcock AL, Forster E, Matthews J, et al. Control of exposure to mite allergen and allergen-impermeable bed covers for adults with asthma. *N Engl J Med.* 2003;349:225–236.

   One of two landmark studies showing that simple interventions for allergen avoidance are not as beneficial as once thought.

51. PHARMACOTHERAPY

Kenneth J. Serio and Timothy D. Bigby

The pharmacologic treatment of asthma involves the administration of multiple agents with varied mechanisms of action in a stepwise approach to the level of response. Prescribed medications include short and long-acting β_2-agonists, anticholinergic agents, theophylline preparations, leukotriene modifiers, corticosteroids, and immunotherapeutic agents. Recent developments include the widespread adoption of inhaled corticosteroids as first-line controller medications, the increasing use of long-acting β_2-agonists and leukotriene modifiers, and the introduction of anti-IgE immunotherapy. National Institute of Health (NIH) asthma guidelines have established a pharmacologic paradigm of agents as either "long-term control" agents (used in asthma maintenance) or "quick-relief" agents (used to treat acute symptoms).

Aerosolized and *inhalational medications* have been the predominant modality in the treatment of asthma. Aerosol delivery is safe, effective, and minimizes systemic side effects, compared with administration by other routes. Factors contributing to optimal aerosol deposition in the distal lung units are airway diameter, particle size (1–5 μm particle size is optimum), gas flow velocity (high velocity increases upper respiratory tract deposition), and breath-holding time (longer times increase particle sedimentation in distal lung units). Commonly used aerosolization techniques include metered-dose inhalers (MDIs), jet nebulization, or ultrasonic nebulization. Available studies indicate that MDIs and nebulizers are equally effective at achieving drug delivery and clinical response in most clinical settings when equivalent doses of medication are administered, proper technique is used, and a "spacer" device (a simple device that connects to an MDI and improves the efficiency of aerosol delivery to the distal lung) is used. As a result, MDIs are the delivery device of choice in most clinical settings, largely owing to their cost-effectiveness. Although legal mandates require the phase-out of ozone layer-depleting chlorofluorocarbon propellants, most gas-powered MDIs in the United States still contain them. Other inhalational delivery methods, such as dry powder inhalers, inspiration-actuated MDIs, and chlorofluorocarbon-free inhalers, are available for some specific medications.

β_2-agonists, which act at β_2-adrenergic receptors located in the conducting airways and peripheral lung units, have been used extensively for the treatment of both asthma and chronic obstructive pulmonary disease (COPD). β_2-Receptor agonism induces bronchodilation, increased mucociliary clearance, suppression of microvascular leakage, inhibition of inflammatory cell-mediator release, and suppression of the cough reflex. Recent evidence indicates that variable individual responses to β_2-agonists may be related to polymorphisms within the gene encoding for the β_2 adrenergic receptor. Common side effects of these medications include muscle tremor (through a direct effect) and tachycardia (through a reflex mechanism). Paradoxical bronchospasm occurs rarely with inhaled β_2-agonists, but the mechanism is unknown.

Short-acting β_2-agonists (including albuterol, pirbuterol, bitolterol, and terbutaline) have an onset of action within 5 to 10 minutes and a short duration of action, typically lasting 3 to 6 hours. Fenoterol (available in Europe) is a more potent, but less selective β_2-agonist that has a somewhat longer duration of action. The short-acting β_2-agonists are used as a sole agent in mild, intermittent asthma and also as additional "quick-relief" treatment for acute symptoms in patients already maintained on a "long-term control" medication. In addition, the short-acting β_2-agonists are effective in prophylaxis against exercise-induced asthma and in the treatment of COPD.

Long-acting β_2-agonists (including salmeterol and formoterol) have a slower onset of action over 15 to 30 minutes (notably longer than the short-acting β_2-agonists), making them less effective for the control of acute symptoms. However, their sustained duration of action, up to 12 hours, make them ideal long-term control medications in asthma. Safety profiles are comparable for both short-acting and long-acting

β_2-agonists. Importantly, studies suggest that there is no increased risk of toxicity or significantly decreased efficacy when the medications are used concomitantly. The long-acting β_2-agonists afford protection against various bronchoconstrictor stimuli, and there has been no observed rebound increase in bronchial reactivity after the cessation of salmeterol therapy. The sustained effects of long-acting β_2-agonists make them particularly well suited to the treatment of nocturnal asthma, exercise-induced asthma, and aspirin-sensitive asthma. Current recommendations indicate that the addition of a long-acting β_2-agonist is preferred over increasing the steroid dose for patients on low-dose to medium-dose inhaled steroids. Salmeterol appears to be better tolerated and more efficacious in the treatment of asthma than the long-acting theophylline preparations. However, adverse events, even death, have been recorded in patients treated with long-acting β_2-agonists in the absence of inhaled corticosteroids. Thus, the recommendation is that long-acting β_2-agonists not be used in the absence of inhaled corticosteroids.

Although early studies cited concerns about the safety of β_2-agonist agents and their association with asthma deaths, such studies were likely confounded by factors such as asthma severity, delay in the initiation of other treatment, mode of drug delivery, and patient age. Current data indicate that the regular use of short-acting agents does not cause significant adverse effects but likely provides no added benefit. Importantly, excessive use of short-acting inhaled β_2-agonists (≥ 1.4 canisters per month) or a pattern of escalating use are markers for increased asthma severity and indicate overreliance on these agents. Studies in exercise-induced asthma suggest that although long-term salmeterol treatment appears to provide sustained bronchodilation, the duration of activity of the drug after a single dose decreases. Although the data are conflicting as to whether significant clinical tolerance occurs with use of the long-acting β_2-agonists, adverse effects on asthma morbidity and overall control of symptoms have not been demonstrated.

Oral β_2-agonists are used infrequently to manage nocturnal asthma. These preparations exhibit less fluctuation in drug levels, less bronchodilation, more prominent side effects than inhaled preparations, and require less frequent dosing. Similarly, terbutaline and epinephrine are available for subcutaneous or intravenous administration, but available studies in the emergency department setting indicate that parenteral β_2-agonist administration results in no significant enhancement of bronchodilation. As these studies also demonstrate significantly greater side effects, the use of parenteral β_2-agonists is not currently recommended.

Anticholinergic medications (including ipratropium and tiotropium) have been used extensively to treat bronchospasm. These atropine-like agents antagonize airway muscarinic receptors, resulting in bronchodilation. Anticholinergic drugs have been demonstrated to block airway constriction in response to gastroesophageal reflux and airway irritants, but not in response to allergen challenge or exercise. Ipratropium bromide has been widely available for delivery through both MDI and nebulizer. It has minimal systemic absorption, is safe and well tolerated, and produces clinical benefits when used alone or as an adjunct to short-acting β_2-agonists. Its use as a quick-relief medication is somewhat limited by its relatively slow onset of action compared to the β_2-agonists. Although most trials have demonstrated efficacy of anticholinergic medications in patients with bronchospasm in association with COPD or β-blocker administration, a subset of asthma patients also demonstrate responsiveness to these agents. The recently introduced long-acting anticholinergic agent, tiotropium, may provide an additional long-term control medication for the treatment of asthma, although its current role in asthma management has not been defined.

Theophylline has been used extensively to treat asthma. It is widely available in immediate-release and sustained-release oral forms, as well as intravenous aminophylline. Theophylline functions through multiple mechanisms, including phosphodiesterase inhibition, adenosine receptor antagonism, inhibition of leukotriene synthesis, and modulation of immune function. Physiologic effects of theophylline include bronchodilation, increased mucociliary clearance, decreased eosinophil infiltration of bronchial mucosa, and increased diaphragmatic muscle contractility. Extended-release oral theophylline preparations are efficacious in the management of nocturnal asthma symptoms, being comparable to the long-acting β_2-agonists. Studies indicate that theophylline does provide significant benefit when added to other standard therapies in the treatment of acute asthma exacerbation. Common side effects of theophylline include insomnia, nausea, arrhythmias, tremor, gastrointestinal symptoms, hypokalemia, gastroesophageal reflux, and central nervous system symptoms. Given the narrow therapeutic range of this drug and the fact that theophylline levels are altered by a number of commonly administered medications, regular monitoring of drug levels is strongly recommended.

Cromolyn sodium and nedocromil, which probably function to block chloride channels and modulate mast cell degranulation and mediator release, have been widely used in the treatment of asthma. These agents inhibit both the early and late asthmatic responses to allergen. After at least 2 to 6 weeks of use, they manifest clinical effects of decreased asthma symptoms and requirement for quick-relief β_2-agonist use. These drugs also are used to treat aspirin-intolerant asthma, an effect attributed to inhibition of cysteinyl leukotriene synthesis. Additionally, they have been used to treat allergen-induced and exercise-induced asthma. These medications remain expensive and produce a substantially less predictable response than inhaled corticosteroids; however, their safety is well established and significant side effects are rare. Cromolyn and nedocromil have no role in the treatment of COPD.

The *leukotriene modifiers* include both 5-lipoxygenase inhibitors (including zileuton) and cysteinyl leukotriene receptor antagonists (including montelukast, zafirlukast, and pranlukast). These agents inhibit synthesis of lipid mediators derived from arachidonic acid through the 5-lipoxygenase pathway in inflammatory cells (5-lipoxygenase inhibitors) or block the action of leukotrienes when binding to their receptors (cysteinyl leukotriene receptor antagonist). These potent mediators function to increase vascular permeability, smooth muscle contraction, mucus hypersecretion, bronchial hyperreactivity, and eosinophil chemotaxis. Leukotriene modifiers have been shown to decrease asthmatic symptoms, decrease requirements for quick-relief therapy with short-acting β_2-agonists, and decrease the need for oral corticosteroid rescue. However, in contrast to inhaled corticosteroids, these medications are efficacious in only about 50% of asthmatics. Likewise, with chronic administration, they are less potent than inhaled corticosteroids and are equipotent to theophylline preparations and the long-acting β_2-agonists. The main use of leukotriene modifiers is to allow a reduction in inhaled and oral corticosteroid doses (so-called "steroid-sparing" effect) without a subsequent loss in asthma control.

The 5-lipoxygenase inhibitor, zileuton, is used as a long-term control medication in asthma, particularly in the management of aspirin-intolerant and exercise-induced asthma. However, its use has been limited by frequent dose requirement (four times per day) and the side effect of elevated liver function tests (in >4% of cases). The cysteinyl leukotriene receptor antagonists (including zafirlukast and montelukast in the United States and pranlukast in Japan) have high oral bioavailability and are administered with once- or twice-daily dosing. These agents are effective in the management of cough-variant asthma, exercise-induced asthma, and aspirin-intolerant asthma. Although cysteinyl leukotriene receptor antagonists are well tolerated, a rare association with the development of the Churg-Strauss syndrome (eosinophilic vasculitis) has been observed. This association has been attributed to withdrawal of corticosteroids and unmasking a previously unrecognized vasculitis. All the leukotriene modifier agents have been reported to cause elevations in serum theophylline levels.

Corticosteroids have been used widely in the treatment of asthma, as they manifest multiple glucocorticoid-mediated anti-inflammatory and other properties that are beneficial. They are known to decrease airway inflammation and hyperresponsiveness, inhibit late response to allergen challenge, decrease frequency of exacerbations, decrease asthma symptom severity, and, possibly, decrease airway remodeling. However, among the most important early effects of corticosteroids are their ability to upregulate the expression and affinity of β_2 receptors in the lung. Side effects depend on the route of administration. Although corticosteroids are effective in a wide variety of asthmatic patients, corticosteroid resistance has been reported in a small subset.

Inhaled corticosteroids (including fluticasone, beclomethasone, budesonide, flunisolide, and triamcinolone—ciclesonide and mometasone are not available in the United States at this time) remain first-line agents for long-term control of asthma that is unresponsive to inhaled short-acting β_2-agonists alone. Inhaled corticosteroids are preferred over long-acting β_2-agonists alone, although their use early in the disease has not been demonstrated to impact the natural course of asthma. These agents function to suppress airway inflammatory responses and are effective in >70% of asthmatics. Recently described polymorphisms in gene encoding for corticotropin-releasing hormone receptor 1 (CRHR1) may play a role in responsiveness to inhaled corticosteroids. These medications decrease the risks of asthma exacerbation, hospital readmission after an acute asthma exacerbation, and asthma mortality. In patients not well controlled on low- to medium-dose inhaled corticosteroids, the addition of a long-acting agent (such as a long-acting β_2-agonist, theophylline, or leukotriene modifier agent) is a better choice than increasing the corticosteroid dose. Inhaled corticosteroids are generally well tolerated, although side effects of cough, dysphonia, and oral thrush may be seen occasionally. These reactions can be minimized by giving the lowest effective dose, using a spacer device, and oral rinsing. At high doses, inhaled corticosteroids may suppress the hypothalamic-pituitary-adrenal axis, but clinically relevant adrenal suppression is rare. These medications may also contribute to the development of cataracts and osteoporosis.

Systemic corticosteroids are used commonly in the treatment of acute exacerbations, as well as for disease refractory to other agents. They can be administered orally (prednisone and prednisolone), intravenously (methylprednisolone), and intramuscularly (triamcinolone). Demonstrated effects include reduction in hospitalizations, shortening the duration of asthma exacerbation, and reduction of disease relapse. Acute asthma exacerbations are typically treated with high-dose (oral or intravenous) corticosteroids, followed by an individualized tapering regimen over 5 to 10 days. However, there is little evidence that tapering these agents after initial improvement decreases the risk of relapse. With prolonged administration of systemic corticosteroids, special attention should be paid to conditions (e.g., diabetes mellitus) that may be exacerbated by their use. Long-term use of systemic corticosteroids may result in myopathy, osteoporosis, hyperglycemia, dermal thinning, cataracts, weight gain, mood disturbance, Cushing's syndrome, and hypothalamic-pituitary-adrenal axis suppression. The corticosteroid withdrawal syndrome also has been reported with tapering corticosteroids in chronically treated patients. Therefore, with long-term administration, a regimen of careful tapering is essential.

Newer generation antihistamines (including fexofenadine, terfenadine, cetirizine, and loratadine) have been advocated as adjunctive therapy for asthma. However, only a few studies have documented clinical benefits and concerns have been raised about the increased doses that may be required. Randomized studies are currently underway to determine the exact role of these newer generation agents in the treatment of asthma.

Omalizumab, a monoclonal anti-IgE antibody that functions to deplete serum IgE, has been shown to improve asthma symptom control, decrease frequency of exacerbations, and decrease requirements for inhaled corticosteroids. This medication is well tolerated and is typically administered by subcutaneous injection on a monthly basis, with a suggested minimum duration of use of at least 12 weeks. Recent studies indicate that the greatest benefits are in patients with high inhaled corticosteroid requirements, frequent emergency department visits, and poor lung function.

Macrolide antibiotics may be useful in the treatment of asthma complicated by persistent airway infection with *Mycoplasma pneumoniae* or *Chlamydia pneumoniae*. However, these agents also have defined anti-inflammatory activities, including membrane-stabilizing effects and the inhibition of eosinophil IL-8 release. Both erythromycin and troleandomycin can decrease corticosteroid requirements in steroid-dependent asthma. However, the role of these agents in the current treatment of asthma remains unclear after more than 20 years.

Corticosteroid-sparing agents that have been used in refractory and corticosteroid-resistant asthma include azathioprine, cyclosporine, methotrexate, immunoglobulins, gold, and hydroxychloroquine. Placebo-controlled trials demonstrate that cyclosporine administration allows for a reduction in corticosteroid use and improves lung function. Similarly, randomized trials with methotrexate have demonstrated modest reduction in corticosteroid use. However, the risk of potential toxicity and further immunosuppression with these agents must be carefully weighed against the risk of continued corticosteroid use.

Novel agents currently being developed for treatment of asthma include the cytokine antagonists/agonists, serotonin-uptake enhancing drugs, cell adhesion inhibitors, platelet-activating factor inhibitors, phosphodiesterase IV inhibitors, and nitric oxide synthase inhibitors. These agents are being investigated and are promising future therapies for asthma.

Reviews and Classic Articles

1. Barnes PJ, Adcock IM. How do corticosteroids work in asthma? *Ann Intern Med.* 2003;139:359–370.

    An exhaustive review of the mechanism of action of corticosteroids in the treatment of asthma.

2. Bernstein B. Cromolyn sodium in the treatment of asthma: Coming of age in the United States. *J Allergy Clin Immunol.* 1985;76:381–388.

    An older, but comprehensive review of cromolyn and its use in asthma.

3. Cocchetto DM, Sykes RS, Spector S. Paradoxical bronchospasm after use of inhalational aerosols: a review of the literature. *J Asthma.* 1991;28:49–53.

    A review of this rare complication of aerosolized medication administration.

4. Drazen JM, Israel E, O'Byrne PM. Treatment of asthma with drugs modifying the leukotriene pathway. *N Engl J Med.* 1999;340:197–206.

    An excellent review of the physiology and role of the cysteinyl leukotriene receptor antagonists and the 5-lipoxygenase inhibitor, zileuton, in the treatment of asthma.

5. Haskell RJ, Wong BM, Hansen JE. A double-blind randomized clinical trial of methylprednisolone in status asthmaticus. *Arch Intern Med.* 1983;143:1324–1327.

    One of only a few double-blind studies clearly demonstrating that parenteral corticosteroids are effective at high doses in the treatment of status asthmaticus.

6. Kips JC, Pauwels RA. Long-acting inhaled beta(2)-agonist therapy in asthma. *Am J Respir Crit Care Med.* 2001;164:923–932.

    Comprehensive review of the pharmacology of long-acting β_2-agonists.

7. Nathan RA, Kemp JP. Efficacy of antileukotriene agents in asthma management. *Ann Allergy Asthma Immunol.* 2001;86(suppl 1):9–17.

    Recent review of the body of literature documenting the efficacy of antileukotriene agents in the treatment of asthma.

8. Nelson HS. β-Adrenergic bronchodilators. *N Engl J Med.* 1995;333:499–506.

    A review of the pharmacology, delivery, clinical role, and side effects of the short- and long-acting β_2-agonists.

9. Newman SP. Aerosol deposition considerations in inhalation therapy. *Chest.* 1985;88:152S–160S.

    A review of the dynamics and determinants of aerosol deposition in the lung.

10. Sin DD, Man J, Sharpe H, et al. Pharmacological management to reduce exacerbations in adults with asthma: a systematic review and meta-analysis. *JAMA.* 2004;292:367–376.

    Excellent review of the overall pharmacologic management of asthma.

11. Spitzer WO, Suissa S, Ernst P, et al. The use of β_2 agonists and the risk of death and near death from asthma. *N Engl J Med.* 1992;326:501–506.

    Based on health insurance data in 12,301 asthmatics, this controversial study reported an increased risk of death or near death with the regular use of aerosolized β_2-agonists, especially fenoterol. This influential study has led to multiple trials that address the safety of these medications and the issue of overreliance on these drugs in the setting of worsening asthma severity.

12. Staresinic AG, Sorkness CA. The use of inhaled corticosteroids in adult asthma. *Med Clin North Am.* 2002;86:1035–1047.

    Recent review of the role of inhaled corticosteroids in the treatment of asthma.

13. Weinberger M, Hendeles L. Theophylline in asthma. *N Engl J Med.* 1996;334:1380–1388.

An excellent review of theophylline pharmacology, its role in the treatment of asthma, and its side effects.

14. Wenzel SE. Antileukotriene drugs in the management of asthma. *JAMA.* 1998; 280:2068–2069.

    A review of the leukotriene modifier agents in the treatment of asthma.

15. Westby M, Benson M, Gibson P. Anticholinergic agents for chronic asthma in adults. *Cochrane Database Syst Rev.* 2004;3:CD003269.

    A meta-analysis of short-acting anticholinergic agents (i.e., ipratropium) that suggests that these agents may add little to other conventional asthma therapies. However, the authors cannot rule out that a subgroup of asthma patients may benefit from these medications. Trials of long-acting anticholinergics were not included in this analysis.

Important Clinical, Diagnostic, or Therapeutic Studies

1. Aaron SD, Dales RE, Pham B. Management of corticosteroid-dependent asthma with methotrexate: a meta-analysis of randomized clinical trials. *Respir Med.* 1998;92:1059–1065.

    This meta-analysis of randomized trials of methotrexate administration in corticosteroid-dependent asthma demonstrated a modest corticosteroid-sparing effect. The study cites that the risk of potentially life-threatening side effects must be weighed carefully against possible benefits.

2. Blake KV, Hoppe M, Harman E, et al. Relative amount of albuterol delivered to lung receptors from a metered-dose inhaler and nebulizer solution. Bioassay by histamine bronchoprovocation. *Chest.* 1992;101:309–315.

    A study addressing the question of the effectiveness of MDI versus nebulizer delivery of β_2-agonists. These authors used histamine bronchoprovocation to evaluate the delivery systems. They found 10 puffs of the MDI to be equivalent to 2.5 mg of nebulized solution. This study suggests the need to use higher doses of MDIs during the treatment of acute asthma exacerbation.

3. Bousquet J, Wenzel S, Holgate S, et al. Predicting response to omalizumab, an anti-IgE antibody, in patients with allergic asthma. *Chest.* 2004;125:1378–1386.

    Multicenter, double-blind, randomized, placebo-controlled phase III trial documenting the benefits of omiluzimab in patients with asthma.

4. Dahlén B, Nizankowska E, Szczeklik A, et al. Benefits from adding the 5-lipoxygenase inhibitor zileuton to conventional therapy in aspirin-intolerant asthmatics. *Am J Respir Crit Care Med.* 1998;157:1187–1194.

    A study demonstrating the efficacy of the 5-lipoxygenase inhibitor, zileuton, in the treatment of aspirin-induced asthma.

5. Dompeling E, van Schayck CP, van Grunsven PM, et al. Slowing the deterioration of asthma and chronic obstructive pulmonary disease observed during bronchodilator therapy by adding inhaled corticosteroids. A 4-year prospective study. *Ann Intern Med.* 1993;118:770–778.

    This study provides compelling evidence that the inhaled corticosteroids inhibit the loss of lung function in asthmatics over time.

6. Drazen JM, Israel E, Boushey HA, et al. Comparison of regularly scheduled with as-needed use of albuterol in mild asthma. *N Engl J Med.* 1996;335:841–847.

    A multicenter, double-blind trial in 255 patients that demonstrated no adverse or beneficial effects of regularly administered versus as-needed albuterol in patients with mild asthma. The authors, therefore, suggest that short-acting β_2-agonists be used on an as-needed basis.

7. Drazen JM, Yandava CN, Dubé L, et al. Pharmacogenetic association between ALOX5 promoter genotype and the response to anti-asthma treatment. *Nat Genet.* 1999;22:168–170.

    An intriguing study demonstrating that the clinical response to the leukotriene modifier agents may be related to mutations within the 5-lipoxygenase gene promoter.

8. Harrison TW, Oborne J, Newton S, et al. Doubling the dose of inhaled corticosteroids to prevent asthma exacerbations: randomised controlled trial. *Lancet.* 2004;363:271–275.

Recent study indicating that increasing inhaled steroid doses in patients with deteriorating asthma control is not of benefit. These data support that of other studies, which suggests that patients in this subset may benefit more from the addition of another medication (such as a leukotriene modifier agent or a long-acting β₂-agonist).

9. Hawkins G, McMahon AD, Twaddle S, et al. Stepping down inhaled corticosteroids in asthma: randomised controlled trial. *BMJ.* 2003;326:1115.

Randomized, double-blind trial documenting that a stepwise reduction in inhaled corticosteroid dose is safe in chronic stable asthma patients.

10. Idris AH, McDermott MF, Raucci JC, et al. Emergency department treatment of severe asthma. Metered-dose inhaler plus holding chamber is equivalent in effectiveness to nebulizer. *Chest.* 1993;103:665–672.

A representative study of this type; the authors examined 35 patients with an average forced expiratory volume in 1 second (FEV₁) of 37% of predicted, comparing MDI albuterol to nebulized albuterol. The study demonstrated no difference in effectiveness and the MDI was found to be delivered more rapidly.

11. Ilowite J, Webb R, Friedman B, et al. Addition of montelukast or salmeterol to fluticasone for protection against asthma attacks: a randomized, double-blind, multicenter study. *Ann Allergy Asthma Immunol.* 2004;92:641–648.

Randomized, double-blind trial demonstrating that the addition of montelukast or salmeterol is equally efficacious in asthmatics with poor control on inhaled corticosteroids.

12. Israel E, Rubin P, Kemp JP, et al. The effect of inhibition of 5-lipoxygenase by zileuton in mild-to-moderate asthma. *Ann Intern Med.* 1993;119:1059–1066.

A randomized, double-blind, placebo-controlled, multicenter study of 139 patients with mild-to-moderate asthma treated with the 5-lipoxygenase inhibitor, zileuton; the authors found both subjective and objective improvement at 1 and 2 hours after drug administration, as well as at 4 weeks.

13. Lock SH, Kay AB, Barnes NC. Double-blind, placebo-controlled study of cyclosporine A as a corticosteroid-sparing agent in corticosteroid-dependent asthma. *Am J Respir Crit Care Med.* 1996;153:509–514.

The authors demonstrated a modest corticosteroid-sparing effect of cyclosporine.

14. Milgrom H, Fick RB Jr, Su JQ, et al. Treatment of allergic asthma with monoclonal anti-IgE antibody. rhuMAb-E25 Study Group. *N Engl J Med.* 1999;341:1966–1973.

Landmark randomized trial documenting the efficacy of anti-IgE therapy in asthma.

15. Nelson JA, Strauss L, Skowronski M, et al. Effect of long-term salmeterol treatment on exercise-induced asthma. *N Engl J Med.* 1998;339:141–146.

A double-blind, crossover trial that addresses the issue of tolerance to the long-acting β₂-agonist, salmeterol, in patients with exercise-induced asthma. The study reported that the duration of drug activity is decreased after a single dose, but that the protection against exercise-induced asthma is sustained.

16. Pauwels RA, Löfdal C-G, Postma DS, et al. Effect of inhaled formoterol and budesonide on exacerbations of asthma. *N Engl J Med.* 1997;337:1405–1411.

A randomized, double-blind, multicenter trial in 852 patients demonstrating superior clinical benefit of the addition of the long-acting β₂-agonist, formoterol, to a regimen of low-dose inhaled corticosteroids when compared with increasing the dose of corticosteroids.

17. Pearlman DS, Stricker W, Weinstein S, et al. Inhaled salmeterol and fluticasone: a study comparing monotherapy and combination therapy in asthma. *Ann Allergy Asthma Immunol.* 1999;82:257–265.

A randomized, double-blind trial demonstrating improved symptom control and pulmonary function with a combined salmeterol and inhaled fluticasone combination, as compared with inhaled fluticasone alone.

18. Reiss TF, Chervinsky P, Dockhorn RJ, et al. Montelukast, a once-daily leukotriene receptor antagonist, in the treatment of chronic asthma: a multicenter, randomized, double-blind trial. Montelukast Clinical Research Study Group. *Arch Intern Med.* 1998;158:1213–1220.

A randomized, double-blind, multicenter trial of the leukotriene receptor antagonist, montelukast, in the treatment of 681 patients with asthma. The authors demonstrated that montelukast decreased the occurrence of asthma exacerbations and improved asthma control. Side effects were minimal in the study population.

19. Salpeter SR, Ormiston TM, Salpeter EE. Meta-analysis: respiratory tolerance to regular β_2-agonist use in patients with asthma. *Ann Intern Med.* 2004;140:802–813.

Recent meta-analysis of 22 trials suggesting that regular β_2-agonist use (for at least 1 week) may contribute to tolerance to bronchodilator effects and may result in poorer disease control. Approximately half the trials in the analysis evaluated short-acting β_2-agonists and half evaluated long-acting β_2-agonists. The data support the current clinical recommendation that short-acting β_2-agonists should be used on an "as-needed" basis only. However, the tolerance that may develop in response to long-acting β_2-agonist use requires further study.

20. Suissa S, Ernst P, Benayoun S, et al. Low-dose inhaled corticosteroids and the prevention of death from asthma. *N Engl J Med.* 2000;343:332–336.

Population-based cohort study from the Saskatchewan Health database documenting an association between inhaled corticosteroid use and a decreased risk of death from asthma. A notable observation in this study was an increase in risk of asthma-related death in patients in the first 3 months after the discontinuation of inhaled corticosteroids.

21. Ververeli K, Chipps B. Oral corticosteroid-sparing effects of inhaled corticosteroids in the treatment of persistent and acute asthma. *Ann Allergy Asthma Immunol.* 2004;92:512–522.

Review of evidence indicating that inhaled corticosteroids exhibit a "steroid-sparing" effect.

Important Case Report

1. Wechsler ME, Garpestad E, Flier SR, et al. Pulmonary infiltrates, eosinophilia, and cardiomyopathy following corticosteroid withdrawal in patients with asthma receiving zafirlukast. *JAMA.* 1998;279:455–457.

One of the initial reports establishing an association between leukotriene receptor antagonist administration and development of the Churg-Strauss syndrome.

---

52. CHRONIC OBSTRUCTIVE PULMONARY DISEASE: DEFINITION AND EPIDEMIOLOGY

Andrew L. Ries

Chronic obstructive pulmonary disease (COPD) refers to a group of disorders that have in common the presence of persistent airflow obstruction that is not fully reversible. The airflow limitation is usually progressive and is associated with an abnormal inflammatory response of the lung to noxious particles or gases, primarily caused by cigarette smoking.

From the viewpoint of the pathologist, chronic bronchitis and emphysema are distinct processes, the former limited to the airways, the latter to the pulmonary parenchyma. From the viewpoint of the clinician, such a distinction is difficult for several reasons: (1) some degree of each may coexist in the same patient; *pure* forms of chronic bronchitis and emphysema are exceptions rather than the rule; (2) both are characterized by expiratory flow obstruction on simple spirometric testing; (3) patients with both processes often present with the same symptom—dyspnea on exertion; and (4) the presence of airway hyperreactivity (*asthma*, acutely reversible airways disease) in many patients with chronic bronchitis or emphysema further complicates the distinction. Faced with such complexities, it is understandable that the clinician often lumps together patients with chronic expiratory obstruction under the label *COPD*.

Nevertheless, distinct advantages are found in attempting to distinguish chronic bronchitis from emphysema, or at least to define the relative extent of each in a given patient. Such advantages relate particularly to the selection of therapy and to the natural history of these disorders, which is reflected in the individual patient's prognosis. For example, recent studies have indicated that mucous gland hypertrophy and mucus hypersecretion—both hallmarks of chronic bronchitis—are not major factors in causing airflow obstruction. Attempts at distinction also are essential to determine the pathogenetic differences between chronic bronchitis and emphysema, although the dominant role of cigarette smoking in both is clear.

The confusion between chronic bronchitis and emphysema has been compounded by the manner in which they have been defined by various scientific societies, in different studies, and in different nations. In defining chronic bronchitis and emphysema, three options are available: pathologic, clinical, and physiologic. In fact, all three options have been used. This is not surprising because pathologic evidence is rarely sought (or advisable) while the patient is alive; the physiologic techniques that allow distinction are still not generally applied; and attempts to provide clinical definitions were useful when neither pathologic nor physiologic criteria were available.

Chronic bronchitis has long been defined in clinical terms. The most widely used definition is that of the American Thoracic Society, which defines chronic bronchitis as "a clinical disorder characterized by excessive mucous secretion ... manifested by chronic or recurrent productive cough ... on most days for a minimum of three months in the year and for not less than two successive years." This clinical definition is now known to have serious deficits. First, other disorders with similar manifestations must be excluded, such as bronchiectasis, tuberculosis, and lung abscess. Furthermore, patients with predominant asthma or emphysema may fit this definition. Finally, many patients with pathologic or physiologic hallmarks of chronic bronchitis may not qualify under this definition (i.e., they do not cough).

If pathologic findings were used to define chronic bronchitis, the task would be relatively easy. Pathologically, the hallmark of chronic bronchitis is the hyperplastic and hypertrophied mucous glands found in the submucosa of large cartilaginous bronchi. The ratio of bronchial gland thickness to bronchial wall thickness (Reid index) is increased. The small airways (noncartilaginous bronchioles <2 mm in diameter) may also be involved, demonstrating mucous plugging, mural fibrosis and narrowing, goblet-cell hyperplasia, and inflammatory cell infiltrates. Thus, in the absence of parenchymal change, these findings in the airways would characterize *pure* chronic bronchitis.

Because such pathologic evidence is not conveniently available, much effort has been devoted to correlating pathologic data with physiologic tests. By physiologic testing, the pure chronic bronchitis patient should demonstrate:

1. Relatively normal total lung capacity (TLC) with modest elevation of the residual volume (RV) and functional residual capacity (FRC).
2. Some degree of expiratory and inspiratory flow obstruction (both flows are abnormal because airway narrowing is fixed anatomically).
3. Flow obstruction not acutely improved by bronchodilator administration.
4. Normal elastic recoil and compliance (pressure–volume curve of the lung).
5. Significant disturbances of gas exchange producing hypoxemia because of ventilation–perfusion imbalance. Hypercapnia can develop with more severe disease.
6. Normal diffusing capacity for carbon monoxide.

In contrast with the clinical description of chronic bronchitis, emphysema has long been defined in anatomic–pathologic terms. The widely used American Thoracic Society definition states that emphysema is present when there is "an anatomical alteration of the lung characterized by an abnormal enlargement of the airspaces distal to the nonrespiratory bronchioles, accompanied by destructive changes of the alveolar walls." Thus, pure emphysema is a parenchymal (airspace) disease in which the bronchi are not involved. In recent years, high-resolution computed tomography has been used to detect emphysema based on anatomic changes in the lung parenchyma.

Pathologically, emphysema is characterized by disruption of the alveolar walls at some location within the acinus, which is the lung division distal to the terminal bronchiole that includes the respiratory bronchioles, alveolar ducts, and terminal alveoli. Depending on the dominant site of involvement, emphysema is defined pathologically as centrilobular (proximal acinar), in which the proximal part of the acinus is involved, or as panacinar, in which the whole acinar structure is involved.

A clinical definition of emphysema is lacking; if one did exist, it would be dominated by the historic finding of effort dyspnea.

Physiologically, patients with pure emphysema demonstrate distinct features:

1. The lung volumes show evidence of hyperinflation, namely, an elevated FRC, RV, and RV:TLC ratio. Often, TLC is increased. Early in the course of disease, vital capacity may be preserved (i.e., concomitant elevation in RV and TLC). With more severe disease, vital capacity (VC) may be reduced in proportion to the elevation in RV. Such measurements are best made in a body plethysmograph, because the lung volume measured by gas dilution techniques (e.g., helium dilution, nitrogen washout) may underestimate the lung volume in emphysema.
2. Significant expiratory flow obstruction is present with preservation of inspiratory flows. This observation is most dramatically demonstrated by flow–volume curves that show normal flow rates during inspiration but severely reduced flow rates on expiration.
3. Expiratory obstruction is not immediately improved by bronchodilator administration.
4. Elastic recoil is low (i.e., low pleural pressures exist at TLC and other specified lung volumes) and compliance is increased (i.e., small pleural pressure changes are associated with large increases in lung volume). These findings are the physiologic correlates of alveolar disruption and are the hallmarks of emphysema.
5. Gas exchange is well preserved in the stable state, despite advanced spirometric abnormalities.
6. The diffusing capacity for carbon monoxide is reduced.

Therefore, to the extent that chronic bronchitis and emphysema exist in pure forms, they can be distinguished from each other and from asthma by physiologic tests that reflect the pathology involved. In practical terms, as already noted, mixed forms are the rule. This is particularly true when advanced disease is present.

Controversy exists about whether asthma itself is part of the spectrum of COPD. Nonspecific airway hyperresponsiveness has been proposed as a risk factor that predisposes smokers to developing COPD (the Dutch hypothesis). Asthmatic bronchitis is one of the recognized epidemiologic patterns of COPD. Asthma can result in chronic airflow obstruction and should probably be included within the clinical spectrum of COPD.

Chronic obstructive pulmonary disease is a major cause of death and disability. Because COPD is insidious, with a long latency period before clinical recognition, official statistics underestimate morbidity and mortality. As of 1990, COPD had moved up to the fourth leading cause of death in the United States. In 2000, COPD was listed as the underlying cause of more than 119,000 deaths and, for the first time, the number of women dying from COPD surpassed the number of men. From 1980 to 2000, the COPD death rate among women increased dramatically from 20.1 to 56.7/100,000, whereas for men there was a more modest increase from 73.0 to 82.6/100,000. It should be noted that mortality rates for COPD significantly underestimate the magnitude of the problem because many decedents with COPD have their deaths attributed to other causes. In 1998 only 45% of death certificates mentioning COPD listed COPD as the underlying cause of death even though people with COPD listed on their death certificate typically have severe disease. Thus, COPD is likely a more important contributor to death than generally recognized.

In the United States, the overall prevalence of COPD is approximately 6% in adults age 25 and older based on self-reports of chronic bronchitis or emphysema. Using extensive questionnaires and physical examination, including spirometry testing, the Third National Health and Nutrition Examination Survey (NHANES III) reported a 14% prevalence of airway obstruction in a representative sample of U.S. adults surveyed from 1988 to 1994.

The impact of COPD on morbidity is even greater than on mortality. In 2000, COPD was responsible for 8 million physician office or hospital outpatient visits, 1.5 million emergency department visits, and 726,000 hospitalizations. As a cause of disability-adjusted life-years (DALYs), in 1996 COPD was estimated to be the eighth among men and seventh among women. Worldwide, COPD is expected to move up from the twelfth leading cause of DALYs in 1990 to fifth in 2020.

Epidemiologic studies have identified two main syndromes, with different risk factors and natural histories. The usual emphysematous form is associated closely with cigarette smoking. Patients develop airflow obstruction insidiously over many years, with minimal symptoms, followed by clinical disease in later years, with progressive symptoms and high morbidity and mortality. The second form of COPD, chronic asthmatic bronchitis, is associated with risk factors of atopy, high serum IgE, and bronchial hyperreactivity. Patients develop chronic airflow obstruction independent of smoking, although smoking can add risk. Asthmatic bronchitis is more amenable to medical therapy and has a better prognosis and survival than the emphysematous type.

Cigarette smoking is the major risk factor, accounting for nearly 90% of COPD cases. Compared with nonsmokers, current smokers have approximately ten times the relative risk of developing COPD. The risk is equal for men and women. Previously, COPD was more common in men because of their higher smoking rates; in recent years, however, the disease has manifested more gender equality, reflecting similar smoking rates for men and women.

Significant individual variation in susceptibility is seen, and host factors play an important role. Only 10 to 15% of smokers develop significant obstructive lung disease. In susceptible persons, smoking is associated with an accelerated decline in lung function over many years that is related to the amount of smoking. Because of the large reserve in healthy lungs, disease is not typically recognized until later in life.

Exposure of nonsmokers to the smoke of others in an indoor environment (secondhand smoke) is associated with an increase in respiratory infections and lung disease in children and with modest changes in lung function in adults. However, it has not been clearly established that passive smoke exposure leads to clinically significant obstructive lung disease.

Some evidence indicates that environmental exposures (e.g., air pollution and occupational dusts and fumes) are harmful for persons with underlying lung disease and may increase the risk for developing COPD. However, it is unclear whether the effects are independent of smoking. Growing evidence also suggests that a history of childhood respiratory infections increases the risk for developing COPD in later life.

One credible theory about the pathogenesis of emphysema is that the disease results from an imbalance between lung proteases and antiproteases, enzymes that, respectively, promote injury and protect the lung against injury. Human neutrophil elastase (HNE) is released from granules of the neutrophil during phagocytosis and after stimulation, chemotaxis, and cell death. Cigarette smoke components appear to promote the release of (1) neutrophil chemotactic factors from alveolar macrophages and (2) HNE from neutrophils. The activity of HNE is mitigated by a serum protein, α_1-antiprotease (α_1-Pi), which is synthesized by the liver and migrates freely into alveoli. Formulation of the protease/antiprotease theory of emphysema was catalyzed by the discovery that emphysema is common among individuals who are severely deficient in α_1-Pi, a globulin that is a potent inhibitor of several enzymes, including trypsin and elastase. It is postulated that elastase, which is found in polymorphonuclear leukocytes and in alveolar macrophages, is normally released from these cells; larger quantities may be released in response to lower respiratory tract infections. When α_1-Pi is present, elastase is inhibited; in its absence, released elastase is free to digest the lung.

The gene for α_1-Pi deficiency is inherited in an autosomal recessive pattern—Pi MM is the normal phenotype, Pi ZZ the most common phenotype of homozygous deficiency. Although heterozygous persons have reduced levels of α_1-Pi, they do not have a clearly increased risk for developing disease. In congenital emphysema, anatomic changes predominate at the lung bases rather than in the upper lung fields. Less than 1 of 2,000 individuals is severely deficient in α_1-Pi. More than 90% of the population—and the vast majority of patients with emphysema—are of the normal (MM) phenotype and have normal serum levels of α_1-Pi. Nevertheless, the same concept of enzyme–inhibitor balance may apply to other patients with emphysema. This possibility is supported by animal experiments in which emphysema-like disorders have been induced by intrapulmonary instillation of papain, elastase, and leukocyte homogenates. Evidence that a protease–antiprotease imbalance exists in the alveoli of patients deficient in α_1-Pi, and that this balance can be restored by intravenous administration of α_1-Pi, adds further weight to this hypothesis, as does the demonstration that certain oxidants (including components of cigarette smoke) can inactivate α_1-Pi, rendering it unable to inhibit elastase and other proteolytic enzymes.

It should be noted that the term *emphysema* is also applied to several conditions in which lung hyperinflation occurs without alveolar destruction. Among these conditions is congenital lobar emphysema, in which overinflation of a lobe (usually the left upper lobe) occurs, which can be life threatening. Pathologically, overdistention of single or multiple lobes is seen. *Compensatory emphysema* is a term applied to overinflation of the remaining lung in the face of collapse, destruction, or resection of other lung zones. Partial obstruction of a major bronchus does not cause tissue destruction characteristic of emphysema, although it does result in overdistention of alveoli. *Senile emphysema* is a term applied to the normal modest overinflation of the lung that occurs with aging and is reflected in an increase in RV:TLC ratio, and is better referred to as the *aging lung*.

---

1. Celli BR, NacNee W, and committee members. Standards for the diagnosis and treatment of patients with COPD: a summary of the ATS/ERS position paper. *Eur Respir J.* 2004;23:982–994.

    Official statement published jointly by the American Thoracic Society and European Respiratory Society that updates official practice guidelines for the diagnosis and treatment of COPD. An online version of the document is available at www.thoracic.org/copd.

2. Pauwels RA, Buist AS, Calverley PM, et al. Global strategy for the diagnosis, management, and prevention of chronic obstructive pulmonary disease. National Heart, Lung, and Blood Institute (NHLBI)/WHO Global Initiative for Chronic Obstructive Lung Disease (GOLD) Workshop summary. *Am J Respir Crit Care Med.* 2001;163:1256–1276.

    International evidence-based review cosponsored by NHLBI and World Health Organization (WHO) providing guidelines for diagnosis and management. Major initiative to raise awareness about the global epidemic of COPD. Full online resources available at www.goldcopd.com *including Workshop Reports, Executive Summaries, Pocket Guides, Patient Guides, and Additional Resources with a slide set.*

3. Similowski T, Whitelaw WA, Derenne J-P, eds. Clinical Management of Chronic Obstructive Pulmonary Disease. New York, NY: Marcel Dekker; 2002.

    Excellent reference and resource in the Lung Biology in Health and Disease series. Comprehensive reviews of many topics related to pathogenesis, diagnosis and management of COPD.

4. Snider GL, Faling LJ, Rennard SI. Chronic bronchitis and emphysema. In: Murray JF, Nadel JA, eds. *Textbook of Respiratory Medicine.* Philadelphia, Pa: WB Saunders; 1994:1331.

    An excellent comprehensive review of the pathogenesis, clinical features, and treatment of COPD.

5. Snider GL. Nosology for our day: its application to chronic obstructive pulmonary disease. *Am J Respir Crit Care Med.* 2003;167:678–683.

    Excellent summary of terminology and definitions for COPD.

6. Snider GL. Emphysema: the first two centuries—and beyond: a historical overview, with suggestions for future research. *Am Rev Respir Dis.* 1992;146:1334,1615.

Distinguished J. Burns Amberson lecture, with an excellent review of the history and pathogenesis of emphysema.

7. Fletcher CM, Peto R. The natural history of chronic airflow obstruction. *BMJ*. 1977;1:1645–1648.

   Classic epidemiologic study of London working men, demonstrating the gradual decline in forced expiratory volume in 1 second (FEV₁) in nonsmokers and an accelerated decline in susceptible smokers.

8. Diener CF, Burrows B. Further observations on the course and prognosis of chronic obstructive lung disease. *Am Rev Respir Dis*. 1975;111:719.

   Long-term survival in a prospective study of 200 patients with COPD. Survival was related to the baseline level of FEV₁.

9. Burrows B. Epidemiologic evidence for different types of chronic airflow obstruction. *Am Rev Respir Dis*. 1991;143:1452.

   Report from the Tucson Epidemiologic Study of Obstructive Airway Diseases of a population sample of 1467 in 1971–1972. Suggests at least two different types of COPD: chronic asthmatic bronchitis and the usual form of emphysematous COPD.

10. Mannino DM. Chronic obstructive pulmonary disease: definition and epidemiology. *Respir Care*. 2003;48:1185–1191.

    Recent summary of epidemiologic data for COPD.

11. Centers for Disease Control and Prevention. Chronic obstructive pulmonary disease surveillance—United States, 1971–2000. *MMWR*. 2002;51/SS-6:1–16.

    Centers for Disease Control and Prevention (CDC) report of trends in COPD over the past 30 years.

12. Auerbach O, Hammond EC, Garfinkel L, et al. Relation of smoking and age to emphysema. *N Engl J Med*. 1972;286:853.

    Of 658 men who smoked 20 or more cigarettes a day, 0.3% had no emphysema, 32.7% moderate, and 19.2% advanced.

13. Eriksson S. Pulmonary emphysema and alpha-1-antitrypsin deficiency. *Acta Medica Scand*. 1964;17:197.

14. Eriksson S. A 30-year perspective on α_1-antitrypsin deficiency. *Chest*. 1996;110:237S.

    Original description of syndrome (11) and a recent perspective (12) from the discoverer of the α_1-antitrypsin deficiency syndrome.

15. American Thoracic Society. Guidelines for the approach to the patient with severe hereditary α_1-antitrypsin deficiency. *Am Rev Respir Dis*. 1989;140:1494–1497.

    Official statement of the American Thoracic Society, describing the background, diagnosis, and treatment of patients with α_1-antitrypsin deficiency.

16. Silverman EK, Pierce JA, Province MA, et al. Variability of pulmonary function in alpha-1-antitrypsin deficiency: clinical correlates. *Ann Intern Med*. 1989;111:982.

    Case series of 52 individuals with α_1-antitrypsin deficiency, many of whom did not have clinically significant abnormalities in lung function. Emphasizes the variable expression of the Pi Z phenotype.

17. DeMeo DL, Silverman EK. Genetics of chronic obstructive pulmonary disease. *Semin Respir Crit Care Med*. 2003;24:151–159.

    Succinct summary of current knowledge about genetics of COPD, emphasizing variability in susceptibility and heterogeneity. Deficiency of α_1-antitrypsin is the only proven genetic risk to date.

18. Nagai A, West WW, Paul JL, et al. The National Institutes of Health IPPB Trial: pathologic studies. I. Interrelationship between morphologic lesions. *Am Rev Respir Dis*. 1985;132:937.

19. Nagai A, West WW, Thurlbeck WM. The National Institutes of Health IPPB Trial: pathologic studies. II. Correlation between morphologic findings, clinical findings, and evidence of air-flow obstruction. *Am Rev Respir Dis*. 1985;132:946.

    These two papers review the lung morphology in nonhypoxemic COPD patients (at autopsy) and the correlation of morphology with other findings (clinical, physiologic). Mucous gland hypertrophy or hypersecretion does not appear, in these patients, to relate directly to airflow obstruction; emphysema does.

53. CHRONIC OBSTRUCTIVE PULMONARY DISEASE: CLINICAL AND LABORATORY MANIFESTATIONS, PATHOPHYSIOLOGY, AND PROGNOSIS

Andrew L. Ries

Chronic obstructive pulmonary disease (COPD) typically appears later in life. Dyspnea is the hallmark symptom that brings the patient to medical attention and leads to a diagnosis. A careful history of the insidious onset of breathlessness on exertion, with or without a history of cough, sputum, or frequent lung infections, often provides the clue to diagnosis.

Because of the slow, progressive course of disease and the large reserve in lung function, a long preclinical period elapses during which the person who has smoked for years "without a problem" begins to note breathlessness with physical activities previously accomplished without difficulty. This may be attributed to "getting older" or "being out of shape." Reduced expiratory flow rates may be detected at this stage. Later, the patient may come to medical attention after a critical event, such as a winter cold from which recovery has been slow. Disease onset is often attributed to this time; in reality, however, this event just pushed the patient over the clinical edge of recognition, much like a rope weakened by progressive fraying breaks when *only* a small weight is attached.

Cough is a frequent symptom, often attributed as a "smoker's cough" early in disease. It is usually productive; sputum is described as mucoid. Often there is a history of frequent respiratory infections associated with increased cough, purulent sputum, and breathlessness. The patient may note that it takes longer than usual to recover from these infections.

Some patients with COPD develop abnormal gas exchange with hypoxemia or hypercapnia. Hypoxemia can be associated with cognitive or personality changes, polycythemia, and cyanosis. Chronic hypercapnia can cause headache, particularly on arising, and increased somnolence. During exercise, the arterial Po_2 may change significantly and unpredictably from the resting level. In many patients, the PaO_2 decreases with physical activity; in others, it does not change or may actually increase.

On physical examination, decreased maximal expiratory flow may be apparent even in early disease. Therefore, it is important to assess maximal expiratory flow in persons at high risk (e.g., smokers). In early disease, the examination may be normal, but later, prolonged expiration or wheezing can be detected on forced exhalation. This can be assessed easily with the forced expiratory time, a useful screening test for expiratory obstruction. In this maneuver, the patient exhales with maximal effort through an open mouth after a full inspiration. The examiner listens with the bell of the stethoscope over the trachea in the suprasternal notch and records the time in seconds until airflow ceases. Normal persons can exhale completely within 4 seconds. A forced expiratory time greater than 6 seconds signifies significant expiratory obstruction.

Other physical signs of COPD often are not present until the disease becomes moderate to severe. Overinflation of the lungs can result in an increased anteroposterior diameter of the thorax and a low, flat diaphragm with reduced respiratory excursion. The flattened diaphragm contributes less to inspiration, placing more burden on the accessory breathing muscles (neck and intercostals) and producing greater respiratory movement in the upper chest. With severe hyperinflation, the diaphragm can even become inverted and move paradoxically—up on inspiration, down on expiration. This can be detected best with the patient supine, noting the inward movement of the lower rib cage and abdomen during inspiration. With advanced emphysema, the breath sounds are diminished because of reduced flow and increased lung inflation. Signs of pulmonary hypertension and right-sided heart failure (e.g., peripheral edema and hepatic congestion) are not usually detected until an advanced stage of disease.

The central diagnostic feature of COPD is reduced expiratory airflow, resulting from increased airway resistance because of airway narrowing. Spirometry is the standard pulmonary function test for measuring maximal airflow and is relatively simple, reliable, and reproducible. It is useful for detecting airflow obstruction, staging severity, and following the disease course. A reduction in the forced expiratory volume in 1 second (FEV_1) in relation to the forced vital capacity (FVC)—the FEV_1:FVC ratio—is a standard measure of obstruction. The FEV_1 is the best measure of disease severity; it correlates with exercise tolerance and survival. Other measures of expiratory airflow can also be helpful.

Measures of lung volumes reveal hyperinflation with an increase in residual volume, functional residual capacity, and, sometimes, total lung capacity. These tests can help to confirm the diagnosis suggested from spirometry. Emphysema causes a greater increase in total lung capacity than other obstructive diseases, as well as a reduced carbon monoxide diffusing capacity (DLCO), primarily because of the loss of alveolar–capillary surface area. However, DLCO is neither specific nor sensitive for emphysema.

Chest radiographs have limited usefulness in diagnosing or staging COPD; early in disease, they may be normal. Their main use is in detecting other parenchymal lung or cardiovascular diseases that can present with similar symptoms. With advanced emphysema, the chest radiograph may reveal overinflation of the lungs with a low, flat diaphragm and an increase in the retrosternal airspace (anterior to the heart) on the lateral film. The emphysematous lungs also may appear radiolucent because of bullous changes and a paucity of vascular shadows. High-resolution computed tomography may be useful in documenting pathologic evidence of emphysema and characterizing its distribution.

Arterial blood gas analysis may reveal hypoxemia and hypercapnia, particularly in advanced disease. The relationship between gas exchange abnormalities and other measures of lung function is poor. Hypoxemia can worsen with exercise, sleep, or changes in body position.

The electrocardiogram is usually normal early in disease; later, signs may appear of right-sided heart strain, including right axis shift, increased R waves over the right precordial leads (V_1 and V_2), and peaked P waves (P pulmonale). These changes do not correlate well with the level of pulmonary hypertension.

Two characteristic clinical patterns of COPD were originally described by Dornholst: the *pink puffer* (type A or emphysematous type) and the *blue bloater* (type B or bronchitic type). Type A patients typically have severe dyspnea, with little cough and sputum. They are usually thin with a hyperinflated chest. Arterial blood gases reveal mild, if any, hypoxemia (i.e., *pink* without cyanosis) and normal to low arterial P_{CO_2} (i.e., *puffing* with increased breathing effort). Type B patients typically have a history of chronic bronchitis with cough, sputum, and recurrent exacerbations with respiratory tract infections. Dyspnea on exertion is a prominent symptom, but is often episodic. On examination, they tend to be overweight and cyanotic (*blue*) and have dependent edema, dilated neck veins, and hepatomegaly because of right ventricular failure (*bloated*). Auscultation of the lungs reveals diffuse expiratory and inspiratory rhonchi. Arterial blood gases demonstrate severe hypoxemia and hypercapnia with CO_2 retention (reflecting low ventilation). These differences may reflect variations in ventilation-perfusion ($\dot{V}/\dot{Q}$) mismatching and central respiratory drive.

In clinical practice, most patients with COPD have a mixture of type A and type B disease and fall between these two extremes. In addition, many patients with COPD have an element of asthma (i.e., reversible airways obstruction with bronchospasm). As discussed in chapter 52, epidemiologic studies of COPD have identified two main syndromes with different risk factors and prognosis: emphysematous form and chronic asthmatic bronchitis.

The pathophysiologic basis of emphysema is a consequence of slowly progressive alveolar fragmentation, loss of lung elasticity, and mechanically related expiratory airflow obstruction. If acute problems (e.g., infection, anesthesia, sedation, left ventricular failure) do not occur, the patient slowly becomes more breathless, inactive, and wasted. This decline can extend over a period of many years. The development of acute respiratory failure is usually an ominous sign, because it occurs near the end stage (i.e., when very advanced parenchymal destruction is present).

On the other hand, the patient with more predominant bronchitis and asthmatic components of disease tends to have a more episodic course punctuated with exacerbations and reactive airway disease. Such patients tend to respond more to medical therapy and have a better prognosis.

1. Anthonisen NR, Wright EC, Hodgkin JE. Prognosis in chronic obstructive pulmonary disease. *Am Rev Respir Dis.* 1986;133:14–20.

    A 3-year follow-up of 985 patients with COPD in the National Institutes of Health—Intermittent Positive Pressure Breathing trial. Age and FEV_1 were best predictors of mortality.

2. Bates DV. The fate of the chronic bronchitic: a report of the ten-year follow-up in the Canadian Department of Veterans' Affairs coordinated study of chronic bronchitis. *Am Rev Respir Dis.* 1963;108:1043.

    In approximately 10% of men who smoke, pulmonary function deteriorates faster than the normal rate of decline. This accelerated deterioration can occur in the absence of chest infections.

3. Burrows B, Bloom JW, Traver GA, et al. The course and prognosis of different forms of chronic airways obstruction in a sample from the general population. *N Engl J Med.* 1987;317:1309.

    The 10-year mortality rate among nonatopic smokers without a history of asthma was close to 60% versus 15% among atopic subjects or nonsmokers with known asthma. The mean rate of decline in FEV_1 was 70 mL/year in the former group and less than 5 mL/year in the latter group.

4. Postma DS, Burema J, Gimeno F, et al. Prognosis in severe chronic obstructive pulmonary disease. *Am Rev Respir Dis.* 1979;119:357.

    Five-year and 10-year cumulative survival rates in 129 patients (initial FEV_1 <1,000 mL) were 69 and 40%, respectively. Best indicators of survival were a decrease in FEV_1/year and an increase in FEV_1 after inhaled bronchodilator.

5. Renzetti AD, McClement JH, Citt BD. The VA cooperative study of pulmonary function. III. Mortality in relation to respiratory function in chronic obstructive lung disease. *Am J Med.* 1968;44:115.

    Excellent correlation found between degree of physiologic abnormality and mortality rate. A higher mortality rate was also noted in the patient group at moderately elevated altitude.

6. Peto R, Speizer FE, Cochrane AL, et al. The relevance in adults of airflow obstruction but not of mucus hypersecretion to mortality from chronic lung disease. *Am Rev Respir Dis.* 1983;128:491.

    A study of 2,718 British men. Death rates were not significantly related to initial mucus hypersecretion among men with similar initial airflow obstruction.

7. Fletcher C, Peto R, Tinker C, et al. *The Natural History of Chronic Bronchitis and Emphysema.* London: Oxford University Press; 1976.

    An important prospective study of nearly 800 working men. The authors emphasize that COPD and mucus hypersecretion are two independent consequences of smoking.

8. Celli BR, Cote CG, Marin JM, et al. The body-mass index, airflow obstruction, dyspnea, and exercise capacity index in chronic obstructive pulmonary disease. *New Engl J Med.* 2004;350:1005–1012.

    Description and development of the BODE index, a simple grading system that was found to be better than the FEV_1 in predicting risk of death from COPD.

9. Murphy TF, Sethi S. Bacterial infection in chronic obstructive pulmonary disease. *Am Rev Respir Dis.* 1992;146:1067.

    A comprehensive review of the role of bacterial infection as a risk factor, cause of acute exacerbation, and promoter of lung damage in COPD.

10. Derenne J-P, Fleury B, Pariente R. Acute respiratory failure in chronic obstructive pulmonary disease. *Am Rev Respir Dis.* 1988;138:1006.

A comprehensive review and discussion of the causes, pathophysiology, and management of acute respiratory failure in patients with COPD.

11. O'Connor GT, Sparrow D, Weiss ST. The role of allergy and nonspecific airway hyperresponsiveness in the pathogenesis of chronic obstructive pulmonary disease. *Am Rev Respir Dis.* 1989;140:225.

    An excellent review of allergy and airway hyperresponsiveness as risk factors for the development of COPD and as influences on the response to therapy and prognosis in patients with COPD.

12. Parker DR, O'Connor GT, Sparrow D, et al. The relationship of nonspecific airway responsiveness and atopy to the rate of decline of lung function. *Am Rev Respir Dis.* 1990;141:589.

    Among 790 men 40 to 79 years of age, airway responsiveness, as measured by methacholine challenge, was associated with a more rapid decline in FEV_1. This relationship was stronger among skin test-negative cigarette smokers and does not support a relationship between atopy and decline in FEV_1.

13. MacNee W. Pathophysiology of cor pulmonale in chronic obstructive pulmonary disease. *Am J Respir Crit Care Med.* 1994;150:833;1158.

    A two-part state-of-the-art review of the pathogenesis of right ventricle failure in COPD, including a discussion of techniques used to assess cardiovascular function and management.

14. Bergin C, Muller N, Nichols DM, et al. The diagnosis of emphysema. A computed tomographic pathologic correlation. *Am Rev Respir Dis.* 1986;133:541.

    Computed tomography (CT) was performed on 32 patients before lung resection surgery. The presence and degree of emphysema were compared with measurements of pulmonary function testing. CT proved to be a better predictor of the degree of emphysema than pulmonary function testing.

15. Knudson RJ, Standen JR, Kaltenborn WT, et al. Expiratory computed tomography for assessment of suspected pulmonary emphysema. *Chest.* 1991;99:1357.

    This study is similar to the one in reference 13 and suggests that CT reduces the subjectivity of diagnosing emphysema in the living patient.

16. Hogg JC, Macklem PT, Thurlbeck WM. Site and nature of obstruction in chronic obstructive lung disease. *N Engl J Med.* 1968;278:1355.

    A major site of obstruction is in small airways.

17. Mitchell RS, Stanford RE, Johnson JM, et al. The morphologic features of the bronchi, bronchioles, and alveoli in chronic airway obstruction: a clinicopathologic study. *Am Rev Respir Dis.* 1976;114:137.

    Chronic airway obstruction best correlated with the severity of destructive emphysema.

54. CHRONIC OBSTRUCTIVE PULMONARY DISEASE: MANAGEMENT

Andrew L. Ries

Chronic obstructive pulmonary disease (COPD) is a chronic, progressive, and largely irreversible disease, so the primary goals of management should be directed toward preventive health strategies to slow progression and reduce complications. Secondary goals are to improve symptoms and function and treat reversible components. Optimal management depends on the stage of disease. For patients with mild to moderate disease, early detection and diagnosis and counseling regarding appropriate preventive health strategies are important. For patients with moderate to severe disease, symptomatic treatment is also indicated.

Teaching the patient and family members how to participate in the patient's management as active partners with the physician is a key goal that affects all other goals. Patients who are adequately informed and motivated can work with the physician and maintain a level of function that the uninformed, poorly motivated, *passive* patient cannot.

Most patients with COPD are former or current cigarette smokers. Controlling smoking behavior is essential, regardless of the stage of disease. Smoking cessation will slow the rate of decline in forced expiratory volume in 1 second (FEV_1) and decrease coughing and sputum production. Naturally, the more advanced the functional loss, the less the impact will be. Therefore, early detection of COPD, particularly in smokers who are at high risk, and smoking cessation should be emphasized. Physicians play an important role by setting a smoke-free example in their lives and workplace. Physician advice is important and effective in inducing smokers to quit and maintain abstinence. Several studies have demonstrated that a physician who spends a few minutes inquiring about smoking status and providing advice to quit can achieve abstinence rates of up to 10 to 20% at 1 year. The use of additional modalities such as a comprehensive smoking cessation program, nicotine replacement therapy (gum, dermal patches, nasal spray or oral inhaler), bupropion, or clonidine (oral or patches) can lead to long-term cessation rates of as high as 50% in motivated patients.

Pulmonary infection is the most common complication in COPD. Prophylactic influenza vaccination should be administered annually, preferably in the early fall. Pneumococcal vaccination, with the expanded version (containing the capsular polysaccharide of 23 serotypes), should be administered every 5 to 10 years. As effective antiviral agents become available (e.g., amantadine), consider their use for the patient with COPD, particularly during epidemics of influenza A.

Another preventive approach is to assess patient exposure to occupational–environmental air pollutants and, if possible, eliminate or reduce that exposure. A final method used to prevent complications is to avoid therapies and drugs that can compromise patient function. Patients with COPD tend to become victims of polypharmacy. To avoid this problem, carefully consider the risk-to-benefit characteristics of each therapy (drug, oxygen, or mechanical device) before it is instituted. Constantly review the treatment regimen, deleting elements that have been of no benefit, particularly if they can induce long-term toxicity.

For patients with recognized COPD, pharmacotherapy is directed toward the reversible component of airway obstruction and control of secretions. Bronchodilators used to improve symptoms and increase airway caliber include sympathomimetic β-agonists, anticholinergics, and methylxanthines (theophylline). The decision to treat a patient with a bronchodilator should not depend on demonstrating an acute response, as many patients respond to regular therapy. Airway hyperreactivity is common in patients with COPD and long-term therapy with bronchodilators can serve to prevent airways constriction caused by inhaled irritants. Also, these medications may have effects beyond just bronchodilation.

Sympathomimetic bronchodilators are used commonly. Newer β_2 agents are more selective and longer acting and have fewer side effects than older, nonselective drugs. The preferred method of administration is by inhalation, usually with a metered-dose inhaler (MDI). This produces more bronchodilation with fewer side effects than oral or other systemic routes. Used properly, an MDI is equally effective and less expensive than a liquid nebulizer and can be used in acute and emergency department settings. Extensions or spacers may help persons who have difficulty coordinating the MDI, particularly children and older adults. The key to MDI use is proper technique. All patients should be instructed and observed in following several key steps in using MDIs: (1) shake inhaler, remove cap, hold upright; (2) exhale to functional residual capacity or below; (3) place inhaler 2 to 4 cm in front of open mouth; (4) activate inhaler just after the start of a slow, deep inhalation; (5) hold breath for 5 to 10 seconds; (6) exhale slowly; and (7) wait at least 1 minute before next puff. In addition to bronchodilation, β-agonists can also reduce airway hyperresponsiveness and enhance mucociliary clearance. The most common side effects are tachycardia and skeletal muscle tremor.

Anticholinergics have recently gained prominence in the treatment of COPD. Although their bronchodilating effects have been known for many years, the selectivity and reduced side effects of newer agents have increased their usefulness. Bronchodilation is thought to be caused by inhibition of cholinergic-mediated bronchomotor tone. The drugs are reported to be more effective in larger airways, making them particularly useful for patients with COPD. They can be used concomitantly with β_2 agonists.

Theophylline preparations have been used in treating patients with COPD for many years, but their use has decreased because of a narrow toxic–therapeutic margin, frequent problems with toxicity, and the advent of newer, more selective bronchodilating agents. The mechanism of bronchodilation from theophylline is still not clearly defined. Theophylline has other potentially beneficial effects, such as improved diaphragmatic function, reduced dyspnea, increased mucociliary clearance, and stimulation of respiratory drive. Because of individual variability in metabolism and the many factors that can alter metabolism (e.g., drugs such as cimetidine, erythromycin, and ciprofloxacin), blood levels must be monitored with chronic therapy. The target therapeutic level is typically 10 to 20 μg/mL. Minor side effects such as tremor, insomnia, irritability, and gastrointestinal upset can occur with levels well below 20 μg/ml. More serious side effects, including vomiting, dysrhythmias, hypotension, and seizures generally develop at higher blood levels. Older patients are particularly susceptible to toxicity.

Corticosteroids can be beneficial for some patients with COPD. The complications of long-term use are well known and chronic use of systemic corticosteroids should be avoided, if possible. A meta-analysis of 16 clinical trials of oral steroid therapy for stable patients found that a 20% improvement in FEV_1 occurred in approximately 10% more patients on steroids than on placebo. Many patients on corticosteroids report subjective symptom improvement, but long-term steroid use is associated with many serious side effects. A limited trial of corticosteroids is probably justified in patients who cannot be managed with standard bronchodilators alone. A single morning dose of prednisone (20–40 mg) for 5 to 7 days is a typical starting point. Treatment beyond a few weeks should be continued only with a significant improvement in pulmonary function and symptoms. For long-term therapy, the dose should be kept as low as possible to minimize side effects.

Inhaled steroids, best used through a spacer device to minimize oral deposition, are safer, but their effectiveness in COPD has not been clearly established. Several multicenter clinical trials have evaluated the role of inhaled corticosteroids in the management of COPD. There is some evidence that inhaled corticosteroids may be associated with clinical benefits, such as reduced exacerbations and hospitalizations, even without documented improvement in lung function. However, prolonged use of these agents, particularly at high doses, may produce systemic side effects (e.g., subcapsular cataracts and decreased bone mineral density).

For patients with chronic cough and sputum, techniques to control secretions are important. Patients should be encouraged to drink several glasses of fluid per day, but excessive hydration is not warranted. They should also be taught the technique of controlled coughing, which involves a deep inspiration, breath-holding for a few seconds, and then coughing two or three times. Postural drainage is effective in patients with heavy sputum production. The use of mucolytic agents to thin secretions and promote clearance is controversial. Theoretically, therapy with drugs such as oral iodinated glycerol, nebulized acetylcysteine, or, more recently, recombinant human deoxyribonuclease, works best in thinning secretions that are thick, mucoid, and heavy. Whether this produces physiologic or symptomatic improvement is unclear. Cough suppressant therapy is generally not recommended, as cough is an essential protective mechanism.

Because of impaired mucociliary clearance and less effective cough, secretions can pool in dependent portions of the lung and be difficult to clear. For acute exacerbations, when sputum changes color and increases in volume, treatment with antibiotics is indicated. In many cases, a specific bacterial pathogen cannot be identified from purulent sputum. For such episodes of acute bronchitis, it is appropriate to institute a course (7–10 days) of antibiotics empirically without a sputum culture. Oral antibiotics such as trimethoprim–sulfamethoxazole, ampicillin, amoxicillin–clavulanate, tetracycline, or erythromycin are commonly chosen to cover pathogens colonizing the respiratory tract, including *Haemophilus influenzae, Streptococcus pneumoniae,* and *Moraxella catarrhalis.*

In the severely hypoxemic patient, oxygen therapy has been shown to improve survival and reduce morbidity from consequences such as right ventricular failure, polycythemia, and psychologic–mental dysfunction. Less clearly defined are the possible benefits of supplemental oxygen for nonhypoxemic patients or for patients with hypoxemia only under certain conditions (e.g., exercise, sleep). The results of two multicenter clinical trials (one in Great Britain, the other in the United States) justify long-term oxygen therapy for patients with significant resting hypoxemia (arterial Po_2 $\leq$55 mmHg or oxygen saturation [So_2] $\leq$88%). For patients with an arterial Po_2 between 56 and 59 mmHg, oxygen is indicated in cases of erythrocytosis (hematocrit 55 or more) or cor pulmonale. The decision for long-term therapy should be made only in stable patients on optimal treatment for at least 30 days. Patients recovering from an acute illness should be reevaluated after a period of stability before committing to this expensive treatment. Several options exist for long-term oxygen therapy. Home-care providers, respiratory therapy personnel, and pulmonary rehabilitation professionals are excellent sources of information about available options, including gas sources (e.g., liquid, compressed gas, concentrators) and delivery devices (e.g., nasal, transtracheal, or conserving catheters and inspiratory demand regulators). Hypoxemic patients living at high altitude may benefit by moving to sea level, where the ambient oxygen tension is higher. If air travel is contemplated, arrangements may be necessary for supplemental oxygen because commercial aircraft cabins are pressurized at 5,000 to 8,000 feet.

Patients with right ventricular failure often respond to gentle diuresis and the initiation of long-term oxygen therapy. Digitalis may be useful if left ventricular failure is present; however, its role, if any, in pure right ventricle failure has not been established. Phlebotomy has long been advocated for the treatment of polycythemia. Patients often report an immediate subjective improvement in their dyspnea and some improvement in their exercise tolerance. However, objective evidence for long-term improvement in lung function and hemodynamic indices is lacking.

Surgery may play a role in a few patients with COPD. Bullectomy may benefit selected patients with large space-occupying bullae. The role of laser ablation of bullae remains to be defined. Lung transplantation for COPD is feasible and has been performed in many centers; criteria for selection and long-term follow-up are still evolving. Lung volume reduction surgery has been found to result in improved survival, exercise tolerance, symptoms, and quality of life compared with medically treated patients in a large, randomized clinical trial (National Emphysema Treatment Trial). The benefits were most evident in patients with a predominance of upper lobe distribution of emphysema and very low exercise tolerance.

Pulmonary rehabilitation is an established preventive health strategy that enhances standard therapy for persons with chronic lung disease to control and alleviate symptoms, optimize function, and reduce the medical and economic burdens of disease. Multidisciplinary programs include education, respiratory and chest physiotherapy instruction, psychosocial support, and exercise training. As with other rehabilitation programs, the primary goal is to restore the patient to the highest possible level of independent function. This can be accomplished by helping patients become more knowledgeable about their disease, more actively involved in their own healthcare, more independent in daily care activities, and less dependent on family, friends, and health professionals and other expensive medical resources. Benefits of pulmonary rehabilitation include improved exercise tolerance and symptoms and reduced hospitalizations and use of expensive medical resources. Patients report improved quality of life with a reduction in respiratory symptoms, an increase in exercise tolerance and ability to perform physical activities of daily living, and improved psychological function, with less anxiety and depression and increased feelings of hope, control, and self esteem.

Breathing retraining techniques include instruction in pursed-lip breathing and breathing patterns. Pursed-lip breathing imparts a subjective relief of dyspnea in some individuals. In theory, it prevents airway collapse during expiration. Pursed-lip breathing is often accompanied by an instantaneous diminution in activity of the accessory muscles of respiration. Slow, deep breathing often provides a subjective sense of improved respiratory control. The increased tidal volume can serve to reduce wasted ventilation.

Formal rehabilitation programs have obvious advantages for both patients and physicians. But, however achieved, patient education is essential. Patients who understand their disease, medications, and the other elements of their regimen are likely to avoid hospitalization and a variety of other untoward events.

1. Celli BR, NacNee W, and committee members. Standards for the diagnosis and treatment of patients with COPD: a summary of the ATS/ERS position paper. *Eur Respir J.* 2004;23:982–994.
   Official statement published jointly by the American Thoracic Society and European Respiratory Society that updates official practice guidelines for the diagnosis and treatment of COPD. An online version of the document is available at www.thoracic.org/copd.
2. Pauwels RA, Buist AS, Calverley PM, et al. Global strategy for the diagnosis, management, and prevention of chronic obstructive pulmonary disease. NHLBI/WHO Global Initiative for Chronic Obstructive Lung Disease (GOLD) Workshop summary. *Am J Respir Crit Care Med.* 2001;163:1256–1276.
   International evidence-based review cosponsored by NHLBI and WHO providing guidelines for diagnosis and management. Major initiative to raise awareness about the global epidemic of COPD. Full online resources available at www.goldcopd.com *including Workshop Reports, Executive Summaries, Pocket Guides, Patient Guides, and Additional Resources with a slide set.*
3. Similowski T, Whitelaw WA, Derenne J-P, eds. *Clinical Management of Chronic Obstructive Pulmonary Disease.* New York: Marcel Dekker; 2002.
   Excellent reference and resource in the Lung Biology in Health and Disease series. Comprehensive reviews of many topics related to pathogenesis, diagnosis, and management of COPD.
4. Anthonisen NR, Connett JE, Kiley JP, et al. Effects of smoking intervention and the use of an inhaled anticholinergic bronchodilator on the rate of decline of FEV_1: the Lung Health Study. *JAMA.* 1994;272:1497.
   Results of the Lung Health Study, a multicenter, randomized trial of smoking cessation and inhaled anticholinergic bronchodilator therapy in 5,887 smokers with early COPD. Over 5 years of follow-up, smoking cessation significantly reduced the age-related decline in FEV_1. Anticholinergic therapy led to a small improvement in FEV_1 but did not influence long-term decline.
5. The Smoking Cessation Clinical Practice Guideline panel and staff. The Agency for Health Care Policy and Research Smoking Cessation Clinical Practice Guideline. *JAMA.* 1996;275:1270.
   Consensus panel recommendations about smoking cessation techniques for primary care clinicians, smoking cessation specialists, and healthcare administrators. Emphasizes the need for systematic practices and a multipronged attack to identify smokers and encourage smoking cessation practices.
6. Nett LM. The physician's role in smoking cessation. *Chest.* 1990;98:28S.
   Emphasizes the physician's role in encouraging, supporting, and facilitating smoking cessation.
7. Tashkin DP, Altose MD, Bleecker ER, et al. The lung health study: airway responsiveness to inhaled methacholine in smokers with mild to moderate airflow limitation. *Am Rev Respir Dis.* 1992;145:301.
   Airway hyperresponsiveness was found in 85% of female and 59% of male smokers with mild to moderate COPD. Emphasizes the importance of airway reactivity in these patients.
8. Mostow SR, Cate TR, Ruben FL. Prevention of influenza and pneumonia. *Am Rev Respir Dis.* 1990;142:487.

Official statement of the American Thoracic Society, emphasizing the importance of influenza and pneumococcal vaccination in patients with chronic lung diseases and other high risk groups.

9. Shapiro ED, Berg AT, Austrian R, et al. The protective efficacy of polyvalent pneumococcal polysaccharide vaccine. *N Engl J Med.* 1991;325:1453.

   The more recent vaccine is effective against the 23 serotypes that are responsible for 90% of serious pneumococcal disease.

10. Sin DD, McAlister FA, Man SFP, et al. Contemporary management of chronic obstructive pulmonary disease: scientific review. *JAMA.* 2003;290:2301.

    Systematic review of long-acting bronchodilators, inhaled corticosteroids, nocturnal noninvasive mechanical ventilation, pulmonary rehabilitation, domiciliary oxygen therapy, and disease management programs in COPD. Concluded that long-acting bronchodilators and inhaled corticosteroids reduced exacerbations, oxygen therapy improved survival in patients with resting hypoxemia, and pulmonary rehabilitation improved health status. Noninvasive ventilation and disease management programs have not been shown to improve outcomes.

11. Kasik JE, Alexander MR. Reversing the irreversible. *Chest.* 1982;82:517.

    The authors present the pros and cons of routine use of bronchodilating agents in patients with COPD. Most evidence suggests that they are worth using, whether or not pulmonary function tests demonstrate acute improvement.

12. Bergofsky EH, ed. Cholinergic pathway and obstructive airways disease. *Am J Med.* 1986;81:1.

    A comprehensive discussion of this topic. Reviews background science, clinical efficacy, safety, and combination therapy with other bronchodilators.

13. Callahan CM, Dittus RS, Katz BP. Oral corticosteroid therapy for patients with stable chronic obstructive pulmonary disease: a meta-analysis. *Ann Intern Med.* 1991;114:216.

    A meta-analysis of published studies of oral corticosteroids in patients with stable COPD. Overall, a more than 20% improvement in FEV_1 was seen 10% more often in patients on steroid therapy compared with controls.

14. Niewoehner DE, Erbland ML, Deupree RH, et al. Effect of systemic glucocorticoids on exacerbations of chronic obstructive pulmonary disease. *N Engl J Med.* 1999;25:1941.

    A randomized clinical trial of systemic corticosteroids in 271 patients hospitalized for exacerbation of COPD in which steroid therapy was associated with improved clinical outcomes.

15. Alsaeedi A, Sin DD, McAlister FA. The effects of inhaled corticosteroids in chronic obstructive pulmonary disease: a systematic review of randomized placebo-controlled trials. *Am J Med.* 2002;113:59–65.

    Summary and systematic review of recently conducted randomized clinical trials of inhaled corticosteroids in COPD. Concludes that there is a beneficial effect on reducing COPD exacerbations. Modest survival benefit was not statistically significant.

16. Highland KB, Strange C, Heffner JE. Long-term effects of inhaled corticosteroids on FEV_1 in patients with chronic obstructive pulmonary disease; a meta-analysis. *Ann Intern Med.* 2003;138:969–973.

    Meta-analysis of randomized clinical trials that did not find a significant relationship between the use of inhaled corticosteroids and the rate of decline in FEV_1 in COPD.

17. Rennard S. New approaches to COPD therapy. *Adv Stud Med.* 2003;3:S408–S415.

    Succinct review of newer classes of agents being evaluated for treatment of COPD, such as phosphodiesterase 4 inhibitors and other anti-inflammatory agents, retinoids, long-acting anticholinergics, and anabolic steroids.

18. Murphy TF, Sethi S. Bacterial infection in chronic obstructive pulmonary disease. *Am Rev Respir Dis.* 1992;146:1067.

    A state-of-the-art review of bacterial infection in COPD, including a discussion of its role in exacerbations, microbiology, and treatment. A treatment algorithm emphasizes use of Gram's stain without sputum culture and empiric choice of antibiotics.

19. Saint S, Bent S, Vittinghoff E, et al. Antibiotics in chronic obstructive pulmonary disease exacerbations. A meta-analysis. *JAMA*. 1995;273:957.

   A meta-analysis summarizing published randomized trials on the effectiveness of antibiotics in treating COPD exacerbations. Results suggest a small but statistically significant improvement.

20. Kirilloff LH, Owens GR, Rogers RM, et al. Does chest physical therapy work? *Chest*. 1985;88:436.

21. Rochester DF, Goldberg SK. Techniques of respiratory physical therapy. *Am Rev Respir Dis*. 1980;122:133.

   References 19 and 20 review the rationale for and use of chest physiotherapy and breathing retraining techniques in patients with chronic lung diseases.

22. Petty TL. The National Mucolytic Study: results of a randomized, double-blind, placebo-controlled study of iodinated glycerol in chronic obstructive bronchitis. *Chest*. 1990;97:75.

   A randomized, double-blind, placebo-controlled multicenter study demonstrating efficacy of iodinated-glycerol (60 mg four times daily) given as an adjunctive therapy. Although dyspnea showed a "trend toward improvement," the physicians' global evaluation did not differ between the two groups. The test agent improved chest symptoms and patient well-being.

23. American Thoracic Society. Pulmonary rehabilitation—1999. *Am J Respir Crit Care Med*. 1999;159:1666.

   An updated official statement of the American Thoracic Society, summarizing the benefits and describing the current practice of pulmonary rehabilitation.

24. Medical Research Council Working Party. Long-term domiciliary oxygen therapy in chronic hypoxic cor pulmonale complicating chronic bronchitis and emphysema. *Lancet*. 1981;1:681.

25. Nocturnal Oxygen Therapy Trial Group. Continuous or nocturnal oxygen therapy in hypoxemic chronic obstructive lung disease: a clinical trial. *Ann Intern Med*. 1980;93:391.

   References 23 and 24 are classic multicenter clinical trials conducted in Great Britain (23) and the United States (24) that demonstrated improved survival from oxygen therapy in hypoxemic patients with COPD.

26. Crockett AJ, Cranston JM, Moss JR, et al. A review of long-term oxygen therapy for chronic obstructive pulmonary disease. *Respir Med*. 2001;95:437–443.

   Systematic review evidence for use of long-term oxygen therapy in COPD.

27. Douglas NJ, Flenley DC. Breathing during sleep in patients with obstructive lung disease. *Am Rev Respir Dis*. 1990;141:1055.

   An excellent review of a relatively common disturbance (particularly hypoxemia and nocturnal wheezing) among patients with COPD.

28. National Emphysema Treatment Trial Research Group. A randomized trial comparing lung-volume reduction surgery with medical therapy for severe emphysema. *New Engl J Med*. 2003;348:2059–2073.

29. National Emphysema Treatment Trial Research Group. Cost effectiveness of lung-volume reduction surgery for patients with severe emphysema. *New Engl J Med*. 2003;348:2092–2102.

   These two references report primary outcomes of the National Emphysema Treatment Trial, a landmark study sponsored by NHLBI, CMS, and AHRQ to evaluate lung volume reduction surgery. Ideal patients were those with predominant upper lobe distribution of emphysema and lowest exercise tolerance. Emphasizes the poor prognosis of medically treated patients.

30. Orens JB, Martinez FJ. Lung and heart-lung transplantation: indications, timing, and results. *Semin Respir Crit Care Med*. 2001;22:477–587.

   Compendium of eight articles related to lung and heart-lung transplantation.

55. PULMONARY REHABILITATION

Andrew L. Ries

Comprehensive pulmonary rehabilitation (PR) programs are well established as a means to enhance standard medical therapy, control and alleviate symptoms, optimize functional capacity, and reduce disability for patients with chronic lung diseases. The primary goal is to restore the patient to the highest possible level of independent function. This can be accomplished by helping patients to become (1) more knowledgeable about their disease, (2) more actively involved in their own healthcare, and (3) more independent in performing daily care activities. Consequently, patients do much better and become less dependent on family, friends, health professionals, and expensive medical resources.

The typical program includes multidisciplinary participation by physicians, nurses, respiratory and physical therapists, exercise specialists, psychologists, and other healthcare professionals with particular expertise. The program should be tailored to the needs of the individual patient. To be successful, it should address important emotional and psychosocial problems as well as help to optimize medical therapy to improve lung function. The role of the rehabilitation program is to provide support for the patient, family, and primary care physician. Any patient with symptomatic chronic lung disease can be a candidate for PR. The greatest experience with PR has been in patients with chronic obstructive pulmonary disease (COPD); however, patients with other chronic lung diseases are also appropriate candidates. PR has also been found to be a beneficial adjunct to surgical programs such as lung transplantation and lung volume reduction surgery. In these settings, PR not only helps to better prepare patients for surgery and facilitate their recovery, but also aids in selection by assisting both patients and staff to better understand and weigh the risks and potential benefits.

Appropriate patients for PR are those who recognize their symptoms are caused by lung disease, perceive impairment or disability related to that disease, and are motivated to be active participants in their own care to improve their health status. Patients should be stabilized on standard medical therapy and evaluated carefully before entering a program so that appropriate and realistic goals can be set. Pulmonary function tests are used to characterize the lung disease and quantify its severity; however, patient selection should be based on symptoms and disability, not on arbitrary criteria based on lung function alone. Exercise testing helps to assess initial exercise tolerance, evaluate possible blood gas changes (e.g., exercise-induced hypoxemia), and plan a safe and appropriate training program.

The components of a comprehensive PR program include education, instruction in respiratory chest physiotherapy techniques, psychosocial support, and exercise training. Educating patients and significant others about lung disease and teaching them specific ways to deal with problems are essential. Educated patients are better able to cope with their disease, easier to deal with, and more likely to avoid unnecessary visits to physicians' offices, emergency departments, and hospitals. Patients should be taught appropriate chest and respiratory therapy techniques. Proper coughing and postural drainage techniques are important for all patients, especially those with excess mucus production. Techniques of pursed-lip and diaphragmatic breathing and relaxation training help to improve ventilatory efficiency and assist patients in gaining control over the frightening symptom of dyspnea. Patients with respiratory therapy equipment should be instructed in its proper use, care, and cleaning. Patients with significant hypoxemia should be evaluated for optimal methods of continuous oxygen therapy and instructed in its proper use because oxygen therapy has been shown to improve survival and to reduce morbidity for these patients. Lightweight portable systems should be emphasized for ambulatory patients.

Patients with chronic lung disease have significant psychosocial problems as they struggle to cope with symptoms that are often poorly understood. They become depressed, frightened, anxious, and dependent on others to care for their needs. Progressive breathlessness leads to a vicious fear–dyspnea cycle in which increasing dyspnea produces more fear and anxiety that, in turn, leads to more dyspnea. In PR, these problems can be dealt with effectively by enthusiastic and supportive staff, who can communicate with, understand, and motivate these patients. Important family members and friends should be included in program activities. Support groups and group therapy sessions are also effective. Patients with severe psychiatric disorders may benefit from individual counseling and psychotherapy. Psychotropic drugs should generally be reserved for patients with severe levels of psychological dysfunction.

Exercise training provides both physiologic and psychological benefits and is an ideal opportunity for patients to practice methods for controlling dyspnea. The exercise program should be safe and designed appropriately for each patient's interest, environment, and level of function. Walking programs are particularly useful and have the added benefit of encouraging patients to expand their social horizons. Other types of exercise (e.g., cycling, swimming) are also effective. Because many patients with chronic lung disease have limited exercise tolerance, emphasis during training should be placed on increasing *endurance,* the time of sustained activity. Exercise training of the upper extremities may be beneficial for the many pulmonary patients who report disabling dyspnea for daily care activities involving the arms (e.g., lifting, grooming) at work levels much lower than for the legs.

In recent years, increased attention has been drawn to peripheral muscle dysfunction in patients with chronic lung disease and the role of muscle fatigue as a limitation to exercise tolerance. This has stimulated new research initiatives in this area. Specific peripheral muscle strength and endurance training regimens have been developed and incorporated into PR programs. The potential role of respiratory muscle fatigue in pulmonary patients has led to attempts to train the ventilatory muscles. Although ventilatory muscles can be trained successfully, the role of this type of training in improving exercise performance has not been clearly established.

Exercise-induced hypoxemia occurs unpredictably in patients with COPD who may not be hypoxemic at rest. Hypoxemia is not a contraindication to exercise training. Such patients can be given convenient, lightweight portable systems for ambulatory oxygen so that exercise can be performed safely.

There is now a substantial body of evidence with well-designed trials that demonstrate the benefits of PR. As an effective, preventive healthcare intervention, PR has proved to be cost effective in decreasing both hospitalization days and the use of expensive medical resources. After rehabilitation, patients have an improved quality of life, reduced symptoms, increased exercise tolerance, more independence, increased ability to perform activities of daily living, and improvement in psychological function, with less anxiety and depression and increased feelings of hope, control, and self-esteem. Even after a short-term intervention, benefits typically last for at least 1 to 2 years.

1. Ries AL, Carlin BW, Carrieri-Kohlman V, et al. ACCP/AACVPR Pulmonary Rehabilitation Guidelines Panel. Pulmonary rehabilitation: joint ACCP/AACVPR evidence-based guidelines. *Chest.* 1997;112:1363 and *J Cardiopulm Rehab.* 1997; 17:371.
   Evidenced-based document developed jointly by the American College of Chest Physicians and American Association of Cardiovascular and PR that reviews the available scientific evidence for PR in patients with COPD. Recommendations are supported by evidence tables summarizing published clinical trials.
2. American Association of Cardiovascular and Pulmonary Rehabilitation. *Guidelines for Pulmonary Rehabilitation Programs.* 3rd ed. Champaign, IL: Human Kinetics; 2004.
   Updated reference that provides recommended guidelines for practice.
3. American Thoracic Society. Pulmonary rehabilitation—1999. *Am J Respir Crit Care Med.* 1999;159:1666.

Official statement of the American Thoracic Society (ATS), summarizing the benefits and describing the current practice of PR.

4. American Thoracic Society. Standards for the diagnosis and care of patients with chronic obstructive pulmonary disease. *Am J Respir Crit Care Med.* 1995;152:S77.

   Official statement of the ATS, providing standards for the management of patients with COPD. Includes a section on the role of PR.

5. Hodgkin JE, Connors GL, Bell CW, eds. *Pulmonary Rehabilitation: Guidelines to Success.* 2nd ed. Philadelphia: JB Lippincott; 1993.

6. Casaburi R, Petty TL, eds. *Principles and Practice of Pulmonary Rehabilitation.* Philadelphia: WB Saunders; 1993.

   Two excellent references that review all aspects of PR.

7. Lacasse Y, Wong E, Quejatt GH, et al. Meta-analysis of respiratory rehabilitation in chronic obstructive pulmonary disease. *Lancet.* 1996;348:1115.

8. Cambach W, Wagenaar RC, Koelman TW, et al. The long-term effects of pulmonary rehabilitation in patients with asthma and chronic obstructive disease: a research synthesis. *Arch Phys Med Rehabil.* 1999;80:103.

   References 7 and 8 are meta-analyses evaluating the effects of rehabilitation on exercise capacity and quality of life. Lacasse and coworkers reviewed 14 controlled clinical trials and found that rehabilitation relieves dyspnea and improves control over COPD. Statistically significant increase in exercise capacity were found, although the magnitude of benefit is of unclear clinical significance. Cambach and coworkers reviewed 18 controlled studies and found significant improvements in 6-minute walking distance, dyspnea, and quality of life. Improvements in maximal exercise capacity were heterogeneous.

9. Ries AL, Kaplan RM, Limberg TM, et al. Effects of pulmonary rehabilitation on physiologic and psychosocial outcomes in patients with chronic obstructive pulmonary disease. *Ann Intern Med.* 1995;122:823.

10. Ries AL, Kaplan RM, Myers R, et al. Maintenance after pulmonary rehabilitation in chronic lung disease: a randomized trial. *Am J Respir Crit Care Med.* 2003;167:880.

    Two randomized clinical trials evaluating PR. Reference 9 demonstrates significant improvements after a short-term intervention that last 1 to 2 years. Reference 10 evaluates a postrehabilitation maintenance program and emphasizes the importance of looking at rehabilitation strategies as longer term interventions and an integral part of chronic disease management.

11. Lacasse Y, Guyatt GH, Goldstein RS. The components of a respiratory rehabilitation program: a systematic overview. *Chest.* 1997;111:1077.

    A systematic review of published literature with a best-evidence synthesis of 22 randomized controlled trials. Concludes that PR is likely to improve exercise capacity and quality of life if it includes exercise training and psychosocial support.

12. Foster S, Thomas HM. Pulmonary rehabilitation in lung disease other than chronic obstructive pulmonary disease. *Am Rev Respir Dis.* 1990;141:601.

    Describes results of PR in 32 non-COPD patients. Improvement in exercise tolerance was similar to that observed in 317 COPD patients.

13. Palmer SM, Tapson VF. Pulmonary rehabilitation in the surgical patient: lung transplantation and lung volume reduction surgery. *Respir Care Clin North Am.* 1998;4:71.

14. Ries AL. Pulmonary rehabilitation and lung volume reduction surgery. In: Fessler HE, Reilly JJ Jr, Sugarbaker DJ, eds. *Lung Volume Reduction Surgery for Emphysema.* New York: Marcel Dekker; 2004:123.

    References 13 and 14 discus the role of PR as an adjunct to surgical programs like lung transplantation and lung volume reduction surgery.

15. Fishman AP. Pulmonary rehabilitation research. *Am J Respir Crit Care Med.* 1994;149:825.

    Summary of a National Institutes of Health workshop that describes state-of-the-art of research in pulmonary rehabilitation. Provides an updated definition of PR.

16. Ries AL, Bullock PJ, Larsen CA, et al. *Shortness of Breath: A Guide to Better Living and Breathing.* 6th ed. St. Louis: Mosby; 2001.

    An excellent book for patient education.

17. Dudley DL, Glaser EM, Jorgenson, BN, et al. Psychosocial concomitants to rehabilitation in chronic obstructive pulmonary disease. Part 1. Psychosocial and psychological considerations; Part 2. Psychosocial treatment; Part 3. Dealing with psychiatric disease (as distinguished from psychosocial or psychophysiologic problems). *Chest.* 1980;77:413, 544, 677.

   A comprehensive three-part review of the psychosocial problems of patients with COPD, including a review of the literature and recommendations for evaluation and treatment.

18. Casaburi R. Exercise training in chronic obstructive lung disease. In: Casaburi R, Petty TL, eds. *Principles and Practice of Pulmonary Rehabilitation.* Philadelphia: WB Saunders; 1993.

   An excellent review of exercise training issues in patients with COPD. Includes a table summarizing literature review of 37 published studies with 933 patients.

19. Belman MJ. Ventilatory muscle training and unloading. In: Casaburi R, Petty TL, eds. *Principles and Practice of Pulmonary Rehabilitation.* Philadelphia: WB Saunders; 1993.

   An excellent review of ventilatory muscle training and rest in the treatment of patients with COPD.

20. California Pulmonary Rehabilitation Collaborative Group. Effects of pulmonary rehabilitation on dyspnea, quality of life and health care costs in California. *J Cardiopulmonary Rehabil* 2004;24:52.

   Collaborative study of 647 patients in 10 centers in California that demonstrated significant improvements in dyspnea and quality of life with substantial reduction in health care utilization over 18 months of follow-up.

21. Ries AL, Farrow JT, Clausen JL. Pulmonary function tests cannot predict exercise-induced hypoxemia in chronic obstructive pulmonary disease. *Chest.* 1988;93:454.

   Reports on blood gas changes with exercise in 40 patients with COPD, indicating that exercise-induced hypoxemia is unpredictable from resting measurements of pulmonary spirometry and gas exchange.

22. Petty TL, Casaburi R. Recommendations of the Fifth Oxygen Consensus Conference. *Respir Care.* 2000;45:940.

   Discussion of use of long-term oxygen therapy for patients with chronic lung disease. Review of scientific rationale based on two classic randomized trials (Nocturnal Oxygen Therapy Trial and British Medical Research Council studies).

---

56. BRONCHIECTASIS

Julian P. Lichter

Bronchiectasis is defined in morphologic terms as persistent and irreversible dilatation, distortion, and thickening of the walls of medium-sized bronchi. The entity was first described by Laennec in 1819. Bronchi can be dilated temporarily (e.g., following pneumonia, tracheobronchitis) and then return to normal size after several weeks or months. This, however, is not true of bronchiectasis.

It is now generally accepted that bronchiectasis is an acquired disease process that develops in early childhood or later on in life, rather than a congenital abnormality present at birth. Bronchiectasis is not a discrete disease entity, but rather the end stage of a variety of unrelated pulmonary insults and antecedent events. However, all forms require an infectious insult and impairment of drainage, airway obstruction, or a defect in host defense.

CLASSIFICATION

Bronchiectasis has been classified in a number of ways: (1) on the basis of putative pathogenetic mechanisms; (2) by gross and microscopic pathologic findings; (3) by bronchographic anatomy; or (4) by predisposing causative factors. The most enduring anatomic classification is that of Reid (1950), who first correlated pathologic changes with bronchography. Three different appearances were described: *Cylindrical bronchiectasis* refers to bronchi that are uniformly dilated and do not taper, but rather end abruptly. This is caused by plugging of smaller bronchi by thick mucus and casts. The bronchi are dilated to greater than 2 mm but can be so large as to admit a finger. *Varicose bronchiectasis* describes dilated bronchi with irregular, bulging contours reminiscent of a varicose vein. They do not taper and terminations are bulbous. Bronchial subdivisions are reduced. *Cystic or saccular bronchiectasis,* the most severe form, is characterized by sharply reduced bronchial subdivisions and dilated bronchi ending in cystic, pus-filled cavities. *Saccules* may occur at the fifth subdivision (normally approximately 20 subdivisions exist), with the more peripheral bronchial branches destroyed and fibrosed. All three forms can be present in the same patient. Each anatomic type of bronchial dilatation has been shown to be potentially reversible, including saccular changes.

Traction bronchiectasis describes bronchial changes (typically seen on chest computed tomography [CT] scans) caused by traction of adjacent extensive interstitial pulmonary fibrosis. This simulates bronchiectasis, but other features of true bronchiectasis are not present.

PATHOGENESIS

The pathogenesis of bronchiectasis has not been fully elucidated, but the key element appears to be inflammatory destruction of the muscle, elastic tissue, and cartilage of the bronchial wall by infected mucopus in close and prolonged contact with the bronchial wall. Mucopurulent material contains neutrophilic products capable of damaging lung tissue (serine proteases and toxic oxygen radicals), as well as nitric oxide, inflammatory cytokines (e.g., interleukin 8, tumor necrosis factor), and substances that interfere with ciliary movement and mucociliary clearance. Buildup of such infected secretions often occurs distal to obstruction by inspissated mucous plugs with accompanying postobstructive atelectasis. An infected mucocele develops with subsequent mechanical dilatation of bronchi already weakened by proteolytic attack. The initial inflammatory insult is followed by secondary bacterial colonization, which produces further bronchial wall damage and predisposes to further colonization, thus setting up a vicious cycle. Eventually fibrosis of bronchial walls and surrounding lung probably results in traction on the weakened flabby bronchial walls and more distention. Distention can also be aggravated by surrounding atelectatic lung, which allows the bronchi to be more affected by intrathoracic pressure swings.

Pathologically, the endobronchial mucosa is denuded and may be replaced by nonciliated, low cuboidal, or squamous epithelium. Fragmentation and destruction of the muscular, elastic, and cartilaginous components of the bronchial wall occurs. Affected airways become tortuous and flabby. Areas of mucosa are eroded and microabscesses form, with the eventual development of cystic sacs of pus. In chronic, long-standing bronchiectasis, marked fibrosis occurs in and surrounding the bronchial walls. Bronchial walls are both dilated and thickened on CT imaging studies. Bronchial arteries may also be considerably enlarged (up to three times normal caliber) and tortuous, forming extensive anastomoses with the pulmonary circulation.

The incidence of the more severe forms of bronchiectasis (multilobar involvement with voluminous purulent or fetid sputum) has declined in the Western world with the development of antibiotics. Symptomatic bronchiectasis, nevertheless, is still prevalent today in less severe forms and especially in patients with underlying congenital diseases. Many patients with diagnosed chronic bronchitis and chronic sputum production, recurrent acute exacerbations, or both may well have underlying undiagnosed bronchiectasis. Clinically, these two pathologic processes may be indistinguishable.

Bronchiectasis is bilateral in approximately 30% of patients. The left lower lobe is involved about three times more often than the right lower lobe, probably because the left mainstem bronchus is slightly narrower. Dependency enhances the likelihood of involvement because drainage of secretions is impaired. The lingula and right middle lobe are the next most common sites.

Predisposing causative factors can be divided into those causing a focal process and those causing diffuse disease involving both lungs and often accompanied by other sinopulmonary diseases. Focal causes are mostly secondary to bronchial obstruction, namely, aspiration of a foreign body, a broncholith, a slow-growing tumor, surrounding lymph nodes, or inspissated viscid secretions. Diffuse bronchiectasis is usually associated with prior recurrent pulmonary infections, although the disease can be caused by a single severe episode of widespread pneumonia. Other causes include chronic granulomatous diseases, hypersensitivity disorders, immunodeficiency disorders, genetic syndromes, and certain rheumatic diseases. Pneumonias are either primary viral or secondary bacterial pneumonias following viral infections (especially during childhood). Pertussis and measles were very common antecedents of follicular bronchiectasis before immunization for these diseases. Severe influenza, varicella pneumonia, and repeated mycoplasma infections can also result in bronchiectasis. Bacteria that cause necrotizing pneumonias, such as *Klebsiella, Staphylococcus aureus, Pseudomonas,* and anaerobes (following aspiration) can cause saccular bronchiectasis.

A number of organisms are associated with colonization and recurrent episodes of superimposed infection in patients with underlying bronchiectasis, namely, *Haemophilus influenza, Staphylococcus aureus, Pseudomonas aeruginosa, Mycobacterium avium complex,* and *Aspergillus* species. Risk factors for colonization with potential pathogenic microorganisms include diagnosis of bronchiectasis before age 14, presence of varicose-cystic disease, and an FEV_1 of less than 80% of predicted.

The majority of patients with allergic bronchopulmonary aspergillosis have diffuse varicoid or cystic bronchiectasis, or both, at the time of diagnosis. The bronchial abnormalities occur in more central airways as a result of type III immune complex reactions.

A frequent cause of bronchiectasis today is the spectrum of granulomatous diseases: tuberculosis, sarcoidosis, histoplasmosis, and coccidioidomycosis. Tuberculosis is classically associated with bronchiectasis affecting mainly the upper lobes. Tuberculosis is also the most common cause of the middle lobe syndrome, in which obstruction of the normally slit-like middle lobe bronchial orifice by inflammatory lymph nodes occurs. Several reports have been published of presumed normal hosts (usually nonsmoking women over the age of 50 years) who have developed bronchiectasis with primary *Mycobacterium avium* complex infections. Chest CT usually shows small irregular nodules.

Bronchiectasis can be a manifestation of congenital (X-linked agammaglobulinemia, IgG_2 subclass deficiency) or acquired (chronic granulomatous disease) immunodeficiency states. The recent recognition of bronchiectasis in AIDS illustrates the accelerated destructive interaction between repeated infections and impaired host defense.

An array of genetic defects are associated with clinical syndromes in which bronchiectasis is often prominent. Cystic fibrosis, Mounier-Kuhn syndrome (tracheobronchomegaly), Williams-Campbell syndrome (bronchial cartilage deficiency), Kartagener syndrome (situs inversus, paranasal sinusitis, and bronchiectasis), Young syndrome (obstructive azoospermia and chronic sinopulmonary infection), and immotile cilia syndrome or primary ciliary dyskinesia (abnormal ciliary ultrastructure and function) are examples. All predispose to recurrent lower respiratory tract infections as a result of poor tracheobronchial clearance.

Two rheumatic diseases, rheumatoid arthritis and Sjögren syndrome, can be complicated by bronchiectasis. The arthropathy and sicca features are usually advanced when the bronchiectasis becomes apparent. Bronchiectasis has also developed in patients with inflammatory bowel disease (ulcerative colitis or Crohn disease).

PRESENTATION

Clinically, it is important to recognize that not all anatomically demonstrable areas of bronchiectasis cause symptoms. In fact, symptomatic bronchiectasis is much less common than asymptomatic anatomic bronchiectasis, which may never require treatment. If there is bilateral or multilobar involvement and the patient is symptomatic, symptoms can be caused by involvement of only one segment or one lobe. Indium-labeled white blood cells may be useful in identifying bronchiectatic segments that are infected and responsible for symptoms.

Clinically, bronchiectasis presents in a number of well-described ways. The classic presentation is with chronic cough and copious purulent or mucopurulent sputum (*wet* bronchiectasis). Sputum production may be continuous with intermittent febrile exacerbations during which both cough and expectoration increase, or the patient can have quiescent periods punctuated by frequent recurrences. Patients often present with frequent bouts of bronchial infection that require repeated courses of antibiotics. Isolation of mucoid *Pseudomonas* organisms suggests a diagnosis of bronchiectasis rather than chronic bronchitis. Alternatively, the patient may present with recurrent, discrete infections arising from the same segment or lobe. This suggests a structural abnormality in the area of the lung, which could be caused by bronchiectasis. A third less common presentation is that of recurrent, dry cough associated with intermittent episodes of hemoptysis (*dry* bronchiectasis). Usually, there is a remote history of granulomatous infection, especially tuberculosis, where the upper lobes are often primarily affected, and good drainage can usually occur. A mild respiratory infection not infrequently precedes the hemoptysis. Episodes of hemoptysis can occur months or years apart. Hemoptysis can be life threatening because bleeding is from bronchial vessels with systemic pressures. Hemoptysis eventually complicates 50% of cases of bronchiectasis. Wheezing and dyspnea can complicate bronchiectasis and become more persistent as the disease progresses. Pleuritic chest pain may be a prominent symptom, indicating a recurrent respiratory infection. Sinusitis is commonly associated with bronchiectasis (~50%).

Physical examination often reveals localized and persistent, coarse, *moist* crackles (70%). In the preantibiotic era, clubbing, cyanosis, cor pulmonale, cachexia, and secondary amyloidosis were common, but these are rarely observed today.

DIAGNOSTIC TESTING

Chest radiograph can be normal in 7 to 20% of patients with established bronchiectasis. Radiographic abnormalities are rarely distinctive or diagnostic. The diagnosis is supported by increased or crowded lung markings, tubular or *ring* shadows (produced by thickened dilated bronchial walls), *gloved finger* shadows, and, especially, cystic air-containing areas with or without fluid levels.

High-resolution CT has become the most reliable modality in the evaluation and noninvasive diagnosis of bronchiectasis. Recently published studies using thinner sections at close interslice intervals indicate that both sensitivity and specificity were higher than 95% in the diagnosis of cylindrical bronchiectasis. An airway diameter of more than 1.5 times the adjacent blood vessel is indicative of cylindrical bronchiectasis. Other anatomic forms are even easier to diagnose on CT.

The diagnostic approach to a patient where bronchiectasis is strongly suggested on the basis of chronic cough, sputum, recurrent focal infection, or hemoptysis includes chest x-ray study, sputum smear and culture, pulmonary function testing (which should show a picture of airflow limitation), immunologic evaluation, especially quantitation of IgG and its subclasses, IgA and IgM, sweat chloride test, chest CT and, possibly, bronchography. A presumptive diagnosis can usually be made on the basis of the clinical history, examination, and the aforementioned tests, although chronic bronchitis may be indistinguishable on purely clinical grounds.

High-resolution CT scanning under static and dynamic (in expiration) conditions shows that the pathophysiologic basis of airflow obstruction in bronchiectasis is primarily linked to intrinsic disease of the small and medium airways and not to bronchiectatic abnormalities in large airways, emphysema, or retained endobronchial secretions. Airway hyperresponsiveness is often present and 40% of patients have 15% or greater improvement in FEV_1 after β-adrenergic agonist administration.

TREATMENT

Medical Management

Treatment and management of bronchiectasis should include identification of acute exacerbations, appropriate antibiotic therapy, suppression of the microbial load, treatment of underlying conditions, promotion of bronchial hygiene, control of hemoptysis, and appropriate surgical intervention. Higher than usual doses of antibiotics may be required for prolonged periods (months) to adequately reduce the colonizing microbial load and to break the vicious circle from buildup of purulent, elastase-positive, ciliotoxic secretions resulting in increasing tissue damage, worsening bronchiectasis, and further predisposition to infection. Preemptive or suppressive antimicrobial treatment may be required at regular intervals or even continuously. Antibiotics should be rotated to reduce the emergence of resistant organisms, although the efficacy of these regimens is less well-studied. Aerosolized antibiotics (especially tobramycin for chronic *Pseudomonas* infection) have been used effectively and safely in bronchiectasis. Ongoing studies are evaluating long-term safety (emergence of resistant organisms). A recent meta-analysis of six trials (302 patients) looking at the potential benefit of prolonged courses (4 weeks to 12 months) of antibiotics for purulent bronchiectasis showed only a small positive effect.

There is still not enough evidence to support or refute the use of bronchopulmonary hygiene (including chest percussion and postural drainage), and the routine use of mucolytics in bronchiectasis. In the past there has been a suggestion of the beneficial effects of various secretion-loosening and enhanced secretion-removal maneuvers in patients with bronchiectasis. These include the use of oral bromhexine, inhaled acetylcysteine, cold-water jet nebulizing humidification of inspired air or oxygen during chest physiotherapy, and aerosolized recombinant human deoxyribonuclease (effective only in patients with cystic fibrosis). More recently, inhaled hypertonic agents such as dry powder mannitol have been tried with some benefit.

Inhaled steroids have also been shown to reduce daily sputum production (by 18%) and to reduce cough significantly.

γ-Globulin infusions can reduce the frequency and severity of respiratory tract infections and thus reduce further lung damage in patients with hypogammaglobulinemia. Newer studies suggest that higher doses (up to 600 mg/kg) are more effective.

Surgical Management

Many patients do well with a tightly controlled program of medical management as described. Some, however, remain significantly symptomatic and debilitated. These patients deserve consideration for surgical options. Resection of multilobar and bilateral disease has been successful with low mortality and morbidity rates in carefully selected patients, especially if the lung tissue being resected is already shrunken and functionless and if compensatory expansion or hypertrophy of the remaining normal lung exists preoperatively. In some cases, resection of severe areas of bronchiectasis on one side resulted in such an improvement in symptoms that subsequent planned resection of contralateral disease was put on hold. In some patients, therefore, there may be a role for resection of a bronchiectatic sump area that is causing severe symptoms, ignoring other, less-involved areas that are not causing significant or any symptoms. This is supported by a recent study where limited surgical removal of a target region in nonlocalized bilateral disease resulted in lasting symptomatic improvement. Nevertheless, most surgical studies recommend that resection should be limited to patients with localized disease and that complete resection should be performed whenever possible to achieve maximal benefit. A recent publication of a large series of patients (238) confirmed that surgical resection for bronchiectasis can be performed with low morbidity and mortality at any age.

High-quality bilateral bronchograms or CT scans should be performed before any resectional surgery to determine the exact extent and severity of the bronchiectatic changes.

All patients should have a preoperative bronchoscopy to rule out obstruction by stricture, foreign body, or neoplasm and to determine the degree of inflammation in the bronchial wall, which, if severe, can negate resection until better infection control has been achieved. If an interventional radiology service is available, bronchial artery embolization is the initial treatment of choice for intractable bleeding caused by bronchiectasis because it preserves lung tissue and eliminates the need for a thoracotomy. Surgery may still be necessary if bleeding persists.

Young patients with severe, progressive bronchiectasis, uncontrolled by conservative measures, and with lung function too severely impaired to tolerate resection may now be candidates for lung transplantation. Multiple antibiotic resistance in patients colonized with *Pseudomonas aeruginosa* or *Burkholderia cepacia* is not an absolute contraindication to transplantation. Removal of both native lungs is mandatory to prevent spillover infection of the transplanted lung by the contralateral lung in patients with generalized bronchiectasis and cystic fibrosis. Currently, bilateral, sequential lung transplantation is the procedure of choice for patients who have bronchiectasis or cystic fibrosis, although evidence suggests that bilateral pneumonectomy and single lung transplantation may be an option in the future. Patients with cystic fibrosis who undergo lung transplantation have survival rates similar to those of patients who are transplanted for other diseases (40 to 60%). Patients with bronchiectasis and cystic fibrosis were included in the results of the Swiss lung transplant registry where the 5-year survival since 1998 is 72%.

PROGNOSIS

The prognosis of patients with bronchiectasis has improved markedly over the past 50 years, owing to the impact of antibiotics. Early in this century, life expectancy for a patient with severe bronchiectasis was no greater than for most untreated malignancies. Since the 1960s, the mean age at death has remained at about 53 years, compared with a death rate of 70% before the age of 40 in a large series published in 1940. In Finland, 842 patients with bronchiectasis were followed from 1982 to 1993 with a death rate of 28%. Patients with bronchiectasis have a 1-year mortality of 40% after a first ICU stay for respiratory failure. Use of long-term oxygen and age above 65 are associated with reduced survival.

1. Barker AF. Bronchiectasis. *N Engl J Med.* 2002;346(18):1383–1393.
   An up-to-date review of pathogenesis, etiology and management.
2. Desai SR, Wells AU, Rubens MB, et al. Traction bronchiectasis in cryptogenic fibrosing alveolitis; associated computed tomographic features and physiological significance. *Eur Radiol.* 2003;13(8):1801–1808.
   Traction bronchiectasis is associated with additional physiologic impairment for a given extent of pulmonary fibrosis.
3. Roberts HR, Wells AU, Milne DG, et al. Airflow obstruction in bronchiectasis; correlation between computed tomography features and pulmonary function tests. *Thorax.* 2000;55(3):198–204.
   Airflow obstruction in bronchiectasis linked to intrinsic disease of small and medium airways on CT scanning.
4. Mitchell TA, Hamilos DL, Lynch DA, et al. Distribution and severity of bronchiectasis in allergic bronchopulmonary aspergillosis (ABPA). *J Asthma.* 2000; 37(1):65–72.
   The majority of patients with ABPA have evidence of central cystic and/or varicoid bronchiectasis in four or five lobes on high-resolution CT.
5. Evans DJ, Bara AI, GreenstoneM. Prolonged antibiotics for purulent bronchiectasis. *Cochrane Database of Systematic Reviews.* 2003;(4):CD001392.
   Evidence available shows only a small benefit from the use of prolonged antibiotics in the treatment of bronchiectasis.
6. Kolbe J, Wells A, Ram FS. Inhaled steroids for bronchiectasis. *Cochrane Database of Systematic Reviews.* 2000;(2):CD000996.

Regular use of inhaled corticosteroids may improve lung function but does not appear to reduce morbidity or prevent progression of underlying bronchiectasis.

7. Mazieres J, Murris M, Didier A, et al. Limited operation for multisegmental bilateral bronchiectasis. *Ann Thorac Surg.* 2003;75(2):382–387.

   Limited operation may be indicated in nonlocalized bilateral bronchiectasis, provided that a target which is cystic and/or functionless can be identified.

8. Prieto D, Bernardo J, Matos MJ, et al. Surgery for bronchiectasis. *Eur J Cardio-Thorac Surg.* 2001;20(1):19–23.

   Surgery for bronchiectasis has a low complication rate and markedly improves symptoms in the majority of patients, especially when complete resection of the disease is achieved.

9. Speich R, Nkod LP, Aubert JD, et al. 10 years of lung transplantation in Switzerland; results of the Swiss lung transplant registry. *Swiss Med Weekly.* 2004;134(1–2):18–23.

   Since 1998, the 5-year survival is 72%. Best results in patients with cystic fibrosis/bronchiectasis, emphysema, and parenchymal disorders. Worse prognosis in pulmonary hypertension and patients over the age of 60.

10. Dupont M, Gacouin A, Lena H, et al. Survival of patients with bronchiectasis after first ICU stay for respiratory failure. *Chest.* 2004;125:1815–1820.

    A study of 48 patients, wherein the 1-year mortality was 40%. Long-term use of oxygen and age above 65 associated with reduced survival.

11. Au J, Scott C, Husan A, et al. Bilateral sequential lung transplantation for septic lung disease: surgical and physiologic advantages over heart-lung transplantation. *Transplant Proc.* 1992;24:2652.

    A recommendation for bilateral, sequential lung transplantation as the procedure of choice for the surgical treatment of end-stage septic lung disease over heart–lung and en bloc double lung transplantation.

12. Bachman AL, Howitt WR, Beckly HC. Bronchiectasis: a bronchographic study of 60 cases of pneumonia. *Arch Intern Med.* 1953;91:78.

    Bronchiectatic changes are commonly seen on bronchograms in patients with pneumonia but are usually reversible.

13. Currie DC, Cooke JC, Morgan AD, et al. Interpretation of bronchograms and chest radiographs in patients with chronic sputum production. *Thorax.* 1987;42:278.

    No clinical difference was seen between patients with bronchographically confirmed bronchiectasis versus chronic bronchitis. Plain chest radiographs are insensitive in diagnosing bronchiectasis.

14. Currie DC, Saverymutt VSH, Peters AM, et al. Indium-111-labelled granulocyte accumulation in respiratory tract of patients. *Lancet.* 1987;1:1335.

    Labeled granulocytes appear to accumulate only in bronchiectatic areas wherein is active inflammation.

15. Fine A, Baum GL. Long-term follow-up of bronchiectasis. *Lancet.* 1966;86:505.

    A 20-year follow-up of patients with limited bronchiectasis. The prognosis is good even without pulmonary resection.

16. Glauser E, Cook CD, Harris GBC. Bronchiectasis: a review of 187 cases in children with follow-up pulmonary function studies in 58. *Acta Paediatr.* 1966;165:2.

    From 1940 through 1960, the incidence of bronchiectasis declined sharply with the advent of antibiotics and the decrease in pertussis. Overall outcome also improved.

17. Hayakawa K, Tanaka F, Torizuka T, et al. Bronchial arterial embolization for haemoptysis: immediate and long term results. *Cardiovasc Intervent Radiol.* 1992;15:154.

    Immediate success rate was 86%; complete remission in 50%; recurrence rate was 28%. Patients with bronchiectasis had best results. Neoplasm had worst results.

18. Hill SL, Burnett D, Hewetson KA, et al. The response of patients with purulent bronchiectasis to antibiotics for four months. *Q J Med.* 1988;66:163.

    Macroscopic clearance of secretions was achieved in all patients, with a significant reduction in sputum elastase content and improvement in well-being and dyspnea.

19. Joharjy IA, Bashi SA, Abdullah AK. Value of medium thickness computed tomography in the diagnosis of bronchiectasis. *AJR*. 1987;149:1133.
    Reports that CT with medium-thickness cuts of 4 mm and medium slice intervals (5 mm) were 100% specific, 100% sensitive for cystic bronchiectasis, and 94% sensitive for cylindrical bronchiectasis.
20. Kharitonov SA, Wells AU, O'Connor BJ, et al. Elevated levels of exhaled nitric oxide in bronchiectasis. *Am J Respir Crit Care Med*. 1995;151:1889.
    Exhaled NO may represent a way to monitor disease activity and assess effects of therapy.
21. Konietzko RW, Carton RW, Leroy EP. Causes of death in patients with bronchiectasis. *Am Rev Respir Dis*. 1969;100:852.
    In contrast with the preantibiotic years, suppurative complications are now uncommon.
22. Lau K, Lieberman J. Young's syndrome: an association between male sterility and bronchiectasis. *West J Med*. 1986;144:744.
    Bronchiectasis was associated with obstructive azoospermia, normal spermatogenesis, normal cilia, and normal sweat test.
23. Le Roux BT, Mohlala ML, Stemmler P, et al. Suppurative diseases of the lung and pleural space. Part II: Bronchiectasis. *Curr Probl Surg*. 1986;23:93.
    The most comprehensive modern-day, surgical experience; insightful discussion of pathogenesis, bronchography, and surgical indications.
24. O'Donnell AE, Barker AF, Ilowite JS, et al. Treatment of idiopathic bronchiectasis with aerosolized recombinant human DNaseI. *Chest*. 1998;113:1329.
    RhDNase was ineffective and potentially harmful in patients with stable idiopathic bronchiectasis in contrast to patients with cystic fibrosis bronchiectasis.
25. Ramsey BW, Dorkin HL, Eisenberg JD, et al. Efficacy of aerosolized tobramycin in patients with cystic fibrosis. *N Engl J Med*. 1993;328:1740.
    Short-term aerosol administration of high-dose tobramycin in patients with cystic fibrosis is efficacious and safe for Pseudomonas bronchitis.
26. Sanderson JM, Kennedy MCS, Johnson MF, et al. Bronchiectasis: results of surgical and conservative management. *Thorax*. 1974;29:407.
    A review of 393 patients, two thirds of whom were treated surgically. Promotes a surgical approach to the problem and makes the point that the current bias toward conservative management may be unjustified.
27. Shadick NA, Fanta CH, Weinblatt ME, et al. Bronchiectasis. A late feature of severe rheumatoid arthritis. *Medicine (Baltimore)*. 1994;73:161.
    Bronchiectasis can complicate severe, long-standing nodular rheumatoid arthritis more frequently than was previously thought.
28. Thomas RD, Blaquiere RM. Reactive mediastinal lymphadenopathy in bronchiectasis assessed by computed tomography. *Acta Radiol*. 1993;34:489.
    Reactive mediastinal lymph nodes are very common in bronchiectasis.
29. Wilson JF, Decker AM. The surgical management of childhood bronchiectasis: a review of 96 consecutive pulmonary resections in children with nontuberculous bronchiectasis. *Ann Surg*. 1982;195:354.
    Surgical management resulted in better outcome than conservative treatment. Diseased segments not resected at surgery deteriorated postoperatively.
30. Reid LM. Reduction in bronchial subdivision in bronchiectasis. *Thorax*. 1950;5:233.
    Classic classification system correlating pathologic and bronchographic findings in bronchiectasis.

V. ACUTE RESPIRATORY FAILURE

57. ACUTE HYPERCAPNIC RESPIRATORY FAILURE

Timothy A. Morris

The principle function of the lungs is gas exchange; *hypercapnia* indicates severe compromise of this vital function. Although disease may substantially affect any of the functional elements of the respiratory system, the term *acute respiratory failure* (ARF) is used only when gas exchange is so severely impaired that arterial hypoxemia or hypercapnia occurs. Hypoxemia may involve a multitude of respiratory and metabolic processes and may occur in the absence of hypercapnia. However, hypercapnia is more directly linked to inadequate gas exchange and dysfunction of one or more elements of the respiratory system (e.g., control of breathing, mechanical performance of the lungs, respiratory muscle function, lung parenchyma, and vasculature). Hypercapnic respiratory failure (HRF) is often referred to as *alveolar hypoventilation* and nearly always involves some level of hypoxemia as well. Specific values of arterial P_{CO_2} (Pa_{CO_2}) that indicate HRF are not well defined, but most experts agree that a Pa_{CO_2} greater than 45 mm Hg (in a previously eucapnic patient) reflects ARF. In patients with chronic hypercapnic lung disease, a sudden increase of 5 mm Hg or more of P_{CO_2} from a previously stable level represents acute HRF superimposed on chronic respiratory failure.

DIAGNOSIS

The hallmark of acute HRF is an elevated Pa_{CO_2}. A rise in Pa_{CO_2} signals that pulmonary "clearance" of carbon dioxide is inadequate; that is, more carbon dioxide is being produced by body metabolism than the respiratory apparatus can clear by ventilation. This relationship is defined by the equation:

$$Pa_{CO_2} = K \, \dot{V}_{CO_2} / \dot{V}_A$$

In this equation, $\dot{V}_{CO_2}$ represents carbon dioxide production; $\dot{V}_A$, alveolar ventilation; and K, a constant. An increase in $\dot{V}_{CO_2}$ secondary to an elevated caloric intake, is almost never the primary cause of hypercapnia because the respiratory system usually can compensate for the higher ventilatory requirement. When other elements of the respiratory system impair alveolar ventilation, however, increases in $\dot{V}_{CO_2}$ (e.g., secondary to fever or sepsis) can contribute to hypercapnia. The central cause of HRF remains inadequate alveolar ventilation.

Alveolar ventilation is a physiologic process described by the equation:

$$\dot{V}_E = \dot{V}_A + \dot{V}_D$$

$\dot{V}_E$ (the volume of gas expired per minute, or "minute ventilation") is a measurable quantity. The equation implies that the minute ventilation is divisible into two separate components: (1) alveolar ventilation ($\dot{V}_A$), which participates in gas exchange, and (2) dead space ventilation ($\dot{V}_D$), which does not participate in gas exchange. $\dot{V}_D$ may also be viewed as "wasted" ventilation, that is, ventilation that does not reach the gas-exchanging areas of the lung. Rearranging this equation,

$$\dot{V}_A = \dot{V}_E - \dot{V}_D$$

This expression of alveolar ventilation makes it clear that hypercapnia may occur via two distinct mechanisms: (1) a reduction in minute ventilation itself (*absolute hypoventilation*), or (2) an increase in dead space ventilation (*relative hypoventilation*).

Although mixed forms of hypoventilation occur, the distinction between absolute and relative hypoventilation is useful in separating patients with HRF into two major categories: those with normal lungs and those with intrinsic disease of the lungs. Patients with normal lungs manifest hypercapnia because of inadequate minute ventilation caused by abnormalities in respiratory control (induced by disease or drugs), neuromuscular disorders, or chest wall abnormalities. Lung function may be normal in this group. Patients with abnormal lungs manifest hypercapnia because of the increased dead space (wasted) ventilation associated with maldistribution of ventilation and perfusion. The net result of these derangements is inadequate carbon dioxide clearance, even though minute ventilation (and respiratory drive) is normal or increased.

Combined forms of hypercapnic respiratory occur occasionally, such as in a patient with chronic obstructive pulmonary disease (COPD) who receives sedatives or narcotics (for anxiety or sleeplessness, or because of a misdiagnosis of left ventricular failure). Similarly, excessive diuretic use or other circumstances may cause hypokalemia, hypomagnesemia, or hypocalcemia and impair diaphragmatic contractility. Somewhat controversial is the relationship of excessive amounts of supplemental oxygen to absolute and relative hypoventilation and acute deterioration of patients with chronic hypercapnia (discussed below).

Regardless of the pathogenesis, the consequences of HRF are the same. All patients with acute hypercapnia have hypoxemia, acidosis, an increase in pulmonary vascular resistance, and dilatation of the cerebral vessels. Arterial hypoxemia is an inevitable consequence of hypercapnia because, as alveolar P_{CO_2} rises, alveolar P_{O_2} (and therefore arterial P_{O_2}) must fall. The alveolar–arterial gradient (A–a gradient) is a useful indicator of how much of a patient's hypoxemia is attributable to hypoventilation itself. The gradient is calculated as

$$P_{(A-a)}O_2 = P_A O_2 - P_a O_2$$

$$= [F_I O_2^*(\text{ambient pressure} - P_A H_2 O) - P_A CO_2/0.8] - P_a O_2$$

$$= [F_I O_2^*(713) - P_a CO_2/0.8] - P_a O_2$$

where $P_A O_2$ is the alveolar oxygen pressure, $P_A O_2$ is the arterial oxygen pressure, $F_I O_2$ is the fraction of oxygen in inspired air, $P_A H_2 O$ is the alveolar water vapor pressure (47 torr), and $P_A CO_2$ is the alveolar CO_2 pressure (which is equal to the arterial CO_2). If hypercapnia alone is responsible for hypoxemia, the $P_{(A-a)}O_2$ is not widened. If this difference is widened, hypoxemia is more severe and indicates the presence of coexistent cardiopulmonary disease. For example, in ARF induced purely by drug overdose, hypoxemia is fully explained by hypercapnia and the $P_{(A-a)}O_2$ is normal. However, if the patient has aspirated, zones of acute lung injury may create low ventilation–perfusion ($\dot{V}/\dot{Q}$) units leading to hypoxemia and an increased $P_{(A-a)}O_2$.

Acidosis

Acidosis is a direct consequence of hypercapnia, although patients with ARF may have other reasons for acidosis. The severity of acidosis attributable to hypercapnia itself can be calculated using the equilibrium expression:

$$Ka = [H_2 CO_3]/[H^+][HCO_3^-]$$

Rearranging the terms yields the Henderson-Hasselbalch equation:

$$pH = [pKa + \log ([HCO_3^-]/[H_2 CO_3])$$

or:

$$pH = 6.1 + \log ([HCO_3^-]/0.03 \times Pa CO_2)$$

If the HCO_3^- concentration were constant (no metabolic acid–base disorder), the Henderson-Hasselbalch equation is approximated (between pH 7.0 and 7.5) by a linear formula:

$$\Delta\,pH = 0.008 \times \Delta\,Pa_{CO_2}$$

Within these limits, an acute change in Pa_{CO_2} of 10 torr changes (in the opposite direction) the blood pH by 0.08. Changes in pH not predicted by this equation must be attributed to causes other than acute hypercapnia.

Alveolar hypercapnia, hypoxemia, and arteriovenous acidosis all contribute to constriction of pulmonary resistance vessels and an increased pulmonary arterial pressure. This can lead to a higher work requirement for the right ventricle and right ventricular failure. These same factors cause dilatation of cerebral resistance vessels and increases in intracranial pressure. Together with hypoxemia and hypercapnia, disorientation, personality changes, coma, headache, papilledema, and asterixis may appear in patients with hypercapnic respiratory failure.

MANAGEMENT

The primary goals of management in acute HRF are to (1) prevent respiratory arrest in patients who are rapidly decompensating; (2) restore adequate gas exchange; and (3) treat the disorder(s) responsible for inducing respiratory failure. These goals can be pursued simultaneously.

Supplemental Oxygen

The development and worsening of hypercapnia strongly suggests that a patient's respiratory system is failing and dangerous degrees of hypoxemia are imminent. Under these circumstances, severe hypoxemia is the greatest danger to patient survival and requires immediate attention. In some cases of mild HRF, supplemental oxygen alone may stabilize the patient. However, oxygen alone may not reverse the respiratory decompensation observed in many cases of severe hypercapnic failure. Furthermore, two potential risks are associated with the administration of high oxygen concentrations to patients with HRF: respiratory depression and worsening of ventilation–perfusion mismatching.

The hazard of respiratory depression with oxygen delivery is confined to patients with HRF in whom the normal stimuli to ventilation are compromised and in whom hypercapnia has been present for at least several days. In these patients, retention of bicarbonate leads to moderation of the acidosis that acute hypercapnia causes in both the arterial blood and cerebrospinal fluid—an acidosis that provides a strong drive to respiration. In acute HRF, these drives are present and oxygen poses no depression hazard. In chronic hypercapnic states, however, particularly if the patient is obtunded or sedated, hypoxemia is the major residual drive to ventilation. Oxygen administration may blunt this drive; the patient ventilates less, and the P_{CO_2} rises. More commonly, however, the Pa_{CO_2} may rise even if the $\dot{V}_E$ does not decrease, because of worsened relative hypoventilation. Excessive supplemental oxygen raises the alveolar P_{O_2} in diseased areas of the lung that are not normally well perfused. In these areas, hypoxic vasoconstriction is reversed by the presence of supplemental oxygen and blood flow to them is increased. Increased perfusion to the diseased areas of the lung worsens ventilation–perfusion mismatching, leading to an apparent increase in $\dot{V}_D/\dot{V}_T$ and worsened hypercapnia. Whatever the mechanisms, the fact remains that excessive oxygen administration to patients with chronic hypercapnia can induce hypercapnic coma and death.

Both excessive oxygen delivery and sedatives should be avoided in patients with chronic hypercapnia. Although oxygen therapy to relieve hypoxemia is essential in any patient with HRF, it should be used judiciously in those with chronic hypercapnia. A reasonable goal of oxygen therapy in these patients is to a P_{O_2} in the 50- to 60-mm Hg range, corresponding to an oxygen saturation of approximately 90%. In these cases, it is imperative to closely monitor the arterial P_{O_2} and P_{CO_2} during therapy with oxygen.

Mechanical Ventilation

If supplemental oxygen fails to provide an adequate Po_2 without inducing marked hypercapnia, or if clinical signs of respiratory decompensation are detected, the next step is use of a mechanical ventilator. This step is a major decision because it generally requires endotracheal intubation, may require sedation or paralysis, and makes patients totally dependent on a "closed system" and the personnel caring for them. Furthermore, this step exposes patients to new risks. Therefore, the decision to initiate mechanical ventilation should not be made until it is clear that simpler measures will not suffice. Despite intensive investigative efforts, no absolute criteria for intubation–ventilation exist. The decision still rests on an overall assessment of the individual patient, particularly the degree of hypoxemia and acidosis and, often, the response to a trial of nonventilator management.

There is a potential intermediate step before intubation–ventilation, namely the use of various nasal or nasal–oral continuous positive airway pressure devices. Some centers have reported success in selected patients using mechanical ventilation through face masks, without controlling the airways with endotracheal tubes. Defining how often and in which patients such approaches will suffice remains an investigative challenge.

Gas exchange aberrations pose an immediate risk to patient survival, and should be corrected. Prompt action must be taken to revert or avoid hazardous levels of hypoxemia, hypercapnia, and acidosis. Such levels must be defined rather arbitrarily, because coexistent conditions modify such definitions. For example, a degree of hypoxemia well tolerated by a young adult with a barbiturate overdose may be hazardous in a person who has recently sustained a myocardial infarction. There is reasonable agreement, however, that Po_2 levels below 40 mm Hg are poorly tolerated by adults; these levels are commonly associated with cardiac arrhythmias and functional or anatomic abnormalities of the heart, brain, kidney, liver, and other organs. The dangerous effects of Pco_2 relate chiefly to the degree of associated acidosis. Thus, a chronically elevated Pco_2 of 60 mm Hg with an essentially normal pH is not dangerous, whereas a sudden rise to 60 mm Hg induces a potentially hazardous acidosis. In the nonintubated patient, a blood pH below 7.2 indicates imminent respiratory arrest and available data indicate that the mortality risk rises with each decrement below 7.2. Once the risk of respiratory arrest has been minimized by intubation and mechanical ventilation, however, the levels at which hypercapnia and respiratory acidosis become harmful are more difficult to establish. Whereas acidosis itself potentiates the functional abnormalities induced by hypoxemia (such as pulmonary hypertension, cerebral vasodilatation, and depression of myocardial contractility), there is no widely accepted "hazardous" level. Indeed, excessive attempts to lower arterial Pco_2 in mechanically ventilated patients, by increasing minute ventilation at the cost of alveolar overdistention and lung damage, are probably misguided. To spare the lungs from trauma during mechanical ventilation, some experts use lower tidal volumes and respiratory rates, allowing the Pco_2 to rise to high (previously considered alarming!) levels. Within limits, this strategy of "permissive hypercapnia" is well tolerated by respiratory failure patients, provided that adequate blood oxygenation is ensured.

Underlying Causes

As the life-threatening alterations in gas exchange are being controlled, attention also is directed toward diagnosis and treatment of the disorder(s) that induced HRF. In some instances, diagnosis of the precipitating disorder may determine decisions regarding institution of mechanical ventilation.

In patients with absolute hypoventilation (reduced $\dot{V}_E$), the primary problem is usually readily identified and treated. For example, respiratory depression due to drug overdose may be treated with specific antagonists or by enhancing drug excretion using dialysis. Myasthenia gravis or myxedema can be treated with specific agents. In patients with Guillain-Barré syndrome, however, ventilatory support is required until the disorder runs its course.

Among patients with relative hypoventilation due to obstructive lung disease, therapy is directed toward the problems that caused acute deterioration in gas exchange. The most frequent reversible problems are accumulation of secretions, infection, and bronchospasm. As these abnormalities are resolved, the mechanical function of the lungs improves, ventilation–perfusion relationships return toward normal, and gas exchange is enhanced. In some patients, recovery depends on these factors alone. In others, the respiratory muscles may have become exhausted from hours or days of respiratory failure and mechanical ventilation may be necessary until they have adequately rested.

Symptomatic Treatment

Secretions are best removed by encouraging the patient to cough and by adequately hydrating the patient. There is little evidence that available "mucolytic" agents are of significant value. However, new agents with greater potency (e.g., DNase) need evaluation in this context. Hydration is best achieved by oral fluid intake; if this intake is not adequate, intravenous administration or aerosolization of water or both can be added. Sputum mobilization can be enhanced by chest percussion and vibration, and by instruction from a skilled respiratory or physical therapist. If necessary, catheters inserted by the nasal or oral route into the trachea can be used to suction secretions, or fiberoptic bronchoscopy can be performed.

The treatment of bronchospasm is an integral part of the management of most patients with HRF associated with COPD because most patients have some degree of reversible bronchoconstriction (see Chapters 47 and 51).

Infection is a frequent cause and a common complication of HRF in patients with COPD and other chronic lung diseases. Treatment with broad-spectrum antimicrobial drugs (ampicillin, tetracycline, trimethoprim-sulfamethoxazole, ciprofloxacin, and others) should be initiated on the presumption that infection is present. However, appropriate samples for smear and culture should be requested so that more specific therapy can be applied if indicated.

Corticosteroids are commonly given during the first few days of therapy, usually in high doses, to reverse airway inflammation and bronchospasm. Most clinicians initiate therapy with the equivalent of 100 to 125 mg of methylprednisolone on presentation, followed by about half this dose every 6 hours. Empiric trials suggest that such therapy has modest positive impact on the course of patients with HRF. Unfortunately, large clinical trials comparing the effects of different corticosteroid doses are unavailable.

It is important to consider and search for other factors that may have induced HRF, particularly left ventricular failure and pulmonary embolism, and attention to the patient's nutritional needs. Left ventricular failure may cause ventilation–perfusion aberrations due to alveolar edema as well as dysfunction of poorly perfused respiratory muscles. Cardiac ischemia is increasingly recognized as a reason for failure of some patients to wean from mechanical ventilation. Pulmonary embolism is common in patients with acute and chronic lung disease. In most patients who die with pulmonary embolism, clinicians had not suspected the diagnosis premortem, possibly because the characteristic signs and symptoms were attributed to other coexisting lung conditions (see Chapter 63). Many patients with COPD are malnourished; correction of nutritional depletion and avoidance of further depletion during a bout of ARF, may enhance recovery and forestall future episodes of ARF (see Chapter 60).

The role of respiratory muscle performance and in respiratory control in the pathogenesis of hypercapnic respiratory failure has generated a great deal of research interest. Treatment for alterations of respiratory control is not yet available, but respiratory muscle performance may be improved by several proposed methods. Putting the respiratory muscles to rest may improve muscle performance in some patients with ARF. Some patients have chronic respiratory muscle dysfunction and may benefit from pharmacologic therapy. Some physicians have advocated the use of theophylline preparations in this setting because these agents are known to modestly enhance diaphragmatic function.

COMPLICATIONS

Patients with HRF are subject to complications associated with both respiratory failure and its treatment. Often such complications lead to acute deterioration in a previously stable or improving patient. Several common complications have been identified: (1) Cardiac arrhythmias of all types are common, relating to diverse factors including hypoxemia, wide swings in pH, electrolyte disturbances, and drugs that may be employed such as β-adrenergic agents, theophylline, and digoxin. (2) Gastrointestinal hemorrhage, chiefly from the stomach and duodenum, is frequent. Again, multiple factors may be involved, and the hemorrhage can be sudden and massive. (3) Pneumothorax occurs in a significant number of patients with respiratory failure, particularly among those who are mechanically ventilated. (4) Bronchial obstruction may occur due to thick, inspissated secretions or improper placement or obstruction of endotracheal tubes. Other complications include acute right or left ventricular failure (or both), pulmonary embolism, and convulsions from hypoxia or even alkalosis following sudden reversion of hypercapnia.

The patient with HRF requires careful initial evaluation and close monitoring throughout management. Such patients are best cared for in a respiratory intensive care unit that is staffed by experienced personnel and properly equipped. In this environment, most patients can be stabilized promptly, decisions regarding the need to intubate and mechanically ventilate can be made properly, and therapy can be applied and monitored appropriately.

1. Dereune JP, Fleury B, Pariente R. Acute respiratory failure of chronic obstructive pulmonary disease. *Am Rev Respir Dis*. 1988;138:1006.
   An exhaustive review of the problem posed by ARF in COPD, with more than 450 references.
2. West WW, et al. The NIH intermittent positive pressure breathing trial: pathology studies. III. The diagnosis of emphysema. *Am Rev Respir Dis*. 1987;135:123.
   This large NIH trial has shed some light on the pathology of COPD and the value of certain interventions (including the nonvalue of intermittent positive pressure breathing).
3. Waldhorn RE. Nocturnal nasal intermittent positive pressure ventilation with bi-level positive airway pressure (Bi PAP) in respiratory failure. *Chest* 1992;101:516.
4. Hill NS, et al. Efficacy of nocturnal positive pressure ventilation in patients with restrictive thoracic disease. *Am Rev Respir Dis*. 1992;145:365.
5. Strumpf DA, et al. Nocturnal positive pressure ventilation via nasal mask in patients with chronic obstructive pulmonary disease. *Am Rev Respir Dis*. 1991;144:1234.
   References 3, 4, and 5 report on alternative approaches to intubation in patients with respiratory failure, employing other systems for enhancing ventilation.
6. Sassoon CS, Hassell KT, Mahuette CL. Hyperoxic-induced hypercapnia in stable chronic obstructive pulmonary disease. *Am Rev Respir Dis*. 1987;135:907.
7. Stadling JR. Hypercapnia during oxygen therapy in airway obstruction: a reappraisal. *Thorax*. 1986;41:897.
   These two papers emphasize that the mechanisms responsible for oxygen exacerbation of hypercapnia involve more than simple "blunting of hypoxic drive."
8. Aubier M, et al. Effect of hypophosphatemia on diaphragmatic contractility in patients with acute respiratory failure. *N Engl J Med*. 1985;313:420.
   Hypophosphatemia is one of several electrolyte disturbances that may impair diaphragmatic function and lead to ARF.
9. Wilson DO, et al. Nutritional intervention in malnourished patients with emphysema. *Am Rev Respir Dis*. 1986;134:672.
10. Pingleton SK, Harinon GS. Nutritional management in acute respiratory failure. *JAMA*. 1987;257:3094.
    Two of many articles emphasizing that the nutritional status of COPD patients, in or out of ARF, should not be neglected.

11. Frostell C, et al. Inhaled nitric oxide. *Circulation*. 1991;83:2038.
12. Rossaint R, et al. Inhaled nitric oxide for the adult respiratory distress syndrome. *N Engl J Med*. 1993;328:399.
    Inhalation of nitric oxide may improve ventilation-perfusion relationships by increasing blood flow to the best ventilated lung zones because of its pulmonary vasodilator activity. The potential clinical role of this new modality remains to be fully defined.
13. Anthonisen NR, et al. Antibiotic therapy in exacerbations of chronic obstructive pulmonary disease. *Ann Intern Med*. 1986;106:196.
    New data dealing with an old question that indicates that antimicrobial therapy often helps. Sometimes "standard practice" is validated. But the controversy is not fully settled.
14. Bolder PM, et al. The extra work of breathing through adult endotracheal tubes. *Anesth Analg*. 1986;65:853.
    One reason some patients do better when the tube is pulled.
15. Ishaaya AM, Nathan SD, Belman MJ. Work of breathing after extubation. *Chest*. 1995;107:204–209.
    A well-performed series of physiologic experiments that suggests the opposite conclusion from the previous reference.
16. Albert RK, Martin TR, Lewis SW. Controlled clinical trial of methylprednisolone in patients with chronic bronchitis and acute respiratory insufficiency. *Ann Intern Med*. 1980;92:753.
    If you feel short-course steroids help, this paper validates your practice; if you do not, you will find fault with the paper.
17. Campbell EJ. The management of acute respiratory failure in chronic bronchitis and emphysema. *Am Rev Respir Dis*. 1967;96:626.
    Classic article emphasizing the rational administration of oxygen.
18. Rochester DF, Arora NS. Respiratory muscle failure. *Med Clin North Am*. 1983;67:573.
    An excellent review of the role respiratory muscles can play in HRF and of strategies that may be useful in avoiding or moderating muscle fatigue.
19. Shapiro BA, et al. Preliminary evaluation of intraarterial blood gas system in dogs and humans. *Crit Care Med*. 1989;17:455.
20. Zimmerman JL, Dellinger LV. Initial evaluation of a new intraarterial blood gas system in humans. *Crit Care Med*. 1993;21:495.
    References 20 and 21 review new approaches to monitoring of arterial blood gases with systems that do not require blood withdrawal.
21. Antonelli M, Conti G, Rocco M, et al. A comparison of noninvasive positive-pressure ventilation and conventional mechanical ventilation in patients with acute respiratory failure. *N Engl J Med*. 1998;339:429–435.
    Non-invasive ventilatory support may be a helpful adjunct to standard medical therapy in selected patients with respiratory failure due to exacerbations of COPD. However, the only COPD patients were entered into the trial, and patients appeared to require immediate intubation and mechanical ventilation were excluded.
22. Wysocki M, Tric L, Wolff MA, Millet H, Herman B. Noninvasive pressure support ventilation in patients with acute respiratory failure. A randomized comparison with conventional therapy. *Chest*. 1995;107:761–768.
    Preliminary study suggesting that respiratory failure due to "non-COPD" causes was not as amenable to non-invasive ventilatory support.

58. THE ACUTE RESPIRATORY DISTRESS SYNDROME

Robert M. Smith

A marked increase in the permeability of the alveolar–capillary membrane to water, solutes, and plasma proteins is the defining characteristic of the acute respiratory distress syndrome (ARDS). The 1972 National Heart, Lung, and Blood Institute Task Force on Respiratory Diseases estimated that approximately 70 cases of ARDS per 100,000 population occur annually in the United States. Although there is some suggestion that the incidence has decreased somewhat in the last decade, ARDS remains a frequent and dreaded problem in modern intensive care units.

ETIOLOGY
Events that have preceded and appear to act as precipitants to ARDS are remarkably diverse (Table 58-1), although sepsis and trauma are the most common associated clinical settings. The wisdom of grouping patients with such disparate precipitating factors together under the umbrella of ARDS has been debated frequently. However, because the biochemical and cellular pathways that lead to ARDS are not understood and because the patients have a number of apparent physiologic and histologic features in common, it has proven useful to consider them together. The probability of developing ARDS increases with multiple risk factors, but it is not known whether different precipitants act independently or via some common pathway leading to lung injury.

PATHOPHYSIOLOGY
There are no specific physical or laboratory findings that identify patients with ARDS. Prior to the development of frank respiratory failure, respirations are rapid and shallow, and the patient may be cyanotic. Auscultation usually reveals bronchial breath sounds; rales are often absent. Serum chemistries and blood cell counts tend to reflect the underlying diseases, rather than ARDS itself. The chest radiograph shows rapidly progressing diffuse infiltrates, often with characteristics suggesting alveolar filling. Occasionally there is a brief early period during which an interstitial infiltrate predominates. Particularly in the early stages, the infiltrates may look patchy or

Table 58-1. Clinical settings associated with the development of ARDS

CLINICAL PROCESSES WHERE ARDS OCCURS IN MORE THAN 1% OF PATIENTS AT RISK
Aspiration of gastric contents
Pneumonia requiring intensive care unit
Severe sepsis
Multiple trauma
Disseminated intravascular coagulation (usually associated with other events)

OTHER CLINICAL PROCESSES ASSOCIATED WITH ARDS
Near drowning
Smoke inhalation
Inhalation of irritant or toxic gases
Fat or air embolism
Pancreatitis
Hypertransfusion
Thermal burn
Cardiopulmonary bypass
Narcotic administration

appear to spare some parts of the lung, leading to a mistaken diagnosis of pneumonia. Arterial blood gas analyses typically show markedly reduced PaO_2 with a normal or reduced $PaCO_2$. It has been suggested that the level of hypoxemia should be used to stage the severity with a PaO_2/F_IO_2 ratio between 200 and 300 corresponding to a diagnosis of acute lung injury and a PaO_2/F_IO_2 ratio of less than 200 corresponding to full-blown respiratory distress syndrome. However, the PaO_2/F_IO_2 ratio can be influenced by other factors such as the mode of mechanical ventilation and the distinction between values above and below 200 does not accurately predict subsequent outcome.

Clinically, physiologically, and pathologically, ARDS typically progresses through successive stages. After exposure to the triggering event, there is often an interval of apparently normal lung function lasting hours to days. With the onset of symptoms, there is rapidly worsening gas exchange with decreasing lung compliance and functional residual capacity over 1 to 3 days. Subsequently, lung compliance decreases further, and increases occur in the proportion of the total ventilation going to unperfused "dead space" lung regions ($\dot{V}_D/\dot{V}_T$) and in pulmonary vascular resistance. Multiple organ system failure, which may include renal dysfunction, hepatic dysfunction, and biventricular cardiac dysfunction, often becomes apparent at this point, although it may occur at any time. It is not known whether impairment in these organ systems is caused by the same process precipitating ARDS (e.g., sepsis) or to distinct pathologic processes. In addition, the interventions used to support gas exchange, such as mechanical ventilation or positive end-expiratory pressure (PEEP) may also have deleterious effects on the function of extrapulmonary organs. From 10 to 30 days after the onset of symptoms, the patient may enter a more chronic stage in which pulmonary function has stabilized although persistent functional impairment remains. If the patient survives the acute events long enough to enter the chronic stage, there is usually a gradual improvement in lung function over weeks to months. The risk of mortality at this point is more often related to nonpulmonary causes.

Histologic examination of pulmonary tissue supports the differentiation of ARDS into acute and chronic stages. In the early stages, termed the *exudative phase,* alveolar type I epithelial cells are focally destroyed, and endothelial cells may appear swollen. Neutrophils are seen clogging capillaries and extravasating into the interstitium. Interstitial edema is found, with cuffs of more intense edema around bronchioles and vessels. The alveoli are filled with proteinaceous exudate containing red blood cells, neutrophils, macrophages, and cell fragments. Increased numbers of cells are recovered in bronchoalveolar lavage fluid, and polymorphonuclear neutrophil leukocytes (normally less than 2% of recovered cells) predominate. A more chronic stage of acute lung injury, termed the *fibroproliferative phase,* is apparent after 1 to 2 weeks. Plasma cells, histiocytes, and lymphocytes are seen in the interstitium and are accompanied by proliferation of pericytes and fibroblasts. Intravascular microthrombi are common. Cuboidal epithelial cells cover the surfaces of alveoli and alveolar ducts, and the acinar architecture of the lung is progressively replaced by thick bands of fibrotic tissue.

The processes responsible for tissue injury in ARDS remain obscure. Neutrophils and their granular products have been implicated in the pathogenesis of ARDS in animal models, and evidence of neutrophil granule release (e.g., the presence of elastase or myeloperoxidase) is often found in lung lavage fluid. Similarly, the production of highly reactive oxygen radical species by neutrophils or by resident lung macrophages may contribute to ARDS either by direct tissue injury or by modification of proteins, lipids, or DNA leading to inactivation (e.g., $\alpha 1$-proteinase inhibitor) or abnormal function. A number of factors may lead to neutrophil accumulation in the lung. Cytokines, elaborated systemically or locally in the lung following sepsis or trauma, may act as chemotactic factors (e.g., interleukin (IL)-8) or can cause upregulation of endothelial and leukocyte adhesion molecules (e.g., IL-1). In preliminary studies, an elevated level of IL-8 in alveolar lavage fluid of patients at risk for ARDS predicts the subsequent development of the full-blown syndrome. However, this finding has not been confirmed in larger studies and the complex interplay between the various cytokines is not yet well understood. The occurrence of ARDS in severely neutropenic patients and the lack of neutrophil participation in some animal models of ARDS suggest that neutrophil-independent mechanisms of tissue injury are also important. Loss of surfactant activity in lung lavage is seen early in ARDS and is a potential explanation for many of the physiologic abnormalities. The loss of surfactant activity is caused in part by alterations in surfactant production by type II pneumocytes and in part by inhibition of surfactant activity by the ingress of plasma proteins.

One novel mechanism for lung injury stems from the observation that application of positive-pressure ventilation in animal models results in diffuse lung injury with histologic features indistinguishable from those of patients with ARDS. This injury occurs in animals with even modest levels of positive pressure (e.g., sustained peak airway pressures of 30 cm H_2O for 24 hours). Data suggest that injury may be a result of cyclic opening and closing of alveoli or overdistension and stretching of the alveolar capillary membrane at peak inflation. Injury is diminished in these models by limiting maximal ventilatory excursion or by the application of PEEP. Further studies have demonstrated the elaboration of pro-inflammatory cytokines and the alteration of surfactant structure and function in the lungs of these animals as a result of positive pressure ventilation. Although these studies do not shed light on the pathophysiologic events initiating ARDS, they do support the hypothesis that the ventilatory support necessary to preserve gas exchange may worsen or modify the course of the underlying lung injury.

MANAGEMENT

Initial management of the patient with ARDS centers on supporting the patient while identifying and treating potentially reversible processes that may exacerbate or mimic ARDS. An aggressive diagnostic approach is warranted in the patient with known or suspected immunocompromise. In particular, bronchoscopy with lavage and brushings may be useful to determine the presence of *Pneumocystis carinii* pneumonia for patients suspected of having AIDS. Transbronchial biopsy may be considered, but the risk of complications in the setting of mechanical ventilation suggests this approach should be used with caution. Open lung biopsy should be considered for those patients in whom no specific diagnosis can be made with less invasive techniques.

Oxygenation of the arterial blood and delivery of that oxygen to peripheral tissues are the primary goals of supportive therapy in ARDS. These goals must be coupled with the limiting of further lung injury possibly resulting from ventilatory support. Initially, supplemental oxygen via face mask or nasal cannula may be adequate. However, tracheal intubation and positive-pressure ventilation are usually needed and should be instituted as soon as it is apparent that an acceptable PaO_2 cannot be maintained with supplemental oxygen alone. The optimal method of supplying ventilatory support remains controversial. However, confirming the findings seen in animal models of lung injury, a recent National Institutes of Health–sponsored trial of low-stretch ventilation (low tidal volume) compared with high-stretch ventilation (high tidal volume) demonstrated marked reduction in ARDS mortality when the low-stretch, "lung-protective" strategy was followed. In this study, patients ventilated with 6 mL/kg tidal volumes had a 30% mortality compared to the 40% mortality experienced by patients subjected to "standard" 12 mL/kg tidal volume ventilation. Although this study used a volume-controlled method of mechanical ventilation, end-inspiratory plateau pressures were limited to 25 cm H_2O and 45 cm H_2O in the low- and high-stretch arms, respectively. It is likely that other ventilatory strategies that limit end-inspiratory pressure to a similar level of 25 cm H_2O (such as pressure-cycled ventilation) would be equally successful.

PEEP at levels from 10 to 15 cm H_2O should be applied when positive-pressure ventilation cannot maintain a PaO_2 greater than 55 to 60 mm Hg using an FiO_2 of 0.6 or less. The physiologic effects of PEEP are thought to result from (1) redistribution of capillary blood flow, resulting in improved ventilation–perfusion matching, and (2) the recruitment of previously collapsed alveoli and prevention of their collapse during exhalation. The net effect of these changes is an improvement in PaO_2, which then allows a reduction in FiO_2. The improvement in lung function due to PEEP may require 30 to 60 minutes to become apparent, but is lost more rapidly if PEEP is removed. PEEP also may have significant deleterious consequences. As end-expiratory pressure is increased, mean thoracic pressure may also increase, compromising venous return. In addition, PEEP may directly impact cardiac function by restricting the filling of the atria or ventricles during diastole. On the plus side, the application of PEEP appears to limit alveolar excursion during positive-pressure ventilation and protects from ventilation-associated lung injury in animal models. Although PEEP is essential for the support of patients at nontoxic F_IO_2, early prophylactic PEEP has been shown ineffective in preventing subsequent ARDS.

It is vital to recognize and to balance the beneficial and deleterious effects of ventilatory support techniques. Improvements in PaO_2 brought about by the incremental application of PEEP must be weighed against any decrement in cardiac output and the resulting drop in oxygen delivery. To achieve this balance, it is important to monitor the variables that determine cardiac function (pulmonary artery and pulmonary artery wedge pressures), as well as those that measure total arterial oxygen delivery (arterial oxygen saturation, hemoglobin, and cardiac output). Measurements of the mixed venous oxygen tension (PvO_2) and the difference between arterial and mixed venous oxygen contents ($C[a-v]O_2$) have also been suggested as useful monitoring techniques. In those patients with hemodynamic instability, it may be advisable to use a pulmonary artery catheter with cardiac output monitoring capability to assess the effectiveness of fluid administration or the use of inotropic agents. Absolute standards to guide therapy should be avoided. The optimum level of PEEP is usually the lowest level allowing a PaO_2 greater than 55 to 60 mm Hg with an acceptable cardiac output. Further increases of PEEP may improve PaO_2, but may significantly increase the risk of barotraumatic injury and impaired cardiac function.

Alternative methods of ventilatory support have been explored with only limited success and none have demonstrated efficacy in controlled trials. However, high-frequency jet ventilation and high-frequency oscillation coupled with positive-pressure ventilation may improve gas exchange in certain patients. Similarly, the use of pressure-cycled inverse ratio ventilation (i.e., inspiratory time greater than expiratory time) may occasionally provide benefit, as may ventilation of patients in the prone position. Although extracorporeal bypass with membrane oxygenation did not improve survival in a large randomized trial, its application in selected patients or the application of extracorporeal carbon dioxide removal through a venovenous bypass circuit may preserve function where other approaches fail. Inhalation of nitric oxide improves PaO_2 acutely, but has not had a measurable impact on survival in a number of well-controlled trials.

Ongoing management of the patient with ARDS requires meticulous attention to detail and careful surveillance for possible complications. As for any critically ill patient, appropriate early attention must be paid both to nutritional support and to prevention of venous thrombosis. For patients with severely compromised lung function, sedation and muscle paralysis may be required to prevent struggling against the ventilator and increased oxygen utilization. Any sudden deterioration in hemodynamic status, increase in peak airway pressure, or drop in PaO_2 should suggest the possibility of a tension pneumothorax and prompt immediate action. Daily chest films and frequent examination of the chest for asymmetric breath sounds should be performed to survey for slowly developing air leaks. In selected patients, pharmacologic agents (e.g., inotropic agents, vasodilators, or both) may be useful if cardiac output cannot be preserved with acceptable low left ventricular filling pressures. However, optimal management of cardiac function is also an area of ongoing debate, because physiologic goal, although reasonable, may lead to conflicting strategies. Maximizing filling pressures to prevent a drop in cardiac output with PEEP conflicts with the strategy of reducing filling pressures to decrease the leak of fluid across the alveolar–capillary membrane. In general, strategies that aim toward reducing lung edema by limiting filling pressures appear more successful, although each situation warrants an individual decision. There does not appear to be any survival advantage conferred by elevating cardiac output and tissue oxygen delivery to supranormal levels.

PROGNOSIS

The mortality of patients who develop moderate or severe ARDS remains distressingly high (~30–40%), although this figure represents an improvement over the 90% mortality reported in the initial studies of ARDS. In general, mortality in ARDS correlates more with the presence of multiple organ failure and with other coexisting or preexisting disease than with the severity of pulmonary impairment. Long-term outlook for survivors of ARDS is relatively good in spite of the severe physiologic impairment and pathologic changes present during or immediately following hospitalization. Lung volumes and compliance often return to predicted levels within 6 to 18 months, and there is often only minimal impairment in exercise capacity compared to premorbid levels. Dyspnea persisting months after recovery should prompt a search for causes other than residual fibrosis from ARDS (e.g., tracheal stenosis). Unfortunately, patients with the most severe derangement of function during their acute illness are more likely to have persistent derangement of pulmonary function and have a persistent decrease in health-related quality of life.

Specific therapy for ARDS is not yet available. Early corticosteroid therapy does not prevent the development of ARDS or alter its outcome. Corticosteroids during the fibroproliferative phase of ARDS may hasten recovery, but their efficacy has not been studied rigorously. Efforts attempting to examine the use of agents to block elements of the inflammatory cascade (e.g., cyclooxygenase inhibitors or protease inhibitors) or attempts to manipulate cytokine cascades (e.g., anti–tumor necrosis factor or IL-1 receptor antagonists) have been disappointing. Manipulation of dietary lipids or administration of glutathione precursors may be useful as part of the support of patients with lung injury. Instillation of animal-derived surfactant products into the airways early in ARDS appeared to improve gas exchange in preliminary studies. However, delivery of surfactant as an aerosol has been unsuccessful, possibly because of the inefficiency of the delivery method, and recent studies examining the instillation of a synthetic surfactant product have similarly not shown benefit.

1. Alberts WM, Priest GP, Moser, KM. The outlook for survivors of ARDS. *Chest.* 1983;84:272.

   The authors compile the results of 21 articles describing the long-term outcome of patients with ARDS. Over 90% had no or minimal dyspnea on exertion, 80% had normal chest films, and 72% had normal static lung volumes. Seventy-three percent had normal arterial blood gases, and the remainder had hypoxemia; 48% had a decline in Pao_2 with exercise. Forty-nine percent had a persistently abnormal DLCO.

2. Bachofen M, Weibel ER. Alterations of the gas exchange apparatus in adult respiratory insufficiency associated with septicemia. *Am Rev Respir Dis.* 1977;116:589.

   A classic description of the electron microscopic findings seen at various stages of ARDS. The authors showed that neutrophil infiltration and interstitial edema occurred before endothelial changes were found.

3. Bernard GR, et al. High-dose corticosteroids in patients with the adult respiratory distress syndrome. *N Engl J Med.* 1987;317:1565.

   Methylprednisolone (30 mg/kg q6h for 4 doses) was administered in a double-blind, randomized trial to patients with ARDS (defined as refractory hypoxemia and bilateral infiltrates). Patients had received mechanical ventilation for an average of 3 days prior to steroid administration. The authors found no significant difference in mortality or in rates of disease remission or infectious complications.

4. Bernard GR, et al. The American-European Consensus Conference on ARDS. Definitions, mechanisms, relevant outcomes, and clinical trial coordination. *Am J Respir Crit Care Med.* 1994;149:818.

   The results of a consensus conference reviewing definitions of ARDS and acute lung injury, and recommending standards for future usage.

5. The Acute Respiratory Distress Syndrome Network. Ventilation with lower tidal volumes as compared with traditional tidal volumes for acute lung injury and the acute respiratory distress syndrome. *N Engl J Med.* 2000;342:1301.

   In this randomized trial of "standard" 12 mL/kg tidal volumes compared to lower (6 mL/kg lean body weight, 5.2 mL/kg total body weight) tidal volumes, the use of lower tidal volumes and reduced respiratory system pressures was associated with a reduction in overall mortality from 40 to 30%.

6. Carroll GC, et al. Minimal positive end-expiratory pressure (PEEP) may be "best PEEP." *Chest.* 1988;93:1020.

Adjustment of PEEP to "minimal effective levels" was compared to optimization of PEEP based on calculated shunt ratios. The former levels of PEEP (mean = 4 cm H₂O) were associated with significantly lower rates of complications than the latter (mean PEEP = 15).

7. Dreyfuss D, Basset G, Soler P, Saumon G. Intermittent positive-pressure hyperventilation with high inflation pressures produces pulmonary microvascular injury in rats. *Am Rev Respir Dis.* 1985;132:880–884.

   One of the initial studies showing that positive pressure ventilation resulted in lung injury and demonstrated the protective effect of PEEP.

8. Elliott CG, Rasmusson BY, Crapo RO. Upper airway obstruction following adult respiratory distress syndrome: analysis of 30 survivors. *Chest.* 1988;94:526.

   Symptomatic laryngeal stenosis was found in 3 of 30 survivors of ARDS. Those with obstruction did not differ from asymptomatic survivors with respect to age, duration of intubation, or maximal level of PEEP.

9. Elliott CG. Prediction of pulmonary function abnormalities after adult respiratory distress syndrome (ARDS). *Am Rev Respir Dis.* 1987;135:634.

   Pulmonary function was examined at least 1 year after ARDS. Residual decreases in vital capacity and total lung capacity were modest but were correlated with the severity of ARDS as measured by lung compliance, pulmonary artery hypertension, highest level of PEEP, and shunt fraction. An abnormal DLCO was found in five of seven survivors who were supported at Fio_2 above 0.6 for more than 24 hours.

10. Gobien RP, Reines HD, Schabel SI. Localized tension pneumothorax: unrecognized form of barotrauma in adult respiratory distress syndrome. *Radiology.* 1982;142:15.

    With severe ARDS, the lung often does not collapse as expected in the presence of a pneumothorax. The radiographic features of pulmonary barotrauma are often subtle.

11. Gregory TJ, et al. Surfactant chemical composition and biophysical activity in acute respiratory distress syndrome. *J Clin Invest.* 1991;88:1976.

    A description of the abnormalities of surfactant composition and function found in the lavage fluid recovered from patients with ARDS.

12. Gregory TJ, et al. Bovine surfactant therapy for patients with acute respiratory distress syndrome: a pilot study. *Am J Respir Crit Care Med.* 1997;155:1309.

    Instillation of a bovine surfactant preparation into the airways resulted in significant improvement in gas exchange and a strong suggestion of reduced mortality.

13. Lewis JF, Jobe AH. Surfactant and the adult respiratory distress syndrome. *Am Rev Respir Dis.* 1993;147:218.

    A comprehensive review of the current knowledge of the role played by surfactant in the pathophysiology of ARDS (181 references).

14. Meduri GU, et al. Effect of prolonged methylprednisolone therapy in unresolving acute respiratory distress syndrome: a randomized controlled trial. *JAMA.* 1998;280:159.

    The administration of methylprednisolone (2 mg/kg per day, n = 16) was compared to placebo (n = 8) in patients with unresolving ARDS. Steroid therapy was associated with improved lung injury score and mortality.

15. Michael JR, et al. Inhaled nitric oxide versus conventional therapy: effect on oxygenation in ARDS. *Am J Respir Crit Care Med.* 1998;157:1372.

    Nitric oxide therapy resulted in short-term improvement in Pao_2, but failed to improve mortality in ARDS. Similar results were reported by a European multicenter trial in the same volume.

16. The National Heart, Lung, and Blood Institute ARDS Clinical Trial Network. Higher versus lower positive end-expiratory pressures in patients with the acute respiratory distress syndrome. *N Engl J Med.* 2004;351:327.

    When patients were ventilated with 6 mL/kg tidal volume ventilation, the routine application of higher levels of PEEP did not improve outcomes when compared with lower levels.

17. Pepe PE, Hudson LD, Carrico CJ. Early application of positive end-expiratory pressure in patients at risk for the adult respiratory distress syndrome. *N Engl J Med*. 1984;311:281.

   The authors performed a randomized trial of the application of 8 cm H_2O of PEEP for 72 hours to patients at risk for ARDS. There was no reduction in the subsequent development of ARDS.

18. Milberg JA, Davis DR, Steinberg DP, Hudson LD. Improved survival of patients with acute respiratory distress syndrome (ARDS): 1983–1993. *JAMA*. 1995;273:306.

   Decreasing ARDS mortality was seen at a single institution over a 10-year period even with consistent data definitions and attempts to eliminate selection bias.

19. Spragg RG, et al. Effect of recombinant surfactant protein c-based surfactant on the acute respiratory distress syndrome. *N Engl J Med*. 2004;351:884.

   In a randomized blinded study of 448 patients with ARDS, the instillation of a synthetic surfactant containing recombinant surfactant protein C improved hypoxemia during the treatment period, but did not change overall mortality.

20. Tsuno K, et al. Histopathologic pulmonary changes from mechanical ventilation at high peak airway pressures. *Am Rev Respir Dis*. 1991;143:1115.

   A description of the histologic and gas exchange abnormalities found in sheep subjected to positive pressure ventilation with peak airway pressure of 30 cm H_2O for 24 to 96 hours.

21. Van Hook CJ, Carilli AD, Haponik EF. Hemodynamic effects of positive end-expiratory pressure: historical perspective. *Am J Med*. 1986;81:307.

   A review of the hemodynamic changes associated with the application of PEEP and a critical appraisal of the impact of PEEP on each of the major determinants of cardiac output.

59. AIRWAY MANAGEMENT

Mark R. Looney and Robert M. Jasmer

Placement of an endotracheal tube can be a life-saving procedure in a variety of clinical circumstances. The indications for tracheal intubation are varied and determined by both clinical and laboratory data. The need for mechanical ventilation is the primary indication for tracheal intubation. Another indication is for the relief of upper airway obstruction.

EMERGENT INTUBATION

During a respiratory arrest, the airway needs to be controlled immediately. It is critical to open the airway by the head tilt–chin lift maneuver to prevent the tongue from collapsing against the posterior pharynx. Ventilation can be temporarily satisfied using effective techniques for mask-to-mouth resuscitation. However, if the need for ventilatory support is not immediately reversed, an artificial airway should be established. Placement of an oral endotracheal tube using direct laryngoscopy is the method of choice in this setting.

Occasionally, placement of an orotracheal tube proves difficult and alternate means of endotracheal intubation must be pursued. For this reason, one should always have back-up methods of endotracheal intubation readily available in case a difficult airway is encountered. Blind nasal intubation using a specially designed endotracheal tube with a guided flexible tip facilitating tracheal placement is a common second option. However, nasal intubation takes time to perform and may not be suitable in emergency settings. Another option is the laryngeal mask airway (LMA). This artificial airway has a fenestrated opening that overlies the larynx and is surrounded by a cuff, which forms a low-pressure seal around the laryngeal inlet. Advantages of the LMA include ease of placement (blindly) and the ability to convert to a secure airway with an endotracheal tube. Disadvantages include potential distention of the stomach with subsequent aspiration of gastric contents and the inability to adequately ventilate poorly compliant lungs. More invasive means of securing the difficult airway in an emergency include (1) the retrograde wire technique, in which a wire is inserted percutaneously between the cricoid cartilage and the first tracheal ring, then up through the trachea into the mouth where it is used as a guide for endotracheal intubation; (2) transtracheal jet ventilation, where a small catheter is inserted into trachea to provide access for jet ventilation; and (3) cricothyroidotomy.

NONEMERGENT INTUBATION
In the less acute setting, tracheal intubation may become necessary as ventilation or oxygenation is progressively compromised. Noninvasive ventilation in some circumstances may be an alternative to tracheal intubation and should be considered. Acute upper airway obstruction also may require tracheal intubation or emergency tracheotomy. If the obstruction is caused by aspiration of a large piece of solid matter (the *cafe coronary* syndrome), an attempt should be made to remove the solid matter manually, followed by forceful compression of the thoracic cage (Heimlich maneuver) in an attempt to dislodge the obstruction. Upper airway obstruction caused by infection (acute epiglottis), edema (burn injury, infection, allergic reaction, or tumor), or stricture (prior endotracheal intubation) may require endotracheal intubation or emergency tracheotomy.

METHODS
Endotracheal intubation can be accomplished with an orotracheal tube, a nasotracheal tube, or a tracheostomy tube, each of which has its particular advantages and disadvantages. The orotracheal tube is used in most patients. Passage through the mouth places less limitation on tube size than passage through the nose; however, it is uncomfortable for the conscious patient and does not allow oral ingestion of food. Placement of a nasotracheal tube requires somewhat greater skill; however, it can often be performed on patients with limited neck mobility, in whom passage of an orotracheal tube is difficult or impossible. If time permits, local anesthesia applied at the nose, nasopharynx, and mouth reduces patient discomfort and facilitates cooperation. Nasotracheal tubes have the disadvantages of being difficult to place quickly and occasionally kinking in the posterior nasopharynx. In addition, the size of the nasopharynx can limit the diameter of the tube that can be placed, making it more difficult to suction through. They also occlude sinus drainage, increasing the risk of sinusitis.

In difficult cases, fiberoptic bronchoscopy may be useful for intubating patients, particularly those with arthritic or traumatic neck disorders. In awake patients, administration of intravenous medications for sedation and muscular paralysis can facilitate tracheal intubation.

The application of pressure to the cricoid cartilage (Sellick maneuver) during laryngoscopy and intubation helps to occlude the esophagus and prevent potential aspiration. Correct placement of an endotracheal tube leaves the tip 2 to 4 cm above the carina; a chest radiograph should be obtained after intubation to confirm placement. Tube position can also be confirmed by direct visualization of the tube passing through the vocal cords or by bronchoscopy.

Tracheostomy
A tracheostomy tube placed through a surgically prepared tracheostomy site or through progressive percutaneous dilatation at the cricothyroid or tracheal level is generally well tolerated and allows excellent suctioning capability. Because a tracheostomy tube does not traverse the larynx, vocal cord injury is minimized. Verbalization can occur during spontaneous breathing through a fenestrated tracheostomy tube with a special one-way valve. During positive-pressure ventilation, some tracheostomy tubes allow flow of an air jet through the vocal cords and, thus, permit

speech, even during mechanical ventilation. Tracheostomy tubes have the obvious disadvantage of requiring a surgical procedure, which is often performed at the bedside in the intensive care unit.

MANAGEMENT

Adult nasotracheal, orotracheal, and tracheostomy tubes use an inflatable cuff to seal the tube within the trachea. A common misconception is that this cuff seal prevents significant aspiration of oropharyngeal contents. In fact, the cuff provides only partial protection against aspiration; oropharyngeal suctioning still is necessary as well as meticulous attention to cuff inflation, not only to try to prevent aspiration, but also to minimize the pressure being transmitted to the tracheal mucosal surface. The high-volume, high-compliance cuffs can seal the trachea with minimal leak and low pressures (<25 mmHg), which results in significantly fewer cuff-related postextubation tracheal problems because tracheal mucosal blood flow is not compromised.

The routine care of patients with tracheal intubation includes frequent suctioning to prevent accumulation of pulmonary secretions, careful nasal and oral hygiene (including suctioning of oropharyngeal contents), and regular monitoring of cuff inflation pressure. In addition, for patients with tracheostomy tubes in place, attention must also be directed to the surgical incision, with appropriate topical treatment, dressing changes, and avoidance of pressure necrosis at the surgical site.

COMPLICATIONS

Mechanically ventilated patients are at risk for potentially catastrophic events that can occur suddenly and can be related to the underlying disorder or malfunction of the ventilator or artificial airway. If a patient cannot be ventilated, the first step is to disconnect the patient from the ventilator and begin hand ventilation with an anesthesia bag containing 100% oxygen. The artificial airway should be checked for evidence of external obstruction (e.g., kinking of tubing) and for patency by passing a suction catheter through the tube to remove mucus plugs or blood clots that may be causing the problem. If the suction catheter can be passed through the entire length of the endotracheal tube and into the chest but ventilation is still difficult, potential causes of the difficulty include major airway obstruction not removed by suctioning, peripheral airways obstruction, or pneumothorax. Physical examination is often useful to distinguish among these possibilities—main bronchial obstruction is indicated by the absence of air entry into the lung distal to the obstruction, causing absent breath sounds and dullness to percussion on the affected side; peripheral airways obstruction is often associated with wheezing; and pneumothorax leads to absent breath sounds and hyperresonance to percussion on the affected side. In an emergency setting, a 14-gauge needle can be inserted into the second anterior intercostal space to restore ventilation and blood pressure in a patient with a tension pneumothorax.

The long-term clinically significant complications of endotracheal intubation are less common today than several decades ago because of the softer, more compliant cuffs now available. Approximately 5 to 8% of extubated patients develop stridor secondary to laryngeal edema, which requires a combination of vasoconstrictors (inhaled racemic epinephrine), anti-inflammatory agents (steroids), or reintubation. Tracheostomy avoids these laryngeal complications but it is associated with its own, often more serious complications (hemorrhage, barotrauma, and tracheal stenosis, especially at the stomal site). A complication unique to nasotracheal intubation is sinusitis, which has been radiographically detected in approximately 50% of patients after prolonged use.

Clinically, the overwhelming majority of patients who have survived prolonged intubation (up to 3 weeks) recover upper airway function completely. No absolute time limit has been set for endotracheal intubation beyond which tracheostomy is necessary. Tracheostomy can help in weaning the patient from mechanical ventilator support by allowing improved mobilization and better suctioning of airway secretions and by promoting easier communication and swallowing. Therefore, if more than 14 to 21 days of intubation are anticipated in a patient who is expected to survive an acute illness (e.g., spinal cord injury), then a tracheostomy after only a few days of mechanical ventilation may minimize the laryngeal complications associated with transglottic intubation. However, if successful extubation is anticipated within 2 to 3 weeks and the patient is tolerating transglottic intubation well, it is prudent to avoid a tracheostomy. Similarly, performing a tracheostomy on a patient who is so critically ill that survival is not expected serves no useful purpose for the patient. If such a patient does survive, the risk of intubation-related complications is sufficiently small that delaying a tracheostomy until the patient shows signs of improvement is justified.

1. Balk RA. The technique of orotracheal intubation. *Journal of Critical Illness.* 1997;12:316.
   A concise review of the indications, contraindications, and technique of orotracheal intubation.
2. Benumof JL. Laryngeal mask airway and the ASA difficult airway algorithm. *Anesthesiology.* 1996;84:686.
   A review article on how the LMA fits into the difficult airway algorithm, with special emphasis on the many ways of using the LMA as a conduit for tracheal intubation.
3. Bishop MJ, Weymuller EA, Fink BR. Laryngeal effects of prolonged intubation. *Anesth Analg.* 1984;63:335.
   A review article that explains why and what laryngeal complications develop (52 references).
4. Butler KH, Clyne B. Management of the difficult airway: alternative airway techniques and adjuncts. *Emerg Med Clin North Am.* 2003;21:259.
   A comprehensive review article detailing the many options for securing the difficult airway including useful algorithms.
5. Colice G. Resolution of laryngeal injury following translaryngeal intubation. *Am Rev Respir Dis.* 1992;145:361.
   A prospective fiberoptic laryngoscopic study of 54 patients who required more than 4 days of translaryngeal intubation. Although laryngeal injury at extubation was common, healing usually occurred within 8 weeks. Length of intubation and subsequent tracheostomy did not adversely affect healing.
6. Dacey MJ. Managing the unstable patient. The first 10 minutes often set the course. *Postgrad Med.* 1999;105:69.
   A nice overview of the approach to the critically ill patient with respiratory compromise. Also reviewed are dosing guidelines and advantages and adverse effects of sedative agents commonly used during intubation.
7. Danzle DF. Tracheal intubation and mechanical ventilation. In: Tintinalli JE, Kelen GD, Statczynski JS, eds. *Emergency Medicine: A Comprehensive Study Guide.* 5th ed. New York, NY: McGraw Hill; 1999.
   A review of various tracheal intubation techniques. Pharmacologic characteristics of sedative or induction and neuromuscular relaxants are nicely summarized in table form.
8. Dellinger RP. Fiberoptic bronchoscopy in adult airway management. *Crit Care Med.* 1990;18:882.
   A well-referenced article describing a technique for intubation with bronchoscopic guidance, including how to position a double-lumen endobronchial tube correctly.
9. Manzano JL, et al. Verbal communication of ventilator-dependent patients. *Crit Care Med.* 1993;21:512.
   A unidirectional valve allowed verbal communication while patients were maintained on mechanical ventilation.
10. Maziak DE, Meade MO, Todd R. The timing of tracheotomy: a systematic review. *Chest.* 1998;114:605.
    A systematic review addressing the issue of the optimal time to perform a tracheotomy in patients with respiratory failure who require an artificial airway.

11. Pedersen J, et al. The effect of nasotracheal intubation on the paranasal si-
    nuses: a prospective study of 434 intensive care patients. *Acta Anaesthesiol
    Scand*. 1991;35:11.
    *Of patients intubated nasotracheally, 49% had radiographic evidence of
    sinusitis.*
12. Stauffer JL, Olson DE, Petty TL. Complications and consequences of endotracheal
    intubation and tracheotomy: a prospective study of 150 critically ill adult patients.
    Am J Med. 1981;70:65.
    *The authors found a 60% complication rate during placement and use of either a
    tracheostomy tube or an endotracheal tube. These complications were more severe
    after tracheostomy, and a strong argument is presented against the arbitrary use
    of tracheostomy after a set number of days of intubation.*

60. MECHANICAL VENTILATION: DEVICES AND METHODS

Timothy A. Morris

The introduction of microprocessor-controlled algorithms to manage ventilator performance has dramatically expanded the potential for a single ventilator to provide
multiple modes of ventilatory support. Ventilators may cycle from inspiration to expiration based on a set pressure, time, inspiratory flow rate, or tidal volume. A variety
of inspiratory flow patterns may be delivered, or inspiratory flow may be adjusted
based on the pressure during inspiration. The ratio of inspiratory to expiratory time
may be inverted to produce very long inspiratory times, very short expiratory times,
or both. Positive end-expiratory pressure (PEEP) may be added at the airway opening
to keep alveoli open throughout exhalation. The choice of appropriate modalities for
ventilatory support is determined by the respiratory care objectives for the patient
at a given point in the disease course (e.g., improved oxygenation, respiratory muscle
rest, weaning). One of the advantages of the newer generation of microprocessor-
based mechanical ventilators is that it is possible to dramatically alter the ventilatory support technique as the patient's requirements change without changing the
ventilator.

The wide variety of ventilatory modalities may be categorized according to how the
following functions are handled: (1) control and adjustment of air movement into the
lungs during inspiration; (2) function during exhalation; (3) scheduling of mandatory (machine-driven) breaths; and (4) function during spontaneous (patient-driven)
breaths. Each function has the goal of improving arterial oxygenation, protecting the
alveoli from overdistension, or reducing the work of breathing by synchronization with
spontaneous patient effort.

CONTROL: VOLUME VS PRESSURE

The most fundamental aspect of mechanical ventilation is how air movement into
the lungs is controlled and adjusted during inspiration. The basic choice is to control
either pressure or flow. The most straightforward model of controlling pressure is a
simple pressure-driven system. In this idealized situation, the patient's airway would
be connected to a large tank of air maintained at a specific pressure. At the start of
inspiration, the pressurized air from the tank would enter the lungs at a flow rate
determined by the resistance and compliance of the respiratory system. As the lung
pressure approached equilibrium with the air in the tank, flow would decelerate at
a rate similarly determined by respiratory resistance and compliance. In this model,
the pressure in the airways would be "controlled" at a constant level, while, at any

given instant, the flow rate would depend on the resistance and compliance of the respiratory system.

A different idealized model of mechanical ventilation would supply a constant flow of air to the lungs, allowing the pressure to change depending on the resistance and compliance of the lungs. A simple, idealized model of flow control might involve a highly pressurized tank of air connected to the patient's airway by a resistant valve used to control airflow, a setup similar to the high-pressure pump used to inflate one's tires at a filling station. In this idealized system, flow is held constant, and the intrapulmonary pressure at any given instant depends on the resistance and compliance of the lungs. The lungs (like tires) are not allowed to reach equilibrium with the high-pressure tanks. The volume of air delivered to the lungs is determined by the flow rate and duration of the breath delivered.

These two idealized systems are, of course, too cumbersome and inflexible for actual clinical use. However, modern ventilator modalities simulate either one of these two basic models by using microprocessor-controlled valves to regulate the output from high-pressure solenoid pumps. The ventilator generates a "volume-controlled" breath by repetitively sampling the flow it is delivering during inspiration and adjusting the solenoid output to provide a precise flow pattern for a specific duration of time (volume = flow × time). To generate a pressure-controlled breath, the microprocessor samples the pressure it is delivering and adjusts the solenoid pump output to achieve and maintain a constant pressure in the airways.

As modern ventilators develop faster methods of monitoring and adjusting their output, as well as more complete control over airway pressure and flow, they increase their versatility and applicability to a variety of clinical needs. For example, if a patient who coughs or "bucks" when an older style ventilator is delivering an inhaled breath (in pressure-control or volume-control mode), the airway pressure may rise rapidly, exposing the lungs to barotrauma before the ventilator detects the high pressure and ends the breath. Modern ventilators, however, can adapt to rapid changes in lung compliance (such as coughing or bucking) by (1) increasing the rapidity with which the flow and pressure in the airway is monitored; and (2) using the microprocessor to constantly adjust both the inhalation valves and exhalation valves in the airway circuit without ending the inspired breath. Thus, barotrauma is minimized, minute ventilation is preserved, and the work of breathing is reduced.

DURATION OF INHALATION AND EXHALATION

Modern ventilators may also vary the duration of the inspiratory and expiratory phases of breathing to suit the needs of the patient. Conscious patients, for example, tolerate mechanical ventilation more readily with relatively brief inhalation times, allowing more time for exhalation (similar to the normal cadence of spontaneous breathing). However, if severe hypoxemia occurs, the patient may require long inspiratory and short expiratory times: a reversal of the normal inspiratory-to-expiratory (I/E) time ratio, termed *inverse ratio ventilation* (IRV). The IRV mode is commonly used with pressure-controlled ventilation, but can be used with volume control as well. The inspiratory time, respiratory rate, and I/E ratio are, of course, interdependent. Some ventilators allow the setting of two parameters (such as I/E and rate) directly; the other parameter is adjusted as needed. Because IRV so distorts the normal pattern of ventilation, the patient usually requires sedation, neuromuscular blockade, or both to avoid patient–ventilator asynchrony. This mode of ventilation is able to achieve acceptable levels of arterial oxygenation at lower peak and end-expiratory airway pressure. It remains controversial whether this effect is the result of the inspiratory pressure plateau preventing alveolar collapse or whether the short expiratory times, which do not allow expiration flow to finish before inspiration begins, simply provide PEEP at the alveolar level that is not measured at the airway opening (alveolar or intrinsic PEEP).

PEEP

During exhalation, the ventilator may either allow the lungs to reach atmospheric pressure or provide positive pressure throughout exhalation (PEEP). The most common use of PEEP is to prevent damaged alveoli from collapsing during exhalation, increasing the proportion of ventilated lung units and decreasing the amount of shunt. Because a large component of gas exchange dysfunction in lung injury is attributed to intrapulmonary shunting, PEEP may relieve hypoxemia in these cases without requiring the use of high oxygen concentrations. Some clinicians also use PEEP for other uses, such as (1) reducing the work of breathing in patients manifesting intrinsic PEEP from obstructive lung disease; and (2) decreasing intrathoracic venous return (preload) in patients with congestive heart failure.

TRIGGERING INHALATION

Ventilator modalities also differ in scheduling when mandatory breaths (driven entirely by the ventilator) are given. A mandatory breath can be triggered by the patient's effort (assisted) or the ventilator breaths may be delivered at a set rate (controlled). The ventilator may be set to assist every breath (continuous mandatory ventilation, also called assist control) or only a set number of breaths per minute (synchronized intermittent mandatory ventilation). Using either mode, if the patient does not trigger assisted breaths at or above a rate specified, the machine delivers controlled breaths at that rate. Usually, the patient receives some combination of assisted and controlled breaths, depending on set ventilator rate and his own intrinsic respiratory rate. Patients receiving only assisted (self-initiated) breaths may become fatigued because, although assisting the breath decreases the work of breathing, it does not entirely rest the muscles of respiration. Once the diaphragm begins an inhalation, it continues to contract throughout the entire inspiratory cycle. One approach to resting the diaphragm is to set the ventilator rate such that a majority of breaths are controlled (machine initiated).

Another approach to reduce the work of breathing uses a nearly opposite strategy: to reduce or eliminate mandatory breaths and aid the patient's spontaneous breathing using pressure support. In pressure support ventilation mode, the ventilator must be triggered by patient effort. Once triggered, it provides a flow rate that varies with the difference between the airway pressure and the preset target pressure. The result is a rapidly rising upward ramp of pressure. Inspiration is terminated when the flow drops below a threshold level or a fraction of the peak inspiratory flow. When ventilated using high-level pressure support, the patient has substantial breath-by-breath control over inspiratory flow rate, tidal volume, inspiratory time, and respiratory rate. Awake patients almost universally describe this mode of ventilation as more comfortable than conventional volume-cycled mechanical ventilation, probably because the increased responsiveness of the ventilator in this mode leads to improved synchronization of the mechanical ventilator to the patient's spontaneous effort. The patient wastes less of his or her energy "fighting the ventilator" and the respiratory muscles are partially unloaded. Pressure support ventilation also allows the patient to vary the inspiratory flow rate, tidal volume, and inspiratory time from breath to breath, and it therefore is perceived by the patient as a much more natural pattern of breathing and more comfortable. This improved synchronization of mechanical ventilation may have the additional benefit of reducing barotrauma in patients who can be ventilated using pressure support. This mode is most effective with patients who have good respiratory muscle strength and high ventilatory drives (e.g., AIDS patients with *Pneumocystis* pneumonia) and allows ventilatory support of these patients without levels of sedation that impair interaction with visitors and staff. The limitations of high-level pressure support ventilation include the inability to use this mode in patients who are not able to maintain a sufficient respiratory rate (those who are obtunded, sedated, or given neuromuscular blocking agents) and the requirements for patient effort on each breath, which does not allow complete respiratory muscle rest and may precipitate respiratory muscle exhaustion.

Whatever modality is chosen, matching the ventilator response to the patient's demand reduces the work performed by the respiratory muscles and may prevent respiratory muscle fatigue. The patient perceives the ventilator's response on each breath in four ways: (1) the energy necessary to begin inspiratory flow, (2) the rate at which inspiration flow actually occurs given the level of muscle effort expended, (3) the duration of inspiratory flow (inspiratory time), and (4) the volume inspired. When the response of the ventilator fails to match the patient's demand in one or more of these aspects, the work performed by the patient increases, ventilatory drive increases, the patient becomes uncomfortable and may begin to fight the mechanical ventilator.

VENTILATOR RESPONSIVENESS

Mechanical ventilators differ in their responsiveness to patient effort in their inspiratory triggering mechanisms, their inspiratory demand values, and their mechanisms of ending the inspired breath. When a mechanical ventilator is assisting the patient's breath, it must "sense" that the patient has begun inhaling and initiate the machine-driven breath using an inspiratory triggering mechanism. For many ventilators, the breath is triggered once the patient's spontaneous efforts exceed a preset negative pressure. For earlier generations of mechanical ventilators, this threshold was –2 cm H_2O or more. Newer generations of mechanical ventilators have thresholds that can be set as slow as –0.5 cm H_2O. In addition, ventilators can also be triggered by a drop in the flow passing by the endotracheal tube. Flow triggering may make the ventilator more sensitive to the patient's inspiratory effort and, by using software to drive the pressure at the airway opening to a slightly positive value, further reduces patient work during spontaneous breathing. The result is a virtual elimination of the ventilatory work added by the mechanical ventilator circuit during spontaneous breathing.

The work performed by the patient increases when the flow provided by the mechanical ventilator lags behind that demanded by the patient. Inspiratory demand valves on older models of many mechanical ventilators required greater effort to produce higher flows. More recently, ventilator inspiratory flow valves have been designed to increase flows with much smaller effort. Pressure support provides an even further reduction in inspiration work by increasing the inspiratory flow in the airway to maintain a positive pressure, allowing the ventilator to provide some of the work of breathing without controlling the patient's breathing pattern.

PROPORTIONAL ASSIST VENTILATION

Synchronization between the patient and the mechanical ventilator is likely to be enhanced in a new generation of mechanical ventilators currently available. Complex software algorithms and rapid feedback mechanisms to control airway pressure and flow allow these ventilators a great deal of flexibility to adjust their function to patient demands. One such strategy made possible by these developments is proportional assist ventilation, which is designed to provide a fixed proportion of the energy required for ventilation regardless of the size of the tidal volume generated or minute ventilation required. The energy required to move the respiratory system during ventilation can be divided into that part required to overcome the elastic recoil of the lung and chest wall and that part required to overcome the resistance to airflow through the airways of the lung. A proportional assist mechanical ventilator continuously adjusts the pressure it provides throughout inspiration, calculating at each adjustment both the pressure required to drive the instantaneous airflow and the pressure required to support the current inspired volume. The clinical benefits of proportional assist ventilation and other new modes of mechanical ventilation are unclear and are topics of ongoing research.

---

1. Ravenscraft SA, et al. Tracheal gas insufflation augments CO_2 clearance during mechanical ventilation. *Am Rev Respir Dis.* 1993;148:345.

   Tracheal gas insufflation in eight patients was a useful adjunct to a pressure-targeted strategy of ventilatory management (in either volume-cycled or pressure-controlled modes).
2. Chan K, Abraham E. Effects of inverse ratio ventilation on cardiorespiratory parameters in severe respiratory failure. *Chest.* 1992;102:1556.

   In 10 patients with severe respiratory failure, pressure-controlled inverse ratio ventilation was associated with significant increases in PaO$_2$, arterial pH, and mean airway pressure. Significant decreases in pulmonary shunt fraction, PaCO$_2$, and cardiac index were also found in comparison to pressure-controlled ventilation without inverse ratios.

3. Chatburn R. Classification of mechanical ventilators. In: N MacIntyre and R. Branson eds. Consensus Conference on the Essentials of Mechanical Ventilators. *Respir Care.* 1992;37(special issue):1009.

   A proposed new classification terminology for mechanical ventilators.
4. Downs J, et al. Intermittent mandatory ventilation: a new approach to weaning patients from mechanical ventilators. *Chest.* 1973;64:331.

   Describes the rationale, circuitry, and advantages of this ventilator mode.
5. Duncan SR, Riak NW, Raffin TA. Inverse ratio ventilation PEEP in disguise. *Chest.* 1987;92:390.

   Editorial that raises the question whether inverse ratio ventilation is effective because of prolonged inspiratory plateaus or because of alveolar PEEP.
6. Forese A, Bryan AC. Effects of anesthesia and paralysis on diaphragmatic mechanics in man. *Anesthesiology.* 1974;41:242.

   An often-quoted and controversial paper describing use of a fluoroscopic technique to compare diaphragmatic function in mechanical ventilation and spontaneous ventilation.
7. Greenbaum DM, et al. Continuous positive airway pressure without tracheal intubation in spontaneously breathing patients. *Chest.* 1976;69:615.

   The authors suggest that this technique can be employed safely and effectively; however, the potential for vomiting and aspiration appears too great for widespread application.
8. Hinson JR, Marini JJ. Principles of mechanical ventilator use in respiratory failure. *Annu Rev Med.* 1992;43:341.

   Recent review of the physiology of respiratory failure and its treatment using mechanical ventilation.
9. MacIntyre NR. Respiratory function during pressure support ventilation. *Chest.* 1986;89:677.

   Pressure support ventilation improves patient comfort, reduces ventilatory work, and tends to normalize the pressure–volume change characteristics of the remaining work of breathing in stable patients recovering from acute respiratory failure.
10. MacIntyre NR. Clinically available new strategies for mechanical ventilatory support. *Chest.* 1993;104:560.

    Recent review of strategies for mechanical ventilation.
11. Marini JJ, Smith TC, Lamb VJ. External work output and force generation during synchronized intermittent mechanical ventilation. *Am Rev Respir Dis.* 1988;138:1169.

    Respiratory muscle work in the synchronized intermittent mechanical ventilation mode is similar for the assisted and the spontaneous breaths.
12. Marini JJ, Rodriguez RM, Lamb VJ. The inspiration workload of patient-initiated mechanical ventilation. *Am Rev Respir Dis.* 1986;134:902.

    Substantial respiratory muscle effort occurs in patients on mechanical ventilators even when the ventilator is set to assist each breath, particularly for older ventilators with less responsive inspiratory flow values.
13. Slutsky AS. Non-conventional methods of ventilation. *Am Rev Respir Dis.* 1988;138:175.

    An excellent review of apneic oxygenation, high-frequency ventilation, and low-frequency positive pressure ventilation with extracorporeal carbon dioxide removal.
14. Suter PM, Fairley HB, Isenberg MD. Effect of tidal volume and positive end-expiratory pressure on compliance during mechanical ventilation. *Chest.* 1978;73:158.

    During mechanical ventilation, both static and dynamic lung compliance are affected by changes in tidal volume and PEEP. Measurements of lung compliance must be made at constant mechanical ventilation settings.
15. Tharratt RS, Roblee PA, Albertson TE. Pressure controlled inverse ratio ventilation in severe adult respiratory failure. *Chest.* 1988;94:755.

    A description of this mode of mechanical ventilation in comparison to conventional ventilation with results that suggest that comparable gas exchange can be achieved with lower minute volume, peak airway pressure, and PEEP.

16. Tobin MJ. Mechanical ventilation. *N Engl J Med*. 1994;330:1056.
    A recent review of mechanical ventilation.
17. Younes M. Proportional assist ventilation: a new approach to ventilatory support.
    Am Rev Respir Dis. 1992;145:114.
    Presents the theoretic justification for proportional assist ventilation and an experimental prototype to implement this form of ventilation.
18. Younes M, et al. Proportional assist ventilation: results of an initial clinical trial.
    Am Rev Respir Dis. 1992;145:121.
    Proportional assist mechanical ventilation was well tolerated in four patients with a 50% reduction in peak airway pressure and a reduction in the spontaneous respiratory rate when compared to synchronized intermittent mechanical ventilation.

61. MECHANICAL VENTILATION: COMPLICATIONS AND DISCONTINUATION

Timothy A. Morris

Mechanical ventilation itself poses an increased risk for serious complications and should be discontinued as soon as it is safe to do so. Unnecessarily prolonged mechanical ventilation may be minimized by (1) frequently assessing the ventilated patient to determine when the patient is capable of breathing without mechanical assistance and (2) progressing the transition to unassisted breathing as rapidly as tolerated by the patient. The term *weaning*, which implies a mandatory stepwise reduction in support, is more appropriately referred to as *liberation* from mechanical ventilation, which implies no such requirement.

In general, the reasons for mechanical ventilation dictate both the complications of mechanical ventilation and the method of liberation. Patients are placed on mechanical ventilators because of (1) failure to maintain adequate arterial oxygenation on supplemental oxygen, (2) failure to maintain adequate alveolar ventilation (excrete carbon dioxide), or (3) therapeutic objectives not directly related to gas exchange (e.g., hyperventilation for head trauma, paralysis for tetanus). More than one indication may coexist; however, one indication usually predominates.

COMPLICATIONS

The complications inherent to mechanical ventilation warrant its discontinuation as quickly as possible. Complications associated with endotracheal intubation itself are common to all ventilated patients and include sinusitis, laryngeal injury, and tracheomalacia (see Chapter 11). In addition, patients with hypoxic ventilatory failure often require high fractional inspiratory oxygen concentrations (F_IO_2) and elevated peak and end-expiratory ventilatory pressures. The inhalation of an F_IO_2 above 0.5 for extended periods of time increases the risk of oxygen toxicity and pulmonary fibrosis. The use of an F_IO_2 of 1.0 (i.e., 100% oxygen) can result in an increased shunt fraction because of resorption atelectasis involving segments of the lung containing low ventilation–perfusion ($\dot{V}/\dot{Q}$) units.

Barotrauma

The problems associated with high inspiratory and expiratory pressures include hemodynamic compromise and barotrauma. High inspiratory pressure and positive end-expiratory pressure (PEEP) may unpredictably diminish cardiac output and blood pressure. Although PEEP reduces intrapulmonary shunting, it also may lead to (1) a fall in left ventricular compliance and right atrial venous return; (2) an increase or decrease in pulmonary vascular resistance; and (3) overdistention and injury of unimpaired ("normal") alveolar units. The net effect on cardiac output and gas exchange is usually impossible to predict for an individual patient. Therefore, most patients with severe hypoxic ventilatory failure who receive high levels of PEEP require systemic arterial and pulmonary artery catheterization for repeated measurements of hemodynamic parameters and gas tensions. During the initial management of patients requiring a very high F_IO_2, systemic oxygen delivery (arterial oxygen content times cardiac output) generally can be maximized by adjusting the levels of PEEP and by simultaneously expanding intravascular volume or pharmacologically enhancing cardiac output. When hemodynamic stability is achieved, efforts should be aimed at decreasing the F_IO_2 to a safer level (below 0.7), while at the same time maintaining oxygen delivery.

The incidence of barotrauma in mechanically ventilated patients is exceptionally high and correlates with mean and peak airway pressures. Pneumothorax may be dramatic and associated with vascular collapse, as in tension pneumothorax, or it may be a subtle radiographic finding because of the limited potential for the severely damaged lung to collapse. The presence of a chest tube (either prophylactic or therapeutic) does not guarantee that another pneumothorax will not develop in the same hemithorax; in fact, patients with severe adult respiratory distress syndrome may require multiple chest tubes bilaterally. If a bronchopleural fistula develops, ventilation may be further compromised.

In hypercapnic ventilatory failure caused by obstructive lung disease, mechanical ventilation also can reduce cardiac output because of the sudden increase in intrathoracic pressure (with decrease in venous return). This reaction is usually limited to patients with at least mild hypovolemia at the time of intubation and responds readily to volume repletion. Barotrauma occurs less often in these patients with hypoxic ventilatory failure and is probably related to localized differentials in alveolar pressure and distention, rather than to absolute transpulmonary pressure. The markedly distorted lung architecture in these patients may lead to barotrauma at much lower pressures.

Infection
Intubated patients of all types are at an increased risk of infection. Bacterial overgrowth of gastric contents following adjustment of gastric pH with antacid or H_2-blocking agents is a major source of nosocomial pneumonias and can be minimized by substitution of sucralfate for these agents as prophylaxis for gastric bleeding. Malnutrition can be a major problem in patients requiring prolonged ventilatory support. Nutritional support should begin as soon as possible in any patient in whom prolonged ventilatory support is contemplated.

In the final group of patients in whom special indications prompt ventilatory support, the complications are often directly related to the therapeutic modalities utilized rather than to the ventilator per se, because these patients often enter the intensive care unit (ICU) with relatively normal lungs. The consequences of ventilators disconnected from the paralyzed patient are tragic; appropriate safeguards, including carefully tested apneic alarms, should be initiated in this situation. The application of barbiturate coma for head trauma patients, particularly in conjunction with rigorous maintenance of the head-up posture, may lead to a greater than normal problem of maintaining bronchial hygiene, even in those patients with normal lungs. This group may develop lobar collapse and gram-negative pneumonia if careful prophylactic measures are not initiated.

In addition, patients on mechanical ventilation also may experience cardiac arrhythmias, seizures, and gastrointestinal bleeding. Arrhythmias may be related to hypoxemia, hypokalemia, or other electrolyte disturbances and the use of drugs (e.g., beta agonists, aminophylline) with an arrhythmogenic potential. Seizures may occur because of prior hypoxia, too rapid reversion of chronic hypercapnia, or theophylline excess. Gastrointestinal bleeding from gastritis or frank gastric ulceration is common; however, the mechanisms responsible are not clear. Antacids and H_2-receptor blockers appear to reduce the incidence of bleeding, particularly in patients with acute central nervous system disease (e.g., head trauma, cerebrovascular accidents).

DISCONTINUATION

Mechanical ventilation should be discontinued as soon as it is safe to do so. Although this usually requires the reversal, to some degree, of the primary causes for mechanical ventilation, the causes need not be entirely resolved before patients can be safely extubated. Furthermore, although the term *weaning* is commonly used to describe the process of ventilator discontinuation, gradual tapering of ventilator support may not be necessary in many patients. Depending on the patient, then, procedure to liberate patients from mechanical ventilation may have two possible purposes: (1) assure the medical team that mechanical ventilation is no longer necessary; and (2) gradually train the respiratory muscles to assume the entire work of breathing.

As much as 40% of the time on mechanical ventilation is spent after gas exchange itself has improved to the point that spontaneous breathing could be possible. Methods to decrease the time it takes to liberate patients from mechanical ventilation may reduce complication rates and save considerable expense. Timing is a major issue. The patient who is extubated too early, requiring reintubation, is subject to difficulties obtaining an airway, laryngeal injury, aspiration pneumonia, and cardiac ischemia, all of which lead to a higher mortality. Conversely, the patient who is left on mechanical ventilation too long risks nosocomial pneumonia, tracheal injury, and the other complications mentioned.

Successful extubation requires that the work required for breathing be substantially less than the capacity to breath. The work of breathing depends on factors such as (1) the amount of gas exchange required, which in turn depends on O_2 consumption and CO_2 production; (2) gas exchange efficiency, including the (A–a) O_2 gradient and $\dot{V}_D/\dot{V}_T$; and (3) the physical work required to inflate the lungs, such as lung and chest wall compliance. The capacity to breath, in turn, depends on (1) neurologic mechanisms to control breathing, (2) respiratory muscle strength, and (3) endurance. Despite a great deal of clinical investigation, it is still difficult to predict when the balance of these factors permits discontinuation of mechanical ventilation in particular patients.

Indications

The good news for clinicians is that complex, time-consuming, and often inconsistent methods of weaning are largely being replaced by simpler algorithms that are at least as effective. Essential to the process is the categorization of patients into one of four basic groups: (1) those in whom immediate extubation is likely to be successful; (2) those in whom weaning is progressing toward the goal of extubation; (3) those who are not progressing, in whom further investigation is necessary; and (4) those in whom weaning of any type is contraindicated.

The first step is to identify patients in the last group, in whom weaning would be likely to cause harm. This group generally has one or more of the following problems: (1) inadequate gas exchange, evidenced by a low Po_2/F_{IO_2} ratio or the requirement for high levels of PEEP; (2) inability to cough or clear secretions during spontaneous breathing; (3) instability such as shock or hypotension; (4) severe muscle weakness or paralysis; (5) sedation or obtundation; (6) major procedures planned in the near future; (7) unstable myocardial ischemia; or (8) elevated intracranial pressure. Patients with these contraindications to weaning should be monitored daily for signs of resolution. Others should begin the process of liberation. This aggressive approach is safe and shortens the duration of mechanical ventilation.

The next step is to distinguish those patients who are ready for immediate discontinuation of mechanical ventilation from those in whom intermediate steps are necessary. The patient's respiratory performance (while receiving minimal support from the ventilator) may predict when extubation will be tolerated. A variety of "weaning parameters" have become popular, such as minute ventilation, respiratory rate, and inspiratory pressures. A simple and accurate predictor is the "rapid shallow breathing index," representing the ratio of the respiratory rate to the tidal volume ($f/\dot{V}_T$). Our preference is to test the $f/\dot{V}_T$ during brief periods of spontaneous breathing (on T-piece or with low amount of pressure support) at least once daily. Patients with low $f/\dot{V}_T$ ratios are allowed to continue spontaneous breathing and, if they tolerate the "sprint" for 1 to 2 hours, are extubated. Those in whom the initial $f/\dot{V}_T$ is high require further steps to be liberated from mechanical ventilation.

For those patients who cannot be extubated immediately, intermediate steps may be necessary. Whether the patient's performance during these weaning steps is the cause of or the result of improved respiratory status is controversial. Options include (1) periodically "sprinting" the patient with intervals where the ventilator provides lower levels of assistance, using IMV, pressure support or T-piece with humidified oxygen flowing past; or (2) intermittently decreasing the assistance from the ventilator allowing the patient to gradually assume the burden of ventilation, using IMV, pressure support, or a combination. Although there is no general consensus on the relative merits of these two strategies, recent evidence appears to favor periodic sprinting. Whatever the modality chosen, a few points should be considered when designing a weaning program. First, patients may improve faster than expected, and any weaning process should include routine screening to identify those who have developed the ability breath without mechanical assistance. Conversely, the patient should not be allowed to work the respiratory muscles to exhaustion, because a prolonged period of rest may then be necessary before the next attempt at weaning. Finally, the clinician must routinely evaluate the patients' progress during weaning, and identify those who are not advancing toward extubation. Patients who fail to progress during weaning should be reassessed to disclose any reversible causes of prolonged dependency on the ventilator.

Procedure

Weaning is best begun early in the morning when the patient is rested and the ICU staff is maximum. The patient should be placed on an F_IO_2 that is 0.1 higher than the maintenance level and observed both clinically and with oximetry. Clinical evidence of respiratory muscle fatigue includes tachycardia, an increase in the respiratory rate to 35 or above, or complaints of severe dyspnea. In most patients these signs indicate the need to return to the prior level of ventilatory support regardless of blood gases. However, a PaO_2 of less than 60 mmHg or a pH less than 7.25 is also a clear indication to stop the weaning interval.

Psychological factors can be a major problem for some patients during weaning. An attempt should be made to carefully explain to the patient the weaning process and the likely sensations. The development of trust between the patient and staff is particularly important. Continued reassurance and confidence often achieve the best results.

Failure to advance toward liberation from the ventilator can generally be traced to insufficiencies of gas exchange, ventilatory drive, muscle strength, or endurance. In general, a PaO_2 greater than 60 mmHg on 35% oxygen or less should be enough to permit spontaneous breathing. True neurologic abnormalities of ventilatory drive are rare and, when present, are usually inconsistent with successful weaning. Secondary abnormalities of respiratory drive are common, however, and are usually reversible. The most common secondary abnormalities are metabolic alkalosis and oversedation. One hallmark of a suppressed respiratory drive is the presence of an elevated $PaCO_2$ during weaning without a corresponding increase in respiratory rate. Muscle strength and mechanical advantage of the muscles also are critical to successful weaning and should be considered in relation to the work the muscles are obligated to perform. The maximum inspiratory pressure (MIP) is a simple measure of muscle strength, and the peak pressure needed by the ventilator to move a tidal volume breath provides a gross approximation of the work the muscles will have to perform. Useful rules of thumb are that the MIP should equal the ventilatory peak pressure and that the vital capacity should at least equal the tidal volume provided by the ventilator.

Careful examination of the patient during weaning may be help explain the reasons for failure to progress. The pattern of muscle fatigue during weaning is usually characterized by a decreasing tidal volume and an increasing respiratory rate. An important warning sign is the development of paradoxical motion of chest and abdomen, in which the abdomen moves inward during inspiration, suggesting diaphragmatic fatigue. These changes may precede $PaCO_2$ elevation and indicate the need to return the patient to a higher level of ventilatory support. A number of factors may contribute to muscle weakness and fatigue: inadequate nutrition, respiratory muscle deconditioning and atrophy, electrolyte depletion (potassium, phosphate, magnesium, and calcium), hormonal imbalance (thyroid or steroid), neural and neuromuscular lesions (including spinal cord lesions), and increased lung volume. Many of these problems are easily detected once they are considered. Correcting them can make a profound difference in a patient's ability to wean.

1. Antonelli M, et al. Risk factors for early onset pneumonia in trauma patients. *Chest.* 1994;105:224.

   In 124 trauma patients, combined severe abdominal and thoracic trauma represented a major risk factor for early-onset pneumonia. Mechanical ventilation administered during the first days after trauma seems to reduce the risk of early-onset pneumonia. Mechanical ventilatory support lasting more than 5 days is associated with an increased risk of late-onset pneumonia.

2. Beach T, Millen E, Grenvik A. Hemodynamic response to discontinuance of mechanical ventilation. *Crit Care Med.* 1973;1:86.

   Approximately 50% of cases showed an increase and 50% showed a decrease in cardiac output, possibly reflecting differences in "myocardial reserve."

3. Bellemare F, Grassino A. Evaluations of human diaphragm fatigue. *J Appl Physiol.* 1982;53:1196.

   Two determinants of respiratory muscle fatigue are the percentage of time spent in inspiration (Ti/Tt) and the strength of muscle contraction on a breath as a fraction of maximal contraction.

4. Craven DE, et al. Risk factors for pneumonia and fatality in patients receiving continuous mechanical ventilation. *Am Rev Respir Dis.* 1985;133:792.

   The use of H_2-blocking agents increased the risk of nosocomial pneumonia, possibly by altering the pH of the stomach contents in patient on mechanical ventilation.

5. Douglass JA, et al. Myopathy in severe asthma. *Am Rev Respir Dis.* 1992;146:517.

   In 19 of 25 (76%) patients mechanically ventilated for exacerbation of asthma who received corticosteroids and aminophylline intravenously and salbutamol both nebulized and intravenously, there was elevation of creatine kinase (CK) levels to a median of 1,575 U/L occurring 3.6 ± 1.5 days after admission. In nine patients, there was clinically detectable myopathy. The presence of either myopathy or CK enzyme rise was associated with a significant prolongation of ventilation time.

6. Elpern EH, et al. Pulmonary aspiration in mechanically ventilated patients with tracheostomies. *Chest.* 1994;105:563.

   Feeding-related aspiration is seen frequently in patients with tracheostomies receiving prolonged positive pressure mechanical ventilation. Advanced age increases the risk of aspiration in this population, and episodes of aspiration are not consistently accompanied by clinical symptoms of distress to alert the bedside observer to their occurrence.

7. Ely EW, et al. Effect on the duration of mechanical ventilation of identifying patients capable of breathing spontaneously. *N Engl J Med.* 1996;335:1864–1869.

   An excellent study demonstrating that protocols to routinely assess patients' ability to tolerate weaning are safe and effective. Three hundred mechanically ventilated patients were screened daily. Those that met four criteria (Po_2/Fio_2 less than 200, PEEP <5, adequate cough and absence of vasopressors and sedative infusions) were randomized to physician-directed weaning versus daily protocolized trials of minimum support "sprints." Patients in the "sprint protocol" group were extubated earlier and reintubated less frequently.

8. Esteban A, et al. Modes of mechanical ventilation and weaning. A national survey of Spanish hospitals. The Spanish Lung Failure Collaborative Group. *Chest.* 1994;106:1188–1193.

   Weaning may account for more than 40% of the time patients spend on mechanical ventilation.

9. Esteban A, et al. A comparison of four methods of weaning patients from mechanical ventilation. Spanish Lung Failure Collaborative Group. *N Engl J Med.* 1995;332:345–350.

In 132 mechanically ventilated patients, once or twice daily sprints using T-piece weaned patients off ventilators more rapidly than gradual reductions in IMV rates or in pressure support.

10. Esteban A, et al. Effect of spontaneous breathing trial duration on outcome of attempts to discontinue mechanical ventilation. Spanish Lung Failure Collaborative Group. *Am J Respir Crit Care Med.* 1999;159:512–518.

Thirty-minute sprints may be just as good a test as 2-hour sprints for predicting the ability to tolerate discontinuing mechanical ventilation.

11. Field S, Kell SM, Macklem PT. The oxygen cost of breathing in patients with cardiorespiratory disease. *Am Rev Respir Dis.* 1982;126:9.

The average oxygen cost of taking over spontaneous ventilation was 75 mL of oxygen per minute and ranged up to 286 mL/min.

12. Gandia F, Blanco J. Evaluation of indexes predicts the outcome of ventilator weaning and value of adding supplemental inspiratory load. *Intensive Care Med.* 1992;18:327.

The ratio of inspiratory airway occlusion pressure at 0.1 second to MIP and the ratio of respiratory frequency to tidal volume were accurate, early predictors of weaning outcome.

13. Gracey DR, et al. Outcomes of patients admitted to a chronic ventilator-dependent unit in an acute-care hospital. *Mayo Clin Proc.* 1992;67:131.

The outcomes in 61 patients admitted to a chronic ventilator-dependent unit are reviewed. Of 58 who survived, 53 weaned from the mechanical ventilator, and 35 were discharged home (5 of these patients required nocturnal mechanical ventilation). Chronic obstructive pulmonary disease was the most common reason for admission to the unit.

14. Kumar A, et al. Pulmonary barotrauma during mechanical ventilation. *Crit Care Med.* 1973;1:181.

Pulmonary barotrauma (e.g., pneumothorax, pneumomediastinum, subcutaneous emphysema) correlated with the presence of chronic lung disease and with peak airway pressure (>35 cm H_2O), but not with PEEP per se.

15. Laggner AN, et al. Oropharyngeal decontamination with gentamicin for long-term ventilated patients on stress ulcer prophylaxis with sucralfate? *Wien Klin Wochenschr.* 1994;106:15.

Despite reduction of bacterial colonization rates of pharyngeal and tracheal secretions, gentamicin administered topically to the oropharynx did not seem to offer additional clinical benefits in long-term mechanically ventilated patients on stress ulcer prophylaxis with sucralfate.

16. Liebler JM, et al. Respiratory complications in critically ill medical patients with acute upper gastrointestinal bleeding. *Crit Care Med.* 1991;19:1152.

Respiratory complications occurred during 22% of serious upper gastrointestinal bleeding episodes.

17. Pingleton SK, Hinthorn DR, Lui C. Internal nutrition in patients receiving mechanical ventilation: multiple sources of tracheal colonization including the stomach. *Am J Med.* 1986;80:827.

Seventy-five percent of the bacteria contaminating the respiratory tract originated in the oropharynx or stomach and suggests that the high gastric pH due to tube feeding may increase gastric colonization.

18. Prod'hom G, et al. Nosocomial pneumonia in mechanically ventilated patients receiving antacid, ranitidine, or sucralfate as prophylaxis for stress ulcer: a randomized controlled trial. *Ann Intern Med.* 1994;120:653.

Stress ulcer prophylaxis with sucralfate reduces the risk for late-onset pneumonia in ventilated patients compared with antacid or ranitidine.

19. Rouby JJ, et al. Histologic aspects of pulmonary barotrauma in critically ill patients with acute respiratory failure. *Intensive Care Med.* 1993;19:383.

Air space enlargement, defined as the presence of either alveolar overdistention in aerated lung areas or intraparenchymal pseudocysts in nonaerated lung areas, was found in 26 of 30 lungs of young critically ill patients (mean age 34 ± 10 years) that were histologically examined in the immediate post mortem period. Patients with severe air space enlargement had a significantly greater incidence of pneumothorax, were ventilated using higher peak airway pressures and tidal volumes, were exposed significantly longer to toxic levels of oxygen, and lost more weight than patients with mild air space enlargement.

20. Tobin MJ, et al. Kono-Mead analysis of ribcage-abdominal motion during successful and unsuccessful trials of weaning from mechanical ventilation. *Am Rev Respir Dis.* 1987;135:1320.

    Paradoxical motion of the rib cage and abdomen can occur due to increased airway resistance or decreased compliance and is not specific for respiratory muscle fatigue. Asynchronous motion with a phase difference between rib cage and abdominal motion was a more sensitive indicator.

21. Tobin MJ, et al. The pattern of breathing during successful and unsuccessful trials of weaning from mechanical ventilation. *Am Rev Respir Dis.* 1986;134:111.

    Patients who failed a weaning trial developed rapid shallow breathing.

22. Warner MA, Warner ME, Weber JG. Clinical significance of pulmonary aspiration during the perioperative period. *Anesthesiology.* 1993;78:56.

    Patients with clinically apparent aspiration who do not develop symptoms within 2 hours are unlikely to have respiratory sequelae.

23. Yang KL, Tobin MJ. A prospective study of indexes predicting the outcome of trials of weaning from mechanical ventilation. *N Engl J Med.* 1991;324:1445.

    Rapid shallow breathing, reflected by the f/VT ratio, was the most accurate predictor of failure, and its absence the most accurate predictor of success, in weaning 64 patients from mechanical ventilation.

24. Zwillic CW, et al. Complications of assisted ventilation. *Am J Med.* 1974;57:162.

    Reports that 314 consecutive patients on mechanical ventilation were studied prospectively for complications. Intubation of right mainstem bronchus, endotracheal tube malfunction, and alveolar hypoventilation were associated with decreased survival.

---

62. OXYGEN THERAPY AND TOXICITY

David H. Kupferberg

Oxygen-enriched air is principally used in medicine to treat tissue hypoxia. Tissue oxygenation, however, cannot be measured directly in most circumstances. Clinicians must rely on indirect but more accessible measures of oxygenation in arterial blood (PaO_2 and hemoglobin–oxygen saturation) or estimates in peripheral tissue (oxygen saturation by pulse oximetry).

INDICATIONS

Supplemental oxygen can reverse the impact of tissue hypoxia and may be required acutely or chronically. Patients with chronic obstructive pulmonary disease (COPD) comprise the largest numbers receiving supplemental oxygen, but oxygen may be needed in any type of lung disease. Chronic oxygen supplementation (15 to 24 hours/d) can prevent and reverse the adverse consequences of hypoxia such as dyspnea, effort intolerance, pulmonary hypertension, heart failure, erythrocytosis, neuropsychiatric abnormalities, and hospital costs as well as prolong survival.

Most patients who require oxygen therapy can be managed by modest supplementation of the inspired oxygen concentrations. The most common modes of delivery are nasal cannula (with flow rates up to 6 L/min) or a mask (with flow rates up to 15 L/min). The flow of oxygen is set empirically, and effectiveness is evaluated using oximetry or arterial blood gas measurements aiming to keep an oxygen saturation of 90 to 92% or PaO_2 above 60 mmHg.

Oxygen therapy is often initiated after an episode of acute respiratory failure. Reevaluation 1 to 3 months after an acute exacerbation is warranted. Decisions about the requirement and dose of oxygen should be based on measurements of arterial oxygen levels during rest, exercise, and sleep. Many patients with COPD develop their greatest hypoxemia during sleep. Most laboratories do not measure oxygenation during sleep; therefore, oxygen flow should be raised by 1.0 L/min over the daytime requirement during this time. No evidence supports the efficacy of patients using oxygen "as needed" for dyspnea. For that reason, the clinician must discuss with the patient and family the basis for the oxygen prescription.

Patients with acute hypoxic respiratory failure usually require high concentrations of oxygen to maintain acceptable levels of arterial oxygenation. When nasal catheters fail to provide adequate oxygen, masks with nonrebreathing bags may be tried. Recently, gas blenders have been introduced that allow delivery of known concentrations of oxygen at flow rates greater than 100 L/min. Several modalities are available for delivery of supplemental oxygen in acute respiratory failure. A patient with an endotracheally tube or tight-fitting mask with straps can be provided a specified fractional concentration of oxygen. Other modes of oxygen delivery enrich the oxygen concentration in inspired air but do not guarantee a constant or precisely specified concentration. A number of devices can deliver a specified concentration of oxygen to the vicinity of the patient"s airway, but the concentration actually received by the patient depends on the amount of room air inspired with the oxygen. The concentration of oxygen received varies with the flow of oxygen, the location and fit of the oxygen delivery device, and the patient's minute ventilation, inspiratory flow rate, and tidal volume.

METHODS OF DELIVERY

Oxygen-conserving devices can improve the efficiency of oxygen delivery. A small reservoir at the nose or in a pendant on the chest increases the amount of oxygen provided during inspiration and decreases the waste of continuous flow oxygen during expiration; thus, lower flow rates may be needed to maintain the same level of oxygen saturation. Also, devices attached to the oxygen source that limit the flow of oxygen to the early inspiratory phase of breathing (*pulse* or *demand delivery* devices) can improve the efficiency of gas delivery and extend the life of portable sources. A transtracheal cannula inserted percutaneously into the neck can also reduce the amount of oxygen needed to sustain adequate saturation and can be particularly useful for patients with high oxygen requirements; however, the care needs for insertion and maintenance of this system are significantly greater than for other devices.

For chronic oxygen therapy, the two most common sources of oxygen are oxygen tanks (liquid oxygen or compressed gas) and oxygen concentrators. Portable oxygen tanks are useful when the patient is away from the home for up to 8 hours at a time, but must be replaced frequently. Liquid oxygen is more compact and can be carried in smaller, more portable tanks. Newer devices that deliver oxygen only on patient inspiration are gaining popularity because they increase the efficiency of oxygen use and extend the usable life of portable tanks. Stationary oxygen reservoirs or oxygen concentrators are used in the home, with variable tubing lengths to allow room-to-room mobility.

The amount of oxygen flow needed by a specific patient can be estimated using either PaO_2 or pulse oximetry measurements. Generally, the goal of oxygen therapy is to sustain a PaO_2 of at least 60 mmHg or a saturation of at least 90% at rest, exercise, and during sleep, although the recommendation can differ in specific clinical situations.

TOXICITY

Oxygen toxicity can complicate the use of high concentrations of supplemental oxygen. The actual incidence is unclear because inflammatory and fibroproliferative changes in the lung caused by oxygen toxicity may be obscured by the underlying primary pulmonary diseases necessitating oxygen therapy. However, evidence suggests that a subclinical alteration in cellular function may result from exposure to oxygen concentrations exceeding 50%, potentially affecting the reparative process following the acute lung disease.

Pathogenesis

The pathogenesis of oxygen-associated lung injury appears to be caused by the excessive generation of free oxygen radicals occurring in the setting of hyperoxia. This could result in a chain of events that interrupts normal cellular function and, if sufficiently severe, leads to cellular death. In animal models of hyperoxia, a cytokine-mediated inflammatory response has been observed.

Four clinical syndromes resulting from exposure to normobaric hyperoxia have been described: (1) acute tracheobronchitis, (2) absorption atelectasis, (3) acute alveolar lung injury (acute respiratory distress syndrome [ARDS]), and (4) bronchopulmonary dysplasia. Although the last is primarily the end result of the neonatal respiratory distress syndrome, similar chronic fibrotic changes have been described in adults exposed to high partial pressures of inspired oxygen. These findings, however, may simply represent the nonspecific result of the reparative phase following an acute alveolar–interstitial injury.

The acute clinical syndromes are better understood after examining the physiologic and pathologic consequences of hyperoxic exposure. In normal subjects breathing 100% oxygen, the earliest manifestation of adverse effects is tracheobronchial irritation. Bronchoscopic evidence of tracheitis has been observed as soon as 6 hours following exposure to 90 to 95% oxygen. This has been accompanied by a reduction in tracheal mucociliary transport, although pulmonary function tests remain normal. After more lengthy exposure (6 to 24 hours), a reduction in vital capacity is seen, believed to be related primarily to absorption atelectasis. Extending the duration of oxygen exposure beyond 24 hours has been associated with a decrement in lung compliance, widening of the $P(A-a)O_2$ gradient, and a decline in carbon monoxide diffusing capacity.

Clinical Manifestations

In the clinical arena, pulmonary physiologic measurements of intubated patients exposed to hyperoxia have been quite variable, likely because of the underlying clinical problems. Some evidence suggests that beyond 48 hours of hyperoxia (inspired oxygen concentration $[F_IO_2] = 1.0$), a decline in PaO_2, an increase in intrapulmonary shunt, and radiographic evidence of interstitial infiltrates can be observed.

The pathologic sequence resulting from oxygen-induced injury parallels that following a number of insults, such as radiation exposure, ARDS, and drug-induced pulmonary disease. Amplification of oxygen's toxic effects has been reported in association with certain medications. Bleomycin, a glycopeptide antibiotic used in chemotherapy, forms a ferrous–DNA complex that generates superoxide anion. In the presence of hyperoxia, the potential adverse effects on the lung become more pronounced. Case reports have described similar findings with amiodarone. Nitrofurantoin and paraquat—both metabolized through free radical intermediates—have similar synergistic toxic effects on the lung when combined with high levels of supplemental oxygen.

Despite the body of evidence describing the damaging effects of hyperoxia, clinical experience and numerous animal studies suggest that a degree of oxygen tolerance can develop in the setting of acute lung injury. A retrospective study found that, in patients with acute respiratory failure, the duration of exposure to an F_IO_2 of 0.9 or greater was no different in survivors versus nonsurvivors; in fact, the total duration of exposure to an F_IO_2 greater than 0.5 was longer in surviving patients. It is speculated that acute lung injury may protect against oxygen toxicity.

Management

With questions remaining about the incidence, modulating factors, and natural history of normobaric hyperoxia in the critically ill patient, definite guidelines about safe levels of supplemental oxygen are difficult to define. However, certain practical guidelines can be suggested: (1) short-term exposure (24 to 36 hours) to an F_IO_2 of 0.6 or above can be tolerated and is probably without long-term sequelae; (2) in the hypoxemic patient, optimization of oxygen-carrying capacity through careful attention to hemoglobin levels and cardiac output should accompany concerns about the level of supplemental oxygen; (3) measures such as positive end-expiratory pressure should be used in the setting of diffuse parenchymal lung disease in an effort to reduce F_IO_2; and (4) F_IO_2 should be reduced below 0.6 as quickly as possible once adequate tissue oxygenation has been ensured.

In summary, in the chronic hypoxemic patient, long-term oxygen supplementation has many well-documented benefits and is very safe. The role of hyperoxic lung damage in the setting of acute respiratory failure is less well defined. Aiming to limit the F_IO_2 <0.6 is a reasonable goal and may limit additive lung toxicity.

1. Anthonisen NR. Long-term oxygen therapy. *Ann Intern Med.* 1983;99:519.
   A comprehensive review of a topic that previously was the subject of a great deal of uncertainty. Includes guidelines for the supplemental use of oxygen in a variety of conditions.
2. Bradley BL, et al. Oxygen-assisted exercise in chronic obstructive lung disease: the effect on exercise capacity and arterial blood gas tension. *Am Rev Respir Dis.* 1978;118:239.
   Endurance was increased by supplemental oxygen, but maximal work rate was not.
3. Morrison DA, Stovall JR. Increased exercise capacity in hypoxemic patients after long-term oxygen therapy. *Chest.* 1992;102:542.
   Exercise capacity was increased by supplemental oxygen, which increased peripheral O_2 delivery but did not relieve hypoxic vasoconstriction.
4. Tarpy SP, Celli BR. Long-term oxygen therapy. *N Engl J Med.* 1995;333:710.
   An excellent review on long-term oxygen therapy.
5. Burrows B, et al. Patterns of cardiovascular dysfunction in chronic obstructive lung disease. *N Engl J Med.* 1972;286:912.
   A longitudinal study of 50 patients with COPD that correlated survival (inversely) with pulmonary vascular resistance.
6. Channick RN, et al. Improvement in pulmonary hypertension and hypoxemia during nitric oxide inhalation in a patient with end-stage pulmonary fibrosis. *Am J Respir Crit Care Med.* 1994;149:811.
   Beneficial responses to inhaled nitric oxide in a single patient with severe interstitial pulmonary fibrosis, hypoxemia, pulmonary hypertension, and cor pulmonale suggest that, even in severe chronic lung disease, reversible pulmonary vasoconstriction is present.
7. Christopher KL, et al. A program for transtracheal oxygen delivery. *Ann Intern Med.* 1989;107:801.
   A review of the safety and efficacy of transtracheal oxygen in 100 patients who tolerated the modality well.
8. Fujimoto K, et al. Benefits of oxygen on exercise performance and pulmonary hemodynamics in patients with COPD with mild hypoxemia. *Chest.* 2002;122:457.
   Oxygen can improve 6-minute walk distance and pulmonary hemodynamics with most improvement in severe COPD.
9. Anonymous. Ventilation with lower tidal volumes as compared with traditional tidal volumes for acute lung injury and the acute respiratory distress syndrome. The Acute Respiratory Distress Syndrome Network. *N Engl J Med.* 2000;342:1301.
   Major must read article on low tidal volume ventilation with strategies to reduce FiO_2 with PEEP. A 6-cc/kg tidal volume group showed lower mortality.
10. Greif R, et al. Supplemental perioperative oxygen to reduce the incidence of surgical-wound infections. *N Engl J Med.* 2000;342:161.
    A randomized, multicentered, double-blind study on the efficacy of perioperative O_2 on the reduction of surgical wound infections after colorectal surgery.
11. Heimlich HJ, Carr GC. Micro-trach. A seven year experience with transtracheal oxygen therapy. *Chest.* 1989;95:1008.
    In this 7-year experience, 87.5% of 200 patients tolerated transtracheal oxygen delivery.

12. Holt JH, Branscomb BV. Hemodynamic responses to controlled 100% oxygen breathing in emphysema. *J Appl Physiol.* 1965;20:215.

    In 13 patients with moderate to severe COPD, 100% oxygen challenge led to a significant reduction in pulmonary vascular resistance.

13. Krop HD, Block AJ, Cohen E. Neuropsychological effects of continuous oxygen therapy in chronic obstructive pulmonary disease. *Chest.* 1973;64:317.

    Demonstrates neuropsychological abnormalities in hypoxic COPD versus non-hypoxic COPD.

14. Eaton T, et al. Ambulatory oxygen improves quality of life of COPD patients: a randomised controlled study. *Eur Respir J.* 2002;20:306.

    Despite short-term improvement in health-related quality of life, patient compliance remains a major issue.

15. Medical Research Council Working Party. Long-term domiciliary oxygen therapy in chronic hypoxic cor pulmonale complicating chronic bronchitis and emphysema. *Lancet.* 1981;1:681.

16. Nocturnal Oxygen Therapy Trial Group. Continuous or nocturnal oxygen therapy in hypoxemic chronic obstructive lung disease: a clinical trial. *Ann Intern Med.* 1980;93:391.

    References 15 and 16 are two landmark, randomized clinical trials conducted in Great Britain and the United States, establishing the survival benefits of long-term oxygen therapy in hypoxemic patients with COPD.

17. Jenkinson SG. Oxygen toxicity. *J Intensive Care Med.* 1988;3:137.

    An excellent review with particular attention paid to the pathophysiology and clinical consequences of hyperoxic exposure.

18. Nash G, Blennerhassett JB, Pontoppidan H. Pulmonary lesions associated with oxygen therapy and artificial ventilation. *N Engl J Med.* 1967;267:368.

    Early description of the exudative and proliferative pathologic findings in ventilated patients exposed to hyperoxia.

19. Tiep BL, Lewis MI. Oxygen conservation and oxygen conservation devices in chronic lung disease. A review. *Chest.* 1987;92:263.

    A basic review on oxygen-conserving devices.

20. Weitzenblum E, et al. Long-term oxygen therapy can reverse the progression of pulmonary hypertension patients with COPD. *Am Rev Respir Dis.* 1985;131:4.

    Sixteen patients with COPD underwent cardiac catheterization to evaluate pulmonary artery pressures. With long-term O_2 therapy, the progression of pulmonary hypertension was ameliorated but reversal to normal was rare. Early description of the exudative and proliferative pathologic findings in ventilated patients exposed to hyperoxia.

21. Kapanci Y, et al. Oxygen pneumonitis in man; light- and electron-microscopic morphometric studies. *Chest.* 1972;62:162.

    Pathologic changes in patients, receiving a F_1O_2 of 0.6 to 1.0 for 14 hours to 13 days included reduction in endothelial volume, increase in interstitial tissue, and decrease in alveolar surface density.

22. Caldwell PRB, et al. Changes in lung volume, diffusing capacity, and blood gases in men breathing oxygen. *J Appl Physiol.* 1966;21:1477.

    Functional abnormalities in four volunteers following hyperoxia for up to 72 hours.

23. Sackner MA, et al. Pulmonary effects of oxygen breathing: a 6-hour study in normal man. *Ann Intern Med.* 1975;82:40.

    A decline in tracheal mucous clearance and onset of tracheitis occur early in the course of hyperoxic exposure.

24. Davis WB, et al. Pulmonary oxygen toxicity: early reversible changes in human alveolar structures induced by hyperoxia. *N Engl J Med.* 1983;309:878.

    Exposure of normal humans to 17 hours of 95% oxygen revealed reversible capillary leak; alveolar macrophages showed increased release of fibronectin and growth factor for fibroblasts.

25. Deneke SM, Fanburg BL. Normobaric oxygen toxicity of the lung. *N Engl J Med.* 1980;303:76.

    A well-referenced review.

26. Singer MM, et al. Oxygen toxicity in man: a prospective study in patients after open-heart surgery. *N Engl J Med*. 1970;283:1474.

    No physiologic evidence for pulmonary oxygen toxicity following 24 hours of 100% oxygen exposure; two patients were followed for 5 and 7 days.

27. De Los Santos R, et al. One hundred percent oxygen lung injury in adult baboons. *Am Rev Respir Dis*. 1987;136:657.

    The development of an ARDS pattern in baboons exposed to 100% oxygen for 5 to 7 days. Bronchoalveolar lavage samples showed evidence of polymorphonuclear neutrophil leukocyte and protease involvement.

28. Crapo JD, et al. Structural and biochemical changes in rat lungs occurring during exposures to lethal and adaptive doses of oxygen. *Am Rev Respir Dis*. 1980;122:123.

    An analysis of alveolar and endothelial cell changes following exposure to 85% and 100% oxygen up to 14 days.

29. Crapo JD. Morphologic changes in pulmonary oxygen toxicity. *Annu Rev Physiol*. 1986;48:721.

    An excellent overview of the cellular and pathologic changes resulting from hyperoxic exposure.

30. Jones R, et al. Oxygen toxicity and restructuring of pulmonary arteries in a morphometric study. *Am J Pathol*. 1985;121:212.

    Describes the pulmonary vascular changes consequent to normobaric hyperoxic exposure in the rat.

31. Goldiner PL. Factors influencing postoperative morbidity and mortality in patients treated with bleomycin. *BMJ*. 1978;1:1664.

    Reports on severe respiratory distress following hyperoxia for brief periods in patients receiving bleomycin 6 to 12 months earlier; experience with F_IO_2 (0.22–0.25) in a similar patient population revealed no subsequent pulmonary problems.

32. Hayatdavoudi G, et al. Pulmonary injury in rats following continuous exposure to 60% O_2 for 7 days. *J Appl Physiol*. 1981;51:1220.

    Less prominent pathologic changes were seen in rats exposed to 60% oxygen for 7 days; changes were primarily in endothelial cells.

33. Yam J, Roberts RJ. Pharmacological alteration of oxygen-induced lung toxicity. *Toxicol Appl Pharmacol*. 1978;47:367.

    Systematic investigation into the mechanisms of oxygen toxicity and the agents that minimize (vitamin E, vitamin C) or enhance (corticosteroids, L-thyroxine) this toxicity in rats.

34. Wagner PD, et al. Protection against pulmonary O_2 toxicity by N-acetylcysteine. *Eur Respir J*. 1989;2:116.

    Lung edema, abnormal $\dot{V}/\dot{Q}$ relationships, and pulmonary vascular resistance were improved following N-acetylcysteine administration in the canine exposed to 100% oxygen for 54 hours.

35. Ehrenlerarz RA, Ablow RC, Warshew JB. Prevention of bronchopulmonary dysplasia with vitamin E administration during the acute stages of respiratory distress syndrome. *J Pediatr*. 1979;95:873.

    This follow-up study failed to demonstrate any protection from bronchopulmonary dysplasia afforded by vitamin E administration in the acute stages of infant respiratory distress syndrome.

36. Flink EB, et al. High-dose magnesium sulfate attenuates pulmonary oxygen toxicity. *Crit Care Med*. 1992;20:1692.

    An animal study demonstrating a protective effect of high-dose magnesium sulfate in the setting of hyperoxic exposure.

37. Capellier G, et al. Oxygen tolerance in patients with acute respiratory failure. *Intensive Care Med*. 1998;24:422.

    A 10-year retrospective study examining high oxygen ($>0.90 \, F_IO_2$) in 74 patients with respiratory failure. Survivors had similar days of high O_2 versus nonsurvivors, suggesting acute lung injury can induce protection from hyperoxia.

38. Wendt CH, et al. Hyperoxia upregulated Na, K-adenosine triphosphate β_1 gene transcription. *Chest*. 1999;116:887s.

Hyperoxia upregulates Na, K-ATPase gene transcription, which plays a critical role in reabsorbing edema fluid and improving gas exchange in lung injury.

39. Smith B, et al. Absence of pulmonary oxygen toxicity in association with high-frequency jet ventilation. *Lancet.* 1984;8375:505.

Neonates tolerated prolonged high FiO_2; in those who died, no evidence was seen of oxygen pulmonary injury.

40. Suzuki Y, et al. Effect of hyperoxia on adhesion molecule expression in human endothelial cells and neutrophils. *Am J Physiol.* 1997;272:L418.

The expression of ICAM-1 on endothelial cells was shown to be operative for neutrophil accumulation during hyperoxia exposure.

41. Jensen JC, et al. Role of tumor necrosis factor in oxygen toxicity. *J Appl Physiol.* 1992;72:1902.

A good overview the role of TNF in oxygen toxicity.

42. Piedboef B, et al. In vivo expression of intercellular adhesion molecule 1 in type II pneumocytes during hyperoxia. *Am J Respir Cell Mol Biol.* 1996;15:71.

Discusses the role of type II pneumocytes in promoting the inflammatory response to hyperoxia.

43. Folz RJ, Abushamaa AM, Suliman HB. Extracellular superoxide dismutase in the airways of transgenic mice reduces inflammation and attenuates lung toxicity following hyperoxia. *J Clin Invest.* 1999;103:1055.

Transgenic mice overexpressing extracellular SOD protects against hyperoxia lung damage, partially that caused by attenuating the neutrophil inflammatory response.

63. PROTOCOL-DRIVEN CARE IN RESPIRATORY THERAPY

Timothy A. Morris and Richard Ford

The success of complex treatment plans for pulmonary patients depends on a clear understanding of the elements by all health care practitioners charged with implementing them. *Patient-driven protocols* are a set of medical staff-approved care plans driven by the patient's condition and response to therapy that allow the respiratory care practitioner to initiate, change, discontinue, or restart treatments and services. Protocols ensure that (1) the physician's intentions are realized; (2) care is appropriate, timely, and driven by the patient's condition; (3) lower cost alternatives are implemented when appropriate; and (4) most important, clinical conditions requiring physician notification are clear. Protocols are simply algorithmic paths that specify what care will be delivered, when it will be discontinued or altered, and when the physician will be contacted for changes in management. They cover only those alterations in care that the hospital physicians agree should always occur when the protocol criteria are fulfilled.

Once the physician establishes the need for treatment, protocols provide a means to ensure that what is supposed to happen to the patient does happen. Access to the program may be structured so the physician can request a specific therapy, specific protocol, or simply "respiratory care protocol." If the therapist identifies the opportunity to use a protocol of care that differs from the initial physician request, he or she contacts the physician to review and approve new or additional care plans. The protocols supplement, but never override, physician instructions; orders that deviate from the protocols continue to define the care delivered.

Physicians who use protocols should be familiar with the protocol path or algorithms and understand the ability of the protocol program to achieve the desired outcomes. On the other hand, they should also recognize exceptionally complicated cases for which protocols may be inappropriate. Protocols should contain clear decision points defining when the therapist should apprise the physician of changes in patient status. The therapist should contact the physician directly if there is any acute deterioration in a patient's condition or document the achievement of therapeutic goals and outcomes on an evaluation form. Advantages to physicians include: (1) the ability to write flexible orders that can adapt to predictable changes in the patient's condition; (2) assurance that the care provided is state of the art; (3) notification when the patient's status changes significantly; (4) freedom from documentation; and (5) the ability to exempt patients who do not fit the protocols.

DEVELOPMENT

Respiratory care protocols are developed by physicians, respiratory care practitioners, and other members of the medical team as a group process and depend on a thorough review of published literature and the savvy of experienced clinicians. Tailored to the specifics of each hospital, the protocols reflect the consensus of the medical team regarding the optimal care plans to be used in most cases for specific respiratory conditions. Protocols allow a physician to have active input into evaluation and treatment algorithms, as well as to specify when a protocol should be stopped and when he or she should be notified. The clarity and detail with which these plans are made far exceed what is possible through written orders for each individual patient. Similarly, the respiratory care practitioner becomes much less an "ancillary service" and more an agent of the physician, ensuring that patients receive timely and appropriate interventions as outlined in the protocol. The respiratory care practitioner is trained to evaluate and quantify the physiologic effects of treatment on each patient. Round-the-clock documentation of physiologic parameters can be invaluable to the care of patients with respiratory conditions. Furthermore, the therapist is able to follow a clear consensus plan on how to adjust therapy based on the "real-time" condition of the patient and previous response to treatment. Finally, the therapist has clear guidelines for when to contact the physician, when to discontinue a protocol, and when to suggest another, more appropriate protocol.

ADVANTAGES

The financial pressures resulting from fixed payment reimbursement and quality care issues make it increasingly important to ensure that respiratory care services are provided only when indicated. Clinical studies have demonstrated a decrease in the utilization of respiratory care services using protocol programs to defer therapy, promote the timely discontinuance of therapy, or make a transition to therapy that does not require the same labor intensity. These reports showed no reduction in the quality of patient care, but vast reductions in overall cost of care with protocolized programs. Medical centers have reduced up to 25% of multimillion dollar annual respiratory care costs by using protocolized program that, for example, adjust the dose and scheduling of bronchodilator administration using therapist-measured physiologic feedback parameters.

Although the hospital or department administrator may realize that protocols have the ability to significantly reduce expenses, the creation of respiratory care protocols more than 20 years ago had little to do with cost reduction. The need arose as technology to support mechanical ventilation was developed and devices were designed to treat and support patients with respiratory impairments. As treatment became more complex and dynamic, caring for the respiratory patient was like hitting a moving target. Patient condition changed continuously, requiring ongoing modifications to treatment. The observation and feedback from the bedside therapist became an important asset to the physician, who could not always be in the room.

Initiating and maintaining a respiratory care protocol program requires a team effort among (1) the medical director of respiratory care; (2) a program leader to oversee planning and keep the program on track; (3) interested physicians to plan and utilize the protocols; and (4) the therapists who will execute them. Step-by-step instructions on how to plan and initiate respiratory care protocol programs, as well as detailed examples of specific protocols, are referenced below. The number of protocols implemented and the timeline for program expansion likely depends on the readiness of the RC department and physician staff. It is essential to provide specific training and competency assessment prior to implementing any protocol. Program development extends well beyond drafting a set of protocols. It includes defining related policies, identifying responsibilities, determining competencies and required training, and establishing mechanisms to monitor activities.

Protocols must be considered statements of what everyone agrees should happen when certain conditions occur. All of the "stakeholders" must be offered the opportunity to modify the protocols prior to acceptance. Although attempts to gain some consensus among physicians in the institution regarding the complex aspects of respiratory care delivery may take considerable time (4 to 12 months), the early "buy-in" is critical. All suggestions should be incorporated or addressed in some way. All applicable medical staff committees should review protocols in the developmental stage, and a one-on-one conference should be conducted with key stakeholders to foster the support needed for implementation. An understanding of the medical center environment, medical staff objectives, and incentives for change may assist in developing a strategy to gain medical staff support of protocols.

BARRIERS

Many barriers are encountered during implementation of complex programs such as these. Despite known benefits of protocol-driven care, therapists can view them as too much work and physicians can perceive them as loss of control over the patient. Such barriers need to be addressed and can be overcome through education, participation, and sharing in the positive outcomes of the program. Establishing a high level of support and intrinsic motivation among respiratory care staff is the most important aspect of implementation and can also be the most difficult, particularly in a program that demands that the therapists learn new skills, enhance communication abilities, and adapt to change. Workgroups and teams consisting of members of the department accelerates planning and implementation.

The adage that "the best evidence of life is growth" is particularly true for respiratory care protocols. To be effective and to reflect the true state of the art in therapy, the protocols must be regularly reappraised. The protocols must be routinely updated as new medical information relevant to respiratory care becomes available. In addition, routine feedback from physicians and other staff members during protocol updating helps to ensure that the protocols remain practical and fosters communication with the entire health care team.

1. Ford RM, Phillips-Clar JE, Burns DM. Implementing therapist-driven protocols. *Respir Care Clin North Am.* 1996;2:51.

   Excellent compendium of information, including the rationale for protocols, logistics for implementing them, and legal considerations. The chapter authored by the UCSD team specifically describes the UCSD experience and the results of implementing a hospital-wide program.

2. Burton G. American Association for Respiratory Care 43rd National Congress. Atlanta, Presentation.

   Dr. Burton is credited with creating the first formalized protocols for Respiratory Care nearly 20 years ago. This lecture provides his unique insight regarding the value of such programs. A tape of this lecture can be obtained from the American Association for Respiratory Care offices in Dallas, Texas.

3. Kester L, Stoller JK. Ordering respiratory care services for hospitalized patients: practices of overuse and underuse. *Cleve Clin J Med.* 1992;59:581–585.

   While the focus of protocols is often to reduce unnecessary care, this study found that 20% of patients needed more intensive respiratory treatment. This demonstrates an important aspect of respiratory care "consult services" in recognizing the need for additional interventions.

4. American Association for Respiratory Care. The AARC clinical practice guidelines. *Respir Care.* 1991:1398–1426 and 1992:882–922.

National standards available through AARC that list the indications, hazards, and considerations in the delivery of many respiratory care procedures. These standards, developed by experts, provide an evidence-based reference to develop protocol programs.

5. Browning JA, Kiaser DL, Durbin CG Jr. The effect of guidelines on the appropriate use of arterial blood gas analysis in the intensive care unit. *Respir Care.* 1989;34:269–276.
   Browning was one of the first to evaluate the impact of respiratory care protocol programs. In an ICU setting, a reduction in the number of blood gases per patient was demonstrated in his early work.
6. Albin RJ, Criner JG, Thomas S, et al. Pattern of non-ICU inpatient supplemental oxygen utilization in a university hospital. *Chest.* 1992;102:1672–1675.
   Demonstrates that programs can be designed specific for oxygen therapy in which respiratory practitioners can insure improved compliance with indications for therapy.
7. Tenholder MF, Bryson MJ, Whitlock WL. A model for conversion from small volume nebulizer to metered dose inhaler aerosol therapy. *Chest.* 1992;101:634–637.
   When lower cost alternatives are available to achieve similar clinical outcomes, they should be considered. This reference is one of the first of many to demonstrate a successful program in which patients were converted from small volume nebulizers to metered dose inhalers.
8. Nielson-Tietsort J, Poole B, Creagh CE, et al. Respiratory care protocol: an approach to in-hospital respiratory therapy. *Respir Care.* 1981;26:430–436.
   Few protocol programs existed in the early 1980s and this review of the impact of such programs suggested that protocols should be the approach to the delivery of respiratory care.
9. Burns DM. When information is key to survival: breathing life into respiratory care. *Healthc Inform.* 1994;11:24–30.
   Protocol programs require that significant information be captured and that reports be available to assist in tracking clinical and cost outcomes. A department information system provides a valuable tool in the development, implementation, and surveillance of protocol programs.
10. Ford R, Phillips J, Burns D. Early results of implementing a patient driven protocol system [abstract]. *Respir Care.* 1993;38:1306.
    Significant reductions in both aerosol therapy and CPT were experienced at UCSD within 90 days of implementing protocols on a single Pulmonary Intensive floor. The results of the pilot program are presented.
11. Phillips JE, Ford RM, Morris TA. *UCSD Patient Driven Protocols.* Daedalus Enterprises Inc; 1998.
    A detailed view of 23 protocols, developed at the UCSD Department of Respiratory Care, including algorithms, policies, and one page reference guidelines.
12. Burton GG, Tietsort JA. *Therapist-Driven Respiratory Care Protocols: A Practitioner's Guide.* Academy Medical Systems; 1993.
    Early protocols were assembled from respiratory care departments throughout the country and assembled in this text for review.
13. American Association for Respiratory Care web site. Dallas, Tex.
    The AARC has assembled numerous documents, guidelines, expert lists, and other resources that can assist in understanding all aspects of protocol programs. Many of these resources are available on line at www.aarc.org.
14. Stoller J, Kester L, eds. Therapist driven protocols. *Respir Clin North Am.* 1996;2(1, special issue).
    This issue is an excellent compendium of information, including the rationale for protocols, the logistics for implementing them, and legal considerations.

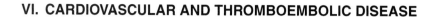

VI. CARDIOVASCULAR AND THROMBOEMBOLIC DISEASE

64. THROMBOEMBOLIC DISEASE: EPIDEMIOLOGY, NATURAL HISTORY, AND DIAGNOSIS

Timothy A. Morris

Venous thromboembolism (VTE) should be entirely preventable or treatable. Yet, it is a persistent and prevalent cause of significant morbidity and mortality in the United States and responsible for an estimated 50,000 deaths and 500,000 nonfatal episodes each year. Despite important diagnostic and therapeutic developments, medical science is only scratching the surface at understanding VTE and clinical strategies have only partially impacted disability and death following VTE.

Venous thromboembolism, by definition, originates in systemic venous thrombosis, and is pathologically distinct from arterial thrombosis. Conditions that favor thrombosis may fall into three categories (as predicted by Virchow over a century ago): (1) venous stasis, (2) injury to the venous intima, and (3) alterations in the coagulation–fibrinolytic system. The potential role of all three factors has been demonstrated in a variety of situations. Venous stasis occurs during bedrest and is associated with deep venous thrombosis (DVT); using intermittent compression stockings to restore venous flow reduces the risk for DVT. Injury to the venous wall is the most likely mechanism of the large number of lower extremity DVTs observed in proximity to sites of trauma and major orthopedic surgery. Coagulation abnormalities that occur alone or in concert with other conditions can promote clinical venous thrombosis. For example, there is an increased risk for VTE associated with mutations in factor V (factor V_{Lieden}) and in the untranslated region of the gene encoding prothrombin (although the procoagulant mechanism of the later mutation is still under investigation). Other less prevalent, but probably more potent, "thrombophilias" include deficiencies of antithrombin III, protein C, and protein S; aberrations in the thrombolytic system; and the presence of the doubly misnamed "lupus anticoagulant." Clinical conditions that involve combinations of these fundamental risk factors are associated with a higher risk of thrombosis.

Many large studies have identified the major risk factors for DVT of the lower extremities. These include (1) surgery involving general anesthesia for more than 30 minutes; (2) injury or surgery involving the lower extremities or pelvis; (3) congestive heart failure; (4) prolonged immobility from any cause; and (5) pregnancy, particularly during the postpartum period. Other conditions that increase risk are cancer, obesity, advancing age, varicose veins, a prior episode of DVT, the use of estrogen-containing compounds, and dehydration. Predictably, these risk factors are cumulative.

The deep veins of the lower extremities are the dominant source of clinically significant pulmonary emboli—an important epidemiologic, diagnostic, and therapeutic consideration. Less commonly, thrombi can arise in superficial veins and in prostatic, uterine, renal, and other veins. They also can occur in the right cardiac chambers in patients with right ventricular failure. However, more than 95% of clinically significant pulmonary emboli arise from DVT in the lower extremities (whether or not such DVT is clinically detectable).

The events initiating venous thrombosis are not fully understood. The valves of the lower extremity veins, especially in the calves, are common sites for the initial event. The development of a small nidus leads to the elaboration of clot-potentiating materials that trigger prolongation of the thrombus with red blood cells (RBCs), fibrin and, to a lesser degree, platelets. Once formed, the thrombus grows by accumulating additional RBC, fibrin and platelet "layers," seen pathologically as the lines of Zahn.

Even as thrombosis is occurring, the process of resolution is beginning. The thrombi resolve by one or both of two mechanisms: fibrinolysis and organization. *Fibrinolysis* refers to actual dissolution of the thrombus by plasma enzymes. It is a relatively rapid process, proceeding over a period of hours to several days. If fibrinolysis is not totally successful, organization finishes the job of resolution. Reparative cells infiltrate the residual thrombus and replace the "thrombotic components" with connective tissue. The fibrotic residuum is then incorporated into the venous wall and re-endothelialized. Organization usually thickens the venous wall, which may provide loci for further thrombus formation. The thickening may also incorporate one or more venous valves, rendering them incompetent. Whatever the fate of a given thrombus, available data indicate that the sequence of resolution is complete within 7 to 10 days. By that time, the initial thrombus is gone or has been incorporated into the venous wall. In the latter case, the pathology is more accurately termed a *venous scar* than an *old clot*.

At any time during the process of resolution, pulmonary embolism (PE) can occur. It is important to recognize that embolism is not a new disorder; it is a serious complication of DVT. Because thrombi are most friable early in their development, embolic risk is highest during the first few days after thrombus formation. Thereafter, dissolution or organization sharply limits embolic risk (as long as no new thrombotic material has been laid down in the interval).

When emboli arise and lodge in one or more pulmonary arteries, hemodynamic and respiratory consequences occur. The hemodynamic consequences include a decrease in the available cross-sectional area of the pulmonary arterial system through both mechanical obstruction and release of vasoconstrictive thrombus metabolites directly into the vascular bed. The pulmonary vascular resistance rises, causing an increased pulmonary arterial pressure, and therefore an increased right ventricular workload. If these consequences are severe, the right ventricle may not tolerate the workload and the cardiac output will fall. Respiratory consequences include (1) altered ventilation–perfusion relationships, which (combined with a fall in cardiac output and resulting lowered venous oxygen concentration) may lead to arterial hypoxemia, (2) development of one or more zones of alveolar dead space (zones that are ventilated but not perfused), (3) transient pneumoconstriction of these same zones, (4) hyperventilation (the reasons for which are debated), and (5) loss of surfactant in the underperfused zones. The first four events occur immediately; the fifth requires approximately 24 hours of total occlusion before alveolar surfactant is depleted. The two major consequences of surfactant depletion are atelectasis and an increase in permeability of the alveolocapillary membrane, causing further problems with gas exchange.

Pulmonary infarction is a rare consequence of embolism; fewer than 10% of emboli lead to infarction. Therefore, embolism is by no means synonymous with infarction.

An important clinical question concerns the hemodynamic deterioration observed in some patients with PE in the first few days after embolization. Although PE can be immediately fatal, a large number of patients who eventually succumb do so 1 or more days after presentation. It stands to reason that these "late fatalities" are caused by either progressively deteriorating myocardial fatigue (right ventricular infarction or other myocyte injury) or to increases in workload because of factors such as recurrent emboli, embolus propagation, or further release of vasoactive mediators from the embolus.

The phenomenon of embolic fragments entrapped in the right atrium and ventricle has been recognized in experimental embolism for some time; as cardiac echocardiography is more extensively utilized, this phenomenon has become more widely recognized in human disease as well. The clinical significance of these sessile cardiac thrombi has not been studied in a controlled fashion. However, it is likely that these thrombi may embolize; therefore, larger cardiac thrombi may warrant emergent surgical removal, especially in the presence of preexisting hemodynamic compromise.

Beyond these acute events, emboli (like venous thrombi) tend to resolve if prevented from propagating by anticoagulants. Precise data on the speed of resolution in humans are not available. The earliest reported time of total embolic resolution is about 2 days; most resolve substantially or completely within a few weeks. A very small number fail to dissolve, for unknown reasons, and form permanent vascular scars within the pulmonary arteries, causing chronic thromboembolic pulmonary hypertension (see Chapter 67).

Signs and symptoms of DVT are inconsistent and are essentially manifestations of its two consequences: inflammation of the venous wall and venous obstruction. The former may lead to local pain, tenderness (tenderness along the vessel wall is particularly suggestive), redness, and warmth; the latter may lead to edema in the leg zones drained by the vein(s) involved. Unfortunately, studies have demonstrated that fewer than half of patients with DVT have signs or symptoms at all and few have sufficient inflammation or edema to allow a clinical diagnosis to be made. Therefore, reliable and early detection requires that laboratory tests be used to supplement history and physical examination.

Three well-validated diagnostic procedures are generally available to diagnose and follow the course of DVT: compression ultrasound, impedance plethysmography, and contrast venography. Radiolabeled fibrinogen, a previously invaluable investigative tool for detecting thrombus presence and propagation, is no longer available. Other tests such as serologic markers of thrombosis/thrombolysis, magnetic resonance imaging (MRI) and, radiolabeled thrombus-specific agents are under development, but have not been completely validated for clinical use.

Compression ultrasonography involves the use of ultrasound visualization and Doppler analysis to distinguish between solid (thrombus) and fluid (blood) contents of the proximal deep veins of the leg. Failure to compress visualized veins suggests that at least part of the lumen is filled with solid material and is the only reliable criterion for DVT diagnosis. Findings such as "echogenic densities" or Doppler blood flow velocity measurements have not proved reliable in clinical studies and should not be used to make the diagnosis. The technique is not reliable in detecting thrombi limited to the calf or iliac veins. In addition, the vessel wall thickening from prior DVTs causes wall thickening in nearly half of cases, which can cause noncompressibility on ultrasound. Even the most rigorously controlled clinical trials, using complex algorithms to compare old and new studies side by side, distinguished new thrombi from old scars only with great difficulty. In its current state, compression ultrasonography should not be used to diagnose recurrent DVT at the site of prior thrombosis.

Impedance phlethysmography (IPG), which measures the rate of venous drainage from the leg, is positive when there is substantial obstruction to venous outflow at any point from the popliteal vein to the inferior vena cava. It is sensitive to above-the-knee thrombi, especially when unilaterally positive. The test has been well-validated in clinical studies and is a relatively inexpensive, standardized method to detect DVT. A great deal of work has been performed comparing the accuracy of IPG to that of compression ultrasound. As a group, these studies show compression ultrasound to be slightly more accurate, although it is more expensive and highly operator dependent. Unlike ultrasound, IPG has the benefit of returning to normal within weeks of an acute DVT, making it useful for diagnosing DVT recurrence. It should be noted that neither of these noninvasive tests reliably detects calf thrombi or asymptomatic proximal vein thrombi.

Contrast venography is an invasive test in which radiopaque contrast is injected into the leg veins, yielding a very complete image of leg DVTs on radiographs, even in the calves. However, it has substantial drawbacks, including expense and discomfort. At the present time, contrast venography is usually reserved for special situations, such as patients suspected of having recurrent DVT, those with equivocal results on IPG or ultrasound testing or in whom those tests cannot be done (e.g., those with extensive lower extremity trauma or casts).

Among the promising newer techniques for DVT diagnosis are serologic tests of thrombosis (fibrinopeptide A and B, prothrombin fragment F1.2, thrombin-antithrombin complexes, and soluble fibrin monomer) and or thrombolysis (D-dimer). A potential advantage of these blood tests is that their results may correlate with the presence of both DVT and PE. At present, these tests are still under investigation. The D-dimer assay is the only one that has been extensively evaluated clinically; however, it suffers from two drawbacks. The first is practical; only carefully performed, precise methods to measure D-dimers can distinguish normal controls from VTE patients, who may have only modestly elevated plasma levels. Furthermore, even when D-dimers are measured using sophisticated enzyme-linked immunoassays, the plasma elevations are so common in medical illnesses that relatively few hospitalized patients have normal values for this assay.

Magnetic resonance imaging has been explored as a diagnostic tool for DVT. The results of initial studies performed by investigators at specialized centers have been encouraging and suggest that the technique can be used to diagnose DVT and PE, and perhaps even distinguish new DVTs from old venous scars. These reports, however, are preliminary and must be interpreted with caution. Large trials comparing MRI results to standard venography have not been performed. Outcome studies have not verified the safety of managing patients based on MRI results. Another consideration is that the interpretative performance of the expert readers who are pioneering this new technology may not be easily matched in general practice.

Radiolabeled thrombus-specific agents, such as antibodies targeted at components of fibrin and platelets, are under investigation. When these agents are systemically injected they bind to acute thrombi, and localize them as "hot spots" on nuclear medicine scans. Like MRI, these scans have the potential for diagnosing both PE and DVT simultaneously. Furthermore, because they are specific for the biochemical components of acute thrombi, they do not bind to venous scars and may distinguish them from recurrent DVTs. Finally, agents specific for propagating thrombi may foster unique insights about the ability of different anticoagulant drugs to "extinguish" active clotting.

As is true for DVT, clinical data are not sufficient to confirm or exclude the diagnosis of PE. This fact notwithstanding, the recognition of signs and symptoms suggestive of PE is the single most important factor in preventing death from this disease. This point is highlighted by the rather chilling observation that, in the vast majority of patients who die with PE, the condition was not diagnosed or even suspected ante mortem. Furthermore, although few patients who succumb to pulmonary emboli manifest all of the "textbook" clinical clues, almost all manifested at least one of them. The clinical impact of sophisticated diagnostic technology in reducing fatality from PE pales in comparison to the role of the astute clinician who maintains a low threshold for suspicion.

Signs and symptoms (even nonspecific ones) unexplained by other pathology should raise the possibility of PE and trigger a workup. Dyspnea of sudden onset is a nonspecific, but common symptom. Pleuritic chest pain and hemoptysis, which indicate infarction, occur in a minority of patients. Other individual symptoms, such as syncope and substernal chest pain, are even less common and suggest myocardial damage or strain. In addition, specific physical findings are usually few. Tachycardia of variable duration is also nonspecific, but observed in the majority of patients. Other cardiac findings (e.g., increased pulmonic valve closure sound, right ventricular S3, right ventricular tap) can be subtle and typically occur only in the (fortunately) rare cases of massive embolism. Examination of the lungs rarely discloses a pleural friction rub or evidence of pleural effusion (because these require infarction). Scattered rales or focal wheezing may be heard but are hardly diagnostic.

Clinical clues are crucial for suggesting the diagnosis of PE, but as is true for DVT, objective testing is necessary to confirm or exclude it. Unfortunately, "routine" tests cannot offer such confirmation. The arterial Po_2 is variable and a low value is commonly observed in other respiratory disorders. The chest x-ray is most often either normal or discloses nonspecific findings such as small pleural effusions. The ECG commonly shows only sinus tachycardia. Although such tests may be highly suggestive and are useful in ruling out other diagnoses (e.g., pneumothorax, myocardial infarction), a definitive diagnosis can be arrived at only through a limited number of specific tests.

The currently available diagnostic techniques include (1) ventilation and perfusion scintiphotography, (2) computer-assisted tomography (computed tomographic [CT] scanning and MRI), DVT studies, and (3) pulmonary angiography. All have potential roles in the workup of a potential PE. Each test has, in turn, been declared the "optimal study;" however, they all have specific values and limitations. It is better to individualize the choice and interpretation of these complimentary imaging studies to the particular clinical situation. Unfortunately, blood tests are not yet capable of diagnosing PE in clinical practice.

The pulmonary perfusion scan is highly sensitive, but nonspecific and is recommended as the first test for most patients suspected of PE. A negative scan is invaluable because it excludes the diagnosis as reliably as a pulmonary angiogram; however, a positive scan may be caused by many disorders other than embolism. Combining perfusion lung scans with ventilation scans and/or chest x-rays enhances the specificity of the procedure. Embolism is most reliably diagnosed when there are segmental or larger perfusion defects (which are normally ventilated) in the presence of a clear chest x-ray. Defects anatomically "matched" by radiographic opacities or ventilation defects should be regarded as nondiagnostic and should prompt further workup. Smaller perfusion defects occur less commonly with PE, but these scan findings, regardless of ventilation results, should be regarded as nondiagnostic. Using "probability" estimates to make treatment decisions is, by definition, a gamble. Careful consideration of the risks of an incorrect decision should guide the decision to continue the workup.

If the diagnosis of PE is in doubt after noninvasive testing, searching for DVT is a sensible strategy. Because the two diagnoses are manifestations of the same disease, the treatments are largely the same. The yield of noninvasive testing for DVT is low (less than 10%) in PE suspects without leg symptoms. However, the potential benefits of making the diagnosis without further thoracic imaging justifies the performance of noninvasive leg testing, even in patients without leg symptoms.

Cross-sectional tomographic imaging of the thorax, using either CT or MRI, is under investigation as a diagnostic tool for PE. Both techniques make use of intravascular contrast to fill the lumen of the pulmonary arteries. (Unfortunately, the initial optimism that noncontrast MR imaging would distinguish thromboemboli based on their specific signal characteristics did not come to fruition.) Currently, CT scanning has the advantages over MRI of higher special resolution, wider availability, and larger clinical series demonstrating its value. Both technologies are constantly advancing and the diagnostic value of each test is likely to improve. In both types of scans, emboli are detected as focal defects in pulmonary artery filling. Both scans, when performed and interpreted correctly, are capable of identifying emboli in the segmental or larger pulmonary arteries. However, certain areas, such as the hila, are prone to false positives. Reading emboli in these areas should be done with special care. Perhaps more importantly, neither scan is of much value in imaging emboli in subsegmental pulmonary arteries. There are insufficient data to support the notion that thromboembolic disease invisible to thoracic tomography does not require treatment. At the present time, a negative thoracic CT scan or MRI does not indicate that withholding treatment is safe, especially in cases where limited cardiopulmonary reserve may make undetected emboli (or recurrent emboli) particularly dangerous. In those cases, negative scans should be followed up with further testing.

If other tests fail to confirm or refute the suspicion of PE, angiography may be indicated. Pulmonary angiography remains the "gold standard" because it can demonstrate the embolus itself, even in subsegmental pulmonary arteries. The procedure is invasive, but can be performed with little risk in most situations, if special care is exercised. The most common serious complications arise from the use of contrast dye: the same amount of contrast dye used for helical CT scanning. The decision to perform angiography in patients with equivocal results from noninvasive studies must be based on the specific clinical situation. The fundamental rule is that the greater the risk involved in making a therapeutic decision, the higher the degree of diagnostic certainty required. The small risk involved with angiography in these patients is minor in comparison to the risks involved with making the wrong diagnosis: unnecessary long-term anticoagulation or, conversely, complications of untreated thromboembolism. It must be kept in mind, however, that if DVT has been diagnosed, it is rarely necessary to proceed to angiography because the need to treat the patient already has been established and—except in rare instances—the treatment regimen is the same.

New procedures to diagnose PE are generally the same as those discussed for DVT, including the use of radiolabeled monoclonal antibodies directed against other thromboembolic components and MRI. These agents are still under investigation and their diagnostic value remains to be defined.

---

1. Bell WR, Simon TL, DeMets DL. The clinical features of submassive and massive pulmonary emboli. *Am J Med*. 1997;62:355.
    A breakdown of the clinical features of the participants in the urokinase–streptokinase trials. Pleuritic chest pain and hemoptysis were more common in submassive than in massive emboli.

2. Dalen J, et al. Pulmonary angiography in experimental pulmonary embolism. *Am Heart J*. 1966;72:509.

   An excellent review of criteria to be used in angiographic diagnosis of PE.
3. De Nardo G, et al. The ventilatory lung scan in the diagnosis of pulmonary embolism. *N Engl J Med*. 1970;282:1334.

   A classic study indicating the enhanced diagnostic specificity achieved by combining ventilation with perfusion scanning in patients with PE.
4. Heijboer H, Beuller HR, Lensing AW, et al. A comparison of real time compression ultrasonography with impedance plethysmography for the diagnosis of deep-vein thrombosis in symptomatic outpatients [see comments]. *N Engl J Med*. 1993;329:1365–1369.

   Ultrasound had a slightly higher sensitivity and specificity for symptomatic proximal DVT than did IPG. However, both of their sensitivities depend on the serial performance of the tests when the first result is negative. Also, the IPG in this trial performed much worse than it had in a previous clinical trial on a similar patient population performed by the same investigators.
5. Hull R, et al. Pulmonary angiography, ventilation lung scanning and venography for clinically suspected pulmonary embolism in the abnormal perfusion scan. *Ann Intern Med*. 1983;98:891.

   A prospective study showing that emboli are present in 86% of patients with segmental or larger Q defects, normal ventilation, and a clear chest x-ray. Other scan patterns are much less commonly associated with emboli; venous studies are important in the initial evaluation.
6. The PIOPED Investigators. The value of the ventilation/perfusion scan in acute pulmonary embolism. *JAMA*. 1990;263:2753.

   A complex scheme for interpreting lung scans was developed by the teams of investigators involved in this study.
7. Hull RD, Raskob GE. Low-probability lung scan findings: a need for change. *Ann Intern Med*. 1991;114:142.

   This report indicates that "low probability" scan interpretations are best deleted from the scan-reporting vocabulary because they confuse rather than clarify.
8. Karwinski ES. Comparison of clinical and postmortem diagnosis of pulmonary embolism. *J Clin Pathol*. 1989;42:135–139.

   A university hospital in Norway with a 75 to 80% autopsy rate (!) did a retrospective analysis of 21,529 cases. In patients who died from PE, the diagnosis was made before death in only 10 to 20% of cases. In addition, the rates of ante mortem diagnosis got worse over the 20-year span of the study.
9. Kearon C, Julian JA, Newman TE, et al. Noninvasive diagnosis of deep venous thrombosis. McMaster Diagnostic Imaging Practice Guidelines Initiative [see comments]. *Ann Intern Med*. 1998;128:663–677.

   A well-written review of previous clinical studies. Although both tests are accurate enough to use as management tools, CUS has a slightly higher accuracy than IPG. However, either test can be in error and should be confirmed with venography if the results are discordant with clinical suspicion.
10. Kakkar V, et al. Natural history of post-operative deep vein thrombosis. *Lancet*. 1969;2:230.

    One of the early studies with radiolabeled fibrinogen, indicating that clinical detection of DVT is unreliable.
11. Kipper MS, et al. Long-term follow-up of patients with suspected pulmonary embolism and a normal lung scan. *Chest*. 1982;82:411.

    Study indicating that a normal perfusion scan has the same value as a normal pulmonary angiogram in ruling out embolism (and the need for anticoagulant therapy).
12. Moser KM, Fedullo PF. Venous thromboembolism: three simple decisions. *Chest*. 1983;83:117, 256.

    A well-referenced review of diagnostic and therapeutic options and controversies.
13. Moser K, et al. In vivo and postmortem dissolution rates of pulmonary emboli and venous thrombi in the dog. *Circulation*. 1973;48:170.

A study that demonstrates the speed with which fresh venous thrombi and pulmonary emboli can resolve in the dog.

14. Prophylactic therapy of deep vein thrombosis and pulmonary embolism. DHEW Publication No. (NIH) 76–866, 1976.
    An excellent review of many aspects of VTE by experts in this field.

15. Quinn PA, et al. A prospective investigation of pulmonary embolism in women and men. *JAMA.* 1992;268:1689.
    Women in the PIOPED study had a somewhat lower frequency of embolism than men but had the same risk factors—except that those on oral contraceptives had a higher postsurgical risk.

16. Stein PD, Henry JW. Prevalence of acute pulmonary embolism among patients in a general hospital and at autopsy. *Chest.* 1995;108:978–981.
    Even during a time when the investigators were recruiting patients for a multicenter trial for PE diagnosis (the PIOPED study), 70% of patients who died with PE had the disease unsuspected premortem.

17. Hoellerich VL, Wigton RS. Diagnosing pulmonary embolism using clinical findings. *Arch Intern Med.* 1986;146:1699.
    The authors indicate that a battery of 92 clinical items, including lung scans, disclosed no one variable of significant power in predicting the diagnosis of embolism by angiography. However, a battery of eight items (including the lung scan) had reasonable diagnostic power.

18. Hull RD, et al. Pulmonary embolism in outpatients with chest pain. *Arch Intern Med.* 1988;148:838.
    Pulmonary embolism was present in only 21% of patients presenting in an emergency room with pleuritic chest pain. Clinical variables were not very sensitive (85%) or specific (36%). They conclude that objective tests (scan, angiogram) were necessary for diagnosis.

19. Huisman MV, et al. Serial impedance plethysmography for suspected deep venous thrombosis in outpatients. *N Engl J Med* 1986;314:823.
    Careful study demonstrating excellent outcomes in outpatients with suspected venous thrombosis who had negative serial IPG tests and were not treated.

20. Huisman MV, et al. Utility of impedance plethysmography in the diagnosis of recurrent deep-vein thrombosis. *Arch Intern Med.* 1988;148:881.
    Initially positive IPGs in patients with acute above-knee DVT return to normal in 95% over 12 months. Serial testing at 3-month intervals may allow detection of recurrence if an IPG that has returned to normal again becomes positive.

21. Davidson BI, et al. Low accuracy of color Doppler ultrasound in the detection of proximal leg vein thrombosis in asymptomatic high-risk patients. *Ann Intern Med.* 1992;117:735.
    Color Doppler ultrasound was found to be insensitive to proximal DVT in asymptomatic high-risk patients.

22. Lensing AW, et al. Detection of deep venous thrombosis by real-time B-mode ultrasonography. *N Engl J Med.* 1989;320:342.
    Using strict diagnostic criteria (ability to compress popliteal and femoral veins), ultrasound had same diagnostic value as IPG in symptomatic patients. Echogenicity was not a useful criterion; calf thrombi were poorly detected. Serial studies, as with IPG, were necessary to rule out thrombus extension.

23. Anderson DR, et al. Limitations of impedance plethysmography in diagnosis of clinically-suspected deep-vein thrombosis. *Ann Intern Med.* 1993;118:25.
    Questions the sensitivity and specificity of IPG versus ultrasound. The following two references point out serious methodologic problems with this study that place its conclusions in question.

24. Raskob GE. Impedance plethysmography and DVT diagnosis: letter to editor. *Ann Intern Med.* 1993;199:247.

25. Wheeler HB, Anderson FA, Jr. Impedance plethysmography and DVT diagnosis: letter to editor. *Ann Intern Med.* 1993;119:246.

26. Rubinstein I, et al. Fatal pulmonary emboli in hospitalized patients. *Arch Intern Med.* 1988;148:1425.

The authors conclude from this autopsy study that embolism is still underdiagnosed. Only 31% of this series with embolism at autopsy had the diagnosis suspected prior to death.

27. Lensing AWA, et al. Detection of deep-vein thrombosis by real-time B-model ultrasonography. *N Engl J Med.* 1989;320:342.

A careful study of this technique. Diagnostic criteria need to be refined and other populations require acute and long-term study before the technique can be fully validated. Currently, as with IPG, detection of calf-limited thromboses is poor (36%).

28. Ludwig JW, et al. Comparison of conventional pulmonary angiography with intravenous digital subtraction angiography for pulmonary embolic disease. *Radiology.* 1983;147:345.

Motion limits diagnostic sensitivity of the technique in embolism beyond the main pulmonary arteries, but its application in selected patients is useful. Technologic advances may improve the results further.

29. Prandoni P, et al. Deep vein thrombosis and the incidence of subsequent symptomatic cancer. *N Engl J Med.* 1992;327:1128.

An old question, much debated, is revisited. These authors conclude that patients with idiopathic DVT, especially those with recurrences, have an increased incidence of cancer during long-term follow-up (7.6% in idiopathic DVT versus 1.9% in those with clear risk factors). A randomized trial is suggested to determine whether the cost and discomfort of excluding cancer in such patients are worthwhile.

30. Ginsberg JS, et al. Anticardiolipin antibodies and the risk for ischemic stroke and venous thrombosis. *Ann Intern Med.* 1992;117:997.

Anticardiolipin antibodies are a definite risk factor for venous thrombosis.

31. Bounameaux H, et al. Measurement of plasma D-dimer for the diagnosis of deep venous thrombosis. *Am J Clin Pathol.* 1989;91:82.

32. Heijboer H, et al. The use of the D-dimer test in combination with non-invasive testing versus serial non-invasive testing alone for the diagnosis of deep vein thrombosis. *Thromb Hemost.* 1992;67:510.

33. Bounameaux H, et al. Measurement of D-dimer in plasma as diagnostic aid in suspected pulmonary embolism. *Lancet.* 1991;337:196.

The previous three references discuss the potential value of D-dimer assays in diagnosis of DVT and PE. The value of this assay to "rule out" these diagnoses remains unsettled.

34. Morris TA, et al. Single photon emission computed tomography of pulmonary emboli and venous thrombi using anti–D-dimer. *Am J Respir Crit Care Med.* 2004;169:987–993.

New approach to the diagnosis of VTE. Further study is needed to determine the value of these and similar "thrombus-targeted" methods.

65. THROMBOEMBOLIC DISEASE: PROPHYLAXIS

Timothy A. Morris

The best way to reduce the morbidity and mortality associated with venous thromboembolic (VTE) disease is to prevent it from occurring in the first place. When performed properly, the risks of VTE prophylaxis are small and the improvements in morbidity and mortality rates are enormous. The ultimate goal of safely preventing VTE has not yet been achieved and is the focus of a great deal of research.

Theoretically, two options exist: (1) to provide prophylaxis for VTE and (2) to monitor with noninvasive tests and treat if VTE develops. In virtually all patients, the first option is the best because venous thrombosis and embolism can develop rapidly, and the first signal of these events can be a sudden, fatal embolic event.

Strategies to prevent VTE must address the mechanisms by which venous thrombi are formed and progress to clinically significant disease. The basic science underlying the pathogenesis and natural history of VTE is only partially understood, a fact that is reflected in our inability to completely prevent this disease. In addition, clinical studies to evaluate prophylactic methods suffer from an incomplete understanding of how best to define and detect "clinically significant VTE." Nevertheless, the prophylactic methods developed and validated have had a tremendous impact on the incidence of this disease.

When considering prophylaxis, deep vein thrombosis (DVT) and pulmonary embolism (PE) should be considered as different manifestations of VTE, rather than as separate disorders. The vast majority (>95%) of clinically significant pulmonary emboli arise from deep veins of the lower extremities. Thus the prevention of PE, for the most part, is really the prevention of lower extremity DVT.

Substantial data suggest that only lower extremity DVTs extending into the proximal deep veins (popliteal and above) cause clinically apparent emboli; thrombi that remain confined to calf veins pose no significant embolic risk. It is not known whether this observation reflects the fact that thrombi restricted to the calf veins do not embolize or that such emboli are so small that clinical disease does not result, although the latter is more likely. Whatever the case, it is now evident that the key to prevention of PE is the prevention of DVT of the lower extremity veins or, failing this, prevention of the extension of calf vein thrombosis into the more proximal venous system.

There are two requirements for developing an effective strategy for preventing any disorder: (1) identification of the patients at risk, and (2) the availability of effective prophylactic modalities. For DVT, both of these requirements have been largely, but again, incompletely satisfied. The risk associated with various patient populations have been well defined, yet we lack an accurate method of assessing the risk for individual patients. Likewise, the efficacy and safety of several prophylactic regimens have been established clinically, although these trials are complicated by the difficulties inherent to detecting asymptomatic DVT and controversies over its clinical importance.

The decision to apply prophylaxis involves weighing the risk of venous thrombosis (and therefore PE) against the risk of a prophylactic regimen. Risk factors are cumulative and the total clinical picture should determine whether prophylaxis is used, and the aggressiveness of the methods to be employed. For example, patients undergoing extensive lower extremity orthopedic surgery are at very high risk for DVT and require aggressive mechanical and moderate-dose anticoagulant prophylaxis. Younger, healthier persons with less severe medical problems and limited immobilization could be adequately protected by lower doses of anticoagulants or by mechanical methods alone.

There are several mechanical and pharmacologic methods available to prevent VTE. The exact prophylactic "recipe" appropriate depends on the risks associated in each clinical situation. Many studies have been performed to compare different methods and drug regimens in VTE prophylaxis. Although these comparative trials may provide useful clinical guidance, they should be interpreted with some care, considering each trial's sponsorship and scientific rigor. For example, the comparator medication should have been dosed optimally (or, in the case of mechanical modalities, optimal devices/methods should have been employed).

The mechanical compressive devices prevent venous stasis by inflating a cuff for several seconds each minute. Some compress the calf alone; others compress the calf and thigh sequentially; there seems to be little difference in efficacy. Although it is unclear if different pressures and speeds of intermittent cuff inflation lead to improved prophylactic efficacy, it is clear that the pattern of rhythmic inflation is helpful because simple elastic stockings have not been shown to be useful (unless patient tailored to provide a gradient of pressures). The intermittent compressive devices are safe, effective, and well-tolerated. The only contraindications to their use are the presence of active venous thrombosis (which should be ruled out prior to their application if suspected), limb ischemia from arterial insufficiency, or the presence of circumstances that prevent their application (e.g., a cast in place). The devices should be applied promptly (e.g., preoperatively) and maintained during the risk period. This approach has particular value in those patient groups for whom antithrombotic drugs are contraindicated (e.g., neurosurgical, head trauma, known hemorrhagic diathesis).

Prophylactic subcutaneous heparin has been studied widely. Doses of 5000 to 7500 U subcutaneously every 8 to 12 hours have proved safe and effective in preventing VTE in most populations. This regimen is effective because of the inhibition of events that occur early in the coagulation cascade, prior to the elaboration of thrombin. After initial screening studies (e.g., platelet count, partial thromboplastin time, prothrombin time, careful history), no further coagulation studies are necessary to monitor the patient. Substantial experience has indicated the low bleeding risk associated with this regimen, even in surgical populations.

Low-molecular-weight heparins (LMWHs), a heterogeneous group of drugs derived by partial depolymerization of heparin, present another option for prophylaxis. Like heparin, they are administered subcutaneously for DVT prophylaxis. They possess certain theoretical advantages over (unfractionated) heparin, such as a reduced incidence of laboratory demonstrated heparin-induced thrombocytopenia during routine use. These medications are 10 times more expensive to use than heparin and would constitute a great increase in pharmaceutical cost if adopted for all prophylactic needs. The high cost of the various LMWHs is justified if each drug represents a true clinical advantage over properly dosed heparin.

Fondaparinux is the first entirely synthetic anticoagulant whose structure is based on the active site of heparin and LMWH. The mechanism of action is similar to heparin-based anticoagulants. It is being tested clinically for both prophylaxis and treatment. After orthopedic procedures, it appears to be comparable to the LMWHs for prophylaxis. Clinical trials have not been reported comparing fondaparinux's safety and efficacy to heparin or LMWHs in a wide range of clinical situations.

Warfarin is an alternative, effective drug for prophylaxis in high-risk subjects. Several regimens have been studied, particularly in very high-risk groups such as hip replacement patients. One approach is to begin prior to surgery with low doses (1–2 mg/d), then escalate to a therapeutic range after surgery. Another is to begin warfarin only after surgery, finally achieving the desired prothrombin range (International Normalized Ratio [INR]: 2.0–3.0) after several days. It is likely that these regimens do not prevent small calf thrombi but do prevent extension into the popliteal veins and above, thereby sharply reducing embolic risk.

Hirudin, a potent thrombin inactivator, has been studied under several clinical conditions for DVT prophylaxis. Results of initial clinical trials have been encouraging for its use in both prophylaxis and treatment of VTE. However, further studies must be performed before it can be recommended for clinical use.

Among other options, aspirin, dipyridamole, sulfinpyrazone, and other antiplatelet drugs have not been shown to be useful for prophylaxis of venous thrombosis. Reports regarding the value of intravenous infusion of low-molecular-weight dextran are mixed, placing this polymer in the category of "probably effective." Dextran does carry the potential risk of volume overload and allergic reactions.

There are always patients who are at high risk but in whom neither antithrombotic agents nor venous compression devices can be applied (e.g., patients with extensive trauma). In such patients, prophylactic placement of an inferior vena caval filter should be considered.

The prophylactic approach selected depends on the magnitude of thromboembolic risk and the relative risks inherent to prophylactic methods. In patients at low or moderate risk, either the application of intermittent pneumatic leg compression devices or prophylactic doses of subcutaneous low-dose heparin or warfarin provide adequate protection. Such patients include those who are immobilized for brief periods, are undergoing general surgical procedures (e.g., cholecystectomy), or have suffered an uncomplicated myocardial infarction. However, none of these individual approaches provides optimal protection in patients at high risk: patients with trauma to the pelvis or lower extremities; patients undergoing extensive surgical procedures on the lower extremities (e.g., hip or knee replacement) or surgical prostatectomy; and patients with multiple risk factors. In these individuals, multiple studies have indicated that the combination of intermittent leg compression with either heparin or warfarin provides optimal protection.

Regardless of the specific regimen selected, it is clear that prophylaxis should be applied to all patients at risk of venous thromboembolism. Failure to apply prophylaxis should be specifically justified. Because prevention of DVT is the best means of preventing PE and death due to embolism, and because the vast majority of venous thrombi arise among hospitalized patients to whom a prophylactic option easily can be applied, widespread use of prophylactic options can, at the current time, considerably reduce the incidence of DVT and PE. Further developments in this field hold the promise of safely preventing it even further, perhaps to the point of eliminating it entirely.

1. Gruber VF, Saldeen T, Brokup B. Incidence of fatal post-operative pulmonary embolism after prophylaxis with dextran-70 and low-dose heparin: an international multicentre study. *Br Med J.* 1980;1:69.

   Dextran-70 was effective in this well-done study; other reports, both positive and negative, leave the efficacy question unresolved.

2. Kakkar VV, Corrigan TP, Fossard DP. Prevention of post-operative embolism by low-dose heparin: an international multi-center trial. *Lancet.* 1975;2:45.

   A large trial documenting a reduction in incidence of DVT, PE, and lethal PE in patients treated with low-dose heparin versus controls.

3. Kakkar VV, et al. Deep vein thrombosis: is there a high-risk group? *Am J Surg.* 1970;120:527.

4. Moser KM, LeMoine JR. Is embolic risk conditioned by location of deep venous thrombosis? *Ann Intern Med.* 1981;94:439.

   The answer to the questions posed in articles 4 and 5 seems to be "yes"; those with thrombi extending into above-knee veins are at high embolic risk.

5. Prophylactic therapy of deep vein thrombosis and pulmonary embolism. DHEW Publication No. (NIH) 76-866, 1976.

   Publication of proceedings of a conference attended by many investigators, at which numerous prophylactic treatment approaches were discussed in depth.

6. Report of the Steering Committee of a trial sponsored by the Medical Research Council. Effect of aspirin on postoperative venous thromboses. *Lancet.* 1972;2:441.

   This article is one of many reports in which aspirin was not effective.

7. Salzman EW, et al. Intraoperative external pneumatic calf compression to afford long-term prophylaxis against deep vein thrombosis in urologic patients. *Surgery.* 1980;87:239.

   One of a large number of reports indicating the efficacy of this prophylactic option.

8. Sevitt S, Gallagher NG. Venous thrombosis and pulmonary embolism: a clinicopathologic study in injured and burned patients. *Br J Surg.* 1961;48:475.

9. Sevitt S, Gallagher NG. Prevention of venous thrombosis and pulmonary embolism in injured subjects: a trial of anti-coagulant prophylaxis with phenindione in middle-aged and elderly patients with fractured femoral necks. *Lancet.* 1959;2:981.

   References 8 and 9 are carefully done landmark studies establishing the efficacy of prothrombinopenic drugs as prophylactic agents in these patient groups. The positive results, based on vein and lung dissection, are not open to debate, a rare event in the thromboembolic literature.

10. Turpie AGG, et al. Prevention of venous thrombosis in patients with intracranial disease of intermittent pneumatic compression of the calf. *Neurologia.* 1977;27:435.

    This prophylactic option was effective in patients with neurologic disease.

11. Collins R, et al. Reduction in fatal pulmonary embolism and venous thrombosis by perioperative administration of subcutaneous heparin. *N Engl J Med.* 1988;318:1162.

An exhaustive review of the many studies regarding prophylaxis with heparin in patients at risk. The authors conclude that the value of this approach has been clearly established in multiple surgical subgroups.

12. Clark-Pearson DL, et al. Prevention of postoperative venous thromboembolism by external pneumatic calf compression in patients with gynecologic malignancy. *Obstet Gynecol.* 1984;63:92.

   The study concludes that application of this device significantly reduces the incidence of postoperative DVT in these patients.

13. Geerts WH, et al. Prevention of venous thromboembolism: The Seventh ACCP Conference on Antithrombotic and Thrombolytic Therapy. *Chest.* 2004;126:338S–400S.

   This is an exhaustively well-referenced review of the various available prophylactic regimens, and the evidence supporting their use in specific clinical situations.

14. Francis CW, et al. Two-step warfarin therapy. *JAMA.* 1983;249:374.

   This approach proved effective, and with low bleeding risk, in patients undergoing hip and knee replacement.

15. Francis CW, et al. Comparison of warfarin and external pneumatic compression in prevention of venous thrombosis after total hip replacement. *JAMA.* 1992;267:2911.

   Both approaches were effective in reducing the frequency of DVT.

16. Levine MN, et al. Prevention of deep vein thrombosis after elective hip replacement: a randomized trial comparing low molecular weight heparin with standard unfractionated heparin. *Ann Intern Med.* 1991;114:543.

   Low-molecular-weight heparin is as effective as standard heparin in prophylaxis of these patients.

17. Huisman MV, et al. Serial impedance plethysmography for suspected deep venous thrombosis in outpatients. *N Engl J Med.* 1986;314:823.

   Excellent study demonstrating that, unless DVT suspects have or develop positive impedance plethysmography (indicating thrombosis in popliteal vein and above), outcomes are excellent without treatment. Thus, without treatment, thrombi that remain calf limited pose no significant embolic risk.

18. Oster G, et al. Prevention of venous thromboembolism after general surgery: cost-effectiveness analysis of alternative approaches to prophylaxis. *Am J Med.* 1987;82:889.

   Prophylaxis not only reduces morbidity and mortality but also is cost effective.

19. Moser KM. Venous thromboembolism: state of the art. *Am Rev Respir Dis.* 1990; 141:235.

   A review of multiple aspects of venous thromboembolism, heavily referenced.

20. Kakkar VV, et al. Low molecular weight versus standard heparin for prevention of venous thromboembolism after major abdominal surgery. *Lancet.* 1993;341:259.

   The two drugs were of equal efficacy.

21. Eriksson BI, Ekman S, Lindbratt S, et al. Prevention of thromboembolism with use of recombinant hirudin. Results of a double-blind, multicenter trial comparing the efficacy of desirudin (Revasc) with that of unfractionated heparin in patients having a total hip replacement. *J Bone Joint Surg Am.* 1997;79:326–333.

   Hirudin performed well as a prophylactic agent in this trial, compared to low-dose heparin.

22. Eriksson BI, Wille-Jorgensen P, Kalebo P, et al. A comparison of recombinant hirudin with a low-molecular-weight heparin to prevent thromboembolic complications after total hip replacement [see comments]. *N Engl J Med.* 1997;337:1329–1335.

   Hirudin performed well, compared to one of the more popular low-molecular-weight heparins.

23. Samama MM, Cohen AT, Darmon JY, et al. A comparison of enoxaparin with placebo for the prevention of venous thromboembolism in acutely ill medical patients. Prophylaxis in Medical Patients with Enoxaparin Study Group. *N Engl J Med.* 1999;341:793–800.

Moderately high doses of enoxaparin compared favorably to placebo in this patient population, although its performance compared to higher dose prophylactic heparin is unknown.

24. Philbrick JT, Becker DM. Calf deep venous thrombosis: a wolf in sheep's clothing? *Arch Intern Med.* 1988;148:2131.

   A review suggesting that calf-limited DVT, followed to ensure that it does not extend, is of no significant morbid or embolic risk.

25. Anderson FA, Jr, et al. Physician practices in the prevention of venous thromboembolism. *Ann Intern Med.* 1991;115:591.

   Although the value of prophylaxis is established, this report indicates that it is still not adequately applied by physicians.

---

66. THROMBOEMBOLIC DISEASE: THERAPY

Timothy A. Morris and C. Jackson Wray

Rational management of venous thromboembolism (VTE) should be guided by the primary goals of treatment, namely to prevent and minimize serious sequelae. These include (1) death from pulmonary emboli (PE); (2) dyspnea, chest pain, and hemodynamic instability from PE; (3) leg discomfort from deep vein thrombosis (DVT); (4) long-term recurrence of VTE; and (5) other long-term problems such as postphlebitic leg swelling and pulmonary hypertension. From a biological perspective, acute therapy should diminish the amount of vascular obstruction in PE and DVT and prevent embolization or, in the case of DVT, further embolization. In the case of hemodynamically significant PE, inhibiting the release of vasoactive substances into the pulmonary circulation and optimizing right ventricular (RV) function also may be important. Such factors as reducing damage to the venous wall and valves are likely to lower long-term complication rates.

In most cases, the treatment of DVT and stable PE are identical. Heparin is the treatment of choice in acute disease; however, low-molecular-weight heparins (LMWH) may be equivalent in some situations. Although the mechanisms of action are somewhat different, both heparin and LMWH catalyze endogenous antithrombin III to stop ongoing thrombosis by inactivation of various clotting factors, thrombin, and factor Xa being the most important of these. By doing so, they immediately inhibit growth of both DVT and PE, allowing the fibrinolytic system to proceed unopposed. Thus, they indirectly speed the resolution of preexisting DVT and PE and reduce the size of potential emboli. Overall, available evidence suggests that some LMWH are comparable to heparin in safety and in efficacy; however, it is important to realize that clinical trials have failed to demonstrate a clear or consistent superiority of LMWH over unfractionated heparin in either regard. The choice between agents depends in large part on their relative cost and ease of administration.

Neither heparin nor LMWH reduces embolic risk or enhances thrombus resolution directly. Treated patients remain at embolic risk until the DVT either dissolves or organizes; consequently, embolization occurring in the first few days of therapy does not reflect "drug failure." The only evidence of heparin (or LMWH) failure is thrombus growth or initiation of a new thrombus during therapy. Furthermore, some 50% of patients with above-knee acute DVT already have had asymptomatic PE; thus, it is important not to misinterpret the presence of preexisting emboli discovered during the course of treatment as evidence of recurrent thromboembolic disease.

DVT confined to calf veins typically does not require anticoagulant therapy because of its low rate of clinically important sequelae (see Chapters 63 and 64). However, DVT occurring in the popliteal or more proximal veins require treatment. Both compression ultrasound and impedance plethysmography (IPG) are convenient, reliable ways to make this distinction. However, if IPG or ultrasound is not available or if the patient cannot be followed by reliable tests for 10 to 14 days to ensure that extension of calf-limited thrombi does not occur (it does in 15–20%), patients with calf-limited thrombi also should be treated. Serial outpatient testing over the course of a week avoids hospitalization and is a useful, cost-effective approach but this method requires a well-organized system for follow-up to ensure that proximal DVT is detected and treated promptly.

Two heparin regimens are available for use in the treatment of VTE: continuous intravenous infusion of approximately 18 U/kg per hour and twice daily subcutaneous injections of approximately 250 U/kg. The question of which regimen is safer and more effective remains unanswered despite a large body of research; however, the continuous intravenous regimen has been the most popular. The subcutaneous route permits more mobility and the possibility of outpatient management, and is gaining popularity in the current milieu of medical cost containment.

The best method for laboratory monitoring of heparin therapy and the necessity for such monitoring remain controversial issues. A myriad of laboratory tests are available but none reliably predicts a safe and effective heparin dosage regimen. Test results can vary widely among laboratories, depending on technical details of sample handling, reagents, and test performance. Furthermore, substantial diurnal variation in tests can occur during continuous intravenous infusion of heparin; for example, an 8 AM test may not reliably predict results several hours later. This applies to the three most widely used tests: (1) whole blood clotting time, (2) plasma recalcification time, and (3) activated partial thromboplastin time (aPTT). The aPTT is the most popular; most experts believe that the aPTT should be maintained at 1.5 to 2.5 times control during continuous intravenous infusion and 1.5 times control just prior to the next dose on an intermittent schedule. Although animal and clinical studies suggest that continuous prolongation of the aPTT above 1.5 times control is associated with less thrombus growth and VTE recurrence, the observed effects may be entirely due to the use of appropriate doses of heparin (as outlined), irrespective of the aPTT test results. Indeed, a meta-analysis has indicated that subcutaneous regimens, with or without monitoring, are at least as safe and effective as intravenous regimens; other studies have noted the vagaries of the aPTT for monitoring therapy.

Fondaparinux is the first drug in a new class of synthetic agents that are based on the active sites of both heparin and LMWH. Fondaparinux can be given once a day and has been shown to be comparable to LMWH and heparin in patients with DVT and stable PE (respectively). Although fondaparinux may be more convenient to use than most currently used regimens for unfractionated heparin and LMWH, it has not been shown to be safer or more effective than either.

The major complication of therapy with heparin and LMWH is hemorrhage. The initial hope that LMWH would be safer than heparin was not borne out in clinical studies; both drugs most likely carry the same risk of bleeding. In fact, host factors appear to be far more important than the type and dose of heparin in determining bleeding risk. These include age (especially beyond the sixth decade); the presence of unsuspected or known bleeding sites (e.g., stomach, bowel, kidney); uremia; and demonstrable hemostatic defects (e.g., thrombocytopenia). Available data indicate that bleeding risk is very low among patients who do not have a significant coexistent disease or coagulopathy. It should also be noted that many hemorrhagic episodes in heparinized patients occur when clotting parameters are in "therapeutic range."

The necessary duration of anticoagulant therapy for VTE is controversial, both in the acute stage and in follow-up. In the acute stage, thrombi contain a high concentration of activated clotting factors and antithrombin III–mediated direct inhibition with heparin, LMWH, or fondaparinux is necessary to halt the thrombotic process. Although clinical data are relatively sparse, most experts agree that at least 5 days of heparin-like drugs or LMWH are necessary for initial treatment. The limited available evidence indicates that venous thrombi resolve or become organized approximately within this timeframe.

Follow-up anticoagulation therapy is necessary in almost all cases to prevent recurrence of VTE. The appropriate type and duration of therapy should be tailored to the clinical situation. Patients at high risk for recurrence, characterized by having unresolved or ongoing risk factors for VTE, are likely to require prolonged (possibly lifelong) anticoagulation. Such risk factors include immobility, heart failure, persistent venous obstruction, and malignancy. In addition, patients with idiopathic VTE have high rates of recurrence and are likely to have persistent "hypercoagulable states," based either on known biochemical disorders or on as yet uncharacterized factors. The duration of follow-up anticoagulation necessary for patients with transient risk factors is controversial. The simple clinical answer is that protection should be continued until the original risk factor(s) have subsided (e.g., the broken leg has healed and the patient is fully ambulatory). Most experts, however, recommend at least 3 to 6 months of anticoagulation for patients with VTE, even those with transient risk factors.

As soon as the diagnosis of VTE is confirmed, one can assume that follow-up treatment will be required beyond hospitalization. Currently, warfarin is the most practical option; it can be initiated as soon as heparin has been started. Heparin is continued until the prothrombin time has been in range (International Normalized Ratio: 2–3) for 2 consecutive days. At that point, heparin can be discontinued and the patient discharged on warfarin. If, for some reason, warfarin cannot be used, high doses of subcutaneous heparin (adjusted to keep the aPTT <1.5 × control) can be started on day 6 and the patient discharged on this regimen. Both approaches are acceptable; the choice involves the patient's desires (e.g., injections versus the need for regular prothrombin times). Direct thrombin inhibitors, currently being developed, may represent an addition to the pharmacologic arena of long-term anticoagulation, and may obviate the need for regular laboratory monitoring.

Approaches specific to DVT therapy have been proposed, but are not commonly used. Surgery (e.g., thrombectomy, ligation) has no role. Thrombolytic agents (streptokinase, urokinase, tissue plasminogen activator) do not appear to offer improved short- or long-term outcome as compared to heparin in patients with DVT and increase the risk of intracranial hemorrhage. Future studies with new or existing thrombolytic agents may modify these views.

The treatment of PE in very stable patients is generally identical to DVT but several issues require extra consideration. The most important one is the recognition that outpatient, subcutaneous treatment regimens in PE have only been tested in the most clinically stable patient populations. Less "healthy" patients merit hospital admission. Additional therapeutic issues specific to PE include (1) the size of the initial dose of heparin and the dosage regimen during the first 24 hours, (2) the need for cardiopulmonary supportive measures, (3) the role of caval filters and surgery, and (4) the role of thrombolytic agents.

The size of the initial heparin dose required following PE is controversial. Animal data indicate that pharmacologically active peptides are released from platelets coating an embolus and that they contribute to the initial severity of the cardiopulmonary symptoms by inducing pulmonary vasoconstriction and bronchoconstriction. These studies have shown that a large initial bolus of heparin is necessary to inhibit platelet aggregation, which initiates release of these agents. Based on these data, we recommend a large initial intravenous bolus (15,000–20,000 U) of heparin, followed by a continuous infusion similar to the intravenous DVT regimens. Dose adjustment is generally the same as for DVT, but with special attention to avoiding low doses or low aPTT values during the first 1 to 2 days of therapy. Some clinicians prefer to use larger dose heparin infusions during the initial 24 hours after an embolic event. This approach is based on the results of coagulation tests and the notion that high levels of thrombin may persist during this period. However, because of the excellent clinical outcomes observed in PE patients treated without the "high initial dose" approach, we do not give larger doses during the first 24 hours in most patients.

Cardiopulmonary supportive measures may be indicated for PE treatment, including administration of oxygen if arterial hypoxemia is present. Systemic hypotension, if present, is usually due to acute RV ischemia and failure. Animal experiments suggest that an important mechanism of RV ischemia is low myocardial perfusion pressure (coronary pressure – RV pressure) occurring as the right heart "strains" to overcome massive pulmonary artery obstruction. For that reason, we prefer systemic vasoconstrictive agents, such as phenylephrine, to raise arterial pressure (and coronary pressure) during PE-associated shock.

Massive PE may require a more aggressive approach, particularly during the first few days of heparin therapy when heparin cannot prevent a recurrence. In this situation, death may be caused by additional embolization of lower limb DVT that occurs while the patient is already hemodynamically compromised. Multiple procedures are available to prevent recurrent embolism of lower limb DVTs. Our current choice is limited to the insertion of a Greenfield (or similar) inferior vena caval filter. These devices are relatively easy to insert, do not interfere with caval blood flow, and have an excellent (95%) record of long-term patency. It is, for us, the "standard" against which other devices and approaches should be measured. When a recurrence may be fatal in the setting of massive PE, we consider filter placement to be a life-saving procedure.

The role of thrombolytic agents in management of PE is unclear. The choice of patients who might benefit from thrombolytics must be made on the basis of indirect information rather than by comparative clinical trials. Multiple studies have established that these agents promote more rapid embolic resolution than heparin alone. Positive effects on morbidity and mortality have not been demonstrated; in addition, the degree of embolic resolution after the first week of anticoagulation is about the same without thrombolytic therapy. Thrombolytic agents are costly and carry significant risks for adverse consequences. We believe that such agents should be used only in the management of patients with massive embolism and persistent hypotension and only by physicians quite familiar with the drugs.

Acute pulmonary embolectomy (by thoracotomy, suction catheter, or balloon catheter) is an aggressive procedure that is performed at some institutions. In our view, it is rarely warranted because medical therapy is so successful, patient selection so difficult, and the results of acute embolectomy so unimpressive. Conceivably, there are special situations in which this surgery is possible (massive embolism fails to respond promptly to medical therapy and the diagnosis is certain). However, the procedure carries a very high mortality and we do not recommend it in most cases.

For follow-up after the immediate treatment period, the use of lung scans in patients with above-knee DVT (to rule out asymptomatic embolism) and in patients with PE (to evaluate resolution) merits comment. Often, in patients with DVT, pleuritic chest pain or other embolic symptoms appear several days after admission, and a scan demonstrates defects. In our experience, these defects were usually present on the admission scan and, therefore, do not merit a change in therapy. Absent the admission scan, such decisions are much more difficult. A follow-up scan during PE treatment not only provides evidence of satisfactory embolic resolution but also alerts the physician to the possibility that the patient may require close follow-up to rule out chronic postembolic pulmonary hypertension (see Chapter 66).

---

1. Alpert JS, et al. Mortality in patients treated for pulmonary embolism. *JAMA.* 1976;236:1477.
   An interesting study that implies, among other things, that embolectomy is not likely to impact on the mortality associated with PE.
2. Basu D, et al. A prospective study of the value of monitoring heparin treatment with the activated partial thromboplastin time. *N Engl J Med.* 1972;287:324.
   Well-designed study discussing the optimum heparin regimen and the value of monitoring the dose with the partial thromboplastin time. Compare with references 7 and 20.
3. Bentley PG, et al. An objective study of alternative methods of heparin administration. *Thromb Res.* 1980;18:177.
   Another approach to heparin administration.

4. Bonnameau XH, et al. Results of the European thrombolysis with rt-PA in venous thrombosis trial. *Thromb Hemost*. 1992;67:306.
   Trial was discontinued because of low efficacy and excessive bleeding.
5. Brandjes DPM, et al. Acenocoumarol and heparin compared with acenocoumarol alone in the initial treatment of proximal vein thrombosis. *N Engl J Med*. 1992; 327:1485.
   Initiation of therapy with heparin is advisable.
6. Brill-Edwards P, et al. Establishing a therapeutic range for heparin therapy. *Ann Intern Med*. 1993;119:104.
   The variability of reagents used for the aPTT test can influence the heparin dose significantly. The authors suggest an alternative (but not generally available) monitoring approach.
7. Crotty GM, Bynum LJ, Wilson JE, III. Heparin therapy in venous thromboembolism. *Clin Res*. 1978;26:135A.
   Well-designed study that proposes guidelines for heparin use that differ from those in references 2 and 20.
8. Fedullo PF, et al. 111-Indium labelled platelets: effect of heparin on uptake by venous thrombi and relationship to the activated partial thromboplastin time. *Circulation*. 1982;66:632.
   In dogs, maintaining an APTT above 1 1/2 times the control does prevent venous thrombus growth, as measured by prevention of platelet accretion to the thrombus.
9. Fihn SD, et al. Risk factors for complications of chronic anticoagulation. *Ann Intern Med*. 1993;118:511.
   By closely monitoring the prothrombin time ratio, safety and efficacy of chronic anticoagulation can be enhanced. Bleeding risk is highest during the first several months of therapy.
10. Hirsh J. Oral anticoagulant drugs. *N Engl J Med*. 1991;324:1865.
11. Hirsh J. Heparin. *N Engl J Med*. 1991;321:1565.
    References 10 and 11 provide detailed reviews of the actions, therapeutic uses, and new developments with regard to heparin and oral anticoagulant drugs.
12. Hommes DW, et al. Subcutaneous heparin compared with continuous intravenous heparin administration in the initial treatment of deep vein thrombosis: a meta-analysis. *Ann Intern Med*. 1992;116:279.
    This meta-analysis concluded that subcutaneous heparin, with or without monitoring, was a bit more effective and safer than monitored, continuous intravenous therapy.
13. Huisman MV, et al. Unexpected high prevalence of pulmonary embolism in patients with deep venous thrombosis. *Chest*. 1989;95:498.
    When treating DVT, one is often treating PE as well; in this series, 51% of patients with DVT—with no symptoms of embolism—had a "high probability" lung scan.
14. Hull R, et al. Adjusted subcutaneous heparin versus warfarin sodium in the long-term treatment of venous thrombosis. *N Engl J Med*. 1982;306:189.
    Efficacy and safety are quite similar with an upward adjustment in heparin dose and a downward adjustment in warfarin "range."
15. Marder VJ. The use of thrombolytic agents: choice of patient, drug administration, laboratory monitoring. *Ann Intern Med*. 1979;90:802.
    An informative review written by a proponent of this form of therapy.
16. Moser KM. Venous thromboembolism: state of the art. *Am Rev Respir Dis*. 1990; 141:235.
    A detailed review of many aspects of the subject.
17. Nelson PH, et al. Risk of complications during intravenous heparin therapy. *West J Med*. 1982;136:189.
    A study and review indicating that coexistent disease, not heparin dose, is the major determinant of hemorrhagic risk.
18. Research Committee of the British Thoracic Society. Optimal duration of anticoagulation for deep vein thrombosis and pulmonary embolism. *Lancet*. 1992;340:873.
    Although arbitrary durations can be suggested, as in this study, establishing specific criteria for individual patients is a preferable approach.

19. Rosenberg RD. Heparin action. *Circulation*. 1974;49:603.
    An excellent comment on how heparin works.
20. Salzman EW, et al. Management of heparin therapy: a controlled prospective study. *N Engl J Med*. 1975;292:1046.
    Well-designed study that reaches conclusions differing from those in references 2 and 7.
21. Hull R, et al. Different intensities of anticoagulation in the long-term treatment of proximal venous thrombosis. *N Engl J Med*. 1982;307:1676.
22. Hull R, et al. Adjusted subcutaneous heparin versus warfarin sodium in the long-term treatment of venous thrombosis. *N Engl J Med*. 1982;306:189.
23. Huisman MV, et al. Utility of impedance plethysmography in the diagnosis of recurrent deep-vein thrombosis. *Arch Intern Med*. 1988;148:681.
    The IPG test can be used effectively to determine whether DVT has recurred and, therefore, additional treatment is necessary. In 67% of patients with proximal DVT, IPG reverts to negative at 3 months; 85% at 6 months; 95% at 12 months.
24. Kirchmaier CM, Wolf H, Scheafer H, et al. Efficacy of a low molecular weight heparin administered intravenously or subcutaneously in comparison with intravenous unfractionated heparin in the treatment of deep venous thrombosis. Certoparin-Study Group. *Int Angiol*. 1998;17:135–145.
25. Meyer G, Brenot F, Pacouret G, et al. Subcutaneous low-molecular-weight heparin fragmin versus intravenous unfractionated heparin in the treatment of acute non massive pulmonary embolism: an open randomized pilot study. *Thromb Haemost*. 1995;74:1432–1435.
26. Fiessinger JN, Lopez-Fernandez M, Gatterer E, et al. Once-daily subcutaneous dalteparin, a low molecular weight heparin, for the initial treatment of acute deep vein thrombosis. *Thromb Haemost*. 1996;76:195–199
27. Lindmarker P, Holmstrom M. Use of low molecular weight heparin (dalteparin), once daily, for the treatment of deep vein thrombosis. A feasibility and health economic study in an outpatient setting. Swedish Venous Thrombosis Dalteparin Trial Group. *J Intern Med*. 1996;240:395–401.
28. Luomanmeaki K, Grankvist S, Hallert C, et al. A multicentre comparison of once-daily subcutaneous dalteparin (low molecular weight heparin) and continuous intravenous heparin in the treatment of deep vein thrombosis. *J Intern Med*. 1996;240:85–92.
29. de Valk HW, Banga JD, Wester JW, et al. Comparing subcutaneous danaparoid with intravenous unfractionated heparin for the treatment of venous thromboembolism. A randomized controlled trial [see comments]. *Ann Intern Med*. 1995;123:1–9.
30. Levine M, Gent M, Hirsh J, et al. A comparison of low-molecular-weight heparin administered primarily at home with unfractionated heparin administered in the hospital for proximal deep vein thrombosis. *N Engl J Med*. 1996;334:677–681.
31. Hull RD, Raskob GE, Pineo GF, et al. Subcutaneous low-molecular-weight heparin compared with continuous intravenous heparin in the treatment of proximal-vein thrombosis [see comments]. *N Engl J Med*. 1992;326:975–982.
32. Prandoni P, Lensing AW, Beuller HR, et al. Comparison of subcutaneous low-molecular-weight heparin with intravenous standard heparin in proximal deep-vein thrombosis. *Lancet*. 1992;339:441–445.
33. Koopman M, Prandoni P, Piovella F. Treatment of venous thrombosis with intravenous unfractionated heparin administered in the hospital as compared with subcutaneous low-molecular-weight heparin administered at home. *N Engl J Med*. 1996;334:682–687.
34. Lopaciuk S, Meissner AJ, Filipecki S, et al. Subcutaneous low molecular weight heparin versus subcutaneous unfractionated heparin in the treatment of deep vein thrombosis: a Polish multicenter trial. *Thromb Haemost*. 1992;68:14–18.
35. Simonneau G, Sors H, Charbonnier B, et al. A comparison of low-molecular-weight heparin with unfractionated heparin for acute pulmonary embolism. The THESEE Study Group. Tinzaparine ou Heparine Standard: Evaluations dans l'Embolie Pulmonaire. *N Engl J Med*. 1997;337:663–669.

References 24 to 35 describe randomized controlled trials of subcutaneous LMWHs to intravenous unfractionated heparin for the treatment of DVT and/or PE. Taken as a whole, the trials demonstrate no differences in efficacy, safety or complications (i.e., thrombocytopenia) between the two types of regimens.

36. Buller HR, Davidson BL, Decousus H, et al. Subcutaneous fondaparinux versus intravenous unfractionated heparin in the initial treatment of pulmonary embolism. *N Engl J Med.* 2003;349:1695–1702.

37. Buller HR, Davidson BL, Decousus H, et al. Fondaparinux or enoxaparin for the initial treatment of symptomatic deep venous thrombosis: A randomized trial. *Ann Intern Med.* 2004;140:867–873.

References 36 and 37 show that the synthetic anticoagulant fondaparinux is comparable (but not superior) in safety and efficacy to heparin and LMWH for the treatment of stable PE and DVT, respectively.

38. Dalen JE, Alpert JS, Hirsh J. Thrombolytic therapy for pulmonary embolism: is it effective? Is it safe? When is it indicated? *Arch Intern Med.* 1997;157:2550–2556.

This well-written review describes the lack of data supporting improved outcome for patients with PE treated with thrombolytics. In addition, the increased incidence of intracranial bleeding with thrombolytics argues against their routine use in PE patients.

67. CHRONIC THROMBOEMBOLIC PULMONARY HYPERTENSION

William Auger and Peter F. Fedullo

Chronic thromboembolic pulmonary hypertension (CTEPH) is an aberrant outcome that occurs in a minority of patients following an acute episode of pulmonary embolism (PE). However, CTEPH may be more prevalent than previously thought. A recent study demonstrated a cumulative incidence of symptomatic CTEPH of 3.8% over the first 2 years in patients surviving an acute PE, far greater than the previous estimates of 0.1 to 0.3%.

The pathophysiologic events leading to CTEPH are not entirely understood. In most cases of acute PE, there is either minimal and clinically insignificant residua or total resolution of pulmonary hemodynamics, gas exchange, and exercise tolerance. Incomplete thrombus resolution and hemodynamic recovery following an acute thromboembolic event, even with appropriate antithrombotic therapy, can occur in some patients, placing them at risk for developing CTEPH. It is also apparent that many patients with CTEPH have had asymptomatic or misdiagnosed acute PE event(s). Because appropriate antithrombotic therapy was not initiated at the time of the initial embolic event, it is possible that endogenous fibrinolytic mechanisms were overcome by the age, extent, or location of the obstructing embolus. Recent data confirm that venous thrombosis and PE are frequently overlooked in the population at large.

Despite extensive investigation, identifying a thrombophilic tendency or a defect in fibrinolytic activity has been elusive in most patients with established chronic thromboembolic disease. The presence of a lupus anticoagulant or anticardiolipin antibodies can be established in 10 to 24% of CTEPH patients. Hereditary thrombophilias such as protein C, protein S, and antithrombin III deficiencies cumulatively appear in less than 5% of patients, whereas factor V_{Leiden} can be seen in 4.0 to 6.5% of individuals with chronic thromboembolic disease. The incidence of other thrombophilic tendencies, such as the prothrombin gene mutation 20210 G/A, elevated factor VIII levels, and hyperhomocysteinemia have not been adequately established in this patient population.

The diagnosis of CTEPH usually is not made until the degree of pulmonary hypertension is advanced. As a result, the exact hemodynamic evolution of the disease has not been established. The symptomatic history has been well described. A patient may carry on relatively normal activities following a pulmonary embolic event, whether clinically apparent or occult, and even when extensive pulmonary vascular occlusion has occurred. Following an asymptomatic period, which may range from months to years, exertional dyspnea worsens and hypoxemia, and right ventricular failure ensue. The basis for this asymptomatic ("honeymoon") period followed by gradual hemodynamic and symptomatic decline has only recently been elucidated.

The progressive nature of the pulmonary hypertension in the majority of patients with chronic thromboembolic disease does not appear to be the result of recurrent embolic events or in situ thrombosis, as initially postulated. The majority of patients with sequential perfusion scans experience symptomatic and hemodynamic decline in the absence of new perfusion defects. As experience with the diagnosis and surgical management of this disease process has evolved, it has become increasingly apparent that the increase in pulmonary artery pressures arises from two different sources: a decrease in the cross-sectional area of the pulmonary vascular bed associated with the unresolved thromboembolic component of the disease; and the development over time of a distal, small-vessel arteriopathy pathologically indistinct from that seen in a wide range of pulmonary hypertensive disorders. It appears that these secondary pulmonary hypertensive changes, perhaps induced by high pulmonary artery pressures or flows, result in an incremental increase in right ventricular afterload, progressive pulmonary hypertension, and, ultimately, right ventricular failure.

Progressive dyspnea is a complaint common to all patients with CTEPH. The subjective complaint of dyspnea must be considered in context of the patient's usual lifestyle. The sensation of dyspnea and development of exercise intolerance are more troubling and lead to earlier evaluation in patients who are normally active than in those who live a sedentary lifestyle. Later in the course of the disease, exertional chest pain, near-syncope or syncope, and lower extremity edema may develop.

Although a history of documented thromboembolism may be absent, many patients provide a history consistent with an acute embolic event such as an episode of "pleurisy," lower extremity "muscle strain," or prolonged, atypical "pneumonia." Alternatively, they may describe a hospitalization or surgical procedure from which they never fully recovered.

Diagnostic delay commonly occurs, particularly in the absence of an acute history of venous thromboembolism. Progressive dyspnea and exercise intolerance from CTEPH are often erroneously attributed to coronary artery disease, cardiomyopathy, interstitial lung disease, asthma, deconditioning, or psychogenic dyspnea. Prior to consideration of a pulmonary vascular problem as a basis for their complaints, many patients with CTEPH have undergone one or more left-sided cardiac catheterizations and coronary angiograms. Others have undergone lung biopsy. Still others have been advised to enroll in an exercise program or to seek psychiatric help. Unfortunately, the period of diagnostic delay does not appear to have shortened substantially over the last several years, emphasizing that an evaluation of the pulmonary vascular bed should be considered in any patient with dyspnea in whom no compelling cause can be established.

Findings on physical examination may be subtle early in the course, thereby contributing to the diagnostic delay. Prior to the development of significant right ventricular hypertrophy or overt right ventricular failure, abnormalities can be limited to a widening of the second heart sound or a subtle accentuation of its pulmonic component. In time, more obvious findings of pulmonary hypertension and right ventricular dysfunction develop, which may include a right ventricular heave, jugular venous distension, prominent A and V wave venous pulsation, fixed splitting of S2, a right ventricular S4 or S3, a murmur of tricuspid regurgitation, hepatomegaly, ascites, and peripheral edema. A distinctive physical finding in certain patients with chronic thromboembolic disease is the presence of flow murmurs over the lung fields. These subtle bruits, which appear to originate from turbulent flow through partially obstructed or recanalized pulmonary arteries, are high pitched and blowing in quality, heard over the lung fields rather than the precordium, accentuated during inspiration, and frequently heard only during periods of breath-holding. Their importance lies in their not having been described in primary pulmonary hypertension, which is the most common alternative diagnostic possibility. The flow murmurs, however, are not unique to chronic thromboembolic disease and may be encountered in congenital stenotic lesions of the pulmonary vasculature, and in major-vessel pulmonary vasculitides.

The diagnostic approach is relatively straightforward once an abnormality of the pulmonary vascular bed has been considered as a basis for the patient's complaints. The goals of diagnostic evaluation are: (1) to establish the presence and degree of pulmonary hypertension; (2) to define its etiology; and (3) to determine if major vessel thromboembolic disease is present and accessible to surgical intervention. Findings on standard laboratory tests are nonspecific, dependent upon the point in the natural history of the disease at which they are obtained, and reflective of the hemodynamic and gas exchange consequences of the thromboembolic obstruction and the accompanying cardiac dysfunction. The chest radiograph is often normal although it may demonstrate one or more of the following findings that suggest the diagnosis: (1) enlargement of both main pulmonary arteries or asymmetry in the size of the central pulmonary arteries; (2) areas of hypoperfusion or hyperperfusion; (3) evidence of old pleural disease, unilaterally or bilaterally; (4) evidence of right ventricular hypertrophy. Pulmonary function testing is often within normal limits although approximately 20 percent of patients demonstrate a mild to moderate restrictive abnormality. The majority of patients have a reduction in the single breath diffusing capacity for carbon monoxide (DLCO); however, a normal value does not exclude the diagnosis. When a spirometric abnormality is present (reflecting either restrictive or obstructive disease), the degree of the abnormality is almost always less impressive than the patient's gas exchange abnormalities, symptomatic complaints, and degree of pulmonary hypertension. Although the arterial Po_2 may be within normal limits, the alveolar-arterial oxygen gradient is typically widened, and the majority of patients have a decline in the arterial Po_2 with exercise. Dead space ventilation ($\dot{V}_D/\dot{V}_T$) is often increased at rest and worsens with exercise. Echocardiography commonly provides the initial objective evidence for pulmonary hypertension. Findings include evidence of right atrial and right ventricular enlargement, abnormal septal position and motion related to the right ventricular pressure and volume overload, and evidence of pulmonary hypertension as determined from the tricuspid regurgitant jet.

Once the diagnosis of pulmonary hypertension has been established, it is essential to determine whether it originates from abnormalities of the small, resistance vessels or from central, chronic thromboembolic obstruction, characteristic of CTEPH. Ventilation–perfusion lung scanning provides an excellent noninvasive means of distinguishing between potentially operable major-vessel thromboembolic pulmonary hypertension and small-vessel pulmonary hypertension. In chronic thromboembolic disease, at least one (and more commonly, several) segmental or larger mismatched ventilation–perfusion defects are present. In primary pulmonary hypertension, perfusion scans are either normal or exhibit a "mottled" appearance characterized by subsegmental defects. However, it is important to recognize that the ventilation–perfusion scan often understates the actual *extent* of central pulmonary vascular obstruction. Channels through or partial flow around partially recannalized or organized central obstructing lesions allow the radioisotopic agent to reach the periphery of the lung. Depending on the distribution of flow, these areas may appear normal or as relatively hypoperfused "grey zones." Ventilation–perfusion scanning, therefore, is capable of suggesting the potential presence of chronic thromboembolic obstruction, but it is unable to determine the magnitude, location, or proximal extent of the disease, information critical to the question of surgical accessibility.

Right-heart catheterization and pulmonary angiography are essential to determine the degree of pulmonary hypertension, to exclude competing diagnoses, and to define the surgical accessibility of the obstructing thrombotic lesions. If hemodynamic measurements at rest demonstrate only modest degrees of pulmonary hypertension, measurements should be obtained following a short period of exercise. In patients with chronic thromboembolic obstruction sufficient to abolish normal compensatory mechanisms, exercise-related increases in cardiac output will be accompanied by an excessive elevation in pulmonary artery pressure.

The angiographic findings in chronic thromboembolic disease bear little resemblance to the sharply defined, intraluminal defects diagnostic of acute embolism. Five distinct angiographic patterns have been described that correlate with the finding of organized thromboembolic material at the time of thromboendarterectomy: (1) defects with a pouch configuration; (2) pulmonary artery webs or bands; (3) intimal irregularities; (4) abrupt narrowing of the major pulmonary arteries; (5) obstruction of lobar or segmental vessels at their point of origin, with complete absence of blood flow to pulmonary segments normally perfused by those vessels. In experienced hands, pulmonary angiography can be safely performed even in patients with severe pulmonary hypertension. The use of nonionic contrast media, provision of supplemental oxygen to avoid hypoxemia, and minimizing contrast volume with separate proximal pulmonary artery injections (i.e., avoiding right ventricular injections) are some of the technical safeguards necessary to prevent adverse outcomes in the evaluation of this patient population.

Pulmonary angioscopy can play a valuable role in confirming the presence of chronic thromboembolic obstruction and in determining whether it is accessible to surgical intervention. The pulmonary angioscope is a fiberoptic device which allows visualization of the pulmonary arteries to the segmental level. The normal pulmonary artery has a round or oval contour with a smooth, pale, glistening appearance to the intima, and with bright red blood filling the lumen. The features of organized chronic emboli consist of roughening or pitting of the intimal surface, bands and webs across the lumen, pitted masses of chronic embolic material within the lumen, and partial recanalization.

Currently, pulmonary angiography and angioscopy remain the cornerstone procedures for the diagnosis of CTEPH and in confirming the surgical accessibility of the obstructing lesions. Computed tomography can be useful in the evaluation of competing diagnostic possibilities such as pulmonary artery sarcoma, fibrosing mediastinitis, and extrinsic vascular compression related to malignancies or inflammatory disease. Large vessel pulmonary arteritis can also mimic certain of the angiographic findings of chronic thromboembolic disease. Arch aortography may be useful if this diagnosis is being considered.

A variety of abnormalities may be appreciated on helical computed tomography (CT) scans obtained in patients with CTEPH, including right ventricular enlargement, chronic thromboembolic material within dilated central pulmonary arteries, bronchial artery collateral flow, and mosaic attenuation of the pulmonary parenchyma. The detection of central disease by CT scanning does not necessarily imply that the patient represents an operative candidate. A syndrome of primary pulmonary hypertension with secondary, central pulmonary artery thrombosis has been described, a situation in which surgical intervention is contraindicated. Furthermore, CT scanning lacks sensitivity in detecting chronic thromboemboli at the segmental level as well as chronic thrombus which is well-endothelialized rather than intraluminal. Both segmental-level disease and endothelialized disease are amenable to surgical intervention. Until more information regarding helical CT scanning is available in this patient population, it should be considered an adjunctive study that may provide information additive to that obtained by angiography/angioscopy.

Several other essential issues must be considered prior to surgery. In our view, it is important that the patient be protected against embolic recurrence, both during the high-risk perioperative period and over the long term. Therefore, an inferior vena caval filter is routinely placed prior to surgery unless an obvious non-leg or non-pelvic source of embolism is present. For those patients at risk of coronary artery disease, coronary angiography is routinely performed prior to surgery, usually at the time of the right heart catheterization and pulmonary angiography. Coronary artery bypass grafting, if necessary, can be performed at the time of the thromboendarterectomy.

The decision to proceed to pulmonary thromboendarterectomy in patients suffering from CTEPH is based upon both objective and subjective factors, which are carefully defined during the preoperative evaluation. The first and most important criterion for potential surgical intervention is the accessibility of the thrombi, as defined by angiography and angioscopy. Present surgical techniques allow removal of chronic thrombi whose proximal location extends to the main, lobar, and segmental arteries. Those that begin more distally are not typically subject to endarterectomy. Failure to remove sufficient embolic material to lower pulmonary vascular resistance, especially in patients with severe pulmonary hypertension and right ventricular dysfunction, may result in inability to wean the patient from cardiopulmonary bypass at the time of thromboendarterectomy and, if the patient does survive, is associated with a negative long-term outcome. The second criterion involves the presence of hemodynamic or ventilatory impairment as a consequence of the chronic thromboembolic pulmonary vascular obstruction. The majority of operated patients have a pulmonary vascular resistance in excess of 300 dynes/sec/cm^5, at rest or with exercise. Occasional patients, especially those with involvement of one main pulmonary artery, have significant exercise impairment due to high minute ventilatory demands, without substantially altered pulmonary hemodynamics. The third criterion involves the presence and severity of comorbid conditions, such as severe parenchymal lung disease, which may adversely affect outcome. Although the presence of other disease processes does not represent an absolute contraindication to the procedure, the risks imposed by any coexistent condition and its potential effect on long-term outcome are carefully reviewed with the patient before a surgical decision is made. Age by itself is not a contraindication to the procedure. Patients up to 84 years of age, if they are otherwise fit, have successfully undergone a pulmonary thromboendarterectomy

The surgical option is also considered in patients with only moderate degrees of pulmonary hypertension at rest but who develop striking levels of pulmonary hypertension with minimal exercise. Because this hemodynamic response reproduces events during the patient's activities of daily living, it may reflect the true work load of the right ventricle. Furthermore, given what is now suspected about the pathophysiologic mechanisms of the disease, it is possible that the exercise-related augmentation of pressure and flow over a sufficient period of time will result in progressive levels of pulmonary hypertension.

Although a thoracotomy approach to CTEPH has been utilized in the past, sternotomy with cardiopulmonary bypass and periods of circulatory arrest currently represent the procedure of choice. The most critical need for sternotomy arises from the bilateral nature of the disease process. Sternotomy allows access to both pulmonary arteries and assures more complete removal of the chronically obstructing material. The use of cardiopulmonary bypass allows periods of complete circulatory arrest, which provides the bloodless operative field essential for meticulous lobar and segmental dissections. Finally, the presence of bronchial artery collateral flow and pleural adhesions makes a transthoracic approach difficult.

It should be emphasized that thromboendarterectomy bears no resemblance to acute pulmonary embolectomy. The neointima in chronic thromboembolic disease is deceptive and often is not easily recognizable as chronic thrombi. The procedure is a true endarterectomy, requiring careful dissection of chronic endothelialized material from the native intima to restore pulmonary arterial patency. Establishing the correct plane is essential and requires a considerable degree of surgical experience and expertise. Too deep a plane will result in perforation of the vessel; too superficial a plane will not result in an adequate endarterectomy.

Periods of circulatory arrest are limited to 20-minute intervals. With experience, the entire unilateral endarterectomy usually can be accomplished within this time. If additional arrest time is necessary to complete the thromboendarterectomy, reperfusion is carried out until the venous saturations reach 90 percent, or for a minimum of 10 minutes. At the completion of the bilateral endarterectomy, circulation is reestablished and the patient rewarmed. The atrial septum is routinely inspected, since an atrial septal defect or persistent foramen ovale is seen (and subsequently repaired) in approximately 25 percent of cases. If additional procedures are required, such as coronary bypass grafting or valve replacement, they are performed during the rewarming period.

Careful postoperative management is essential for a successful outcome following pulmonary thromboendarterectomy. Although pulmonary hemodynamics immediately improve in the majority of patients, the postoperative course can be complex. In addition to complications common to other forms of cardiac surgery (arrhythmias, atelectasis, wound infection, pericardial effusions, delirium), patients undergoing pulmonary thromboendarterectomy often experience three unique postoperative conditions capable of significantly impairing gas exchange and hemodynamic stability: pulmonary artery "steal," reperfusion pulmonary edema, and persistent pulmonary hypertension.

Pulmonary artery "steal" represents a postoperative redistribution of pulmonary arterial blood flow away from previously well perfused segments and into the newly endarterectomized segments. Although the basis for this phenomenon remains speculative, it is likely related to the temporary development of differential resistances and the loss of normal vasoregulation in the pulmonary vascular bed following thromboendarterectomy. Long-term follow up has demonstrated that pulmonary vascular steal resolves in the majority of patients.

Reperfusion pulmonary edema appears to represent a form of high-permeability lung injury (acute respiratory distress syndrome) which is limited to those areas of lung from which proximal thromboembolic obstructions have been removed. It may appear up to 72 hours after surgery and is highly variable in severity, ranging from a mild form of edema resulting in postoperative hypoxemia to an acute, hemorrhagic and fatal complication. When associated with pulmonary artery steal, reperfusion pulmonary edema can represent a significant challenge in terms of postoperative gas exchange since pulmonary blood flow is directed toward edematous, noncompliant areas of lung, which contribute poorly to gas exchange.

Management of reperfusion edema, as with other forms of acute lung injury, is supportive until resolution occurs. As is the case in patients with ARDS, low volume ventilatory strategies are routinely practiced. The judicious use of inverse ratio ventilation has proven useful in improving ventilation/perfusion relationships and gas exchange when conventional ventilatory support has failed. Nitric oxide, delivered at a concentration of 20 ppm, has also proven beneficial in improving gas exchange although its effect on mortality remains unclear. Finally, extracorporeal support has been utilized successfully when conventional measures have failed.

Patients posing the most difficult management problem in the postoperative period are those with persistent pulmonary hypertension following thromboendarterectomy. This outcome is the result of either distal, surgically inaccessible thromboembolic disease or to a secondary, small vessel arteriopathy and is associated with a poor short-term and long-term outcome. Unless right ventricular afterload is substantially reduced at the time of surgery, even patients with well compensated right ventricular function prior to the procedure may experience postoperative hemodynamic instability and a low output state as a result of the depressant effects of cardiopulmonary bypass, deep hypothermia, acidosis and hypoxemia.

The initial step in management of these patients should occur in the operating room. In patients with severe pulmonary hypertension in whom an inadequate thromboendarterectomy is achieved, a patent foramen ovale, if present, is not closed. In patients in whom difficulty is encountered upon attempted discontinuation of cardiopulmonary bypass due to right ventricular failure, enlargement of an existing patent foramen ovale or creation of an atrial sepal communication may prove valuable. The potential benefits of such an intervention include a decrease in right atrial pressure, an increase in cardiac output and systemic oxygen transport, and improved right coronary artery perfusion. Of course, such an intervention is an irrevocable one associated with severe postoperative hypoxemia and should only be attempted when weaning from cardiopulmonary bypass cannot be achieved in the setting of maximal pharmacological support and when other potentially reversible conditions (hypothermia, electrolyte imbalance) responsible for the right ventricular dysfunction have been addressed.

The early intensive care management goals for the patient with persistent pulmonary hypertension and right ventricular failure following attempted thromboendarterectomy should be directed toward minimizing systemic oxygen consumption, optimizing right ventricular preload, and providing aggressive inotropic support. The use of afterload reduction in this patient population is fraught with difficulty. Pulmonary vascular resistance is commonly fixed and attempts at pharmacologic manipulation of right ventricular afterload (sodium nitroprusside, calcium channel blockers, epoprostenol) may simply decrease systemic blood pressure and right coronary artery perfusion pressure. Inhaled nitric oxide at a concentration of 20 to 40 ppm is theoretically ideal for this circumstance since it has negligible systemic effects. Experience with this intervention in the setting of persistent postoperative pulmonary hypertension, however, has been disappointing.

At the University of California—San Diego Medical Center, the operative and perioperative mortality rate in the 196 patients who underwent pulmonary thromboendarterectomy prior to 1990 was 15.8 percent. During development and early experience with this procedure, mortality was related to many causes. Since 1990, however, with greater clinical experience and with changes in operative techniques, perioperative mortality rates have steadily declined. Between 1994 and 1998, in-hospital mortality in the 500 patients operated during this time period was 8.8%, declining further to 4.4% for the 500 patients operated on between 1998 and 2002. During this latter time frame, the major causes of death were related to reperfusion pulmonary edema and to residual postoperative pulmonary hypertension and right ventricular failure when pulmonary thromboendarterectomy failed to achieve substantial improvement in pulmonary hemodynamics. Other centers involved with this procedure have experienced the same learning curve. The need for a coordinated, multidisciplinary team to manage the care of these patients cannot be emphasized too strongly. Experience and expertise in the evaluative, surgical, and postoperative aspects of care are essential to minimize the substantial morbidity and mortality associated with the surgical correction of this disease state.

Among survivors of thromboendarterectomy, the immediate hemodynamic improvement observed has been dramatic, with marked reductions in pulmonary artery pressures and pulmonary vascular resistance. Echocardiography demonstrates a decrease in right atrial and right ventricular chamber size, normalization of the interventricular septum, and improvement or resolution of tricuspid regurgitation. This improvement is reflected in the patient's postoperative physical examination and symptomatic status.

The long-term hemodynamic and symptomatic outcomes have been equally dramatic. Symptomatic improvement continues for periods as long as nine to 12 months following surgery. This long-term improvement probably involves resolution of the patients' postoperative anemia and deconditioned state as well as an improvement in the ventilation/perfusion balance as the postoperative pulmonary artery steal resolves. In addition, resolution of the pulmonary hypertensive changes within the pulmonary vascular bed, suggested by preliminary scan and angiographic data, further reduces right ventricular afterload. The majority of patients, who were initially in NYHA Class III or IV status preoperatively return to NYHA Class I or II status and are able to resume normal activities. One follow-up of 308 patients surveyed a mean of 3.3 years after surgery found that 62 percent of patients who were unemployed prior to thromboendarterectomy had returned to work.

Pulmonary thromboendarterectomy is helpful, but not "curative" in approximately 5 to 10 percent of patients undergoing the procedure. This group includes patients whose disease involves a substantial component of distal, surgically inaccessible thromboemboli and patients who have developed severe, irreversible secondary pulmonary hypertensive changes in their distal pulmonary vascular bed. In certain carefully selected patients with a significant component of surgically inaccessible disease, thromboendarterectomy is capable of improving pulmonary hemodynamics, functional status, and survivorship. The use of primary pulmonary vasodilators, such as epoprostenol and endothelin antagonists, as well as lung transplantation remain viable options for those patients in whom significant pulmonary hypertension persists following attempted endarterectomy.

All patients are maintained on lifelong anticoagulation with warfarin. Thromboembolic recurrence has not occurred in any patient maintained on therapeutic levels of anticoagulation although it has occurred in several patients in whom anticoagulation was discontinued or was allowed to fall to a subtherapeutic level.

In summary, experience over the past 20 years has demonstrated that CTEPH represents a potentially treatable form of pulmonary hypertension, and that pulmonary thromboendarterectomy, when performed at a center experienced in the management of these patients, is capable of restoring severely compromised patients to a near-normal or normal hemodynamic and symptomatic status.

---

1. Auger WR, Kerr KM, Kim NHS, et al. Chronic thromboembolic pulmonary hypertension. *Cardiol Clin*. 2004;22:453–466.
   Comprehensive review of chronic thromboembolic disease, and its evaluation and management.
2. Pengo V, Lensing AWA, Prins MH, et al. Incidence of chronic thromboembolic pulmonary hypertension after pulmonary embolism. *N Engl J Med*. 2004;350:2257–2264.
   The 2-year cumulative incidence of CTEPH was 3.8% in 223 pulmonary embolic survivors.
3. Benotti JR, Dalen JE. The natural history of pulmonary embolism. *Clin Chest Med*. 1984;5:403–410.
   Concise discussion of the natural history of PE.
4. Wartski M, Collignon M-A. Incomplete recovery of lung perfusion after 3 months in patients with acute pulmonary embolism treated with antithrombotic agents. *J Nucl Med*. 2000;41:1043–1048.
   Residual perfusion scan abnormalities after 3 months were observed in 66% of patients experiencing an acute embolic event, with 8% of patients having defects greater than 50% of the total pulmonary vascular bed.
5. Meignan M, Rosso J, Gauthier H, et al. Systematic lung scans reveal a high frequency of silent pulmonary embolism in patients with proximal deep venous thrombosis. *Arch Intern Med*. 2000;160:159–164.
   Regardless of the interpretive criteria used for assessing lung scans, the frequency of silent PE is 40 to 50% in patients with deep venous thrombosis.
6. Riedel M, Stanek V, Widimsky, Prerovsky I. Longterm follow-up of patients with pulmonary thromboembolism. Late prognosis and evolution of hemodynamic and respiratory data. *Chest*. 1982;81:151–158.
   Pulmonary hypertension occurred most frequently in patients with occult embolism. Pulmonary hypertension progressed further in patients with mean pulmonary artery pressure greater than 30 mm Hg.
7. Wolf M, Soyer-Neumann C, Parent F, et al. Thrombotic risk factors in pulmonary hypertension. *Eur Resp J*. 2000;15:395–399.
   Incidence of prothrombotic tendencies in CTEPH patients.
8. Auger WR, Permpikul P, Moser KM. Lupus anticoagulant, heparin use and thrombocytopenia in patients with chronic thromboembolic pulmonary hypertension: a preliminary report. *Am J Med*. 1995;99:392–396.
   Of patients referred for thromboendarterectomy, 10.6% had a lupus anticoagulant.
9. Moser KM, Bloor CM. Pulmonary vascular lesions occurring in patients with chronic major vessel thromboembolic pulmonary hypertension. *Chest*. 1993; 103:685–692.
   A description of the small-vessel changes that occur in patients with CTEPH.
10. Morris TA, Auger WR, Ysrael MZ, et al. Parenchymal scarring is associated with restrictive spirometric defects in patients with chronic thromboembolic pulmonary hypertension. *Chest*. 1996;110:399–403.
    Of patients referred for thromboendarterectomy, 22% had a restrictive ventilatory pattern. The presence of parenchymal scarring was highly associated with lung restriction.
11. Fishmann AJ, Moser KM, Fedullo PF. Perfusion lung scans vs pulmonary angiography in evaluation of suspected primary pulmonary hypertension. *Chest*. 1983;84:679–683.
    The presence of one or more segmental defects was present in patients with CTEPH. No patient with primary pulmonary hypertension had segmental or larger defects.

12. Ryan KL, Fedullo PF, Davis GB, et al. Perfusion scan findings understate the severity of angiographic and hemodynamic compromise in chronic thromboembolic pulmonary hypertension. *Chest.* 1988;93:1180–1185.

   Perfusion scans consistently understated the degree of pulmonary artery obstruction as defined by pulmonary angiography.

13. Nicod P, Peterson K, Levine M, et al. Pulmonary angiography in severe chronic pulmonary hypertension. *Ann Intern Med.* 1987;107:565–568.

   Pulmonary angiography can be performed safely in patients with severe pulmonary hypertension secondary to chronic thromboembolic disease.

14. Auger WR, Fedullo PF, Moser KM, et al. Chronic major-vessel thromboembolic pulmonary artery obstruction: appearance at angiography. *Radiology.* 1992; 182:393–398.

   A discussion of the angiographic patterns encountered in CTEPH.

15. Shure D, Gregoratos G, Moser KM. Fiberoptic angioscopy: role in the diagnosis of chronic pulmonary arterial obstruction. *Ann Intern Med.* 1985;103:844–850.

   A description of pulmonary angioscopy.

16. Bergin CJ, Sirlin CB, Hauschildt JP, et al. Chronic thromboembolism: diagnosis with helical CT and MR imaging with angiographic and surgical correlation. *Radiology.* 1997;204:695–702.

   Computerized chest CT findings in chronic thromboembolic disease. The yield of CT scanning was higher than that of MR imaging. Neither CT or MR imaging was as accurate as angiography.

17. Moser KM, Fedullo PF, Finkbeiner WE, et al. Do patients with primary pulmonary hypertension develop extensive central thrombi. *Circulation.* 1995;91:741–745.

   Three pulmonary hypertensive patients with massive central thrombi are described.

18. Kerr KM, Auger WR, Fedullo PF, et al. Large vessel pulmonary arteritis mimicking thromboembolic disease. *Am J Respir Crit Care Med.* 1995;152:367–373.

   Case report of four patients with Takayasu's arteritis affecting the major pulmonary arteries.

19. Moser KM, Daily PO, Peterson K, et al. Thromboendarterectomy for chronic major-vessel thromboembolic pulmonary hypertension. Immediate and long-term results in 42 patients. *Ann Intern Med.* 1987;107:560–565.

   Landmark publication describing the short- and long-term outcomes in 42 patients undergoing pulmonary thromboendarterectomy.

20. Jamieson SW, Kapelanski DP, Sakakibara N, et al. Pulmonary thromboendarterectomy: experience and lessons learned in 1,500 cases. *Ann Thorac Surg.* 2003;76:1457–1464.

   Discussion of the updated surgical approach and outcome in 1500 patients undergoing thromboendarterectomy.

21. Thistlethwaite PA, Auger WR, Madani MM, et al. Pulmonary thromboendarterectomy combined with other cardiac operations: Indications, surgical approach, and outcome. *Ann Thorac Surg.* 2001;72:13–19.

   Report of 90 patients safely undergoing other cardiac surgical procedures at the time of their pulmonary thromboendarterectomy.

22. Olman MA, Auger WR, Fedullo PF, et al. Pulmonary vascular steal in chronic thromboembolic pulmonary hypertension. *Chest.* 1990;98:1430–1434.

   A description of the pulmonary artery steal phenomenon occurring after thromboendarterectomy.

23. Moser KM, Metersky ML, Auger WR, et al. Resolution of vascular steal after pulmonary thromboendarterectomy. *Chest.* 1993;104:1441–1444.

   Pulmonary artery steal occurred in 79% of patients undergoing thromboendarterectomy; 96% demonstrated complete or partial resolution within 11 months of surgery.

24. Levinson R, Shure D, Moser KM. Reperfusion pulmonary edema after pulmonary artery thromboendarterectomy. *Am Rev Respir Dis.* 1986;134:1241–1245.

   A description of reperfusion pulmonary edema occurring after thromboendarterectomy.

25. Dittrich HC, Nicod PH, Chow LC, et al. Early changes of right heart geometry after pulmonary thromboendarterectomy. *J Am Coll Cardiol.* 1988;11:937–943.
    Echocardiographic findings obtained on 30 patients within 6 days of thromboendarterectomy.
26. Hartz RS, Byrne JG, Levitsky S, et al. Predictors of mortality in pulmonary thromboendarterectomy. *Ann Thoracic Surg.* 1996;62:1255–1259.
    At one center, patients with severe hemodynamic compromise had a substantially higher mortality following thromboendarterectomy.
27. Mayer E, Dahm M, Hake U, et al. Mid-term results of pulmonary thromboendarterectomy for chronic thromboembolic pulmonary hypertension. *Ann Thorac Surg.* 1996;61:1788–1792.
    Short- and long-term hemodynamic outcome following thromboendarterectomy.
28. Kramm T, Mayer E, Dahm M, et al. Long-term results after thromboendarterectomy for chronic pulmonary embolism. *Eur J Cardiothorac Surg.* 1999;15:579–583.
    Hemodynamic and symptomatic follow-up in 22 patients, 48 to 72 months after thromboendarterectomy demonstrating persistent improvement.
29. Archibald CJ, Auger WR, Fedullo PF, et al. Long-term outcome after pulmonary thromboendarterectomy. *Am J Respir Crit Care Med.* 1999;160:523–528.
    Long-term symptomatic, quality-of-life, and functional follow-up in 308 patients undergoing thromboendarterectomy.

68. UNUSUAL FORMS OF EMBOLISM

Peter F. Fedullo and Beat Walder

Because the lung receives all of the blood flow returned from the venous system, the pulmonary vascular bed serves as a "sieve" for all particulate substances entering the venous blood and is the first vascular bed to be exposed to any toxic substance injected intravenously. As a result of its strategic position, the pulmonary vascular bed is, therefore, exposed to a wide variety of potentially obstructing and injurious agents.

SCHISTOSOMIASIS

The most common agent to obstruct the pulmonary vascular system worldwide is schistosomiasis, although it is not common within the United States, Schistosomiasis is caused by one of a variety of blood flukes, *Schistosoma haemotobium* (Africa and Middle East), *Schistosoma japonicum* (Japan, China, Philippines), *Schistosoma mansoni* (Africa, Arabia, South America), *Schistosoma mekongi* (Laos, Thailand), and *Schistosoma intercalatum* (Africa) being among the most common. Limited data suggest that cardiopulmonary schistosomiasis is seen most often in *S. mansoni* and *S. Japonicum* infection.

Infection occurs after contact with water containing the infective stage of the parasite, the cercaria. The cercaria penetrate unbroken skin and subcutaneous tissue and migrate through the lungs and then to the portal vein, probably by an intravascular route. The maturing schistosomes pair in the portal vein and then migrate to the venules of the mesentery, bladder, or ureters and begin to deposit eggs, many of which are subsequently swept back to the liver. During acute infection (Katayama fever), nonspecific influenza-like symptoms, abdominal pain, lymphadenopathy, hepatosplenomegaly, and blood eosinophilia associated with fleeting chest radiographic abnormalities can occur.

Pulmonary hypertension occurs in fewer than 5% of infected patients. Cor pulmonale related to schistosomal infection usually does not occur in the absence of concomitant liver schistosomal liver disease, because the liver is usually quite extensively involved before the lung is affected. Pulmonary vascular obstruction appears to be induced by two mechanisms: anatomic obstruction by the organism itself and an intense, granulomatous, inflammatory vasculitic response to shunted and embolized schistosomal eggs. In endemic areas, schistosomal disease is the most common cause of cor pulmonale.

The premortem diagnosis of cardiopulmonary schistosomiasis depends on the detection of viable schistosomal ova in stool, urine, or tissue (rectal mucosa or lung) along with evidence of hepatic fibrosis and pulmonary hypertension. Currently utilized serologic tests only indicate past or present infection, although promising serologic markers capable of differentiating acute from chronic disease are being investigated. Treatment with praziquantel can effectively eradicate schistosomal infections in the acute phase of the disease with minimal toxicity. However, chronic cardiopulmonary manifestations are not likely to be reversible once fibrotic changes are present.

VENOUS AIR EMBOLISM

An increasingly common form of nonthrombotic embolism in the United States is venous air embolism. The rising frequency of the problem reflects the wide variety of invasive surgical and medical procedures now available, the broad use of indwelling central venous catheters, the use of positive-pressure ventilation with high levels of positive-end expiratory pressure, and the frequency of thoracic and other forms of trauma. The simple inadvertent transection or loss of closure of a large-bore intravenous catheter, particularly in the jugular or subclavian veins, can result in ingress of substantial quantities of air. Air bubbles enter the pulmonary vascular bed and, from there, can enter the arterial system and disseminate throughout the body by way of either an intracardiac shunt (atrial septal defect, patent foramen ovale) or, more likely, through microvascular pulmonary shunts.

Physiologic consequences include an abrupt rise in pulmonary artery pressure. Noncardiogenic pulmonary edema may develop, lung compliance falls, and hypoxemia ensues. The symptoms of venous air embolism are variable and nonspecific, and may include alterations in sensorium, chest pain, dyspnea, or a sense of impending doom. These and other consequences appear to be caused by two phenomena: actual lodgment of the bubbles in capillary beds, which interfere with nutrient supply to the affected organs, and the formation of platelet–fibrin aggregates, which create diffuse microthrombi. Thrombocytopenia may be seen as a consequence of this latter event. The most serious consequences result from cerebral or coronary artery air embolism; the severity depends on the rate and volume of air gaining access to the circulation.

The best approaches to air embolism are prevention and early detection. Treatment consists of measures designed to restore flow and to promote reabsorption of the intravascular air. In massive, life-threatening air embolism, techniques to restore flow include patient positioning (Trendelenburg position with the left side down), removal of air through central venous catheters or direct needle aspiration, and closed chest cardiac massage. Techniques to increase absorption of the air collections themselves include the use of 100% oxygen and the institution of hyperbaric oxygen therapy as early as possible. Recovery even after delayed institution of hyperbaric oxygen has been reported. Utilizing such aggressive measures, mortality from venous air embolism has been dramatically reduced.

FAT EMBOLISM

Another reasonably frequent and dramatic form of nonthrombotic embolism is fat embolism. A rather characteristic syndrome follows entry of neutral fat into the vascular system, consisting of the onset of dyspnea, hypoxemia, petechiae, and mental confusion. Seizures and focal neurologic deficits have been described. There is a variable lag time of 24 to 72 hours in the onset of the syndrome following the inciting event; rarely, cases occur within 12 hours or as late as 2 weeks after the event.

By far, the most common inciting event is traumatic fracture of long bones, with incidence rising with the number of fractures. However, orthopedic procedures and trauma to other fat-laden tissues (e.g., fatty liver) occasionally can be followed by the same syndrome. Although considerably less common, fat embolism syndrome has been reported following both liposuction and lipoinjection procedures.

The variability in incidence of the syndrome after apparently comparable injuries has not been well-defined; neither has the reason for the delay in clinical presentation been explained. The pathophysiologic consequences appear to derive from two events: (1) actual vascular obstruction by neutral particles of fat, and (2) the injurious effects of free fatty acids released by the action of lipases on the neutral fat. The latter effect is probably the more important, causing diffuse vasculitis with leakage from cerebral, pulmonary, and other vascular beds. The time necessary to produce toxic intermediaries may explain the delay from the inciting event to clinical presentation.

The diagnosis of fat embolism syndrome is a clinical one suggested by the onset of dyspnea, neurologic abnormalities, petechiae, and fever in the proper clinical context. Petechiae, typically distributed over the head, neck, anterior chest, and axillae, are present in only 20 to 50% of cases. Their absence, therefore, should not preclude consideration of the disease. No laboratory test is diagnostic of the syndrome. Fat can be demonstrated in the serum of a majority of fracture patients with evidence of fat embolism syndrome. The finding of lipid-laden cells in bronchoalveolar lavage fluid appears to occur commonly in patients with traumatic injuries irrespective of the presence of fat embolism syndrome.

Although a variety of treatments have been suggested (e.g., intravenous ethanol, albumin, dextran, heparin), none has proven effective. The role of corticosteroid therapy to prevent the onset of fat embolism syndrome after an inciting event remains controversial. Supportive treatment, including mechanical ventilatory support when necessary, is the primary approach, and survival is now the rule with meticulous support.

AMNIOTIC FLUID EMBOLISM

Another special form of embolism is amniotic fluid embolism, a rare but unpredictable and catastrophic complication of pregnancy that represents the third leading cause of maternal mortality. This disorder occurs during or after delivery when amniotic fluid gains access to uterine venous channels and, therefore, to the pulmonary and general circulations. The delivery may be either spontaneous or by cesarean section and usually has been uneventful. Most cases occur during labor, but delayed onset of symptoms up to 48 hours after delivery can occur. Advanced maternal age, multiparity, premature placental separation, fetal death, and meconium staining of amniotic fluid have been associated with increased risk of amniotic fluid embolism.

Amniotic fluid embolism syndrome is primarily a clinical diagnosis. There is, unexpectedly, sudden onset of severe respiratory distress, cyanosis, hypotension, cardiovascular collapse, and, often, disseminated intravascular coagulation. Occasionally, seizure activity occurs. It has been postulated that there is a biphasic pattern of hemodynamic disturbance: an initial period of pulmonary hypertension, commonly seen in animal models, followed by left ventricular dysfunction and cardiogenic shock. Patients who survive the first several hours develop noncardiogenic pulmonary edema coincident with improvement in left ventricular function.

Amniotic fluid contains particulate materials that can cause pulmonary vascular obstruction, but the major pathogenetic mechanism of the syndrome remains uncertain. Amniotic fluid has thromboplastic activity that leads to extensive fibrin deposition in the lung vasculature and, occasionally, in other organs. As a consequence of fibrin deposition, a severe consumptive coagulopathy develops, including marked hypofibrinogenemia and thrombocytopenia. Following the acute event, an enhanced fibrinolytic state often occurs.

The diagnosis of amniotic fluid embolism is based on a compatible clinical picture, often enhanced by finding amniotic fluid components in the pulmonary circulation. The presence of squamous cells in pulmonary arterial blood, once considered pathognomonic, has proven to be a nonspecific finding. Serologic assays and immunohistochemical staining techniques have been described as having high sensitivity for amniotic fluid embolism. Validation is required prior to being introduced into clinical practice.

Although various forms of therapy have been suggested (e.g., antifibrinolytic agents such as aminocaproic acid, cryoprecipitate), the best approach is supportive. Pulmonary artery catheterization is essential to monitor left ventricular function and volume status, and to guide the appropriate utilization of inotropic and vasoactive agents. Even in the setting of aggressive supportive measures, however, maternal mortality has approached 80%.

SEPTIC EMBOLISM

Septic embolism is another special disorder that, unfortunately, is also increasing in frequency owing to widespread intravenous drug abuse and the expanding use of indwelling intravenous catheters. Previously, septic embolism was almost exclusively a complication of septic pelvic thrombophlebitis because of both septic abortion and postpuerperal uterine infection. However, almost any venous structure can be involved, either as a focus of primary infection or from intravascular or contiguous spread. Examples include septic cavernous sinus thrombosis resulting from meningitis, sinusitis, or facial cellulitis; septic portal vein thrombosis resulting from diverticulitis or liver abscess; and septic tonsillar or internal jugular vein thrombosis (Lemierre syndrome) resulting from oropharyngeal infection. Increasingly common causes are those related to intravenous drug use and those that are iatrogenic; namely, infections secondary to indwelling catheters inserted for a variety of diagnostic or therapeutic purposes.

Microscopically, septic phlebitis consists of purulent material admixed with fibrin thrombus. When the material embolizes, it can obstruct small pulmonary vessels, but the major consequence is pulmonary infection. Characteristically, the chest radiograph displays scattered pulmonary infiltrates that undergo cavitation. More infiltrates develop over periods of hours to a few days. Symptoms and signs include a septic temperature course, dyspnea, cough, pleuritic chest pain, and hemoptysis. Initial treatment consists of appropriate antimicrobial drugs. If an indwelling catheter is the source of the infection, it should be removed. If there is not a prompt response to this regimen, surgical isolation or resection of the septic vein, if present, should be considered. The role of systemic anticoagulation remains uncertain. Endocarditis may complicate septic phlebitis, or mimic it, particularly in drug addicts.

TUMOR EMBOLISM

Involvement of the pulmonary vascular bed by tumor cells is common, as suggested by the frequency with which circulating tumor cells can be identified in patients with malignancies and the frequency with which tumor emboli are discovered as an incidental finding at autopsy. Tumor embolism becomes clinically apparent, however, in only a minority of patients with malignancy.

Microvascular tumor embolism is associated with a wide range of malignancies, the most common sites of origin being the breast, lung, prostate, stomach, and liver. Tumor embolism of large fragments occurs rarely and may mimic acute thromboembolic disease. In this setting, survival following tumor embolectomy has been reported.

The clinical presentation of microvascular tumor embolism is typically subacute and involves progressive dyspnea, tachycardia, and tachypnea. Jugular venous distention, a prominent P_2, tricuspid regurgitation, or a right-sided S_3 may be present on physical examination if the extent of pulmonary vascular obstruction is sufficient to cause pulmonary hypertension.

The development of pulmonary hypertension is a common accompaniment of symptomatic microvascular tumor embolism and remains a major cause of mortality. Pulmonary hypertension appears to result from both an obliteration of the pulmonary vascular bed by an admixture of tumor cells and thrombus as well as the development of medial hypertrophy, intimal fibrosis, and fibrinoid necrosis encountered in other variants of pulmonary hypertension.

Hypoxemia and a compensated respiratory alkalosis are common. The chest radiograph is most often normal but focal or diffuse infiltrates, which may be fleeting, have been described. Ventilation–perfusion scanning most commonly demonstrates a mottled appearance or peripheral, subsegmental defects; segmental or larger defects, indistinguishable from those associated with thromboembolic embolism, may occur in those rare instances of large-vessel involvement. Computed tomography may demonstrate peripheral, wedge-shaped defects consistent with infarcts; a pattern of multifocal dilatation and beading of the peripheral pulmonary arteries has been described. In the setting of pulmonary hypertension, echocardiographic findings reflect that diagnosis and include evidence of right atrial and right ventricular hypertrophy, abnormal septal position and motion, and a tricuspid regurgitant envelope consistent with elevated pulmonary artery pressures.

Pulmonary angiographic findings are most commonly normal. Delayed vascular filling, pruning, and tortuosity, similar to that seen in other forms of small-vessel pulmonary hypertension, may be encountered. The angiographic findings in large fragment tumor embolism may be indistinguishable from those seen in acute thromboembolic disease.

Pulmonary microvascular cytology on specimens aspirated through a wedged pulmonary artery catheter may demonstrate malignant cells. Positive cytologies, however, can also be obtained in the setting of lymphangitic carcinomatosis. It should also be emphasized that the misidentification of megakaryocytes obtained in this manner has been reported to lead to false-positive results.

Although diagnosis by transbronchial biopsy has been reported, diagnostic confirmation may require open-lung biopsy. Before proceeding to that step, however, it must be stressed that the impact of early diagnosis on outcome is uncertain. This intervention should only be considered in the setting of a primary malignancy for which effective chemotherapeutic options are available.

The differential diagnosis of tumor embolism includes thrombotic embolism, parenchymal metastasis, lymphangitic carcinomatosis, malignant pericardial effusion, and chemotherapy-related lung toxicity. The premortem diagnosis is often one of exclusion. Parenchymal metastasis, lymphangitic carcinomatosis, and chemotherapy-related lung toxicity can be differentiated from tumor embolism by findings on high-resolution computed tomography. Differentiation of tumor embolism from thrombotic embolism may be somewhat more problematic, especially if there is large-vessel involvement. Under most circumstances, however, pulmonary angiography is capable of differentiating thrombotic embolism from microvascular tumor embolism.

OTHER EMBOLI

Because of the lung's sieve-like quality, a wide variety of other materials may embolize into it. Trophoblastic tissue can escape the uterus and lodge in the pulmonary circulation during pregnancy. After head trauma, brain tissue has been found in the lungs; the same is true of liver cells following abdominal trauma and of bone marrow after cardiopulmonary resuscitation.

Finally, in this era of intravenous drug abuse, noninfectious vasculitic–thrombotic complications are being seen with increasing frequency in association with the intravenous use of drugs intended for oral use. Medications implicated with pulmonary complications include methylphenidate hydrochloride, oral opiates (pentazocine, meperidine), and antihistamines. Particulate and irritant drug carriers (e.g., talc, cellulose) and occasionally the drugs themselves may cause vascular inflammation and secondary thrombosis. The clinical presentation may be diverse and includes lower lobe emphysema, diffuse interstitial fibrosis, and progressive massive fibrosis. Repetitive insults may lead to severe and irreversible pulmonary hypertension. In many intravenous drug users, perfusion scans demonstrate segmental or smaller defects. Distinguishing these defects from those caused by venous thromboembolism may be difficult.

The diagnosis is often suggested by the clinical history. Radiographic findings include small, diffuse, well-defined nodular densities. These nodules can progress and massive fibrosis may ensue. Lower lobe emphysematous changes may also be present.

Diagnostic confirmation often requires lung biopsy, either open or transbronchial. The prognosis is poor, with progressive pulmonary disease being the rule.

1. King MB, Harmon KR. Unusual forms of pulmonary embolism. *Clin Chest Med.* 1994;15:561–580.
   A comprehensive, well-referenced review.
2. Dudney TM, Elliott CG. Pulmonary embolism from amniotic fluid, fat and air. *Prog Cardiovasc Dis.* 1994;36:447–474.
   A comprehensive, well-referenced review.
3. Morris W, Knauer CM. Cardiopulmonary manifestations of schistosomiasis. *Semin Resp Infect.* 1997;12:159–170.
   Concise review of the cardiopulmonary manifestations of schistosomal disease.
4. Palmer PE. Schistosomiasis. *Semin Roentgenol.* 1998;33:6–25.
5. Orebaugh SL. Venous air emboli: Clinical and experimental considerations. *Crit Care Med.* 1992;20:1169–1177.
   A comprehensive, well-referenced review.
6. Tibbles PM, Edelsberg JS. Hyperbaric-oxygen treatment. *N Engl J Med.* 1996;334: 1642–1648.
   Review of the indications for hyperbaric oxygen treatment, including air embolism.
7. Morris WP, Butler BD, Tonnesen AS, et al. Continuous venous air embolism in patients receiving positive end-expiratory pressure. *Am Rev Respir Dis.* 1993;147: 1034–1037.
   Description of three patients in who continuous air embolism in the inferior vena cava that persisted for days was detected. The bubbles appeared to arise from splanchnic veins, and they were associated with barotrauma and positive airway pressure.
8. Alvaran SB, Tuong JK, Graff TE, et al. Venous air embolism: Comparative merits of external cardiac massage, intracardiac aspiration, and left lateral decubitus position. *Anesth Analg.* 1978;57:166–170.
   In an animal model of venous air embolism, intracardiac aspiration was not superior to either external cardiac massage of left lateral decubitus position despite the shorter resuscitation time.
9. Armon C, Deschamps C, Adkinson C, et al. Hyperbaric treatment of cerebral air embolism sustained during an open-heart surgical procedure. *Mayo Clin Proc.* 1991;66:565–571.
   Hyperbaric treatment, begun 30 hours after the occurrence of air embolism, resulted in good immediate and long-term recovery.
10. Ely EW, Hite RD, Baker AM, et al. Venous air embolism from central venous catheterization: a need for increased physician awareness. *Crit Care Med.* 1999; 27:2113–2117.
    Awareness of venous air embolism or its prevention did not correlate with the level of physician training, experience, or specialty.
11. Parisi DM, Koval K, Egol K. Fat embolism syndrome. *Am J Orthop.* 2002;31:507–512.
    Review of current literature on fat embolism syndrome with regard to its causes, pathophysiology, clinical presentation, diagnosis, and treatment.
12. Roger N, Xzaubet A, Agusti C, et al. Role of bronchoalveolar lavage in the diagnosis of fat embolism syndrome. *Eur Respir J.* 1995;8:1275–1280.
    BAL oil red O positive macrophages were frequently observed in trauma patients irrespective of the presence of fat embolism syndrome.
13. Kallenbach J, Lewis M, Zaltman M. "Low dose" steroid prophylaxis against fat embolism. *J Trauma.* 1987;27:1173–1176.
    Controlled study demonstrating that 1.5 mg/kg of methylprednisolone given every 8 hours for 6 doses after skeletal trauma dramatically lowered the incidence of fat embolism syndrome.

14. Schonfeld SA, Ploysongsang Y, DiLisio R, et al. Fat embolism prophylaxis with corticosteroids. A prospective study in high risk patients. *Ann Intern Med.* 1983;99:438–443.
    Supports the value of corticosteroid treatment in patients at high risk for the fat embolism syndrome, particularly if unfavorable predictors are present.

15. Davies S. Amniotic fluid embolism: a review of the literature. *Can J Anaesth.* 2001;48:829–830.
    Review of the pathophysiology, clinical presentation, diagnosis, and therapy of amniotic fluid embolism.

16. Oi H, Kobayashi H, Hirashima Y, et al. Serological and immunohistochemical diagnosis of amniotic fluid embolism. *Semin Thromb Hemost.* 1998;24:479–484.
    Both TKH-2 immunostaining and serum TRH-2 levels appear to be sensitive methods to diagnose patients with amniotic fluid embolism.

17. Clark SL, Montz FJ, Phelan JP. Hemodynamic alterations associated with amniotic fluid embolism: a reappraisal. *Am J Obstet Gynecol.* 1985;151:617–621.
    Presentation of a theoretical model of hemodynamic changes accompanying amniotic fluid embolism that incorporates both experimental and clinical observations.

18. Clark SL, Hankins GD, Dudley DA, et al. Amniotic fluid embolism: analysis of the national registry. *Am J Obstet Gynecol.* 1995;172:1158–1167.
    In a review of 61 cases of amniotic fluid embolism, maternal mortality was 61%, with neurologically intact survival seen in only 15% of women. Of fetuses in utero at the time of the event, only 39% survived.

19. Julander I. Staphylococcal septicaemia and endocarditis in 80 drug users. *Scand J Infect Dis.* 1983;41:49–54.
    Descriptive report of 80 patients with staphylococcal sepsis. Endocarditis was documented or suspected in 65% of patients.

20. Pittet D, Hulliger S, Auckenthaler R. Intravascular device-related infections in critically ill patients. *J Chemother.* 1995;7(suppl 3):55–66.
    A comprehensive review.

21. Oim GM, Jeffrey RB Jr, Ralls PW, et al. Septic thrombophlebitis of the portal vein: CT and clinical observations. *J Comput Assist Tomogr.* 1989;13:656–658.
    Review of the CT and clinical findings in seven patients with septic thrombosis of the portal vein.

22. Thatai D, Chandy L, Dhar KL. Septic cavernous sinus thrombophlebitis: a review of 35 cases. *J Indian Med Assoc.* 1992;90:290–292.
    Review of 35 cases of septic cavernous sinus thrombophlebitis. Even with appropriate antibiotic therapy, the overall mortality was 34%.

23. Kniemeyer HW, Grabitz K, Buhl R, et al. Surgical treatment of septic deep venous thrombosis. *Surgery.* 1995;118:49–53.
    In complicated cases of septic deep vein thrombosis without improvement after conservative management, venous thrombectomy can be a life-saving procedure.

24. Plemmons RM, Dooley DP, Longfield RN. Septic thrombophlebitis of the portal vein (pylephlebitis): diagnosis and management in the modern era. *Clin Infect Dis.* 1995;21:1114–1120.
    Case report and review of the literature.

25. Brown CE, Stettler RW, Twickler D, et al. Puerperal septic pelvic thrombophlebitis: incidence and response to heparin therapy. *Am J Obstet Gynecol.* 1999;181:143–148.
    Women given heparin in addition to antimicrobial therapy for septic thrombophlebitis did not have a better outcome than did those for whom antimicrobial therapy alone was continued.

26. Kubik-Huch RA, Hebisch G, Huch R, et al. Role of duplex color Doppler ultrasound, computed tomography, and MR angiography in the diagnosis of septic puerperal ovarian vein thrombosis. *Abdom Imaging.* 1999;24:85–91.
    Magnetic resonance angiography is recommended in patients with inconclusive duplex color Doppler ultrasound findings and persistent suspicion for septic puerperal ovarian vein thrombosis.

27. Chan ED, Hermanoff MH, Connick E. Lemierre's syndrome: review of the English literature over the past 25 years. *Clin Pulm Med*. 1999;6:333–338.

A comprehensive, well-referenced review.

28. Ebright JR, Pace MT, Niazi AF. Septic thrombosis of the cavernous sinuses. *Arch Intern Med*. 2001;161:2671–2676.

A comprehensive, well-referenced review.

29. Roberts KE, Hamele-Bena D, Saqi A, et al. Pulmonary tumor embolism: a review of the literature. *Am J Med*. 2003;115:228–232.

A comprehensive, well-referenced review of pulmonary tumor embolism.

30. Goldhaber SZ, Dricker E, Buring JE, et al. Clinical suspicion of autopsy-proven thrombotic and tumor pulmonary embolism in cancer patients. *Am Heart J*. 1987;114:1432–1435.

Of 73 patients with solid malignant tumors and PE, 56 had major thrombotic PE and 17 had major tumor embolism to the lungs. Of the 56 with cancer and thrombotic PE, 45% had the correct diagnosis suspected antemortem. By contrast, in only 6% of patients with tumor embolism was the diagnosis made correctly ante mortem.

31. Lukl P. Pulmonary microvascular cytology in the dyspneic cancer patient: merits and caution. *Arch Pathol Lab Med*. 1992;116:129–130.

Megakaryocytes obtained by wedge aspiration cytology may be misinterpreted as malignant cells.

32. Soares F, Pinto AP, Landell GA, et al. Pulmonary tumor embolism to arterial vessels and carcinomatous lymphangitis. A comparative clinicopathological study. *Arch Pathol Lab Med*. 1993;117:827–831.

A prospective study of 222 consecutive autopsies of cancer cases, which concluded that carcinomatous lymphangitis and arterial tumor embolism of the lungs, though clinically similar, are different clinicopathologic entities.

33. Shepard JA, Moore EH, Templeton PA, et al. Pulmonary intravascular tumor emboli: dilated and beaded peripheral pulmonary arteries at CT. *Radiology*. 1993;187:797–801.

Description of the chest CT scan findings in four patients with intravascular tumor emboli.

34. Arnett EN, Battle WE, Russo JV, et al. Intravenous injection of talc-containing drugs intended for oral use. A cause of pulmonary granulomatosis and pulmonary hypertension. *Am J Med*. 1976;60:711–718.

Description of two patients with pulmonary talc granulomas and review of the literature.

35. Pare JP, Cote G, Fraser RS. Long-term follow-up of drug abusers with intravenous talcosis. *Am Rev Respir Dis*. 1989;139:233–241.

Long-term follow-up of six patients with pulmonary talcosis. All developed severe respiratory disability and three died from their disease.

36. Padley SP, Adler BD, Staples CA, et al. Pulmonary talcosis: CT findings in three cases. *Radiology*. 1993;186:125–127.

Computed tomographic findings in three patients with pulmonary talcosis. Widespread ground-glass attenuation was present in one case and massive fibrosis in two.

69. PULMONARY HYPERTENSION: PATHOGENESIS AND ETIOLOGY

Kelly M. Chin, Richard N. Channick, and Lewis J. Rubin

Pulmonary hypertension encompasses several distinct disease processes affecting the cardiopulmonary system. Understanding the physiology of the normal pulmonary vasculature and the pathophysiologic derangements that can arise is essential in formulating an organized approach to the diagnosis and management of these varied disorders.

Under normal conditions, the pulmonary arterial bed is a high-flow, low-pressure, low-resistance circuit, allowing the relatively thin-walled right ventricle to maintain adequate cardiac output, even in the face of high demand. Pulmonary capillaries are capable of distending to accommodate increased flow and previously closed capillary beds are recruited in situations associated with increased output, such as exercise. As a result, pulmonary vascular resistance decreases and pulmonary arterial pressure rises only minimally despite large increases in flow.

The common finding in all pulmonary hypertensive states is a reduction in the effective cross-sectional area of the pulmonary vascular tree. Initially, this derangement may be manifested solely by a loss of recruitability and distensability of small resistance vessels. Pulmonary arterial pressures and vascular resistance, thus, can remain normal under resting conditions. With increases in flow, however, pulmonary arterial pressure increases. As the pulmonary hypertensive process progresses, and the cross-sectional area is further compromised, resting pulmonary hypertension ensues. To sustain the increased pulmonary arterial pressure, the right ventricle must transform itself into a more muscular chamber. In practical terms, markedly elevated pulmonary arterial pressures always indicate a chronic process in which the right ventricle has had an opportunity to hypertrophy.

In all forms of pulmonary hypertension, the clinical manifestations depend on the degree to which the right ventricle can compensate for the high afterload. With mild pulmonary hypertension, cardiac output is appropriately augmented in response to increased demand (e.g., exercise); symptoms, thus, may be minimal. In more severe pulmonary hypertension, however, the right ventricle is unable to achieve an appropriate rise in cardiac output. These patients typically have exertional symptoms (dyspnea, fatigue), but no manifestations of right-sided heart failure. Eventually, if the right ventricular afterload is great enough, right-sided heart failure develops, manifesting as resting dyspnea, jugular venous distension, hepatic congestion, ascites, and dependent edema.

A reduction in the pulmonary vascular cross-sectional area can result from three fundamental pathologic processes: vasoconstriction, obstruction, and obliteration. In most forms of pulmonary hypertension, more than one of these processes is present. For example, pulmonary vasoconstriction, which can be present in primary pulmonary hypertension, chronic hypoxia, cardiac disease, and parenchymal lung disease, leads to hypertrophy of the pulmonary arterial medial layer. This structural change results in further compromise of the vessel lumen. As a result, vascular wall tension increases, leading to proliferation and scarring in the intima and further obliteration of the peripheral vessels and fixed pulmonary hypertension. In fact, small-vessel structural lesions, including muscular hypertrophy, intimal proliferation, and fibrosis are common end points in virtually all forms of long-standing pulmonary hypertension.

The pathways leading to vasoconstriction and the various histopathologic lesions described are complex and vary significantly in different forms of pulmonary hypertension. A delicate balance exists between mediators that maintain the pulmonary vascular bed in a relatively dilated, nonproliferating, nonthrombotic state (prostacyclin, nitric oxide, and heparin-like growth inhibitors) and those that promote constriction, proliferation, and thrombosis (thromboxane A_2, platelet-activating factor, endothelin-1, angiopoietin-1, and growth factors). Perturbations in this balance lead to the development and progression of hypertensive arteriopathic changes in the pulmonary vasculature.

Pulmonary hypertension can be grouped into one of five general categories based on similar pathophysiologic processes and treatment: (1) pulmonary arterial hypertension (PAH); (2) pulmonary venous hypertension; (3) pulmonary hypertension associated with lung diseases and/or hypoxemia; (4) pulmonary hypertension caused by chronic thrombotic or embolic disease; and (5) miscellaneous disorders associated with pulmonary hypertension. A 2003 symposium on the clinical classification of pulmonary hypertension recommended use of this clinically based classification system, and also proposed elimination of the word *primary,* favoring use of *idiopathic* to describe PAH without associated conditions (see Chapter 70).

Elevation in pulmonary venous pressure can occur with any disorder impairing pulmonary venous outflow, including systolic and diastolic left ventricular dysfunction, mitral stenosis, and, less commonly, disorders of the pericardium or pulmonary veins themselves. The elevated pulmonary venous pressure causes mild pulmonary hypertension, augmented to some degree by vasoconstriction. Over time, microvascular changes (e.g., muscular hypertrophy and intimal proliferation) can occur, leading to sustained pulmonary hypertension, even after the pulmonary venous pressure is reduced (e.g., by repair of the mitral stenosis).

Pulmonary parenchymal diseases, including chronic obstructive pulmonary disease (COPD), interstitial lung disease, and widespread parenchymal destructive processes (tuberculosis), can lead to pulmonary hypertension. Both obliteration of the pulmonary vascular bed and hypoxic vasoconstriction can contribute to the pulmonary hypertensive state.

In COPD, the degree of pulmonary hypertension generally reflects the severity of gas exchange impairment rather than the extent of parenchymal destruction. Pulmonary hypertension in this group is generally modest (i.e., mean pulmonary artery pressures are typically <40 mmHg). Suspicion for a superimposed process should be raised by pulmonary hypertension out of proportion to the degree of gas exchange derangement or a rapid worsening of previously mild pulmonary hypertension in a patient with COPD.

Interstitial lung disease can lead to pulmonary hypertension through both vasoconstriction and obliteration of small pulmonary arteries. However, severe restriction typically is necessary before pulmonary hypertension develops (i.e., lung volume reduction of ≥50%). The same is true of destructive lung disorders. Therefore, severe pulmonary hypertension should not be attributed to mild restrictive lung disease. In fact, in both idiopathic PAH and thromboembolic pulmonary hypertension, a mild pulmonary restrictive defect (mean forced vital capacity and total lung capacity of approximately 80% of predicted) is often encountered.

Hypoventilation syndromes, including sleep apnea, central alveolar hypoventilation, and obesity–hypoventilation, syndrome can be associated with mild pulmonary hypertension induced by hypoxemia, hypercapnia, or acidosis. The degree of pulmonary hypertension in these disorders appears to correlate with the magnitude of gas exchange abnormalities, most notable the presence of daytime hypoxemia. Although structural vascular changes can occur with chronic hypoventilation, they are mainly limited to muscular hypertrophy and, typically, reverse after resolution of the ventilatory derangement.

Chronic thromboembolic pulmonary hypertension (CTEPH) is a distinct entity characterized by obstruction of large, elastic (main, lobar, and segmental) pulmonary arteries by chronic, unresolved, organized pulmonary emboli. Pulmonary hypertension results from the obstruction and, in some patients, secondary changes that develop in the small resistance arteries. This entity is discussed in detail in Chapter 67.

Patients who have pulmonary hypertension (mean PA pressure >25) without evidence of increased wedge pressure, parenchymal lung disorders, or thromboembolic disease are considered to have PAH. PAH can be idiopathic or related to an associated condition, and the idiopathic form can be sporadic or familial. Familial PAH is transmitted in an autosomal dominant pattern with variable penetrance and accounts for approximately 7% of idiopathic cases. The most common associated conditions include

HIV, connective tissue disease, portal hypertension, congenital systemic–pulmonary–cardiac shunts, and certain drugs (including the diet drug fenfluramine that was removed from the market in 1997).

Pulmonary hypertension associated with these diverse conditions has similarities in response to medical therapies and in pathologic findings, including a spectrum of microvascular lesions found in the small, resistance arteries: medial hypertrophy, intimal fibrosis, plexiform lesions (multichanneled outpouchings from arterioles and small arteries), and microthrombotic lesions. However, despite the common end point, the exact mechanisms through which these diverse conditions result in pulmonary hypertension are unknown.

For patients with congenital heart disease, it is known that increased flow across the pulmonary vascular bed increases the risk of PAH, and that once PAH occurs, the resulting microvasculature changes are similar to those noted in other forms of PAH. Risk is greatest for patients with congenital heart conditions that increase both pressure and flow (i.e., ventricular septal defects, patent ductus arteriosus); for patients with atrial septal defects and small ventricular septal defects risk is much lower. A hallmark of advanced septal defect-associated pulmonary hypertension is augmented right-to-left intracardiac shunting (Eisenmenger physiology), resulting in significant arterial hypoxemia. Under these circumstances, closure of the septal defect can worsen pulmonary hemodynamics and induce overt right ventricular failure.

Mutations in the BMPR2 gene (a member of the TGF-β superfamily) have been found in pulmonary hypertension including approximately 60% of those with familial PAH, 10 to 30% of those with idiopathic PAH, and 9% of dexfenfluramine-associated PH. The mechanism through which BMPR2 is linked to pulmonary hypertension is unknown, although BMP proteins in general play a role in the regulation of growth, differentiation, and apoptosis in various cell types. Another protein implicated in the development of pulmonary hypertension is the serotonin transporter protein. Serotonin is a pulmonary vasoconstrictor and can promote smooth muscle cell hyperplasia. Expression of the serotonin transporter protein is increased in PAH, with the highest levels seen in the idiopathic form. Interestingly, the diet drugs associated with PAH, dexfenfluramine and fenfluramine, interact with this protein.

Pulmonary venoocclusive disease (PVOD) is another form of idiopathic pulmonary hypertension, characterized by widespread occlusion of the small pulmonary veins. The presentation in PVOD may mimic that of other forms of PAH. Unlike PAH, however, pulmonary edema often develops after treatment with vasodilating medications, because of increased pulmonary blood flow with "fixed" outflow (pulmonary vein) obstruction. Wedge pressures are typically normal. Overlap with the more usual forms of PAH exists. Although PVOD may respond to medications approved for PAH, prognosis is worse and the potential for pulmonary edema makes treatment difficult.

The diagnostic workup, outlined in Chapter 66, can distinguish between PAH and other forms of pulmonary hypertension with a high level of certainty. Distinguishing PAH from other forms of pulmonary hypertension is critical because treatment strategies differ markedly. Accurately identifying CTEPH is also important, because it is potentially curable through pulmonary thromboendarterectomy surgery.

1. Abenhaim L, Moride Y, Brenot F, et al. Appetite-suppressant drugs and the risk of primary pulmonary hypertension. *N Engl J Med.* 1996;335:609–116.
   The first case-control study clearly describing an association between primary pulmonary hypertension (PPH) and prior anorexigen drug use. The association strengthened with longer use (≥3 months) and with use within the preceding year.
2. Atkinson C, Stewart S, Upton PD, et al. Primary pulmonary hypertension is associated with reduced pulmonary vascular expression of type II bone morphogenetic protein receptor. *Circulation.* 2002;105:1672.
   BMPR-II protein levels were found to be reduced in patients with PPH, and this reduction was greatest in those patients heterozygous for a mutations in the

BMPR-II gene. In normal patients, BMPR-II mRNA was predominately found in endothelial cells, with a lower level of expression in vascular smooth muscle.

3. Chaouat A, Wesitsenblum E, Krieger J, et al. Pulmonary hemodynamics in the obstructive sleep apnea syndrome. Results in 220 consecutive patients. *Chest.* 1996;109:380.

    Pulmonary hypertension in obstructive sleep apnea (OSA) is mild and is not predicted by the severity of the sleep apnea. OSA patients with elevated pulmonary arterial pressures have more daytime hypoxemia and hypercapnia, and have greater airway obstruction by spiromtery (reduced FEV_1 and FEV_1/FVC ratio).

4. Cool CD, Rai PR, Yeager ME, et al. Expression of human herpesvirus 8 in primary pulmonary hypertension. *N Engl J Med.* 2003;349:1113–1122.

    Found that 10 of 16 patients with idiopathic PAH but none of 14 with secondary pulmonary hypertension had plexiform lesions positive for LANA-1 (HHV-8 Antigen).

5. Christman BW, McPherson CD, Newman JH, et al. An imbalance between the excretion of thromboxan and prostacyclin metabolites in pulmonary hypertension. *N Engl J Med.* 1992;327:70.

    Stable urinary metabolites of thromboxane and prostacycline were measured in normals, patients with PPH, and patients with secondary pulmonary hypertension. An increase in the ratio of thromboxane:prostacyclin was found in the PPH group, suggesting a role for this imbalance (favoring vasoconstriction and smooth muscle proliferation) in either the development or maintenance of PPH.

6. Dev V, Shrivastava S. Time course of changes in pulmonary vascular resistance and the mechanism of regression of pulmonary arterial hypertension after balloon mitral valvuloplasty. *Am J Cardiol.* 1991;67:439.

    Following balloon valvuloplasty, an initial decrease occurred in pulmonary arterial pressures, corresponding to decreases in wedge pressure. A second gradual further decrease in pulmonary arterial pressures occurred thereafter because of decreased pulmonary vascular resistance, presumably as a result of the pulmonary arteriopathic changes

7. Du Lingling, Sullivan CC, Chu D, et al. Signaling molecules in nonfamilial pulmonary hypertension. *N Engl J Med.* 2003;348:500–509.

    Showed that the expression of angiopoietin-1 and TIE2 were upregulated in pulmonary hypertension and correlated with disease severity. Also demonstrated that angiopoietin-1 shut off expression of BMPR1A, a protein required for BMPRII signaling.

8. Enrique-Sarano M, et al. Determinants of pulmonary hypertension in left ventricular dysfunction. *J Am Coll Cardiol.* 1997;29:153.

    Pulmonary hypertension is frequent but variable in severity in patients with left ventricular dysfunction. It is strongly associated with diastolic dysfunction and with mitral valve regurgitation, but is not independently related to left ventricular systolic function.

9. Levin ER. Mechanisms of disease. Endothelins. *N Engl J Med.* 1995;333:356–363.

    Good review of the physiology and pathophysiology of the endothelins.

10. Gurtner HP. Aminorex and pulmonary hypertension. *Cor et Vasa.* 1985;27:160.

    An outbreak of PPH occurred in Europe between 1967 and 1973 and was traced to ingestion of the anorexigen aminorex.

11. Hadengue A, et al. Pulmonary hypertension complicating portal hypertension: prevalence and relation to splanchnic hemodynamics. *Gastroenterology.* 1991: 100–520.

    Pulmonary hypertension was found on right heart catheterization in 2% of patients with portal hypertension, significantly higher than estimates for the general population. The cause of this association is unknown.

12. Hong Z, et al. Sub-acute hypoxia decreases Kv channel expression and function in pulmonary artery myocytes. *Am J Respir Cell Molec Biol.* 2004:240:163.

    Moderate hypoxia in rats resulted in reduced expression and activity of voltage-activated K^+ channels in pulmonary artery smooth muscle cells, resulting in a more depolarized resting membrane potential and an increased cytosolic calcium.

This suggests a role for these channels in chronic hypoxemia associated pulmonary hypertension.

13. Kuo PC, et al. Distinctive clinical features of portopulmonary hypertension. *Chest.* 1997;112:980.

   Thirty patients with portopulmonary hypertension were compared with 30 patients with PPH and 30 patients with liver disease alone. Portopulmonary hypertension is characterized by higher cardiac indices than found in PPH.

14. Loyd JE, et al. Familial primary pulmonary hypertension: clinical patterns. *Am Rev Respir Dis.* 1984;129:194.

   In the NIH registry, 7% of cases were familial. A spectrum of histopathologic lesions can be seen in members of the same family. No differences in presentation, hemodynamics, or natural history were noted between familial and nonfamilial cases.

15. Machado RD, et al. BMPR2 Happloinsufficiency as the inherited molecular mechanism for primary pulmonary hypertension. *Am J Hum Genet.* 2001;68:92.

   Heterozygous mutations in the BMPR-2 gene were found in 23 of 47 families with pulmonary hypertension. BMPR-2 mutations have also been seen at lower rates in sporadic PAH and anorexigen-associated PAH.

16. Marcos E, Fadel E, Sanchez O, et al. Serotonin-induced smooth muscle hyperplasia in various forms of human pulmonary hypertension. *Circ Res.* 2004;94:1263–1270.

   Found increased expression of the serotonin transporter protein (5-HTT) in pulmonary hypertension, and increased rates of the LL-polymorphism of the 5-HTT gene (which leads to increased expression). Rates were intermediate in secondary pulmonary hypertension and lowest in controls.

17. Mesa RA, et al. Human immunodeficiency virus infection and pulmonary hypertension: two new cases and a review of 86 reported cases. *Mayo Clin Proc.* 1998;73:37.

   A nice review of the increasingly recognized association between PAH and HIV. Development of PAH does not correlate with CD4 count, and survival in these patients at 1 year was only 51%. However, evidence from other studies suggests that some of these patients may respond well to treatment.

18. Pietra GG, et al. Histopathology of primary pulmonary hypertension: a qualitative and quantitative study of pulmonary blood vessels from 58 patients in the National Heart, Lung, and Blood Institute primary pulmonary hypertension registry. *Circulation.* 1989;80:1198.

   A landmark study describing the histologic lesions seen in PPH.

19. Proceedings of the Third World Symposium on Pulmonary Arterial Hypertension. *J Am Coll Cardiol.* 2004;43:1S–90S.

   This supplement reviews advances in the pathogenesis of pulmonary hypertension with articles on cellular and molecular pathobiology, histopathology, and genetics, as well as diagnosis and treatment.

20. Rich S, et al. Primary pulmonary hypertension: a national prospective study. *Ann Intern Med.* 1987;107:216.

   An important study that summarizes the results of the NIH PPH registry, which collated 194 cases from 32 centers between 1981 and 1985. Reported that 6% of cases were familial.

21. Salvaterra CG, Rubin LJ. Investigation and management of pulmonary hypertension in chronic obstructive pulmonary disease. *Am Rev Respir Dis.* 1993;148:1414.

   Review article; pulmonary hypertension caused by COPD is typically mild (mPAP <40 mmHg).

22. Smith P, et al. The ultrastructure of plexogenic pulmonary hypertension in HIV infection. *J Pathol.* 1990;160:111.

   A histopathologic paper discussing mechanisms for the development of intimal proliferation and plexiform lesions.

23. Trembath RC, Harrison R. Insights into the genetic and molecular basis of primary pulmonary hypertension. *Pediatr Res.* 2003;53:883–888.

Reviews genetic studies investigating BMPR2, 5-HTT transporter and clinical applications.

24. Yuan JX, et al. Dysfunctional voltage-gated K$^+$ channels in pulmonary artery smooth muscle cells of patients with primary pulmonary hypertension. *Circulation.* 1998;98:1400.

Smooth muscle cells from patients with pulmonary hypertension have decreased potassium currents resulting in membrane depolarization level and a higher resting calcium level. Because intracellular calcium regulates both contractility and cell growth, this finding suggests a potential role for potassium channels in the development of pulmonary hypertension.

---

70. PULMONARY HYPERTENSION: DIAGNOSIS AND TREATMENT

Kelly M. Chin, Richard N. Channick, and Lewis J. Rubin

The first challenge in the diagnosis of pulmonary hypertension is recognizing that pulmonary hypertension is, in fact, present. Historical information is often nonspecific. For example, dyspnea on exertion is present in virtually all patients with pulmonary hypertension and may be the only presenting symptom. Other common symptoms include cough (30%), chest pain (21%), hemoptysis (10%), and easy fatigability (25%). These nonspecific symptoms often suggest other, more common, diagnostic considerations (asthma, coronary artery disease, psychogenic dyspnea) rather than pulmonary arterial hypertension (PAH). More specific historical information, such as a history of venous thromboembolism or childhood heart murmurs, should arouse suspicion for a specific pulmonary hypertensive disorder.

Physical findings can also be relatively subtle. Classic signs of pulmonary hypertension include accentuation of the pulmonic component of the second heart sound (S$_2$), fixed splitting of S$_2$, murmurs of tricuspid regurgitation or pulmonic insufficiency (in some cases), and a left parasternal lift, indicative of right ventricular hypertrophy. One notable physical examination finding observed in some patients with chronic thromboembolic pulmonary hypertension (CTEPH) is the presence of pulmonary artery flow murmurs. These are bruits auscultated over the lung fields, heard best during breath holding at mid-inspiration. These sounds indicate flow through partially occluded central pulmonary arteries and are highly suggestive of chronic large-vessel pulmonary embolic disease.

Chest radiography may be unrevealing. If pulmonary hypertension is severe, enlargement of the right ventricle and pulmonary arteries is apparent. Chest radiography, however, can be useful in searching for secondary causes of pulmonary hypertension (interstitial lung disease, chronic obstructive pulmonary disease [COPD]). One notable radiographic finding is the presence of interstitial edema (Kerley B lines) in the setting of right ventricular failure and pulmonary artery enlargement. This constellation of x-ray findings should raise suspicion for pulmonary venoocclusive disease.

In patients in whom pulmonary hypertension is suspected, echocardiography is a very useful initial test that is likely to be abnormal in the presence of moderate or severe pulmonary hypertension. Two-dimensional echocardiography demonstrates varying degrees of right atrial and right ventricular enlargement. Paradoxical movement of the interventricular septum indicates right ventricular pressure overload. Doppler echocardiography can also estimate the pulmonary artery systolic pressure (PASP) using the velocity of the tricuspid regurgitant jet (if present) and the formula PASP = $4*v^2$ + right atrial pressure. Pulmonary hypertension that occurs only during exercise is becoming an increasingly recognized entity, and may present with a normal echocardiogram. Exercise with a pulmonary artery catheter in place is recommended when this entity is suspected.

Five major diagnostic categories of pulmonary hypertension are now recognized:

1. PAH
   a. Idiopathic
   b. Familial
   c. Associated with collagen vascular disease, congenital systemic to pulmonic shunts, portal hypertension, HIV, drugs and toxins, other
   d. Associated with significant venous or capillary involvement: pulmonary venooc-clusive disease, pulmonary capillary hemangiomatosis
2. Pulmonary hypertension with left-sided heart disease
3. Pulmonary hypertension associated with lung diseases or hypoxemia: COPD, inter-stitial lung disease, sleep-disordered breathing, alveolar hypoventilation disorders, chronic exposure to high altitude, developmental abnormalities
4. Pulmonary hypertension caused by chronic thrombotic or embolic disease
5. Miscellaneous: sarcoidosis, histiocytosis X, lymphangiomatosis, compression of the pulmonary vessels

Once a patient is identified as likely to have pulmonary hypertension, additional tests are required to confirm the diagnosis and to determine which type is present. These tests include (1) echocardiography to exclude the presence of congenital heart disease (atrial septal defect, ventricular septal defect, patent ductus arteriosus) and left-sided heart disease (valvular or ventricular dysfunction); (2) pulmonary function testing to determine if significant obstructive or restrictive lung disease is present, although parenchymal disease must be severe to cause pulmonary hypertension; (3) ventilation–perfusion scanning and possibly pulmonary angiography to identify CTEPH; (4) arterial blood gases to define a hypoventilation syndrome; (5) sleep stud-ies, if clinically indicated; (6) chest radiograph and high-resolution computed tomog-raphy scanning if the diagnosis of interstitial lung disease–associated pulmonary hy-pertension is contemplated.

With these noninvasive studies, multiple disorders can be excluded and patients with PAH can be identified. Further studies to identify conditions associated with PAH include blood tests for antibodies to HIV and antinuclear antibody titer to screen for collagen vascular disease. Patients should also be asked about a family history of pulmonary hypertension, a history of anorexigen use, or a history of use of stimulant drugs (methamphetamines, cocaine). Once a diagnosis of PAH is made, one should proceed with right heart catheterization to confirm the diagnosis (including exclu-sion of an elevated wedge pressure), assess disease severity, and determine whether vasoreactivity is present.

The outcome of patients with untreated idiopathic PAH is generally unfavorable. In the National Institutes of Health Registry, median survival from the time of recogni-tion was 2.9 years. Factors associated with a worse prognosis include severity of right ventricular failure (high right atrial pressure, low cardiac index), poor functional class, and poor exercise capacity as assessed by a 6-minute walk test.

Because outcome depends on the severity of pulmonary hypertension and the ade-quacy of right ventricular compensation, it is critical to determine the ability of the pulmonary vascular bed to vasodilate in response to pharmacologic agents. Agents that have been used for acute vasodilator testing include prostacyclin, inhaled ni-tric oxide, and adenosine; longer acting agents should not be used. An acute fall in pulmonary arterial pressures toward normal (mean PAP <40 mmHg) identifies a sub-group that may do well on long-term calcium channel blockers. Unfortunately, only 6% of patients fall into this acute "vasoreactor" subgroup.

Specific, highly effective medical therapy is now available for most patients with PAH. Therapies currently available in the United States include (1) epoprostenol, an intravenous prostacyclin analog requiring continuous administration; (2) trepros-tinil, a subcutaneously administered prostacyclin analog; and (3) bosentan, an oral endothelin antagonist.

Choice of treatment depends on the severity of the pulmonary hypertension and the side effect and complication profile of the medications. Epoprostenol therapy is invasive, has numerous side effects, and requires an indwelling catheter for administration. However, it is still highly effective, works quickly, and improves exercise capacity, pulmonary hemodynamics, and survival even in the most severely compromised patients with PAH. Epoprostenol is generally felt to be the drug of choice in PAH patients who are World Health Organization (WHO) functional class IV. Of interest is that the beneficial effects of epoprostenol are noted even in the absence of favorable acute hemodynamic responses to the agent, suggesting nonvasodilator effects such as vascular remodeling and inotropy.

Bosentan, an orally administered dual endothelin receptor antagonist has also been shown to improve hemodynamics and exercise capacity in patients with PAH; long-term follow-up also suggests a mortality benefit. Bosentan is generally well tolerated, with its main complication being reversible liver function abnormalities in up to 11% of patients. Bosentan can be considered the drug of choice for PAH patients who are WHO functional class III. Treprostinil, a prostacyclin analog administered subcutaneously by a small continuous pump, is also effective if an adequate dose can be achieved, but pain at the infusion site may limit its utility

Therapies currently under investigation include selective endothelin-A antagonists, phosphodiesterase type 5 inhibitors (sildenafil, alone and in combination with epoprostenol), inhaled forms of prostacyclin such as iloprost (approved in Europe) and several trials of combination therapies.

In addition to the primary treatments described, warfarin is recommended based on retrospective data indicating a significant survival benefit in idiopathic PAH. Diuretics are frequently required to control symptoms such as hepatic congestion and leg edema, and in some they may also improve dyspnea, for unclear reasons. Diuretics must, however, be used with caution, because excessive reductions in blood volume can adversely affect the preload-dependent right ventricle and lead to systemic hypotension. Digoxin is generally not beneficial in the treatment of right ventricular failure, but can be considered in patients who develop supraventricular arrhythmias.

Other supportive measures occasionally considered for patients with progressive right ventricular failure include low-dose inotropic therapy and balloon septostomy. Inotropic support with low-dose dopamine, dobutamine, or milrinone can improve cardiac output and symptoms, and has been used long term in a small number of patients. Balloon septostomy creates a small atrial septal defect that allows blood, albeit deoxygenated, to reach the left ventricle, thereby improving cardiac output and, it is hoped, oxygen delivery. Of course, the downside is the resultant hypoxemia. The size of the defect created appears to be critical in balancing improvement in cardiac output against severe hypoxemia.

Lung and heart–lung transplantation are now reserved for patients who do not show significant improvement with medical therapy. This is best assessed through evaluation of posttreatment hemodynamic data in combination with 6-minute walk distance and functional class. Single or double lung transplantation is considered acceptable in most patients with pulmonary hypertension; heart–lung transplantation is generally reserved for complex congenital heart abnormalities that cannot be corrected at the time of lung transplantation. Successful transplantation results in marked hemodynamic and functional improvement. However, beneficial long-term outcomes with lung transplantation have been somewhat tempered by the prevalence of chronic rejection (manifested by bronchiolitis obliterans) in approximately one third of patients.

1. Aguilar RV, Farber HW. Epoprostenol (prostacyclin) therapy in HIV-associated pulmonary hypertension. *Am J Respir Crit Care Med.* 2000;162:1846.

Six consecutive patients with HIV-associated PAH underwent treatment with epoprostenol and were followed for 12 to 47 months. Hemodynamics improved significantly between baseline and 1 year, and functional class improved in all patients.

2. Badesch DB, et al. Continuous intravenous epoprostenol for pulmonary hypertension due to the scleroderma spectrum of disease. *Ann Intern Med.* 2000;132: 425.

   In 111 patients with scleroderma-associated PAH, those treated with intravenous epoprostenol had significantly improved hemodynamics, functional class, and exercise capacity vs. conventionally treated patients, and showed a trend toward less Raynaud's phenomenon and fewer digital ulcers.

3. Barst RJ, et al. A comparison of continuous intravenous epoprostenol (prostacyclin) with conventional therapy for primary pulmonary hypertension. The PPH Study Group. *N Engl J Med.* 1996;334:296.

   A landmark study demonstrating the efficacy of continuous prostacyclin in improving both exercise capacity and survival in PPH.

4. Channick RN, et al. Effects of the dual endothelin-receptor antagonist bosentan in patients with pulmonary hypertension: A randomized placebo-controlled study. *Lancet.* 2001;358:1119.

   Demonstrates the benefits of bosentan in the treatment of PAH, with improved 6-minute walk distance and hemodynamics in bosentan treated patients versus those receiving placebo.

5. D'Alonzo GE, et al. Comparison of progressive exercise performance of normal subjects and patients with primary pulmonary hypertension. *Chest.* 1987;92: 57.

   Exercise limitation in patients with PPH is predominately due to cardiac limitations with an inability to maintain oxygen delivery during exercise.

6. D'Alonzo GE, et al. Survival in patients with primary pulmonary hypertension. Results from a national prospective registry. *Ann Intern Med.* 1991;115:343.

   Documents poor survival in untreated PPH (median survival 2.9 years), which is strongly influenced by hemodynamics such as right atrial pressure, mean pulmonary artery pressure, and cardiac index.

7. Diagnosis and management of pulmonary arterial hypertension: ACCP evidence-based clinical practice guidelines. *Chest.* 2004;126(1 Suppl):1S–92S.

   This supplement to Chest *consists of evidence-based practice guidelines on topics ranging from diagnosis to treatment of patients with pulmonary hypertension.*

8. Fishman AJ, et al. Perfusion lung scans vs. pulmonary angiography in evaluation of suspected primary pulmonary hypertension. *Chest.* 1983;84:679.

   Lung scanning is highly accurate in distinguishing PPH from large-vessel thromboembolic disease. A normal or mottled appearing scan is consistent with PPH.

9. Frank H, et al. The effect of anticoagulant therapy in primary and anorectic drug-induced pulmonary hypertension. *Chest.* 1997;112:714.

   This and other retrospective studies suggest a survival benefit for PAH patients receiving anticoagulation.

10. Higenbottam T, et al. Long-term intravenous prostaglandin (epoprostenol or iloprost) for treatment of severe pulmonary hypertension. *Heart.* 1998;80: 151.

    Confirms the long-term survival benefit of prostacyclin infusions. Benefit was greatest in patients with worse cardiac function (SvO$_2$ <60%, median survival 585 days versus 239 days with conventional therapy).

11. Hopkins WE, et al. Comparison of the hemodynamics and survival of adults with severe primary pulmonary hypertension or Eisenmenger syndrome. *J Heart Lung Transplant.* 1996;15:100.

    Adult patients with Eisenmenger syndrome, as a group, have better maintained cardiac function and improved long-term survival compared with PPH patients.

12. Langleben D, et al. Continuous infusion of epoprostenol improves the net balance between pulmonary endothelin-1 clearance and release in primary pulmonary hypertension. *Circulation.* 1999;99:3266.

    Previous studies by this group demonstrated net production of endothelin-1 (ET-1) in the lungs of PPH patients (arterial:venous ET-1 ratio >1). This study of 11 patients treated with long-term epoprostenol infusion demonstrated that 82% of *patients had arterial:venous ET-1 ratios <1 by day 88 of therapy, suggesting that chronic epoprostenol helps normalize endothelial function.*

13. McLaughlin VV, et al. Survival in primary pulmonary hypertension. The impact of epoprostenol therapy. *Circulation.* 2002;106:1477–1482.

    Intravenous epoprostenol improves long-term survival versus predicted survival, with outcome dependent on posttreatment variables including functional class, hemodynamics, and exercise capacity.

14. Mukerjee D, et al. Prevalence and outcome in systemic sclerosis associated pulmonary arterial hypertension: application of a registry approach. *Ann Rheum Dis.* 2003;62:1088.

    Seven hundred twenty-two patients with scleroderma were screened for PAH by echocardiogram and PFTs; those with suspicious findings underwent catheterization. Twelve percent (89/722) showed evidence of pulmonary hypertension by right heart catheterization, confirming the high risk of disease in this patient population.

15. Olschewski H, et al. Inhaled iloprost for severe pulmonary hypertension. *N Engl J Med.* 2002;347:322.

    This placebo-controlled trial evaluated inhaled iloprost, a prostacyclin analog, in the treatment of pulmonary hypertension including PPH, anorexigens associated, scleroderma associated, and nonoperable CTEPH. At 12 weeks, patients receiving iloprost (2.5–5.0 μg, 6–9 times daily) showed greater improvement in 6-minute walk distance, hemodynamics, and functional class versus placebo.

16. Raymond RJ, et al. Echocardiographic predictors of adverse outcomes in primary pulmonary hypertension. *J Am Coll Cardiol.* 2002;39:1214.

    Pericardial effusion, right atrial enlargement, and septal displacement predict adverse outcomes in patients with advanced PAH.

17. Proceedings of the Third World Symposium on Pulmonary Arterial Hypertension. *J Am Coll Cardiol.* 2004;43:1S–90S.

    PAH symposium; includes articles on the revised clinical classification of pulmonary hypertension, an overview of current treatment, and several articles on classes of medications used for therapy including prostanoids, endothelin-receptor antagonists, nitric oxide, and phosphodiesterase inhibitors.

18. Rich S, et al. The effect of high doses of calcium channel-blockers on survival in primary pulmonary hypertension. *N Engl J Med.* 1992;327:76.

    The first study to demonstrate improved survival in PPH patients who responded acutely to high-dose calcium channel blockers and were then continued on these agents.

19. Rosenzweig EB, et al. Long-term prostacyclin for pulmonary hypertension with associated congenital heart defects. *Circulation.* 1999;99:1858.

    This report of 20 patients with different congenital heart diseases and PAH demonstrated significant benefit of long-term epoprostenol on hemodynamics, exercise capacity, and functional class.

20. Rothman A, et al. Atrial septostomy as a bridge to lung transplantation in patients with severe pulmonary hypertension. *Am J Cardiol.* 1999;84:682.

    Twelve patients with severe pulmonary hypertension were treated with graded balloon dilation to make a small atrial septal defect. Mean oxygen delivery improved, and six patients had clinical improvement, five of whom subsequently underwent lung transplantation.

21. Rubin LJ, et al. Bosentan therapy for pulmonary arterial hypertension. *N Engl J Med.* 2002;346:896.

    Second and larger placebo-controlled trial of bosentan. Confirmed the findings of the earlier study showing improvement in 6-minute walk distance, WHO class, and Borg dyspnea index in the bosentan-treated patients.

22. Sastry BK, et al. Clinical efficacy of sildenafil in primary pulmonary hypertension: a randomized, placebo controlled, double-blind, crossover study. *J Am Coll Cardiol.* 2004;43:1149.

    In this study, 22 patients received either placebo or sildenafil (25–100 mg tid, based on body weight) for 6 weeks, and were then crossed over to the other treatment (placebo or sildenafil) for an additional 6 weeks. Sildenafil led to improved exercise time, cardiac index, and quality-of-life scores.

23. Setaro JF, et al. The right ventricle in disorders causing pulmonary venous hypertension. *Cardiol Clin.* 1992;10:165.
    An excellent review article describing the physiologic and clinical consequences of pulmonary venous hypertension.
24. Simonneau G, et al. Continuous subcutaneous infusion of treprostinil, a prostacyclin analogue, in patients with pulmonary arterial hypertension. *Am J Respir Crit Care Med.* 2002;165:800.
    Showed improved hemodynamics and 6-minute walk distance in treprostinil-treated patients versus placebo. Improvement was greater with higher treprostinil dose achieved.
25. Sitbon O, et al. Long-term intravenous epoprostenol infusion in primary pulmonary hypertension. Prognostic factors and survival. *J Am Coll Cardiol.* 2002;40:780.
    Prospective study of 178 class III/IV PPH patients undergoing treatment with epoprostenol. Persistence of WHO functional class III/IV symptoms, failure to show a decrease in TPR of at least 30%, and any history of right ventricular failure were all independent predictors of mortality when analyzed by multivariate analysis.
26. Soler M, et al. Long-term oxygen therapy for cor pulmonale in patients with chronic obstructive pulmonary disease. *Respiration.* 1991;58(Suppl 1):52.
    Reviews several studies evaluating the mechanisms of the survival effect of oxygen in this group. It appears that patients with COPD and mild pulmonary hypertension have improved survival with oxygen supplementation, whereas those with more severe pulmonary hypertension do not gain a survival benefit.

---

71. HEART–LUNG AND LUNG TRANSPLANTATION

Gordon L. Yung

Although the first human lung transplant was performed in 1963, it was not until the early 1980s that it became an acceptable treatment for end-stage lung diseases following the introduction of cyclosporine as a safe and efficacious immunosuppressive drug. From 1985 to 2001, 14,574 lung transplantations were reported to the Registry of the International Society for Heart and Lung Transplantation. The majority are performed in the United States; 1041 lung transplantations were recorded in 2002. The demand for thoracic transplantation continues to grow, as long-term results improve; however, the number of operations has lagged due primarily to a lack of suitable donor organs. Only 15 to 20% of all potential donors have lungs suitable for transplant, reflecting the fragility of lungs as donor organs. Recent improvements in donor management have resulted in significant increases in organ availability in some regions.

Heart–lung transplantations (the transplant of heart and two lungs en bloc) are seldom performed now; the number reported has decreased by more than 50% since 1995 with only 31 cases in the United States in 2002. In fact, the Registry of the International Society for Heart and Lung Transplantation reported in 2001 that only 35 of 101 lung transplantation centers worldwide were still performing heart–lung transplants. Combined heart–single lung transplantation recently has been reported.

Until recently, lung transplantations were performed in the order patients were listed; the earlier a patient was listed the higher up he or she would be on the waiting list. Experience in other solid organ transplantations suggested that a valid priority system would allow better allocation of organs, resulting in lower mortality for patients on the waiting list. Beginning in 2005, the lung transplantation allocation system in the United States was changed to one based on a priority system. The new system classifies patients into four groups:

A: chronic obstructive pulmonary disease, α-1 antitrypsin deficiency, lymphangiomyomatosis, and sarcoidosis without pulmonary hypertension
B: pulmonary vascular diseases
C: cystic fibrosis and other immunodeficiency states; and
D: restrictive lung diseases, including pulmonary fibrosis, sarcoidosis with pulmonary hypertension, and nontransplant obliterative bronchiolitis.

Patients are then given a lung allocation score that is calculated from the wait list urgency (predicted mortality risk during the waiting time) and 1-year posttransplant survival. This complex system is designed to compare severity among different lung diseases, while accounting for the fact that the sickest patients often have the worst posttransplant outcomes. Unfortunately, the system does not consider the better outcome in individual transplant centers that have expertise in managing specific patient groups.

Guidelines for the optimal timing of recipient referral have been developed based on the underlying lung disease (Table 71-1). Different lung conditions progress at different rates. Therefore, the guidelines in Table 71-1 should only be used as a general guideline; each patient should be considered individually based on the nature of the underlying lung disease and its severity and likelihood of progressing. Other factors that may affect the wait time include ABO blood groups and body/lung size. Decisions about listing a patient should, therefore, be the responsibility of physicians familiar with the local transplant environment.

In the past, patients were only considered for transplant when expected survival without surgery was less than 1 to 2 years, despite optimal medical therapy. The

Table 71-1. Referral guidelines for selected diseases

CHRONIC OBSTRUCTIVE PULMONARY DISEASE
FEV_1 <20–25% predicted or $\leq$500 mL
CO_2 retention ($PaCO_2$ $\geq$55 mmHg)
Pulmonary hypertension
Severe hypoxemia (PaO_2 <55–60 mmHg)
Rapid deterioration

CYSTIC FIBROSIS
FEV_1 <30% predicted
CO_2 retention ($PaCO_2$ $\geq$50 mmHg)
Pulmonary hypertension
Severe hypoxemia (PaO_2 <55 mmHg)
Rapid deterioration

IDIOPATHIC PULMONARY FIBROSIS
Vital capacity or total lung capacity <70% predicted
DLCO <60% predicted
Pulmonary hypertension
Resting hypoxemia
Deterioration despite therapy

PRIMARY PULMONARY HYPERTENSION
NYHA functional class III or IV
Cardiac index <2 L/min/m^2
Right atrial pressure >10–15 mmHg
Mean pulmonary artery pressure $\geq$50–55 mmHg

prognosis following lung transplantation has improved significantly because of advances in medications, surgical techniques, and posttransplant care. Currently, the overall survival after single-lung transplantation is about 3.6 years, and after bilateral lung transplantation, about 4.5 years. Therefore, patients with life expectancy of up to 2 to 3 years when donor lungs become available may also be considered for transplantation.

Lung transplantation has been performed for almost any condition that results in severe isolated lung disease. The commonest indications are chronic obstructive pulmonary disease, primary pulmonary hypertension, cystic fibrosis, and idiopathic pulmonary fibrosis. A vigorous selection process for suitable recipients is crucial to a successful outcome that benefits the largest number of patients because of the significant perioperative and postoperative morbidity and mortality, as well as limitation in organ supplies. The ideal patient should be healthy enough to go through surgery safely with the fewest postoperative complications (both immediate and long term), yet sick enough to justify the considerable risks and expense. Every patient is, therefore, required to undergo an extensive evaluation to determine transplant candidacy. This includes a detailed history and physical examination; blood, urine, and skin testing for latent infections or organ dysfunction; cardiac and pulmonary function testing; chest radiograph and computed tomography scan, as well as a careful psychosocial assessment. Every transplant center has its own set of guidelines regarding recipient selection. Important conditions that affect outcome are discussed in the following section.

1. *Absolute contraindications:* These include (a) HIV infection; (b) extrapulmonary irreversible major organ dysfunction such as concomitant renal or liver disease; patients with irreparable cardiac disease who are otherwise suitable candidates may be considered for heart–lung transplant; (c) hepatitis B antigenemia; and (d) hepatitis C infection, especially with histologically proven liver disease. However, individual centers may have experience in certain disease that may allow for exceptions.

2. *Relative contraindications:* (a) Age: statistically, older patients have worse survival outcome after lung transplantation. In general, the age limit is no older than 65 years for single lung transplant, 60 years for double lung transplant, and 55 years for heart–lung transplant. Chronological and biological/functional age may differ significantly in individuals and some centers are willing to consider patients above these age limits. (b) Preoperative severe osteoporosis has been associated with increased long-term morbidity and may compromise the objective of lung transplantation in improving the quality of life in recipients. (c) Steroid use is no longer an absolute contraindication, because of improvement in surgical techniques in airway anastomosis; many centers now accept patients taking up to a daily dose of 10 to 20 mg of prednisone. (d) History of recent neoplasm, especially within the past 2 years, represents a significant risk of tumor recurrence. The actual disease-free interval depends on the type of tumor and the associated risk of recurrence. Five-year documented disease-free interval may be more suitable in cases where neoplasm presents at a more advance stage. (e) Many centers put patients with active extrapulmonary infection on hold, until the condition is treated. The presence of certain organisms, such as *Burkholderia cepacia* and pan-resistant *Pseudomonas spp*, has been associated with adverse outcome, whereas colonization of *Aspergillus* or nontuberculous mycobacterium does not appear to impact mortality. (f) Severe musculoskeletal disease such as severe kyphoscoliosis may increase intraoperative difficulty and perioperative complications. (g) Ventilator dependence at the time of transplant has been associated with higher postoperative mortality. (h) Previous thoracic surgery, pleurodesis (especially by mechanical means), and pleurectomy all increase surgical difficulties and operative risks. (i) Extreme body weights ($\pm 20\%$ of ideal body weight) are associated with worse outcome and aggressive approaches, including dietary restriction or placement of a feeding tube, are often necessary. (j) High levels of HLA-typed lymphocyte panel (panel reactive antibodies), often from previous blood transfusions or pregnancies, may predispose patients to hyperacute rejection after transplantation. Strategies such as pretransplant HLA typing, plasmapheresis, or treatment with immunosuppressants and immunoglobulins

have been employed, although the efficacy is not known. (k) Psychosocial problems, such as recent or current substance abuse, history of noncompliance, and poorly controlled major affective disorders should be resolved prior to listing. Most centers require patients with history of substance abuse to undergo at least 3 to 6 months of supervised abstinence program. Refusal of blood products, as in the case of a Jehovah Witness, is usually considered a significant contraindication. Finally, all patients should be able participate in the complicated posttransplant care and have the necessary social support after they are discharged home.

PRETRANSPLANT FOLLOW-UP
Patients are generally followed up at regular intervals and transplant physicians have to work closely with referring physicians to ensure that the patient remains a suitable transplant candidate. Because of the specific needs of pretransplant care and long waiting times, transplant physicians increasingly play an active role in patient care for transplant candidates once they are listed. It is common for patients to be placed on hold temporarily when, for instance, there are extreme body weight changes or when patients require temporary mechanical ventilation. Other patients may develop conditions after listing that make transplantation unacceptable, such as airway colonization of B. cepacia in patients with cystic fibrosis. Conversely, patients may become "too healthy" for transplantation, as in some patients with primary pulmonary hypertension who respond well to medical therapies. Health maintenance is an important part of pretransplant care to ensure optimal health prior to surgery. This includes yearly dental, eye, and gynecologic examinations, and up-to-date immunizations for influenza, pneumococcus, hepatitis B, and tetanus. Some transplant physicians initiate aggressive pretransplant treatment of osteoporosis in high-risk patients, such as those on long-term steroid treatment and patients with cystic fibrosis. With the new allocation system, patients who are actively on the transplant list would be required to have periodic assessment of not more than 6 months. In each follow-up, both clinical and laboratory tests (such as pulmonary function tests, 6-minute walk test, echocardiogram or even right heart catheterization) are used to determine the up-to-date allocation score, hence priority to transplant.

DONOR SELECTION
It is clear that proper donor selection and organ preservation improve transplant outcome. After being accepted on the waiting list, patients are matched with donors according to their ABO blood group and lung size. In theory, donors with O blood type may be considered as universal donors, although this may present potential issues of fairness with organ distribution. The choice between matching cytomegalovirus (CMV) status versus prophylactic anti-CMV treatment depends on institutional practice. Donor organs are routinely evaluated for function and to exclude active or latent infections. General guidelines for donors include age under 65 years old, no significant history of lung disease or smoking, normal chest radiograph, good lung compliance and oxygenation, and normal gross and bronchoscopic appearance. The use of marginal donor lungs should be a decision made only after careful consideration supported by informed consent from individual patient.

TYPE OF TRANSPLANTATION PROCEDURES
There are three types of lung transplantation: single lung (SLT), bilateral (sequential) lung (BLT), and living donor transplantation. Heart-lung transplantation (HLT) is sometimes considered a form of lung transplantation, although it should only be done in centers with experience in this type of surgery. The type of transplantation performed depends on the underlying disease, associated conditions (e.g., previous thoracic or pleural surgeries), and institutional practice. Because of the limited number of suitable donors, SLT is preferred whenever feasible. It is also technically the simplest and, unlike other types of transplantation, can usually be performed via a thoracotomy without cardiopulmonary bypass. The disadvantages of SLT are that the recipients are left with one diseased lung, and patients generally have poorer results on pulmonary function testing even after recovery. Practically, however, patients with successful SLT have little functional disability in almost all normal daily activities.

BLT is performed through an anterior thoracosternotomy and is usually reserved for patients at risk of recurrent pulmonary infections if the native lung is left behind. It is, therefore, recommended primarily for patients with cystic fibrosis or generalized bronchiectasis. Perioperative management of patients with primary pulmonary hypertension after BLT appears to be simpler than after SLT, because of their decreased intraoperative hemodynamic disturbances and better pulmonary perfusion distribution. There is also evidence that patients with primary pulmonary hypertension may have better long-term outcomes after BLT, although the better results may be affected by the fact that BLT patients tend to be younger. Balancing this consideration is the fact that the waiting time for BLT may be longer in some centers where organ supply is limited. Finally, as long as there is significant donor organ shortage, the ethics of giving one donor's lungs to two recipients to provide a small additional survival benefits should also be considered.

The incidence of HLT has decreased dramatically. HLT utilizes a median sternotomy approach and is reserved mostly for patients with end-stage lung disease who have irreparable cardiac conditions, as in some cases of Eisenmenger syndrome. Cystic fibrosis represents the third commonest diagnosis leading to HLT, although BLT is much more commonly used for this condition.

Because of the lack of donors, living donor transplantation has become increasing popular. Most cases have been performed on pediatric patients with cystic fibrosis, for whom the donors are close family members. Two donors are required, each donating the lower lobe of one lung (right and left) to the respective chest cavity of the recipient. This procedure has the advantage of allowing extensive donor evaluation and can potentially improve HLA matching. Criteria for living donor transplant recipients should be the same for other types of lung transplantation and the procedure should not be performed as a rescue operation for patients in extremis. Aside from an increase in technical difficulties, there are ethical considerations of subjecting two healthy adults to an operation that does not directly benefit their own health. To date, there have been no deaths attributed to being a living donor and preliminary results suggest that living donor transplantation may be a reasonable option in selected patients.

POSTTRANSPLANT MANAGEMENT

Most centers use a regimen of three immunosuppressive agents beginning immediately before or just after surgery. A typical combination includes cyclosporine or tacrolimus, azathioprine or mycophenolate mofetil, and prednisone. Induction therapy with a cytolytic agent like OKT-3 monoclonal antibody or antithymocyte antibody may also be added during the first weeks after transplantation. Immediate complications after transplantation include bleeding, bronchial anastomosis dehiscence, reimplantation pulmonary edema, acute rejection, graft failure, and infection. Because mortality is highest in the first year after lung transplantation, frequent follow-ups are required during this period. Lung function normally improves gradually after transplant and plateaus at about 2 to 3 months postsurgery.

Besides graft failure, bacterial infection, especially by *Pseudomonas spp*, is the commonest cause of death during the first 3 months after transplantation, and it continues to be a significant problem throughout the life of the recipients. Fungal infections, predominately from *Candida* and *Aspergillus* species, can occur both early and late after lung transplantation and should be treated aggressively. With the advent of oral antifungal agents, many centers now empirically treat patients with evidence of airway colonization by fungi, both before and after transplantation. Prophylactic antiviral therapy after transplantation may reduce infections by viruses like CMV.

Acute lung rejections occur most commonly in the first year, but can occur several years after transplantation. Clinical presentation is similar to that of pneumonia and treatment with short courses of high-dose corticosteroids is often effective. Bronchoscopic examinations with or without transbronchial biopsies are usually required to differentiate between infection and acute rejection.

Chronic allograft rejection, or obliterative bronchiolitis, occurs in 34 to 41% of patients and usually presents with progressive shortness of breath and evidence of airflow obstruction in lung function. It usually occurs months to years after transplantation and is often preceded by an episode of infection or acute rejection. Unlike acute rejection, chronic rejection is often refractory to treatment and some centers advocate routine surveillance bronchoscopic examinations for early disease detection and treatment. Retransplantation remains a controversial option for patients with severe irreversible allograft failure.

Most other long-term complications after transplantation are related to the use of immunosuppressive therapy. Osteoporosis, renal insufficiency, myelosuppression, and malignancy (especially skin cancer and lymphoproliferative disease) occur commonly after lung transplantation. Narrowing of airways at the site of anastomosis is not uncommon and may require bronchoscopic dilatation and stent placement. A high index of suspicion for these complications ensures early detection and early treatment.

1. Trulock EP. State of the art. Lung transplantation. *Am J Respir Crit Care Med.* 1997;155:789–818.
   Overview of lung transplantation, with sufficient details for most clinicians.
2. Arcasoy SM, Kotloff RM. Lung transplantation. *New Engl J Med.* 1999;340:1081–1091.
   A review on lung transplantation that offers fairly detailed and up-to-date information for practicing physicians.
3. Maurer JR, ed. Surgical approaches to end-stage disease: Lung transplantation and volume reduction. *Clin Chest Med.* 1997;18:173–419.
   One of the most comprehensive review of all aspects of lung transplantation.
4. Norman DJ, Suki WN, eds. *The ASTP Primer on Transplantation,* American Society of Transplant Physicians, Thorofare, NJ, 1998.
   A general "primer" for all solid organ transplantation, with good discussion on the immunology aspects of transplantation.
5. Trulock EP, Edwards LB, Taylor DO, et al. The registry of the international society for heart and lung transplantation: Twentieth official report—2003. *J Heart Lung Transplant.* 2003;22:625–635.
   A yearly update with current statistics on survival and analysis of risk factors of heart and lung transplantations performed worldwide. Results are reported according to the type of transplantation.
6. International guidelines for the selection of lung transplant candidates. The joint statement of the American Society for Transplant Physicians/American Thoracic Society/European Respiratory Society/International Society for Heart and Lung Transplantation. *Am J Respir Crit Care Med.* 1998;158:335–339.
   Consensus statement on recipient selection, with good guidelines on timing of referral, and contraindications to transplantation.
7. Shennib H, Massard G. Airway complications in lung transplantation. *Ann Thorac Surg.* 1994;57:506–511.
   Review of airway complications after lung transplantation showed 2 to 3% fatal cases and 7 to 14% late stricture. The authors also proposed a classification of airway complications.
8. Schäfers HJ, Wagner TO, Demertzis S, et al. Preoperative corticosteroids. A contraindication to lung transplantation? *Chest.* 1992;102:1522–1525.
   No increase in post-transplant morbidity and mortality in fourteen patients on longterm preoperative prednisolone (0.1 to 0.3 mg/kg per day).
9. Shane E, Papadopoulos A, Staron RB, et al. Bone loss and fracture after lung transplantation. *Transplantation.* 1999;68:220–227.
   Prospective evaluation of 30 patients after lung transplantation for one year showed preoperative use of steroid and low bone mineral density are risks factors for post-transplantation fractures.
10. Conte JV, Gaine SP, Orens JB, et al. The influence of continuous intravenous prostacyclin therapy for primary pulmonary hypertension on the timing and outcome of transplantation. *J Heart Lung Transplant.* 1998;17:679–685.

Retrospective analysis 37 patients with primary pulmonary hypertension. Use of prostacyclin delayed or obviated the need of lung transplantation in 70% of patients.

11. Starnes VA, Barr ML, Cohen RG, et al. Living-donor lobar lung transplantation experience: Intermediate results. *J Thorac Cardiovasc Surg.* 1996;112:1284–1289.
    Results of a 14-month follow-up of 38 patients (27 adults, 10 pediatrics) who received living-donor lobar lung transplantation. There were 14 deaths in the recipients and 76 donor complications.

12. Sundaresan S, Semenkovich J, Ochoa L, et al. Successful outcome of lung transplantation is not compromised by the use of marginal donor lungs. *J Thorac Cardiovasc Surg.* 1995;109:1075–1079.
    Forty-four lung transplantations with "marginal donor lungs" showed comparable short-term results to controls.

13. Novick RJ, Stitt LW, Al-Kattan K, et al. Pulmonary retransplantation: Predictors of graft function and survival in 230 patients. Pulmonary Retransplantation Registry. *Ann Thorac Surg.* 1998;65:227–234.
    Survival of 230 patients after retransplantation of lungs was 47%, 40%, and 33% at 1, 2, and 3 years, respectively, after surgery. Although survival was better in ambulatory, nonventilated patients, results were still inferior to statistics from first-time transplantations.

14. Kaiser LR, Pasque MK, Trulock EP, et al. Bilateral sequential lung transplantation: The procedure of choice for double-lung replacement. *Ann Thorac Surg.* 1991;52:438–445.
    This study demonstrated the efficacy and safety of sequential lung transplantation over the old en bloc double-lung technique, and is now the procedure of choice for double-lung transplantation.

15. Penn I. The effect of immunosuppression on pre-existing cancers. *Chest.* 1993;55:742–747.
    Follow-up of 913 patients with preexisting malignancies who underwent renal transplantation. The study identified the risks of tumor recurrence, based on type of cancer, and effect of treatment prior to transplantation.

16. Penn I. Incidence and treatment of neoplasia after transplantation. *J Heart Lung Transplant.* 1993;12:S328–336.
    The study looked at 6798 patients who underwent different organ transplantations and showed a higher incidence of lymphoma in heart or heart and lung recipients.

17. Glotz D, Haymann JP, Sansonetti N, et al. Suppression of HLA-specific alloantibodies by high-dose intravenous immunoglobulins. *Transplantation.* 1993;56:335–337.
    Intravenous immunoglobulins suppressed panel reactive anti-HLA antibodies in four of five patients waiting for renal transplantation.

18. Guilinger RA, Paradis IL, Dauber JH, et al. The importance of bronchoscopy with transbronchial biopsy and bronchoalveolar lavage in the management of lung transplant recipients. *Am J Respir Crit Care Med.* 1995;152:2037–2043.
    Retrospective analysis of 1124 bronchoscopies in 161 lung transplant patients showed unsuspected rejection and infection in 25% cases, of which 68% occurred in first 6 months.

19. Sundaresan RS, Trulock EP, Mohanakumar T, et al. Prevalence and outcome of bronchiolitis obliterans syndrome after lung transplantation. *Ann Thorac Surg.* 1995;60:1341–1347.
    High incidence of bronchiolitis obliterans with significant mortality. Most common presentation was decline in spirometry.

20. Ettinger NA, Bailey TC, Trulock EP, et al. Cytomegalovirus infection and pneumonitis: Impact after isolated lung transplantation. *Am Rev Respir Dis.* 1993;147:1017–1023.
    High incidence of CMV pneumonitis after transplantation, especially in CMV-positive donors. Only one third of cases of CMV pneumonitis had chest radiograph changes.

VII. CONGENITAL AND PEDIATRIC LUNG DISEASE

72. PULMONARY MANIFESTATIONS OF SICKLE CELL DISEASE

Stephen P. Bradley

Sickle cell disease (SCD) is a clinical syndrome common to a group of hemoglobinopathies in which the primary defect is the tendency of deoxygenated hemoglobin S to form large polymers that deform erythrocytes. Consequently, capillary blood flow is blocked and tissue ischemia occurs. Pulmonary involvement in SCD is common and often severe; acute chest syndrome is the second leading cause of hospitalization (after pain crisis), and the leading cause of death in adults with SCD. Patients with SCD who survive into adulthood are at risk for developing sickle chronic lung disease, which is associated with marked disability and decreased survival.

Pulmonary function testing in patients with SCD reveals a variety of abnormalities. Asthma is common and present in approximately one half of patients. Twenty percent of patients have mixed obstructive and restrictive abnormalities, and 20% have restrictive defects only.

INFECTION

Patients with SCD, particularly children, are at increased risk of infection. Functional asplenia occurs early in the course (before recurrent infarction leads to involution of the organ), resulting in poor bacterial clearance from the blood stream. In addition, patients with SCD may have defects in polymorphonuclear leukocyte function (defective degranulation and intracellular killing) and deficient serum opsonizing activity, leading to recurrent infections. In the lung, microvascular occlusion probably leads to local impairment of phagocytic activity. As a result of these defects in immune function, children with SCD have a 20- to 100-fold increased risk of developing pneumonia.

Streptococcus pneumoniae is the most frequently identified organism causing pneumonia in SCD, accounting for 58% of such cases in children younger than 2 years of age, and 25% in patients older than 10 years of age. *Haemophilus influenzae* is isolated in approximately 18% of patients; other important causes of pneumonia are *Staphylococcus aureus, Escherichia coli, Salmonella* species, *Mycoplasma* species, and other gram-negative organisms. Pneumonia, particularly with bacteremia, is an important cause of death in children with SCD before the age of 4 years. Thereafter, the decline in the incidence of pneumonia and, particularly, bacteremic pneumonia (14% in children <2 years versus 1.8% in patients >10 years) is attributed to the development of specific antibodies to the offending organisms.

The clinical presentation of pneumonia in patients with SCD is not unique; however, the severity of the illness tends to be greater and the response to therapy is slower, than in otherwise healthy individuals. A combination of third-generation cephalosporin and macrolide therapy is the most common initial empiric therapy; however, the addition of anti-staphylococcal therapy should be considered in some patients.

PULMONARY THROMBOEMBOLISM

The epidemiology of pulmonary thromboembolism in patients with SCD has not been well characterized. These patients probably are at increased risk based on observations of the natural history and the results of autopsy studies. Establishing the diagnosis can be problematic; ventilation–perfusion scans can be difficult to interpret in the setting of acute and chronic SCD-related lung disease, and intravenous contrast dye can both precipitate sickling and cause a deterioration in renal function. Conversely, empirical anticoagulation is generally not recommended because of an increased risk of intracranial and renal hemorrhage.

ACUTE CHEST SYNDROME

The acute chest syndrome (ACS) is defined as the development of a new area of pulmonary consolidation, chest pain, fever, and additional symptoms of dyspnea, wheezing or cough in patients with SCD. The physical examination may be normal in about one third of patients with ACS; rales are the most common abnormal finding. Earlier studies described a normal initial chest radiograph in up to 46% of cases; however, these patients typically developed focal or diffuse pulmonary infiltrates within 1 to 2 days. Pleural effusions are seen in 55% of cases, and are more common in adults than children.

Although the term *acute chest syndrome* was originally used to describe patients in whom a noninfectious cause for their presentation was postulated, distinguishing infectious from noninfectious causes of the described signs and symptoms is clinically quite difficult. The problem is clearly worsened by the insensitivity of currently available diagnostic tests for pneumonia; thus, patients with ACS are almost always empirically treated with antibiotics. For these reasons, recent studies of ACS have included both groups. Characteristics that suggest a noninfectious cause include (1) upper or middle lobe disease; (2) associated pain crisis; (3) older age; (4) negative sputum smears and sputum or blood cultures for usual bacterial pathogens; (5) rapid improvement in chest roentgenography (<72 hours); and (6) associated neurologic symptoms.

Etiology and Pathophysiology

Several causes of ACS have been proposed, and each probably plays a role in different clinical situations. These include infection, lung infarction, bone marrow embolization, thoracic bone infarction, and bronchoconstriction.

Young children often have an infectious organism isolated from blood or sputum. The incidence of ACS in children (and less so in adults) follows a seasonal pattern, with the greatest incidence in the fall and winter, suggesting a causative role for respiratory tract infections by otherwise poorly virulent organisms such as viruses or *Chlamydia*.

Lung infarction, from a variety of causes, is probably an important cause of ACS. The deoxygenated blood entering the pulmonary circulation is susceptible to sickling, making the lung particularly vulnerable to in situ microvascular thrombosis and tissue infarction. Local ischemia, as would occur in the setting of pneumonia or atelectasis, can accelerate this process. The incidence of large-vessel pulmonary embolism resulting from deep vein thrombosis as a cause of ACS is not well characterized.

Several lines of evidence suggest that bone marrow embolization to the lung, occurring as a result of bone infarction during an acute pain crisis, is an important cause of ACS. A syndrome of fatal fat embolism occurring in pregnant women with SCD is well described. Autopsies of these patients disclose necrotic marrow fragments occluding the pulmonary arteries. In addition, an autopsy study of patients with advanced SCD disease dying from any cause disclosed bone marrow fragments in the pulmonary circulation in 13%. Many of the patients with marrow fragments died suddenly and without another explanation, and had a history of a recent episode of ACS. Clinically, acute pain (bony) crisis often precedes the onset of ACS by several days, and bone scintigraphy performed during ACS frequently demonstrates evidence of acute long bone infarction; occasionally, the bone involvement is asymptomatic. A recent study of bronchoalveolar lavage fluid from adults with ACS demonstrated the presence of a high percentage of lipid-laden alveolar macrophages in 77% of patients. This is similar to the finding in fat embolism syndrome secondary to traumatic long bone fracture. As in the fat embolism syndrome, patients with ACS had a high incidence of neurologic abnormalities such as depressed consciousness, seizures, or focal neurologic signs on examination, adding further evidence that marrow embolization is a common cause of ACS.

Thoracic bone infarction is another probable cause of ACS. Infarction involving the ribs, sternum, or thoracic spine can be demonstrated on bone scintigraphy in some patients. Local soft tissue reaction involving the chest wall, pleura, and subpleural lung, as well as atelectasis secondary to splinting, could lead to local ischemia, erythrocyte sickling, and pulmonary infiltrates. Bronchoconstriction, leading to regional hypoxemia and subsequent sickling, is another commonly recognized cause of ACS.

Incidence

ACS occurs in 30 to 45% of patients with SCD over their lifetimes. In the largest retrospective study, approximately 55% of patients who experienced ACS had a single event over their lifetimes, and only 9% had experienced five or more episodes. A recent prospective study, involving 671 episodes of ACS at 30 centers, has greatly advanced our understanding of ACS. Approximately half of the patients were admitted for reasons other than ACS, most commonly vasoocclusive crisis. ACS developed on average 2.5 days after admission in these patients. Complications were common. Thirteen percent of all patients required mechanical ventilation, and neurologic events (altered mental status, seizures, and neuromuscular abnormalities) occurred in 11%. The mean hospital stay was 10.5 days. Eighteen patients died; the most common causes of death were pulmonary emboli (bone marrow, fat, or thrombotic) and bronchopneumonia. Infection contributed to 56% of deaths. Despite an aggressive approach to diagnosis, the cause of ACS could not be determined in approximately 46% of patients. A presumptive diagnosis of infarction was made in 16% of patients, followed by fat embolism (established by demonstrating lipid-laden macrophages in bronchoalveolar lavage fluid) in 8.8%, *Chlamydia* (7.2%), *Mycoplasma* (6.6%), virus (6.4%), bacteria (4.5%), and mixed infections (3.7%).

Management

Patients in this study were managed using a treatment algorithm. Oxygen therapy was administered to maintain an oxygen saturation of 90%. Antibiotics, consisting of a cephalosporin and erythromycin, were given for 7 to 10 days. Fluid administration was maintained at 1.0 to 1.5 times daily fluid requirements, to avoid dehydration (to decrease the rheologic effects of sickled red cells) or overhydration (and hydrostatic pulmonary edema). Incentive spirometry, which has been demonstrated to decrease the risk of pulmonary complications, including development of pulmonary infiltrates or atelectasis, and to shorten hospital stay in ACS secondary to thoracic bone infarcts, was used in all patients. Pain control was accomplished with a combination of patient-controlled analgesia, and nonsteroidal agents, with the goal of avoiding both respiratory splinting (due to pain) and hypoventilation (due to oversedation). Bronchodilators were given to the 61% patients with evidence of reactive airways disease. Transfusion, both simple and exchange, was left to the discretion of the treating physicians; 72% of patients received transfusion, with resulting improvement in oxygenation. Of note was the finding that bronchoscopy, used to establish bone marrow embolization or infectious etiologies, was associated with a high complication rate in patients with ACS. Other studies have questioned the utility of bronchoscopy in this setting; at this time bronchoscopy should not be considered standard of care in ACS.

Other studies have clearly shown transfusion therapy as a means of preventing ACS in one group of patients. A 10% risk of postoperative ACS is seen in patients with SCD undergoing surgical procedures under general anesthesia. Preoperative transfusion to a hemoglobin level greater than 10 g/dl decreases this risk substantially.

Outcomes

Despite aggressive support, up to 25% of deaths in SCD are attributed to ACS. The risk increases with age; whereas the overall mortality during an episode of ACS is 1.8%, in adults it is 4.3%. Other risk factors for death include respiratory failure developing within 48 hours of presentation, bacterial sepsis, and associated pain crisis. However, several authors have noted that the initial presentation can be a poor predictor of outcome; some patients presenting with relatively mild symptoms rapidly develop progressive pulmonary infiltrates and intractable respiratory failure.

Sickle Cell Chronic Lung Disease

Patients who survive repeated episodes of ACS are at risk of developing sickle cell chronic lung disease (SCCLD). SCCLD is characterized by progressive dyspnea with exercise limitation, and chest pain of increasing severity. These patients progress through a series of stages:

- Stage 1: Recurrent chest pain and cough with mild restriction on pulmonary function testing. Oxygen saturation is normal; increased interstitial markings noted on chest radiograph.
- Stage 2: Greater chest pain, moderate restriction on pulmonary function testing, normal oxygen saturation, and diffusely increased interstitial markings.
- Stage 3: Severe chest pain, severe restriction, hypoxemia, marked interstitial infiltrates.
- Stage 4: Intractable chest pain, persistent dyspnea, hypoxemia at rest, severe pulmonary fibrosis pattern on chest radiograph, cor pulmonale.

The average age at diagnosis of SCCLD is 25 years, and life expectancy from initial presentation is just over 7 years. However, careful evaluation of at-risk patients reveals that abnormalities are demonstrable on pulmonary function tests for several years before clinical presentation. Although a clustering of ACS episodes occurring before the onset and throughout the course of SCLD is well documented, the mechanisms by which the acute events lead to irreversible lung damage are not well understood. Therapeutic interventions have not yet been able to change the outcome of this devastating disease. Some patients have been reported to have an improved sense of well-being from chronic transfusion therapy to maintain a hemoglobin S level below 30%.

Pulmonary hypertension, occurring independently of SCCLD, is being increasingly recognized in adults with SCD, and carries a poor prognosis. An obliterative vasculopathy is found in one third of all patients with SCD at autopsy. Prospectively, pulmonary hypertension can be detected in 32% of stable adults with SCD by echocardiography. In these patients, despite only modest elevations in pulmonary artery systolic pressures, and high cardiac output consistent with chronic anemia, survival was markedly lower in SCD patients with pulmonary hypertension than those with normal pulmonary artery pressures. Patients with pulmonary hypertension had not experienced more episodes of ACS than controls, suggesting a different mechanism of disease than for SCCLD. However, markers of hemolysis were higher in pulmonary hypertensive patients. One mechanism by which chronic hemolysis may lead to pulmonary hypertension is through a decrease in levels of the pulmonary vasodilator nitric oxide (NO). Hemolyzed red cells release both free hemoglobin, which scavenges NO, and arginase, which inactivates the NO precursor arginine. Oral administration of L-arginine led to 15% decrease in pulmonary artery pressures in an acute study of pulmonary hypertensive SCD patients. Reports of improved survival in patients treated with inhaled NO, prostacyclin analog infusion, and aggressive exchange transfusion need to be confirmed in prospective studies before such measures are recommended for routine clinical use in SCD patients with pulmonary hypertension.

1. Minter KR, Gladwin MT. Pulmonary complications of sickle cell anemia. A need for increased recognition, treatment, and research. *Am J Respir Crit Care Med.* 2001;164:2016.
    A concise review of the pulmonary manifestations of SCD, including what is known about the pathogenesis of those disorders and recommendations for further areas of research.
2. Charache S, Scott J, Charache P. 'Acute chest syndrome' in adults with sickle cell anemia. Microbiology, treatment, and prevention. *Arch Intern Med.* 1979;139:67.
    The original report suggesting that pulmonary infarction, rather than infection, is a major cause of ACS in adults.
3. Bromberg PA. Pulmonary aspects of sickle cell disease. *Arch Intern Med.* 1974;133:652.
    An excellent review of the pulmonary complications of SCD, including the abnormalities in pulmonary physiologic testing.
4. Haynes JC, Kirkpatrick MB. The acute chest syndrome of sickle cell disease. *Am J Med Sci.* 1993;305:326.
    A concise and fairly up-to-date review.

5. Barrett-Connor E. Bacterial infection and sickle cell anemia: An analysis of 250 infections in 166 patients with a review of the literature. *Medicine.* 1971;50:97.

Of childhood deaths in SCD, 75% were felt to be related to bacterial infections. Impaired splenic function, decreased lung defenses caused by thrombi and ischemia, and deficiency of opsonizing activity against encapsulated bacteria are noted.

6. Smith JA. Cardiopulmonary manifestations of sickle cell disease in childhood. *Semin Roentgenol.* 1987;22:160.

General review of pulmonary manifestations of sickle cell disease, including discussion of infection, pulmonary function, acute chest manifestations, and radiographic findings.

7. Moser KM, Luchsinger PC, Katz S. Pulmonary and cardiac function in sickle cell lung disease: Preliminary report. *Diseases of the Chest.* 1960;37:637.

A discussion of the possible mechanisms for pulmonary vascular occlusion and cor pulmonale in SCD; rest and exercise right ventricular catheterization data are presented in 10 patients, with exercise values for mean pulmonary arterial pressure exceeding normal in 6.

8. Moser KM, Shea JG. The relationship between pulmonary infarction, cor pulmonale and the sickle states. *Am J Med.* 1957;22:561.

Case presentations and discussion emphasizing the occurrence of cor pulmonale in sickle cell anemia and other sickle cell diseases.

9. Haupt HM, Moore GW, Bauer TW, et al. The lung in sickle cell disease. *Chest.* 1982;81:332.

An autopsy study of 72 patients with advanced SCD. The main pulmonary findings were alveolar wall necrosis secondary to vascular obstruction, focal parenchymal scars, and necrotic bone marrow emboli.

10. Wilimas JA, Flynn PM, Harris S, et al. A randomized study of outpatient treatment with ceftriaxone for selected febrile children with sickle cell disease. *N Engl J Med.* 1993;329:472–476.

With the use of conservative eligibility criteria, half of the febrile episodes in children with SCD could be treated safely on an outpatient basis. Patients with segmental or larger pulmonary infiltrates were excluded.

11. Bhalla M, Abboud MR, McLoud TC, et al. Acute chest syndrome in sickle cell disease: CT evidence of microvascular occlusion. *Radiology.* 1993;187:45.

In this thin section CT study, 9 of 10 patients with ACS were found to have small vessel attenuation in the lung, consistent with microvascular obstruction, surrounded by areas of ground glass infiltrate.

12. Bellet PS, Kalinyak KA, Shukla R, et al. Incentive spirometry to prevent acute pulmonary complications in sickle cell diseases. *N Engl J Med.* 1995;333:699.

Of patients with ACS, 39.5% had evidence of thoracic bone infarcts; in these patients, hospital duration and the development of pulmonary complications were significantly reduced by the use of incentive spirometry when compared with controls.

13. Vichinsky E, et al. Pulmonary fat embolism: A distinct cause of severe acute chest syndrome in sickle cell disease. *Blood.* 1994;83:3107.

Of patients with ACS, 12 of 27 had lipid-laden macrophages on bronchoalveolar lavage. Those with evidence of fat embolism had a distinct clinical course, with a higher frequency of concomitant bone pain and neurologic symptoms, a greater degree of hematologic abnormalities, and longer hospitalization.

14. Vichinsky EP, Neumayr LD, Earles AN, et al. Causes and outcomes of the acute chest syndrome in sickle cell disease. *N Engl J Med.* 2000;342:1855.

Large, multicenter study describing the causes and complications of ACS. Management of these patients is also discussed.

15. Santoli F, Zerah F, Vasile N, et al. Pulmonary function in sickle cell disease with or without acute chest syndrome. *Eur Respir J.* 1998;12:1124.

In contrast with most studies demonstrating restrictive physiology, these authors found evidence of obstruction and elevated diffusion capacity on pulmonary physiology testing, both of which correlated with the number of episodes of ACS.

16. Haynes J, Allison RC. Pulmonary edema. Complication in the management of sickle cell pain crisis. *Am J Med.* 1986;80:833.

Of 51 patients treated for acute pain crisis, 4 developed pulmonary edema. The authors postulate that the administration of both hypotonic saline solutions and parenteral narcotics may have been contributing factors in this complication. Less vigorous hydration and more judicious use of short-acting narcotics is recommended for management of such patients.

17. Vichinsky EP, Haberkern CM, Neumayr L, et al. A comparison of conservative and aggressive transfusion regimens in the perioperative management of sickle cell disease. *N Engl J Med.* 1995;333:206.

    A conservative transfusion regimen (to a hemoglobin concentration of 10 g/dL) was as effective as a more aggressive regimen in reducing postoperative complications, and resulted in half as many transfusion-related complications.

18. Castro O, Brambilla DJ, Thorington B, et al. The acute chest syndrome in sickle cell disease: Incidence and risk factors. *Blood.* 1994;89:643.

    Details from the Cooperative Study of Sickle Cell Disease, involving 3751 patients, with 19,867 years of follow-up.

19. Vichinski EP, Styles LA, Colangelo LH, et al. Acute chest syndrome in sickle cell disease: Clinical presentation and course. *Blood.* 1997;89:1787.

    From the same cooperative study are details on the presentation and course of 1722 ACS episodes in 939 patients. Clearly demonstrates the differences in cause, presentation, and course of ACS between adults and children with ACS.

20. Martin L, Buonomo C. Acute chest syndrome of sickle cell disease: Radiographic and clinical analysis of 70 cases. *Pediatr Radiol.* 1997;27:637.

    In 87% of ACS episodes, no bacterial cause was found; these patients typically were older, had a dramatic improvement in radiographic findings within 24 hours of therapy, and had a more favorable clinical course.

21. Horton DP, Ferriero DM, Mentzer WC. Nontraumatic fat embolism syndrome in sickle cell anemia. *Pediatr Neurol.* 1995;12:77.

    A case report of a 14-year-old patient with SCD who presented with bone pain and developed pulmonary edema, coma, seizures, and bilateral flaccid paralysis. Fat embolism syndrome was diagnosed on magnetic resonance imaging; all symptoms resolved by 3 months.

22. Rucknagel DL, Kalinyak KA, Gelfand MJ. Rib infarcts and acute chest syndrome in sickle cell diseases. *Lancet.* 1991;337:831.

    Segmental rib infarction was demonstrated by bone scintigraphy during 11 episodes of ACS in adults.

23. Sutton LL, Castro O, Cross DJ, et al. Pulmonary hypertension in sickle cell disease. *Am J Cardiol.* 1994;74:626.

    Significant pulmonary hypertension was found in 20% of patients referred for echocardiography with suspected cardiac disease (10% had clinically suspected pulmonary hypertension). Mortality rate over 22 months was 42% in the pulmonary hypertensive group, versus 8% in others. Pulmonary hypertensive patients died of intractable right ventricular failure and sudden death.

24. Delatte SJ, Hebra A, Tagge EP, et al. Acute chest syndrome in the postoperative sickle cell patient. *J Pediatr Surg.* 1999;34:188.

    Despite careful perioperative management, including transfusion to hemoglobin greater than 10 g/dL, the incidence of ACS was 10.2%. Most ACS cases occurred after laparoscopic procedures.

25. Platt OS, Brambilla DJ, Rosse WF, et al. Mortality in sickle cell disease. Life expectancy and risk factors for early death. *N Engl J Med.* 1994;330:1639.

    The acute chest syndrome, renal failure, seizures, baseline white cell count above 15,000/mm³ cells, and a low level of fetal hemoglobin were associated with an increased risk of early death.

26. Aquino DL, Gamsu G, Fahy JV, et al. Chronic disorders in sickle cell disease: Findings at thin-section CT. *Radiology.* 1994;193:807.

    Thin-section CT abnormalities in these patients with a previous history of ACS correlated with the number of episodes of ACS, but not with pulmonary function abnormalities.

27. Powars D, Weidman JA, Odom-Maryon T, et al. Sickle cell chronic lung disease: Prior morbidity and the risk of pulmonary failure. *Medicine.* 1988;67:66.

Describes in detail the natural history of sickle cell chronic lung disease, and underscores the importance of recurrent episodes of ACS in its development.

28. Cunningham FG, Pritchard JA, Mason R. Pregnancy and sickle cell hemoglobinopathies: Results with and without prophylactic transfusions. *Obstet Gynecol.* 1983;62:419.

No maternal mortality and a sevenfold decrease in morbidity, including a significant improvement in pulmonary complications, were the findings in patients who were prophylactically transfused. Guidelines for transfusion therapy are given.

29. Yater WN, Hansmann GH. Sickle cell anemia: A new cause of cor pulmonale. *Am J Med Sci.* 1936;471:474.

The first report stressing the occurrence of cor pulmonale in sickle cell anemia.

30. Gladwin MT, Sachdev V, Jison ML, et al. Pulmonary hypertension as a risk factor for death in patients with sickle cell disease. *N Engl J Med.* 2004;350:886.

Large, prospective, controlled study demonstrating that pulmonary hypertension is common in adults with SCD, and that it carries a poor prognosis despite modest elevations in pulmonary artery pressures. The accompanying editorial explains the pathophysiology of pulmonary hypertension in SCD.

31. Kark JA, Posey DM, Schumacher HR, et al. Sickle-cell trait as a risk factor for sudden death in physical training. *N Engl J Med.* 1987;317:781.

A 30-fold increased risk of exercise-related sudden death was found in recruits with sickle cell trait.

32. Castro O, Brown BD. Pulmonary hypertension in sickle cell disease: Cardiac catheterization results and survival. *Blood.* 2003;101:1257.

The poor prognosis of pulmonary hypertension in SCD is demonstrated.

33. Maitre B, Habibi A, Roudot-Thoraval F, et al. Acute chest syndrome in adults with sickle cell disease. Therapeutic approach, outcome, and results of BAL in a monocentric series of 107 episodes. *Chest* 2000;17:1386.

Fat embolism was found to be a common cause of ACS in adults. Patients with fat embolism did not have a more severe course, and bronchoscopy to establish the diagnosis did not affect management.

34. Morris CR, Morris SM, Hagar W, et al. Arginine therapy. A new treatment for pulmonary hypertension in sickle cell disease? *Am J Respir Crit Care Med.* 2003;168:63.

Pulmonary artery pressure decreased by a mean 15.2% after 5 days of treatment with oral L-arginine.

---

73. CYSTIC FIBROSIS

Douglas J. Conrad

Cystic fibrosis is a systemic disease characterized by acute and chronic sinusitis, progressive bronchiectasis, and pancreatic malabsorption. Other frequently encountered manifestations include hemoptysis, pneumothorax, focal biliary fibrosis, pancreatitis, azoospermia, and obstructive colonopathy. In the past, patients with cystic fibrosis rarely survived through childhood and were cared for almost exclusively by pediatricians. However, aggressive treatment and newer therapies have dramatically improved prognosis: the current predicted median age of survival of cystic fibrosis patients is approximately 32 years. Mild or atypical forms of cystic fibrosis are diagnosed somewhat commonly in adults because of recent advances in cystic fibrosis pathophysiology and genetics. For these reasons, primary care providers and adult pulmonologists diagnose and manage cystic fibrosis patients more frequently than in previous years.

ETIOLOGY AND PATHOPHYSIOLOGY

The cystic fibrosis gene and the most common mutations associated with the disease were identified in 1989. These studies also characterized the cystic fibrosis gene product, a protein termed the *cystic fibrosis transmembrane conductance regulator* (CFTR). Cystic fibrosis is inherited as an autosomal recessive. Mutations in CFTR gene are common in the general population (1:29 in North American whites), but the incidence varies significantly among different ethnic populations. The disease occurs in 1 of 3,300 North American whites, 1 of 15,300 African-Americans, 1 of 9,500 Hispanics, and 1 of 32,000 Asian-Americans. Carriers of a single mutated CFTR allele are asymptomatic and have a normal prognosis.

The CFTR protein is located primarily on the apical membranes of epithelial cells of the respiratory, hepatobiliary, and pancreatic tracts, as well as in the crypts of the large intestine and sweat gland ducts. It forms a large pore in the cell membranes, which functions as a chloride channel. Dysfunction of CFTR-dependent ion transport is believed to be responsible for the pulmonary manifestations of cystic fibrosis. The ion transport properties of airway epithelial cells are critical for maintaining the hydration and normal function of the airway lining fluid. When these processes are disturbed, the mucociliary clearance mechanism is diminished and bacteria chronically colonize the airways. Recent studies suggest that the abnormal ion concentration of the epithelial lining fluid alters the immune response by inactivating antimicrobial peptides normally produced by airway epithelial cells or by decreasing airway surface fluid pH.

Bacterial colonization of the airways leads to bronchiectasis, airway obstruction, and, eventually, respiratory failure through a self-perpetuating cycle of inflammation and decreased airway clearance. The bacteria stimulate neutrophil recruitment into the airways. The neutrophils are ineffective in clearing the infection and die, leaving large quantities of cellular DNA and proteases in the airways. The DNA dramatically increases airway secretion viscosity, further impairing airway clearance. The neutrophil proteases stimulate submucosal gland hypertrophy and secretion, and eventually result in a breakdown of the airway architecture and bronchiectasis. The bronchiectasis is progressive and leads to respiratory failure in 85% of patients with cystic fibrosis. The pathophysiology of cystic fibrosis in the gastrointestinal tract involves pancreatic duct obstruction that leads to destruction of the pancreas, pancreatic malabsorption, and insulin deficiency.

CLINICAL PRESENTATION

Patients with cystic fibrosis can present with a wide variety of respiratory and gastrointestinal complaints that are typically evident in childhood. The more common manifestations include nasal polyps, sinusitis, bronchospasm, recurrent bronchitis or pneumonia, airway colonization with *Staphylococcus aureus*, *Haemophilus influenza*, or *Pseudomona aeruginosa*, steatorrhea, pancreatic malabsorption, meconium ileus, failure to thrive, rectal prolapse, distal intestinal obstructive syndrome, and hepatic cirrhosis (focal biliary fibrosis). Undiagnosed adults frequently present with recurrent bronchitis (in a nonsmoker), asthma associated with the radiographic evidence of diffuse bronchiectasis, chronic sinusitis, allergic bronchopulmonary aspergillosis (ABPA), airway bacterial colonization with atypical mycobacteria or mucoid *P. aeruginosa*, cirrhosis, idiopathic pancreatitis, or male infertility.

Typically, the physical examination discloses nonspecific findings. Acute or chronic sinusitis with nasal polyps is common. Chest examination reveals an increase in the anteroposterior diameter, with decreased diaphragmatic excursion. Diffuse rales, rhonchi, and bronchospasm are evident in most patients, although breath sounds are occasionally normal. Digital clubbing is frequent. Most patients have pancreatic insufficiency and, thus, have some degree of protein-calorie malnutrition.

Taken individually, the findings on history and physical examination are nonspecific; however, the particular combination of sinusitis, diffuse bronchiectasis, pancreatic malabsorption with malnutrition, obstructive colonopathy, and male infertility is very specific for cystic fibrosis. Although primary ciliary dysfunction (Kartegener syndrome) and other immunoglobulin deficiencies syndromes can mimic some of the pathophysiologic consequences, they are not usually associated with gastrointestinal symptoms. In patients with mild or atypical clinical presentations, laboratory confirmation is helpful to confirm the diagnosis early in the disease process.

DIAGNOSTIC TESTING

The sweat chloride test remains the standard in the laboratory diagnosis of cystic fibrosis. This test should be performed by experienced laboratory personnel. Pilocarpine iontopheresis is used to stimulate secretion of sweat, which is collected, weighed, and analyzed for its chloride and sodium concentrations. A chloride concentration greater than 60 mEq/L is diagnostic of cystic fibrosis, with most positive tests falling in the 90 to 120 mEq/L range. Positive or indeterminate results (values between 40 and 60 mEq/L) should be repeated at least once.

Since the identification of the gene for cystic fibrosis in 1989, more than 800 disease-causing mutations have been identified. Most laboratories screen for 40 of the most common mutations, which account for nearly 90% of North American patients with cystic fibrosis. The most common mutation is delta F508, which accounts for nearly 70% of the mutated alleles in the North American white cystic fibrosis populations. Homozygosity for delta F508 is the most common genotype in this population and occurs in approximately 50% of patients. Several commercial laboratories now offer complete sequencing of the CFTR gene. Combined CFTR sequencing and sweat chloride testing may be particularly helpful in evaluating patients with atypical presentations.

Standard hematologic, physiologic, and radiographic studies are useful in characterizing the severity and progression of the disease. Pulmonary function testing in the setting of cystic fibrosis is frequently abnormal but not specific. Spirometry reveals airway obstruction and lung volumes frequently demonstrate air trapping. Pulmonary function tests, however, are useful for following the course of the disease or monitoring the effectiveness of therapy. Chest radiographs usually show changes consistent with bronchiectasis or demonstrate evidence of mucus plugging or atelectasis. They may also identify pneumonia, pneumothorax, or manifestations of bronchial arterial bleeding. Bronchiectasis is best evaluated on thin-cut thoracic computed tomography scanning, which has replaced bronchography. Blood counts and serum chemistries can help to identify some common complications of the disease. White blood counts are frequently normal or slightly elevating during exacerbations, but rise much higher during pneumonia or steroid therapy. Hemoglobin levels may help to explain unexpected dyspnea, because many patients are anemic because of chronic inflammation or gastrointestinal blood loss. Serum chemistries can be affected if the patient has renal tubular dysfunction from aminoglycoside use or chronic respiratory acidosis or uses diuretic therapy. Liver-associated enzymes are frequently elevated with a cholestatic pattern, but are typically no greater than three times normal. In patients with abdominal pain, serum lipase and amylase levels may be helpful to rule out pancreatitis. Prealbumin levels can help to guide nutritional therapy. Oral glucose tolerance testing (2-hour testing after a 75-g fasting glucose load) and fasting blood glucose levels are obtained to monitor glucose intolerance. Glucose intolerance and diabetes are associated with lower weights and worse clinical outcomes. Finally, serum levels of vitamins A, E, and D are helpful to monitor the success of dietary supplementation of the fat-soluble vitamins.

MANAGEMENT

Management of cystic fibrosis is focused on (1) maintaining optimal nutritional status; (2) promoting airway clearance of inflammatory cells; (3) decreasing bacterial colonization; and (4) minimizing the impact of respiratory and gastrointestinal complications.

Chronic sinusitis is evident in most patients with the disease; symptoms are managed initially with antibiotics and topical steroids. Although conservative management can be helpful, many patients are eventually referred for surgical polypectomies, sinus antrectomies, and tissue debridement. This aggressive therapy frequently relieves symptoms and, in some cases, is associated with an improvement in pulmonary function.

Management of progressive bronchiectasis focuses on diminishing airway inflammation and promoting airway clearance. Antibiotics are used to decrease the level of bacterial colonization. Although chronic antibiotic suppressive therapy with anti-staphylococcal antibiotics was standard in previous years, more recent randomized clinical studies do not support their general use. Stronger clinical research supports the use of inhaled antibiotics, particularly tobramycin. Recent studies have shown that inhaled tobramycin (3,000 mg, twice daily, every other month) is safe, improves pulmonary function, and decreases the use of IV antibiotics. Other antibiotics that have been used as inhaled medications include gentamicin, colistin, and the β-lactam antibiotics. In general, inhaled antibiotics are best used as prophylactic therapies and are less useful during acute exacerbations.

Several pharmacologic therapies may improve airway clearance and reduce airflow obstruction. The concentration of DNA in respiratory secretions of patients with cystic fibrosis is high and has been shown to dramatically increase the viscosity of the sputum and to impair its clearance. Aerosolized deoxyribonuclease (DNase), a pancreatic-derived enzyme that degrades DNA, may be inhaled to diminish the effect DNA has on respiratory secretion viscosity. Clinical studies have demonstrated improvement in pulmonary function, decreased use of antibiotics, and subjective improvement in symptoms with inhaled DNase.

Airway clearance and airflow obstruction in patients with marked bronchospasm can be improved with corticosteroids and bronchodilators. Inhaled bronchodilator therapy with a β-agonist or ipratropium is helpful for many patients to relieve symptoms secondary to bronchospasm and to facilitate airway clearance. Oral bronchodilators including theophylline and β-agonist preparations are used in the pediatric setting where inhaled therapies are sometimes ineffective, in patients who are not compliant with inhaled therapy, and as an adjunct to optimally delivered inhaled therapy.

A great deal of clinical investigation has focused on anti-inflammatory therapy in cystic fibrosis. The use of steroids in cystic fibrosis is controversial largely because of the risk of adverse effects. They are generally not used in the chronic outpatient management of cystic fibrosis patients, but are helpful in selected patients with severe lung disease and bronchospasm. Selected patients with prominent airway hyperreactivity may improve significantly with inhibitors of the 5-lipoxygenase pathway, particularly the newer leukotriene receptor antagonists. Chronic use of nonsteroidal anti-inflammatory drugs, specifically ibuprofen, has been demonstrated to preserve lung function. These effects were most prominent in children and in patients with mild lung function abnormalities. Several randomized clinical trials in pediatric and adult cystic fibrosis patients have demonstrated that the anti-inflammatory effects of macrolides, particularly azithromycin, improve pulmonary function, decrease antibiotic use, and improve quality of life.

Chest physiotherapy is the major mechanical means of augmenting airway clearance. This is typically delivered manually or with a mechanical percussor two to four times a day. Other airway clearance techniques, such as autogenic drainage, positive expiratory pressure masks, and flutter valves, are helpful. A newer therapy uses a vest attached to a pressure oscillator to generate airway-shearing forces and dislodge inspissated secretions.

Many providers encourage patients to perform strenuous aerobic exercise daily. Exercise improves cardiovascular conditioning, promotes airway clearance, and, importantly, benefits patients psychologically. Patients who perform routine aerobic exercise are also able to notice a decline in their performance, which can be an early indicator of pulmonary illness requiring therapy.

Lung transplantation is an option for some patients with severely depressed lung function whose lifestyles have been significantly limited by the disease (see Chapter 71). Lung transplant candidates are carefully selected, with consideration given to other medical comorbidities, psychosocial support, and patient motivation. In most centers, the mortality rate in patients with cystic fibrosis after lung transplant is similar to that of other lung transplant patients. Most centers that perform lung transplantation for patients with cystic fibrosis report a 1-year survival rate of approximately 70 to 80% and a 3-year survival rate of 50%.

COMPLICATIONS

Commonly encountered pulmonary complications that are frequently managed on an outpatient basis include ABPA and airway colonization with atypical mycobacteria. ABPA is a hypersensitivity reaction to aspergillus in the airway, which has been demonstrated in 5 to 20% of patients with cystic fibrosis. Atypical mycobacteria frequently colonize the airways, causing no harm. On occasion, however, these mycobacteria can invade the lung parenchyma, causing progressive airway destruction and volume loss. Standard therapy has not been established for nontuberculous mycobacterial disease but multiple drug therapy (e.g., clarithromycin, ethambutol, and rifampin) for 12 months is usually recommended.

Pancreatic malabsorption and protein-calorie malnutrition should be aggressively managed. Thorough reviews of daily caloric intake and monitoring of body weight are important to maintaining nutritional goals. Intermittently, protein stores should be evaluated. Fat-soluble vitamins (vitamins A, D, E, and K) are not readily absorbed through the gastrointestinal tract of patients with cystic fibrosis. These vitamin levels should be monitored annually and dietary supplements provided. Adequate pancreatic enzyme replacement is the key to maintaining the nutritional status of the patients and to avoid the symptoms of pancreatic malabsorption. As a general rule, most patients who have insufficient pancreatic function require between 1,000 and 2,000 U/kg body weight per meal of lipase activity. In patients who are compliant with the nutritional regimen but whose body weight remains less than 80% of the ideal body weight, the oral diet should be augmented with nocturnal gastrostomy tube feedings of nutritional supplements. Cystic fibrosis–related diabetes (CFRD) is common in adults with cystic fibrosis and is diagnosed either by an abnormal 2-hour oral glucose tolerance test or persistent elevation of fasting serum glucose values. Patients with untreated diabetes may have significant problems with gaining weight and preserving lung functions. Clinicians are increasingly treating CFRD more aggressively with insulin to assist in the treatment of nutritional therapy and to preserve lung function.

Occasionally patients with cystic fibrosis develop an obstructive colonopathy such as meconium ileus or distal intestinal obstructive syndrome. Frequently, they complain of constipation and right-sided abdominal pain. This abdominal pain needs to be distinguished from peptic ulcer disease, cholelithiasis, pancreatitis, colitis, or appendicitis. Initial management should include the administration of pancreatic enzymes, along with mild laxatives and an increase in dietary fiber. Gastrograffin enemas may help to relieve the obstruction in some cases; surgery is rarely needed.

The most common reasons for hospital admissions are pulmonary exacerbations of infectious bronchiectasis. Patients often present with worsening exertional capacity, diminished pulmonary function, and increased cough and sputum production. Inpatients are typically treated with two antibiotics targeting organisms observed in sputum cultures. In vitro sensitivity data may help to guide the antibiotic selection; however, clinical improvement is frequently observed even when the cultured bacteria have demonstrated significant in vitro resistance. In most cases, patients are treated empirically with two anti-pseudomonal antibiotics and an antibiotic targeting S. aureus if it is present in the airway secretions. In addition to antibiotics, patients typically receive aggressive chest physiotherapy four times daily and frequent bronchodilators. Pancreatic malabsorption is treated the same as it is in the outpatient setting. Although home IV antibiotic administration is an option for treatment of pulmonary exacerbations in some patients, these patients must be carefully selected. Those who are most likely to have successful outcomes with outpatient IV antibiotics typically have had good responses to antibiotics in the past, are very motivated, and have adequate support in the home. IV antibiotics should be continued as long as the patient's clinical status is improving. If stabilization occurs before reaching the patient's functional baseline, then changing antibiotic therapy based on sensitivities should be considered.

The use of mechanical ventilation to treat respiratory failure is particularly controversial. All decisions regarding mechanical ventilatory support should be individualized. Some patients who are cooperative and motivated may respond temporarily to noninvasive ventilatory support. In general, patients who develop respiratory failure despite optimal treatment should not be mechanically ventilated because of the progressive nature of this disease. However, patients who have not received optimal therapy or who have respiratory failure secondary to reversible complications (e.g., hemoptysis, pneumothorax, etc.) should be considered for mechanical ventilation.

Massive hemoptysis (>250 mL/24 hours) is common in patients with cystic fibrosis. Most patients can be treated conservatively, using supportive measures such as IV antibiotics, oxygen supplementation, temporary suppression of cough, avoidance of chest physiotherapy during active bleeding, transfusions of platelets or packed red blood cells, when appropriate, and the correction of any clotting abnormalities with either vitamin K or fresh frozen plasma. Occasionally, these measures are inadequate because of progressive respiratory failure or ongoing bleeding. In these cases, medical stabilization should be followed with bronchial arterial embolization, which usually controls active bleeding quickly. Surgery is very rarely needed for control but should be considered if embolization does not control life-threatening bleeding and the patient is an adequate surgical candidate.

Pneumothorax occurs frequently in patients with severe lung disease caused by cystic fibrosis. Conservative therapy with oxygen supplementation, antibiotics, and bronchodilators is usually successful in patients with small, asymptomatic pneumothoraces. In patients with larger, symptomatic or nonresolving pneumothoraces, a more aggressive approach is warranted. A chest tube should be placed under fluoroscopy or by an experienced individual because the pleural space can be complicated by cystic fibrosis. Chest tube drainage is frequently successful in reexpanding the lung and allows the option of chemical pleurodesis. Surgical pleurodesis is rarely needed.

ONGOING RESEARCH

Cystic fibrosis is an area of active clinical research. Some of the more promising areas of research are aimed at developing inhaled antibiotics or identifying novel anti-inflammatory agents. A promising area of research involves reversing the ion transport abnormalities, using compounds such as uridine triphosphate, amiloride, and other compounds identified by high throughput screening strategies. Other approaches attempt to boost CFTR transport and activity in mutations that have residual activity. Finally, gene therapy offers a chance of curative therapy in selected patients, or of arresting the decline in pulmonary function in patients with existing disease. Successful therapy for cystic fibrosis is likely to involve multiple therapies targeting the pathophysiologic process at several steps.

1. Davis PB, Drumm M, Konstan MW. Cystic fibrosis. *Am J Respir Crit Care Med.* 1996;154:1229.
2. Gibson RL, Burns JL, Ramsey BW. Pathophysiology and management of pulmonary infections in cystic fibrosis. *Am J Respir Crit Care Med.* 2003;168:918–951.
   Two very important reviews covering many basic scientific and clinical issues involved with the clinical care of patients with cystic fibrosis.
3. Kerem B, Rommens JM, Buchanan JA, et al. Identification of the cystic fibrosis gene: Genetic analysis. *Science.* 1989;245:1073.
4. Riordan JR, Rommens JM, Kerem B, et al. Identification of the cystic fibrosis gene: Cloning and characterization of complementary DNA. *Science.* 1989;245:1066.
5. Rommens JM, Iannuzzi MC, Kerem B, et al. Identification of the cystic fibrosis gene: Chromosome walking and jumping. *Science.* 1989;245:1059.
   References 3 and 5 are the classic articles identifying the cysticfibrosis gene, the most common disease causing mutations and the initial characterizationof the gene product CFTR.
6. Goldman MJ, Anderson GM, Stolzenberg ED, et al. Human beta-defensin-1 is a salt-sensitive antibiotic in lung that is inactivated in cystic fibrosis. *Cell.* 1997;88:553.
7. Smith JJ, Travis SM, Greenberg EP, et al. Cystic fibrosis airway epithelia fail to kill bacteria because of abnormal airway surface fluid. *Cell.* 1996;85:229.

References 6 and 7 are important articles linking the molecular defect in cystic fibrosis with a specific pathophysiologic event.

8. Fuchs HJ, Borowitz DS, Christiansen DH, et al. Effect of aerosolized recombinant human DNase on exacerbations of respiratory symptoms and on pulmonary function in patients with cystic fibrosis. The Pulmozyme Study Group [see comments]. *N Engl J Med.* 1994;331:637.

9. Konstan MW, Byard PJ, Hoppel CL, et al. Effect of high-dose ibuprofen in patients with cystic fibrosis [see comments]. *N Engl J Med.* 1995;332:848.

10. Ramsey BW, Pepe MS, Quan JM, et al. Intermittent administration of inhaled tobramycin in patients with cystic fibrosis. Cystic Fibrosis Inhaled Tobramycin Study Group. *N Engl J Med.* 1999;340:23.

11. Saiman L, Marshall BC, Mayer-Hamblett N, et al. Azithromycin in patients with cystic fibrosis chronically infected with *Pseudomonas aeruginosa. JAMA.* 2003;290:1749–1756.

References 8 through 11 are important clinical research studies establishing the roles for rhDNase I, ibuprofen, inhaled tobramycin, and azithromycin in the clinical care of patients with cystic fibrosis.

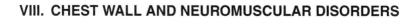

VIII. CHEST WALL AND NEUROMUSCULAR DISORDERS

74. DISORDERS OF THE THORACIC SPINE

Ann M. Romaker

The thorax is normally characterized by (1) a stable volume and (2) the ability to alter that volume. Volume is determined by the height of the thoracic spine and the width and depth of the rib cage. The musculature of the thorax, the diaphragm, and the muscles of respiration provide the ability to change thoracic volume. Disorders that adversely affect the thoracic vertebral column can compromise respiratory function. The most common of these disorders are scoliosis, kyphosis, kyphoscoliosis, and ankylosing spondylitis.

ETIOLOGY AND PATHOPHYSIOLOGY

Scoliosis is a lateral deviation of the spine; *kyphosis* is a posterior angulation. In scoliosis, the initiating curve is called the *primary curve,* and the compensatory curve, which restores postural balance, is called the *secondary curve.* The angle of the scoliosis, defined by the converging limbs of the primary curve, is expressed in degrees (the Cobb angle). In general, the greater the angle, the shorter the hemithorax on the concave side of the curve becomes. The degree of kyphosis is defined by the angle between the upper limb of the spine and the vertical plane. Separately and in combination, scoliosis and kyphosis effect a number of changes on the thorax and its contents, resulting in gross distortion of thoracic configuration and volume. Even mild curves can affect lung function and work capacity. However, significant respiratory and cardiovascular compromise are noted most often when Cobb angles are greater than 100°, when onset of scoliosis occurs prior to age 9, and when kyphosis and scoliosis occur concomitantly, namely, kyphoscoliosis.

The cause of kyphoscoliosis is unknown in approximately 80% of cases. In the remaining cases, the most common causes (in decreasing frequency) are neuromuscular disease (e.g., poliomyelitis, syringomyelia, neurofibromatosis), congenital defects of the spine, vertebral disease (e.g., tuberculosis, tumor, osteomalacia), and thoracic disease (e.g., emphysema, thoracoplasty). Idiopathic deformity is more common in women (4:1) and is usually not severe. In contrast, the deformity in poliomyelitis, tuberculosis, and congenital spine defects is often marked. Now that patients with cystic fibrosis are living into adulthood, an increased incidence of kyphosis secondary to osteoporosis is occurring. This osteoporosis is related to poor nutrition, use of corticosteroids, lower levels of sex steroids, and increased levels of circulating osteoclase-activating factors.

The age of onset has been identified as the major predictor of increased mortality in several long-term follow-up studies. These studies of patients followed for 50 to 60 years also demonstrate that the more common adolescent scoliosis is rarely a cause of mortality. Infantile scoliosis (onset 0 to 3 years) and juvenile scoliosis (onset 4 to 9 years) are more likely to be associated with Cobb angles greater than 100°, as well as other skeletal problems such as fused or absent ribs, rotation of the spine with secondary rib deformity, or restriction of rib motion. Because lung growth is limited by the thoracic cage, any boney abnormalities that reduce thoracic volume early in life may affect the size of the lungs at skeletal maturity. Alveolar multiplication ends at age 8, making these early years the most vulnerable to the development of permanent change. Individuals who reach skeletal maturity with a vital capacity of less than 45% of predicted (using arm span to determine predicted height) have an increased risk of respiratory failure when their lung function is further reduced by the aging process.

Patients with severe thoracic deformity can live for many years without developing respiratory insufficiency. In fact, development of respiratory failure from a remediable cause does not imply a grim prognosis, as was once believed. Currently, median survival after a first bout of respiratory failure is 9 years. Although compression and kinking of pulmonary arteries can lead to some elevation of pulmonary vascular resistance, most cases of significant pulmonary hypertension are a consequence of alveolar hypoventilation. Evidence indicates that patients with kyphoscoliosis have a higher incidence of disordered breathing during sleep compared to normals, which may contribute to pulmonary vasoconstriction. If hypoventilation persists, cor pulmonale develops.

MANAGEMENT

Individuals with severe thoracic deformity are at great risk for respiratory decompensation with minor insults such as viral or bacterial infections and sedation. Treatment is preventive and supportive in the adult. The primary objective is prevention with appropriate immunizations, maintenance of good hydration, prompt attention to respiratory infection, and avoidance of sedatives. Supplementary oxygen may alleviate the vasoconstrictive element of pulmonary hypertension secondary to regional or global alveolar hypoventilation. Some patients can benefit from respiratory muscle training. Many others with persistent respiratory failure benefit from nocturnal mechanical ventilation. This increases lung compliance, decreases the work of breathing, and allows fatigued respiratory muscles to rest. It is now possible to provide positive pressure mechanical ventilation via face mask, alleviating the need for a tracheostomy in most patients. Both nasal continuous positive airway pressure masks and customized foam nose pieces have been used successfully. Nocturnal noninvasive mechanical ventilation has been shown to improve endurance during exercise tests and gas exchange after only 3 months.

Young patients in whom the spine is more flexible may benefit from internal fixation of the spine by a rod (Harrington rod); however, this benefit has not been consistently demonstrated. Adults gain no significant improvement in pulmonary function after corrective surgery. External corrections are considered less effective. Indications for surgery in young patients include (1) progression of disease despite good external brace care; (2) deformity that is too advanced to respond to external bracing; (3) scoliosis greater than 50°; (4) intractable pain; (5) nonalignment of occiput over sacrum; and (6) psychiatric disturbances. However, both bracing and internal fixation can be associated with complications including further reductions in vital capacity. In many patients, however, disease progression is halted.

Ankylosing spondylitis is an uncommon arthritic condition that occurs predominantly in males (4–8:1) aged 20 to 40 years. Approximately 90% of affected individuals have the histocompatibility antigen HLA-B27; 20% of those with HLA-B27 develop ankylosing spondylitis. In approximately one fifth of cases, peripheral joint manifestations are also present. Chest wall pain, usually pleuritic, is noted in more than 60%. Thoracic spine involvement can result in fixation of the chest wall in an inspiratory position. Clinical manifestations, which can be insidious, include intermittent lower back pain, weight loss, anorexia, and fever; dyspnea is unusual. When dyspnea is present, it is more commonly caused by cardiac involvement than by pulmonary involvement. In a large Mayo Clinic study, the incidence of pleuropulmonary involvement was 1.35%. Severe respiratory symptoms are rare as long as diaphragmatic function is normal. Effective treatment for ankylosing spondylitis is not available; treatment in the early stages with steroids, immunosuppressive agents, or both has been proposed, but no data supporting their efficacy are available.

A distinctive upper lobe fibrobullous or fibrocavitary pulmonary process complicates a minority of cases of ankylosing spondylitis; its incidence has been reported to be between 1 and 30%. A marked male predominance is seen, far exceeding that of ankylosing spondylitis per se. The upper lobe changes usually develop many years after the initial skeletal manifestations. The cause is unknown. An unsatisfactory theory relates its pathogenesis to a vertical traction on the lung apices, caused by elongation of the thorax by diaphragmatic excursion in the face of a fixed, noncompliant chest wall. The peculiar apical and subapical location makes aspiration (caused by esophageal motility abnormalities) an unlikely reason for the process. The process bears no temporal relationship to axial radiotherapy (once commonly employed), as it lies outside the radiation ports and occurs in the absence of radiotherapy. Although no large-scale study is available, the process appears to occur equally in individuals with or without HLA-B27 positivity.

Clinically, patients may have a minimally productive cough and exertional dyspnea; these symptoms occur in patients with ankylosing spondylitis with chest wall restriction but no apparent pulmonary parenchymal abnormality. Hemoptysis is common but appears to be related to the presence of aspergillomas within the cavitary lesions. An increased incidence of spontaneous pneumothoraces has been reported.

The chest roentgenogram initially shows a nodular or reticular pattern in the apical or subapical lung zones. This pattern tends to coarsen and become confluent, eventually appearing as dense consolidation. Upward retraction of hilar structures attests to upper lobe volume loss. Involvement may be initially unilateral, but most lesions progress to bilateral involvement. The apical lesions usually cavitate; in those appearing as dense fibrosis, tomography often demonstrates otherwise inapparent cavities. Findings typical of aspergillomas are eventually present in one third to one half of all cavitary lesions.

The clinical course of ankylosing spondylitis is generally one of slow progression seen roentgenographically over months to years. In a few cases, extensive fibrosis eventually affected the upper one third of both lungs, but many tend to stabilize or apparently "burn out." Symptoms from aspergillomas frequently dominate the clinical picture. Colonization of cavities with types I and III atypical mycobacteria has been reported.

Attempts at therapeutic intervention have not been systematically evaluated. Resection of the involved lung has been complicated by an unusually high incidence (50%) of bronchopleural fistulas and empyema, often sterile. Progressive involvement of remaining ipsilateral or contralateral lung is not infrequent. No drug has been identified that actually modifies the disease; however, nonsteroidal anti-inflammatory drugs, methotrexate, and sulfasalazine are frequently used.

1. Aris RM, Renner JB, Wonders AD, et al. Increased rate of fractures and severe kyphosis: Sequelae of living into adulthood with cystic fibrosis. *Ann Intern Med*. 1998;128:186.
   The first article to examine the clinical impact of osteoporosis associated with cystic fibrosis.
2. Bergofsky EH. Respiratory failure in disorders of the thoracic cage. *Am Rev Respir Dis*. 1979;119:643.
   An excellent state-of-the-art review.
3. Campbell RM Jr., Smith MD, Mayer TC, et al. The characteristics of thoracic insufficiency syndrome associated with fused ribs and congenital scoliosis. *J Bone Joint Surg*. 2003;85-A(3):399–408.
4. Crompton GK, Cameron SJ, Langlands AO. Pulmonary fibrosis, pulmonary tuberculosis and ankylosing spondylitis. *Br J Dis Chest*. 1974;68:51.
   Of 225 patients with ankylosing spondylitis, 14 (6%) had chest films consistent with apical pulmonary fibrosis; 3 had been reported as having pulmonary tuberculosis without bacteriologic confirmation.
5. DiRocco PJ, Vaccaro P. Cardiopulmonary functioning in adolescent patients with mild idiopathic scoliosis. *Arch Phys Med Rehabil*. 1988;69:198.
   Changes in pulmonary function and diminished work capacity were demonstrated with curves of only 25°.
6. Ellis ER, Grunstein RR, Chan S, et al. Noninvasive ventilatory support during sleep improves respiratory failure in kyphoscoliosis. *Chest*. 1988;94:811–815.
7. Haslock I. Ankylosing Bailliére's spondylitis. *Clin Rheumatol*. 1993;7:99.
   An excellent review of the respiratory effects of ankylosing spondylitis.
8. Kafer ER. Idiopathic scoliosis: Mechanical properties of the respiratory system and ventilatory response to CO_2. *J Clin Invest*. 1975;55:1153.
   The body size and the degree of deformity were the major determinants of lung mechanics and ventilatory response to carbon dioxide.
9. Libby DM, Briscoe WA, Boyce B, et al. Acute respiratory failure in scoliosis or kyphosis. *Am J Med*. 1982;73:532.

An excellent description of the clinical correlates and prognosis of patients with severe disease.

10. Linderholm H, Lindgren U. Prediction of spirometric values in patients with scoliosis. *Acta Orthop Scand.* 1982;49:469.

    Discusses methods to correct for the degree of scoliosis in predicting lung volumes (which are height dependent).

11. Luthra HS. Extraarticular manifestations of ankylosing spondylitis [Editorial]. *Mayo Clin Proc.* 1977;52:655.

    An editorial that briefly reviews the incidence of extraarticular syndromes in ankylosing spondylitis.

12. Melzon BL, West P, Israels J, et al. Sleep breathing abnormalities in kyphoscoliosis. *Am Rev Respir Dis.* 1980;122:617.

    Interesting findings; however, the clinical significance is not yet clear.

13. Pehrsson K, Larsson S, Oden A. et al. Long term follow up of patients with untreated scoliosis. *Spine.* 1992;17:1091–1096.

    One hundred fifteen patients followed for more than 45 years via a national Swedish registry demonstrate increased mortality between ages 40 and 50 in those with onset within 9 years.

14. Pehrsson K, Bake B, Larsson S, et al. Lung function in adult idiopathic scoliosis. A 20 year follow up. *Thorax.* 1991;46:474–478.

    Looks at time- and disease-related changes in lung function over time in 45 patients with untreated scoliosis.

15. Rosenow EC III, Strimlan CV, Muhm JR, et al. Pleuropulmonary manifestations of ankylosing spondylitis. *Mayo Clin Proc.* 1977;52:641.

    Of 2,080 patients with ankylosing spondylitis, 28 (1.3%) had typical chest roentgenograms; 5 of 28 (18%) had aspergillomas; 3 had transient exudative pleural effusions with normal glucose levels.

16. Sawicka EH, Branthwaite MA. Respiration during sleep in kyphoscoliosis. *Thorax.* 1987;42:801.

    Confirms and extends the findings of Melzon et al. (reference 15).

17. Schenhafe B, Wallstein S, Wiese C, et al. Noninvasive mechanical ventilation improves endurance performance in patients with chronic respiratory failure due to thoracic restriction. *Chest.* 2001;119:1371–1378.

    An excellent study demonstrating improvements in both respiratory and peripheral muscle endurance with 3 months of nocturnal ventilation.

18. Shannon DC, Riseborough EJ, Kazemi H. Ventilation perfusion relationships following correction of kyphoscoliosis. *JAMA.* 1971;217:579.

    The first article to report on functional improvement with surgery.

19. Stewart RM, Ridyard JB, Pearson JD. Regional lung function in ankylosing spondylitis. *Thorax.* 1976;31:433.

    Studies with xenon ventilation showed decreased apical ventilation, which possibly plays a causative role in the pathogenesis of apical fibrosis.

20. Weber B. Pulmonary function in asymptomatic adolescents with idiopathic scoliosis. *Am Rev Respir Dis.* 1975;111:389.

    Discusses the statistical relationships between the degree of scoliosis and pulmonary function.

21. Weinstein SL, Dolan LA, Spratt KF, et al. Health and function of patients with untreated idiopathic scoliosis. A 50 year natural history study. *JAMA.* 2003;289:559–567.

    One hundred seventeen patients with untreated adolescent scoliosis followed for 50 years demonstrate little physical impairment.

75. DIAPHRAGMATIC DISORDERS

Andrew L. Ries and David M. Burns

The diaphragm is the principal muscle of respiration during quiet breathing. Disorders of the diaphragm include paralysis, eventration, herniation, and diaphragmatic dysfunction; these events can be an important part of the pathophysiology of respiratory failure.

PARALYSIS

Paralysis is the most important clinical condition affecting the diaphragm. It can be unilateral or bilateral and either transient or permanent. Each hemidiaphragm is innervated by a phrenic nerve, originating with fibers from the third, fourth, and fifth cervical roots. Diaphragmatic paralysis can result from interruption or dysfunction of the phrenic nerve anywhere from its origins in the neck to the neuromuscular junction. Paralysis can also result from disruption of the spinal cord at or above the level of the phrenic nerve roots. The most common causes of unilateral diaphragmatic paralysis are invasion by bronchogenic carcinoma, surgical section, thoracic trauma, and (presumed) postinflammatory neuropathy.

Bilateral diaphragmatic paralysis is usually the result of spinal cord trauma. Occasionally, idiopathic or postinfection neuropathy can present as bilateral paralysis, particularly when there has been preexisting unilateral diaphragmatic paralysis. Following cardiac surgery, certain patients may develop unilateral or bilateral diaphragmatic paralysis. This paralysis is probably caused by thermal injury to one or both phrenic nerves during cooling of the heart; however, intraoperative trauma to the nerve also can cause phrenic paralysis. Improved intraoperative cooling techniques have made this phenomenon less common.

Patients with unilateral diaphragmatic paralysis are usually asymptomatic, whereas those with bilateral diaphragmatic paralysis experience orthopnea and dyspnea with exertion. With diaphragmatic paralysis, the intercostal and the accessory muscles become the chief muscles of inspiration. Orthopnea occurs when these patients are supine because the abdominal contents push on the flaccid diaphragm, elevating the rib cage. The increase in supine rib cage volume severely compromises the ability of the intercostal and accessory muscles to generate an inspiratory volume. On physical examination, patients with bilateral diaphragmatic paralysis often show prominent activity of the accessory muscles of inspiration (i.e., intercostals, scalene, and sternocleidomastoids), because their inspiration results primarily from elevation of the rib cage by these muscles. Patients often favor the upright position, from which they can fixate their pectoral girdle and use their pectoral muscles to elevate the chest wall and breathe more efficiently. When supine, they display a classic paradoxic inward motion of their anterior abdominal wall during quiet inspiration.

Pulmonary function testing in diaphragmatic paralysis reveals a reduced total lung capacity, vital capacity, inspiratory capacity, and maximal inspiratory pressure. Unilateral paralysis reduces total lung capacity and maximal inspiratory pressure by 20 to 25%. A low inspiratory capacity that falls still further in the supine position suggests diaphragmatic paralysis.

The definitive diagnosis of diaphragmatic paralysis has traditionally rested on fluoroscopic demonstration of diminished, absent, or paradoxic upward motion during normal inspiration. The sniff maneuver is used to enhance this paradoxic upward movement during a quick inspiration; however, fluoroscopy can fail to identify bilateral diaphragmatic paralysis in patients who have learned to breathe by actively expiring below functional residual capacity with forceful contraction of their abdominal muscles. Such a maneuver displaces the flaccid diaphragm upward and compresses the thoracic cavity, thus allowing the elastic recoil of the rib cage and the weight of the abdominal contents to passively assist with the subsequent inspiration. Fluoroscopically, this passive downward motion of the diaphragm is easily misinterpreted as an active contraction. Diaphragmatic performance is more reliably assessed with fluoroscopy by performing a maximum inspiratory maneuver from functional residual capacity against a closed airway. The normal diaphragm moves slightly downward, but the paralyzed diaphragm moves paradoxically upward. A more comprehensive evaluation can be made by recording gastric and esophageal pressures together with rib cage and abdominal motions. The pressure across the diaphragm (Pdi) can be estimated by the difference between gastric and esophageal pressures. Pdi should increase with inspiration and with a maximal inspiratory pressure maneuver, and the abdomen should move outward. The failure to increase Pdi or the generation of a Pdi by inward motion of the abdomen suggests diaphragmatic paralysis. The functional integrity of the phrenic nerves can also be assessed by electromyography.

The therapy and prognosis of diaphragmatic paralysis relate to the underlying disorder. When interruption of the neural control of the diaphragm has occurred centrally, leaving the phrenic nerve intact, considerable improvement in pulmonary status can be achieved by electronic pacing. Electrodes are surgically implanted around the phrenic nerve, and electronic signals are generated using an external radiowave source worn by the patient. Following installation of such a device, weeks or months may be required to achieve full effect if diaphragmatic atrophy has antedated pacing. Patients with bilateral diaphragmatic paralysis are usually paced using one side at a time, because this maintains adequate alveolar ventilation and prevents diaphragmatic fatigue. Patients whose paralysis is postviral or postcardiac surgery often recover function, but this recovery can take 2 to 6 months.

FATIGUE

Diaphragmatic fatigue is a common clinical problem in patients requiring mechanical ventilation. It occurs when the energy expenditure of the diaphragm exceeds the capacity of the blood supply to provide oxygen and nutrients. An increase in the fraction of the maximal contractile pressure developed by the diaphragm during a breath and the fraction of ventilatory time spent in inspiration (i.e., with the diaphragm contracting) both independently increase the likelihood of diaphragmatic fatigue. The multiple of these two fractions, which is called the *tension time index,* predicts the development of fatigue when a value exceeds 0.15. The blood flow to the diaphragm is also an important determinant of fatigue. The threshold for fatigue is reduced under hypotensive or hypoxemic conditions.

Muscle rest is the primary therapy for respiratory muscle fatigue; however, a number of agents, most notably aminophylline, increase diaphragmatic contractility and endurance in the experimental setting. The significance of these findings for therapy of clinical respiratory muscle fatigue remains uncertain, but the complications of these agents probably outweigh their clinical utility in patients with respiratory muscle fatigue.

EVENTRATION

Eventration of the diaphragm is a rare congenital malformation consisting of failure of muscular development of all or part of the diaphragm. It is more common in men. Complete eventration is almost always left sided, whereas partial eventration is more common on the right. The term *eventration* has become synonymous with long-standing elevation of the diaphragm from any cause, although strictly speaking the term should be reserved for the congenital malformation. On chest roentgenogram, eventration is apt to be confused with a diaphragmatic hernia or pleuropericardial cyst. In the adult, the abnormality is frequently discovered as an incidental roentgenographic finding. Individuals are usually asymptomatic; however, with obesity considerable respiratory compromise may be noted. In neonates, involvement of an entire hemidiaphragm can lead to severe respiratory and cardiac compromise from thoracic compression by displaced abdominal contents. This constitutes a surgical emergency.

HERNIATION

Herniation of abdominal contents through the diaphragm can occur through regions of congenital defect or weakness, including the esophageal hiatus, the posterolateral or pleuroperitoneal foramen of Bochdalek (in infants), and the retrosternal (parasternal) foramen of Morgagni (any age). Hiatal hernia (via the esophageal hiatus) is relatively common in adults. It is usually asymptomatic, but can cause retrosternal burning and pain, which are aggravated by lying flat and relieved by antacids. Occasionally, hiatal hernia can be associated with nocturnal aspiration and recurrent pneumonia.

Herniation through the posterolateral aspect of the diaphragm (foramen of Bochdalek) is the most common and serious hernia in infants. It usually presents as an acute respiratory emergency at or shortly after birth and requires immediate surgical repair.

Herniation through the foramen of Morgagni is more common in adults and is often asymptomatic. Obesity is an important predisposing factor. On chest roentgenogram, the abnormal shadow appears retrosternally, usually along the right sternal border, and can mimic a pericardial cyst.

TEARS AND RUPTURE

Tears or rupture of the diaphragm can occur with blunt or penetrating trauma. Use of single-point, lap-belt restraint systems in high-speed motor vehicle accidents is associated with diaphragmatic rupture. Although trauma statistics support an increase in the frequency of right-sided rupture, this injury usually occurs on the left. Herniation of the abdominal contents can cause respiratory distress and substernal pain. This injury can be missed in the unconscious trauma victim until an upright chest roentgenogram shows absence of the affected diaphragmatic outline.

FUNCTIONAL DISORDERS

The most common functional disorder of the diaphragm is the mechanical disadvantage that results from an extreme degree of hyperinflation with severe airways obstruction or advanced emphysema. During the course of chronic obstructive pulmonary disease (COPD), the diaphragm is displaced inferiorly and flattened out, thereby reducing the pressure that can be generated as the diaphragm contracts. Some adaptation of the diaphragm occurs with emphysematous change to make the diaphragm more fatigue resistant, but mechanical disadvantage is more important than fatigue in causing ventilatory limitation. Lung volume reduction surgery can reduce lung volume in selected patients, restoring mechanical advantage to the diaphragm and improving exercise tolerance.

Other functional diaphragmatic disorders include hiccup (singultus) and diaphragmatic flutter. Hiccup is usually a benign disorder that results from repetitive, abrupt inspiratory spasm of the diaphragm, with associated closure of the glottis. It commonly follows transient diaphragmatic irritation, such as occurs with gastric distention caused by aerophagia or overeating, and treatment of acute gastritis can be an effective means of reducing the frequency of hiccups. Protracted episodes may follow upper abdominal surgery, cardiac surgery, or inferior myocardial infarction. Hiccup can also be associated with mediastinitis, tumor invasion, pericarditis, pleuritis, gastritis, and peritonitis. In patients with cardiac pacemakers, hiccup can signal perforation of the right ventricle by the pacing electrode.

Diaphragmatic flutter (respiratory myoclonus or Leeuwenhoek disease) is a rare disorder characterized by dyspnea associated with frequent diaphragmatic contractions ($\sim$100/min) superimposed on the normal respiratory excursion and by prominent epigastric pulsations. The attacks are paroxysmal. Diphenylhydantoin may be helpful.

---

1. Bellemare F, Grassino A. Evaluation of human diaphragm fatigue. *J Appl Physiol*. 1982;53:1196.
   The fraction of maximal contraction and the time spent in inspiration influences the endurance time; a tension time index of 0.15 or greater predicts fatigue.
2. Canbaz S, Turgut N, Halici U, et al. Electrophysiological evaluation of phrenic nerve injury during cardiac surgery—a prospective, controlled, clinical study. *BMC Surgery*. 2004;4:2.

Prospective study of phrenic nerve injury in 78 patients undergoing cardiac surgery. Three weeks after surgery, left phrenic nerve function was absent in 5 of 49 patients who underwent hypothermic cardiopulmonary bypass. None of the 29 patients undergoing normothermic surgery for coronary artery bypass grafting or peripheral vascular surgery developed phrenic nerve injury.

3. Celli B. The diaphragm and respiratory muscles. *Chest Surg Clin North Am.* 1998;8:207.

   A good review of the functional anatomy and function of the diaphragm in the context of the other respiratory muscles.

4. Chervin RD, Guilleminault C. Diaphragm pacing for respiratory insufficiency. *J Clin Neurophysiol.* 1997;14:369.

   A review of diaphragm pacing by electrical stimulation of the phrenic nerve, outlining the preoperative evaluation and procedures for surgical implantation.

5. Criner G, Cardova FC, Leyenson V, et al. Effect of lung volume reduction surgery on diaphragm strength. *Am J Respir Crit Care Med.* 1998;157:1578.

   Lung volume reduction surgery significantly improves diaphragm strength that is associated with a reduction in lung volumes and an improvement in exercise performance.

6. Deslauriers J. Eventration of the diaphragm. *Chest Surg Clin North Am.* 1998;8:315.

   A review of eventration of the diaphragm, which is rare, seldom symptomatic, and often requires no treatment. In symptomatic patients, plication of the diaphragm can relieve the symptoms when present.

7. De Troyer A, Leeper JB, McKenzie, et al. Neural drive to the diaphragm in patients with severe COPD. *Am J Respir Crit Care Med.* 1997;155:1335.

   Patients with severe COPD have an increased neural drive not only to the rib cage inspiratory muscles, but also to the diaphragm. The reduced inspiratory expansion of the abdomen in severe COPD results predominantly from mechanical factors in stable, severe COPD.

8. Dureuil B, Viires N, Cantineau JP, et al. Diaphragmatic contractility after upper abdominal surgery. *J Appl Physiol.* 1986;61:1775.

   Diaphragmatic dysfunction does occur after upper abdominal surgery, but is mediated by central inhibition of phrenic activity rather than decreased muscle contractility.

9. Dureuil B, Matuszczak Y. Alteration in nutritional status and diaphragm muscle function. *Reprod Nutr Dev.* 1998;38:175.

   In cachectic subjects, the diaphragm muscle mass and thickness are reduced in proportion to the reduction in body weight. Respiratory muscle strength and endurance are reduced more dramatically than the weight loss. This finding suggests that malnutrition induces a reduction in muscular mass that is associated with a decrease in contractility.

10. Fromageot C, Lofaso F, Annane D, et al. Supine fall in lung volumes in the assessment of diaphragmatic weakness in neuromuscular disorders. *Arch Phys Med Rehabil.* 2001;82:123.

    Measurement of changes in vital capacity and maximal inspiratory pressure from sitting to supine positions were helpful in detecting diaphragmatic weakness.

11. Hughes PD, Polkey MI, Harrus ML, et al. Diaphragm strength in chronic heart failure. *Am J Respir Crit Care Med.* 1999;160:529.

    Mild reduction in diaphragm strength occurs in chronic heart failure, possibly because of an increased proportion of slow fibers, but overall strength of the respiratory muscles remains well preserved.

12. Johnson BD, Babcock MA, Suman OE, et al. Exercise induced diaphragmatic fatigue in healthy humans. *J Physiol.* 1993;460:385.

    Significant diaphragmatic fatigue can be caused by the ventilatory requirements imposed by heavy endurance exercise. The magnitude of the fatigue and the likelihood of its occurrence increase as the relative intensity of the exercise exceeds 85% of $\dot{V}PO_{2max}$.

13. LaRoche C, Carroll N, Moxham J, et al. Clinical significance of severe isolated diaphragm weakness. *Am Rev Respir Dis*. 1988;138:862.

   All patients studied had normal resting gas exchange, and nocturnal hypercapnia did not develop. Dyspnea with exertion and orthopnea were common to all patients.

14. Lando Y, Boiselle PM, Shade D, et al. Effect of lung volume reduction surgery on diaphragm length in severe chronic obstructive pulmonary disease. *Am J Respir Crit Care Med*. 1999;159:796.

   Lung volume reduction surgery leads to a significant increase in diaphragm length, especially in the area of apposition of the diaphragm with the rib cage. Diaphragm lengthening after this surgery is most likely the result of a reduction in lung volume. Increases in diaphragm length after surgery correlate with postoperative improvements in diaphragm strength, exercise capacity, and maximal voluntary ventilation.

15. Laghi F, Jubran A, Topeli A, et al. Effect of lung volume reduction surgery on neuromechanical coupling of the diaphragm. *Am J Respir Crit Care Med*. 1998;157:475.

   Lung volume reduction surgery improves diaphragmatic function greater than can be accounted for by a decrease in operating lung volume, and enhances diaphragmatic neuromechanical coupling.

16. Laghi F, D'Alfonso N, Tobin MJ. Pattern of recovery from diaphragmatic fatigue over 24 hours. *J Appl Physiol*. 1995;79:539.

   Induction of diaphragmatic fatigue with an experimental protocol produced a marked decrease in diaphragmatic contractility that persisted for at least 24 hours, suggesting that prolonged rest may be necessary for full recovery of diaphragmatic muscle strength after development of fatigue.

17. Levine S, Kaiser L, Leferovich J, et al. Cellular adaptations in the diaphragm in chronic obstructive pulmonary disease. *N Engl J Med*. 1997;337:1799.

   Severe COPD increases the slow-twitch characteristics of the muscle fibers in the diaphragm, an adaptation that increases resistance to fatigue.

18. Matthews BD, Bui H, Harold KL, et al. Laparoscopic repair of traumatic diaphragmatic injuries. *Surg Endosc*. 2003;17:254.

   Description of the use of laparoscopy to repair traumatic diaphragmatic lacerations and hernias in 17 patients. Large traumatic diaphragmatic injuries should be treated with laparotomy.

19. Mihos P, Potaris K, Gakidis J, et al. Traumatic rupture of the diaphragm: Experience with 65 patients. *Int J Care Injured*. 2003;34:169.

   Descriptive case series of 65 patients with traumatic diaphragmatic rupture over 11 years in a trauma center in Greece. Rupture was left sided in 66%, right sided in 32%, and bilateral in 2%. Blunt trauma accounted for 80% of cases. Emphasizes importance of high index of suspicion and early diagnosis, which can be missed in the acute trauma setting despite use of CT scanning.

20. Oh KS, Newman B, Bender TM, et al. Radiologic evaluation of the diaphragm. *Radiol Clin North Am*. 1988;26:355.

   One of those "everything you wanted to know but were afraid to ask" reviews. Especially good on congenital and traumatic disorders of the diaphragm.

21. Phillips JR, Elderidge FL. Respiratory myoclonus (Leeuwenhoek's disease). *N Engl J Med*. 1973;289:1390.

   Clinical features as well as pulmonary function test, electrocardiographic, and electromyography findings are presented. Still the best review of this rare disorder.

22. Polkey MI, Harris ML, Hughes PD, et al. The contractile properties of the elderly human diaphragm. *Am J Respir Crit Care Med*. 1997;155:1560.

   Aging is associated with a reduction in diaphragm strength. However, the magnitude of the reduction is small and may be offset by a leftward shift of the force–frequency relationship.

23. Reber A, Nylund U, Hedenstierna G. Position and shape of the diaphragm: Implications for atelectasis formation. *Anaesthesia*. 1998;53:1054.

   Compared with conscious, spontaneous breathing, mechanical ventilation decreases the inspiratory displacement of the dependent part of the diaphragm. This change in movement of the diaphragm can play an additional role in atelectasis formation.

24. Roussos C. Function and fatigue of respiratory muscles. *Chest.* 1985;88:124S.

Blood flow to respiratory muscles is relatively high and fixed even in the presence of cardiac failure, a point to be remembered when timing interventions such as intubation and mechanical ventilation in cardiac patients.

25. Ruel M, Deslauriers J, Maltais F. The diaphragm in emphysema. *Chest Surg Clin North Am.* 1998;8:381.

Concise review of pathophysiology and surgical treatment options of diaphragmatic dysfunction related to hyperinflation in emphysema.

26. Weksler B, Ginsberg RJ. Tumors of the diaphragm. *Chest Surg Clin North Am.* 1998;8:441.

A review of primary tumors of the diaphragm, more than half of which are benign. Diaphragmatic tumors arise from mesenchymal tissue because of their mesodermal origin, and all varieties of these tumors have been reported.

76. NEUROMUSCULAR DISEASES AND SPINAL CORD INJURY

David A. Bradshaw and Christopher M. Stafford

Neuromuscular disorders directly and indirectly impair respiratory function. A heterogeneous group of disorders can be classified by the primary site of pathology: brain (stroke, trauma, tumor, multiple sclerosis), spinal cord (poliomyelitis, amyotrophic lateral sclerosis), peripheral nerves (Guillain-Barré syndrome, critical illness polyneuropathy), neuromuscular junction (myasthenia gravis, Eaton–Lambert syndrome, botulism), and skeletal muscle (muscle dystrophy, drug-induced myopathy, polymyositis). Although the underlying pathophysiology, response to treatment, and prognosis vary considerably, all neuromuscular disorders may cause pulmonary insufficiency with predictable clinical symptoms and complications.

In normal tidal breathing, lung inflation is achieved primarily by contraction of the diaphragm and expansion of the thorax. Intrathoracic pressure decreases and the lungs fill; exhalation is essentially passive. As the diaphragm shortens, abdominal contents are compressed and the abdominal wall moves outward in synchrony with the chest wall. Weakness or reduced compliance in either the thoracic or abdominal compartments may be appreciated by direct observation. For example, abdominal wall stiffening or spasticity results in greater rib cage elevation and less abdominal compartment displacement for any degree of diaphragm shortening. Chest wall restriction, on the other hand, results in exaggerated movement of the abdominal wall. Although tidal exhalation to functional residual capacity (FRC) is passive, abdominal wall contraction is necessary to further empty the lungs. Neuromuscular disorders may affect the diaphragm, accessory muscles, and abdominal muscles equally or selectively, and the pattern of involvement can be determined by pulmonary function testing. Coughing, an essential protective mechanism that clears mucus-trapped inhalants and maintains airway patency, is achieved by a short vigorous inspiration followed by a forceful exhalation against a transiently closed glottis. Neuromuscular weakness can reduce lung expansion and/or the force of exhalation, thereby impairing cough and increasing the risk for aspiration, atelectasis, and pneumonia.

Patients with respiratory neuromuscular weakness generally assume a rapid shallow breathing pattern, characteristic of patients with a variety of restrictive disorders. Potential respiratory system manifestations of neuromuscular disease include fatigue, dyspnea, impaired swallowing and aspiration, recurrent lower respiratory tract infections, acute or chronic respiratory failure, sleep disruption, pulmonary hypertension, and cor pulmonale. Mild weakness may only be evident when patients lay supine, bend over, sleep, or exercise; however, progressive weakness eventually can lead to symptoms at rest, gas exchange abnormalities, and overt respiratory failure.

PULMONARY FUNCTION TESTING

Pulmonary function testing confirms neuromuscular weakness-associated pulmonary insufficiency, may predict complications, and is extremely valuable in monitoring the clinical course. Initial testing should include spirometry, static lung volumes, and maximal inspiratory and expiratory pressures (MIP and MEP). Neuromuscular weakness is characterized by "restriction," although the pattern varies depending on which muscles are affected (inspiratory or expiratory). Vital capacity (VC) is reduced due either to a loss of inspiratory volume (reduced total lung capacity), expiratory volume (elevated residual volume), or both. FRC, the end-tidal lung volume representing the balance of static lung and chest wall elastic recoil, may be unaffected. The most sensitive tests of respiratory muscle weakness are maximum inspiratory pressure (MIP) and maximum expiratory pressure (MEP). To perform these tests, the patient is encouraged to inspire or expire with maximal effort against an occluded external airway from residual volume (MIP) or from total lung capacity (MEP). The pressures are easily recorded with a manometer. The MIP and MEP can be abnormal early in the course of disease, even when the static lung volumes are normal.

Additional pulmonary function tests may also be helpful in diagnosis. (MVV) may be more sensitive in identifying muscle fatigue than the MIP or MEP. The MVV is performed by asking the patient to breath as hard and fast as possible for 12 seconds, recording the expired volume, and then extrapolating this value to a total volume expired per minute. Diffusing capacity for carbon monoxide, corrected for alveolar volume, is normal, unless there is associated atelectasis or parenchymal disease (e.g., from repeated aspiration). Arterial blood gas analysis is not useful as a screening test because hypoxemia and hypercapnia are relatively late manifestations of respiratory muscle weakness, typically not present until the vital capacity (VC) is <30% of predicted. In the setting of progressive respiratory insufficiency, serial measurements of VC may predict impending respiratory failure; a VC of less than 15 mL/kg generally indicates the need for intubation.

SLEEP APNEA

Sleep-related breathing problems are common in patients with neuromuscular diseases and generally precede awake manifestations and overt respiratory failure. Normal non–rapid eye movement (REM) sleep results in a drop in minute ventilation with an associated decrease in oxyhemoglobin saturation and rise in carbon dioxide. Causes of this physiologic sleep-induced hypoventilation include loss of a "wakefulness drive" (from reduced chemoreceptor and mechanoreceptor responsiveness) and concurrent pharyngeal muscle relaxation, which increases upper airway resistance. REM or "dream" sleep is characterized by active inhibition of motoneurons, sparing only the diaphragm and extraocular muscles. Physiologic loss of intercostal and accessory muscle tone makes REM sleep a time of profound ventilatory vulnerability for patients with diaphragmatic weakness.

Neuromuscular patients are at risk for upper airway obstruction (obstructive sleep apnea), sleep-related hypoventilation, or both depending on the relative strength of the pharyngeal dilator muscles and diaphragm. For example, patients with diaphragmatic paralysis may profoundly hypoventilate during sleep, and patients with predominantly bulbar weakness are more likely to develop upper airway obstruction. Additionally, patients with obstructive apneas during non-REM sleep may paradoxically maintain airway patency during REM sleep because a weak diaphragm is unable to generate sufficient negative intrathoracic pressure to collapse the upper airway. Patients with sleep-related breathing disorders frequently complain of impaired sleep quality and daytime symptoms such as sleepiness, headaches, difficulty concentrating, and fatigue. Consequently, all patients with neuromuscular weakness should be carefully queried regarding sleep-related symptoms.

Noninvasive positive-pressure ventilation delivered through a mask has become a widely accepted treatment for patients with chronic respiratory failure or sleep-related breathing disturbances because of neuromuscular weakness. General indications for initiating noninvasive ventilatory support, based largely on expert consensus, include the presence of symptoms and (1) gas exchange abnormalities, such as $PaCO_2$ of at least 45 mm Hg or nocturnal desaturation (SaO_2 <88% for 5 consecutive minutes) or (2) forced vital capacity of less than 50% of predicted. Potential contraindications to noninvasive ventilation include the inability to adequately protect the upper airway, excessive secretions and ineffective cough, uncooperative or poorly motivated patient or family, and lack of resources. Although some physicians have expressed ethical concerns regarding use of ventilatory support for patients with progressive, irreversible disorders (e.g., amyotrophic lateral sclerosis [ALS]), recent studies have reported prolonged survival and clinically significant quality-of-life improvements in this population that should be considered when discussing treatment with patients and their caregivers.

Although oral mouthpieces or orthotics are often used by neuromuscular patients requiring daytime ventilation, they are poorly tolerated during sleep. Currently, a wide variety of mask interfaces are available for patients requiring nocturnal or continuous ventilatory assistance. The choice of nasal or oronasal mask depends on facial morphology and ability to seal, patient preference, and clinician familiarity. In patients with progressive bulbar dysfunction, tracheotomy is eventually necessary if long-term support is elected. The goals of ventilation can be met with either pressure or volume preset ventilators and require close interaction between the patient and physician in selecting the appropriate mode and specific ventilator settings to satisfy ventilatory demands and promote consolidated sleep.

GUILLAIN-BARRÉ SYNDROME

The most common acute neuropathy to affect the respiratory system is Guillain-Barré syndrome (GBS), with an annual incidence of 1 to 3 per 100,000 persons. Patients typically present with ascending motor weakness (although sensory symptoms may also be present to a lesser degree), often following a viral respiratory or gastrointestinal illness. Areflexia, increased cerebrospinal fluid protein without leukocytosis, and electromyogram evidence of demyelination establish the diagnosis. Respiratory compromise is common, and mechanical ventilation is required in approximately 30% of patients. The rate of progression may be dramatic, with acute respiratory failure occurring within 24 to 48 hours of symptom onset. Serial bedside measurements of the VC provide objective data on which to base intubation and ventilatory assistance decisions. A VC of less than 30 mL/kg compromises cough, and atelectasis with hypoxemia may develop when the VC falls below 25 mL/kg. Intubation should be strongly considered when the VC reaches 15 mL/kg, especially when there is clinical evidence of fatigue or difficulty handling secretions. Other supportive treatments include IV fluids, electrolyte and nutrition management, physical therapy including passive joint movement, meticulous skin care with frequent turning or use of specialized beds, and deep venous thrombosis prophylaxis. Intravenous immunoglobulin and plasmapharesis have been shown to be equally efficacious; combining treatments appears to confer no additional benefit. Approximately 20% of patients experience autonomic complications such as dysrhythmias and volatile blood pressures. Over two thirds of all patients with GBS recover with only minor neurologic deficits.

SPINAL CORD INJURY

More than 200,000 patients in the United States have significant spinal cord injury and approximately 10,000 new injuries occur each year. The anatomic level of spinal cord injury is critical in determining respiratory system impairment. High cervical cord lesions (C1–C2) cause complete paralysis of all muscles of respiration and result in respiratory arrest and need for immediate ventilatory support. Middle cervical cord lesions (C3–C5) cause variable loss of phrenic nerve function, and the prognosis improves with lower lesions: 40%, 14%, and 11% of C3, C4, and C5 lesions, respectively, are chronically ventilator dependent. Lower cervical (C6–C8) and upper thoracic lesions (T1–T6) spare the diaphragm and neck accessory muscles, but chest wall (intercostal muscles) and abdominal muscle function are lost. The nadir of lung function occurs immediately after a spinal cord injury due to flaccid paralysis of the affected respiratory muscles. In the acute setting, during inspiration, the chest wall contracts instead of expands, resulting in a substantial (up to 70%) reduction in maximal inspiratory forces. After several months, the intercostal and abdominal muscles become spastic, no longer collapse with inspiration, and ventilatory function improves to approximately 60% of predicted preinjury levels. VC in tetraplegics decreases with age and duration of spinal cord injury, regardless of age of injury, gender, or severity of injury. Electric pacing of the diaphragm with implanted electrodes is an option for patients with intact phrenic nerves; however, it is a costly procedure and not widely available.

Chronic management issues in spinal cord injury include prevention of pneumonia, atelectasis, and respiratory failure. Despite preservation of the cough reflex, loss of innervation to the expiratory muscles leads to an ineffective cough. To overcome this deficiency, intensive training of the resistive inspiratory muscles can mildly increase MVV and MIP, and in some patients, reduces elements of sleep-disordered breathing, such as $ETco_2$ and nocturnal desaturation. Manually assisted cough techniques have been shown to increase peak cough expiratory flow and mucous clearance. Placement in the supine position (opposed to upright) is an important mechanical factor for quadriplegics. In the supine position, passive pressure from the abdominal contents helps to position the diaphragm optimally; this effect is lost in the upright position because of the flaccid abdominal wall.

1. Bach JR. Amyotrophic lateral sclerosis. Prolongation of life by noninvasive respiratory aids. *Chest*. 2002;122:92–98.
    Retrospective review of patients with ALS from a single medical center. Of patients in this series, 20% used mechanically assisted cough and noninvasive positive pressure ventilation for mean of 14 to 17 months (over 6 years in one case) prior to death or converting to tracheotomy.
2. Ball PA. Critical care of spinal cord injury. *Spine*. 2001;26(24 Suppl):s27–30.
    Brief review of the pathophysiology of pulmonary and hemodynamic derangements after acute spinal cord injury.
3. Baydur A, Adkins RH, Milic-Emili J. Lung mechanics in individuals with spinal cord injury: Effects of injury level and posture. *J Appl Physiol*. 2001;90:405–411.
    Generally FVC and FEV_1 increase with descending spinal injury levels down to level T10. FEV_1 and FVC do not significantly change with position; however, inspiratory capacity increases in the supine position likely because of the effect of gravity on the abdominal contents.
4. Bourke SC, Gibson GJ. Sleep and breathing in neuromuscular disease. *Eur Respir J*. 2002;19:1194–1201.
    Good review of normal breathing and muscle function during sleep in normal individuals and patients with neuromuscular weakness. Individual disorders including isolated diaphragmatic paralysis, ALS, Duchenne muscular dystrophy, myotonic dystrophy, and myasthenia gravis are reviewed.
5. Chatwin M, Ross E, Hart N, et al. Cough augmentation with mechanical insufflation/exsufflation in patients with neuromuscular disorders. *Eur Respir J*. 2003;21:502–508.
    Peak cough flows were compared at baseline and using three augmentation techniques: standard physiotherapy-assisted cough; cough after noninvasive positive pressure inhalation; exsufflation-assisted cough; and combination insufflation/exsufflation-assisted cough. Neuromuscular patient peak cough flows were highest with insufflation/exsufflation. Insufflation/exsufflation consists of positive pressure to achieve maximal lung inflation followed by an abrupt shift to negative pressure, thereby simulating the flow changes characteristic of a spontaneous cough.
6. DePalo VA, McCool FD. Respiratory muscle evaluation of the patient with neuromuscular disease. *Semin Respir Crit Care Med*. 2002;23:201–209.

An in-depth review of the standard and novel pulmonary function tests in neuromuscular disease.

7. Dicpinigaitis PV, Grimm DR, Lesser M. Cough reflex sensitivity in subjects with cervical spinal cord injury. *Am J Respir Crit Care Med.* 1999;159:1660–1662.

   Small trial demonstrating that sensitivity of cough reflex is preserved in spinal cord injury. Given intact reflex, ineffective cough is likely caused by loss of innervation of the respiratory muscles.

8. Gelinas DF. Pulmonary function screening. *Semin Neurol.* 2003;23:89–96.

   Review of the utility, advantages, and disadvantages of pulmonary function tests in neuromuscular disease.

9. Gilchrist JM. Overview of neuromuscular disorders affecting respiratory function. *Semin Respir Crit Care Med.* 2002;23:191–200.

   A general overview of the common neuromuscular diseases by anatomic site.

10. Laghi F, Tobin MJ. Disorders of the respiratory muscles. *Am J Respir Crit Care Med.* 2003;168:20–36.

    State of the art review of the pathophysiology of neuromuscular disease.

11. Langevin B, Petitjean T, Philit F, et al. Nocturnal hypoventilation in chronic respiratory failure (CRF) due to neuromuscular disease. *Sleep.* 2000;23:S204–S209.

    Ventilatory drive during sleep is decreased because of loss of a behavioral stimulus. Concurrently, upper airway muscle tone decreases, resistance increases, and respiratory load compensation is compromised. REM sleep is a particularly vulnerable time because ventilation completely depends on an intact diaphragm; patients with diaphragmatic weakness may profoundly desaturate.

12. Linn WS, Spungen AM, Gong HJ, et al. Forced vital capacity in two large outpatient populations with chronic spinal cord injury. *Spinal Cord.* 2001;39:263–268.

    Development of an equation to predict FVC for patients with nonacute spinal cord injury based on level of injury.

13. Lyall RA, Donaldson N, Fleming T, et al. A prospective study of quality of life in ALS patients treated with noninvasive ventilation. *Neurology.* 2001;57:153–156.

    Prospective cohort study of 16 ALS patients found improvement in the "vitality" domain of the SF-36 questionnaire despite overall disease progression. Other functional domain measures fell with disease progression in both treated patients and a control group; therefore, the authors rejected the hypothesis that improved quality of life obtained from ventilatory assistance would be negated by increasing disability afforded by prolonged survival.

14. Markstrom A, Sundell K, Lysdahl M, et al. Quality-of-life evaluation of patient with neuromuscular and skeletal diseases treated with noninvasive and invasive home mechanical ventilation. *Chest.* 2002;122:1695–1700.

    Home ventilator patients reported good overall health as measured by three different questionnaires. Patients with tracheostomy seemed to do better than noninvasively ventilated patients; however, the authors pointed out that the marked disparity in management routines and social support (monthly versus annual follow-up) may explain the difference.

15. Mehta S, Hill NS. State of the art: Noninvasive ventilation. *Am J Respir Crit Care Med.* 2001;163:540–577.

    Exhaustive overview of the role of noninvasive ventilation in acute and chronic respiratory failure.

16. Piper A. Sleep abnormalities associated with neuromuscular disease: Pathophysiology and evaluation. *Semin Respir Crit Care Med.* 2002;23:211–219.

    A simple relationship between awake pulmonary function tests and sleep-related breathing events does not exist. The importance of studying neuromuscular patients during REM sleep is emphasized.

17. Schönhofer B, Sortor-Leger S. Equipment needs for noninvasive mechanical ventilation. *Eur Respir J.* 2002;20:1029–1036.

    Reviews the important equipment-related issues for noninvasive mechanical ventilation including ventilator selection, ventilator settings, interfaces, leak management, humidification, oxygen supplementation, and medication nebulization.

18. The Plasma Exchange/Sandoglobin Guillain-Barré Trial Group. Randomized trial of plasma exchange, intravenous immunoglobulin, and combined treatments in Guillain-Barré syndrome. *Lancet.* 1997;349:225–230.

   Multicenter, randomized trial of 383 patients demonstrated that IV immunoglobulin and plasmapharesis are equally efficacious when given within the first 2 weeks after onset of neuropathic symptoms; the combination of both treatments did not confer additional benefit.

19. Tow AM, Graves DE, Carter RE. Vital capacity in tetraplegics twenty years and beyond. *Spinal Cord.* 2001;39:139–144.

   Vital capacity in tetraplegics decreases with age and duration of spinal cord injury, regardless of age of injury, gender, or severity of injury.

20. Wang AY, Jaeger RJ, Yarkony GM, et al. Cough in spinal cord injured patients: The relationship between motor level and peak expiratory flow. *Spinal Cord.* 1997;35:299–302.

   Demonstration of a direct relationship between motor level and peak expiratory flow produced during coughing.

21. Wang TG, Wang YH, Tang FT, et al. Resistive inspiratory muscle training in sleep-disordered breathing of traumatic tetraplegia. *Arch Phys Med Rehabil.* 2002;83:491–496.

   Home-based resistive inspiratory muscle training for 6 weeks can mildly enhance MVV and MIP and in some, reduce some elements of sleep disordered breathing (ETCO$_2$ and nocturnal desaturation).

22. Winslow C, Rozovsky J. Effect of spinal cord injury on the respiratory system. *Am J Phys Med Rehabil.* 2003;82:803–814.

   Review of epidemiology and pathophysiology of acute and chronic spinal cord injury.

23. Yavagal DR, Mayer SA. Respiratory complications of rapidly progressive neuromuscular syndromes: Guillain-Barré syndrome and myasthenia gravis. *Semin Respir Crit Care Med.* 2002;23:221–229.

   Thorough review of GBS and myasthenia gravis.

77. SLEEP APNEA, ALVEOLAR HYPOVENTILATION, AND OBESITY HYPOVENTILATION

José S. Loredo

The spectrum of sleep-disordered breathing ranges from intermittent snoring, which is primarily a nuisance, to obesity-hypoventilation syndrome, which is associated with severe morbidity and very high mortality. In between these extremes are disorders of gradually increasing impact on morbidity and mortality including chronic snoring, upper airway resistance syndrome, and sleep apnea.

OBSTRUCTIVE SLEEP APNEA

Obstructive sleep apnea (OSA) is the most common form of sleep-disordered breathing documented in the sleep laboratory. Both children and adults may be affected; however, the prevalence of obstructive apnea is highest among middle-aged men. The prevalence of symptomatic OSA in the middle-aged working population is 4% in men and 2% in women and the prevalence of asymptomatic sleep apnea is 24% in men and 9% in women. OSA is characterized by repetitive upper airway obstructions during sleep. The immediate consequences of OSA include micro-arousals from sleep, full awakenings, hypoxemia, hypercapnia, rises in systemic and pulmonary pressures, nocturia from rises in atrial natriuretic peptide levels, and sleep fragmentation. The most common presenting symptoms are excessive daytime somnolence and chronic loud snoring. However, it is not uncommon for the OSA patient to present complaining of daytime fatigue, decreased cognitive function, sexual dysfunction, depression, and even sleep maintenance insomnia caused by frequent nocturnal awakenings. The bed partner often notes loud snoring, choking spells, leg kicks, and more specifically observed apneas. These patients also have higher rates of automobile accidents than normal individuals. In children, OSA often presents with snoring and hyperactivity, and it is often misdiagnosed as attention deficit hyperactivity disorder.

The etiology of OSA is not well understood, but obesity, a narrowed upper airway, loss of upper airway motor tone during sleep, abnormalities of central control of ventilation, high CO_2 sensitivity, and cardiac function have been implicated in the pathophysiology. There are strong epidemiologic and experimental evidences that link OSA with the development of systemic hypertension and other cardiovascular complications. The mechanism for this association is unclear but chronic intermittent hypoxia and frequent arousals leading to hyperactivity of chemoreceptors and sympathetic nervous system may be involved.

There are three basic types of sleep-disordered breathing: (1) apnea, a 90% or more decrease in airflow in 10 seconds or more, (2) hypopnea, a 50 to more than 90% decrease in airflow in 10 seconds or more associated with either an arousal or oxyhemoglobin desaturation, and (3) respiratory effort–related arousals, the upper airway resistance syndrome (UARS).

Three types of apnea have been described: (1) *obstructive apnea,* in which oronasal airflow is blocked and diaphragmatic efforts continue; (2) *central apnea,* in which diaphragmatic and intercostal efforts cease; and (3) *mixed apnea,* an obstructive apnea with an initial central component. In the majority of symptomatic patients with sleep apnea, all three types of apneas are found commonly, but obstructive events predominate by far. The syndromes of obstructive and mixed sleep apnea are clinically similar and therefore are grouped together. UARS differs in that oxyhemoglobin desaturation and obvious apneas or hypopneas are not evident in the standard polysomnogram.

On physical examination 70% of sleep apnea patients have truncal obesity and it is not unusual to find them snoring in the waiting room. Hypertrophy of the tonsils and adenoids appears to be the cause of the upper airway obstruction in children. Malformations of the jaw and maxilla such as retrognathia, micrognathia, and narrow high arching palate are occasionally noted. More commonly the adult patient with sleep apnea presents with an erythematous enlarged edematous uvula, prominent tonsillar pillars, and drape-like soft palate, reducing the caliber of the oropharyngeal opening. However, in some patients the physical examination may be entirely normal.

Despite having a narrow oropharyngeal opening, airway obstruction during the waking state is absent secondary to neuromuscular compensation. During sleep this neuromuscular compensation is lost, predisposing the patient to upper airway obstruction. In the waking state, pulmonary function tests, arterial blood gases, and ventilatory response to carbon dioxide are usually normal, unless the separate effects of morbid obesity or another disease are present. Systemic hypertension is present in up to 50% of patients. Pulmonary arterial hypertension may occur in up to 40% of cases of uncomplicated OSA; however, this is generally not clinically significant. The diagnosis of the sleep apnea syndromes can be most accurately made by documenting apneic episodes during attended polysomnography. However, unattended home cardiorespiratory recordings are also commonly used to diagnose sleep apnea in patients with classical symptoms. To be considered significant, apneic episodes must last at least 10 seconds and occur repetitively. The Apnea/Hypopnea Index (AHI) is used to determine the severity of sleep apnea. The AHI represents the number of apneas plus hypopneas per hour of sleep. An AHI less than 5 is considered normal, and an AHI greater than 30 is considered severe.

The pathophysiology and hemodynamic consequences of the sleep apnea syndromes have been studied extensively. During an obstructive episode, the posterior wall of the hypopharynx collapses, and the strap muscles of the neck become hypotonic as documented by electromyographic recordings. As the apneic episode continues, hypercapnia and hypoxemia develop. Progressive increases in negative intrathoracic pressure develop with the increasing efforts to breathe against the obstruction. Systemic and pulmonary hypertension, sinus bradycardia, and a variety of arrhythmias and conduction disturbances may occur. A loud snort may signal the end of the obstruction and correlates with an EEG pattern of arousal from sleep. Subsequently, abnormalities of gas exchange and hemodynamics resolve rapidly, unless repetitive apneic episodes occur, a frequent situation in severely affected individuals.

Treatment of patients with OSA should always include behavioral interventions: weight reduction, avoidance of alcohol and sedatives, avoidance of sleep deprivation, avoidance of the supine sleep position, and smoking cessation. Weight reduction to optimum levels can be curative in some cases. However, even modest weight reductions may result in significant reductions in sleep apnea severity. Pharmacologic therapy for sleep apnea has been disappointing. Nocturnal nasal oxygen therapy can improve arterial oxygen saturation, but it does not significantly change the AHI. Continuous positive airway pressure (CPAP) has become the preferred method of treatment for sleep apnea. CPAP maintains upper airway patency during sleep by creating a pneumatic splint. It can effectively control sleep apnea arousals and reverse oxyhemoglobin desaturation in the majority of cases. CPAP remains a cumbersome therapy despite significant technological advances. Oral appliances are an alternative to CPAP in patients with mild to moderate sleep apnea, although not as effective as CPAP in controlling apneic events. Many types of oral appliances are available. The most effective are those that are adjustable and advance the jaw, enlarging the upper airway. Temporomandibular joint pain is a common complaint from the use of jaw advancement devices. Surgical procedures that increase upper airway size (uvulopalatopharyngoplasty) have been found to effectively eliminate snoring, but frequently they fail to control sleep apnea adequately, especially when the sleep apnea is more severe. Unfortunately, there is no way to predict which patients will benefit from surgical treatment. Extensive surgery to advance the entire mouth forward has been as successful as CPAP in controlling sleep apnea in highly selected populations. Recently, radiofrequency volume reduction of the base of the tongue has been successful in improving apnea severity in sleep apnea patients with isolated tongue base obstruction. Tracheostomy is a last resort that is rarely applied but consistently effective in relieving signs and symptoms of OSA. Finally, an effort should be made to identify associated conditions that may worsen sleep apnea, (hypothyroidism, use of testosterone) because their treatment can sometimes also cure their sleep apnea. In children, removal of obstructing tonsils and adenoids is usually curative.

Pure central sleep apnea is often associated with advanced age, neurologic disorders, congestive heart failure, and sleeping at high altitude. It may be associated with high sensitivity to carbon dioxide and conditions that promote hypocapnia. Oral acetazolamide and nasal CPAP have both been successful in treating patients with central sleep apnea. Supplemental oxygen may also be of benefit, especially in central sleep apnea associated with high altitude.

Alveolar hypoventilation is defined as an elevation in the $PaCO_2$ to levels greater than 45 mm Hg due to a reduction in minute ventilation. Because the alveolus is a finite space, a rise in alveolar PcO_2 leads to a decrease in alveolar PO_2 and results in hypoxemia. Alveolar hypoventilation can occur with a number of disorders, referred to as the *hypoventilation syndromes*. Although hypercapnia and hypoxemia can be evident during wakefulness, these are usually more severe during deep sleep in most cases of alveolar hypoventilation.

PRIMARY ALVEOLAR HYPOVENTILATION

The syndrome of primary alveolar hypoventilation (Ondine's curse) is a rare disorder characterized by hypercapnia and hypoxemia that develops mostly in young adult men without abnormalities of the lung parenchyma, chest wall, respiratory muscle function, or voluntary control of ventilation. *Central alveolar hypoventilation* is a term used for those patients whose alveolar hypoventilation is caused by an identified neurologic process such as destructive lesions in the medullary chemoreceptor. Congenital central hypoventilation is a rare disorder of ventilation control diagnosed in early childhood that may have a familial component. In all cases of primary alveolar hypoventilation, there is a failure of the central autonomic regulation of ventilation and inability to integrate the neural input from peripheral chemoreceptors.

Invariably, these children have multisystemic involvement, with significant developmental problems and common occurrence of congenital megacolon.

The clinical manifestations of alveolar hypoventilation include lethargy, somnolence, and morning headaches. Dyspnea is remarkably absent unless congestive heart failure supervenes. Apnea during sleep is often prominent. Cyanosis with a normal alveolar–arterial O_2 gradient is the most common physical finding and it can usually be reversed by voluntary hyperventilation. Polycythemia and cor pulmonale are present in 50% of cases. Although hypercapnia and hypoxemia at rest are noted in the vast majority, arterial blood gases may occasionally be normal, and an unexplained metabolic alkalosis may be a clue to previous chronic hypercapnia. Pulmonary function testing reveals normal lung volumes and flow rates; however, there is a greatly diminished or absent ventilatory response to carbon dioxide inhalation. The response to hypoxia is frequently impaired as well. Breath-holding time is often prolonged, and exercise may result in worsening of hypoxemia and hypercapnia because of impaired chemoreceptor response.

Several forms of therapy have been proposed. Respiratory stimulants are generally ineffective. Rocking beds or mechanical ventilatory assistance (bilevel positive airway pressure via a nasal mask) have been useful in severe cases, particularly at night when the hypoventilation is most severe. Nocturnal phrenic nerve pacing has been described as safe and effective therapy and may be the treatment of choice in severely affected individuals. However, noninvasive ventilation is the most common therapy for congenital central hypoventilation syndrome, usually through a tracheostomy.

OBESITY HYPOVENTILATION SYNDROME

The obesity hypoventilation syndrome is characterized by obesity and alveolar hypoventilation not explained by a neuromuscular, mechanical, or metabolic reason for hypoventilation. This syndrome is often associated with OSA. It was originally described as the "Pickwickian syndrome" by Burwell and Robin, named after a character in Dickens's Pickwick Papers ("the fat boy Joe") who was obese and continually falling asleep.

The etiology of the obesity hypoventilation syndrome is complex and probably results from an imbalance between ventilatory drive and ventilatory load. Not all obese individuals develop alveolar hypoventilation. Currently there are no data supporting an inherited mechanism for decreased ventilatory drive in obesity hypoventilation syndrome. The factors depressing ventilation and gas exchange in these patients include (1) obesity with its increased work of breathing and interference with the mechanical efficiency of ventilation, (2) heart failure, (3) diffuse airway obstruction, and (4) OSA, especially when severe. The obesity hypoventilation syndrome patient is at a high risk of in-hospital mortality and morbidity, often experiencing sudden unexpected death.

The findings on history and physical examination define this syndrome. Patients are severely hypersomnolent and fall asleep at the most inappropriate times. Although snoring is not a universal finding, these patients often have a long history of loud and disruptive snoring. On physical examination, the patients are obese, often greater than 50% above their predicted weights. They may have a ruddy complexion or cyanosis caused by hypoxemia and secondary erythrocytosis. They often have a short, thick neck, an enlarged uvula, and a small oropharyngeal opening. They may have crackles or wheezes on chest examination and demonstrate hepatomegaly, peripheral edema, and other findings of right ventricular heart failure.

Chest radiographs show an enlarged heart and small lung fields with pulmonary congestion. Electrocardiograms often demonstrate right atrial and ventricular enlargement. Arterial blood gases show hypoxemia and hypercapnia, with widened alveolar–arterial oxygen gradient. However, these patients can voluntarily hyperventilate and normalize their P_{CO_2}. Approximately one half of these patients have erythrocytosis. Spirometry demonstrates a lower than normal forced vital capacity (FVC) and forced expiratory volume in 1 second (FEV_1), with some patients having evidence of superimposed airway obstruction, that is, FEV_1/FVC of less than 75%. The total lung capacity is 20% smaller and the maximal voluntary ventilation is 40%

lower than that of patients with simple obesity. Tests of ventilatory control show a diminished response to both hypercapnia and hypoxemia. Polysomnography demonstrates moderate to severe OSA often with prolonged and severe hypoxemia in the great majority of these patients. Only a minority of patients demonstrate pure obesity hypoventilation syndrome.

Clinical evaluation includes a careful history and complete physical examination, arterial blood gases, spirometry, maximal inspiratory and expiratory pressures, thyroid function tests, and overnight polysomnography. The evaluation focuses on any conditions that could contribute to persistent daytime hypoventilation such as hypothyroidism, severe OSA, or respiratory muscle weakness. In addition, this evaluation needs to consider other sources of ventilatory impairment, such as left ventricular heart failure and diffuse airway disease.

These patients should be thoroughly evaluated and treated to avoid serious complications, which include pulmonary arterial hypertension, cor pulmonale, acute ventilatory decompensation, and sudden death. Therapy should focus on reducing ventilatory loads and increasing ventilatory drive. Weight loss invariably results in improvement in hypoventilation and clinical symptoms. Unfortunately, permanent weight loss in these patients is difficult, and may require bariatric surgery. Progestational ventilatory stimulants in high doses (medroxyprogesterone 20 mg PO tid) may be helpful in weaning the obesity hypoventilation syndrome patient from mechanical ventilation. However, side effects limit their long-term use in most patients. The risk of deep venous thrombosis and pulmonary embolism is great in these obese patients, and when nonambulatory, prophylactic measures should be taken with use of subcutaneous heparin and or lower extremity intermittent compression stockings. Sedatives, alcohol, and other ventilatory depressants should be avoided. Nocturnal and daytime oxygen supplementation must be used with caution to avoid further ventilatory depression and worsening hypercapnia. The goal is to maintain an oxyhemoglobin saturation of at least 88% to avoid cardiopulmonary complications. Nocturnal nasal bilevel positive airway pressure should be instituted to correct worsened nocturnal hypoventilation and to abolish sleep apnea. The expiratory positive airway pressure should be titrated to abolish obstructive apneas and the inspiratory pressure should be high enough to augment ventilation and reduce P_{CO_2}.

1. Young T, Palta M, Dempsey J, et al. The occurrence of sleep disordered breathing among middle-aged adults. *N Engl J Med.* 1993;328:1230.

    In a random sample of working adults, 2% of women and 4% of men had a clinically important degree of sleep apnea. Twenty-four percent of men and 9% of women had sleep apnea by laboratory criteria.

2. Umlauf MG, Chasens ER, Greevy RA, et al. Obstructive sleep apnea, nocturia and polyuria in older adults. *Sleep.* 2004;27:139.

    Subjects with higher AHI had higher atrial natriuretic peptide levels and greater nocturia.

3. Findley L, Levinson M, Bonnie R. Driving performance and automobile accidents in patients with sleep apnea. *Clin Chest Med.* 1992;13:427.

    A review of the studies demonstrating poor driving performance and high automobile accident rates in drivers with untreated sleep apnea. Legal and liability questions are also addressed.

4. Gottlieb DJ, Yezina RM, Chase C, et al. Symptoms of sleep-disordered breathing in 5-year-old children are associated with sleepiness and problem behaviors. *Pediatrics.* 2003;112:870.

    Children with symptoms of sleep-disordered breathing had more parent-reported daytime sleepiness and problem behaviors (hyperactivity, inattention, aggressiveness), suggestive of attention deficit hyperactivity disorder.

5. Mezzanote WS, Tangel DJ, White DP. Waking genioglossal electromyogram in sleep apnea patients versus normal controls (a neuromuscular compensatory mechanism). *J Clin Invest.* 1992;89:1571.

*OSA patients demonstrate neuromuscular overcompensation during wakeful-
ness to maintain a patent upper airway. This overcompensation is lost during
sleep, predisposing them to upper airway obstruction.*

6. Resnick HE, Redline S, Shahar E, et al. Diabetes and sleep disturbances: Findings
    from the Sleep Heart Health Study. *Diabetes Care.* 2003;26:702.
    *Diabetics had a higher prevalence of periodic breathing, which is associated with
    abnormalities in the central control of ventilation. Diabetes may be a risk factor
    for OSA.*

7. Javaheri S. A mechanism of central sleep apnea in patients with heart failure.
    N Engl J Med. 1999;341:949.
    *This study concludes that enhanced sensitivity to carbon dioxide may predispose
    patients with heart failure to the development of central sleep apnea.*

8. Garrigue S, Bordier P, Jais P, et al. Benefit of atrial pacing in sleep apnea syn-
    drome. *N Engl J Med.* 2002;346:404.
    *Atrial overdrive pacing decreased the frequency of central and obstructive ap-
    neas.*

9. Sharabi Y, Dagan Y, Grossman E. Sleep apnea as a risk factor for hypertension.
    Curr Opin Nephrol Hypertens. 2004;13:359.
    *Review of the epidemiological data and other factors that link OSA to the devel-
    opment of hypertension and the benefits of treatment.*

10. Loredo JS, Ziegler MG, Ancoli-Israel S, et al. Relationship of arousals from sleep
    to sympathetic nervous system activity and BP in obstructive sleep apnea. *Chest.*
    1999;116:655.
    *Movement arousals independently contribute to daytime sympathetic nervous
    system activity.*

11. Guilleminault C, Chowdhuri S. Upper airway resistance syndrome is a distinct
    syndrome. *Am J Respir Crit Care Med.* 2000;161:1412.
    Excellent review of the physiologic and clinical evidences for the UARS.

12. Sajkov D, Wang T, Saunders NA, et al. Daytime pulmonary hemodynamics in
    patients with obstructive sleep apnea without lung disease. *Am J Respir Crit
    Care Med.* 1999;159:1518.
    *Pulmonary arterial hypertension is common in OSA; however, in most cases, the
    systolic pulmonary pressures are only mildly elevated.*

13. Kansanen M, Vanninen E, Tuunainen A, et al. The effect of a very low-calorie diet-
    induced weight loss on the severity of obstructive sleep apnoea and autonomic
    nervous function in obese patients with obstructive sleep apnoea syndrome. *Clin
    Physiol.* 1998;18:377.
    *Weight loss with a very low-calorie diet in 15 obese patients resulted in significant
    improvement of sleep apnea and favorable effects on blood pressure and baroreflex
    sensitivity.*

14. Loredo JS, Ancoli-Israel S, Dimsdale JE. Effects of CPAP vs placebo-CPAP in sleep
    quality. *Chest.* 1999;116:1545.
    *CPAP was an effective therapy to correct the RDI, oxyhemoglobin desaturation,
    and arousals in OSA. However, CPAP was not as effective in correcting sleep ar-
    chitecture abnormalities after 1 week of treatment*

15. Means MK, Edinger JD, Husain AM. CPAP compliance in sleep apnea patients
    with and without laboratory CPAP titration. *Sleep Breath.* 2004;8:7.
    *In this series CPAP compliance was as high as 75% in patients that received
    face-to-face CPAP instruction and support.*

16. Marklund M, Stenlund H, Franklin KA. Mandibular advancement devices in 630
    men and women with obstructive sleep apnea and snoring: Tolerability and pre-
    dictors of treatment success. *Chest.* 2004;125:1270.
    *A prospective study of the use of a jaw advancement device in mild sleep-
    disordered breathing. The authors concluded that jaw advancement devices are
    recommended for women with sleep apnea, men with supine-dependent sleep ap-
    nea, and for snorers without sleep apnea.*

17. Sher AE, Schechtman KB, Piccirillo JF. The efficacy of surgical modifications of the
    upper airway in adults with obstructive sleep apnea syndrome. *Sleep.* 1996;19:156.

A meta-analysis: only 41% of patients undergoing uvulopalatopharyngoplasty responded with a reduction of the RDI to less than 20.

18. Li KK, Riley RW, Powell NB, et al. Maxillomandibular advancement for persistent obstructive sleep apnea after phase I surgery in patients without maxillomandibular deficiency. *Laryngoscope.* 2000;110:1684.

    Maxillomandibular advancement surgery was effective in correcting OSA after failure of uvulopalatopharyngoplasty.

19. Riley RW, Powell NB, Li KK, et al. An adjunctive method of radiofrequency volumetric tissue reduction of the tongue for OSAS. *Otolaryngol Head Neck Surg.* 2003;129:37.

    Radiofrequency volumetric reduction of the base of the tongue was effective in decreasing sleep apnea severity by more than 50% in sleep apnea patients with isolated tongue base obstruction.

Primary Hypoventilation Syndrome

1. Guilleminault C, Stoohs R, Schneider H, et al. Central alveolar hypoventilation and sleep: Treatment by intermittent positive pressure ventilation through nasal mask in an adult. *Chest.* 1989;96:1210.

   Discusses the successful treatment of central alveolar hypoventilation during sleep in an adult by ventilation through a nasal mask.

2. Kerbl R, Litscher H, Grubbauer HM, et al. Congenital central hypoventilation syndrome (Ondine's curse syndrome) in two siblings: Delayed diagnosis and successful noninvasive treatment. *Eur J Pediatr.* 1996;155:977.

   Primary alveolar hypoventilation, which may have a familial component, can be successfully treated with noninvasive ventilation via a mask in children.

3. Flageole H, Adolph VR, Davis GM, et al. Diaphragmatic pacing in children with congenital central hypoventilation syndrome. *Surgery.* 1995;118:25.

   Successful treatment of congenital central hypoventilation in children with diaphragmatic pacing.

4. Vanderlaan M, Holbrook CR, Wang M, et al. Epidemiologic survey of 196 patients with congenital central hypoventilation syndrome. *Pediatr Pulmonol.* 2004;37:217.

   In this survey, congenital central hypoventilation was associated with multisystem involvement among all participants: 16.3% had congenital megacolon; 61.7% of the children had a tracheotomy. Use of noninvasive ventilation was common.

5. Krachman S, Criner GJ. Hypoventilation syndromes. *Clin Chest Med.* 1998;19:139.

   An excellent and succinct review of the hypoventilation syndromes.

6. Bickelman AG, Burwell CS, Robin ED, et al. Extreme obesity associated with alveolar hypoventilation: A pickwickian syndrome. *Am J Med.* 1956;21:811.

   A classic case report.

7. Kessler R, Chaouat A, Schinkewitch P, et al. The obesity-hypoventilation syndrome revisited: A prospective study of 34 consecutive cases. *Chest.* 2001;120:369.

   In this series, pure obesity hypoventilation syndrome was rare. It was usually associated with OSA. Patients with obesity hypoventilation syndrome had severe diurnal hypoxemia and 58% had pulmonary hypertension as compared with 9% for patients with sleep apnea alone.

8. Jokic R, et al. Ventilatory responses to hypercapnia and hypoxia in relatives of patients with the obesity hypoventilation syndrome. *Thorax.* 2000;55:940.

   This article discusses the hypotheses for the development of obesity hypoventilation syndrome. In this study of relatives of patients with obesity hypoventilation syndrome, no evidence of familial abnormality of chemoresponsiveness was found.

9. Rapoport DM, Garay SM, Epstein H, et al. Hypercapnia in the obstructive sleep apnea syndrome: A re-evaluation of the pickwickian syndrome. *Chest.* 1986;89:627.

   Successful treatment of sleep apnea corrected daytime hypercapnia in approximately one half of patients with OSA and daytime hypercapnia.

10. Saaresranta T, Polo. Kantola P, Irjala K, et al. Respiratory Insufficiency in post-menopausal women. Sustained improvement of gas exchange with short-term medroxyprogesterone acetate. *Chest.* 1999;115:1581.

   Medroxyprogesterone at a dose of 60 mg / day was effective in improving arterial blood gases in women with hypoventilation.

11. Smyth A, Riley M. Chronic respiratory failure: An unusual cause and treatment. *Thorax.* 2002;57:835.

   Case report of successful treatment of alveolar hypoventilation with prolonged use of medroxyprogesterone at 20 mg PO tid.

12. Koenig SM. Pulmonary complications of obesity. *Am J Med Sci.* 2001;321:249.

   A review of the effects of obesity on pulmonary function, morbidity, and mortality.

13. Masa JF, et al. The obesity hypoventilation syndrome can be treated with nonin-vasive mechanical ventilation. *Chest.* 2001;119:1102.

   Use of bilevel positive pressure ventilation for 4 months during sleep was effective in reversing the respiratory failure of obesity hypoventilation syndrome and improving symptoms.

IX. ENVIRONMENTAL AND OCCUPATIONAL DISEASES

78. APPROACHES TO OCCUPATIONAL-ENVIRONMENTAL LUNG DISEASE

William G. Hughson

Occupational-environmental lung disease (OELD) describes a diverse group of conditions that are caused or aggravated by exposures in the workplace or environment; Table 78-1 lists some examples. Correct assessment of OELD requires systematic collection of data from multiple sources. Table 78-2 outlines the general approach to these patients, which begins with a careful review of the symptoms, with special emphasis on their relationship to patient activities. It is important to determine whether symptoms are worse at work and improve when away on weekends or holidays. Cigarette smoking and preexisting conditions such as asthma or allergies must be recorded. Nonrespiratory causes of dyspnea, including obesity or cardiac disease, should be evaluated as part of the general medical history.

A unique aspect of OELD is the crucial importance of the occupational-environmental history (Table 78-3); failure to reach a correct diagnosis usually begins with insufficient attention to collecting and evaluating this information. It is essential to obtain a complete chronology of all jobs held by the patient. Many conditions (e.g., asbestosis) have a long latency between exposure and disease; enquiries limited to the current occupation may fail to identify the culpable exposures.

After completing the history, a workplace or environmental cause may be suggested. Data are then collected to narrow the differential diagnosis. The physical examination should seek not only respiratory signs but also nonpulmonary causes of dyspnea such as heart disease and obesity. Chest radiographs are always important and can be central to the diagnosis of certain conditions (e.g., silicosis). However, the radiographs may be normal (e.g., occupational asthma) or the findings nonspecific. For example, cigarette smoking increases the profusion of irregular densities in the parenchyma, confounding the diagnosis of asbestosis. Confusion can be avoided if the radiologist is a National Institute for Occupational Safety and Health-certified B reader experienced in OELD. Pulmonary function tests are used to determine the general pattern (e.g., restrictive or obstructive) and degree of impairment. Exercise testing is often included to assess work capacity. Bronchial hyperreactivity can be identified using nonspecific agents (e.g., methacholine or histamine) or specific agents from the workplace. Special studies (e.g., skin tests, radioallergosorbent test assays) can be useful in identifying sensitization to workplace or environmental antigens. Invasive techniques (e.g., bronchoscopy, bronchoalveolar lavage, and open lung biopsy) may be necessary in selected cases.

After data have been collected from the patient, the focus then shifts to the workplace and environment. Industrial hygiene information can be obtained from the employer. This includes material safety data sheets for all agents used by the patient. The employer is legally obligated to provide these safety data sheets, which describe chemical constituents and toxicity. In some cases, they can be supplemented with air testing data or results of previous inspections by government agencies. Often, the workers' compensation insurance company has information, including health effects in other workers. When possible, a site visit to the workplace can provide first-hand observation of workplace practices, ventilation, and personal protective equipment. Recommendations may then be made for additional air quality or other industrial hygiene testing. After exhausting all these sources, it is frequently necessary to perform a literature review concerning specific exposures and their known health effects. Consultation with experts such as industrial hygienists and toxicologists may be required.

Many cases of OELD involve litigation, and a formal report containing the clinician's opinions is needed for dispute resolution (see Chapter 83). The clinician may be asked to rate the pulmonary disability using systems such as the American Medical

Table 78-1. Examples of occupational-environmental lung disease

Disorder	General agent	Examples
Industrial bronchitis	Irritants	Gases
		Smoke
		Fumes
Occupational asthma	Chemicals	Isocyanates
	Animal proteins	Laboratory animals
Hypersensitivity pneumonitis actinomycetes	Biologic dusts	Thermophilic
Pneumoconiosis	Mineral dusts	Asbestos
		Coal
		Silica
Lung cancer	Mineral dust	Asbestos
	Metal dust	Arsenic
	Radiation	Radon

Table 78-2. General approach to the patient suspected of having occupational-environmental lung disease

Medical and respiratory history
    Symptoms (e.g., dyspnea, cough, sputum, wheezing)
    Smoking
    Past medical history (e.g., asthma, atopy, cardiorespiratory diseases)
Detailed occupational history (see Table 78-3)
Physical examination
    Respiratory (e.g., wheezing, rales, rhonchi)
    Cardiac (e.g., coronary artery disease, congestive heart failure)
    Other (e.g., obesity, neuromusculoskeletal conditions, clubbing)
Laboratory data
    Chest radiographs (e.g., pneumoconiosis)
    Pulmonary function tests
    Special studies (e.g., serology, skin tests)
Industrial hygiene data
    Material Safety Data Sheets
    Air sampling data
    Site visit
Research—literature review
Report preparation—disability evaluation
Prevention

Table 78-3. Essential features of an occupational-environmental history

Chronologic list of all jobs, beginning with the first
Job activities and materials used for each position
Duration and intensity of exposure in each position
Protective equipment (e.g., respirators, gloves, aprons)
Adequacy of ventilation in workplace
Activities and materials used by coworkers
Health effects in coworkers
Part-time jobs
Domestic exposures (e.g., pets, hobbies)
Chronology of disease in relationship to work or environmental exposures

Association Guides to the Evaluation of Permanent Impairment or the Black Lung Benefits Act. It is important to become familiar with the relevant rating systems and to use appropriate terms when describing disability caused by OELD. Reports that are imprecise or do not contain the appropriate language cannot be used to provide benefits.

The issues of occupational exposure and subsequent disease in a particular patient may provide the basis for interventions or screening programs to prevent or identify OELD in others. Recognition of a specific risk factor for OELD has often begun with an unusual case report. If involved with patients with OELD, consider whether hazardous exposures or working conditions could be altered and make recommendations when appropriate.

1. Balmes JR. Occupational lung diseases. In: Ladou J, ed. *Current Occupational & Environmental Medicine,* 3rd ed. New York: Lange Medical Books/McGraw Hill; 2004,p. 320.

    An excellent review chapter.
2. Cone JE, Ladou J. The occupational medical history. In: Ladou J, ed. *Current Occupational & Environmental Medicine,* 3rd ed. New York: Lange Medical Books/McGraw Hill; 2004, p. 7.

    Includes websites for important data bases such as Toxline and the EPA Integrated Risk Information System.
3. Greenberg GN. Internet resources for occupational and environmental health professionals. *Toxicology.* 2002;178:263.

    Gives web sites for many important data bases providing information concerning hazardous exposures.
4. Guidotti TL, Abraham JL, Hughson WG, et al. Taking the occupational history. *Ann Intern Med.* 1983;99:641.

    Discusses how to take a detailed occupational history. Includes a 1-page history form that can be completed by the patient.
5. Marshall L, Weir E, Abelsohn A, et al. Identifying and managing adverse environmental health effects: 1. Taking an exposure history. *CMAJ.* 2002;166:1049.

    Excellent review article.
6. Parkes WR, ed. *Occupational Lung Disorders,* 3rd ed. Oxford: Butterworth–Heinemann; 1994.

    Comprehensive textbook with detailed reviews and excellent illustrations.
7. Politi BJ, Arena VC, Schwerha J, et al. Occupational medical history taking: how are today's physicians doing? A cross-sectional investigation of the frequency of occupational history taking by physicians in a major U.S. teaching center. *J Occup Environ Med.* 2004;46:550.

    Most physicians fail to obtain an adequate occupational history.
8. Rom WN, ed. *Environmental and Occupational Medicine,* 2nd ed. Philadelphia: Lippincott-Raven; 1998.

    Textbook that deals with all aspects of occupational medicine. Excellent chapters on occupational lung disease.
9. Singh N, Davis GS. Review: occupational and environmental lung disease. *Curr Opin Pulm Med.* 2002;8:117.

    Reviews recent developments in OELD, including increased concern for low-level exposures.

79. SILICOSIS

Richard D. Drucker

Silicosis is a fibrotic disease of the lungs caused by inhalation of crystalline silicon dioxide. Silicon dioxide is a ubiquitous material that is a major component of the earth's crust. Three major crystalline forms are associated with lung injury: quartz, cristobalite, and tridymite. These forms are termed *free silica,* in contrast to silicates, which are crystals of silicon dioxide complexed with inorganic cations such as calcium, iron, magnesium, or aluminum. Silicates are also capable of inducing lung injury. Inhaled free silica particles greater than 10 microns in diameter are trapped in the upper respiratory tract; particles 0.5 to 5.0 microns in diameter deposit in the alveoli and are pathogenic.

The classic occupations at risk for silicosis are mining (quarrying, tunneling), manufacturing (glass, pottery, porcelain, abrasives), and sandblasting. The development of disease appears to be related to the duration, concentration, and structure of the free silica dust in the environment as well as the incompletely characterized individual susceptibility to silica inhalation. With improved dust control, the prevalence of the disease appears to be decreasing. Only a minority of workers at risk actually develop silicosis.

PATHOGENESIS AND ETIOLOGY

The pathogenesis of silicosis is unclear. Abundant evidence indicates that the pulmonary alveolar macrophage plays an important role in mediating lung damage. Early studies suggested that silica particles were isolated within the intracellular phagosomes of the macrophage, which then acquired lytic enzymes from intracellular lysosomes. Within hours of particle ingestion, this phagolysosome ruptured and released enzymes within the macrophage, thereby causing autodigestion of the macrophage, cell lysis, and release of the previously ingested silica particle. This cycle could then be repeated.

More recent observations demonstrate silica-induced release of cytokines and fibrogenic mediators from the intact pulmonary macrophage. Pulmonary alveolar macrophages isolated from bronchoalveolar lavage fluid of silica-exposed animals and human workers are viable and appear to function normally. It is hypothesized that silica stimulates the alveolar macrophage to release mediators of inflammation that affect lymphocytes, polymorphonuclear leukocytes, and other macrophages. These inflammatory mediators may include tumor necrosis factor-α, interleukin-1, and arachidonic acid metabolites. The interplay of these mechanisms is presumed to stimulate the proliferation of type II pneumocytes, fibroblasts, collagen, and eventual fibrosis. The properties of the silica particle that catalyze these later events are still under investigation. Possibilities include the surface properties of the silica crystal and the formation of oxygen free radicals.

The classic pathologic lesion of silicosis is the hyaline nodule, consisting of concentric whorls of connective tissue and an acellular central zone containing free silica. The middle zone has fibroblasts and collagen, and the active peripheral zone contains macrophages, fibroblasts, and free silica. The nodules are scattered throughout the lungs with a predominance in the upper lobes. Simple nodules rarely compress airways or blood vessels, but large coalescent masses in the advanced stage of silicosis can involve these structures. Regional lymphadenopathy and pleural adhesions are common, particularly in more severe cases of silicosis.

CLINICAL PRESENTATION

Three major clinical presentations of silicosis are described: chronic silicosis, accelerated silicosis, and acute silicosis. Chronic silicosis becomes clinically apparent 20 or more years after exposure to free silica. Accelerated silicosis becomes clinically apparent 5 to 15 years after exposure to heavier concentrations of silica. The presentations of chronic and accelerated silicosis are similar. Roentgenographic abnormalities usually antedate the development of symptoms such as cough, sputum production, and dyspnea on exertion. The third clinical presentation, acute silicosis, develops within 6 months to 2 years of massive exposure to free silica. It tends to have a fulminant course with cough, weight loss, rapidly progressive dyspnea, and early death. The disease was initially described as an interstitial fibrosis with minimal nodularity. Histologically, the alveoli are filled with a periodic acid-Schiff–positive acellular material that is similar to that seen in pulmonary alveolar proteinosis (silicoproteinosis). Extrapulmonary involvement (kidney and liver) has been described in acute silicosis.

COMPLICATIONS

Patients with silicosis have an increased incidence of mycobacterial infections. In one series of silicotic sandblasters, 25% had mycobacterial disease, and one half of these were due to nontuberculous mycobacteria. Tuberculosis has been found in up to one third of South African goldmines with silicosis. It is important for the clinician to have a high index of suspicion for possible tuberculosis in patients with silicosis.

Compared with the general population, there is an increased incidence (10%) of connective tissue diseases in patients with silicosis. Particularly prevalent are progressive systemic sclerosis, rheumatoid arthritis, and systemic lupus erythematosus. Clinically, the course of the connective tissue disease is similar whether or not silicosis is present; however, the clinical course of silicosis is less favorable in those patients who also have a connective tissue disease. In silicosis, there is also an increased incidence of hypergammaglobulinemia, antinuclear antibodies, rheumatoid factor, and circulating immune complexes. There is no demonstrated correlation, however, between these serologic abnormalities and the clinical, roentgenographic, or physiologic presentation of the silicotic patient.

An unresolved issue is whether inhaled silica is carcinogenic. Although some studies suggest a correlation between silica exposure and an increase in the incidence of bronchogenic carcinoma, alternative explanations have not been excluded. In 1996, the International Agency for Research on Cancer classified crystalline silica as a group I carcinogen. A subsequent review of the available literature casts doubt on this conclusion based on a lack of consistent association between the development of lung cancer and exposure to crystalline silica as well as the lack of consistent association between those patients with lung cancer with and without silicosis.

There are three main patterns of roentgenographic abnormalities in silicosis. In simple silicosis, reticular and nodular patterns are frequent. The nodules range from 1 mm to less than 10 mm in diameter, predominate in the upper lobes, and usually have sharp margins. Hilar adenopathy is common. Five percent of these lymph nodes have the characteristic "eggshell calcification," which, although once considered to be pathognomonic of silicosis, has also been reported in sarcoidosis and tuberculosis. Progressive massive fibrosis (also termed conglomerate or complicated silicosis) is characterized by densities that are 10 mm or larger in diameter and often seem to coalesce into larger masses. In chronic silicosis, the involvement is primarily in the upper lobes, in contrast to the lower and middle lobe predominance in the accelerated variant. Retraction is common in the involved lobes, with compensatory overexpansion of the remaining lobes. Superimposed mycobacterial disease should be suspected in the presence of cavitation, pleural thickening, or rapid increase in nodule size. In silicoproteinosis, the chest roentgenogram has either a diffuse alveolar filling pattern similar to pulmonary alveolar proteinosis or, less commonly, a reticulonodular pattern.

Pulmonary function abnormalities in silicosis are variable. Asymptomatic patients with simple silicosis usually demonstrate no abnormalities. Patients with progressive massive fibrosis show restriction, obstruction, or a mixed pattern. Reductions in diffusing capacity, compliance, and arterial oxygenation with exercise have been shown in patients with advanced stages of silicosis. Some studies have suggested an association between obstructive pulmonary physiology and silica exposure in the absence of radiographic evidence of silicosis.

DIAGNOSIS

The diagnosis of silicosis is based on a history of exposure to free silica and a characteristic chest roentgenogram. Biopsy is indicated only in patients with atypical roentgenograms or in a medicolegal dilemma (such as a compensation case involving multiple dust exposures). Surgical lung biopsy is preferred to percutaneous or bronchoscopic approaches. Hyaline nodules in various stages of development are characteristic. Doubly refractile particles can be seen with polarizing light microscopy, but these particles are not diagnostic of silicosis. In certain cases, x-ray energy spectrometry or scanning electron microscopy is needed for diagnosis.

TREATMENT

No effective treatment of silicosis exists. Current efforts are aimed at disease prevention by limiting free silica exposure and by removing patients with silicosis from further exposure. The efficacy of corticosteroids is unproved, although an uncontrolled clinical trial has shown short-term improvement in chronic silicosis and a case report has shown improvement in acute silicosis. The use of whole lung lavage in silicosis has been employed successfully to remove dust, but the clinical utility is not yet proven. In the preantibiotic era, most deaths from silicosis resulted from mycobacterial infections. Most current deaths from silicosis are attributed to progressive respiratory insufficiency. Patients with a significantly reactive tuberculin skin test should receive isoniazid chemoprophylaxis. Patients with concomitant connective tissue disease may require corticosteroids, whereas those with obstructive lung disease may require appropriate therapy for that disorder.

1. Ziskind M, Jones RW, Weill H, et al. Silicosis. *Am Rev Respir Dis*. 1976;113:643.
   Classic comprehensive review article.
2. Lapp NL, Castranova V. How silicosis and coal workers' pneumoconiosis develop: a cellular assessment. *Occup Med*. 1993;8:35.
   Excellent review of the cellular mechanisms involved in the development of silicosis.
3. Fujimura N. Pathology and pathophysiology of pneumoconiosis. *Curr Opin Pulm Med*. 2000;6:140.
   Succinct review of the cellular and molecular mechanisms in silicosis.
4. Langer A. Crystal faces and cleavage planes in quartz as templates in biologic processes. *Q Rev Biophys*. 1978;11:543.
   Discussion of the physicochemical properties of quartz and its polymorphs that might be associated with the pathogenesis of silicosis.
5. Katsnelson B, Polzik EV, Privalova LI, et al. Some aspects of the problem of individual predisposition to silicosis. *Environ Health Perspect*. 1986;68:175.
   Wide variation of susceptibility to silicosis that depends on intrinsic characteristics of the host as well as extrinsic environmental factors.
6. Buechner H, Ansari A. Acute silico-proteinosis. *Dis Chest*. 1969;55:274.
   Article describes sandblasters who have acute silicosis and a symptomatology similar to pulmonary alveolar proteinosis.
7. Bailey W, Brown M, Buechner HA, et al. Silico-mycobacterial disease in sandblasters. *Am Rev Respir Dis*. 1974;110:115.
   Association of mycobacterial and other granulomatous diseases in patients with accelerated silicosis.
8. Davies J. Silicosis and tuberculosis among South African goldminers—an overview of recent studies and current issues. *S Afr Med J*. 2001;91:562.
   Discussion of the relationship between silicosis and tuberculosis.
9. Doll N, Stankus RP, Hughes J, et al. Immune complexes and autoantibodies in silicosis. *J Allergy Clin Immunol*. 1981;68:281.
   Investigation of the humoral immune system in 53 patients with silicosis.
10. International Agency for Research on Cancer. Silica, some silicates, coal dust and para-aramid fibrils. *IARC Monogr Eval Carcinog Risks Hum*. 1997;68:1.
    Report that classifies silica as a class I carcinogen.

11. Hessel P, Gamble JF, Gee JB, et al. Silica, silicosis, and lung cancer: a response to a recent Working Group Report. *J Occup Environ Med.* 2000;42:704.
    Literature review that questions the conclusions of the International Agency for Research on Cancer that classified silica as a class I carcinogen.
12. Dee P, Suratt P, Winn W. The radiographic findings in acute silicosis. *Radiology.* 1978;126:359.
    Spectrum of radiographic findings is described.
13. Hertzberg V, Rosenman KD, Reilly MJ, et al. Effect of occupational silica exposure on pulmonary function. *Chest.* 2002;122:721.
    Epidemiologic study showing an association between pulmonary function test abnormalities and estimated silica exposure.
14. Mason G, Abraham JL, Hoffman L, et al. Treatment of mixed-dust pneumoconiosis with whole lung lavage. *Am Rev Respir Dis.* 1982;126:1102.
    Case report of a patient treated with whole lung lavage.
15. Sharma S, Pande J, Verma K, et al. Effect of prednisolone treatment in chronic silicosis. *Am Rev Respir Dis.* 1991;143:814.
    Uncontrolled study in patients with chronic silicosis of corticosteroid effects on lung function and bronchoalveolar lavage.
16. Goodman G, Kapla PD, Stachura I, et al. Acute silicosis responding to corticosteroid therapy. *Chest.* 1992;101:366.
    Case report of improvement in acute silicosis with corticosteroid treatment.

80. COAL WORKERS' PNEUMOCONIOSIS

William G. Hughson

Coal workers' pneumoconiosis (CWP), formerly called *anthracosis* or *anthracosilicosis,* exists in two forms: simple and complicated. Simple CWP is diagnosed by a history of exposure to coal dust and chest radiographs showing an increased profusion of small, round parenchymal densities (categories 0, 1, 2, and 3 as rated by the International Labor Office system for grading radiographs for pneumoconiosis). Complicated CWP is known as *progressive massive fibrosis* (PMF). The diagnosis of PMF requires densities larger than 1 cm in diameter; some authorities require lesions larger than 2 cm.

PATHOPHYSIOLOGY

The basic pathologic lesion in simple CWP is the coal macule. This is a collection of coal dust-laden macrophages, reticulin, and collagen located within the walls of respiratory bronchioles and adjacent alveoli. Macules range in size from 1 to 5 mm in diameter and are located predominantly in the upper lobes. As the number of macrophages grows, fibrosis increases, creating micronodules (<7 mm) and macronodules (7–20 mm). A zone of focal emphysema is usually seen around macules and nodules, possibly caused by mechanical traction on adjacent parenchyma or digestion of alveolar walls by proteolytic enzymes released from macrophages. A tendency is seen for nodules to cluster and eventually to coalesce to produce PMF lesions. There is some evidence that coal workers may be at risk for chronic interstitial pneumonia, even when CWP is not present.

PATHOGENESIS

The pathogenesis of CWP is unclear. Silica in coal dust was thought to be the cause; it is now recognized that CWP is a pathologic entity distinct from silicosis, although the two conditions can coexist. Coal is composed predominantly of elemental carbon and varying amounts of minerals, metals, and organic compounds. Electrically charged surface radicals on coal dust damage biologic membranes. Regional differences in the frequency and severity of CWP may be caused by the content of Fe^{2+} and buffering capacity of the dust. Higher rank (hardness) coals are associated with increased risk of simple CWP and PMF. Anthracite is the highest rank, followed by bituminous and lignite. Experimentally, high-rank coals are cleared more slowly from the lungs and are more cytotoxic. The attack rate for PMF rises with increasing total lung dust; PMF usually occurs in the setting of advanced simple CWP (categories 2 and 3). Increased silica content of inhaled dust also increases the incidence of PMF. Historically, tuberculosis has been considered as a risk factor for PMF; its role has diminished in recent decades, although this organism should always be sought in a patient with expanding upper lobe lesions. Cavitation of PMF lesions usually results from tissue necrosis, not tuberculosis. Coal miners do not have a greater incidence of tuberculosis compared with the general population.

The pulmonary macrophage plays a central role in the pathogenesis of CWP by releasing inflammatory factors, recruiting polymorphonuclear leukocytes into the lung, and stimulating fibroblast production of collagen. A number of immunologic abnormalities have been found in miners with CWP. Their causative role, if any, is unknown and their prevalence has varied in different studies. Miners with CWP have elevated serum levels of IgA, IgG, C3, antinuclear antibodies, rheumatoid factor, and α_1-proteinase inhibitor; similar findings are seen in other forms of pneumoconiosis.

COMPLICATIONS

No clear correlation is found between these serologic factors and the risk or severity of CWP except for rheumatoid pneumoconiosis (Caplan's syndrome), which describes coal miners with rheumatoid arthritis. The characteristic radiographic features of rheumatoid pneumoconiosis are rapidly enlarging, evenly distributed nodules ranging in size from 0.3 to 5.0 cm in diameter, occurring in lungs that otherwise show little evidence of pneumoconiosis. Microscopically, the active lesions are similar to subcutaneous rheumatoid nodules; vasculitis is a common feature. Coal mining does not predispose to rheumatoid arthritis.

The risk of development and progression of CWP increases with cumulative dust exposure. Most affected miners worked before 1969, when the Federal Coal Mine Health and Safety Act (known as the *Coal Act*) was passed. It required that a coal worker's exposure to respirable dust be maintained at or below 2 mg/m^3. The Federal Mine Safety and Health Act of 1977 (known as the *Mine Act*) consolidated all federal health and safety regulations of the mining industry under a single statutory scheme, and created the Mine Safety and Health Administration for enforcement. Annual deaths from CWP have declined. However, new cases of CWP are still occurring, raising the issue of whether the current exposure limit is too high, or if enforcement is inadequate. The National Institute for Occupational Safety and Health is considering a reduction in the exposure limit to 1 mg/m^3.

The issue of impairment and disability caused by CWP is controversial. Most authorities agree that clinically significant pulmonary impairment does not occur in nonsmoking patients with simple CWP, although small reductions in spirometric values are common. Conversely, PMF is associated with significant morbidity and premature death. Cough and sputum production, often described as industrial bronchitis, usually have little effect on lung function in the absence of smoking. Cigarette smoking, although responsible for most pulmonary impairment among coal miners, does not increase the incidence of simple CWP or the risk of progression to PMF. The Mine Act and Black Lung Benefits Program established guidelines for rating disability based on reduction of the forced expiratory volume in 1 second (FEV_1) and maximal voluntary ventilation. Decrements in spirometric values are based on a miner's height, but not age, and do not consider the effects of smoking. Should a miner have either a normal ventilatory capacity or a slight decrement, that person can still qualify for benefits if the PaO_2 is reduced below a certain level with an alveolar–arterial oxygen gradient greater than 45 mm Hg breathing room air at rest. Exercise testing is not included in the rating system.

Today, the life expectancy of a coal worker approximates that of the general population. Excess deaths are seen for nonmalignant respiratory disease, accidents, and possibly stomach cancer. Approximately 4% of coal worker deaths are directly attributable to pneumoconiosis, usually PMF; most studies have not shown an excess mortality for simple CWP. These excess deaths are counterbalanced by decreased mortality from lung cancer and ischemic heart disease. Employed populations typically have morbidity and mortality rates 10 to 20% lower than the general population, which contains individuals disabled by chronic diseases. This deficit of disease is referred to as the *healthy worker effect*. Cor pulmonale and right ventricular hypertrophy do not occur in the absence of cigarette smoking or PMF. No specific treatment exists for CWP except limiting dust exposure.

1. Bang KM, Althouse RB, Kim JH, et al. Recent trends of age-specific pneumoconiosis mortality rates in the United States, 1985-1996: coal workers' pneumoconiosis, asbestosis, and silicosis. *Int J Occup Environ Health*. 1999;5:251.
   CWP mortality rates declined in miners more than 45 years old, but not in the age group 15 to 44.
2. Attfield MD, Castellan RM. Epidemiological data on US coal miners' pneumoconiosis, 1960 to 1988. *Am J Public Health*. 1992;82:964.
   Describes sequential surveys for CWP. Rates have declined with reduced dust exposure. Other articles by this author in the same journal volume describe origin of U.S. standard based on British studies and radiographic data.
3. Attfield MD, Hodous TK. Pulmonary function of US coal miners related to dust exposure estimates. *Am Rev Respir Dis*. 1992;145:605.
   Coal mine dust has an adverse effect on pulmonary function even in the absence of radiographically detected pneumoconiosis. Smoking accelerates a decline in lung function.
4. Attfield MD, Seixas NS. Prevalence of pneumoconiosis and its relationship to dust exposure in a cohort of US bituminous coal miners and ex-miners. *Am J Ind Med*. 1995;27:137.
   Prevalence of CWP and PMF increases with cumulative dust exposure, coal rank, and age. Current standard of 2 mg/m^3 does not completely prevent disease.
5. Brichet A, Tonnel AB, Brambilla E, et al. Chronic interstitial pneumonia with honeycombing in coal workers. *Sarcoidosis Vasc Diffuse Lung Dis*. 2002;19:211.
   Describes a possible association between chronic interstitial pneumonia and coal dust exposure, with or without associated CWP.
6. Cohen R, Velho V. Update on respiratory disease from coal mine and silica dust. *Clin Chest Med*. 2002;23:811.
   Good review article.
7. Fields CL, Roy TM, Dow FT, et al. Impact of arterial blood gas analysis in disability evaluation of bituminous coal miners with simple pneumoconiosis. *J Occup Med*. 1992;34:410.
   Arterial blood gases identify a subset of miners who would not qualify for disability benefits by spirometric criteria.
8. Fisher BE. Between a rock and a healthy place. *Environ Health Perspect*. 1998;106:A544.
   A review of legislation and agencies intended to prevent CWP.
9. Goodwin S, Attfield M. Temporal trends in coal workers' pneumoconiosis prevalence. Validating the National Coal Study results. *J Occup Environ Med*. 1998;40:1065.
   Prevalence of CWP and PMF has diminished with time, but new cases still occur despite current exposure standard for coal dust of 2 mg/m^3. National Institute for Occupational Safety and Health has recommended reducing the exposure limit for coal dust to 1 mg/m^3.
10. Henneberger PK, Attfield MD. Respiratory symptoms and spirometry in experienced coal miners: effects of both distant and recent coal mine dust exposures. *Am J Ind Med*. 1997;32:268.

Frequency of respiratory symptoms decreased after the U.S. Coal Mine Health and Safety Act of 1969, but 2 mg/m³ standard did not eliminate CWP.

11. Heppleston AG. Fournier J, Koenig K, Coal workers' pneumoconiosis: a historical perspective on its pathogenesis. *Am J Ind Med.* 1992;22:905.
    An interesting review of the history of CWP and the theories concerning its cause.

12. Huang X, Fournier J, Koenig K, et al. Buffering capacity of coal and its acid-soluble Fe^{2+} content: possible role in coal workers' pneumoconiosis. *Chem Res Toxicol.* 1998;11:722.
    Frequency of CWP is greater when coal has high acid-soluble Fe^{2+}, and low buffering capacity, which may explain regional differences in frequency and severity of CWP.

13. Joyce S. Major issues in miner health. *Environ Health Perspect.* 1998;106:A538.
    An excellent review of miner health problems and legislation to prevent CWP.

14. Lapp NL, Castranova V. How silicosis and coal workers' pneumoconiosis develop: a cellular assessment. *Occup Med.* 1993;8:35.
    Reviews the role of macrophage in CWP and silicosis. Coal dust is less cytotoxic than silica.

15. Lapp NL, Parker JE. Coal workers' pneumoconiosis. *Clin Chest Med.* 1992;13:243.
    An excellent general review article.

16. Parkes WR. Pneumoconiosis associated with coal and other carbonaceous materials. In: Parkes WR, ed. *Occupational Lung Disorders,* 3rd ed. Oxford: Butterworth–Heinemann; 1994:340.
    An excellent review chapter.

17. Prince TS, Frank AL. Causation, impairment, disability: an analysis of coal workers' pneumoconiosis evaluations. *J Occup Environ Med.* 1996;38:77.
    The relationship of exposure, impairment, and awarded disability in CWP is unclear in many cases. Miners with normal radiographs and spirometry often receive compensation.

18. Richman SI, Smith CJ. Legal aspects of impairment and disability in pneumoconiosis. *Occup Med.* 1993;8:71.
    Reviews legislation concerning definitions and assessment of work-related pulmonary disability.

19. Seixas NS, Robins TG, Attfield MD, et al. Exposure-response relationships for coal mine dust and obstructive lung disease following enactment of the Federal Coal Mine Health and Safety Act of 1969. *Am J Ind Med.* 1992;21:715.
    Concludes that exposure to respirable coal mine dust since 1970 continues to affect respiratory health in underground miners.

20. Stenton SC, Hendrick DJ. Airflow obstruction and mining. *Occup Med.* 1993;8:155.
    Coal mining causes a slight decrement in pulmonary function.

21. Wagner GR, Attfield MD, Parker JE. Chest radiography in dust-exposed miners. *Occup Med.* 1993;8:127.
    Discusses International Labor Office system for rating pneumoconiosis.

22. Vallyathan V, Brower PS, Green FH, et al. Radiographic and pathologic correlation of coal workers' pneumoconiosis. *Am J Respir Crit Care Med.* 1996;154:741.
    Compares whole lung sections with radiographic findings. Radiographs were insensitive to minimal CWP lesions, but correlated fairly well to pathology with International Labor Office (generally referred to as ILO) ratings of 0/1 or greater. For PMF lesions, radiographic and pathologic findings often did not correlate.

23. Wang X, Yano E, Nonaka K, et al. Respiratory impairments due to dust exposure; a comparative study among workers exposed to silica, asbestos, and coalmine dust. *Am J Ind Med.* 1997;31:495.
    Spirometry was reduced in all three groups, even when radiographs did not show pneumoconiosis.

81. ASBESTOS-RELATED DISEASE

William G. Hughson

The term *asbestos* refers to a group of naturally occurring, fibrous hydrated silicates that share characteristics of heat and chemical resistance. *Chrysotile*, or serpentine asbestos, is characterized by curvilinear fibrils. The other types have straight fibers, and are referred to as *amphibole asbestos*. The most important amphiboles are amosite and crocidolite. Asbestos has been used for multiple purposes including textiles, thermal insulation, building materials, and friction products such as brake linings.

The risk of asbestos-related disease is related to the amount of exposure, described using the term *fiber/cc-year*, which is the amount of asbestos that would be inhaled by working for a year in an atmosphere where the time-weighted average level of asbestos was 1 fiber per cubic centimeter of air. The *year* in this term is a working year (8 hours/day for 240 days), and only fibers longer than 5 microns are counted. Historically, exposure levels were very high. For example, insulators working in shipyards and commercial construction were exposed to approximately 10 fibers/cc. Exposures for chrysotile miners and textile workers were in the range of 10 to 100 fibers/cc. In contrast, automobile mechanics doing brake repair had an average exposure of 0.1 fibers/cc. The threshold limit value for asbestos was 5 million particles per cubic foot (approximately 15 fibers/cc) until 1968. Since then, it has been progressively lowered to the current permissible exposure limit of 0.1 fiber/cc.

The risk of asbestos-related disease is also related to fiber type. Chrysotile asbestos is cleared rapidly from the lungs. In contrast, amphibole asbestos is retained to a much greater extent. As a result, the risk of disease in chrysotile-exposed populations is lower on a fiber/cc-year basis. For example, the chrysotile miners and millers of Quebec had little evidence of increased mortality up to a cumulative exposure of approximately 1,000 fiber/cc-years. In contrast the risk of mesothelioma from crocidolite or amosite is increased by exposures in the range of 2 to 5 fiber/cc-years. Approximately 90% of the asbestos used in North America was chrysotile. Amosite was used primarily in insulation products, and crocidolite was used mainly for asbestos cement. In Europe and Australia, amphibole use was more common. Those areas have experienced a much higher rate of asbestos-related malignancies.

Although the high exposure levels of the 1900s are a thing of the past, the widespread use of asbestos-containing construction materials has led to concern that occupants of public buildings and schools may be harmed. Asbestos fibers are present in the air of many buildings, typically in the range of 0.001 to 0.0001 fibers/cc. Most are chrysotile, and there is no evidence that the general public is at increased risk from these environmental or background levels of exposure. There have been reports of family members developing asbestos-related diseases caused by exposure to fibers brought home on the clothes of asbestos workers. Most of those cases involved amphibole asbestos, and lung tissue analysis has demonstrated that the family members had lung tissue concentrations similar to people with occupational exposures.

Regulatory agencies such as the Occupational Safety and Health Agency and Environmental Protection Agency (EPA) use a linear no-threshold model for risk assessment. An inevitable consequence of this model is that any level of asbestos exposure, no matter how small, can be calculated to cause some degree of risk. However, there is ample evidence that low levels of exposure, particularly to chrysotile asbestos, do not cause an increased risk of asbestos-related disease. For example, residents in the Quebec chrysotile mining townships were exposed to ambient levels between 0.1 and 3 fibers/cc prior to 1970. The estimated lifetime exposure at these levels would be approximately 100 fiber/cc-years. There is no evidence of increased lung cancer risk in the townships, and almost all the reported cases of mesothelioma had either occupational exposure in the mining industry, or lived with family members who were employed in the industry. The EPA's model significantly overestimated the risk of lung cancer and mesothelioma in the Quebec mining townships.

The term *asbestosis* refers to parenchymal fibrosis caused by asbestos, and is characterized by the presence of interstitial fibrosis and an increased number of asbestos ferruginous bodies and uncoated asbestos fibers in lung tissue. The ferruginous body is an asbestos fiber coated with proteinaceous iron-staining material; it is visible on light microscopy. Using lung digestion techniques, uncoated fibers can be identified and counted. Patients with asbestosis typically have concentrations of ferruginous bodies and uncoated fibers that are 100 to 1,000 times higher than the general population. Asbestosis usually begins subpleurally in the lung bases. As the disease progresses, it can involve both lungs diffusely as a fine fibrosis. In the final stages, the lungs can acquire a cystic honeycomb appearance and can be indistinguishable radiographically from other forms of severe interstitial fibrosis.

Patients with asbestosis usually present with dyspnea on exertion, and may have a nonproductive cough. A clinical diagnosis of asbestosis requires an appropriate exposure history. Asbestosis requires a high level of exposure, and is now a rare disease. The latency period (the number of years from the initial exposure) is 20 years or longer for most patients. Chest radiographs show an increased profusion of bibasilar irregular densities. The American Thoracic Society (ATS) criteria for a diagnosis of asbestosis require a rating of 1/0 or higher using the International Labor Office system. It is possible, though uncommon, to have histologic evidence of asbestos in a patient with a normal chest radiograph. Other criteria include a restrictive pattern on the pulmonary function tests, reduction in the diffusing capacity for carbon monoxide, and the presence of rales. High-resolution, thin-section computed tomography scans with supine and prone views may demonstrate interstitial disease in the presence of normal, equivocal, or mild parenchymal abnormalities on chest radiographs.

Exercise testing is useful in identifying the cause of dyspnea in patients with relatively normal pulmonary function. The level of dyspnea often does not correlate with a single pulmonary function test value or with a specific radiographic profusion score. The degree of impairment and disability should be noted according to subjective and objective criteria established by the ATS and the American Medical Association.

Pleural disease or *pleural fibrosis* is the most common form of asbestos-related pulmonary injury. It occurs at relatively low levels of exposure, far less than is required for asbestosis. Pathologically, localized areas of pleural scarring (the pleural plaque) are seen. Calcification can occur, and is an index of chronicity rather than severity. Pleural plaques viewed on a plain chest radiograph are usually bilateral and involve the middle and lower thirds of the thoracic cage. They are often seen on the diaphragm. Pleural plaques are generally found on the parietal pleural surface, but can occur on the visceral pleura and mediastinum. Usually, pleural plaques do not lead to abnormal lung function; however, studies of groups of workers with plaques have shown a mild but statistically significant decrement in vital capacity and FEV_1. Extensive pleural plaques can cause restrictive lung disease. Diffuse pleural thickening is distinct from localized pleural plaques, with fibrosis of the visceral and parietal pleura. If extensive and severe enough, it results in lung entrapment and can lead to severe impairment and ventilatory failure. The most likely cause of benign diffuse pleural thickening is an initial asbestos-related pleural effusion. Pleural effusions caused by asbestos are exudative, and may be chronic and recurrent. Infection and malignancy must be excluded before attributing the effusion to asbestos.

Rounded atelectasis is characterized by localized pleural thickening and lung entrapment. Before advances in CT scanning, biopsy was necessary to distinguish this process from mesothelioma and lung cancer.

Populations with high levels of exposure to asbestos have an increased risk of lung cancer. For example, the insulators described by Selikoff had a relative risk of approximately fivefold if they did not smoke regularly. Insulators who smoked had a risk of 50- to 90-fold compared with nonsmoking members of the general public because of a synergistic interaction between the risk of asbestos and smoking. Subsequent studies by Kipen and others demonstrated that the insulators who developed lung cancer had asbestosis. Although there is some controversy on this subject, the preponderance of data suggest that the risk of lung cancer is increased when clinical or pathologic asbestosis is present, and that asbestos exposure alone does not increase the risk in the absence of pulmonary fibrosis. Approximately two thirds of asbestos-related lung cancers occur in the lower lobes, in contrast to the predominantly upper lobe distribution of most lung cancers. The distribution of cell types is similar to smoking-related lung cancers, and is not helpful in identifying tumors caused by asbestos. Many studies do not control adequately for smoking. Because blue collar workers smoke more than the general population, failure to control for smoking can lead to the erroneous conclusion that occupational exposures are causing an increased risk of lung cancer. Lung cancer is discussed in detail in Chapter 102.

Mesothelioma is a rare tumor, arising in the pleura and peritoneum. Approximately 75% of men and 10% of women with mesothelioma have a history of occupational exposure to asbestos. Some cases have been reported in family members of asbestos workers. Fiber type is very important in the etiology of mesothelioma. Although chrysotile can cause mesothelioma, it does so rarely, and only after levels of exposure similar to those necessary to cause asbestosis. In contrast, amphibole asbestos causes mesothelioma at low doses. There is no evidence that the general public is at increased risk of mesothelioma because of ambient levels of asbestos. Mesothelioma is discussed in detail in Chapter 108.

No specific therapy exists for asbestos-related pleural or pulmonary disease. Every effort should be made to eliminate smoking. Other measures include early treatment of lung infections, influenza and pneumonia vaccinations, careful surveillance, and treatment of complications of respiratory failure.

---

1. Camus M, Siemiatycki J, Meek B. Nonoccupational exposure to chrysotile asbestos and the risk of lung cancer. *N Engl J Med*. 1998;338:1565.
   The EPA's model overestimated the risk of lung cancer by at least a factor of 10 in the chrysotile mining areas of Quebec.
2. Camus M, Siemiatycki J, Case BW, et al. Risk of mesothelioma among women living near chrysotile mines versus US EPA asbestos model: preliminary findings. *Ann Occup Hyg*. 2002;46(Suppl):95.
   The EPA's model overestimated the risk of mesothelioma by a factor of about 100 in the chrysotile mining areas of Quebec.
3. Case BW, Camus M, Richardson L, et al. Prelimary findings for pleural mesothelioma among women in the Quebec chrysotile mining regions. *Ann Occup Hyg*. 2002;46(Suppl):128.
   Most of the women diagnosed with mesothelioma had occupational exposures, or lived with employees who worked in the industry.
4. Churg A. Nonneoplastic diseases caused by asbestos, neoplastic asbestos-induced diseases. In: Churg A, Green FHY, eds. *Pathology of Occupational Lung Disease,* 2nd ed. Baltimore: Williams & Wilkins; 1998:277.
   An excellent textbook covering all occupational lung diseases.
5. Churg A. Asbestos-related disease in the workplace and the environment: controversial issues. In: Churg A, Katzenstein AA, eds. *The Lung: Current Concepts.* Baltimore: Williams & Wilkins; 1993:54.
   Good review of the issue of asbestos, asbestosis, and lung cancer.
6. Craighead JE, Abraham JL, Churg A, et al. The pathology of asbestos-associated diseases of the lungs and pleural cavities: diagnostic criteria and proposed grading schema. *Arch Pathol Lab Med*. 1982;106:544.
   Position paper of the College of American Pathologists and NIOSH for the pathological diagnosis of asbestosis.
7. Cugell DW, Kamp DW. Asbestos and the pleura: a review. *Chest*. 2004;125:1103.
   Comprehensive review article.
8. Gevenois PA, de Maertelaer V, Madani A, et al. Asbestosis, pleural plaques, and diffuse pleural thickening: three distinct benign responses to asbestos exposure. *Eur Respir J*. 1998;11:1021.
   An excellent review of radiographic pleural abnormalities caused by asbestos.
9. Guidotti TL, Miller A, Christiani D, et al. Diagnosis and initial management of nonmalignant diseases related to asbestos. *Am J Respir Crit Care Med*. 2004; 170:691.
   Position paper of the American Thoracic Society.

10. Hodgson JT, Darnton A. The quantitative risks of mesothelioma and lung cancer in relation to asbestos exposure. *Ann Occup Hyg*. 2000;44:565.
    Review of epidemiologic studies. The risk of lung cancer and mesothelioma is greater for amphibole asbestos than for chrysotile.
11. Kipen HM, Lilis R, Suzuki Y, et al. Pulmonary fibrosis in asbestos insulation workers with lung cancer: a radiological and histopathological evaluation. *Br J Ind Med*. 1987;44:96.
    Important study of 138 insulators with lung cancer demonstrating that all had pathological evidence of asbestosis, and chest radiographs with an ILO rating of 1/1 or greater identified the excess number of lung cancers. Subsequent reports of 415 cases demonstrated that 99% had pathological asbestos, and virtually all were smokers or ex-smokers.
12. Lanphear BP, Buncher CR. Latent period for malignant mesothelioma of occupational origin. *J Occup Med*. 1992;34:718.
    Latent period for mesothelioma is 20 years or longer in 96% of cases.
13. Lee DJ, Le Blanc W, Fleming LE, et al. Trends in the U.S. smoking rates in occupational groups: the national health interview survey 1987–1994. *J Occup Environ Med*. 2004;46:538.
    Smoking is more common in blue collar workers than the general public.
14. Liddell FDK, McDonald AD, McDonald JC. The 1891–1920 birth cohort of Quebec chrysotile miners and millers: development from 1901 and mortality to 1992. *Ann Occup Hyg*. 1997;41:13.
    Heavily exposed miners and millers had little evidence of increased mortality with cumulative exposures to 1,000 fiber/cc-years.
15. Mossman BT, Churg A. Mechanisms in the pathogenesis of asbestosis and silicosis. *Am J Respir Crit Care Med*. 1998;157:1666.
    Good review article.
16. Roggli VL, Sanders LL. Asbestos content of lung tissue and carcinoma of the lung: a clinicopathologic correlation and mineral fiber analysis of 234 cases. *Ann Occup Hyg*. 2000;44:109.
    Cases with asbestosis had markedly elevated asbestos levels in the lungs, most of which were amphiboles. An amphibole burden sufficient to cause lung cancer is usually accompanied by histologic evidence of asbestosis.
17. Roggli VL, Sharma A, Butnor KJ, et al. Malignant mesothelioma and occupational exposure to asbestos: a clinicopathological correlation of 1445 cases. *Ultrastruct Pathol*. 2002;26:55.
    Commercial amphiboles are responsible for most mesotheliomas in the United States.
18. Roggli VL, Oury TD, Sporn TA, eds. *Asbestos-Associated Diseases*. New York: Springer; 2004.
    Comprehensive textbook with excellent illustrations.
19. Weiss W. Asbestosis: a marker for the increased risk of lung cancer among workers exposed to asbestos. *Chest*. 1999;115:536.
    This article reviews lung cancer risk and exposure to asbestos.
20. Selikoff IJ, Hammond EC. Asbestos and smoking. *JAMA*. 1979;242:458.
    Insulators who smoked had a 50 to 90-fold increased risk of lung cancer.

82. OCCUPATIONAL ASTHMA

William G. Hughson

Asthma is a disorder of lung function characterized by widespread obstruction of the airways that (1) varies in severity; (2) is reversible, either spontaneously or as a result of treatment; and (3) is not caused by cardiovascular disease. Occupational asthma (OA) is related causally to exposure to airborne dusts, gases, vapors, or fumes in the working environment. Some definitions of OA require an immune-mediated sensitivity to a specific agent; however, nonspecific irritants also should be considered because aggravation of preexisting non-OA is usually compensable under workers' compensation guidelines.

ETIOLOGY

Asthma is a common disease. Approximately 10% of people are diagnosed with asthma during their lifetime (i.e., the incidence of asthma). Some cases resolve, but approximately 5% of the population has active asthma (i.e., the prevalence of asthma). OA is responsible for 2 to 15% of asthma prevalence; the actual frequency varies widely among occupations and within industries at different levels of exposure. The true occurrence of OA is probably greater than that reported because affected workers often terminate their employment, leaving unaffected survivors. This type of self-selection is common in studies of working individuals that compare morbidity and mortality rates to those of the general population. Employed populations typically have morbidity and mortality rates 10 to 20% lower than the general population, which contains individuals disabled by chronic diseases. This deficit of disease is referred to as the *healthy worker effect*. Because asthma is common in the general population and the clinical findings in OA are identical to those of non-OA, the challenge is to understand the nature and degree of workplace exposures and to make a temporal association between the asthma and occupation. Diagnosis can be difficult, given the inherent variability of asthma and the fact the patient can have early, late, dual, or recurrent late onset of symptoms.

PATHOGENESIS

The pathogenetic mechanisms of OA can be classified as reflex, inflammatory, pharmacologic, and allergic. *Reflex bronchoconstriction* involves irritant receptors in the airway that are stimulated by agents such as cold air, inert dust particles, gases, and fumes. The reaction does not involve immune mechanisms and is nonspecific. Many patients have a history of asthma. *Inflammatory bronchoconstriction* begins as a nonspecific reaction following inhalation of high concentrations of nonspecific irritants. Most individuals recover, but a few develop chronic asthma. This condition is often referred to as *reactive airways dysfunction syndrome*. Vocal cord dysfunction characterized by hoarseness, cough, and dyspnea is also caused by irritant exposures, and can be mistaken for asthma. *Pharmacologic bronchoconstriction* occurs when agents in the work environment exert a specific pharmacologic effect on the lung. An example is cholinesterase inhibition by organophosphate pesticides causing bronchoconstriction because of excessive parasympathetic stimulation.

Allergic bronchoconstriction is the most common cause of OA. Susceptible workers develop IgE or IgG antibodies following exposure to workplace antigens such as animal or plant proteins. If high-molecular-weight compounds are responsible (e.g., baker's asthma), individuals who are atopic become sensitized more readily than workers who are nonatopic. However, atopy is not a predisposing factor when low-molecular-weight compounds are involved (e.g., isocyanate manufacturing). Sensitization takes time, and the latency period between exposure and the onset of symptoms can be weeks to years. Several hundred workplace agents have been shown to cause OA, and the list grows every year. Cigarette smoking doubles the risk of OA, possibly by recruiting inflammatory cells into the lung where they are available to react with irritants and sensitizers.

DIAGNOSIS

When considering OA as a diagnosis, two questions must be answered: First, does my patient actually have asthma? Second, is the asthma related to work? The general approach to diagnosing asthma is discussed elsewhere in this manual (see Chapter 49). Methods for answering the second question include a detailed clinical and occupational history, physical examination, chest radiographs, pulmonary function tests (PFTs), inhalation challenge tests, and immunologic tests.

The clinical history of the patient with OA typically reveals shortness of breath, chest tightness, cough, and wheezing at work or within several hours after leaving work. Respiratory symptoms are often accompanied by rhinitis or conjunctivitis.

Recurrent attacks of *bronchitis* are often reported. Improvement on weekends, vacations, or when away from work is an important clue. Patients who develop symptoms immediately after exposure or whenever they work with the same material usually recognize a causal relationship. However, a large number of substances, particularly low-molecular-weight organic and inorganic compounds, may give rise to late asthmatic reactions. Nocturnal attacks of dyspnea and cough may be the only manifestation of OA; thus, be aware that the onset of symptoms may not be simultaneous with workplace exposure. Key elements influencing the pattern of symptoms and airflow obstruction seen in workers with OA are the recovery time and the effects of cumulative exposures. Some individuals improve rapidly after leaving work, and recovery is virtually complete before the next workday. Such workers show a similar deterioration during each shift. At the other extreme are those who need more than 2 days to recovery. Repeated exposures over several weeks, even with weekends off, result in a steady deterioration of pulmonary function. Clinical features can be indistinguishable from chronic obstructive lung disease because of nonoccupational causes. The reactive nature of the disease can be masked by a fixed reduction in expiratory flow rates seemingly unrelated to work activities. In such cases, the true relationship between the patient's occupation and asthma becomes apparent only after prolonged cessation of exposure allows sufficient time for recovery of normal pulmonary function. When the patient finally returns to work, the simultaneous reappearance of symptoms and airflow obstruction makes the link obvious.

The occupational history is crucial for the diagnosis of OA. Obtain a detailed description of the patient's work practices, including the agents used, protective equipment such as respirators and gloves, and the adequacy of ventilation. In addition to the patient's own work, information concerning other processes and chemicals used by coworkers should be obtained; bystander exposures can cause reactions in sensitized individuals. It is often helpful to ask whether coworkers have similar problems. Patients usually have only limited knowledge of the agents they use. Material Safety Data Sheets should be obtained from the employer, who is legally required to provide them to the worker. If the clinician is careful to avoid a confrontational situation, the employer or the workers' compensation insurance company may provide industrial hygiene data concerning the nature and degree of exposures. Site visits are often helpful, and the clinician must be prepared to search the medical literature to complete the assessment.

The physical examination may reveal conjunctivitis, rhinitis, and wheezing; however, these signs are often absent, particularly when the patient has been away from work for some time. The chest radiographs are usually normal in patients with OA, although parenchymal infiltrates and hyperinflation may be seen.

PFTs should demonstrate expiratory obstruction and hyperinflation, with improvement following inhalation of bronchodilator medication. However, variability of airway obstruction is a key feature of asthma, and the PFT may be normal. In this situation, the demonstration of bronchial hyperreactivity (BHR) depends on provocation tests using methacoline, histamine, cold air, or exercise as a stimulus. These nonspecific promoters of BHR cannot identify a workplace cause. The gold standard for diagnosing OA in the pulmonary laboratory is a specific inhalation challenge using the suspected agent. However, it is often difficult to select the correct chemical from among many used in the typical, complicated workplace environment. In addition, practical difficulties exist to administering the correct concentration of the agent and few facilities have sophisticated environmental chambers. Pre- and postshift PFT measurements may demonstrate expiratory obstruction after workplace exposures. Another approach is serial measurement of peak flow rates. The patient is provided with an inexpensive flow meter and maintains a diary during the workweek, evenings, and weekends. At least 2 weeks of observation are needed. This requires considerable patient cooperation, and the results of self-administered tests are often suspect in the setting of potential litigation and secondary gain. Some authors have recommended serial measurements of BHR using methacholine before and after work shifts; decreased provocative dose following exposure is supportive of OA.

Skin tests and serology may be useful in identifying specific sensitization. However, selection and preparation of agents for skin testing is difficult, and nonspecific irritation can lead to false-positive findings. Antibody assays are available for only a limited number of workplace chemicals; positive serology indicates previous exposure, but is not diagnostic of asthma caused by that agent. Skin tests and serology may suggest the cause of OA but are not definitive.

TREATMENT

The treatment of OA is identical to that for non-OA. Emphasis should be placed on avoidance of the agent responsible in sensitized individuals and reduction in exposure to nonspecific irritants. The prognosis of patients with OA is guarded. More than 50% remain symptomatic 1 year after removal from exposure. The clinician is often asked to define disability caused by OA. This requires a careful assessment of the degree of airflow obstruction and BHR and whether the patient could return to work with certain restrictions or job modifications. If return to work is not feasible, vocational rehabilitation is required. These decisions require input from the clinician, patient, employer, and the agency responsible for administering workers' compensation claims.

1. Alberts WM, do Pico GA. Reactive airways dysfunction syndrome. *Chest.* 1996;109:1618.
   Reviews the clinical features of this syndrome.
2. Alberts WM. Getting the most from the "gold standard." *Chest.* 2003;123:987.
   Editorial discussing the diagnosis of OA, including the specific inhalation challenge test.
3. Arnaiz NO, Kaufman JD. New developments in work-related asthma. *Clin Chest Med.* 2002;23:737.
   Good review article.
4. Balmes J, Becklake M, Blanc P, et al. American Thoracic Society Statement: occupational contribution to the burden of airway disease. *Am J Respir Crit Care Med.* 2003;167:787.
   Official statement of the American Thoracic Society. Good review article.
5. Banks DE. Use of the specific challenge in the diagnosis of occupational asthma: a 'gold standard' test or a test not used in current practice of occupational asthma? *Curr Opin Allergy Clin Immunol.* 2003;3:107.
   Discusses the difficulty of specific inhalation challenge tests, including the lack of fellowship training and the limited number of centers with inhalation chambers.
6. Bardana EJ. Occupational asthma and allergies. *J Allergy Clin Immunol.* 2003;111(2 Suppl):S530.
   A comprehensive review article.
7. Bresnitz EA, Beckett W, Chan-Yeung M, et al. Guidelines for assessing and managing asthma risk at work, school and recreation. *Am J Respir Crit Care Med.* 2004;169:873.
   Official statement of the American Thoracic Society. Good review article. Includes electronic databases and web sites.
8. Campo P, Lummus ZL, Bernstein DI. Advances in methods used in evaluation of occupational asthma. *Curr Opin Pulm Med.* 2004;10:142.
   Good review of diagnostic tools for OA.
9. Chan-Yeung M, Harber P, Bailey W, et al. Guidelines for the evaluation of impairment/disability in patients with asthma. *Am Rev Respir Dis.* 1993;147:1056.
   American Thoracic Society criteria for rating impairment and disability for asthma.
10. Chan-Yeung M. Assessment of asthma in the workplace. *Chest.* 1995;108:1084.
    American College of Chest Physicians consensus statement concerning OA.
11. Chan-Yeung M. Christie Memorial lecture. Occupational asthma—the past 50 years. *Can Respir J.* 2004;11:21.
    Provides an interesting historical perspective on our understanding of OA.
12. Dykewicz MS. Occupational asthma: a practical approach. *Allergy Asthma Proc.* 2001;22:225.
    A good review of the clinical and medicolegal aspects of assessing OA.

13. Malo JL, Ghezzo H. Recovery of methacholine responsiveness after end of expo-
    sure in occupational asthma. *Am J Respir Crit Care Med.* 2004;169:1304.
    *Responsiveness to methacholine continues to improve 2 and more years after
    cessation to agents causing OA.*
14. Moscato G, Rampulla C. Costs of occupational asthma and of occupational chronic
    obstructive pulmonary disease. *Curr Opin Allergy Clin Immunol.* 2003;3:109.
    *Interesting review of the economic impact of OA and occupational chronic ob-
    structive pulmonary disease.*
15. Newman-Taylor AJ, Pickering CAC. Occupational asthma and byssinosis. In:
    Parkes WR, ed. *Occupational Lung Disorders,* 3rd ed. Oxford: Butterworth–
    Heinemann; 1994:710.
    An excellent review chapter.
16. Perkner JJ, Fennelly KP, Balkissoon R, et al. Irritant-associated vocal cord dys-
    function. *J Occup Environ Med.* 1998;40:136.
    Vocal cord dysfunction can mimic asthma in patients following irritant exposures.
17. Ross DJ, McDonald JC. Health and employment after a diagnosis of occupational
    asthma: a descriptive study. *Occup Med.* 1998;48:219.
    *Reviews outcomes following diagnosis of OA. Fewer than one half of patients
    recover completely.*
18. Tarlo SM, Liss GM. Occupational asthma: an approach to diagnosis and manage-
    ment. *CMAJ.* 2003;168:867.
    Concise review article with good summary tables.

83. DISABILITY AND MEDICOLEGAL EVALUATION

William G. Hughson

Many physicians dislike writing medicolegal reports. They are more comfortable with
their traditional role of diagnosing and treating disease. However, providing clearly
written reports is essential in ensuring that their patients receive appropriate workers' compensation and other benefits following disease and injury. These reports are
read by nonmedical personnel such as disability raters, insurance claims adjusters,
and workers' compensation judges and often require the use of special forms and
obscure terms to achieve specific legal and administrative goals.

It is important to distinguish between impairment and disability. *Impairment* describes an anatomic or functional loss caused by a disease process. *Disability* describes
the effects of the impairment on the patient's life, including the ability to work. It can
be defined as the inability to perform at a specified level of activity, or as undue distress during the performance of that task. The degree of disability is directly related to
the physical requirements of the job. For example, a teacher with a forced expiratory
volume in 1 second (FEV_1) of 1 L might have no disability, whereas a general laborer
would need retraining for another job. Nonmedical people who rely on the physician's
opinions make the final decision regarding disability.

The medicolegal report should contain all of the sections found in a typical medical
consultation plus a detailed occupational history. A patient-generated form that is
completed before an examination can facilitate the latter. The assessment section of
the report should contain answers to all of the questions listed in Table 83-1. We favor
a question-and-answer format because it saves time and allows a clearer explanation
of the issues and the physician's opinion. The key points that should be discussed
require a very specific vocabulary with legal implications.

WHAT IS THE DIAGNOSIS?

This is generally the easiest question to answer. Each lung condition should be
listed along with the evidence supporting its diagnosis. For example, the diagnosis of

Table 83-1. Questions to be answered in a disability evaluation report

1. What is the diagnosis?
2. Is the diagnosis work related by causation, aggravation, acceleration, or precipitation?
3. Is there evidence of impairment? If so, how severe is the impairment? What rating system is used, and how do the patient's findings correspond to this system?
4. Is temporary disability present? If so, is it partial or total? What is the anticipated time of recovery?
5. Can the patient return to his or her previous occupation? Could the patient return to the job if it were modified? Are there any work restrictions or preclusions?
6. Is permanent disability present? If so, is the patient stationary for rating purposes? When did the patient become permanent and stationary?
7. How severe is the permanent disability? What rating system is used, and how do the patient's findings correspond to this system?
8. Are there permanent work restrictions? If so, what are they?
9. Is there any basis for apportionment of the permanent disability? If the work injury had not occurred, would a preexisting condition contribute to the disability?
10. Is vocational retraining indicated? If so, which types of jobs are appropriate?
11. Is further medical treatment needed? If so, what is the nature, frequency, and duration of the treatment?

asbestosis is based on a history of exposure, appropriate latency, the presence of interstitial markings on the chest radiograph, pulmonary function tests showing a restrictive pattern and reduction in the diffusing capacity, and crackles on physical examination. Nonpulmonary diagnoses should also be listed, particularly those affecting impairment or disability.

IS THE DIAGNOSIS WORK RELATED?
This requires a judgment that the disease was caused, aggravated, accelerated, or precipitated by a workplace exposure. *Causation* is defined as a new disease that has been caused by work (e.g., an insulator with asbestosis). *Aggravation* means a preexisting condition that did not interfere with work or usual activities that is now worse because of employment (e.g., chronic obstructive pulmonary disease in a smoker exposed to industrial dusts). *Acceleration* means a preexisting condition that would naturally worsen with time and that deteriorated more rapidly because of employment (e.g., airway obstruction in a patient with emphysema exposed to fumes). *Precipitation* means a preexisting condition that became manifest for the first time because of employment (e.g., asthma in an atopic patient exposed to flour). The time sequence of the disease in relation to employment is very important. For example, pneumoconiosis takes years to develop, and immune-mediated reactions require weeks to months before sensitization occurs. It is important to note whether symptoms are worse at work, and then improve on weekends or vacations. The presence of similar problems in coworkers is highly suggestive. The nature and severity of exposure should be determined by obtaining Material Safety Data Sheets and available industrial hygiene information. The use of protective devices (e.g., respirators) and adequacy of ventilation should be described.

IS THERE EVIDENCE OF IMPAIRMENT? IF SO, HOW SEVERE IS THE IMPAIRMENT?
Subjective data (e.g., dyspnea, weakness, and pain) must be differentiated from objective data because symptoms are often unreliable measures of disease in the setting of litigation. The physical examination and chest radiographs provide diagnostic information, but are not useful in measuring function. Basic spirometry remains the cornerstone for assessing impairment. Other techniques (e.g., exercise testing)

are added as necessary. It is important to know which rating system applies to the patient's case. The American Medical Association's (AMA) *Guides to the Evaluation of Permanent Impairment* is the one most commonly used. The referral source should give clear instructions and provide the rating system to the physician when necessary.

IS DISABILITY PRESENT?

If so, is it partial or total, temporary or permanent? The key question is "Can the patient return to the usual and customary activities of employment?" This requires a clear understanding of the patient's work, including the physical effort needed and the potentially harmful exposures. The work history can be obtained from the patient, and supplemented with a written job description provided by the employer. Partial disability exists when the patient can perform some, but not all, of the usual job responsibilities. Useful questions include: Could the patient return to the job if it were modified? Are there any work restrictions or preclusions? In most states, the employer is required to make reasonable accommodations. However, job modification is often difficult, and the definition of *reasonable* can be contentious. Total disability exists if the patient is completely unable to perform the job, even with accommodation. If the disability is temporary (either partial or total), it is important to provide both the patient and the employer with an estimate of the time needed for recovery. This allows assignment of tasks to other workers. If permanent disability is likely, it is wise to advise both the employer and patient as soon as possible. This facilitates realistic planning for the patient's future.

IS DISABILITY PERMANENT?

If permanent disability is present, is the patient stationary for rating purposes? How severe is the disability? The patient is permanent and stationary for rating purposes after maximal medical improvement has been achieved and no prospect is seen for further recovery. The report should include a lucid description of the patient's impairment and its impact on work capacity. This includes any permanent restrictions and preclusions, but caution is warranted. Sweeping statements such as "No further exposure to dusts or fumes" may make the patient unemployable. Precision is needed, with a description of any specific precluded exposures (e.g., allergens or sensitizers) and consideration of dose (e.g., respirator use, ventilation requirements, Occupational Safety and Health Administration-permissible exposure limits). For example, an insulator with mild asbestosis might be able to continue working under current regulations, because permissible dust levels are now very low. The description of permanent disability must contain terminology appropriate for the rating system that applies. For example, in California words such as *minimal* or *moderate, occasional* or *frequent* have specific meanings when used to describe dyspnea. The California Labor Code has categories such as *Disability precluding heavy work* and *Standard ratings* with percent disability caused by pulmonary disease. Copies of rating systems can be obtained from the referral source or from state and federal regulatory agencies.

IS THERE ANY BASIS FOR APPORTIONMENT?

Apportionment is only considered when permanent disability is present. It is used to describe the relative contribution of occupational and nonoccupational lung diseases to the total disability. However, the medical concept of apportionment differs from the legal principle, just as impairment differs from disability. For example, whereas most physicians would consider preexisting asthma as a factor in a painter with pulmonary impairment, the legal concept of apportionment is concerned only with preexisting disability. A useful question is: If the work injury had not occurred, would the preexisting condition contribute to disability? In the case of the painter, if no evidence was found of disability before the injury at work (e.g., work restrictions, prior job loss because of the condition), no basis would be seen for apportionment, and the entire disability would be considered work related. If a preexisting condition causing disability is aggravated or accelerated by employment, the increment in disability is apportioned and is compensable. The best way to deal with apportionment is to dictate two paragraphs describing the permanent disability. The first describes existing disability factors (subjective and objective) and work restrictions. The second describes disability factors and work restrictions that would have existed without the occupational injury. The hearing officer then decides the extent of disability represented by each of the two paragraphs and, by subtraction, allocates the disability caused by employment.

IS VOCATIONAL RETRAINING APPROPRIATE?

Patients with severe impairment may be totally disabled from any type of employment. Those with better function are suitable for retraining, which is a worker's compensation benefit. The physician should describe the types of jobs and work preclusions suitable for the patient. The physician may be asked to communicate with vocational rehabilitation counselors regarding the patient's condition.

IS FURTHER MEDICAL TREATMENT NEEDED?

It is important to describe the nature, frequency, and anticipated duration of all treatment. In most instances, the cost of medical care is paid by workers' compensation if employment has contributed to disability, even when nonoccupational factors are present. Apportionment of medical costs is usually not allowed.

---

1. American Medical Association. *Guides to the Evaluation of Permanent Impairment,* 5th ed. Chicago: American Medical Association; 2000.
   This book describes the AMA rating system.
2. Brigham CR, Babitsky S. Independent medical evaluations and impairment ratings. *Occup Med.* 1998;13:325.
   A detailed review of medicolegal report writing.
3. Demeter SL. Disability evaluation. *Occup Med.* 1998;13:315.
   Discusses various rating systems, including the AMA Guides.
4. Guidotti TL, Martin CJ. Evaluation of the worker with suspected occupational lung disease. *Occup Med.* 1998;13:279.
   Reviews the approach to occupational lung diseases, including issues of causation and disability.
5. Lentz G, Christian JH, Tierman SM. Disability prevention and management. In: Ladou J, ed. *Current Occupational and Environmental Medicine,* 3rd ed. New York: Lange Medical Books/McGraw-Hill; 2004:21.
   Good review of the concept of disability, and the general approach to its assessment and management. Other chapters in this book deal with the occupational history, and worker's compensation.
6. Plumb JM, Cowell JWF. An overview of workers' compensation. *Occup Med.* 1998;13:241.
   A detailed review of all aspects of workers' compensation.
7. Rondinelli RD, Beller TA. Impairment rating and disability evaluation of the pulmonary system. *Phys Med Rehabil Clin North Am.* 2001;12:667.
   A review of the diagnostic procedures and assessment criteria for pulmonary disability evaluations.
8. Sood A, Beckett WS. Determination of disability for patients with advanced lung disease. *Clin Chest Med.* 1997;18:471.
   Discusses various rating systems, and the approach to report writing.
9. Sood A, Redlich CA. Pulmonary function tests at work. *Clin Chest Med.* 2001; 22:783.
   Excellent review of pulmonary function tests used to diagnose occupational lung diseases, and assess impairment.
10. Taiwo OA, Cain HC. Pulmonary impairment and disability. *Clin Chest Med.* 2002;23:841.
    Detailed review article, including a discussion of pulmonary function tests, and disability rating systems.

84. PULMONARY COMPLICATIONS IN BURN PATIENTS

Stephen H. Lee

Respiratory compromise from smoke inhalation is the leading cause of death in fire-injured victims and significantly increases morbidity and mortality in patients with cutaneous burns. Burns can indirectly cause lung injury and acute respiratory distress syndrome (ARDS) even in patients without inhalation injury via the action of inflammatory mediators.

Inhalation injury consists of four entities that may be present solely or in combination: oxygen depletion, thermal injury, irritating chemical injury, and systemic poisoning. Oxygen depletion occurs as a consequence of combustion and can reduce room air oxygen concentration to dangerously low levels (<5%) that may act additively or synergistically with other toxic fumes to produce harm.

Thermal injury from the heat of fire is usually confined to the supraglottic region, whereas chemical injury from toxic fumes of combustion products can affect both the supra- and infraglottic areas. Although initial injury may look mild, it is critical to remember that dramatic changes take place during the postinhalation period. Delayed intense inflammatory reactions add to the direct effects of mucosal and epithelial injury. Dramatic fluid shifts from the intravascular space, edema, and infection all contribute to the complexity of care. Constant vigilance for pulmonary complications is necessary.

Inhalation injury should be suspected based on history (closed space, duration of exposure) and physical examination (unconsciousness, singed nasal hairs, carbonaceous sputum, stridor, hoarseness, wheezing, and burns, especially to the face). Evaluation for intubation is the initial critical decision as airway patency can be lost quickly. Flexible bronchoscopy or laryngoscopy may be used to directly visualize the upper airway, but the findings should be interpreted with caution. Despite the initial appearance of mild upper airway injury, progressive edema and airway obstruction can develop quickly, especially in the first 24 hours. Frequent serial examinations are necessary. If there is concern that the airway may be lost or that securing the airway may become difficult, immediate intubation should be considered. Thermal injury below the glottis is uncommon because heated air is effectively cooled by the oro- and nasopharynx.

Irritating, toxic compounds in smoke include ammonia, aldehydes, nitrogen dioxide, and hydrogen chloride. These chemicals can damage mucosa, impair mucociliary function, and incite inflammation, bronchorrhea, bronchospasm, and acute lung injury. Mucosal sloughing may develop within a few days after the initial inhalation, forming casts resulting in obstructive atelectasis and loss of lung volume. Bacterial colonization of necrotic tissue may progress to tracheobronchitis or pneumonia. Resultant ventilation and perfusion abnormalities lead to impaired gas exchange. Chest radiographic findings are variable, ranging from normal to interstitial edema, consolidation, atelectasis, or diffuse bilateral infiltrates consistent with ARDS. Although radiographic abnormalities can be seen as early as postburn day 1, the majority tends to occur later (postburn day 5).

Treatment of pulmonary complications and respiratory insufficiency is multifaceted. Aggressive pulmonary toilet, which may include repeated flexible bronchoscopy, may be required to remove pooled secretions and sloughed or necrotic tissue. Postural drainage via a rotational bed may be helpful. Bronchodilators to treat bronchospasm and the application of positive end-expiratory pressure to maintain lung volume are used commonly to treat patients with lower airway inhalation injury. In cases of persistent, severe hypoxemia, successful use of inhaled nitric oxide and high-frequency ventilation has been reported although the effect on overall mortality is less clear. Despite the high risk of pulmonary infection, prophylactic antibiotics are not recommended; however, early, prompt treatment is indicated when infection is suspected. Data regarding the use of corticosteroids in inhalation injury is inconclusive; several older studies show no differences in a variety of outcome measures.

Inhaled, systemic toxins such as carbon monoxide (CO) and hydrogen cyanide can be life threatening. CO is a product of carbon combustion and is always present in fires. Formation of cyanide depends on the presence of nitrogen-containing materials in the fire. A high index of suspicion is necessary to make the diagnosis of cyanide intoxication, because presenting symptoms are very similar to that of CO poisoning.

CO competitively and preferentially binds hemoglobin while displacing oxygen, thus forming carboxyhemoglobin. CO shifts the oxygen–hemoglobin dissociation curve to the left, thereby impairing release of hemoglobin-bound oxygen to the tissues. The end result is tissue hypoxia. CO can also act extravascularly, impeding cellular respiration at the level of the mitochondria. Acute symptoms of CO toxicity primarily reflect tissue hypoxia. The most common are headache, dizziness, and weakness. With increasing toxicity more serious neurologic sequalae can develop, including delirium, hallucinations, lethargy, seizures, and coma. Myocardial ischemia, arrhythmias, lactic acidosis, and shock may also be manifest. Although blood carboxyhemoglobin levels roughly correlate to symptoms of CO toxicity, there is wide variability. In general, carboxyhemoglobin is considered to be potentially lethal at levels greater than 50 to 60%. Administration of 100% oxygen is the mainstay of therapy for CO toxicity and should be given to all patients suspected of inhalation injury until the carboxyhemoglobin level in arterial blood has been measured by co-oximetry. With 100% oxygen, the half-life of carboxyhemoglobin falls to 60 to 80 minutes, compared with about 5 hours when breathing ambient room air. Carboxyhemoglobin levels are not detected by cutaneous oximeters. In fact, oxygen saturation from a pulse oximeter can be misleading because it does not distinguish between carboxyhemoglobin and O_2-hemoglobin. One hundred oxygen supplementation should be continued until carboxyhemoglobin levels fall to the normal range (<5%). Criteria for the use of hyperbaric oxygen (HBO), 100% oxygen at supra-atmospheric pressures (2–4 atm), are not definitive, but HBO, if available, should be considered for serious cases of CO poisoning in which the patient is unconscious, when the carboxyhemoglobin level is not decreasing at an appropriate rate despite administration of atmospheric 100% oxygen, in pregnancy, or in the presence of severe metabolic acidosis or underlying cardiovascular disease. The half-life of carboxyhemoglobin is decreased to 15 to 30 minutes with HBO. There is evidence that HBO may reduce long-term neurocognitive sequelae of CO poisoning.

Cyanide acts by binding cytochrome oxidase, a critical enzyme in the electron transport chain, thus inhibiting cellular respiration. Exposure to high levels can lead to immediate death. In cases of lower level exposure, empiric treatment should be strongly considered in situations in which the clinical suspicion is high for cyanide poisoning: headache, restlessness, seizures, coma, persistent metabolic acidosis despite high levels of supplemental oxygen, and reduced arteriovenous oxygen difference. Blood levels of cyanide cannot usually be obtained quickly enough to be useful. The standard treatment contained within the Cyanide Antidote Kit consists of 300 mg of sodium nitrite injected over 2 to 3 minutes, followed immediately by 12.5 g of sodium thiosulfate. Treatment of cyanide poisoning in fire victims with significant carboxyhemoglobin levels can be complicated because nitrites induce the formation of methemoglobin, further compromising oxygen delivery. In these situations, carboxyhemoglobin and methemoglobin levels should be monitored closely during treatment, or sodium thiosulfate as a sole agent for treatment should be considered.

Respiratory failure may result from causes other than smoke inhalation in burn victims. Chest wall compliance can be significantly reduced with circumferential thoracic third-degree burns, especially as subcutaneous edema progresses in the first 24 hours. Chest wall escharotomy may be necessary to relieve the restriction. Respiratory failure may also occur because of the severe catabolic state induced by major burns. The increase in carbon dioxide production requires an adequate ventilatory response to prevent significant hypercapnia and respiratory acidosis.

1. Ryan CM, Schoenfeld DA, Thorpe WP, et al. Objective estimates of the probability of death from burn injuries. *N Engl J Med*. 1998;338:363–366.

A retrospective review of 1,665 patients with burn injuries identifying age greater than 60 years, inhalation injury, and body surface area burn greater than 40% as the three significant risk factors associated with mortality.

2. Turnage RH, Nwariaku F, Murphy J, et al. Mechanisms of pulmonary microvascular dysfunction during severe burn injury. *World J Surg.* 2002;26:848–853.

A review of the basic science literature and theories regarding the mediators and mechanisms for indirect, burn-induced lung injury.

3. Alarie Y. Toxicity of fire smoke. *Crit Rev Toxicol.* 2002;32:259–289.

A thorough review of the toxic threats of fire, including thermal, chemical, and oxygen depletion. Also evaluates data from major historical fires, highlighting critical learning points by emphasizing the time course, evolution, fire dynamics, and mechanisms of the specific toxic threats.

4. www.burnsurgery.org

A comprehensive educational web site focused on the care of the burn patient. The site is divided into five separate educational modules: initial management of the burn patient, the burn wound, metabolism and nutrition, anabolic strategies, and pulmonary problems. Each educational module is further subdivided. Links to other relevant web sites are provided. No literature reference list for the contents or recommendations of this web site is given.

5. George A, Gupta R, Bang RL, et al. Radiological manifestation of pulmonary complications in deceased intensive care burn patients. *Burns.* 2003;29:73–78.

A retrospective review of chest radiographic findings in 46 deceased burn/inhalation injury patients from one burn intensive care unit.

6. Levine BA, Petroff PA, Slade CL, et al. Prospective trials of dexamethasone and aerosolized gentamicin in the treatment of inhalation injury in the burned patient. *J Trauma.* 1978;18:188–193.

A prospective, randomized trial that showed no significant difference in mortality, pulmonary complications, or pulmonary function between the group treated with steroids versus the control group.

7. Muehlberger T, Kunar D, Munster A, et al. Efficacy of fiberoptic laryngoscopy in the diagnosis of inhalation injuries. *Arch Otolaryngol Head Neck Surg.* 1998;124:1003–1007.

A small prospective study highlighting the contribution of direct upper airway visualization compared to clinical criteria in determining the need for intubation.

8. Cartotto R, Ellis S, Gomez M, et al. High frequency oscillatory ventilation in burn patients with the acute respiratory distress syndrome. *Burns.* 2004;30:453–463.

A retrospective review of 28 patients with ARDS secondary to burn injury. Patients had an average PaO_2/F_IO_2 of 98 who changed to high-frequency oscillatory ventilation after initial management with conventional mechanical ventilation. There was significant improvement in oxygenation parameters after institution of high-frequency oscillatory ventilation.

9. Reper P, Wibaux O, Van Laeke P, et al. High frequency percussive ventilation and conventional ventilation after smoke inhalation: a randomized study. *Burns.* 2002;28:503–508.

A randomized trial of 35 patients with both burn and inhalation injury. PaO_2/F_IO_2 was significantly higher in the high-frequency percussive ventilation group compared to the conventional ventilation control group; however, the difference remained significant for the first 72 hours only. No difference in mortality was seen between the two groups.

10. Ernst A, Zibrak JD. Carbon monoxide poisoning. *N Engl J Med.* 1998;339:603–1607.

A concise review article about CO poisoning.

11. Weaver LK, Howe S, Hopkins R, et al. Carboxyhemoglobin half-life in carbon monoxide-poisoned patients treated with 100% oxygen at atmospheric pressure. *Chest.* 2000;117:801–808.

Calculation of carboxyhemoglobin half-life was based on a retrospective chart review of 93 patients with CO toxicity who were treated with 100% oxygen via a nonrebreather facemask or endotracheal tube.

12. Cummings TF. The treatment of cyanide poisoning. *Occup Med.* 2004;54:82–85.
    A short, concise review of cyanide treatment options used around the world.
13. Baud FJ, Barriot P, Toffis V, et al. Elevated blood cyanide concentrations in victims of smoke inhalation. *N Engl J Med.* 1991;325:1761–1766.
    A prospective study of 109 fire victims showing elevated cyanide levels in fire victims, with cyanide levels being significantly higher in those who died compared to those who survived. There was a significant correlation between cyanide and CO levels. In addition, admission lactate levels correlated better with cyanide levels than CO levels in those without severe burns.
14. Kirk MA, Gerace R, Kulig KW. Cyanide and methemoglobin kinetics in smoke inhalation victims treated with the cyanide antidote kit. *Ann Emerg Med.* 1993;22:1413–1418.
    Four patients with severe inhalation injury and CO poisoning were treated with the cyanide antidote kit. Methemoglobin levels peaked at a mean of 50 minutes following administration of sodium nitrite.

85. HYPERSENSITIVITY PNEUMONITIS

Dominic A. Munafo, Jr.

ETIOLOGY

Hypersensitivity pneumonitis (HP), also known as *extrinsic allergic alveolitis,* results from the immunologic response to various inhaled biologic and chemical antigens. The classic example of HP is farmer's lung, which results from the inhalation of spores of thermophilic actinomycetes, usually *Saccharopolyspora rectivirgula.* Additional antigens include fungi, various animal and insect proteins, and chemicals such as isocyanates and anhydrides. New inciting antigens are reported regularly in the literature. Inhaled antigens are typically 1 to 5 μm; therefore, the site of lung injury is the distal airway and alveolus. An antigen's ability to trigger an immune response depends on its solubility, resistance to digestion by macrophages, and properties as an immunologic adjuvant.

PATHOPHYSIOLOGY

As many as 50% of heavily exposed individuals may develop antibodies to an inhaled antigen, but a smaller percent actually develop disease. Most cases occur through occupational, environmental, or avocational exposures. Examples of HP include farmer's lung (thermophilic actinomycetes in moldy hay), pigeon breeder's lung (serum proteins in pigeon droppings), bagassosis (bagasse in sugar cane), maple bark disease (fungi in moldy bark), and humidifier lung (amoebae in humidifier water). Prevalence rates vary widely (1–30%) in an exposed population and appear to depend on intensity and duration of exposure as well as antigen type and host susceptibility. HP is more prevalent among pigeon breeders than farmers, perhaps in part because of the more chronic nature of the exposure in pigeon breeding.

HP has classically been categorized as acute, subacute, or chronic in presentation. However, the HP Study Group has suggested that patients be considered as having either active or residual disease. *Active disease* includes the acute and subacute presentations and occurs after a previous sensitizing exposure to a particular antigen. Approximately 4 to 8 hours following re-exposure, the individual experiences the abrupt onset of a flu-like syndrome. Symptoms include a nonproductive cough, fever, chills, dyspnea, myalgias, and malaise. The most prominent physical findings are tachypnea, tachycardia, and bibasilar inspiratory crackles. Wheezing is uncommon. Symptoms typically peak within 24 hours and remit spontaneously within

72 hours. Symptoms recur with subsequent exposures and their severity depends on the intensity and duration of exposure as well as a particular individual's sensitivity. Chronic exposure to lower levels of antigen may be accompanied by mild or absent symptoms and disease progression can be insidious. Continued exposure is associated with increasing dyspnea, cough, anorexia, and weight loss. *Residual disease* refers to the end-stage findings of emphysematous change or fibrosis present long after the acute inflammatory reaction has dissipated.

The immunologic mechanisms responsible for HP are complex and are incompletely understood. Although both humoral and cellular immunity are involved, more recent investigations indicate that cell-mediated immunity is likely the more consequential. The acute alveolitis seen hours after antigen exposure is thought secondary to precipitation of immune complexes in the alveoli and interstitium. This type III immune response activates complement, resulting in an increase in vascular permeability and recruitment of additional inflammatory cells. Activated macrophages secrete a variety of proinflammatory cytokines, including tumor necrosis factor-α (TNF-α), macrophage inflammatory protein-1α (MIP-1α), interleukin-1β (IL-1β), IL-8, and IL-12. MIP-1α is chemotactic for CD8$^+$ T cells. A murine model of HP has shown that interferon-γ (IFN-γ) is essential in the formation of granulomatous inflammation. IL-10 inhibits expression of IFN-γ and appears to mitigate the inflammatory response to antigen. Conversely, IL-12 enhances IFN-γ production thus promoting granulomatous inflammation. Additional factors that may enhance the lymphocytic inflammation include increased expression of the adhesion molecule L-selectin by lymphocytes in BALF and the observation that HP lymphocytes demonstrate decreased apoptosis. All these data, coupled with studies showing adoptive transfer of HP using Th1-type cells, suggest that differences in regulation of this type IV immune response may help explain the varying clinical presentations of disease. Bronchus-associated lymphoid tissue can serve as a site of induction and amplification of the local immune response. Interestingly, common respiratory viruses have been found in the lower airways of patients with HP with increased frequency. A murine model suggests that a preceding viral infection can augment the inflammatory response in HP. Approximately 80 to 95% of HP patients are nonsmokers. Smoking may be immunosuppressive and therefore confer some degree of protection. Nicotine has been found to reduce TNF-α release from alveolar macrophages in a murine model. In addition, smokers have a lower incidence of antibody production. A significant active smoking history speaks against a diagnosis of HP.

CLINICAL FINDINGS

Laboratory findings are largely nonspecific. IgG serum precipitating antibodies to the offending antigen are present in most patients. IgA and IgM antibodies may also be seen. Immunoglobulin levels are usually elevated in both serum and bronchoalveolar lavage fluid (BALF); however, IgE levels remain normal. The presence of antibodies is not diagnostic of disease but only indicates previous significant exposure. Leukocytosis with a left shift typically accompanies acute episodes. Eosinophilia is uncommon and should suggest the possibility of another diagnosis. BALF shows a dramatic increase in the number of T lymphocytes recovered. Selective expansion of the CD8$^+$ subset typically occurs, as does reversal of the CD4$^+$:CD8$^+$ ratio. This is in contrast with the findings in sarcoidosis in which the cells are predominantly CD4$^+$. Elevation of CD8$^+$ cells may be associated with less chance of progressive fibrosis. Although the percentage of alveolar macrophages recovered is markedly reduced, the absolute number of macrophages is elevated. BALF findings are not diagnostic of HP but rather serve to support the diagnosis and help to rule out other processes. A normal BALF lymphocyte count would only be found in residual disease.

Histologically, neutrophilic alveolitis in the first 24 hours gives way to an intense peribronchial inflammatory infiltrate of lymphocytes, plasma cells, macrophages, and giant cells. Noncaseating granulomas are often seen in the interstitium. In chronic disease, both granulomas and interstitial fibrosis are seen. Bronchiolitis obliterans is found frequently (25–50%) with or without organizing pneumonia (15–25%). Vasculitis is not present.

Chest radiographic findings of HP are highly variable. Acutely, radiographs may be normal (20%) or show bilateral, ill-defined alveolar and interstitial nodular infiltrates. The distribution can be patchy or diffuse, with some predilection for the lower lobes. Hilar adenopathy and pleural effusions are rare. In chronic disease, the chest radiograph shows a reticulonodular pattern with interstitial fibrosis, honeycombing, and loss of lung volume. The fibrotic changes are often more prominent in the upper lobes and periphery of the lung. High-resolution computed tomography (HRCT) is more sensitive than chest radiography in demonstrating the characteristic centrilobular nodules and emphysematous changes; however, its sensitivity and specificity appear to vary, depending on disease severity and chronicity.

Pulmonary function tests during an acute episode usually show a restrictive defect. Mild to moderate hypoxemia, hypocapnia, and a decrease in the diffusing capacity of the lung for carbon monoxide (D_{LCO}) are often present. As many as 60% of patients may demonstrate airway hyperreactivity, as detected by methacholine challenge. Patients who experience recurring attacks most commonly develop airway obstruction and a persistent decrement in D_{LCO}. Progressive restriction secondary to interstitial fibrosis may also be seen. Early cessation of exposure leads to gradual resolution of the pulmonary function abnormalities over days to weeks. In advanced disease, progressive pulmonary insufficiency, chronic hypoxemia, and cor pulmonale may develop.

DIAGNOSIS

The diagnosis of HP is suggested by a history that relates symptoms to exposure, but may be particularly difficult in those patients with chronic low-level exposure. Most of the signs and symptoms of disease are nonspecific. The HP Study Group published a logistic regression model that identified six significant predictors of HP: (1) exposure to a known offending antigen, (2) precipitating antibodies to the offending antigen, (3) recurrent symptoms, (4) inspiratory crackles on examination, (5) symptoms within 4 to 8 hours of exposure, and (6) weight loss. Depending on the constellation of findings, a probability of disease can be determined from the published chart.

Inhalation challenge, either in a laboratory setting or by returning the patient to the site of exposure, is the most specific diagnostic test. In the absence of an identifiable cause and in more chronic presentations, lung biopsy may be necessary to define the pathology and rule out other possibilities. Skin tests are not helpful. Differential diagnosis in the acute setting includes atypical and viral pneumonia, collagen vascular disease, lymphocytic interstitial pneumonia, organic dust toxic syndrome, and other acute inhalational injuries. In patients who wheeze, consider occupational asthma, allergic bronchopulmonary aspergillosis, and byssinosis. Chronically, miliary tuberculosis, sarcoidosis, fungal infection, eosinophilic granuloma, and idiopathic pulmonary fibrosis can mimic HP. As many as 10% of referrals to some tertiary centers for idiopathic pulmonary fibrosis demonstrate pathology suggestive of HP. Therefore, a detailed exposure history in a patient with interstitial lung disease is essential.

TREATMENT

The mainstay of therapy is avoiding exposure to the offending antigen. A less desirable alternative is the use of a mask or other filtration technique to substantially reduce or prevent exposure. The symptoms of subacute and chronic progressive disease can be indolent. Thus, if continued exposure is unavoidable, close follow-up with pulmonary function tests and radiographic studies is essential to assess disease activity. The use of corticosteroids in the acute setting often speeds recovery and decreases symptoms. In addition, some patients treated with corticosteroids develop less radiographic evidence of fibrosis. To date, however, no clear evidence indicates that corticosteroids have a beneficial effect on lung function. Inhaled corticosteroids may be of some benefit, however, other nonsteroidal anti-inflammatory therapies (e.g., inhaled cromolyn) have not been found effective.

PROGNOSIS

The prognosis of HP is quite variable. Some patients with farmer's lung may tolerate continued exposure without persistent symptoms or disease progression. However, other patients with pigeon breeder's lung have developed progressive disease despite complete antigen avoidance. Chronic low-level exposures appear to confer a worse prognosis than short-term intermittent exposures. The presence of fibrosis on lung biopsy has been associated with reduced survival. Patients should be advised to avoid antigen exposure to the greatest extent possible.

1. Vourlekis JS, Schwarz MI, Cherniack RM, et al. The effect of pulmonary fibrosis on survival in patients with hypersensitivity pneumonitis. *Am J Med.* 2004;116:662.
    Study of 72 patients with HP. Those with fibrosis on lung biopsy exhibited increased mortality.
2. Yi ES. Hypersensitivity pneumonitis. *Crit Rev Clin Lab Sci.* 2002;39:581.
    A comprehensive review with emphasis on several important types of HP as well as a detailed description of the immune pathogenesis of HP.
3. Lacasse Y, Selman M, Costabel U, et al. Clinical diagnosis of hypersensitivity pneumonitis. *Am J Respir Crit Care Med.* 2003;168:952.
    Details the HP study group's prediction rule and the six significant predictors of HP.
4. Girard M, Israel-Assayag E, Cormier Y. Pathogenesis of hypersensitivity pneumonitis. *Curr Opin Allergy Clin Immunol.* 2004;4:93.
    Succinct review of the many factors influencing the immune pathogenesis of HP.
5. McSharry C, Anderson K, Bourke SJ, et al. Takes your breath away—the immunology of allergic alveolitis. *Clin Exp Immunol.* 2002;128:3.
    Reviews immunology of HP with emphasis on pigeon breeder's lung and farmer's lung.
6. Navarro C, Mendoza F, Barrera L, et al. Up-regulation of L-selectin and E-selectin in hypersensitivity pneumonitis. *Chest.* 2002;121:354.
    Suggests that L-selectin is upregulated in HP and may enhance lymphocytic inflammation.
7. Laflamme C, Israel-Assayag E, Cormier Y. Apoptosis of bronchoalveolar lavage lymphocytes in hypersensitivity pneumonitis. *Eur Respir J.* 2003;21:225.
    Pulmonary lymphocytes from patients with HP showed decreased apoptosis compared to normal controls. This suggests another mechanism for the accumulation of lymphocytes in the lung.
8. Schuyler M, Gott K, Cherne A, et al. Th1 CD4$^+$ cells adoptively transfer experimental hypersensitivity pneumonitis. *Cell Immunol.* 1997;177:169.
    Reviews the cytokine profile of Th1 and Th2 subsets. Documents that CD4$^+$ cells with a Th1 profile can adoptively transfer experimental HP in a murine model.
9. Gudmundsson G, Hunninghake GW. Interferon-γ is necessary for the expression of hypersensitivity pneumonitis. *J Clin Invest.* 1997;99:2386.
    Interferon-deficient (knockout) mice did not develop granulomatous inflammation in response to inhaled antigen.
10. Suda T, Chida K, Hayakawa H, et al. Development of bronchus-associated lymphoid tissue in chronic hypersensitivity pneumonitis. *Chest.* 1999;115:357.
    Reports the presence of bronchus-associated lymphoid tissue in three of five patients with chronic HP. The authors postulate that this tissue plays an important role in the mucosal immune response.
11. Blanchet MR, Israel-Assayag E, Cormier Y. Inhibitory effect of nicotine on experimental hypersensitivity pneumonitis in vivo and in vitro. *Am J Respir Crit Care Med.* 2004;169:893.
    Murine model demonstrating the inhibitory effect of nicotine on the immune response.
12. Erkinjuntti-Pekkanen R, Rytkonen H, Kokkarinen JI, et al. Long-term risk of emphysema in patients with farmer's lung and matched control farmers. *Am J Respir Crit Care Med.* 1998;158:662.

A 14-year follow-up study of patients with HP. The study documents an increased risk of developing emphysema using pulmonary function tests and high-resolution computed tomography. Interestingly, no increase in fibrosis was seen in patients with HP compared with matched controls.

13. Erkinjuntti-Pekkanen R, Kokkarinen JI, Tukiainen HO, et al. Long-term outcome of pulmonary function in farmer's lung: a 14-year follow-up with matched controls. *Eur Respir J.* 1997;10:2046.

A persistent decrement in D_{LCO} was the most important sequela of farmer's lung disease. Chronic farmer's lung disease can lead to an obstructive pulmonary defect.

14. Yoshizawa Y, Miyake S, Sumi Y, et al. A follow-up study of pulmonary function tests, bronchoalveolar lavage cells, and humoral and cellular immunity in bird fancier's lung. *J Allergy Clin Immunol.* 1995;96:122.

This 5-year follow-up study in five patients documents the variability of the course of bird fancier's lung. The patients demonstrated persistence of sensitized lymphocytes and continued antibody production. Despite antigen avoidance, these patients should be followed closely for evidence of disease progression.

15. Dakhama A, Hegele RG, Laflamme G, et al. Common respiratory viruses in lower airways of patients with acute hypersensitivity pneumonitis. *Am J Respir Crit Care Med.* 1999;159:1316.

An interesting report using polymerase chain reaction to document the presence of influenza A in the BALF of 6 of 13 patients with HP; two of six controls also had evidence of virus. The ultimate significance of this finding has yet to be determined.

16. Hansell DM, Wells AU, Padley SP, et al. Hypersensitivity pneumonitis: correlation of individual CT patterns with functional abnormalities. *Radiology.* 1996;199:123.

The analysis of thin-section CT in 22 patients demonstrated that the most commonly found pattern was decreased attenuation and mosaic perfusion. Ground glass opacification and nodules were also commonly seen. The radiographic appearance was thought suggestive of bronchiolitis.

17. Kokkarinen JI, Tukiainen HO, Terho EO. Effect of corticosteroid treatment on the recovery of pulmonary function in farmer's lung. *Am Rev Respir Dis.* 1992;145:3.

A double-blind, randomized, placebo-controlled trial in 36 patients with acute farmer's lung, using 8 weeks of systemic corticosteroids. At 1 month, the corticosteroid group showed a significantly higher D_{LCO}. At 3 months, 6 months, 1 year, and 5 years, no significant differences were seen in any of the measures of pulmonary function.

18. Monkare S. Influence of corticosteroid treatment on the course of farmer's lung. *Eur J Respir Dis.* 1983;64:283.

Prospective study of no steroids (in less severe cases) versus 4 and 12 weeks of therapy in 93 Finnish farmers. Treatment had no significant effect on the course of lung function; however, steroids improved acute symptoms and decreased fibrotic changes on chest radiographs.

19. Lynch DA, Rose CS, Way D, et al. Hypersensitivity pneumonitis: sensitivity of high-resolution CT in a population-based study. *AJR.* 1992;159:469.

A population-based study of 31 symptomatic patients, 11 of whom met diagnostic criteria for HP. High-resolution computed tomography scanning was more sensitive than chest radiography. Of the 11 patients, 5 had abnormal CT scans, but only 1 had an abnormal chest radiograph.

86. NEAR-DROWNING AND DIVING ACCIDENTS

Ian R. Grover and Tom S. Neuman

Accidental drowning occurs in all age groups but is most common in children aged 1 to 4 years. Despite a recent decline in the number of deaths, drowning remains the second leading cause of injury-related death for children aged 1 to 14 years. In the year 2000, there were 3,482 unintentional drowning-related deaths, and approximately 90,000 episodes of near drowning in the United States. A recent decline in the number of fatalities may reflect better prevention because of enhanced private pool safety. In adults, alcohol is the most important single factor in drowning incidents.

PATHOPHYSIOLOGY
Historically, the pathophysiology of near drowning was attributed to an electrolyte disturbance induced by aspiration of fluid. Current data suggest aspiration-related hypoxemia as the major pathophysiologic abnormality. The earlier notion that death could result from drowning without aspiration was based on misinterpretation of seminal documents. In 10 to 15% of drowning cases, hypoxemia appeared to be secondary to simple asphyxia. In these cases, termed *dry drowning*, with little or no aspiration the hypothesis was that reflex laryngospasm prevented aspiration. However, no experimental evidence support this hypothesis. Most experts believe that dry drowning does not occur and that other causes for in water fatalities should be sought, such as sudden cardiac death. The sine qua non of drowning is the aspiration of fluid.

The hypoxemia observed in drowning cases is related to aspiration. The exact volume of fluid aspirated by victims remains unclear but animal experiments that seem to duplicate human injury require fluid in the range of 1 to 10 mL/kg. The mechanism of hypoxemia depends on the nature of the fluid aspirated. In seawater aspiration, osmotic and irritative effects from sand, diatoms, algae, and other particles provoke an exudative response. This exudate fills alveoli and results in ventilation/perfusion ($\dot{V}/\dot{Q}$) mismatch and hypoxemia. In fresh water aspiration, pulmonary surfactants are also lost from the lung, leading to focal collapse, $\dot{V}/\dot{Q}$ mismatch, and hypoxemia. When water is instilled into the trachea of experimental animals, pathologic studies reveal damage to alveolar and endothelial cells, as well as disruption of the capillary basement membrane.

CLINICAL MANIFESTATIONS
The clinical manifestations of near drowning vary with the duration and severity of the hypoxemia. The neurologic presentation reflects the degree of cerebral anoxia. Pulmonary injury ranges from mild, manifesting as cough and mild shortness of breath to severe, presenting with extreme dyspnea, pulmonary edema, and acute respiratory distress syndrome.

Laboratory studies generally reveal hypoxemia, metabolic acidosis and, perhaps, superimposed respiratory acidosis. Minor changes in electrolytes are seen frequently; however, clinically significant alterations in serum sodium or potassium are distinctly unusual in near drowning in either freshwater or seawater. Chest radiographs may display a spectrum of abnormalities, ranging from patchy infiltrates to dense pulmonary edema. Rarely, massive particulate aspiration can also occur. It has been hypothesized that the pulmonary edema occasionally seen in near drowning victims is caused by negative pressure inspiration (attempting to breathe against a closed glottis) or to neurogenic factors.

MANAGEMENT
The management of near drowning patients is mainly supportive. Arterial blood gases should be monitored frequently and mechanical ventilatory support should be instituted if acute respiratory failure and refractory hypoxemia develop. Patients with acute respiratory failure may require high ventilator pressures to provide adequate

oxygenation and ventilation, reflecting the marked reduction in pulmonary compliance. The application of positive end-expiratory pressure (PEEP) during mechanical ventilation reduces morbidity and mortality. In most cases, ventilatory support is necessary for only a short time. Less invasive methods of ventilatory support such as nasal continuous positive airway pressure and bilevel positive airway pressure may reduce the need for intubation and the risks associated with mechanical ventilation. The routine administration of hypertonic or hypotonic intravenous fluids is not warranted. The use of antibiotics in the near-drowning victim is usually restricted to those who develop fever, new pulmonary infiltrates, or purulent secretions. Prophylactic antibiotics do not improve mortality or decrease morbidity. Most pulmonary infections in near-drowning victims are secondary to hospital-acquired organisms; prophylactic antibiotics may only select more resistant organisms. Rarely the victim may aspirate water that is heavily contaminated with a known organism. Prophylactic antibiotics may be appropriate in this situation.

Routine bronchoscopy to search for particulate matter causing airway obstruction is generally unnecessary. Adrenocortical steroids are not indicated to treat the lung injury associated with near drowning. Experimental evidence strongly suggests that steroids do not improve the long-term outcome or short-term morbidity. One uncontrolled report (four cases), however, suggests high-dose steroids may be beneficial in near-drowning victims who present with pulmonary edema. The use of surfactants to treat near-drowning victims has been reported recently. It is unclear whether such therapy alters the outcome. In an experimental model, surfactant therapy did not offer any benefit over traditional supportive approach.

COMPLICATIONS

Pneumothorax, lung abscess, and empyema occasionally complicate the course in near-drowning patients if severe respiratory failure occurs. Hypothermia at the time of the immersion incident can also complicate the picture. Although renal failure and disseminated intravascular coagulation have been reported, they are probably sequelae of prolonged acidosis, hypoxemia, and hypotension, rather than specific complications of near drowning.

PROGNOSIS

The victim's prognosis depends primarily on the extent and duration of the hypoxemic episode. Age and prior illnesses can be modifying factors. Epidemiologic data do not support the hypothesis that cold water immersion improves the prognosis of the near-drowning victim. However, in rare, well-documented cases, victims who fully recover after prolonged submersion in cold water have been reported. Many empiric studies have attempted to better define prognostic factors for the near-drowning victim. Unfortunately, no factors seem to be completely reliable. In general, patients who present with a normal chest radiograph or normal mental status are likely to survive without sequelae.

Most large studies indicate that 5 to 10% of all victims suffer varying degrees of permanent neurologic dysfunction, although some suggest a higher percentage with long-term neurologic sequelae. Not surprisingly, those who sustain a cardiorespiratory arrest persisting to the time of presentation in an emergency room have a poor chance of survival and a high incidence of neurologic sequelae. However, children who sustain a "cardiorespiratory arrest" that responds to first aid measures at the scene of the accident do not necessarily have a poor prognosis. In the late 1970s after a small experience of near-drowning victims with a high percentage of long-term neurologic sequelae, it was suggested that the incidence of neurologic dysfunction following near-drowning episodes could be lowered by aggressive attempts at cerebral salvage. This HYPER therapy included barbiturate coma, controlled hyperventilation, diuretics, paralysis, intentional hypothermia, and adrenocortical steroids. The rationale for this therapy was to lower intracranial pressure (ICP), reduce cerebral edema, and lower cerebral oxygen demand in order to prevent further (secondary) neurologic damage. This mode of therapy presumes that further damage occurs after the initial anoxic insult and that further damage can be prevented by these measures.

Unfortunately, after more than two decades of experience, it is not clear that morbidity and mortality have changed appreciably with this mode of therapy. The largest study, performed by the group that originally advocated this therapy, reported a 7% incidence of neurologic morbidity. This was not appreciably different from multiple studies performed before the advent of this therapy. Additionally, although very high ICP is associated with poor outcome, other studies suggest that normal ICP does not ensure neurologic recovery and that HYPER therapy does not necessarily prevent elevation of ICP. Indeed, it appears that elevation of ICP is the result, not the cause, of brain injury. Certainly, most authorities agree that if this therapy is indicated at all, it should be reserved for the most severely affected patients in whom ICP is being monitored, and then only in an intensive care unit setting that is staffed, equipped, and experienced with this therapy. Even in such a setting, the aspects of this therapy that are associated with significant morbidity should be reserved for victims whose ICP cannot be controlled by other more conventional means (e.g., hyperventilation, head elevation, osmotic diuretics).

The decision to admit the near-drowning victim to the hospital is somewhat controversial. Any victim with significant respiratory symptoms, an abnormal chest radiograph, or an abnormal arterial oxygenation (signs or symptoms suggesting aspiration) should probably be admitted to the hospital, because pulmonary damage may not reach its peak for several hours after the accident. It is less clear whether patients who have suffered solely a loss of consciousness and present with normal neurologic function and no cardiopulmonary signs or symptoms require hospital admission.

SPECIAL CIRCUMSTANCES
Scuba Diving

In scuba diving accidents, the most common cause of death is reported to be drowning. However, problems exist with data collection. Barotraumatic systemic gas embolism may, in fact, be a more common cause of death. The physiologic mechanism is related to Boyle's law, which states that in a closed system the product of pressure and volume remains constant at a given temperature ($P_1V_1 = P_2V_2$). If a submerged diver fills his or her lungs from a compressed gas source and then rises in the water column, that gas must expand because of the reduction in barometric pressure. If the egress of gas is blocked (i.e., a closed glottis), intrapulmonary blood vessels can rupture, allowing gas to enter the pulmonary venous circulation resulting in systemic embolism. The most common symptoms are attributable to embolization of air in the cerebral vessels. Sudden unconsciousness with subsequent aspiration can then occur. The expanding gas can also dissect through the interstitium of the lung to the hila, producing pneumomediastinum and subcutaneous emphysema at the base of the neck. Rarely, pneumothorax may occur. Treatment of pulmonary barotrauma is supportive unless air embolism develops. In that case, recompression is indicated. A variety of hematologic and biochemical abnormalities have also been reported from arterial gas embolism. Pulmonary barotrauma with cerebral air embolism is seen only in divers breathing from a compressed gas source. Swimmers who descend below the surface following inspiration to total lung capacity initially compress the gas in their chest. On surfacing, that gas expands, but it does not expand to a volume greater than the initial total lung capacity, and therefore, barotrauma does not occur.

Decompression sickness also affects divers but rarely causes pulmonary problems. Shortness of breath occurs in fewer than 1% of cases. Most patients present with limb pain or spinal cord lesions. These patients also require recompression therapy. The pathophysiology of decompression sickness is related to absorption of an inert gas (nitrogen) with subsequent reduction in barometric pressure sufficient to generate a gas phase within the tissues. The precise pathophysiologic mechanisms of the different forms and presentations of decompression sickness are still unclear. Prophylaxis for deep venous thrombosis in paralyzed divers may be problematic because hemorrhage into the spinal cord secondary to bubble damage is thought to be a mechanism involved in the generation of paralytic symptoms. As a result, these patients must be monitored extremely carefully if heparin prophylaxis is not administered.

Although not generally reported in diving fatality statistics, there is strong evidence that intentional hyperventilation prior to breath-hold diving is associated with both drowning and near-drowning episodes. Hyperventilation reduces the partial pressure of arterial carbon dioxide ($PaCO_2$) so that the breath-hold break point is prolonged sufficiently for hypoxemia to occur before the individual is forced to breathe. Hypoxemia, in turn, may cause the individual to lose consciousness, resulting in a drowning or near-drowning incident.

Submersion-Induced Pulmonary Edema

Another interesting phenomenon reported recently is swimming- or submersion-induced pulmonary edema (SIPE) that usually occurs with strenuous swimming activities, especially in cold water. It appears to have many features similar to exertional pulmonary edema. The pathophysiologic mechanism resulting in SIPE is not currently known. It is known, however, that it is not caused by aspiration or negative pressure inspiration against a closed glottis. It has been postulated that the effects of immersion in water, especially cold water, lead to an increase in central vascular volume, redistribution of pulmonary blood flow, and change in lung volumes. When these changes occur with an increased cardiac output from heavy exertion, it may expose the pulmonary capillary bed to high pressures. This high pressure may cause extravasation of fluid by hydrostatic forces and stress failure of pulmonary capillaries, resulting in pulmonary edema and frank hemorrhage.

These patients then present with dyspnea, cough, hypoxemia, tachypnea, and hemoptysis. Chest radiographs show an infiltrate or frank pulmonary edema. These patients usually require admission for observation and supportive treatment. Recovery is usually quite rapid and diuretics are generally not required.

---

1. Anker AL, Santora T, Spivey W. Artificial surfactant administration in an animal model of near drowning. *Acad Emerg Med*. 1995;2:204.
   No benefit is seen of surfactant administration over standard ventilation in this animal model of near drowning.
2. Bell TS, Ellenberg L, McComb JG. Neuropsychological outcome after severe pediatric near drowning. *Neurosurgery*. 1985;17:604.
   Children who recover from even severe near-drowning episodes generally show average cognitive functioning and only mild gross motor and coordination deficits.
3. Brubank AO, Neuman TS. *Bennett and Elliott's Physiology and Medicine of Diving*, 5th ed. Elsevier Science Limited; 2003.
   A comprehensive, well-written text regarding the physiology of diving and diving medicine.
4. Bohn DJ, Biggar WD, Smith CR, et al. Influence of hypothermia, barbiturate therapy, and intracranial monitoring on morbidity and mortality after near drowning. *Crit Care Med*. 1986;14:529.
   Essentially, a retraction of their earlier work advocating HYPER therapy.
5. Bove AA, Davis JC. *Diving Medicine*, 4th ed. Philadelphia: WB Saunders; 2004.
   An excellent, well-written introductory text to all aspects of diving medicine.
6. Calderwood H, Modell J, Ruiz B. Ineffectiveness of steroid therapy for treatment of fresh water and near drowning. *Anesthesiology*. 1975;43:642.
   Strong evidence that steroids are not routinely useful in cases of near drowning.
7. Conn AW, Edmonds J, Barker G. Cerebral resuscitation in near drowning. *Pediatr Clin North Am*. 1979;26:691.
   An uncontrolled study suggesting decreased long-term morbidity in patients aggressively treated for anoxic encephalopathy.
8. DeNicola LK, Falk JL, Swanson ME, et al. Submersion injuries in children and adults. *Crit Care Clin*. 1997;13:477.
   Comprehensive review of near drowning (125 references).
9. Dubowitz DJ, Blumi S, Arcinue E, et al. MR of hypoxic encephalopathy in children after near drowning: correlation with quantitative proton MR spectroscopy and clinical outcome. *AJNR Am J Neuroradiol*. 1998;19:1617.

An attempt to use magnetic resonance imaging as an aid to prognosis in nearly drowned children.

10. Ender PT, Dolan MJ. Pneumonia associated with near drowning. *Clin Infect Dis.* 1997;25:896.
    A review of the bacteriology of pneumonias associated with near drowning episodes (102 references).

11. Golden F, Tipton MJ, Scott RC. Immersion, near drowning and drowning. *Br J Anaesth.* 1997;79:214.
    A comprehensive review of the pathophysiology and treatment of near drowning and drowning, especially in cold water.

12. Gonzalez-Rothi RJ. Near drowning: consensus and controversies in pulmonary and cerebral resuscitation. *Heart Lung.* 1987;16:474.
    A comprehensive review of the problem of cerebral resuscitation in the near drowning victim (62 references).

13. Grausz H, Amend WJ, Early LE. Acute renal failure in seawater near drowning. *JAMA.* 1971;217:207.
    Concludes that acute renal failure represents acute tubular necrosis secondary to the combination of hypoxemia and hypotension.

14. Huckabee HCG, Craig PL, Williams JM. Near drowning in frigid water: a case study of a 31-year-old woman. *J Int Neuropsychol Soc.* 1996;2:256.
    A case study describing neurologically intact survival after 30 minutes of submersion in cold water.

15. Lavelle JM, Show KN. Near drowning. Is emergency department cardiopulmonary resuscitation or intensive care unit cerebral resuscitation indicated? *Crit Care Med.* 1993;21:368.
    Discussion of 54 pediatric cases showing no apparent benefit of cerebral resuscitation, but approximately 5% of victims arriving at emergency department requiring cardiopulmonary resuscitation (CPR) and cardiotonic drugs went on to full recovery.

16. Lund KL, Mahon RT, Tanen DA, et al. Swimming-induced pulmonary edema. *Ann Emerg Med.* 2003;41:251.
    A discussion of three cases of SIPE.

17. Martin CM, Barrett O. Drowning and near drowning: a review of 10 years experience in a large army hospital. *Mil Med.* 1971;136:439.
    No clinically significant hemoconcentration or hemodilution was noted; no difference in clinical or radiographic recovery occurred in those given antibiotics or steroids.

18. Modell JH, Bellefleur M, Davis JH. Drowning without aspiration: is this an appropriate diagnosis? *J Forensic Sci.* 1999;44:1119.
    An excellent review article looking at animal drowning studies to determine if the entity of "dry drowning" is a possibility.

19. Modell JH. Drowning. *N Engl J Med.* 1993;328:253.
    A classic review article authored by the researcher who defined much of our understanding of the pathophysiology of drowning (53 references).

20. Modell J, Davis J. Electrolyte changes in human drowning victims. *Anesthesiology.* 1969;30:414.
    One of several classic articles refuting the importance of electrolyte changes in drowning victims.

21. Modell J, Graves S, Ketover A. Clinical course of 91 consecutive near drowning victims. *Chest.* 1976;70:231.
    A large series, now mostly of historical interest.

22. Modell J, Calderwood HW, Ruiz BC, et al. Effect of ventilatory patterns on arterial oxygenation after near drowning in seawater. *Anesthesiology.* 1974;40:376.
    Suggests PEEP should be used in victims of near drowning in seawater.

23. Neuman TS. Arterial gas embolism and decompression sickness. *News Physiol Sci.* 2002;17:77.
    A summary of the pathophysiology and treatment of AGE and DCS (14 references).

24. Nichter MA, Everett PB. Childhood near drowning: is cardiopulmonary resuscitation always indicated? *Crit Care Med.* 1989;17:993.

Of 93 pediatric near-drowning cases, two thirds requiring CPR went on to intact survival; however, all patients requiring cardiotonic drugs in association with CPR either died or had severe neurologic damage.

25. Nussbaum E, Maggi JC. Pentobarbital therapy does not improve neurologic outcome in nearly drowned, flaccid-comatose children. *Pediatrics.* 1988;81:630.
    Discusses 31 patients in sequential treatment groups.

26. Orlowski JP. Drowning, near drowning, and ice water submersions. *Pediatr Clin North Am.* 1987;34:75.
    A good review with a fine section on ice water submersion (53 references).

27. Pearn J. The management of near drowning. *BMJ.* 1985;291:1447.
    Although somewhat dated, still an interesting review (107 references).

28. Pearn J. Neurological and psychometric studies in children surviving fresh water immersion accidents. *Lancet.* 1977;1:7.
    Indicates good long-term neurologic outcome of children receiving CPR at the time of rescue.

29. Pearn J, Nixon J, Wilkey I. Freshwater drowning and near drowning accidents involving children: a five-year total population study. *Med J Aust.* 1976;2: 942.
    An excellent, epidemiologic review.

30. Peterson B. Morbidity of children near drowning. *Pediatrics.* 1977;59:364.
    Neurologic outcome of children still requiring CPR on arrival in the emergency room is dismal.

31. Schench H, McAniff JJ. United States underwater fatality statistics, 1970–1981. NOAA Report No. URI-SSR-83-16, University of Rhode Island, Rhode Island, USA.
    Describes all scuba fatalities in the United States during the years 1970–1981 and is the only complete epidemiologic report of its kind. An annual report is published yearly as well.

32. Shupak A, Weiler-Ravell D, Adir Y, et al. Pulmonary oedema induced by strenuous swimming: a field study. *Respir Physiol.* 2000;121:25.
    A prospective study that looked at the incidence and recurrence rate of strenuous SIPE in healthy young men in a fitness-training program.

33. Slade Jr JB, Hattori T, Ray CS, et al. Pulmonary edema associated with Scuba diving. *Chest.* 2001;120:1686.
    A case report of eight scuba divers who developed pulmonary edema after diving.

34. Sladen A, Zander H. Methylprednisolone therapy for pulmonary edema following near drowning. *JAMA.* 1971;215:1793.
    Weak evidence that steroids may be of benefit in patients presenting with pulmonary edema.

35. Smith RM, Neuman TS. Elevation in serum CK in divers with arterial gas embolism. *N Engl J Med.* 1994;330:19.

36. Smith RM, Neuman TS. Abnormal serum biochemistries in association with arterial gas embolism. *J Emerg Med.* 1997;15:285.
    These two articles are representative of several delineating the laboratory abnormalities seen in victims of arterial gas embolism.

37. Spack L. Gedeit R, Splaingard M, et al. Failure of aggressive therapy to alter outcome in pediatric near drowning. *Pediatr Emerg Care.* 1997;13:98.
    The most recent article demonstrating that the currently available aggressive therapies do not alter outcome.

38. Staudinger T, Bankier A, Strohmaier W, et al. Exogenous surfactant therapy in a patient with adult respiratory distress syndrome after near drowning. *Resuscitation.* 1997;35:179.
    The most recent of several case reports using surfactant to treat near-drowning victims.

39. Suominen PK, Korpela RE, Silfvast TG, et al. Does water temperature affect outcome of nearly drowned children. *Resuscitation.* 1997;35:111.
    The only recent article to examine the effect of water temperature on outcome. The data seem to indicate cold water near drownings do no better than others and that duration of immersion is the critical factor.

40. Swann HG, Bruce M. The cardiorespiratory and biochemical events during rapid anoxic death. VI. Fresh water and sea water drowning. *Tex Rep Biol Med.* 1949;7:604.
41. Swann HG, Brucer M, Moore C, et al. Fresh water and sea water drowning: a study of the terminal cardiac and biochemical events. *Tex Rep Biol Med.* 1947;5: 423.
    References 39 and 40 are the basis for 15 years of misunderstanding concerning the pathophysiology of near drowning.
42. van Berkel M, Bierens JJ, Lie RL, et al. Pulmonary oedema, pneumonia and mortality in submersion victims; a retrospective study in 125 patients. *Intens Care Med.* 1996;22:101.
    A retrospective series of 125 victims that evaluates the development of pulmonary edema and the need for hospitalization in near-drowning victims.
43. Zuckerman GB, Gregory PM, Santos-Domaini SM. Predictors of death and neurologic impairment in pediatric submersion injuries. *Arch Pediatr Adolesc Med.* 1998;152:134.
    The most recent of many articles trying to determine factors that can be used to make prognoses on nearly drowned children. Contains 34 references, most of which are to other articles relating to the prognosis of near-drowning victims.

87. AIR TRAVEL AND HIGH-ALTITUDE MEDICINE

Timothy M. Clark

For most people, ascent to high altitude usually means a trip in the pressurized cabin of a commercial airliner. For others, it may come as the swift ride of a ski lift, or the more prolonged exposure of mountaineering. Although the fraction of inspired oxygen (Fio_2) remains relatively constant at any altitude, the partial pressure of inspired oxygen (Pio_2) is directly related to barometric pressure, which is in turn inversely related to elevation above sea level. Thus, for persons with lung disease, even relatively minor changes in Pio_2 may have important consequences. An ever-growing surge of both air travel and high-altitude sojourns increases the need to understand normal adaptation to altitude, problems that may accompany commercial air travel for patients with limited cardiopulmonary reserve, and issues related to high-altitude exposure and the management and prevention of related complications.

AIR TRAVEL

Most commercial airlines fly at altitudes between 22,000 ft (6,706 m) and 44,000 ft (13,411 m). At those elevations, ambient barometric pressure falls from the normal 760 mm Hg at sea level to between 326 and 140 mm Hg, respectively. This causes a decrease in the Pio_2. ($Pio_2 = (P_B - P_{H_2O}) * (F_IO_2)$, where P_B = ambient barometric pressure and P_{H_2O} = vapor pressure of water in the atmosphere). The result is the equivalent of breathing between 8 and 3% F_IO_2. Compressing ambient air makes commercial travel possible at those altitudes, resulting in a cabin pressure between 627 and 565 mm Hg, or 6,000 (1,829 m) to 8,000 ft (2,438 m), respectively, or an Fio_2 equivalent to 15 and 16% at sea level.

Most healthy persons tolerate such altitude exposure without difficulty and the incidence of known in-flight problems remains low. In-flight complaints were estimated at 260 per 8.7 million passengers during a 6-month period of incoming flights to Los Angeles. Also, 577 deaths per 245 million passengers were reported between 1977 and 1984 by multiple international carriers. The Federal Aviation Administration mandated reporting of in-flight medical kit usage found 2,322 cases among an estimated 900 million passengers between 1986 and 1988. Most (85%) of those were by physician passengers assisting other passengers for complaints of chest pain, loss of consciousness, nausea, vomiting, and dyspnea.

Even with preflight screening, a few problems can be anticipated. One study showed that of 1,115 patients referred for screening, 1,011 were cleared for travel and none had significant in-flight problems. The 104 who did not meet clearance criteria either had unstable disease or violated airline policy such as requiring IV drug therapy. Regardless, recognizing the need for preflight evaluations and management requires some understanding of the risks involved for a variety of specific disease states.

Most patients with chronic obstructive pulmonary disease (COPD) can fly safely with little to no intervention. Nevertheless, there is considerable individual variation. Even the moderate altitudes reached in commercial aircraft can lead to changes in ventilatory function. After 60 minutes at 8,000 ft (2,438 m, Pb = 565 mm Hg), pulmonary function changes reported in both normals and patients with severe COPD include a fall in forced vital capacity (FVC), increase in residual volume, and variable changes in airway resistance. Despite these changes, even patients with severe COPD often fly without difficulty. Only 18.2% of one cohort of 100 such patients flying for a median time of 3 hours over a 28-day period reported symptoms during flight. Complaints were primarily dyspnea, edema, wheezing, and cyanosis. Only two patients requested supplemental oxygen, and none required hospital admission. Other studies have shown similar results.

Pulmonary hypertension also poses a significant risk for air travel, although generally not insurmountable. Because hypoxia is known to induce increases in both pulmonary artery (PA) pressure and pulmonary vascular resistance, patients should be carefully selected and evaluated before travel. These patients may be limited by an inability to increase their cardiac output sufficiently to meet an increased demand, and even a mild increase in the level of hypoxia could mean a substantial increase in PA pressure.

Although some authors, including the Aerospace Medical Association, state that severe pulmonary hypertension is an absolute contraindication to flight, this may actually be a relative contraindication. Most authors agree that patients with mild to moderate pulmonary hypertension can travel with between 2 and 4 L/min of supplemental oxygen, and continue all medications including anticoagulation. At the University of California, San Diego, where many patients with pulmonary hypertension fly for medical care, adverse outcomes have been rare as long as supplemental oxygen was used, even with mean PA pressures approaching systemic values. A study of patients referred for transplant or pulmonary thromboendarterectomy, all with severe hypoxemia or pulmonary hypertension (mean PA pressure of at least 30 mm Hg), found that all but one arrived safely at destinations ranging 4 to 21 hours away. The one patient who died was mechanically ventilated with an FiO_2 of 80% and was hemodynamically unstable.

Other pulmonary disorders warrant special consideration. Asthma, among the most common pulmonary diagnoses reported to have exacerbations during flight, can often be managed with the usual medications. Patients with severe disease, such as those requiring frequent oral corticosteroids, may require a pulse of steroids prior to flight. The presence of pneumothorax is an absolute contraindication to air travel; recommendations are to wait at least 2 to 3 weeks after resolution before flying. Any air in the chest cavity, such as that following thoracic surgery for any reason, should follow the same guidelines, because the decreased pressure of even moderate altitude may cause expansion and a life-threatening tension pneumothorax.

Anticoagulation is also strongly encouraged for patients at risk for development of deep vein thrombosis (DVT) or pulmonary embolism (PE). Commercial air travel is a well-known risk factor for DVT, accounting for up to 10% of all cases. Extrinsic risk factors include immobility, dehydration, increased venous pressure from cramped seating, endothelial damage from seat edges, and hemoconcentration from fluid shifts to the interstitial space from decreased cabin pressure. Intrinsic risk factors that contribute to the development of DVT from air travel include history of DVT or PE, post-thrombotic syndromes, malignancy, pregnancy, and chronic venous insufficiency.

High-risk patients should be treated with compression stockings and either warfarin or subcutaneous heparin before and after travel.

Finally, cardiac issues comprise the bulk of in-flight medical problems—and many pulmonary patients have limited cardiac reserve. Moderate hypobaric hypoxia, such as that occurring during flight, increases heart rate and cardiac output (stroke volume remains relatively constant). Patients with baseline hypoxemia or respiratory muscle weakness may decompensate as a result of acute exposure to moderate altitude. Similar to primary pulmonary problems, however, most stable cardiac disorders do not preclude flight. In most cases, a brief waiting period of several weeks is likely to suffice to prove stability of disease. For example, stable angina requires little if any change in management. For patients with more severe angina, such as chest pain with minimal exertion, supplemental oxygen should be considered. Compensated congestive heart failure, even classes 3 and 4, follows the same guidelines. Per current recommendations, myocardial infarction (MI) requires 3 weeks of recovery and evidence of stable disease with exercise before travel, and complicated MI requires 6 weeks before clearance.

Decompensated heart failure and unstable angina are considered absolute contraindications to air travel by the Aerospace Medical Association. Other cardiac disorders that exclude travel by commercial airliner include (1) uncontrolled systemic hypertension, (2) less than 2 weeks following coronary artery bypass grafting, percutaneous transvenous coronary angioplasty, or cerebral vascular accident, (3) poorly controlled supraventricular or ventricular tachycardias, (4) Eisenmenger's syndrome, and (5) severe symptomatic valvular disease.

Supplemental oxygen can often circumvent most barriers to flight among patients with limited cardiopulmonary function. The ground-level PaO_2 has been the most useful predictor for which patients require supplemental oxygen in flight. Oxygen should be considered for patients with a sea level PaO_2 of less than 70 mmHg. For those with a PaO_2 more than 70 mmHg, a number of preflight evaluations have been used to predict the oxygen requirement for the airborne patient with COPD. Some authors suggest simply adding 2 L/min of flow to baseline requirements to keep the PaO_2 above 50 mmHg. Others use more complicated prediction equations. Such equations should be used with caution, because they are derived from specific populations. More subjective issues such as cardiopulmonary reserve or muscle weakness are not included in the equations. Prediction equations also tend to overestimate PaO_2 values for healthy controls. Below is one such equation that resulted in a high predictive value ($r^2 = 0.99$, p < .001) at moderate altitude:

$$PaO_2 \text{ alt} = 0.19(FEV_1 * PaO_2 \text{ grnd}) - 11.51[\ln(\text{max alt} - \text{grnd alt})]$$

where PaO_2 alt = PaO_2 at expected altitude achieved, PaO_2 grnd = PaO_2 at baseline elevation, ln = natural log, max alt = maximum altitude achieved in meters, and grnd alt = baseline elevation in meters.

The hypoxia-altitude simulation test (HAST) can also assist in assessing oxygen demands for patients with a sea-level PaO_2 between 60 and 70 mmHg. This test, which requires a pulmonary function laboratory and trained personnel, involves breathing hypoxic gas mixtures that simulate the altitude of a commercial aircraft (either 17.1% or 15.0% F_IO_2). The test has been validated by both comparing PaO_2 values between normobaric hypoxia and hypobaric hypoxia, as well as comparing sea-level arterial blood gases with those in flight in a nonpressurized cabin. The test allows for subjective variation in hypoxic response, but does not account for any changes from exercise, acceleration, humidity, or temperature.

In summary, few medical problems occur during flight, and most can be circumvented with supplemental oxygen. The moderate altitude achieved in a pressurized aircraft cabin can affect lung function, but rarely significantly enough to produce clinically important sequelae. Patients with a resting PaO_2 less than 70 mmHg at sea level should use supplemental oxygen, usually 2 L/min flow above baseline requirements. For persons with less clear indications for oxygen, the HAST or several prediction equations can serve as a guideline for oxygen therapy.

HIGH-ALTITUDE ILLNESS

Altitudes exceeding those typically simulated by pressurized cabins can produce a unique set of disorders that range from benign to fatal. Fortunately, the more serious problems arise with considerable less frequency. However, increasingly publicized accidents in remote locales reflect a surge of interest in high-altitude adventure and altitude-related disorders. Although most of these represent 12,000,000 annual skiers, increasing numbers of people are adventuring into extreme environments at altitudes exceeding 14,000 ft (4,267 m).

Ski resorts constitute the bulk of recreational destinations at high altitude, and many are located above 9,842 ft (3,000 m), at which people frequently arrive rapidly from low altitudes. There are also commercial activities at altitudes such as 19,520 ft (5,950 m) in Chile and 13,779 ft (4,200 m) at the Mauna Kea Observatory in Hawaii. Some 6,000 people climb Mt. Rainier at 14,408 ft (4,392 m) per year, and 800 climb Denali, the highest peak in North America at 20,320 ft (6,193 m). Nearly 50% of all travelers to these altitudes experience some symptoms of mountain sickness. Reports have noted that 66% of climbers on Mt. Rainier, 47% on Mt. Everest, and 30% on Denali develop symptoms of altitude illness.

Factors contributing to the development of altitude-related illnesses include maximum altitude achieved, rate of ascent, level of exercise, viral illnesses, alcohol consumption, sleep-enhancement drugs, and individual susceptibility. Other factors may include age and gender. Considerable evidence suggests that the incidence of mountain sickness increases substantially above about 10,000 ft (3,000 m) and with rates of ascent greater than approximately 1,000 ft (300 m) per day. A number of extrinsic factors may also contribute by way of lowering barometric pressure. Latitude, temperature, low-pressure storm systems, and winter season may result in lower barometric pressure than expected and, therefore, predispose to altitude-related illness.

Ascent to high altitude can produce a continuum of altitude-related illnesses including acute mountain sickness (AMS) and two uncommon, but potentially fatal, complications, high-altitude pulmonary edema (HAPE) and high-altitude cerebral edema (HACE). A number of other altitude disorders can arise, but exceed the scope of this review. These include snow blindness, retinal hemorrhages, hypothermia, and high-altitude flatus expulsion (a serious concern for climbers trapped in the closed confines of a tent during inclement weather), and problems associated with chronic exposure.

Acute adaptation to high altitude is similar to that discussed at moderate altitude. At higher altitudes, FVC declines by about 4% at 15,000 ft (4,572 m) and about 13% at 29,000 ft (8,839 m), probably due to increases in interstitial edema. Other changes occurring as a result of acute exposure include increased minute ventilation and decreased lung compliance. At rest, ventilation/perfusion matching becomes more homogenous but probably worsens with exercise. Diffusion limitation becomes a major determinant to adaptation, especially at extreme altitudes. Hemodynamically, cardiac output and cerebral blood flow increase, as does pulmonary vascular resistance from hypoxia-induced vasoconstriction. Although hemoglobin concentrations rise within 1 to 2 days from hemoconcentration, the role of oxygen affinity remains unclear (increases in 2,3-diphosphoglycerate may be offset by a respiratory alkalosis resulting from increased ventilation). Finally, acute hypobaric hypoxia results in a proportional significant decrease in maximum oxygen consumption and exercise performance.

AMS represents the most common altitude-related illness. Symptoms may appear immediately on arrival at altitude, or develop as many as 3 days after ascent, and usually resolve spontaneously. Among the chief complaints are headache, occurring in as many as 70% of visitors above 8,000 ft (2,438 m). Sleep-disordered breathing (e.g., Cheyne-Stokes respirations) and poor sleep are also quite common and may contribute to worsening disease. Other symptoms of AMS include nausea, vomiting, dyspnea, peripheral edema, malaise, anorexia, and fatigue. There are no specific laboratory markers of AMS, leaving the diagnosis to historical details in the appropriate setting.

The mechanism behind AMS is likely multifactorial. Chief among them are hypobaric hypoxia and individual response to the insult. Many, though not all, persons suffering from AMS have been found to have relatively low hypoxic ventilatory responses. In addition, many people experience an alteration in body fluid mechanics with retention and redistribution. Evidence also continues to mount suggesting increased cerebral blood flow and, possibly, capillary leak mediated by hypoxia-induced growth factors.

The self-limited nature of AMS usually requires only conservative management, even allowing for continued ascent after brief recovery periods. Prevention plays an important role as well, if feasible (e.g., among rescue workers). A gradual rate of ascent (less than 1,000 ft/d above 10,000 ft), avoidance of alcohol and other soporifics, and both acetazolamide and dexamethasone have all been shown to prevent AMS. Gingko biloba recently showed promise as well, but subsequent studies have failed to prove benefit. Treatment of AMS consists primarily of symptomatic measures, using acetaminophen or nonsteroidal anti-inflammatory drugs for headache or antiemetics (preferably prochloperazine because it increases hypoxic ventilatory response). For refractory or more severe cases, further ascent should be postponed and descent of at least 1,000 ft (300 m) considered. Alternatively, sulfa-based acetazolamide has an established track record for both treatment and prevention. Most authors suggest either 500 mg of a long-acting preparation taken orally once daily or 250 mg taken orally twice daily, until symptoms resolve. Dexamethasone has also been successful in treating symptoms of AMS, usually at doses of 4 mg every 6 hours (some suggest a loading dose of 8 mg). Failure to resolve after 1 to 2 days of conservative or medical management could indicate progression to HAPE or HACE and require prompt attention, usually descent by whatever means possible, including helicopter evacuation as necessary.

Despite a considerably lower incidence of HAPE (between about 2 and 15%), the disorder carries a risk of potentially serious outcomes. As with AMS, HAPE typically occurs in young, fit men ascending rapidly to sleeping altitudes above 2,500 m, more commonly after the second night at altitude. The pathogenesis, although not fully understood, likely involves a variety of changes in the pulmonary vascular system. Among them are hypoxia-induced vasoconstriction, hypertrophy of vascular muscle layers, altered pulmonary hemodynamics and blood flow heterogeneity, and increased capillary permeability. These changes lead to extravasation of proteins, blood, and fluid from the pulmonary capillaries into interstitial tissue and alveolar units, causing a potentially cascading scenario of worsening inflammation and alveolar flooding.

Clinically, patients with HAPE invariably have symptoms of AMS, but will also have progressive dyspnea on exertion or at rest, and, initially, a nonproductive cough that may progress to pink frothy sputum. Signs include increasing tachypnea, tachycardia, and cyanosis. Rales typically arise first in the right midaxillary line and spread diffusely with worsening disease, especially while sleeping. Chest radiographs reveal diffuse patchy infiltrates, with prominence of pulmonary arteries. Notably absent are Kerley B lines or other evidence of pulmonary venous congestion, because pulmonary capillary wedge pressures remain normal.

HAPE is the most common cause of death due to altitude-related illnesses, and, therefore, requires immediate treatment. Numerous studies have attempted to delineate methods to prevent HAPE as well, but only AMS prevention strategies have been advocated until recently. A 2002 study showed a significant improvement in HAPE prevention using the long-acting β-agonist salmeterol. The authors speculated that improved alveolar clearance of fluids may explain the decreased incidence of HAPE among previously susceptible climbers. Descent remains the most important aspect of successful treatment of HAPE, with most authors recommending 2,000 to 3,000 ft (600 to 1,000 m). Supplemental oxygen also plays a major role in the treatment of HAPE, if available. However, HAPE victims are often unable to descend secondary to their physical condition or poor weather. In these cases, the calcium-channel blocker nifedipine is suggested at doses of 20 mg orally every 6 hours for 1 to 2 days. Portable hyperbaric chambers (e.g., the Gamow bag) can also simulate a descent of about 1,476 ft (450 m), but are usually only found on large expeditions to very remote destinations.

HACE occurs even more rarely than HAPE, but may be a harbinger of death. Symptoms indicating HACE include worsening ataxia, changes in level of consciousness, coma, severe lassitude, seizures, cranial nerve palsies, retinal hemorrhages, cyanosis, and hallucinations superimposed on symptoms of AMS or HAPE. Studies have shown elevated cerebral spinal fluid pressures (up to 300 mmHg). Autopsies have also often revealed clinically indolent pulmonary edema. The disorder requires prompt recognition and immediate descent, if possible. In addition, dexamethasone and oxygen remain important adjuncts. Dexamethasone is often given in doses of 4 mg, intravenously, intramuscularly, or orally, followed by 4 mg every 6 hours. Portable hyperbaric chambers are also useful, when available.

In summary, increasing numbers of persons are traveling to high altitude for a variety of reasons. Many of these persons suffer symptoms of mild altitude illness, usually AMS. A few will experience HAPE or HACE, which require prompt attention and descent to prevent life-threatening progression.

Air Travel
1. Aerospace Medical Association, Air Transport Medicine Committee. Medical guidelines for air travel. *Aviat Space Environ Med.* 1996;67:B1–B16.
   A comprehensive monograph of current recommendations regarding air travel for the most common disease states thought to be potentially exacerbated by commercial aviation. Thoroughly referenced.
2. Gong HJ. Air travel and oxygen therapy in cardiopulmonary patients. *Chest.* 1992;101:1104–1113.
   A concise review of flight pathophysiology, medical clearance procedures, and in-flight oxygen issues.
3. Gong HJ, Mark JA, Cowan MN. Preflight medical screenings of patients. Analysis of health and flight characteristics. *Chest.* 1993;104:788–794.
   Analysis of patient characteristics referred for preflight screening based on 1,115 patients mostly referred for in-flight oxygen use.
4. Rosenberg CA, Pak F. Emergencies in the air: problems, management, and prevention. *J Emerg Med.* 1997;15:159–164.
   Reviews the incidence of in-flight emergencies, the onboard medical kit, and some in-flight medical problems and treatments.
5. Dillard TA, Beninati WA, Berg BW. Air travel in patients with chronic obstructive pulmonary disease. *Arch Intern Med.* 1991;151:1793–1795.
   A prospective study of the frequency and outcome of air travel among a cohort of military COPD patients. The authors noted an 18.9% annual frequency of air travel with an 18.2% incidence of transient in-flight complaints.
6. Dillard TA, Rosenberg AP, Berg BW. Hypoxemia during altitude exposure. A meta-analysis of chronic obstructive pulmonary disease. *Chest.* 1993;103:422–425.
   Prospective study using altitude simulation chamber to predict in-flight PaO_2 among patients with severe COPD using sea-level PaO_2 and FEV_1.
7. Schwartz JS, Bencowitz HZ, Moser KM. Air travel hypoxemia with chronic obstructive pulmonary disease. *Ann Intern Med.* 1984;100:473–477.
   Correlation between 17% oxygen arterial blood gas and direct measurement in unpressurized cabin at 5,000 ft (1,650 m) in patients with severe COPD. Validates HAST in this cohort.
8. Vohra KP, Klocke RA. Detection and correction of hypoxemia associated with air travel. *Am Rev Respir Dis.* 1993;148:1215–1219.
   Used Venturi device to assess in flight oxygen requirement in COPD patients.
9. Cramer D, Ward S, Geddes D. Assessment of oxygen supplementation during air travel. *Thorax.* 1996;51:202–203.
   Used body plethysmograph to determine in-flight oxygen requirements for normals and those with either obstructive or restrictive lung disease. The authors found that 2 to 3 L/min supplemental O_2 corrected PaO_2 values obtained in 15% F_IO_2 to that obtained in room air in all subjects.
10. Mercer A, Brown JD. Venous thromboembolism associated with air travel: a report of 33 patients. *Aviat Space Environ Med.* 1998;69:154–157.
    Recent chart review of 134 patients admitted for DVT. Among them, air travel was the only risk factor for 12 subjects (36%); all experienced at least 4 hours of flight time within the preceding 31 days prior to admission.
11. Gong HJ, Tashkin DP, Lee EY, et al. Hypoxia-altitude simulation test. Evaluation of patients with chronic airway obstruction. *Am Rev Respir Dis.* 1984;130:980–986.

Classic study outlining design and validation of simulation test using hypoxic gas mixtures. The authors also derived a regression equation and nomogram to estimate Pao$_2$ at altitudes between 5,000 to 10,000 feet in patients with normocapnic COPD.

12. Dillard TA, Berg BW, Rajagopal KR, et al. Hypoxemia during air travel in patients with chronic obstructive pulmonary disease. *Ann Intern Med.* 1989;111:362–367.
    Increased sensitivity of in-flight Pao$_2$ prediction equation by combining FEV$_1$ with ground-level Pao$_2$ in hypobaric chamber in patients with severe COPD (FEV$_1$ 31 ± 10% of predicted) to aid in supplemental oxygen requirement prediction.

13. Berg BW, Dillard TA, Rajagopal KR, et al. Oxygen supplementation during air travel in patients with chronic obstructive lung disease. *Chest.* 1992;101:638–641.
    The authors outline the capability of oxygen delivery devices to increase Pao$_2$ to levels sufficient for tissue oxygenation in severe COPD patients during acute moderate simulated altitude exposure (8,000 ft, 2,438 m).

14. Dillard TA, Rajagopal KR, Slivka WA, et al. Lung function during moderate hypobaric hypoxia in normal subjects and patients with chronic obstructive pulmonary disease. *Aviat Space Environ Med.* 1998;69:979–985.
    The authors found a slight change in FVC in some, but not all, normals and COPD patients following exposure to a simulated 8,000 ft (2,438 m).

15. Kramer MR, Jakobson DJ, Springer C, et al. The safety of air transportation of patients with advanced lung disease. Experience with 21 patients requiring lung transplantation or pulmonary thromboendarterectomy. *Chest.* 1995;108:1292–1296.
    Outcomes of patients traveling by air with severe lung disease.

16. Naughton MT, Rochford PD, Pretto JJ, et al. Is normobaric simulation of hypobaric hypoxia accurate in chronic airflow limitation? *Am J Respir Crit Care Med.* 1995;152:1956–1960.
    Study showing no significant difference between normobaric and hypobaric hypoxia altitude simulation tests.

17. Gong HJ. Advising patients with pulmonary diseases on air travel. *Ann Intern Med.* 1989;111:349–351.
    Editorial with practical advice.

High-Altitude Medicine

1. Hackett PH, Roach RC, Sutton JR. High altitude medicine. In: Auerbach PS, Geehr EC, eds. *Management of Wilderness and Environmental Emergencies,* 2nd ed. St. Louis: CV Mosby; 1989:1–34.
    Textbook chapter with comprehensive review of adaptation, pathophysiology, and altitude-related illnesses. Includes practical advice and thorough references.

2. Schoene RB, Hornbein TF. High altitude adaptation. In: Murray JF, Nadel JA, eds. *Textbook of Respiratory Medicine,* 2nd ed. Philadelphia: W.B. Saunders Company; 1987:196–220.
    Textbook chapter detailing the physiology of adaptation to high altitude. Very thorough with extensive references.

3. Hultgren HN, Spickard WB, Hellriegel K, et al. High altitude pulmonary edema. *Medicine.* 1961;40:289–313.
    First detailed account and classic characterization of the disorder.

4. Houston CS. Operation Everest one and two. Studies of acclimatization to simulated high altitude. *Respiration.* 1997;64:398–406.
    Review of the classic physiologic studies of acclimatization conducted first on Mt. Everest and later in a hypobaric altitude simulation chamber with comprehensive analysis of the results.

5. Wagner PD, Sutton JR, Reeves JT, et al. Operation Everest II: pulmonary gas exchange during a simulated ascent of Mt. Everest. *J Appl Physiol.* 1987;63:2348–2359.
    Classic physiologic study showing increasing ventilation-perfusion mismatch with long-term exposure to both altitude and exercise, thought to be related to interstitial edema because of the relationship to pulmonary arterial pressure.

6. Hackett PH, Rennie D, Grover RF, et al. Acute mountain sickness and the edemas of high altitude: a common pathogenesis? *Respir Physiol.* 1981;46:383–390.

   Study of Nepal trekkers looking at body weight correlations with AMS symptom scores as a gauge of fluid retention. The authors conclude that rapid ascent combined with fluid retention may identify a common pathogenesis for peripheral, pulmonary, and cerebral edema.

7. Schoene RB. Control of ventilation in climbers to extreme altitude. *J Appl Physiol.* 1982;53:886–890.

   Study comparing ventilatory responses to hypoxia between mountaineers, middle- and long-distance runners, and controls. The authors concluded that extreme high-altitude climbers may succeed because of an enhanced ventilatory response to hypoxia.

8. Schoene RB, Lahiri S, Hackett PH, et al. Relationship of hypoxic ventilatory response to exercise performance on Mount Everest. *J Appl Physiol.* 1984;56:1478–1483.

   Study examined the change in ventilation at sea level, 5,400 m, and 6,300 m. The authors conclude that hypoxic ventilatory response (HVR) predicts exercise ventilation at sea level and high altitude; that the drop in $SaO_2\%$ that occurs with exercise is inversely related to HVR; and persons with a high HVR may perform better at extreme altitude.

9. Hackett PH, Rennie D, Hofmeister SE, et al. Fluid retention and relative hypoventilation in acute mountain sickness. *Respiration.* 1982;43:321–329.

   Study showing correlation between fluid retention and AMS scores in 42 healthy subjects between Katmandu, Nepal (4,518 ft, 1,377 m) and Pheriche (13,921 ft, 4,243 m) within 6 days of exposure.

10. Eldridge MW, Podolsky A, Richardson RS, et al. Pulmonary hemodynamic response to exercise in subjects with prior high-altitude pulmonary edema. *J Appl Physiol.* 1996;81:911–921.

    The authors develop a multiple regression analysis showing a greater pulmonary arterial pressure reactivity to exercise in HAPE-susceptible compared to controls at sea level. The response, however, was not affected by ascent to an altitude of 3,810 m, suggesting an intrinsic pattern among HAPE-susceptible individuals.

11. Podolsky A, Eldridge MW, Richardson RS, et al. Exercise-induced VA/Q inequality in subjects with prior high-altitude pulmonary edema. *J Appl Physiol.* 1996;81:922–932.

    The authors found a higher exercise-induced ventilation-perfusion mismatch (assessed by log standard deviation of perfusion distribution) at sea level, but not at 3,810 m, among HAPE-susceptible individuals.

12. Schoene RB, Hackett PH, Henderson WR, et al. High-altitude pulmonary edema. Characteristics of lung lavage fluid. *JAMA.* 1986;256:63–69.

    Classic description showing elevated total proteins and products of inflammation in lung lavage fluid among patients with HAPE. Direct evidence characterizing HAPE as a high-permeability, rather than hydrostatic, form of pulmonary edema.

13. Hackett PH, Rennie D. The incidence, importance, and prophylaxis of acute mountain sickness. *Lancet.* 1976;2:1149–1155.

    Landmark study of AMS and prevention with gradual ascent or acetazolamide.

14. Johnson TS, Rock PB, Fulco CS, et al. Prevention of acute mountain sickness by dexamethasone. *N Engl J Med.* 1984;310:683–686.

    Key study documenting effectiveness of dexamethasone versus placebo in preventing AMS in a simulated ascent to 15,000 ft (4,570 m) as determined by questionnaire.

15. Hornbein TF, Townes BD, Schoene RB, et al. The cost to the central nervous system of climbing to extremely high altitude. *N Engl J Med.* 1989;321:1714–1719.

    Landmark study of neurobehavioral changes after either actual or simulated ascent to altitudes between 18,005 ft (5,488 m) and 29,028 ft (8,848 m) at 1 to 30 days. The authors found a decline in visual long-term memory and twice as many aphasic errors compared to controls. Interestingly, both correlated with a more vigorous ventilatory response to hypoxia after returning to lower elevations.

16. Severinghaus JW. Hypothetical roles of angiogenesis, osmotic swelling, and ischemia in high-altitude cerebral edema. *J Appl Physiol*. 1995;79:375–379.

   Thorough discussion of potential role of vascular endothelial growth factor in the pathogenesis of HACE.

17. Honigman B, Theis MK, Koziol-McLain J, et al. Acute mountain sickness in a general tourist population at moderate altitudes. *Ann Intern Med*. 1993;118:587–592.

   Documents incidence of altitude-related disorders among cohort of travelers to Colorado sleeping between 6,300 and 9,700 ft (1,920 and 2,957 m).

18. Gilbert DL. The first documented report of mountain sickness: the China or Headache Mountain story. *Respir Physiol*. 1983;52:315–326.

   Detailed historical account of widely believed first documented reports of altitude-related sickness.

88. RADIATION-INDUCED LUNG DISEASE

Mark M. Fuster

Radiotherapy used to treat various thoracic neoplasms frequently injures lung tissue. In such cases, the normal lung is a sensitive innocent bystander in the radiation field. The development of clinical pulmonary syndromes with radiographic infiltrates following exposure to thoracic radiation was first recognized in the early 1920s. The progression of classic radiation pneumonitis, characterized by an acute pneumonitis followed by chronic fibrotic changes, was described in that decade as well.

PATHOPHYSIOLOGY

Acute radiation pneumonitis results from the ability of incident high-energy irradiation to excite electrons in lung tissue near or in the field of the target neoplasm. Free radicals and secondary reactive oxygen species resulting from these electrons can cause intracellular protein denaturation, membrane disruption, and DNA alterations. Immediate pathophysiologic effects of radiation on nongenetic macromolecules, including constituents of endothelial cell membranes and type II cell lamellar bodies (containing surfactant), manifest as dose-related cytotoxicity. Animal models have shown that capillary endothelial disruption occurs within 1 week of radiotherapy. Most symptomatic pulmonary injury, however, results from damage to DNA, and occurs in specific cell types in relation to their respective rates of turnover. Bronchial epithelia are affected early (within days) postradiation, because they have a relatively rapid turnover rate. On the other hand, type I pneumocytes normally are nonproliferating cells; these are replaced by rapidly proliferating type II cells in response to radiation injury. In the first 2 to 3 months after radiation, these changes result in the acute exudative phase of radiation pneumonitis. The nonspecific pathologic changes include endothelial cell swelling, variable capillary occlusion caused by microthrombi, as well as a fibrin-rich exudate (containing sloughed type I cells and acute inflammatory cells) in the interstitial or alveolar spaces. This is accompanied by hyalin-membrane change and decreased surfactant. The endothelial injury can persist for months, and can have profound influence on gas exchange and ventilation–perfusion matching.

Inflammatory cells in the acute phase of radiation pneumonitis induce a cytokine cascade, which ultimately mediates a host response characterized by fibrosis. The cytokine transforming growth factor-β (TGF-β) appears to play an important role in fibrotic progression—particularly as a signaling mediator between macrophages, type II cells, and collagen-producing fibroblasts. Other important chemotactic effectors for fibroblasts include platelet-derived growth factor and fibronectin. The late, fibrotic phase of radiation pneumonitis develops 6 to 12 months following radiation, with the development of septal fibrosis, capillary loss, and obliteration of gas-exchanging units.

Several radiation-delivery variables affect the degree of lung injury caused by local thoracic irradiation. The most important are related to the radiotherapy program and include dose, fractionation, and volume of lung irradiated. With a single dose of radiation, the dose range required to achieve tumor control significantly overlaps the range for significant toxicity, resulting in a narrow therapeutic window. Fractionation addresses this issue, and allows a several times higher total dose to be delivered over any given area with the same probability of lung injury, provided delivery occurs in installments—typically, daily over several weeks. For example, a single dose of 30 Gy can lead to severe clinical radiation pneumonitis and extensive lung fibrosis, whereas a similar dose given in 15 fractions may induce no clinical effects and minimal fibrotic change confined to the irradiated area. This fractionation allows the therapist to augment total delivered dose. However, for any given fractionation schedule, the effect of increasing total dose on progression to radiation pneumonitis still remains. For instance, pneumonitis is virtually never reported following 20 Gy split into 2 Gy/d, whereas it is common once 35 Gy is delivered with the same fractionation schedule. Delivery of any given dose per schedule over a larger lung volume increases the probability of injury. Also, whereas acute infiltrates are confined to the irradiated volume of lung, some nonclassic out-of-field changes can occur in the nonirradiated lung. Radiation planning with computed tomography (CT) scanning techniques allows for optimization of radiation delivery to the minimal volume. Armstrong has demonstrated 3-D conformal radiotherapy as a technique that can reduce radiation outside the target volume significantly.

A number of clinical risk factors play important roles in the development and progression of radiation pneumonitis. Baseline hypoxemia is a significant risk factor. Other recently identified clinical risk factors include low performance status, smoking history, and comorbid lung disease with reduced baseline pulmonary function. A concern specific to lung neoplasms is atelectasis (or even consolidated lung) encountered near the tumor, which appears to suffer more injury per unit of irradiated volume compared to normal adjacent lung. Drug-related variables also play an important role in radiotherapy for any type of thoracic neoplasm. Chemotherapy can compound radiation toxicity, and clinical data strongly suggest avoidance of concurrent administration of adriamycin or actinomycin D with thoracic radiotherapy. Rather, sequential delivery of these drugs with radiation appears to be the safest option. In high-dose chemotherapy (HDCT)/stem cell rescue protocols, delaying radiotherapy (e.g., >2 months) following HDCT reduces the high associated incidence of pneumonitis. Cisplatin, busulfan, bleomycin, and cyclophosphamide may worsen radiation injury. Interestingly, these drugs have been implicated in recall pneumonitis, whereby drug treatment weeks to months following radiation can precipitate an acute radiation pneumonitis-like syndrome within hours of drug delivery. Furthermore, rapid withdrawal of corticosteroids (often used to treat radiation pneumonitis) following radiotherapy can precipitate a flare of acute radiation pneumonitis.

Historically, the incidence of radiation pneumonitis has been reported using either radiographic data alone, or any combination of clinical, radiographic, and pulmonary physiologic data from case series. In general, symptomatic acute radiation pneumonitis occurs less frequently (range of 1–34% in most series) than radiographic manifestations of radiation pneumonitis (e.g., >50% in several series for Hodgkin's disease, breast cancer, and mesothelioma). Symptomatic radiation pneumonitis, or at least postirradiation radiographic change, is especially prevalent following use of large direct radiation ports. Although most patients (>85% overall) have no clinical sequelae from use of limited radiation ports with modern dosing techniques, most do sustain at least a small degree of eventual fibrotic change on the chest film. Thus, radiation fibrosis frequently occurs in the absence of clinically overt radiation pneumonitis.

CLINICAL PRESENTATION

The clinical features of radiation lung injury can be divided into two syndromes: acute radiation pneumonitis and chronic radiation fibrosis. The onset of acute radiation pneumonitis is insidious, usually occurring 2 to 3 months after the completion of radiation therapy, although cases have been reported as early as 1 month after irradiation. Early onset of symptoms generally correlates with a more severe and protracted course. Symptoms secondary to tumor swelling or necrosis can occur within days, and symptoms reflecting bronchial epithelial alterations can occur within 1 week. The symptoms of acute radiation pneumonitis include cough, dyspnea, and occasional fever or pleuritic chest pain. The cough is typically paroxysmal and minimally productive, with occasional streaky hemoptysis. Dyspnea is usually exertional but can progress rapidly to resting shortness of breath. Physical examination is frequently unremarkable, but crackles, signs of consolidation, and pleural and pericardial rubs have been described. Skin changes usually occur over the irradiated field, but do not correlate with the presence or severity of acute radiation pneumonitis. Patients receiving intraluminal endobronchial irradiation occasionally develop symptomatic radiation bronchitis and bronchial stenosis. The clinical course of acute radiation pneumonitis varies from days to weeks, with resolution common within 1 to 2 months. Rarely, rapid progression to respiratory failure and death has been noted. Radiographic improvement usually lags behind clinical improvement, with eventual fibrotic radiographic changes often remaining.

Radiation fibrosis develops to some degree in all patients who experience acute radiation pneumonitis, but it can appear radiographically in many that do not. If clinical pneumonitis does occur, the severity of radiation fibrosis correlates well with the severity of the pneumonitis episode. Most patients are asymptomatic or have minimal symptoms. On the other hand, in cases of a relatively large degree of pulmonary fibrosis, disease may progress to severe exertional dyspnea and signs of cor pulmonale. In the absence of other underlying lung disease, symptoms tend to be mild when less than 25% of the lung parenchyma is involved. The physical findings of radiation fibrosis are those of interstitial fibrosis with volume loss; specific findings may include inspiratory crackles, elevated hemidiaphragms, cyanosis, clubbing, and elevated venous pressure.

Laboratory findings include modest polymorphonuclear leukocytosis, elevated erythrocyte sedimentation rate, and hypoxemia with a widened alveolar–arterial oxygen gradient. The chest radiograph may show a ground-glass haze or indistinct bronchovesicular markings in the irradiated treatment area. Over time, the infiltrate may progress to nodularity; occasionally it becomes dense and confluent, containing air bronchograms. Most radiographic findings are seen within the borders of the treatment area and have sharp margins correlating with the treatment port (straight-edge effect). This helps to distinguish acute radiation pneumonitis from infection or lymphangitic spread of malignancy, the two most likely alternative entities in the differential diagnosis. Hilar or mediastinal lymphadenopathy, or areas of cavitation, should also prompt a search for such diagnoses. High-resolution CT and magnetic resonance imaging are particularly useful in differentiating these processes. Recent research shows that perfusion abnormalities can precede roentgenographic or physiologic impairment. Perfusion studies using ^{99M}Technetium-labeled macro albumin aggregates and 3-D single photon emission CT scanning (SPECT) can detect such abnormalities in the patient who is symptomatic during the early postirradiation period and can also be used to define areas of good perfusion (in the healthy lung) during preradiation planning. Radiographic progression to fibrosis is characterized by a linear interstitial pattern, volume loss, and often pleural thickening. Pulmonary function tests may show reduced lung volumes, decreased lung compliance, and increased work of breathing during the chronic phase of radiation pneumonitis. Decreased diffusing capacity of lung for carbon monoxide (D_{LCO}) is the most sensitive finding during the 2- to 9-month period postradiation. If the volume of irradiated lung is large, gas exchange abnormalities, including hypercapnia, can be seen as well.

COMPLICATIONS

Several other complications attributed to radiation injury can also occur. Pleural effusions attributed to radiation pneumonitis are characteristically small, asymptomatic, and coincident with the onset of acute radiation pneumonitis. They usually resolve, but some effusions may persist for years. Recurrence or sudden increase in an effusion suggests malignancy or infection. Some less common complications include spontaneous pneumothorax, bronchial obstruction, rib fracture, pericardial effusion (rarely, constrictive pericarditis), superior vena cava syndrome, and tracheoesophageal fistula. Tracheoesophageal fistula leading to aspiration pneumonitis is usually seen in patients irradiated for carcinoma of the esophagus. Cystic and bronchiectatic changes can develop following large volume(s) of irradiation. Finally, involvement in the upper lung zones can mimic tuberculosis, with associated volume loss and occasional pleural thickening.

Other important clinical manifestations of lung irradiation have been described. Radiographic changes have been reported outside the zone of lung irradiation with a variety of clinicopathologic patterns. One such pattern is a migratory form of bronchiolitis obliterans with organizing pneumonia (BOOP). Patients experience the onset of symptomatic migratory infiltrates months, or even years, following irradiation; histology of such infiltrates shows an organizing, granulation-tissue pattern consistent with BOOP. The infiltrates tend to respond well to systemic corticosteroids and do not appear to leave a significant degree of fibrosis after resolution. A particularly important response pattern is generalized lymphocytic alveolitis involving both lungs, despite radiographic findings confined to the zone of initial irradiation. Morgan and others have shown that this out-of-field hypersensitivity type of response, termed *sporadic pneumonitis,* is characterized by significantly elevated bronchoalveolar lavage (BAL) lymphocyte counts from both lungs, and reductions in vital capacity and D_{LCO} in asymptomatic patients. An immunopotentiating effect of thoracic irradiation is suspected, although the molecular steps leading to the apparent T-lymphocyte activation are still under investigation. This response may also explain why postradiation pulmonary symptom severity may appear out of proportion to that expected for the amount of lung volume originally irradiated.

Prevention of radiation pneumonitis is a primary concern in radiation planning. Because curative treatment of most radiosensitive malignancies requires total doses in the range above pulmonary tolerance, the volume of tissue irradiated must be minimized. In patients with limited pulmonary function, symptomatic radiation pneumonitis can develop even when the volume of irradiated lung is limited. The patients at highest risk have hypoxemia or a pretreatment FEV_1 less than 40% of predicted. CT scanning and calculation of a dose volume histogram (DVH) are becoming important modalities to limit toxicity. These tools are valuable in predicting distribution of radiation over lung volume while attempts are made to limit irradiation of healthy lung. Finally, pharmacologic radioprotection has been achieved using angiotensin-converting enzyme inhibitors in animals, although such drugs as yet have no clinical use for humans. Amifostine, however, is a radioprotective agent that is showing some promise in recent human chemoradiation trials.

TREATMENT

Therapy for acute radiation pneumonitis is primarily supportive. Patients who are asymptomatic with radiographic abnormalities do not require therapy. Usual measures for patients who are mildly to moderately symptomatic include the use of cough suppressants, antipyretics, analgesics, and supplemental oxygen when indicated for hypoxemia.

Corticosteroids appear to be most effective at the onset of clinically obvious radiation pneumonitis, and approximately 80% of patients respond with improvement in symptoms. Marked symptomatic relief may be observed with a decrease in cough, chest tightness, and fever along with coincident resolution of hypoxemia and radiographic abnormalities. However, lack of response and continued deterioration despite corticosteroid therapy has been reported. Corticosteroids are usually given in doses of 60 mg/d of prednisone for several weeks, followed by a slow taper. Guidelines for dosing and tapering of corticosteroid therapy are not uniformly established, and no data show that prophylactic corticosteroids are effective in preventing radiation pneumonitis. Some experimental work suggests that nonsteroidal anti-inflammatory drugs may be used in the treatment of radiation pneumonitis. Prophylactic antibiotics are of no use and may predispose patients to infection with aggressive, antibiotic-resistant organisms. Empiric treatment of suspected infection should be guided by culture and other clinical information. Prevention of progression to radiation fibrosis is an area of active research.

1. Movsas B, Raffin JA, Ebstein AH, et al. Pulmonary radiation injury. *Chest.* 1997;111:1061.

    An excellent review of clinical syndromes and pathophysiology of classic radiation pneumonitis, as well as modern radiation planning strategies and key factors predisposing to radiation pneumonitis.
2. McDonald S, Rubin P, Phillips TL, et al. Injury to the lung from cancer therapy: clinical syndromes, measurable endpoints, and potential scoring systems. *Int J Radiat Oncol Biol Phys.* 1995;31:1187.

    A detailed summary of the effects of thoracic radiation on lung cell types at various time-points after radiation. The article also illustrates the role of TGF-β in multicellular interactions initiating and sustaining the fibrogenic process.
3. Moosavi H, McDonald S, Rubin P, et al. Early radiation dose–response in lung: an ultrastructural study. *Int J Radiat Oncol Biol Phys.* 1977;2:921.

    A classic study in dog lungs, revealing that capillary endothelium is the first cell type to sustain damage after thoracic irradiation.
4. Prato FS, Kurdyak R, Saibil EA, et al. Regional and total lung function in patients following pulmonary irradiation. *Invest Radiol.* 1977;12:224.

    Radioxenon techniques, spirometry, and lung volume measurements, indicate the functional value that changed the most following radiation was regional blood flow.
5. Davis SD, Yankelevitz DF, Henschke CL, et al. Radiation effects on the lung: clinical features, pathology, and imaging findings. *AJR.* 1992;159:1157.

    A review focusing on imaging findings.
6. Morgan GW, Breit SN. Radiation and the lung: a reevaluation of the mechanisms mediating pulmonary injury. *Int J Radiat Oncol Biol Phys.* 1995;31:361.

    Includes discussion of the steep dose–response relationship between thoracic irradiation and radiation pneumonitis. The review also discusses the nonclassic bilateral lymphocytic alveolitis response as a generalized hypersensitivity response to radiation-damaged lung.
7. VanDyk J, Keane TJ, Kan S, et al. Radiation pneumonitis following large single-dose irradiation: a reevaluation based on absolute dose to lung. *Int J Radiat Oncol Biol Phys.* 1981;7:461.

    Describes the incidence of radiation pneumonitis in a group of 303 patients, based on absolute dose to lung. The onset of pneumonitis occurred at approximately 7.5 Gy.
8. Mah K, Van Dyk J, Keane T, et al. Acute radiation-induced pulmonary damage: a clinical study on the response to fractionated radiation therapy. *Int J Radiat Oncol Biol Phys.* 1987;13:179.

    Study on dosing or fractionation strategies to minimize radiation lung injury. Summary of a number of dose and fractionation schedules is presented in relation to incidence of radiation lung injury.
9. Emirgil C, Heineman HO. Effects of irradiation of chest on pulmonary function in man. *J Appl Physiol.* 1961;16:331.

    A classic article demonstrating a reduction in lung volumes, diffusing capacity, and lung compliance.
10. Heiken JP, Lee JK, Levitt RG, et al. Radiation fibrosis: differentiation from recurrent tumor by MR imaging. *Radiology.* 1985;156:721.

    Indicates that magnetic resonance imaging can assist in narrowing the differential diagnosis of radiographic–clinical findings after radiation.
11. Ikezoe J, Morimoto S, Takashima S, et al. Acute radiation-induced pulmonary injury: computed tomography evaluation. *Semin Ultrasound CT MR.* 1990;11:409.

    Evaluation of CT and high-resolution CT in radiation lung injury.

12. Monson JM, Stark P, Reilly JJ, et al. Clinical radiation pneumonitis and radiographic changes after thoracic radiation therapy for lung carcinoma. *Cancer.* 1998;82:842.
    Clinical radiation pneumonitis developed in 20% (n = 83) of lung carcinoma patients treated with more than 30 Gy of thoracic radiotherapy. Risk factors included low performance status, comorbid lung disease, smoking history, low pulmonary function values, and the absence of a surgical resection. Posttreatment radiograph changes were common, progressed with time, and often extended outside the radiation treatment field (67%).
13. Pass HI, Mitchell JB, Johnson DH, et al. *Lung Cancer: Principles and Practice.* Philadelphia: Lippincott-Raven; 1996:706.
    A detailed review of the clinical spectrum of radiation lung injury. The scoring criteria for varying degrees of radiation lung injury—early and late effects—are reviewed.
14. Roberts CM, Foulcher E, Zaunders JJ, et al. Radiation pneumonitis: a possible lymphocyte-mediated hypersensitivity reaction. *Ann Intern Med.* 1993;118:696.
    A study demonstrating that in most patients receiving unilateral radiation therapy, a lymphocytic alveolitis develops in both lung fields. The effect is most pronounced in patients developing clinical or symptomatic pneumonitis.
15. Polansky SM, Ravin CE, Prosnitz LR, et al. Pulmonary changes after primary irradiation for early breast carcinoma. *AJR.* 1980;134:101.
    Outlines the patterns of radiographic abnormalities after irradiation for primary breast carcinoma in 37 patients.
16. Speiser BL, Spratling L. Radiation bronchitis and stenosis secondary to high dose rate endobronchial irradiation. *Int J Radiat Oncol Biol Phys.* 1993;85:589.
    Radiation bronchitis and stenosis are clinical entities that are identified in patients undergoing bronchial brachytherapy.
17. Ward WF, Lin PJ, Wong PS, et al. Radiation pneumonitis in rats and its modification by the angiotensin-converting enzyme inhibitor captopril evaluated by high-resolution computed tomography. *Radiat Res.* 1993;135:81.
    Captopril spares acute radiation pneumonitis in rats assessed by high-resolution CT.
18. Nakayama Y, Makino S, Fukuda Y, et al. Activation of lavage lymphocytes in lung injuries caused by radiotherapy for lung cancer. *Int J Radiat Oncol Biol Phys.* 1996;34:459.
    Irradiation can induce accumulation of activated T cells in the lung. Increased expression of immunologic markers on T cells (including HLA-DR and ICAM-1) is noted in this BAL study in postradiotherapy lung cancer patients.
19. King TE. BOOP: an important cause of migratory pulmonary infiltrates? [Editorial]. *Eur Respir J.* 1995;8:193.
    Pearl editorial on case reports of migratory BOOP resulting from thoracic irradiation.
20. Arbetter KR, Prakash UB, Tazelaar HD, et al. Radiation-induced pneumonitis in the "nonirradiated" lung. *Mayo Clin Proc.* 1999;74:27.
    A description of six cases of radiation-induced organizing pneumonitis occurring outside the direct radiation field. Reviews clinical, radiologic, and histologic aspects of this entity.
21. Bayle JY, Nesme P, Bejui-Thivolet F, et al. Migratory organizing pneumonitis "primed" by radiation therapy. *Eur Respir J.* 1995;8:322.
    Two cases of migratory BOOP that presented 4 and 7 months following thoracic radiation for breast cancer. Refer to the editorial by King (reference 19) for a review of the entity.
22. Gibson PG, Bryant DH, Morgan GW, et al. Radiation-induced lung injury: a hypersensitivity pneumonitis? *Ann Intern Med.* 1988;109:288.
    Original case report on bilateral lymphocytic alveolitis following thoracic irradiation for breast cancer. Changes noted on imaging, pulmonary function, and BAL are described in four patients.
23. Abratt RP, Morgan GW. Lung toxicity following chest irradiation in patients with lung cancer. *Lung Cancer.* 2002;35:103.

Updated review describing importance of sporadic pneumonitis as a common generalized lung response to thoracic irradiation. Clinical progression and objective measures of injury are reviewed, and the importance of the DVH as a predictive tool is discussed.

24. Komaki R, Lee JS, Milas L, et al. Effects of amifostine on acute toxicity from concurrent chemotherapy and radiotherapy for inoperable non–small-cell lung cancer: report of a randomized comparative trial. *Int J Radiat Oncol Biol Phys.* 2004;58:1369.
    Promising use of a radioprotective agent (and free-radical scavenger) in a human trial.

25. Armstrong J, McGibney C. The impact of three-dimensional radiation on the treatment of non-small cell lung cancer. *Radiother Oncol.* 2000;56:157.
    Discusses the ability of 3-D radiation therapy to deliver high-dose radiation with minimal underdosing, and concomitant relative sparing of normal tissues in non-small cell lung cancer.

89. DRUG-INDUCED LUNG DISEASE

Shazia M. Jamil

The overall incidence of drug-induced lung disease is unknown. More than 200 medications have been implicated in adverse reactions within the respiratory system. However, almost any medication can cause an adverse pulmonary effect in a so-called idiosyncratic reaction that may have not been reported. It is important for physicians to be aware of all current and past medications, including over-the-counter preparations, vitamins, supplements, ophthalmic solutions, illicit drugs, topical creams, medicinal plants, and ointments (vaginal). Medical records and pharmacy data are particularly helpful in obtaining information about medication identity, doses, and duration of treatment.

The clinical presentation and laboratory findings including chest radiographs, blood and pulmonary function tests, nuclear medicine studies, and even lung biopsies in patients with drug-induced lung disease can be nonspecific. However, these can be helpful in supporting the diagnosis or limiting the differential diagnoses. In the absence of a simple confirmatory test, discontinuation of the putative drug is the first step in both diagnosis and treatment. Unfortunately, the response to discontinuing the drug may not be immediate, and the physiologic and pathologic changes in some cases may be irreversible.

Drug-induced lung disease can be categorized by pathophysiologic and clinical syndromes. In this discussion, each pathophysiologic syndrome is reviewed briefly and includes a description of only the most common and clinically significant drugs. Some drugs cause a variety of pulmonary disorders and are listed in multiple categories.

Aspiration of mineral oil laxatives or an oily eye lubricant is often asymptomatic but typically presents as a chronic infiltrate or nodule in the dependent areas of the lung. Occasionally, a computed tomography (CT) scan may show fat density within the lesion and biopsy may demonstrate oil within the lung parenchyma.

Angioedema is an uncommon fatal complication of angiotensin-converting enzyme inhibitors, and is seen more commonly in obese individuals with a past history of intubation or head and neck surgery. Angioedema is also reported with the use of losartan and paclitaxel (Taxol).

Alveolar hemorrhage has been reported with anticoagulant therapy; when this occurs, the possibility of an underlying pulmonary lesion should be considered. D-Penicillamine may rarely cause a Goodpasture's-like, pulmonary–renal syndrome with alveolar hemorrhage in patients who had received the medication for a long period of time. The presentation is acute, with dyspnea, hemoptysis, and hematuria; however, unlike Goodpasture's syndrome, immunofluorescence of biopsy tissue fails to demonstrate linear deposition of immunoglobulin. Plasmapheresis has been used successfully in a few reported survivors. Some cephalosporin antibiotics are reported to cause alveolar hemorrhage by hypoprothrombinemia, which appears to be a consequence of inhibition of hepatic vitamin K epoxidereductase enzyme. Concurrent therapy with vitamin K, especially in patients receiving parenteral nutrition, helps to prevent this complication. Diffuse alveolar hemorrhage has been reported following smoking of cocaine, use of nitrofurantoin, thrombolytics, sirolimus, and, after multiple intravenous doses of amiodarone.

Bronchospasm can be precipitated by oral, intravenous, or ophthalmic administration of nonselective β-adrenergic antagonists. Timolol ophthalmic solution has been reported to be responsible for more than 100 deaths because of aggravation of asthma or emphysema. Bronchospasm has also been reported with atenolol, which is relatively β_1-selective; therefore, this drug should be avoided if possible in patients with obstructive lung disease. Inhaled ipratropium bromide is the drug of choice in treating the bronchospasm induced by β blockade. Sulfiting agents used as preservatives can provoke bronchospasm in susceptible individuals. Aspirin and other nonsteroidal anti-inflammatory drugs (NSAIDs) are the most common cause of drug-induced bronchospasm (reported in 5–10% of asthmatics). These patients may have aspirin-sensitive asthma, a triad of aspirin sensitivity, nasal polyposis, and asthma. Bronchospasm generally develops within minutes of ingestion. Approximately 8% of asthmatic admissions in the intensive care unit may be precipitated by inadvertent aspirin or other NSAID usage. These agents should be avoided in all patients with moderate to severe persistent asthma. Inert materials in corticosteroid and cromolyn preparations can also cause paradoxical bronchospasm in asthmatics. Drug-induced histamine release from mast cells has been implicated in bronchospasm occurring with morphine and muscle relaxants (D-tubocurarine and atracurium). Slower administration of these intravenous medications or alternative drugs (e.g., fentanyl and vecuronium) should be considered. Bronchospasm can also occur with contrast media injection, cholinesterase inhibitors, aerosolized pentamidine, and protamine.

Bronchiolitis obliterans with organizing pneumonia secondary to drugs is histologically and radiologically indistinguishable from non–drug-induced disease, especially in the case of gold and penicillamine, where distinction from the underlying rheumatic disease may not be possible.

Calcification is a rare complication reported following prolonged treatment with busulfan. Hypervitaminosis D or inorganic phosphorus administration for hypercalcemia can cause metastatic calcification within the lung. Intravenous calcium gluconate has been reported to cause calcifications within the lung. Technetium 99m diphosphonate scans and dual-energy digital chest radiography may help to confirm the diagnosis.

Cough is a recognized complication of all angiotensin-converting enzyme inhibitors; hence, switching from one to another does not help. This cough has been linked to accumulation of bradykinin or tachykinins in the airways with consequent stimulation of vagal afferents. It can take several weeks to resolve after drug withdrawal. Concomitant use of inhaled cromolyn may minimize the cough in some patients. Methotrexate-induced pneumonitis commonly produces a dry cough; therefore, a productive cough warrants search for pulmonary infection; patients on methotrexate are susceptible to opportunistic infections.

Chest pain (acute) during bleomycin infusion has been reported in approximately 3% of patients. Acute chest pain syndrome has also reported with methotrexate therapy. Chest pain, the single most common presenting symptom of patients abusing cocaine, could be caused by bronchial irritation, Valsalva maneuver during inhalation, coronary artery spasm, or myocardial infarction.

Churg–Strauss syndrome has been associated with zafirlukast, a leukotriene receptor antagonist used by asthmatics. It is unclear whether this is secondary to increased case finding in patients receiving a new drug, reduction in corticosteroid doses, or an idiosyncratic reaction.

Granuloma formation has been described with bacillus Calmette–Guerin, methotrexate, nitrosureas, fluoxetine, oil aspiration, and talc. Talc granulomatosis is reported to occur in intravenous drug abusers mixing illicit drugs with talc (magnesium silicate) containing fillers. Talc is identified as strongly birefringent crystals within the granuloma on biopsy.

Hilar adenopathy occurs rarely in association with phenytoin or hydantoin analog (mephenytoin and ethotoin) therapy. Hydantoin-related adenopathy is usually seen 1 to 4 months after initiating therapy and regresses within 1 to 2 weeks after withdrawal of the medication. Hilar adenopathy is a common feature of methotrexate-induced hypersensitivity pneumonitis.

Hypersensitivity reactions are characterized by the acute onset of fever, nonproductive cough, dyspnea, urticaria, arthralgias, and peripheral eosinophilia. Pleuritic chest pain, pulmonary infiltrates, and pleural effusions may be present. A large number of drugs have been implicated, most notably ampicillin, azothioprine, phenytoin, sulfasalazine, and hydrochlorthiazide. The reactions are not dose related. A short course of corticosteroids may promote rapid improvement.

Hypoventilation can be caused by central nervous system (CNS) depression from narcotics, sedatives, anxiolytics or psychotropic medications, and by neuromuscular blockade. The degree of neuromuscular blockade can be tested with a nerve stimulator or, in a cooperative patient, by asking the patient to elevate the head for 5 seconds or more. Neuromuscular blockade is also seen with aminoglycosides, macrolides, and, rarely, calcium channel blockers.

Interstitial lung disease (acute interstitial pneumonitis, chronic pneumonitis, and fibrosis) is a common manifestation of drug-induced lung disease. Diagnosis in an immunocompromised host is challenging because a similar picture can develop with recurrence of underlying disease, metastasis, and opportunistic infections. Drug-induced lung disease from chemotherapeutic agents is almost always associated with fever. Bleomycin can cause pulmonary disease in 10% of patients, of whom 10% die of pulmonary sequelae. Clinically, acute pneumonitis, chronic pneumonitis, and fibrosis are well described. Risk factors for developing lung disease from bleomycin are (1) total dose greater than 400 to 450 mg; (2) increased age; (3) higher inspired oxygen concentrations; (4) radiation therapy; and (5) multidrug cytotoxic regimens. Lung volumes and diffusing capacity (D_{LCO}) should be measured regularly during treatment. Treatment consists of discontinuing the drug, although dramatic responses to steroids have also been reported. Busulfan lung toxicity is usually seen after a total dose of 2 g. Busulfan pulmonary fibrosis often progresses after discontinuation of treatment, does not respond to corticosteroids, and is associated with high mortality. Carmustine (BICNU) lung toxicity is reported with cumulative doses greater than 1,000 mg/m^2. Both carmustine and cyclophosphamide can cause pulmonary fibrosis years after discontinuation.

Amiodarone is a potent phospholipase inhibitor that results in intense cellular phospholipid accumulation. The incidence of drug-induced lung disease is 10 to 15% with mortality of 10 to 20%. Both chronic pneumonitis and fibrosis can occur. Known risk factors are a high maintenance dose (>400 mg/d) and, possibly, preexisting pulmonary disease. Proposed mechanisms include phopholipidosis, altered calcium ion regulation, generation of oxygen species, formation of an amiodarone aryl radical, and perturbation of cellular energy production. Diagnosis can be difficult, even with lung biopsy, because phopholipid-laden lamellar body inclusions in macrophages are seen commonly in all patients on treatment without lung toxicity. CT scanning can be helpful if it shows areas of high attenuation, owing to amiodarone being an iodinated compound. The current approach is to change the antiarrhythmic therapy, if possible, or reduce the dose and treat with corticosteroids. However, because of tissue accumulation, the elimination half-life after discontinuation is 30 to 60 days, requiring a prolonged treatment with corticosteroids.

Gold-induced lung disease is difficult to diagnose in patients with rheumatoid arthritis. Criteria favoring interstitial lung disease from the drug rather than the disease are (1) female gender; (2) fever; (3) peripheral eosinophilia; (4) absence of clubbing and subcutaneous nodules; (5) skin rash; (6) liver dysfunction; (7) bronchioalveolar lavage lymphocytosis with CD4$^+$:CD8$^+$ ratio of less than 1; (8) pleural involvement (rarely); and (9) nonbasilar predominance of lung infiltrates. Complete clinical remission has been reported in 71% of patients following drug discontinuation and treatment with corticosteroids.

Methotrexate is known to cause severe pulmonary toxicity, in both high and low doses used in the treatment of malignancy or rheumatoid arthritis, respectively. Pneumonitis (both hypersensitivity and nonhypersensitivity) and pulmonary fibrosis are described. Low-dose methotrexate is also a risk factor for opportunistic infection leading to pneumonia, *Pneumocystis carinii* being one of the most common. In methotrexate pneumonitis, chest radiographs reveal bilateral, diffuse interstitial and alveolar infiltrates. Bronchioalveolar lavage usually shows a predominance of helper T-cell lymphocytosis and lung biopsy reveals a lymphocytic interstitial pneumonitis, bronchiolitis, and giant cell formation. Treatment is drug discontinuation; high-dose corticosteroids are indicated in severe cases.

Acute nitrofurantoin pneumonitis occurs a few hours to days after initiation of treatment. The chest radiograph usually reveals an asymmetric or unilateral alveolar or interstitial infiltrate, and is often confused with bacterial pneumonia. Chronic nitrofurantoin use is the classic example of noncytotoxic, drug-induced pulmonary fibrosis that is indistinguishable from idiopathic pulmonary fibrosis. Lung disease almost always reverses following discontinuing the drug, although one half of cases may require the addition of corticosteroids.

A Lupus-like syndrome with lung involvement occurs most commonly from procainamide, hydralazine, phenytoin, penicillamine, and isoniazid. Fever, pleuritis, pleural effusions, and arthralgias can occur. Symptoms may develop as early as 1 month or as late as 12 years from the start of treatment. Renal and CNS involvement are rare. Antinuclear antibody (ANA) is usually positive; antihistone antibodies are positive, whereas anti-dsDNA antibody is negative, and complement levels are normal. ANA positivity can persist for several months, but the symptoms usually resolve within 2 months of discontinuing the drug. Steroids may be beneficial.

Mediastinal lipomatosis is an unusual reaction to chronic corticosteroid use. Fat is deposited in the mediastinum, mimicking a mediastinal tumor. A CT scan is helpful in detecting fat rather than tissue density throughout the mediastinum. Tapering steroids is usually not necessary.

Obliterative bronchiolitis without parenchymal involvement has been reported with gold, penicillamine, and amphotericin B.

Pulmonary hypertension has been reported with intravenous and nasal cocaine abuse. Drug-related thrombosis, particulate embolization (talc and starch granules), and talc granulomatosis around pulmonary arterioles can cause pulmonary hypertension. Funduscopic examination reveals a characteristic white, glistening, refractile particle (talc) within the small vessels near the macula in about 50% of these patients. Appetite suppressants fenfluramine and dexfenfluramine have recently been associated with development of pulmonary hypertension, the pathology of which is reminiscent of primary pulmonary hypertension. The use of fenfluramine-related anorexigens for more than 3 months increases the risk of developing pulmonary hypertension about 23 times. The pathogenesis is not entirely clear, but hypotheses have implicated serotonin and direct vasoconstrictor effects of amphetamine-like substances contained in anorexic agents. Recent evidence suggests that persons with relative nitric oxide deficiency may be predisposed to develop pulmonary hypertension. Pulmonary hypertension has also been reported with chronic methamphetamine use. Protamine can cause the acute onset of pulmonary vasoconstriction, leading to pulmonary hypertension and is seen most commonly during heparin reversal therapy following cardiopulmonary bypass surgery.

Pleural effusion, pleural thickening, and pleuritis can occur because of drug-induced serositis, cardiac decompensation with associated pulmonary edema, constrictive pericarditis, pulmonary emboli, or vasculitis. The esophageal variceal sclerotherapeutic agents (sodium morrhuate and absolute alcohol) are common causes of pleural effusions. Pleural effusion is usually right sided and resolves spontaneously within 7 days. The proposed mechanism is transmediastinal inflammation from the esophagus to the mediastinal pleura and pleural space. Drug-induced lupus pleural effusions are exudative, with nucleated cell counts of 200 to 15,000/μL, and may demonstrate a pleural fluid:ANA ratio greater than 1; however, the presence of lupus erythematosus cells is the only diagnostic finding. Drug-induced lupus pleuritis improves rapidly after discontinuing the drug; NSAIDs or a short course of corticosteroids may be beneficial for severe or prolonged symptoms. Pleural fluid eosinophilia (>10% of nucleated cells) is seen with nitofurantoin, dantrolene, valproic acid, propylthiouracil, and isotretinoin.

Pneumothorax and pneumomediastinum have been well documented in crack cocaine abusers as a result of attempting to increase the alveolar–capillary absorption with a Valsalva maneuver. Nitrorsureas are also known to cause pneumothorax.

Pulmonary infiltrates with eosinophilia syndrome is attributed to many drugs. It is similar to Löffler's syndrome, although frequently more severe. Cough and dyspnea, with or without fever, can begin abruptly or insidiously. Chest roentgenograms typically reveal unilateral patchy alveolar infiltrates, which are frequently migratory. Peripheral eosinophilia (4–80%) often peaks as the infiltrate wanes. Recovery occurs rapidly after discontinuation of the offending drug. Steroids may hasten recovery.

Pulmonary nodules have been reported with the use of amiodarone, bleomycin, fludarabine, and mineral oil. In patients with malignancy being treated with bleomycin or fludarabine, such a finding warrants early biopsy and pathologic diagnosis. Amiodarone can also cause mass lesions with cavitations.

Pulmonary edema, both cardiogenic and noncardiogenic (acute lung injury/acute respiratory distress syndrome [ALI/ARDS]), can be induced by a number of drugs. Cancer chemotherapeutic agents clearly associated with ALI/ARDS are cytarabine, interleukin-2, gemcitabine, as well as all-*trans*-retinoic acid (tRA) in acute promyelocytic leukemia patients. Opiates, including heroin, methadone, codeine, buprenorphine, and the narcotic antagonist, naloxone, both in therapeutic doses and in overdose, can cause noncardiogenic edema. Patients typically present with stupor, depressed respiration, and miotic pupils. Prognosis is excellent with supportive care. Aspirin-induced noncardiogenic pulmonary edema almost always occurs with serum levels above 40 mg/dL. Clinical presentation includes acute dyspnea, fever, obtundation, a high anion gap metabolic acidosis, and respiratory alkalosis. The prognosis is good with supportive treatment, and early detection is important to prevent long-term sequelae of salicylate ingestion. Tocolytics, namely terbutaline, albuterol, and ritodrine, have also been reported to cause pulmonary edema. Tocolytic agents are started to halt premature labor and produce vasodilation and increased intravascular volume. It is proposed that on discontinuation and reversal of vasodilation, the lungs may be subjected to a large intravascular volume leading to pulmonary edema. This could be multifactorial as these patients are often also started on intravenous fluids and corticosteroid therapy to accelerate fetal lung maturation. Transfusion-related acute lung injury is a pulmonary leukoagglutinin reaction to sensitized lymphocytes from multiparous female donors. ALI/ARDS occurs within minutes to a few hours of blood transfusion and may be associated with fever, hypotension, and rash. Treatment is supportive and recovery is dramatic, usually within 48 hours to a week. The donor and recipient should be tested for leukoagglutinating antibodies to confirm the diagnosis. Finally, 10 to 25% of patients receiving amiodarone may develop ALI/ARDS in the postoperative period, usually after angiography and cardiothoracic surgery, and typically occurs after 18 to 72 hours. The mechanism is unknown and treatment is supportive.

Septic pulmonary emboli are seen most commonly in intravenous drug users as a consequence of septic thrombophlebitis and right-sided endocarditis caused by contaminated needles.

Pulmonary thromboembolism and deep venous thrombosis occur with increased frequency in patients taking oral contraceptives. The risk is greatest during the first year and is probably associated with other risk factors like smoking.

Pulmonary venoocclusive disease has been reported with carmustin (BICNU), bleomycin, mitomycin, cyclophosphamide, and zinostatin.

Respiratory dyskinesia is an irregular tachypneic pattern of breathing caused by respiratory muscle involvement by the tardive dyskinesia associated with neuroleptic medications. Interestingly, this can occur in the absence of usual dyskinetic movements of tongue, face, and neck. Presentation includes an irregular breathing pattern, tachypnea, and dyspnea that worsens with anxiety and pain. Pulmonary function tests are normal; arterial blood gases show a high PaO_2 and a low $PaCO_2$ and, hence, are usually mistaken for psychogenic hyperventilation. Unfortunately, symptoms may persist after discontinuation of the offending drug.

Pulmonary vasculitis, usually accompanying a systemic vasculitis, has been reported with the use of sulfonamides, penicillin, thiouracil, hydralazine, phenylbutazone, quinidine, promazine, and the hydantoins. Illicit use of intravenous drugs contaminated with insoluble particulates can induce a localized vasculitis when trapped within the lung. Hypersensitivity angiitis can occur from serum sickness (antivenom) or secondary to a drug-induced small vasculitis.

Rare syndromes of drug-induced pulmonary disease include lymphoma from low-dose methotrexate; alveolar proteinosis from busulfan; sarcoidosis with nitrosureas; microangiopathic hemolytic anemia, renal failure, and noncardiogenic pulmonary edema from mitomycin-C; pulmonary manifestations of eosinophilic myalgia syndrome with L-tryptophan ingestion; and noncardiogenic pulmonary edema after intrathecal methotrexate administration.

1. Morelock SY, Sahn SA. Drugs and the pleura. *Chest.* 1999;116:212.
   A retrospective review of literature from 1966 to 1998, identifying drugs associated with pleural disease, and detailing clinical, radiographic, and pleural fluid findings.
2. Cooper Jr JA. Drug-induced lung disease. *Adv Intern Med.* 1997;42:231.
   This review focuses primarily on drugs in which more complete studies have been performed to determine the incidence and pathogenesis of side effects (149 references).
3. Wesselius LJ. Pulmonary complications of cancer therapy. *Compr Ther.* 1999; 25:272.
   An update on the clinically important lung diseases induced by chemotherapy.
4. Rosenow EC III, Limper AH. Drug-induced pulmonary disease. *Semin Respir Infect.* 1995;10:86.
   The article reviews important drugs that cause lung disease, focusing on evaluation of drug-induced lung disease in the immunocompromised host and chemotherapeutic agents.
5. Limper AH, Rosenow EC III. Drug-induced interstitial lung disease. *Curr Opin Pulm Med.* 1996;2:396.
   A review article emphasizing the importance of awareness of all the potential adverse effects of drugs on the lung to prevent a high rate of morbidity and mortality.
6. Cannon GW. Methotrexate pulmonary toxicity. *Rheum Dis Clin North Am.* 1997;23:917.
   This article reviews different types and clinical features of methotrexate-induced pulmonary disease, reports different proposed diagnostic criteria, and suggests a management plan.
7. Worthy S, Kang EY, Muller NL. Acute lung disease in the immunocompromised host: differential diagnosis at high-resolution CT. *Semin Ultrasound CT MR.* 1995;16:353.
   A review of CT findings of complications seen in AIDS and other immunocompromised patients, including drug-induced lung disease, infections, pulmonary hemorrhage, pulmonary edema, Kaposi's sarcoma, and AIDS-related lymphoma.
8. Pisani RJ, Rosenow EC III. Drug-induced pulmonary disease. In: Simmons DH, Tierney DF, eds. *Current Pulmonology.* St. Louis: Mosby Year Book; 1992:13, 311.
   A review of patterns, mechanisms, clinical features, differential diagnosis, and recommendations regarding treatment. Referenced with 218 citations.
9. Hunt Jr LW, Rosenow EC III. Drug-induced asthma. In: Weiss EB, Stein M, eds. *Bronchial Asthma: Mechanisms and Therapeutics.* Boston: Little, Brown, and Company; 1993:621.

This chapter includes a comprehensive list of drugs causing or exacerbating asthma.

10. Rice KL. Pulmonary infiltrates associated with noncytotoxic drugs. *Semin Respir Infect*. 1988;3:229.

    A concise, well-written review with a useful table of noncytotoxic drug-induced lung disease.

11. Zitnik RJ, Cooper Jr JA. Pulmonary disease due to antirheumatic agents. *Clin Chest Med*. 1990;11:139.

12. Goldiner PL, et al. Factors influencing postoperative morbidity and mortality in patients treated with bleomycin. *BMJ*. 1978;1:16648.

    Bleomycin-treated patients who subsequently underwent surgery developed clinically apparent pneumonitis with FiO_2 greater than 0.39. When the FiO_2 was less than 0.24, pneumonitis did not occur.

13. Van Barneveld PWC, et al. Natural course of bleomycin-induced pneumonitis: a follow-up study. *Am Rev Respir Dis*. 1987;135:48.

    Reports on the resolution of radiographic abnormalities and normalization of lung ventilation and perfusion scans in patients with bleomycin-induced pneumonitis with 2 years of diagnosis.

14. Weinstein A. Drug-induced lupus erythematosus. *Prog Clin Immunol*. 1980;4:1.

    A comprehensive, in-depth review of drug-induced lupus erythematosus.

15. Miller Jr WT. Drug-related pleural and mediastinal disorders. *J Thorac Imag*. 1991;6:36.

    Reviews the full range of mediastinal and pleural changes secondary to the toxic effects of drugs.

16. Liebow AA, Carrington CB. The eosinophilic pneumonias. *Medicine* (Baltimore). 1969;48:251.

    A review of pulmonary infiltration with eosinophilia and related drug-induced syndromes.

17. Hertzman PA, et al. The eosinophilic-myalgia syndrome: status of 205 patients and results of treatment 2 years after onset. *Ann Intern Med*. 1995;122:851.

    A multicenter follow-up of 205 patients with this syndrome who were monitored for 18 to 24 months showed that pulmonary symptoms were present in 67% at onset, with 13% manifesting interstitial process; 4% were found to have pulmonary hypertension.

18. Wechsler M, et al. Pulmonary infiltrates, eosinophilia, and cardiomyopathy following corticosteroid withdrawal in patients with asthma receiving zafirlukast. *JAMA*. 1998;279:455.

19. Nicolls MR, et al. Diffuse alveolar hemorrhage with underlying pulmonary capillaritis in the retinoic acid syndrome. *Am J Respir Crit Care Med*. 1998;158:1302.

    A case report and discussion of alveolar hemorrhage and other pulmonary toxicity caused by all-trans-retinoic acid.

20. Archer SL, et al. Nitric oxide deficiency in fenfluramine and dexfenfluramine-induced pulmonary hypertension. *Am J Respir Crit Care Med*. 1998;158:1061.

    A prospective case-control study in patients diagnosed with anorexigenic-induced pulmonary hypertension, demonstrating that nitric oxide deficiency may play a role in the pathogenesis.

21. Massey TE, et al. Mechanisms in the pathogenesis of amiodarone-induced pulmonary toxicity. *Can J Physiol Pharmacol*. 1995;73:1675.

    An excellent review that examines the experimental model systems used to study amiodarone toxicity and summarizes the current state of knowledge regarding the processes.

22. Angle P, et al. Bronchiolitis obliterans with organizing pneumonia and cold agglutinin disease associated with phenytoin hypersensitivity syndrome. *Chest*. 1997;112:1697.

    This is the first case report identifying this type of pneumonia in a patient with hypersensitivity reaction to phenytoin.

23. Tomioka R, King Jr TE. Gold-induced pulmonary disease; clinical features, outcome, and differentiation from rheumatoid lung disease. *Am J Respir Crit Care Med*. 1997;155:1011.

A review of cases of gold-induced pulmonary toxicity, and analysis of diagnostic criteria, outcome, and clinical features distinguishing it from rheumatoid arthritis-induced lung disease.

24. Iskander S, Raible DG, Brosena SC, et al. Acute alveolar hemorrhage and orthodeoxia induced by intravenous amiodarone. *Catheter Cardiovasc Interv.* 1999;47:61.

    A case report followed by a review of literature describing pulmonary hemorrhage after multiple intravenous boluses of amiodarone to treat ventricular tachycardia.

25. Mecker DP, Wiedemann HP. Drug-induced bronchospasm. *Clin Chest Med.* 1990;11:163.

26. Dunn TL, et al. The effect of topical ophthalmic instillation of timolol and betaxolol on lung function in asthmatic subjects. *Am Rev Respir Dis.* 1986;133:264.

    Betaxolol ophthalmic instillation was well tolerated in eight timolol-sensitive patients.

27. Sebastian JL, et al. Angiotensin-converting enzyme inhibitors and cough: prevalence in an outpatient medical clinic population. *Chest.* 1991;99:36.

28. Briasoulis E, Pavlidis N. Noncardiogenic pulmonary edema: an unusual and serious complication of anticancer therapy. *Oncologist.* 2001;6:153.

29. Cooke CR, Hyland JW. Pathological calcification of the lungs following intravenous administration of calcium. *Am J Med.* 1960;29:363.

    Calcification occurred after the patient received a large amount of both calcium and vitamin K.

30. Murray RJ, et al. Diffuse alveolar hemorrhage temporally related to cocaine smoking. *Chest.* 1988;93:427.

31. Cuellar ML. Drug induced vasculitis. *Curr Rheumatol Rep.* 2002;4:55.

32. Heitzman ER. Lymphadenopathy related to anticonvulsant therapy: roentgen findings simulating lymphoma. *Radiology.* 1967;89:311.

    Extremely rare complication of a commonly prescribed medication.

33. Eramus JJ, et al. Drug-induced lung injury. *Semin Roentgenol.* 2002;37:72.

    Discusses radiological findings of drug-induced lung injury, including pulmonary edema, bronchiolitis obliterans with organizing pneumonia, and pulmonary hemorrhage, among many others.

X. IDIOPATHIC, IMMUNOLOGIC, AND GRANULOMATOUS DISEASES

90. SARCOIDOSIS

Antine E. Stenbit

Sarcoidosis is a multisystem, noncaseating granulomatous disease affecting people worldwide of all races, ages, and genders. It predominantly affects adults ages 20 to 40; patients older than 40 have a more chronic form and worse prognosis. The presentation of sarcoidosis varies from an incidental finding on a routine chest radiograph in an asymptomatic individual to life threatening cardiac or neurologic disease. An international consensus conference in 1999 proposed the adoption of standard diagnostic criteria for the assistance of clinical evaluation and standardization of research. The criteria include the presence of typical radiographic and clinical findings, histopathologic evidence of noncaseating granulomas as well as the exclusion of other known causes of granulomatous disease. The epidemiology of sarcoidosis remains problematic because of its variable presentation, diverse prevalence, and insensitive and nonspecific diagnostic tests. In the U.S., sarcoidosis has a higher prevalence among African-Americans, especially in women. Sarcoidosis also occurs more frequently in Scandinavia and in Irish women in England. Several epidemiologic studies have shown temporal, seasonal, and geographic clustering of sarcoidosis cases, suggesting a common etiologic origin; however, after years of study and improved diagnostic criteria, the etiology of sarcoidosis remains elusive.

PATHOPHYSIOLOGY

Most experts believe that sarcoidosis develops from a complex interplay between causative organisms (e.g. mycobacteria, *Propionbacteria,* or Chlamydia) or environmental exposures and host immunologic responses. Several genes have been identified that may predispose or protect individuals from the development of sarcoidosis. A majority of these genes are involved in the host immune response. Because of the complexity of finding the causative organisms and exposures, the precise etiology of a given patient's sarcoidosis may never be determined. Regardless of the initial trigger, the immune response to these antigens begins a cascade of events leading to granuloma formation.

The development of sarcoidosis involves three events: (1) exposure to the antigen; (2) presentation of the antigen (by macrophages via HLA class II molecules to T lymphocytes); and (3) immune effector cells promoting the development of noncaseating granulomas, the pathologic hallmark of sarcoidosis. The release of cytokines, such as IL-2 and interferon-γ, by activated CD4 T lymphocytes (indicating a Th-1 immunologic response) eventually leads to enhanced fibroblast replication and granuloma formation. Despite the increased local immunologic activity, cutaneous anergy is commonly present, probably reflecting the depletion of immunologic factors responsible for local reactions.

Using microsatellite markers, the most prominent genetic linkage was associated within a major histocompatibility complex region on the short arm of chromosome 6. Several alleles have been shown to confer susceptibility for the disease (HLA DR 11, 12, 14, 15 and 17) and several are protective (HLA DR1 and 4). In addition, polymorphisms in the promoter region of TNF-α have been associated with Lofgren's syndrome, a form of sarcoidosis characterized by erythema nodosum, hilar adenopathy, uveitis, and a good prognosis. Insertion/deletions in the promoter of angiotensin-1 converting enzyme have also been identified; however, the association with sarcoidosis remains controversial.

The diagnosis of sarcoidosis is made by clinical correlation of nonspecific symptoms with biochemical, pathologic, and radiologic confirmation. The clinical manifestations of sarcoidosis are protean, reflecting multisystem involvement and can be just as important as the pathology in making a diagnosis of sarcoidosis. The most common presentations include respiratory symptoms (cough, chest pain, and dyspnea), musculoskeletal symptoms (arthralgias and myalgias), ocular symptoms (visual changes and pain), systemic B symptoms, and skin manifestations (erythema nodosum, nodules, plaques, and papules). The common feature of this disease is its multiorgan involvement. The clinical presentation ranges from asymptomatic to life-threatening organ involvement (e.g., neurologic or cardiac).

CLINICAL PRESENTATION
Pathologically, the most commonly involved organ systems are the lungs (90%), peripheral lymphatics (50–75%), skin (10–30%), liver (60–80%), eye (17%), spleen (15%), bone (1–35%), salivary glands (5%), joints (10–15%), and heart (30%). Often, sarcoidosis lesions are present in some organs without affecting their function. Pulmonary sarcoidosis can present as (1) asymptomatic or isolated constitutional symptoms; (2) interstitial lung disease; (3) asthma-like syndrome; (4) bullous lung disease; or (5) isolated hilar adenopathy. Cough and dyspnea are the most common respiratory complaints; chest pain, sputum production, and hemoptysis can also occur. Cor pulmonale occurs in 1 to 4% of cases, usually in the presence of severe fibrocystic sarcoidosis. Erythema nodosum is seen occasionally with the typical presentation of bilateral hilar adenopathy and indicates a good prognosis. Pleural disease occurs uncommonly and can be associated with lymphocytic exudative or transudative effusions.

Between 30 and 60% of patients are asymptomatic and present with incidental findings on chest radiographs. By international convention, the chest radiograph is staged as follows: *stage 0,* clear chest roentgenogram (5–16% of cases at presentation); *stage 1,* bilateral hilar adenopathy (25–40%); *stage 2,* bilateral hilar adenopathy with pulmonary infiltrate (24–49%); and *stage 3,* pulmonary infiltrates without hilar adenopathy (6–15%). Some investigators characterize a stage 4, in which pulmonary fibrosis or destruction occurs without adenopathy. The staging system is not believed to reflect chronologic stages of the disease, but provides a framework for clinical classification of pulmonary pathology.

DIAGNOSIS
Several imaging modalities have been evaluated for the diagnosis of sarcoidosis; each with particular limitations. Routine computed tomography (CT) of the chest is more sensitive than a standard chest radiograph in evaluating thoracic lymph node enlargement, the pattern of parenchymal disease, and the presence of pleural involvement, but lacks specificity for sarcoidosis and, therefore, remains controversial for routine assessment. High-resolution thin section CT may identify a pattern of parenchymal involvement relatively specific for sarcoidosis: nodular infiltrates adjacent to central bronchovascular structures. The importance of magnetic resonance imaging (MRI) with gadolinium and nuclear imaging has recently been evaluated to aid in the diagnosis, monitor disease activity, and determine the optimal site for biopsy. MRI with gadolinium has significantly improved the evaluation of sarcoidosis involving the nervous system, heart, muscle, bone and, to some extent, thorax. PET scanning with various markers can identify intra- and extrathoracic disease activity; however, one of its limitations is differentiating sarcoidosis from lymphoma. [99]Technetium, administered either by injection or inhalation, is useful in diagnosing intrathoracic (inhalation), bone involvement, and, in conjunction with [67]gallium, cardiac sarcoidosis. The modalities described can all help the clinician to determine the optimal site for biopsy. When tissue diagnosis is required, biopsy of an abnormal lymph node, parotid gland, nasal mucosal lesion, or other involved site almost always is diagnostic. Other methods of diagnosis are transbronchial lung biopsy (91% yield), mediastinoscopy (96%), open lung biopsy (100%), liver biopsy (70%), blind scalene-node biopsy (40–70%), blind bronchial mucosal biopsy (50%), and blind subconjunctival biopsy (50%). The selection of any of these procedures should be guided by the clinical presentation, with careful consideration of the risks and benefits for an individual patient.

The diagnosis of sarcoidosis is based on (1) a compatible clinical picture; (2) exclusion of other granulomatous disease; and (3) histologic evidence of noncaseating granulomas on tissue biopsy. The histologic picture is not pathognomonic; therefore, diseases such as tuberculosis, fungal infection, beryllium exposure, drug reactions, and local sarcoid-like reactions must be excluded. Bilateral hilar adenopathy in the presence of erythema nodosum or uveitis, or in the asymptomatic patient (Lofgren's syndrome), strongly suggests sarcoidosis rather than an infectious or neoplastic process. Laboratory tests are generally not helpful in making a diagnosis. Levels of angiotensin-1 converting enzyme are increased in 60 to 80% of patients with sarcoidosis, but this finding is not specific because increased levels are also found in other disorders such as Gaucher's disease, leprosy, lymphangiomyomatosis, diabetes mellitus with severe retinopathy, alcoholic cirrhosis, and hyperthyroidism. This test should not be used for screening; rather, it should be interpreted in light of the other clinical conditions in which it can be elevated. Bronchoalveolar lavage (BAL) fluid demonstrates increased numbers of CD4 T-helper lymphocytes.

COMPLICATIONS

A variety of pulmonary function changes may be observed. Spirometry and lung volumes most commonly reveal a restrictive pattern, although a subset of patients may demonstrate airway obstruction, particularly if endobronchial disease is present. A reduction in lung compliance and diffusing capacity is common. Hypoxemia may be present at rest and during exercise. The degree of functional impairment cannot be accurately predicted from the radiograph, and vice versa. Serial pulmonary function testing is often useful, both in selecting patients for therapy and following them while on medication.

TREATMENT

Most patients (80%) require no therapy and many expereince spontaneous remission and radiographic resolution. Systemic therapy is mandatory when evidence of significant vital organ involvement or severe systemic symptoms are present. The most urgent indications for treatment are symptomatic ocular, myocardial, and central nervous system disease. Other relative indications are persistent hypercalcemia, disfiguring cutaneous lesions, persistent or progressive symptomatic respiratory disease, thrombocytopenia, and occasionally, severe constitutional symptoms. The difficult treatment dilemma arises in an asymptomatic individual with stable lung infiltrates persisting for a period of time (1–2 years) without reduction in pulmonary function. Some pulmonologists treat the patient with corticosteroids for a few months to assess the disease reversibility and diminish the prospect of permanent fibrosis, whereas others reserve treatment for those who demonstrate declining function.

Corticosteroids remain the drugs of choice for pulmonary sarcoidosis with significant functional impairment. Most therapeutic regimens use prednisone (30–60 mg/d), with tapered doses over a period of 6 months or longer until a response is observed. In the presence of a positive tuberculin reaction or complete anergy, it may be reasonable to give isoniazid concomitantly with corticosteroids. Exacerbations can occur when prednisone is decreased below 15 mg/d. Therapy is best monitored by serially evaluating the clinical resolution of the original therapeutic indication (e.g., pulmonary function deficits, uveitis, arthritis), because the effect is radiographically inconsistent. Serial assessments of angiotensin-1 converting enzyme, ^{67}Ga scanning, and BAL to monitor the course of sarcoidosis and the response to steroid therapy are of unproved benefit.

Inhaled corticosteroids have been used but their role is unclear. Immunosuppressive agents and specific TNF-α inhibitors recently have been evaluated in more depth. Methotrexate, azathioprine, and cyclosporine have been studied with varying results. These are usually used in treating chronic sarcoidosis as steroid-sparing agents. Methotrexate has also been shown to be beneficial in acute sarcoidosis as a steroid-sparing agent. Azathioprine is used in corticosteroid-resistant sarcoidosis. Chloroquine, intradermal steroids, methotrexate, and retinoids appear to be effective in managing skin disease. Topical steroids may be effective in treating uveitis.

With further understanding of the role of macrophages and TNF-α in the development and progression of sarcoidosis, specific TNF-α inhibitors are beginning to be evaluated for sarcoidosis treatment. Phosphodiesterase inhibitors, such as pentoxifylline, have been shown to be beneficial in patients with acute, mild, or moderate sarcoidosis; however, it is unclear how many of those patients would have improved without treatment. Infliximab, developed for the treatment of sepsis, has been shown to be beneficial in refractory sarcoidosis. The optimal drug and the appropriate patients for treatment remains to be elucidated. Organ transplantation has been successfully for lung, heart, kidney, and liver disease in a small number of patients. Noncaseating granulomas have recurred in the transplanted organ in a few of these cases.

PROGNOSIS

The prognosis of sarcoidosis is generally favorable. About two thirds of patients who present with an abnormal chest radiograph completely clear or improve within 2 years. The other one third follow a gradually declining course over a period of a decade or more. About one half of those with persistent activity may progress to fatal outcomes, usually from pulmonary insufficiency and cor pulmonale. The worst prognosis is experienced by patients with significant pulmonary disease, such as those classified as stage 3 by radiographic criteria. Death from sarcoidosis is a rare outcome among patients with minimal or radiographic stage 1 disease.

1. Statement on sarcoidosis. Joint Statement of the American Thoracic Society (ATS), the European Respiratory Society (ERS) and the World Association of Sarcoidosis and Other Granulomatous Disorders (WASOG) adopted by the ATS Board of Directors and by the ERS Executive Committee, February 1999. *Am J Respir Crit Care Med*. 1999;160:736.
   Sarcoidosis is descriptively defined by the International Conference on Sarcoidosis. This article also reviews the clinical and radiological diagnosis of sarcoid in addition to reviewing the etiology and genetics.
2. Johns CJ, Michelle TM. The clinical management of sarcoidosis. *Medicine*. 1999;78:65.
   Review of Johns Hopkins Hospital Sarcoid Clinic experience over the past 40 years. Excellent discussion of diagnostic tools, treatment indications, follow-up, and unusual manifestations, including extrathoracic manifestations of sarcoidosis.
3. Thomas KW, Hunninghake GW. Sarcoidosis. *JAMA*. 2003;289:3300.
   Comprehensive state-of-the-art review pertaining to the clinical aspects of sarcoidosis, including cause, laboratory findings, diagnosis, and treatment.
4. Baughman RP, Lower EE, du Bois RM. Sarcoidosis. *Lancet*. 2003;361:1111.
   An excellent review of all aspects of pulmonary and extrathoracic sarcoidosis in addition to a review of the genetics and etiology of sarcoidosis.
5. Lofgren S. Primary pulmonary sarcoidosis. Early signs and symptoms. *Acta Med Scand*. 1953;145:424.
   In the author's population was found a high frequency of erythema nodosum, articular symptoms, and elevated sedimentation rate.
6. Reich JM. What is sarcoidosis? *Chest*. 2003;124:367.
7. Moller DR. Cells and cytokines involved in the pathogenesis of sarcoidosis: vasculitis and diffuse lung disease. *Sarcoidosis Vasc Diffuse Lung Dis*. 1999;16:24.
8. Rybicki BA, et al. The major histocompatibility complex gene region and sarcoidosis susceptibility in African Americans. *Am J Respir Crit Care Med*. 2003;167:444.
9. Schurmann M, et al. Results from a genome-wide search for predisposing genes in sarcoidosis. *Am J Respir Crit Care Med*. 2001;164:840.
   References 7 to 9 review the complex mechanisms involved in the pathogenesis etiology and genetics of sarcoidosis.
10. Mana J. Magnetic resonance imaging and nuclear imaging in sarcoidosis. *Curr Opin Pulm Med*. 2002;8:457.
    Excellent review of the different imaging modalities and their limitations in both intra- and extrathoracic sarcoidois.
11. Winterbauer R, Belic N, Mooses KD. A clinical interpretation of bilateral adenopathy. *Ann Intern Med*. 1973;78:65.
    The authors suggest that tissue biopsy for diagnosis is not necessary for patients with bilateral hilar adenopathy who are either asymptomatic or have erythema nodosum or uveitis. The diagnosis a priori is sarcoidosis.

12. Fong KF, Israel CW. Conjunctival biopsy in the diagnosis of sarcoidosis. *South Med J*. 1979;72:124.

Suggests that this test is a simple office procedure (for an ophthalmologist) and should be considered even in the absence of conjunctival follicles or nodules when sarcoidosis is clinically suspected.

13. Kantrow SP, et al. The CD4/CD8 ratio in BAL fluid is highly variable in sarcoidosis. *Eur Respir J*. 1997;10:2716.

Finding indicated that BAL-derived CD4:CD8 ratios failed to distinguish the presence of sarcoidosis among 86 patients with biopsy-proven disease.

14. Beekman JF, et al. Spectrum of pleural involvement in sarcoidosis. *Arch Intern Med*. 1976;136:323.

A literature review of 73 cases of pleural effusion, only 2 of which were bloody.

15. Levinson RS, et al. Airway function in sarcoidosis. *Am J Med*. 1977;62:51.

Abnormal airway function was demonstrated in all patients.

16. Paramothayan S, Jones PW. Corticosteroid therapy in pulmonary sarcoidosis: a systematic review. *JAMA*. 2002;287:1301.

17. Baughman RP, Lower EE. Infliximab for refractory sarcoidosis. *Sarcoidosis Vasc Diffuse Lung Dis*. 2001;18:70.

18. Gottlieb JE, et al. Outcome in sarcoidosis: the relationship of relapse to corticosteroid therapy. *Chest*. 1997;111:623.

19. Winterbauer R, et al. Treatment with corticosteroids. *Clin Chest Med*. 1997;18:843.

20. Baughman RP, Lower EE. Steroid-sparing alternative treatments for sarcoidosis. *Clin Chest Med*. 1997;18:853.

References 18 and 20 discuss the role and methods for implementing corticosteroid and alternative therapies to relieve and control disabling symptoms. Steroids remain the drug of choice for treatment.

91. WEGENER'S GRANULOMATOSIS

Kevin M. Murray

Wegener's granulomatosis (WG) is a systemic vasculitis that may involve any organ system, but most frequently affects the upper respiratory tract, the lungs, and the kidneys. A class of autoantibodies known as antineutrophil cytoplasmic antibodies (ANCA) is closely associated with WG and other forms of vasculitis, and likely contributes to the pathogenesis of these disorders. Most patients with WG have involvement of the upper or lower respiratory tracts. Upper respiratory symptoms in WG include chronic sinusitis, rhinorrhea, bloody nasal drainage, sinus pain, otitis media and nasal or oral ulcerations. Tracheal involvement can lead to obstruction and stridor. Pulmonary symptoms may include cough, pleuritic chest pain, dyspnea, or hemoptysis. Rarely, WG can present as fulminating pulmonary hemorrhage leading to respiratory failure, or as an acute lung injury syndrome. Up to one third of patients with pulmonary findings may be asymptomatic.

Radiographic findings in pulmonary WG include areas of consolidation, solitary, or multiple nodules that may cavitate, pleural effusions, and localized interstitial infiltrates. Involvement of mainstem bronchi can cause lobar consolidation or atelectasis. Hilar adenopathy does not occur. One characteristic roentgenographic finding is the simultaneous waxing and waning of different infiltrates as inflammation occurs and resolves in different lung regions. Computed tomography may detect lesions that are not well visualized on plain chest radiographs. Sinus radiographs may show air–fluid levels.

Renal involvement is very common in WG, occurring in up to 80% of patients. Microscopic hematuria and red cell casts may be seen on urinalysis, and renal biopsies show varying degrees of inflammation, from a focal or segmental glomerulitis to a rapidly progressing necrotizing glomerulonephritis. Immunofluorescence shows this to be a "pauci-immune" glomerulonephritis, with absent or nearly absent immunoglobulin deposits. Glomerulonephritis may precede pulmonary WG by a period of months to years.

Other manifestations of WG include arthralgias or myalgias, mono- or polyarthritis, fever, weight loss, neurologic symptoms including mononeuritis multiplex, skin lesions, and pericarditis. Lesions of WG have been found in nearly all organs, testifying to the systemic nature of this disease.

In the 1980s, a new class of autoantibodies to specific antigens in neutrophils was discovered: ANCA. They were found in patients with several forms of systemic vasculitis, including WG, Churg-Strauss syndrome, and microscopic polyangiitis.

Two patterns of indirect immunofluorescence have been described: a diffuse cytoplasmic pattern (cANCA) and a perinuclear pattern (pANCA). Occasionally, other nonspecific ANCA patterns are seen in some conditions. The specific antigens involved have been identified. Proteinase 3 (PR3) is the usual target of cANCA, and myeloperoxidase (MPO) is the most common target of pANCA. Antibodies against a number of other neutrophilic antigens can cause cANCA or pANCA immunofluorescence. ELISA assays for antibodies against specific antigens are more sensitive and specific for active disease.

Approximately 90% of patients with active WG are ANCA positive. The cANCA associated with WG is almost always an anti-PR3 antibody. Therefore, it is prudent to confirm a finding of cANCA by a specific ELISA assay for anti-PR3 or anti-MPO. Inactive disease is much less likely to manifest ANCA, and up to 10% of patients with WG and one third of patients with limited WG do not show evidence of ANCA. The contribution of ANCA to the pathogenesis of WG is unclear, but they appear to be responsible for some portion of the immune response that leads to disease. Passive transfer of ANCA in mice causes vasculitis. ANCA may be formed in response to an initiating exposure or infection and may subsequently cause the activation of neutrophils and monocytes, leading to tissue damage.

Titers of ANCA rise and fall in relation to disease activity in two thirds of patients. However, this correlation is not precise enough to allow adjustment of disease management based solely on ANCA levels. Therefore, a rising ANCA level should not be used as the sole reason for reinstituting therapy for a patient in clinical remission. However, such patients should be followed closely for clinical signs of relapse.

The definitive diagnosis of WG is made by tissue biopsy. Biopsies of lesions in the upper respiratory tract are relatively easy to obtain and are frequently diagnostic, but pathologic findings in severely inflamed or infected tissue may be nonspecific. In the presence of impaired renal function or active urinary sediment, renal biopsy can demonstrate a characteristic pattern of segmental necrotizing glomerulonephritis, and is less invasive than open lung biopsy. Transbronchial lung biopsy is of limited usefulness, and most authorities recommend open or thoracoscopic lung biopsy as the invasive procedure of choice for the diagnosis of pulmonary disease in the absence of renal or upper airway disease.

Historically, untreated patients with WG had a 2-year mortality of 90%. Combination therapy with prednisone and cyclophosphamide has been well established as the gold standard of therapy based on some 30 years of experience. An initial oral dose of cyclophosphamide (2 mg/kg per day) is usually given in combination with prednisone (1 mg/kg per day). Prednisone is then tapered over 3 months to 0.25 mg/kg per day, and continued for at least one year. Fulminant or life-threatening disease has been treated with higher doses of steroids, including pulse doses of intravenous methylprednisolone, as well as higher doses of cyclophosphamide. Plasmapheresis has been used to treat renal disease requiring dialysis and has been recommended in patients with severe pulmonary hemorrhage. Patients receiving cyclophosphamide and prednisone are at risk for *Pneumocystis carinii* pneumonia, and prophylactic therapy is recommended. Most clinicians use trimethoprim-sulfamethoxazole, one double-strength tablet three times weekly.

Remission is reflected by absence of clinical symptoms, resolution of radiographic abnormalities, and reduction or elimination of ANCA. Following remission, most authorities have advocated continuing therapy for at least 12 months at lower doses. Because cyclophosphamide therapy is associated with significant adverse affects, including hemorrhagic cystitis and an increased risk of bladder cancer, myelodysplasia, and lymphoproliferative disorders, alternative agents have been explored, especially for patients in remission. Azathioprine or low-dose methotrexate has been effective in maintaining remission when administered with continued low-dose prednisone. Each drug is begun after 3 months of cyclophosphamide therapy. Trimethoprim-sulfamethoxazole prophylaxis has been used during therapy of less severe cases as well.

Relapses of WG are treated by resuming or increasing doses of cyclophosphamide and prednisone until clinical remission is attained. Fulminant relapses may require the reinstitution of induction therapy. If cyclophosphamide cannot be used because of toxicity, alternative agents such as azathioprine, methotrexate, mycophenolate mofetil, cyclosporine, and etoposide may be effective. Anti-tumor necrosis factor agents also show promise for the treatment of WG. The overall median survival of patients with WG is now over 20 years, a remarkable statistic for a disease that was once uniformly fatal.

1. Csernok E. Anti-neutrophil cytoplasmic antibodies and pathogenesis of small vessel vasculitidies. *Autoimmun Rev.* 2003;2:158.
   Review of work to date establishing that ANCA are directly involved in the pathogenesis of WG and related disorders.
2. Cordier J, Valeyre D, Guilevin L, et al. Pulmonary Wegener's granulomatosis: a clinical and imaging study of 77 cases. *Chest.* 1990;97:906.
   Review of the experience in a French hospital. Computed tomographic scans were useful to detect opacities or cavities not seen on plain radiographs.
3. Daum T, et al. Tracheobronchial involvement in Wegener's Granulomatosis. *Am J Respir Crit Care Med.* 1995;151:522.
   A review of the Mayo Clinic experience including the use of interventional bronchoscopy for localized airway stenosis.
4. DeGroot K, Reinhold-Keller E, Tatsis E, et al. Therapy for the maintenance of remission in sixty-five patients with generalized Wegener's granulomatosis: methotrexate versus trimethoprim/sulfamethoxazole. *Arthritis Rheum.* 1996;39:2052–2061.
   Methotrexate maintained remissions in 86% of patients compared to 58% given trimethoprim-sulfamethoxazole.
5. Del Buono E, Flint A. Diagnostic usefulness of nasal biopsy in Wegener's granulomatosis. *Hum Pathol.* 1991;22:107.
   Nasal biopsies were diagnostic in 53% of cases. Emphasizes the importance of large biopsies.
6. Fahey AS, Haynes BF, Katz P. Wegener's granulomatosis. *Am J Med.* 1954;17:168.
   Classic article that defines the disease as a distinct clinicopathologic entity. Seven cases define the classic triad.
7. Fauci AS, et al. Wegener's granulomatosis: prospective clinical and therapeutic experience with 85 patients for 21 years. *Ann Intern Med.* 1983;98:76.
   Reports the National Institutes of Health (NIH) experience and confirms the efficacy of cyclophosphamide as a potentially curative agent.
8. Girard T, et al. Are antineutrophil cytoplasmic antibodies a marker predictive of relapse in Wegener's Granulomatosis? A prospective study. *Rheumatology (Oxford).* 2001;40:147.
   Rising levels of ANCA are not sufficient evidence of relapse to warrant treatment without clinical disease.
9. Hoffman G, et al. Wegener granulomatosis: an analysis of 158 patients. *Ann Intern Med.* 1992;116:488.

Long-term follow-up of the NIH trials, confirming the benefit of cyclophosphamide, but raising concerns about the frequency of relapse and toxicity of treatment.

10. Hoffman GS, Specks U. Antineutrophil cytoplasmic antibodies. *Arthritis Rheum.* 1998;41:1521.

    An excellent, comprehensive review of ANCA, including their clinical utility and the evidence for their involvement in the pathogenesis of WG.

11. Jayne D, et al. A randomized trial of maintenance therapy for vasculitis associated with antineutrophil cytoplasmic antibodies. *N Engl J Med.* 2003;349:36.

    Documents the efficacy of azathioprine as maintenance therapy after induction of remission. Of patients receiving azathioprine, 15.5% suffered relapses.

12. Kyndt X, Reumaux D, Bridoux F, et al. Serial measurements of antineutrophil cytoplasmic antibodies in patients with systemic vasculitis. *Am J Med.* 1999;106:527.

    The predictive value of a rise in cANCA for a subsequent relapse of WG was only 28%.

13. Landman S, Burgener F. Pulmonary manifestations of Wegener's granulomatosis. *AJR.* 1974;122:750.

    Extensive review with radiologic emphasis.

14. Langford C, et al. Use of a cyclophosphamide-induction methotrexate-maintenance regimen for the treatment of Wegener's granulomatosis: extended follow-up and rate of relapse. *Am J Med.* 2003;114:463.

    Methotrexate given for maintenance therapy was well tolerated but had a 52% rate of relapse.

15. Liebow A. The J. Burns Amberson Lecture: pulmonary angiitis and granulomatosis. *Am Rev Respir Dis.* 1973;108:1.

    Reviews classic and limited Wegener's granulomatosis.

16. Niles J, et al. The syndrome of lung hemorrhage and nephritis is usually an ANCA-associated condition. *Arch Intern Med.* 1996;156:440.

    Of 88 patients with this syndrome, 55 had ANCA. Only 8 had WG.

17. Nishino H, et al. Neurological Involvement in Wegener's granulomatosis: an analysis of 324 consecutive patients at the Mayo Clinic. *Ann Neurol.* 1993;33:4.

    Neurologic involvement was found in 33.6% of patients with WG.

18. Ognibene F, et al. Pneumocystis carinii pneumonia: a major complication of immunosuppressive therapy in patients with Wegener's granulomatosis. *Am J Respir Crit Care Med.* 1995;151:795.

    Six percent of patients treated for WG developed P. carinii pneumonia.

19. Pretorius E, et al. Wegener's Granulomatosis: CT evaluation of pulmonary parenchymal lesions in treated disease. *Crit Rev Comput Tomogr.* 2004; 45:67.

    Although most CT abnormalities improve or resolve with therapy, some nodules became larger, and lobar atelectasis did not improve, suggesting fixed endobronchial lesions.

20. Reinhold-Keller E, et al. An interdisciplinary approach to the care of patients with Wegener's granulomatosis: long-term outcome in 155 patients. *Arthritis Rheum.* 2000;43:1021.

    Review of patients treated with cyclophosphamide and prednisone; complete remission occurred in 83 of 155. Drug toxicity was a significant problem, especially when total cyclophosphamide dose equaled 100 g.

21. Reinhold-Keller E, et al. High rate of renal relapse in 71 patients with Wegener's granulomatosis under maintenance of remission with low-dose methotrexate. *Arthritis Rheum.* 2002;47:326–332.

    One third of 71 patients receiving weekly intravenous methotrexate relapsed.

22. Seo P, Stone J. The antineutrophil cytoplasmic antibody-associated vasculitides. *Am J Med.* 2004;117:39.

    Comprehensive review of clinical manifestations, diagnosis and treatment of WG and other ANCA-associated diseases.

23. Savige J, et al. Antineutrophilcytoplasmic antibodies and associated diseases: a review of the clinical and laboratory features. *Kidney Int.* 2000;57:846.

Discusses testing for ANCA, clinical features, and treatment of various vasculitides associated with ANCA.

24. Stegemen CA, Tervaert JWC, deJong PE, et al. Trimethoprim-sulfamethoxazole for the prevention of relapses of Wegener's granulomatosis. *N Engl J Med.* 1996;335:16.

Eighty-one patients were randomized to receive either trimethoprim-sulfamethoxazole or placebo. Relative risk of relapse for patients given SPM/SMX was 0.40 over 24 months.

25. Sullivan E, Hoffman G. Pulmonary vasculitis. *Clin Chest Med.* 1998;19:759.

Excellent, comprehensive review of pulmonary involvement in vasculitides.

26. Rottem M, et al. Wegener granulomatosis in children and adolescents: clinical presentation and outcome. *J Pediatr.* 1993;122:26.

Compares 23 cases of childhood-onset WG with 135 cases of adult-onset WG. Subglottic stenosis and nasal deformity are more common; however, overall treatment-related morbidity is less common among children.

27. Schnabel A, Holl-Ulrich K, Dalhoff K, et al. Efficacy of transbronchial biopsy in pulmonary vasculitides. *Eur Respir J.* 1997;10:2738.

Transbronchial biopsy had a low yield in WG, but bronchoscopic biopsy of upper airway lesions was useful. Biopsy of upper respiratory tract lesions had the highest yield in WG.

28. Wiik A. Antineutrophil cytoplasmic antibodies in Wegener's granulomatosis. *Clin Exp Rheum.* 1993;11:191.

A comprehensive review of ANCA in Wegener's and evidence for the role of ANCA in the pathogenesis of the disease.

29. Woodworth T, et al. Severe glomerulonephritis with late emergence of classic Wegener's granulomatosis. *Medicine* (Baltimore). 1987;66:181.

Reports 4 cases and reviews 15 others from the literature. Pulmonary manifestations developed 4 to 78 months after the onset of glomerulonephritis and renal failure.

30. Xiao H, et al. Antineutrophil cytoplasmic auto-antibodies specific for myeloperoxidase cause glomerulonephritis and vasculitis in mice. *J Clin Invest.* 2002;110:955.

Supports causative role of ANCA in WG and other vasculitides. Passive transfer of anti-MPO IgG caused typical lesions in mice kidneys.

92. GOODPASTURE'S SYNDROME

Beat Walder and Donna Tigno

PATHOPHYSIOLOGY

Goodpasture's syndrome refers to a clinical entity of pulmonary hemorrhage, glomerulonephritis, and the presence of antiglomerular basement membrane (anti-GBM) antibodies. Historically, the eponym, *Goodpasture's syndrome,* has been applied inconsistently, referring to any syndrome of glomerulonephritis and alveolar hemorrhage, regardless of cause or mechanism. This chapter focuses on the syndrome associated with anti-GBM antibodies. The target of the antibodies is the α-3 chain of type IV collagen found in the basement membranes of lungs and kidneys. It is likely that patients described in the 1950s and 1960s, before the development of the anti-GBM antibody assay (1970s), represented a mixture of causes and mechanisms.

ETIOLOGY

A rare disorder, anti-GBM antibody disease has an estimated incidence of about 0.1 patients per 1 million population. It is more frequent in men than in women, with reported gender ratios ranging from 1.2:1 to 8:1. The disease has a bimodal peak in age of presentation; most patients present in their third or fourth decade, whereas a smaller number present in the fifth and sixth decades. It is most often idiopathic, although it can follow pulmonary infections or hydrocarbon exposure. A unique setting in which this can also occur is in 5 to 10% of renal transplant patients with underlying hereditary nephritis.

Approximately 60% of patients with anti-GBM antibody disease have the pulmonary and renal manifestations of Goodpasture's syndrome. Pulmonary involvement can precede renal involvement by up to 12 months. Patients both with and without pulmonary hemorrhage seem to have similar antibodies against the α-3 chain. The variable presence of pulmonary involvement reflects the limited access that the antibodies have to the alveolar basement membrane. It appears that pulmonary injury allows this access, whether by smoking, infection, or hydrocarbon exposure. Less commonly, nephritis precedes the onset of pulmonary hemorrhage. Isolated renal involvement is seen in approximately 40% of patients; isolated pulmonary involvement is unusual. The usual duration of symptoms preceding the diagnosis of anti-GBM antibody disease is weeks to months.

CLINICAL MANIFESTATIONS

Clinically, patients with Goodpasture's syndrome complain of minimal to massive hemoptysis (72–82%), dyspnea (44–64%), and gross hematuria (up to 41%). Systemic symptoms such as malaise, weight loss, fever, and arthralgia are uncommon; the presence of such features suggests that the patient has concurrent vasculitis. Patients with isolated glomerulonephritis present most commonly with nonspecific symptoms (55%) and gross hematuria (44%). The most common clinical signs in Goodpasture's syndrome include pallor (76%) and pulmonary crackles (47%). Pallor in patients with isolated glomerulonephritis is seen in approximately 53% of patients.

Laboratory examination in anti-GBM antibody disease discloses anemia in 77% of patients, with a mean hemoglobin level at the time of presentation of 8.6 g/dL. Abnormal urinalysis (hematuria, proteinuria, or nephritic sediment) is common (71–100%).

The chest radiographic findings in patients with Goodpasture's syndrome are often nonspecific and are of limited value in the differential diagnosis. The chest radiograph most frequently shows bilateral, symmetric air space filling in the middle and lower lung zones. Less common are asymmetric, focal, or interstitial abnormalities. Resolution of infiltrates generally occurs over days. Pleural effusions in the absence of infection or volume overload are rare. The chest radiograph can be normal, even in the presence of hemoptysis. Long-term radiographic abnormalities have not been reported.

Pulmonary function testing often reveals mild restriction and decreased diffusing capacity for carbon monoxide/alveolar ventilation (D$_{LCO}$/VA). However, elevated D$_{LCO}$/VA values occur during pulmonary hemorrhage, even in the absence of either hemoptysis or abnormal chest radiograph findings. Serial measurements of D$_{LCO}$/VA have been advocated as a noninvasive diagnostic tool to detect recurrent pulmonary hemorrhage. At long-term follow-up, patients with anti-GBM antibody disease with pulmonary hemorrhage have lower D$_{LCO}$/VA values than patients without hemorrhage and controls.

The pulmonary histopathologic findings in anti-GBM antibody disease are nonspecific. Neutrophilic capillaritis can be seen. Immunofluorescent studies may demonstrate characteristic linear deposition along the alveolocapillary basement membrane of IgG and (often) complement.

The finding of bloody pulmonary secretions and hemosiderin-laden macrophages obtained by bronchoscopy with bronchoalveolar lavage can provide indirect evidence of alveolar hemorrhage. Assessment of the major airways and collection of specimens for microbiologic studies can also be accomplished at the time of bronchoscopy. Transbronchoscopic lung biopsy for immunofluorescent studies in patients with anti-GBM antibody disease and hemoptysis has had variable success, the yield ranging from 30 to 100%.

Mendenhal, PA

The renal pathologic findings typically demonstrate focal or diffuse proliferative glomerulonephritis with crescent formation, although other forms of glomerulonephritis have been described. Immunofluorescent studies of the glomerular basement membrane are of key diagnostic importance. Although IgG deposits along the basement membranes are characteristic, they are considered diagnostic only in the context of serologic confirmation of anti-GBM antibody. In their absence, elution studies of IgG deposits from kidneys may demonstrate their specificity against the glomerular basement membrane.

The likely auto-antigen in anti-GBM antibody disease has been localized to the noncollagenous (NCL) domain of the 3 chain of type (IV) collagen. Type (IV) collagen is one of the main structural components in basement membranes. Each type (IV) collagen molecule consists of three α chains that form a triple helix except in the C-terminal end where they form separate globular structures, the NCL domains.

Antibodies directed against the α 3(IV)NCL domain were found in all sera tested in several studies, whereas specificities against other chains were also detected. Isolated α 3(IV) chains probably contain no additional epitopes beyond the NCL domain. Mounting evidence points to the N-terminal region of α 3(IV)NCL as carrier of the important epitope(s).

The pathogenetic potential of anti-GBM antibodies has been shown in a classic transfer experiment in which antibodies eluted from patients induced glomerulonephritis in recipient monkeys. More recent investigations have focused on the interaction of neutrophils, cytokines, adhesion molecules, and complement in the pathogenesis of the disease. The role of T-cell immunity in this disorder is also being investigated.

More than 90% of patients with Goodpasture's syndrome have circulating anti-GBM antibodies. Different assays using a variety of glomerular basement membrane antigenic preparations are available: indirect immunofluorescent study, radioimmunoassay, and, more recently, ELISA and immunoblotting. Both radioimmunoassay and ELISA are very sensitive and specific and more sensitive than indirect immunofluorescent study. Immunoblotting serves as a confirmatory test. Attempts at correlating anti-GBM antibody titers with specific clinical or laboratory findings have shown contradictory results. Anti-GBM antibody titers decrease faster with therapy than without and are used to monitor response to therapy.

The cause of anti-GBM antibody disease remains unknown. It is likely that a combination of genetic predisposition and environmental stimuli are responsible. In terms of the genetic background, a strong association with certain HLA antigen class II genes has been found. HLA-DRw15, a subspecificity of DR2, was present in 76% of patients with anti-GBM antibody as compared with 31% of controls; HLA-DR4 may also contribute to the genetic risk. The list of associated environmental factors is extensive and includes cocaine use, extracorporeal shock wave lithotripsy, exposure to hydrocarbons and hard metal dust, cigarette smoking, and influenza A2 virus infections.

The diagnosis of anti-GBM antibody disease is established by a compatible clinical presentation (alveolar hemorrhage, glomerulonephritis, or both) and demonstration of either circulating or tissue-bound anti-GBM antibody. Kidney biopsies are frequently performed and have a very high diagnostic yield if renal abnormalities are present. Even in the presence of circulating anti-GBM antibody, kidney biopsies can add to the evaluative process: (1) anti-GBM antibody can be demonstrated with direct immunofluorescent studies; (2) accompanying or alternative lesions can be assessed; and (3) additional prognostic information (e.g., the percentage of crescent glomeruli) may be obtained. Lung biopsy, which usually does not add to the information obtained from documenting anti-GBM antibody disease serologically or by renal biopsy, is rarely indicated.

DIAGNOSIS

The differential diagnosis for patients presenting with diffuse alveolar hemorrhage or Goodpasture's syndrome is broad and a combination of clinical and laboratory data is often needed to establish a definitive diagnosis. The most common competing diagnoses are Wegener's granulomatosis (WG), microscopic polyarteritis (systemic necrotizing vasculitis), systemic lupus erythematosus, and idiopathic glomerulonephritis with alveolar hemorrhage. Determination of serum autoantibodies such as ANCA, anti-GBM antibody, and antinuclear antibodies as well as complement levels may be invaluable in the diagnostic process. Rapid screening assays for anti-GBM antibody and ANCA have been developed. Less common underlying conditions include rheumatoid arthritis, Behçet's disease, Henoch-Schöenlein purpura, antiphospholipid antibody syndrome, mixed cryoglobulinemia, pulmonary cholesterol emboli, pulmonary hemorrhage after bone marrow transplantation, idiopathic pulmonary hemosiderosis, certain localized and metastatic tumors, drug reactions (e.g., penicillamine, cocaine), mitral stenosis, and pulmonary venoocclusive disease.

Goodpasture's syndrome may also overlap with WG. Therefore, it is important to test for both anti-GBM antibodies and ANCA. The two disorders present similarly, and between 10% and 38% of patients with anti-GBM antibody disease also test positive for ANCA and may have signs of systemic vasculitis. The anti-GBM antibodies, in patients who also have ANCA, have the same antigen specificities as those who test positive solely for anti-GBM antibodies. The combined serologies signify a prognostic difference because the patients who are ANCA positive appear to have a more treatable disease in comparison to patients who have only anti-GBM antibodies.

TREATMENT

The treatment of choice for anti-GBM antibody disease is plasmapheresis combined with prednisone and cyclophosphamide. Plasmapheresis removes circulating anti-GBM antibodies and other mediators of inflammation, namely, complement, and the immunosuppressive medications suppress new antibody formation. The recommended initial plasmapheresis regimen is either daily or alternate day, 4-L exchanges for 2 to 3 weeks. Albumin is given as the replacement fluid unless the patient has had a recent renal biopsy or has pulmonary hemorrhage; in which case the replacement fluid is 1 to 2 L of fresh frozen plasma at the end of the procedure. This would replace any pheresis-induced depletion of coagulation factors. The patient should be reassessed at the end of the initial regimen. Further plasmapheresis may not be necessary if the patient clinically improves and there is a decline in the anti-GBM antibodies. On the other hand, further treatments may be necessary if the patient still has hemoptysis and the antibody titers remain elevated. Plasmapheresis is accompanied by corticosteroids and cyclophosphamide. Pulse methylprednisolone, administered at 30 mg/kg or 1,000 mg, is given every other day for three doses and is then followed by daily oral prednisone (1 mg/kg per day), which is then tapered once remission is achieved.

Immunosuppressive therapy is usually continued for 6 to 12 months, the time associated with spontaneous cessation of autoantibodies. Most patients are switched at 3 to 4 months from cyclophosphamide to azathioprine, which is less toxic.

OUTCOMES

The clinical outcome of patients with Goodpasture's disease appears to depend largely on severity at presentation. In the largest retrospective review of patients treated for confirmed anti-GBM disease, 71 patients were treated with plasma exchange, prednisone, and cyclophosphamoride. In that review, among the 42 patients with pulmonary hemorrhage, 90% stopped bleeding with therapy. Regarding renal dysfunction, patients who presented with a plasma creatinine concentration of less than 5.7 mg/dL, had survival and renal preservation of 100 and 95% at 1 year, respectively, and 84 and 74% at last follow-up (median of 90 months). Patients who presented with a plasma creatinine concentration greater than 5.7 mg/dL, but who did not require immediate dialysis (within 72 hours at presentation), had survival and renal preservation of 83 and 82% at 1 year and 72 and 69% at last follow-up. Among those who required immediate dialysis, survival and renal preservation were 65 and 8% at 1 year and 36 and 5% at last follow-up. Those who required immediate dialysis but recovered renal function had tubular necrosis, in addition to crescentic glomerulonephritis. This underscores the utility of renal biopsy in identifying patients who would benefit from aggressive therapy.

Patients with anti-GBM disease and severe renal failure who do not require immediate hemodialysis should be considered for aggressive therapy, namely, immunosuppression and plasma exchange. Patients who present with dialysis-requiring renal failure are less likely to benefit, but may occasionally. Furthermore, patients who require immediate dialysis and have 100% crescents on renal biopsy are very unlikely to recover renal function.

Chronic variants of Goodpasture's syndrome, with relapses (worsening clinical manifestations while anti-GBM antibody still present) and recurrences (manifestations after an interval of clinical quiescence and normalized anti-GBM antibody titer) have been described. Relapses have been attributed to resumption of smoking and bacterial infections. The rare recurrences are usually accompanied by elevated anti-GBM antibody titers, especially when testing is done using sensitive assays. Treatment is the same as that described for the initial presentation.

Renal transplantation is a promising therapeutic option for patients with end-stage renal disease secondary to anti-GBM antibody disease. Renal transplants are usually delayed until anti-GBM antibody titers have normalized for 9 to 12 months. A 5-year graft survival of 44% has been reported. Recurrent disease in transplanted kidneys was responsible for 14% of graft failures.

1. Goodpasture EW. The significance of certain pulmonary lesions in relation to the etiology of influenza. *Am J Med Sci*. 1919;158:863.
   The original description of Goodpasture's syndrome. The patient probably had a vasculitis.
2. Ball JA, Young Jr KR. Pulmonary manifestations of Goodpasture's syndrome. Antiglomerular basement membrane disease and related disorders. *Clin Chest Med*. 1998;19:777.
   References 2 through 4 are comprehensive reviews.
3. Bolton WK. Goodpasture's syndrome. *Kidney Int*. 1996;50:1753.
   The author outlines specific treatment options.
4. Kelly PT, Haponik EF. Goodpasture's syndrome: molecular and clinical advances. *Medicine* (Baltimore). 1994;73:171.
5. Stanton MC, Tange JD. Goodpasture's syndrome. *Australasian Annals of Medicine* 1958;7:132.
   The origin of the term Goodpasture's syndrome.
6. Wilson CB, Dixon FJ. Anti-glomerular basement membrane antibody-induced glomerulonephritis. *Kidney Int*. 1973;3:74.
   The first large series on patients with anti-glomerular basement membrane antibody-induced glomerulonephritis (AGBMA).
7. Lockwood CM, Rees AJ, Pearson TA, et al. Immunosuppression and plasma-exchange in the treatment of Goodpasture's syndrome. *Lancet*. 1976;1:711.
   The first article using plasmapheresis in AGBMA disease.
8. Daly C, Conlon PJ, Medwar W, et al. Characteristics and outcome of anti-glomerular basement membrane disease: a single-center experience. *Ren Fail*. 1996;18:105.
   A recent patient series.
9. Merkel F, Pullig O, Marx M, et al. Course and prognosis of anti-basement membrane antibody (anti-BM-Ab)-mediated disease: report of 35 cases. *Nephrol Dial Transplant*. 1994;9:372.
   Morbidity and mortality data for the chapter were taken from references 9 through 15.
10. Herody M, Bobrie G, Gouarin C, et al. Anti-GBM disease: predictive value of clinical, histological and serological data. *Clin Nephrol*. 1993;40:249.
11. Savage CO, Pusey CD, Bowman C, et al. Antiglomerular basement membrane antibody mediated disease in the British Isles 1980–4. *BMJ* (Clin Res Ed). 1986;292:301.
12. Walker RG, Scheinkestel C, Becker GJ, et al. Clinical and morphological aspects of the management of crescentic anti-glomerular basement membrane antibody (anti-GBM) nephritis/ Goodpasture's syndrome. *Q J Med*. 1985;54:75.
13. Johnson JP, Moore JR, Austin HA, et al. Therapy of anti-glomerular basement

membrane antibody disease: analysis of prognostic significance of clinical, pathologic and treatment factors. *Medicine* (Baltimore). 1985;64:219.

   The only prospective, randomized trial of immunosuppression versus immunosuppression plus plasma exchange (n = 17). The percent crescents on initial renal biopsy and serum creatinine correlated better with outcome than therapeutic modality.

14. Simpson IJ, Doak PB, Williams LC, et al. Plasma exchange in Goodpasture's syndrome. *Am J Nephrol.* 1982;2:301.

15. Briggs WA, Johnson JP, Teichman S, et al. Antiglomerular basement membrane antibody-mediated glomerulonephritis and Goodpasture's syndrome. *Medicine* (Baltimore). 1979;58:348.

16. Levy JB, Turner AN, Rees AJ, et al. Long-term outcome of anti-glomerular basement membrane antibody disease treated with plasma exchange and immunosuppression. *Ann Intern Med.* 2001;134:1033.

   The largest report of long-term outcome of patients with anti-GBM disease.

17. Kaplan AA. The use of apheresis in immune renal disorders. *Ther Apheresis Dial.* 2003;7:165.

18. Boyce NW, Holdsworth SR. Pulmonary manifestations of the clinical syndrome of acute glomerulonephritis and lung hemorrhage. *Am J Kidney Dis.* 1986;8:31.

   In 45 patients with Goodpasture's syndrome, the underlying diseases were AGBMA disease, WG, panarteritis nodosa, SLE, microscopic polyarteritis, tumor, endocarditis, and idiopathic glomerulonephritis with idiopathic lung hemorrhage.

19. Bowley NB, Steiner RE, Chin WS. The chest x-ray in antiglomerular basement membrane antibody disease (Goodpasture's syndrome). *Clin Radiol.* 1979;30:419.

   The chest radiograph study was normal in 18% of episodes of pulmonary hemorrhage.

20. Ewan PW, Rees AJ, et al. Detection of intrapulmonary hemorrhage with carbon monoxide uptake. Application in Goodpasture's syndrome. *N Engl J Med.* 1976;295:1391.

   A rise of D_{LCO}/VA over 30% correlated with pulmonary hemorrhage; 22% of bleeding episodes were not suspected on clinical grounds. Mean baseline DLCO/VA was 28% below normal.

21. Conlon Jr PJ, Walshe JJ, Daly C, et al. Antiglomerular basement membrane disease: the long-term pulmonary outcome. *Am J Kidney Dis.* 1994;23:794.

   The AGBMA group with pulmonary involvement had a significantly lowered mean DLCO/VA as the only difference between the groups. It did not translate into a lower $V_{O_{2max}}$ with exercise.

22. Colby TV. Pulmonary pathology in patients with systemic autoimmune diseases. *Clin Chest Med.* 1998;19:587.

   A general review. References 22 and 23 show that capillaritis is commonly seen in a variety of pulmonary–renal hemorrhage syndromes.

23. Travis WD, Colby TV, Lombard C, et al. A clinicopathologic study of 34 cases of diffuse pulmonary hemorrhage with lung biopsy confirmation. *Am J Surg Pathol.* 1990;14:1112.

   A detailed analysis of 34 patients with diffuse alveolar hemorrhage. Causes included probable or definite WG; systemic necrotizing vasculitis; SLE; rheumatoid arthritis; AGBMA disease; idiopathic IgA nephropathy; idiopathic glomerulonephritis; and unclassified pulmonary renal syndrome.

24. Hellmark T, Johansson C, Wieslander J. Characterization of anti-GBM antibodies involved in Goodpasture's syndrome. *Kidney Int.* 1994;46:823.

   Of IgG antibodies against (IV)NCL, 90% are directed against α3(IV)NCL; all patients had antibodies directed against α3(IV)NCL, but antibodies against other α(IV) chains were also found.

25. Leinonen A, Netzer KO, Boutaud A, et al. Goodpasture antigen: expression of the full-length α(IV) chain of collagen IV and localization of epitopes exclusively to the noncollagenous domain [see comments]. *Kidney Int.* 1999;55:926.

   Plasmapheresis fluid of five patients with AGBMA disease reacted exclusively with the NCL domain out of the entire α(IV) chain.

26. Netzer KO, Leinonen A, Boutard A, et al. The Goodpasture autoantigen. Mapping

the major conformational epitope(s) of alpha3(IV) collagen to residues 17–31 and 127–141 of the NC1 domain. *J Biol Chem.* 1999;274:11267.

References 26 and 27 highlight the importance of the N-terminus of the α(IV)NCL domain.

27. Ryan JJ, Mason PJ, Pusey CD, et al. Recombinant alpha-chains of type IV collagen demonstrate that the amino terminal of the Goodpasture autoantigen is crucial for antibody recognition. *Clin Exp Immunol.* 1998;113:17.

28. Lerner RA, Glassock RJ, Dixon FJ. The role of anti-glomerular basement membrane antibody in the pathogenesis of human glomerulonephritis. *J Exp Med.* 1967;126:989.

A classic article describing a transfer experiment of human AGBMA eluted from patients that induced glomerulonephritis in recipient monkeys.

29. Burns AP, Fisher M, Li P, et al. Molecular analysis of HLA class II genes in Goodpasture's disease. *Q J Med.* 1995;88:93–100.

Of patients with AGBMA disease, 91% had either HLA-DR2, subspecificity DRw15, or HLA-DR4.

30. Rees AJ, Peters DK, Amos N, et al. The influence of HLA-linked genes on the severity of anti-GBM antibody-mediated nephritis. *Kidney Int.* 1984;26:445.

31. Peces R, Navascues RA, Baltar J, et al. Antiglomerular basement membrane antibody-mediated glomerulonephritis after intranasal cocaine use. *Nephron.* 1999;81:434.

32. Xenocostas A, Ghayur T, Setrakian JC, et al. Anti-glomerular basement membrane glomerulonephritis after extracorporeal shock wave lithotripsy. *Am J Kidney Dis.* 1999;33:128.

One of several similar reports.

33. Westman KW, Ericsson UB, et al. Prevalence of autoantibodies associated with glomerulonephritis, unaffected after extracorporeal shock wave lithotripsy for renal calculi, in a three-year follow-up. *Scand J Urol Nephrol.* 1997;31:463.

A study of 66 patients who underwent lithotripsy treatment. At 3-year follow-up, no patient had developed elevated AGBMA titers.

34. Bombassei GJ, Kaplan AA. The association between hydrocarbon exposure and anti-glomerular basement membrane antibody-mediated disease (Goodpasture's syndrome). *Am J Ind Med.* 1992;21:141.

35. Lechleitner P, Defregger M, Lhotta K, et al. Goodpasture's syndrome. Unusual presentation after exposure to hard metal dust. *Chest.* 1993;103:956.

36. Donaghy M, Rees AJ. Cigarette smoking and lung haemorrhage in glomerulonephritis caused by autoantibodies to glomerular basement membrane. *Lancet.* 1983;2:1390.

37. Wilson CB, Smith RC. Goodpasture's syndrome associated with influenza A2 virus infection. *Ann Intern Med.* 1972;76:91.

38. Calderon EJ, Wichmann I, Vareta JM, et al. Presence of glomerular basement membrane (GBM) antibodies in HIV-patients with *Pneumocystis carinii* pneumonia. *Clin Exp Immunol.* 1997;107:448.

Found AGBMA in 75% of patients who were human immunodeficiency virus (HIV)-negative with Pneumocystis carinii pneumonia (PCP), but not in five patients HIV-positive with PCP. Immunoblot was not performed.

39. Kalluri R, Meyers K, Mogyorosi A, et al. Goodpasture's syndrome involving overlap with Wegener's granulomatosis and anti-glomerular basement membrane disease. *J Am Soc Nephrol.* 1997;8:1795.

Up to 30% of patients with AGBMA disease have ANCA and up to 8% of ANCA-positive patients have AGBMA.

40. Hellmark T, Niles JL, Collins AB, et al. Comparison of anti-GBM antibodies in sera with and without ANCA. *J Am Soc Nephrol.* 1997;8:376.

41. Bosch X, Mirapeix E, Font J, et al. Prognostic implication of anti-neutrophil cytoplasmic autoantibodies with myeloperoxidase specificity in anti-glomerular basement membrane disease. *Clin Nephrol.* 1991;36:107.

Of 37 consecutive patients with AGBMA, 12 were dual positive for ANCA/AGBMA. With therapy, 5 of 12 (42%) recovered renal function, all 5 of whom had serum creatinine values above 6.8 mg/dL.

42. Levy JB, Lachmann RH, Pusey CD. Recurrent Goodpasture's disease [see comments]. *Am J Kidney Dis*. 1996;27:573.
    Report of a patient and review.
43. Rees AJ, Lockwood CM, Peters DK. Enhanced allergic tissue injury in Goodpasture's syndrome by intercurrent bacterial infection. *BMJ*. 1977;2:723.
    Bacterial infections (mostly shunt related) were associated with relapses.
44. Briggs JD, Jones E. Renal transplantation for uncommon diseases. Scientific Advisory Board of the ERA-EDTA Registry. European Renal Association-European Dialysis and Transplant Association. *Nephrol Dial Transplant*. 1999;14:570.
45. Saxena R, Bygren P, Arvastson B, et al. Circulating autoantibodies as serological markers in the differential diagnosis of pulmonary renal syndrome. *J Intern Med*. 1995;238:143.
    Of 40 patients with Goodpasture's syndrome, 27 (68%) had ANCA, 9 (22%) had AGBMA.
46. Green RJ, Ruoss SJ, Kraft SA, et al. Pulmonary capillaritis and alveolar hemorrhage. Update on diagnosis and management [published erratum appears in *Chest*. 1997;112:300]. *Chest*. 1996;110:1305.
    A general review on diffuse alveolar hemorrhage.
47. Westman KW, Bygren P, Eilert I, et al. Rapid screening assay for anti-GBM antibody and ANCAs; an important tool for the differential diagnosis of pulmonary renal syndromes. *Nephrol Dial Transplant*. 1997;12:1863.
48. Zamora MR, Warner ML, Tudor R, et al. Diffuse alveolar hemorrhage and systemic lupus erythematosus. Clinical presentation, histology, survival, and outcome. *Medicine* (Baltimore). 1997;76:192.
    References 49 through 53 include some of the differential diagnoses.
49. Tanoue LT. Pulmonary manifestations of rheumatoid arthritis. *Clin Chest Med*. 1998;19:667.
50. Sullivan EJ, Hoffman GS. Pulmonary vasculitis. *Clin Chest Med*. 1998;19:759.
51. Asherson RA, Cervera R, Piette JC, et al. Catastrophic antiphospholipid syndrome. Clinical and laboratory features of 51 patients. *Medicine* (Baltimore). 1998;77:195.
52. Sabatine MS, Oelberg DA, Mark EJ, et al. Pulmonary cholesterol crystal embolization. *Chest*. 1997;112:1687.
53. Kalluri R, Pertrides S, Wilson CB, et al. Anti-alpha1 (IV) collagen autoantibodies associated with lung adenocarcinoma presenting as the Goodpasture syndrome. *Ann Intern Med*. 1996;124:651.

93. IDIOPATHIC PULMONARY HEMOSIDEROSIS

William L. Ring

ETIOLOGY

Idiopathic pulmonary hemosiderosis (IPH) is a rare disease of unclear etiology and pathogenesis characterized by the abnormal collection of hemosiderin in the lungs. It is primarily a disease of the first decade of life, but may be diagnosed in adults. Equal gender distribution is seen and at least some cases have a genetic predisposition. A number of reports have noted an association between celiac disease and IPH, and in some cases treatment of the celiac disease seemed to improve the course of the IPH. However, a pathogenetic link between the celiac disease and IPH remains controversial. Some reports have suggested that IPH may be associated with low socioeconomic status, toxic exposure (insecticides, hydrocarbons), seasonal clustering (spring and fall), viral agents, or diet (cow's milk allergy). Exacerbations of IPH have been reported with pregnancy. Despite these associations, the etiology of IPH remains obscure.

PRESENTATION

The presentation of IPH is highly variable. Iron deficiency anemia and recurrent or chronic pulmonary symptoms (e.g., cough, hemoptysis, and dyspnea) characterize IPH. Patients may present with hemoptysis, which tends to be episodic. Although hemoptysis can be massive, it is often mild and can be absent despite significant intrapulmonary bleeding. Intrapulmonary bleeding may initially be clinically silent. An iron deficiency anemia can overshadow clinical or roentgenographic pulmonary abnormalities. Chronic cough, fatigue, dyspnea, and pallor are frequent. Occasionally, pulmonary hypertension develops.

DIAGNOSIS

The diagnosis of IPH is one of exclusion and generally requires ruling out a coagulopathy, hemodynamic abnormalities (congestive heart failure, mitral stenosis), and infection, as well as systemic disorders such as vasculitis, immune-complex disease, or antibasement membrane antibody disease.

CLINICAL FINDINGS

Chest radiographs in IPH are generally abnormal and demonstrate diffuse parenchymal infiltrates. At the time of an acute hemorrhage, chest radiographs may show diffuse mottled densities, which are particularly prominent in the perihilar regions and lower lung fields. After 2 to 3 days, the consolidation is replaced by a reticular pattern that resolves over 10 to 14 days. With repeated bleeding episodes, progressive interstitial changes can develop into a pattern of interstitial fibrosis, which can become massive. Hilar lymph nodes may be enlarged, particularly during acute episodes. Computed tomography (CT) findings confirm the chest roentgenogram findings. Magnetic resonance imaging may specifically diagnose a new hemorrhage because of the paramagnetic effect of ferric iron. Pulmonary function studies show a restrictive pattern, with an elevation of the carbon monoxide diffusing capacity during an episode of bleeding. A transient obstructive component also may be present.

The histologic findings are nonspecific, but an open lung biopsy is often required to exclude other diagnoses. The dominant histopathologic features are intra-alveolar hemorrhage and hemosiderin-laden macrophages. Hyperplasia of the alveolar epithelium and variable degrees of fibrosis can be seen, but vasculitis, necrosis, and granuloma formation are absent. Immunofluorescent stains are negative for immune deposits at the basement membranes, and inflammatory changes are minimal.

TREATMENT AND PROGNOSIS

The prognosis of IPH is highly variable, ranging from decade-long periods of remission to sudden death from massive hemoptysis. The median survival is usually reported to be approximately 3 years after diagnosis, although at least one recent study reports much better prognosis. Treatment of IPH is controversial and largely supportive. The results of therapy are difficult to interpret because of the natural variation in the clinical course of the disease and the small number of patients reported. No controlled therapeutic trials have been conducted. Corticosteroids remain the primary line of treatment, supported by clinical improvement in a number of case reports. However, the efficacy of high-dose corticosteroids during acute bleeding episodes remains unclear, and chronic steroid therapy may not alter the disease course. Case reports suggest that long-term treatment with moderate doses of inhaled steroids after stabilization with systemic steroids helps to control IPH. Claims have also been made of responsiveness of the disease to other immunosuppressants, particularly azathioprine and chloroquine. However, separation of drug effects from spontaneous remission is difficult to ascertain.

1. Soergel KH, Sommers SC. Idiopathic pulmonary hemosiderosis and related syndromes. *Am J Med*. 1962;32:499.
   A classic description of IPH.

2. Leatherman JW, Davies SF, Hoidal JR. Alveolar hemorrhage syndromes: diffuse microvascular lung hemorrhage in immune and idiopathic disorders. *Medicine* (Baltimore). 1984;63:343.

   An excellent review of all alveolar hemorrhage syndromes, including IPH.

3. Buxton-Thomas M, et al. Adult idiopathic pulmonary haemosiderosis: a comparison of lung function changes and the distribution of pulmonary disease in patients with and without coeliac disease. *Br J Dis Chest*. 1983;77:282.

   Results of chest radiographs, pulmonary function studies, CT scans, and ventilation–perfusion scans are reported in seven patients.

4. Cassimos CD, Chryssanthopoulos C, Panagiotidou C. Epidemiologic observations in idiopathic pulmonary hemosiderosis. *J Pediatr*. 1983;102:698.

   An epidemiologic survey of 30 children from northern Greece. The incidence of newly diagnosed cases decreased with improved living conditions and prohibition of certain insecticides, suggesting that environmental factors may contribute to the pathogenesis.

5. Breckenridge RL, Ross JS. Idiopathic pulmonary hemosiderosis: a report of familial occurrence. *Chest*. 1979;75:636.

   Reports on two siblings with IPH and speculates on familial or genetic factors.

6. Pacheco A, et al. Long-term clinical follow-up of adult idiopathic pulmonary hemosiderosis and celiac disease. *Chest*. 1991;99:152.

   A typical case report of the association between IPH and celiac disease, including improvement of the IPH when the patient was placed on a gluten-free diet, with 4 years of disease-free follow-up.

7. Helman D, et al. Management of idiopathic pulmonary haemosiderosis in pregnancy: report of two cases. *Respirology*. 2003;8:398.

   Review of the treatment of IPH during pregnancy.

8. Buschman DL, Ballard R. Progressive massive fibrosis associated with idiopathic pulmonary hemosiderosis. *Chest*. 1993;104:293.

   A case report of a patient diagnosed with IPH during pregnancy at age 30 years, who over the next 23 years developed massive pulmonary fibrosis, felt to be secondary to the IPH.

9. Akyar S, Ozbek SS. Computed tomography findings in idiopathic pulmonary hemosiderosis. *Respiration*. 1993;60:63.

   A case report on the CT findings in a patient with IPH.

10. Rubin GD, et al. Diagnosis of pulmonary hemosiderosis by MR imaging. *AJR*. 1989;152:573.

    Suggests magnetic resonance imaging may have a role in the diagnosis of occult pulmonary hemorrhage.

11. Kiper N, et al. Long-term clinical course of patients with idiopathic pulmonary hemosiderosis (1979–1994): prolonged survival with low-dose corticosteroid therapy. *Pediatr Pulmonol*. 1999;27:180.

    Reports the experience at a university hospital in Turkey, following 23 patients with IPH for between 6 months and 10 years. Seven patients were lost to follow-up; only one death was confirmed. The authors felt that long-term, low-dose steroids explained the improved survival.

12. Rossi GA, et al. Long-term prednisone and azathioprine treatment of a patient with pulmonary hemosiderosis. *Pediatr Pulmonol*. 1992;13:176.

    A case in which immunosuppressive agents appeared to lead to remission.

13. Zaki M, Saleh QA, Mutari GA. Effectiveness of chloroquine therapy in idiopathic pulmonary hemosiderosis. *Pediatr Pulmonol*. 1995;20:125.

    A case report of 7-month remission with chloroquine treatment, recurrence within 2 months of discontinuing chloroquine, and finally 18 months of remission with restarting chloroquine.

14. Tutor JD, Eid NS. Treatment of idiopathic pulmonary hemosiderosis with inhaled flunisolide. *South Med J*. 1995;88:984.

    A case report of treating an adult with inhaled flunisolide 750 µg twice per day, after weaning off systemic corticosteroids, associated with at least 4 years of remission.

15. Cohen S. Idiopathic pulmonary hemosiderosis. *Am J Med Sci.* 1999;317:67.
    Reports on two children, 5 and 13 years of age, with IPH who ultimately died of this disease. This study reported peripheral blood neutropenia and eosinophilia before acute exacerbations of IPH.

94. IDIOPATHIC INTERSTITIAL PNEUMONIA

Tony Han, J. Scott Parrish, and Cecilia M. Smith

Idiopathic interstitial pneumonias (IIP) comprise a group of diffuse parenchymal lung diseases characterized by various degrees of inflammation and fibrosis leading to destruction of lung architecture. The primary area of damage involves the space between the alveolar epithelium and the capillary basement membrane (interstitium), but other areas become involved as the disease progresses.

Idiopathic denotes an unknown etiology; therefore known causes must be excluded by careful history and exam. There are many secondary causes of *interstitial pneumonia* including systemic drugs (bleomycin, methotrexate), inhaled agents (silica, isocyanates), connective tissue diseases (lupus, scleroderma), and viral illnesses. Other major criteria for diagnosing IIP are impaired gas exchange with hypoxemia at rest or with exercise, restrictive pulmonary function with reduced lung volumes, and reticular changes on high-resolution computed tomography (HRCT) or chest radiographs. Other distinct diffuse lung diseases such as lymphangioleiomyomatosis, Langerhan's cell histiocytosis, eosinophilic pneumonia, and sarcoidosis are excluded from this category.

The diagnostic approach to the patient presenting with dyspnea, cough, and interstitial radiographic changes should begin with a thorough history, with special attention focused on (1) the clinical progression of symptoms such as cough, dyspnea, and exercise tolerance; (2) an environmental and occupational history, including exposure to drugs; (3) tobacco use; (4) connective tissue diseases; and (5) exposures or familial predisposition such as family history for similar symptoms.

Based on the recent 2001 ATS/ERS classification, the seven clinicopathologic entities within the IIP are idiopathic pulmonary fibrosis, nonspecific interstitial pneumonia, cryptogenic organizing pneumonia, acute interstitial pneumonia, respiratory bronchiolitis-associated interstitial lung disease, desquamative interstitial pneumonia, and lymphoid interstitial pneumonia.

IDIOPATHIC PULMONARY FIBROSIS

Idiopathic pulmonary fibrosis (IPF) is a chronic fibrosing interstitial pneumonia and is the most common form of IIP. It was previously known as cryptogenic fibrosing alveolitis (CFA or lone CFA), but the definition of IPF has become more specific with the recent changes in classification of IIP. Diagnosis is made after excluding all known causes of interstitial pneumonia and is based on a pattern of usual interstitial pneumonia (UIP) on surgical lung biopsy. Alternatively, diagnosis can be made based on a compatible clinical picture, functional lung abnormalities, and a typical appearance on HRCT.

IPF has a male predominance and a reported prevalence of 20.2 per 100,000 population for men and 13.2 per 100,000 for women. Mean age at diagnosis is 66 years old, and there is no predilection for race or ethnicity. Cases of familial IPF have been described, but no specific genetic markers have been identified.

IPF presents with insidiously progressive nonproductive cough and dyspnea lasting months. On physical examination, 25 to 50% of patients exhibit digital clubbing.

Dry, end-inspiratory crackles are commonly heard on chest auscultation, and are referred to as "Velcro" crackles. Some findings (e.g., evidence of pulmonary hypertension and cor pulmonale) may occur in late disease. Chest roentgenograms typically disclose basilar and bilateral reticular opacities that may predate symptoms. HRCT often reveals patchy, bilateral, peripheral and subpleural reticular opacities. Subpleural honeycombing and traction bronchiectasis are also seen in more severe cases. Small areas of ground-glass opacity can be seen; however, extensive ground glass appearance suggests another diagnosis. Pulmonary function tests disclose reduction in static lung volumes (i.e., restrictive lung disease) and reduced carbon monoxide diffusing capacity (DLCO). In the setting of significant obstructive disease (i.e., emphysema), lung volumes can appear normal. Arterial blood gases demonstrate hypoxemia with a widened (A–a) gradient during rest or exercise. Finally, serologic examination for hypersensitivity pneumonia and connective tissue disease may be helpful in ruling out other causes in certain patients.

Histopathologic samples obtained by thoracoscopic lung biopsy may distinguish IIP subsets and predict the patient's response to immunosuppressive therapy. Multiple samples should be obtained from separate lobes. Unfortunately, transbronchial biopsy does not provide sufficient tissue to allow an accurate analysis. The histologic pattern of UIP is the sine quo non of IPF. UIP features temporal and geographic heterogeneity within the same lung, containing zones of inflammation, interstitial fibrosis, collagen deposition, and thickened alveolar septa. Focal nests of proliferating fibroblasts are characteristic. Honeycombing with distorted alveolar architecture is found adjacent to areas of normal lung parenchyma.

The clinical course is insidious and, although survival and prognosis vary, the mean survival after diagnosis is around 2.8 years. Although older studies suggest a favorable response to immunosuppression in IPF, these older studies probably included other types of IIP that typically respond to steroids. There have been no controlled trials to definitively support immunosuppressive therapy in IPF. Some experts now debate the role of inflammation in IPF and consider abnormal fibrosis regulation as a primary mechanism of disease. There are current studies looking into fibrosis regulation as a possible target for treatment. A large, recent multicenter trial involving gamma interferon was negative; however, there was a trend toward improved mortality in a smaller subgroup with milder disease. A previous open-label study looking at pirfenidone seemed to show disease stabilization in end-stage IPF. The main diagnostic task is distinguishing IPF from other types of IIP, because the other types respond more favorably to steroid therapy.

NONSPECIFIC INTERSTITIAL PNEUMONIA

Nonspecific interstitial pneumonia (NSIP) is a form of IIP that is clinically similar to IPF, but with a different histologic pattern and a better prognosis. The term was previously used to describe lung disease in immunocompromised patients, but now refers to a subacute, progressive inflammatory lung disorder with varying amounts of fibrosis. This disorder was previously lumped together with IPF, and some cases of NSIP with prominent fibrosis may indeed be early IPF. The inflammatory type of NSIP appears to be a distinct entity. NSIP has a slight female predominance with a slightly younger mean age of onset than IPF. Compared to IPF, NSIP has a more subacute progression over weeks and months and fever is more common. Prognosis is related to the amount of fibrosis present on histology with good response to immunosuppressive therapy when a cellular pattern is prominent.

Chest radiographs are almost always abnormal with patchy parenchymal opacities being the most common finding. HRCT shows predominant ground glass opacities in a bilateral, symmetric distribution. Honeycombing and consolidation are not commonly seen.

Histopathologically, the inflammatory pattern is temporally homogeneous with a patchy distribution suggestive of a response to a single insult. A variable amount of inflammatory infiltrate is seen, but fibrosis is mild. Fibroblastic foci and honeycombing which are hallmarks of UIP are typically absent.

CRYPTOGENIC ORGANIZING PNEUMONIA

Cryptogenic organizing pneumonia (COP), which was previously described as *bronchiolitis obliterans organizing pneumonia*, is the term used to describe a distinct idiopathic clinical entity with characteristic patchy consolidation on radiographs and histopathology of granulation tissue filling alveoli and bronchioles. Organizing pneumonia is a histopathologic finding common to a number of diseases including infections. It should be considered in the patient presenting with a flulike illness, with patchy infiltrates on chest radiograph not responsive to antibiotics. No gender predominance and no association with tobacco use are seen. Organizing pneumonia can be found in a number of different clinical settings such as postinfectious syndromes (e.g., cytomegalovirus, adenovirus, influenza, chlamydia, malaria); reactions to drugs (e.g., gold, sulfasalazine, methotrexate, bleomycin, amiodarone, cephalosporins, cocaine, phenytoin); collagen vascular diseases (rheumatoid disease, polymyositis); bone marrow, lung, and renal transplantation; and radiation therapy. The idiopathic form (COP) is diagnosed by excluding secondary causes and can occur in childhood as well as adulthood.

Radiographically, COP is characterized by migratory bilateral patchy alveolar infiltrates. HRCT demonstrates bilateral consolidation, predominantly in subpleural or peribronchial areas. Lung biopsy reveals an alveolar filling process with polypoid granulation tissue plugs that fill bronchial lumens. Distal bronchiolar inflammation is also seen.

The prognosis and response to immunosuppressive therapy is generally good. Recovery rates range from 65 to 85%. Treatment can begin with up to 1 mg/kg or 60 mg daily of prednisone for 1 to 3 months; the dose is then tapered according to clinical parameters.

RESPIRATORY BRONCHIOLITIS INTERSTITIAL LUNG DISEASE AND DESQUAMATIVE INTERSTITIAL PNEUMONIA

Respiratory bronchiolitis interstitial lung disease (RB-ILD) and desquamative interstitial pneumonia (DIP) are interstitial inflammatory lung diseases closely associated with significant smoking history. They are part of a continuum of smoking-related conditions with DIP being more severe. Clinically, RB-ILD and DIP patients are less symptomatic than IPF and NSIP patients. Histologically, the alveoli contain pigmented macrophages and there is peribronchiolar thickening of alveolar septae. The pattern is uniform and thought to be reactive. Historically, macrophages were thought to be desquamating epithelial cells leading to the term *DIP*. Macrophage accumulation can also be a nonspecific incidental finding in lungs of smokers. Honeycombing and fibroblastic foci are rare. The disorder occurs in the fourth and fifth decades of life and has a male predominance. The clinical course is insidious, but has a good prognosis and high rate of spontaneous resolution if the patient stops smoking. It may also respond to steroid therapy.

ACUTE INTERSTITIAL PNEUMONIA

An acute variant of ILD is described as *acute interstitial pneumonia* (AIP), *diffuse alveolar damage* (DAD), and the *Hamman–Rich* syndrome. Considerable overlap is seen in the description of these entities, both clinically and histopathologically. AIP can be thought of as idiopathic acute respiratory distress syndrome with a similar presentation and clinical course. The histopathology is called DAD, and demonstrates uniform, diffuse, active, massive, interstitial fibrosis with hyaline membrane formation in the early phases. Clinically, patients have acute, rapidly progressive respiratory failure requiring mechanical ventilation with a low incidence of recovery. The syndrome is often preceded by an acute viral illness, but the exact etiology is unknown. The ongoing lung damage and respiratory failure respond poorly to immunosuppressive therapy. The lungs undergo various stages of injury starting with exudates, followed by proliferation, and finally fibrosis.

LYMPHOID INTERSTITIAL PNEUMONIA

Lymphoid interstitial pneumonia (LIP) is characterized by a prominent lymphocytic interstitial inflammation. It is usually related to an underlying systemic disease such as HIV infection, low-grade lymphoma or autoimmune disorders. Transbronchial biopsy can be diagnostic, with histopathology showing a dense lymphoid infiltrate with follicles and granulomas. Management involves identifying and treating the underlying lymphoma, immunodeficiency state, or autoimmune disease.

Because of the poor response to therapy in patients with IPF, and the risk of significant adverse reactions to immunosuppression, routine therapy cannot be recommended at this time. If therapy is warranted, the current recommendations for treatment consists of prednisone (0.5–1 mg/kg per day) combined with an immunosuppressive agent such as cyclophosphamide (2 mg/kg per day) or azathioprine (2 mg/kg per day) based on ideal body weight. Serially performed objective tests (e.g., rest and exercise arterial blood gases, pulmonary function tests, and HRCT scans) can greatly enhance the clinical assessment of therapy response. These can be followed at 3-month intervals, unless symptoms warrant more frequent testing. Research is ongoing to seek new therapies for IPF. Of particular interest are therapies directed at those factors involved in fibroblast propagation, collagen synthesis, and the release of proliferative cytokines. Pirfenidone, an inhibitor of transforming growth factor-β, inhibits collagen synthesis. In a preliminary study, pirfenidone appeared to stabilize lung function in a small group of patients with IPF. Interferon γ-1b combined with low-dose prednisolone initially showed some promise in a small study, but a larger multicenter trial failed to show overall benefit in lung function or quality of life.

The drug regimen of choice for non–UIP IIP is also evolving and depends the histopathology identified. A reasonable strategy is to initiate therapy with oral corticosteroids (e.g., prednisone) in a dose of 0.5 to 1.0 mg/kg per day (not to exceed 100 mg/d), for 4 to 6 weeks. Response is assessed at the end of this period and the dose is adjusted accordingly. If no response is noted, the steroid therapy is tapered off. If a response occurs, the same or a slightly modified dose is maintained and reevaluation is carried out in 4 weeks. Thereafter, dosing is determined by evaluating patient response and steroid side effects. The usual sequence is to taper slowly to an alternate day regimen of 15 to 20 mg for 3 to 6 months. An attempt is then made to taper the steroids off. Often discontinuation is not possible and steroids are maintained long term (months to years), with periodic slow withdrawal to determine whether the patient is in remission.

Other therapeutic approaches include the use of bronchodilators in those patients who may have combined obstructive and restrictive disease. Infection prophylaxis with the influenza vaccine, pneumococcal vaccine, and *Pneumocystis carinii* prophylaxis in those patients on immunosuppressive regimens are beneficial.

Lung transplantation should be anticipated early in the disease course for patients who are deemed candidates, because the waiting list for transplantation often exceeds the survival of the patient with IPF. Single lung transplantation is usually performed for symptomatic disease when the FVC is less than 60% or DLco is less than 50%. Long-term survival after transplant is around 40% at 5 years.

---

1. Alasaly K, et al. Cryptogenic organizing pneumonia—a report of 25 cases and a review of the literature. *Medicine* (Baltimore). 1995;74:201.

    A review of the clinical presentation and radiographic and histopathologic features of COP.

2. Bjoraker, et al. Prognostic significance of histopathologic subsets in idiopathic pulmonary fibrosis. *Am J Respir Crit Care Med.* 1998:157:199.

    A histopathologic review defining subsets with improved prognosis when compared with classic usual IP.

3. Coultas D, et al. The epidemiology of interstitial lung diseases. *Am J Respir Crit Care Med.* 1994;150:967.

    A broad review of the many causes of ILD: infectious, collagen vascular, and other etiologies.

4. Daniil ZD, et al. A histologic pattern of nonspecific interstitial pneumonia is associated with a better prognosis than usual interstitial pneumonia in patients with cryptogenic fibrosing alveolitis. *Am J Respir Crit Care Med.* 1999;160:899.
   One hundred thirteen cases of CFA (IPF) were reviewed and reclassified as NSIP and IPF using more current criteria. There was a distinct improvement in survival in NSIP patterns.
5. Fujita J, et al. Clinical features of non-specific interstitial pneumonia. *Respir Med.* 1999;93:113.
   A histopathologic description of NSIP that distinguishes outcome compared with UIP.
6. Epler G. Heterogeneity of bronchiolitis obliterans organizing pneumonia. *Curr Opin Pulm Med.* 1998;4:93.
   Reviews clinical presentation, causes, radiographic features, and treatment of COP.
7. Gay S, et al. Idiopathic pulmonary fibrosis—predicting response to therapy and survival. *Am J Respir Crit Care Med.* 1998;157:1063.
   Emphasizes the importance of lung biopsy cellularity as well as the use of a clinical, radiographic, and physiologic scoring system to determine response to therapy.
8. Johnson MA, et al. Randomised controlled trial comparing prednisolone alone with cyclophosphamide and low dose prednisolone in combination in cryptogenic fibrosing alveolitis. *Thorax.* 1989;44:280.
   Suggests that combination therapy may be a steroid-sparing alternative; however, many patients still failed either outcome. The study is small, which may have an impact on the lack of achieving statistical significance in terms of outcomes.
9. Katzenstein A, Myers J. Idiopathic pulmonary fibrosis. *Am J Respir Crit Care Med.* 1998;157:1301.
   A detailed description of histopathologic subsets and clinical outcomes.
10. Myers J. NSIP, UIP, and the ABCs of idiopathic interstitial pneumonias [EDITORIAL]. *Eur Respir J.* 1998;12:1003.
    Distinguishes and compares NSIP with UIP.
11. Nagai S, et al. Idiopathic nonspecific interstitial pneumonia/fibrosis: comparison with idiopathic pulmonary fibrosis and BOOP. *Eur Respir J.* 1998;12:1010.
    Reviews 31 patients with NSIP, described as a separate entity from IPF and COP.
12. Orens J, et al. The sensitivity of high-resolution CT in detecting idiopathic pulmonary fibrosis proved by open lung biopsy—a prospective study. *Chest.* 1995;108:109.
    In patients with dyspnea and abnormal pulmonary function tests, a normal HRCT was found not to exclude ILD. Physiologic testing was thought to be more sensitive than HRCT in detecting mild abnormalities in biopsy-proved disease in the presence of a normal HRCT.
13. Raghu G, et al. Azathioprine combined with prednisone in the treatment of idiopathic pulmonary fibrosis: a prospective double-blind, randomized, placebo-controlled clinical trial. *Am Rev Respir Dis.* 1991;144:291.
    Twenty-seven patients diagnosed with IPF were randomized in a prospective, double-blind, placebo-controlled study comparing combination therapy with azathioprine and prednisone to prednisone and placebo. Lung function evaluated after 1 year demonstrated slight improvement that did not reach statistical significance. Survival seemed better for the patients on combined therapy compared with those on prednisone alone.
14. Raghu G, et al. Treatment of idiopathic pulmonary fibrosis with a new antifibrotic agent, pirfenidone: results of a prospective, open label phase II study. *Am J Respir Crit Care Med.* 1999;159:1061.
    A small study describing stabilization of lung function in patients with biopsy-proven IPF who had experienced deterioration on standard immunosuppressive therapies.
15. Reynolds H. Diagnostic and management strategies for diffuse interstitial lung disease. *Chest.* 1998;113:192.

An algorithmic approach to the patient with diffuse ILD in a resource-efficient way, as well as variables predicting outcomes.

16. Ziesche R, et al. A preliminary study of long-term treatment with interferon gamma-1b and low-dose prednisolone in patients with idiopathic pulmonary fibrosis. *N Engl J Med.* 1999;341:1264.
    A 12-month treatment in patients with IPF who had prior documented failure to respond on prednisone therapy found improvement in total lung capacity and arterial oxygenation at rest and with exercise.

17. King TE Jr, et al. IPF: guidelines for diagnosis and treatment. ATS IPF Statement. *Am J Respir Crit Care Med.* 2000;161:646.

18. Raghu G, et al. A placebo-controlled trial of interferon gamma-1b in patients with idiopathic pulmonary fibrosis. *N Engl J Med.* 2004;350:125–133.
    A large, multicenter study of interferon gamma for IPF failed to show any benefit in survival, disease progression or lung function.

19. Honoré I, et al. Acute respiratory failure after interferon-γ therapy of end-stage pulmonary fibrosis. *Am J Respir Crit Care Med.* 2003;167:953–957.
    Four patients with IPF apparently develop DAD and respiratory failure shortly after IFN treatment.

20. American Thoracic Society/European Respiratory Society. International Multidisciplinary Consensus Classification of the Idiopathic Interstitial Pneumonias. *Am J Respir Crit Care Med.* 2002;165:277–304.
    This article is the current, definitive, multidisciplinary report on classification of IIP with diagnostic criteria and treatment recommendations.

21. Crystal R, et al. Future research directions in idiopathic pulmonary fibrosis: summary of a National Heart, Lung, and Blood Institute Working Group. *Am J Respir Crit Care Med.* 2003;166:236–246.
    This is a summary report suggesting future goals for research in the diagnosis and treatment of IPF. Suggestions include early detection methods, apoptosis mediators, fibroblast activity modifiers.

22. Ryu J, et al. Bronchiolar disorders. *Am J Respir Crit Care Med.* 2003;168:1277–1292.
    This is a comprehensive review of bronchiolar disorders including RB-ILD, DIP, and COP.

23. Flaherty K, et al. Fibroblastic foci in usual interstitial pneumonia: idiopathic versus collagen vascular disease. *Am J Respir Crit Care Med.* 2003;167:1410–1415.
    Increased profusion of fibroblastic foci in idiopathic UIP is associated with a poorer prognosis than UIP associated with collagen-vascular disease suggesting a marker for disease activity.

24. Nicholson A, et al. The relationship between individual histologic features and disease progression in idiopathic pulmonary fibrosis. *Am J Respir Crit Care Med.* 2002;166:173–177.
    Fibroblastic foci seem to correlate with DLCO, FVC, and mortality in IPF in this retrospective review.

25. Lama V, et al. Prognostic value of desaturation during a 6-minute walk test in idiopathic interstitial pneumonia. *Am J Respir Crit Care Med.* 2003;168:1084–1090.
    Desaturation on 6-minute walk was predictive of increased mortality and was seen more commonly in IPF versus NSIP patients.

26. Latsi P, et al. Fibrotic idiopathic interstitial pneumonia: the prognostic value of longitudinal functional trends. *Am J Respir Crit Care Med.* 2003;168:531.
    Retrospective analysis of IPF (CFA) shows that prognosis is related to DLCO decline and that a histologic pattern of fibrotic NSIP has a similar poor prognosis compared to UIP pattern.

27. Collard H, et al. Changes in clinical and physiologic variables predict survival in idiopathic pulmonary fibrosis. *Am J Respir Crit Care Med.* 2003;168:538–542.
    Prospective evaluation of changes in clinical and physiological variables over 6 and 12 months seem to provide a more accurate prognosis than baseline values alone.

28. Flaherty K, et al. Prognostic implications of physiologic and radiographic changes in idiopathic interstitial pneumonia. *Am J Respir Crit Care Med.* 2003;168:543–548.
    Decline in FVC at 6 months was the best predictor for mortality in patients with UIP and NSIP on surgical lung biopsy. HRCT changes and D_{LCO} were less useful.

29. Wells A, et al. Idiopathic pulmonary fibrosis: a composite physiologic index derived from disease extent observed by computed tomography. *Am J Respir Crit Care Med.* 2003;167:962–969.
    A composite physiologic index based on CT appearance, D_{LCO}, FVC. and FEV_1 was found to be useful for prognosis and prediction of mortality. This index was derived to account for changes caused by underlying COPD.

30. Saydain G, et al. Outcome of patients with idiopathic pulmonary fibrosis admitted to the intensive care unit. *Am J Respir Crit Care Med.* 2002;166:839–842.
    Of patients requiring ICU admission, 92% died at amedian of 2 months after discharge. The authors conclude that patients with idiopathic pulmonary fibrosis requiring admission to anintensive care unit have poor short- and long-term prognoses.

31. Strieter R. Mechanisms of pulmonary fibrosis: conference summary. *Chest.* 2001;120:77S–85S.
    This article is summary of recent molecular biology findings in IPF.

32. Nadrous H, et al. Impact of angiotensin-converting enzyme inhibitors and statins on survival in idiopathic pulmonary fibrosis. *Chest.* 2004;126:438–446.
    This retrospective study reported no beneficial effect of ACE inhibitors or statins on survival in IPF patients based on 52 patients on ACE inhibitors and 35 patients on statins.

33. Collard H, et al. Combined corticosteroid and cyclophosphamide therapy does not alter survival in idiopathic pulmonary fibrosis. *Chest.* 2004;125:2169–2174.
    One hundred sixty-four patients with IPF based on new consensus criteria did not appear to benefit from combination therapy in this retrospective study. This suggests inflammation may not be a major factor in disease progression.

34. Hunninghake G, et al. Radiologic findings are strongly associated with a pathologic diagnosis of usual interstitial pneumonia. *Chest.* 2003;124:1215–1223.
    Lower lobe honeycombing and irregular upper lobe lines were strongly associated with UIP on surgical biopsy in this multivariate analysis of 91 referred patients.

35. Wahidi M, et al. Progression of idiopathic pulmonary fibrosis in native lungs after single lung transplantation. *Chest.* 2002;121:2072–2076.
    Honeycombing and fibrosis progressed in the native lungs of five patients despite cyclosporine treatment for single lung transplant.

36. Timmer S, et al. Predicting survival of lung transplantation candidates with idiopathic interstitial pneumonia: does PaO_2 predict survival? *Chest.* 2002;122:779–784.
    This article predicts survival after transplant using PaO_2 and FEV_1/FVC ratios in IPF patients.

37. Travis W, et al. Idiopathic nonspecific interstitial pneumonia: prognostic significance of cellular and fibrosing patterns. *Am J Surg Pathol.* 2000;24:19–33.
    A retrospective review of NSIP seemed to show improved prognosis for cellular patterns of NSIP.

38. Gross T, Hunninghake G. Idiopathic pulmonary fibrosis. *N Engl J Med.* 2001;345:517–525.
    A review of IPF.

39. Wittram C. CT-histologic correlation of the ATS/ERS 2002 classification of idiopathic interstitial pneumonias. *Radiographics.* 2003;23:1057–1071.
    An extensive review of CT and histopathology in IIP.

95. PULMONARY MANIFESTATIONS OF RHEUMATOID ARTHRITIS

Frank D. Bender

Rheumatoid arthritis (RA) is a systemic inflammatory disorder whose pulmonary effects can be grouped into eight categories: (1) pleural disease; (2) interstitial pneumonitis; (3) drug-related pulmonary disease; (4) pulmonary nodules; (5) airways disease; (6) pulmonary vascular disease; (7) apical fibrocavitary disease; and (8) miscellaneous effects. Although frequently present as distinct entities, more than one manifestation can occur simultaneously or in sequence in an individual with rheumatoid disease.

PLEURAL DISEASE
Pleural disease is the most frequent pulmonary manifestation; it occurs as pleurisy in 20% of cases or as pleural effusion in 3 to 5%. In addition, asymptomatic pleural involvement is probably common, because autopsy series show pleural fibrosis or pleural effusion in approximately 50% of patients with RA. Despite the fact that RA itself is more common among women, pleural disease has a striking predominance for middle-aged men. It can occur at any time during the course of the RA; in 20% of cases, however, it immediately precedes or occurs at the onset of arthritis. The presence of pleural disease appears to bear no definite relationship to the activity of the arthritis or to the titer of rheumatoid factor but correlates to some extent with the presence of subcutaneous nodules. Pathologically, the pleura shows chronic (mononuclear cell) inflammation; pleural or subpleural rheumatoid nodules may occasionally be seen.

Symptoms, which are usually minimal, are absent at least one third of the time. When present, symptoms can include pleuritic pain or cough. Rarely, a large effusion causes dyspnea, especially in individuals with underlying parenchymal lung disease. Fever is uncommon. The chest roentgenogram reveals pleural thickening or effusion, which is unilateral in 80% of cases with a right-sided predominance.

A diagnostic thoracentesis is indicated to rule out malignancy or infection. The pleural fluid is characteristically a yellow-green color, although long-standing effusions may have an opalescent or milky quality from cholesterol crystals. Rheumatoid effusions are exudative and have elevated protein levels and lactate dehydrogenase levels frequently above 1000 U/L. The pH and glucose levels are low. The glucose is less than 50 mg/dL in 80% of cases and is less than 25 mg/dL in 66% of patients. The pleural fluid glucose fails to rise during intravenous infusions of glucose—a characteristic that distinguishes rheumatoid effusions from low glucose effusions caused by other diseases. The hyaluronidase level may be elevated. The differential cell count is usually lymphocytic, but granulocytes can predominate if the thoracentesis is done early on in the inflammatory process. Rheumatoid factor is present in higher concentrations than in the serum, but this is a nonspecific finding that occurs in effusions from other causes as well. Complement levels in pleural fluid can be sharply reduced in comparison with blood levels, a finding that distinguishes rheumatoid effusions and effusions secondary to systemic lupus erythematosus from those of other causes. A characteristic pleural fluid cytologic triad of elongated macrophages, giant multinucleated macrophages, and granular cell debris is felt to be diagnostic and should be sought. Mesothelial cells are nearly always absent.

The pleural effusions in RA tend to resolve spontaneously over the course of several months and frequently leave residual pleural thickening. Rarely, such thickening is sufficient to cause significant lung restriction and lead to consideration of pleural stripping. If the pleural disease causes significant dyspnea or other symptoms, therapeutic options include (1) nonsteroidal anti-inflammatory drugs, (2) drainage by thoracentesis, (3) a trial of oral corticosteroids if the effusion recurs, and (4) pleurodesis. Approximately 20% of RA-associated pleural effusions are persistent. Most of these, however, resolve within 1 to 5 years. Empyema has been reported to complicate rheumatoid pleural effusion, possibly because of impaired local defense mechanisms in conjunction with necrosis of a subpleural necrobiotic nodule. Systemic steroids, if used, could contribute to or mask the presence of an empyema, and those undergoing this treatment should be monitored carefully.

INTERSTITIAL PNEUMONITIS

Interstitial pneumonitis, historically and clinically indistinguishable from the idiopathic variety, occurs with greater than expected frequency in patients with RA. Conversely, 15 to 20% of patients with idiopathic interstitial pneumonitis either have a positive rheumatoid factor or develop symmetric polyarthritis consistent with RA during their clinical course. As with pleural disease, men are overrepresented. Interstitial pneumonitis occasionally precedes the onset of arthritis. Patients are generally seropositive, but the activity of the arthritis bears no relationship to the occurrence or severity of the interstitial pneumonitis.

The exact incidence of interstitial pneumonitis in RA is unclear. Characteristic roentgenographic findings of interstitial pneumonitis, a diffuse reticulonodular infiltrate with basilar predominance, occurred in 1.6% in a series of 516 patients with RA. Other series show characteristic plain chest film abnormalities in up to 6% of patients. High-resolution computed tomography (HRCT) is more sensitive than a plain chest roentgenogram in detecting interstitial disease. Various series report interstitial abnormalities in 10 to 40% of patients. Pulmonary function test abnormalities occur frequently. One report describes abnormal pulmonary function in 41% of an unselected series of patients with RA, the majority of whom had no pulmonary symptoms. The carbon monoxide diffusing capacity (DLCO) is believed to be more sensitive than spirometry in detecting interstitial disease. A recent study concluded that a diffusing less than 54% of predicted at presentation is a sensitive predictor of progressive interstitial lung disease.

With a combination of imaging techniques, physiologic testing, and bronchoalveolar lavage, abnormalities suggesting interstitial lung disease can be seen in up to 58% of patients with recent onset RA. In 14%, the changes are clinically significant. Cigarette smoking is an important risk factor in the development of interstitial disease. Serologic testing for circulating levels of KL-6 (a MUC1 mucin) has been proposed as a sensitive marker for active rheumatoid interstitial pneumonitis as well as other forms of interstitial lung disease.

Nonproductive cough, exertional dyspnea, and easy fatigability are the most frequent symptoms. Clinical stability may be present for years or, rarely, a rapid progression toward respiratory failure is seen. Examination reveals characteristic fine "Velcro" bibasilar crepitation. Subcutaneous nodules occur in most cases, and finger clubbing is quite common. Symptomatic individuals demonstrate hypoxemia (worsened by exercise), diminished DLCO, and reduced static lung volumes. The course of rheumatoid interstitial pneumonitis is variable.

The decision to treat rheumatoid-associated interstitial disease is based on the initial severity of symptoms and of physiologic impairment, as well as on the rate of deterioration over time. Initial treatment is usually with corticosteroids. Immunosuppressive agents (e.g., cyclophosphamide or methotrexate) can be tried in those who are unresponsive to corticosteroids or who are at risk for severe side effects from them. Infliximab, the tumor necrosis factor-α inhibitor, may have a role in treating RA-associated pulmonary fibrosis as detailed in a recent case report. A poor prognosis for patients with RA hospitalized for evaluation or treatment of interstitial pneumonitis has been reported, with a median survival of 3.5 years and a 5-year survival of 39%.

DRUG-RELATED PULMONARY DISEASE

The possibility of drug-induced interstitial pneumonitis and of other pulmonary reactions to treatment must be kept in mind when evaluating patients with RA. Methotrexate causes pulmonary reactions in 1 to 5% of patients. An acute hypersensitivity interstitial pneumonitis is most common. Other reactions include pleuritis, hilar adenopathy, and nodules. An eosinophilia may be seen up to 50%. Cough not associated with interstitial disease can occur, which is felt to be an irritant effect of methotrexate.

Risk factors for the development of methotrexate-associated pulmonary toxicity include advanced age, diabetes, low serum albumin, preexisting interstitial abnormalities, and previous adverse reactions to disease-modifying antirheumatic drugs. Low-dose methotrexate is not associated with the development of chronic interstitial lung disease.

Gold can produce interstitial pneumonitis. Factors that can help in distinguishing gold-induced interstitial pneumonitis from rheumatoid-associated interstitial disease are a female predominance, the presence of a skin rash or fever, low titers of rheumatoid factor, a lymphocytosis in bronchoalveolar lavage fluid, and gold-specific chest CT findings. With both methotrexate and gold, treatment of pulmonary toxicity involves withdrawal of the drug and administration of corticosteroids.

Ibuprofen has been associated with hypersensitivity pneumonitis, pleural effusions, and exacerbation of asthma. Corticosteroids are associated with opportunistic pulmonary infections that can resemble an interstitial pneumonitis.

Infliximab is associated with the development of opportunistic infections. *Mycobacterium tuberculosis* is the most frequent, and may occur early in treatment and present with extrapulmonary disease.

In general, the evaluation and management of possible drug-related pulmonary toxicity requires (1) excluding progression of rheumatoid interstitial disease and infection; (2) withdrawing the potentially offending drug (and not rechallenging); and (3) treating with corticosteroids, as appropriate.

A lung biopsy should be considered in cases (1) of rapidly progressive interstitial disease; (2) where concern exists regarding drug-induced disease or opportunistic lung infection; or (3) of unexplained fever.

PULMONARY NODULES

Necrobiotic nodules in the lung parenchyma, either single (34% of cases) or multiple (66%), can occur at any time during the course of RA. They sometimes occur coincident with an exacerbation of joint symptoms. Necrobiotic nodules are more common in men and correlate with the presence of subcutaneous nodules. Histologically identical to subcutaneous rheumatoid nodules, they are characterized by palisading epithelial cells surrounding a central core of fibrinoid necrosis. These lesions tend to be asymptomatic unless they become very large, when they can cause compressive symptoms. They infrequently undergo cavitation, at which time minimal hemoptysis may be present. Few become infected. Nodules can rupture into the pleural space, resulting in bronchopleural fistulas, pleural effusions, pneumothoraces, or pyopneumothoraces. On chest radiographs, the nodules appear as rounded, homogenous densities 0.3 to 7.0 cm in diameter, typically located in the peripheral lung fields. They can persist unchanged, cavitate, or resolve spontaneously; frequently, they wax and wane with disease activity. Although reports attest to steroids hastening their resolution, most nodules require no specific therapy; however, a single nodule requires the same evaluation as any solitary pulmonary nodule.

Caplan's syndrome was initially described as the appearance of nodular pulmonary opacities in coal miners with simple pneumoconiosis who had symmetric polyarthritis consistent with rheumatoid disease, a positive rheumatoid factor, or both. The syndrome has subsequently been described in individuals with occupational exposure to silicates, asbestos, iron, and aluminum powder. Histologically, the nodules resemble necrobiotic nodules except that a zone of inflammatory cells containing the offending dust is interposed between the palisading epithelial cells and the central necrosis. The nodules tend to occur in crops, which may herald the onset or worsening of arthritis symptoms. Roentgenographically, the nodules are multiple, 0.5 to 5.0 cm in diameter, and peripherally located. They frequently undergo cavitation and occasionally calcify. No specific therapy currently exists.

AIRWAYS DISEASE

Distal airways involvement in RA can manifest as small airways disease with expiratory airflow obstruction, bronchiectasis, bronchiolitis obliterans with organizing pneumonia (BOOP), or obliterative bronchiolitis.

Small airways disease resulting in expiratory airflow obstruction occurs in 16 to 30% of nonsmokers and 60% of smokers with RA. Airflow obstruction is caused by a peribronchiolar mononuclear cell infiltration, which can progress to an obliterative bronchiolitis. Small airways disease is associated with the presence of rheumatoid factor in high titer, rheumatoid nodules, keratoconjunctivitis sicca (Sjögren's syndrome), and specific HLA alloantigens.

Pathologically, *BOOP* is defined as granulation tissue in terminal bronchioles with distal organizing pneumonia. BOOP is associated with restrictive pulmonary function tests, cough, fever, weight loss, dyspnea, and bilateral pulmonary infiltrates. Corticosteroids are useful for treatment.

Obliterative bronchiolitis is pathologically a constrictive peribronchiolar fibrosis involving small airways. Despite the similar sounding name, this disorder is pathologically and prognostically distinct from BOOP. Obliterative bronchiolitis is associated with obstructive pulmonary function tests, female gender, more advanced rheumatoid disease, use of gold and penicillamine, and Sjögren's syndrome. Rapidly progressive dyspnea with cough is seen. Corticosteroids are used in treatment.

Bronchiectasis is seen in 35% of patients on HRCT scan and may reflect the result of small airways disease and recurrent infections.

PULMONARY VASCULAR DISEASE

Severe pulmonary vascular involvement in RA is rare. Several cases of progressive pulmonary hypertension with resultant cor pulmonale have been reported in young women with long-standing RA. Although lung tissue from individuals with rheumatoid interstitial pneumonitis occasionally contains a minor component of vasculitis, lung histology from these women predominantly reveals pulmonary arteritis with fibrotic intimal proliferation and medial hypertrophy within small muscular pulmonary arteries and negligible interstitial pneumonitis. Whether such cases represent a distinct variant of rheumatoid lung disease rather than a coincidental association of pulmonary arteritis with RA remains unclear. Patients with this syndrome have a poor prognosis and look and behave similarly to those with primary pulmonary hypertension.

Pulmonary hypertension (pulmonary artery systolic pressure of 30 mm Hg or more by Doppler echocardiography) was detected in 31% of a group of patients with RA. Two thirds of this group had no clinical evidence of heart disease or pulmonary function test abnormalities.

Pulmonary capillaritis and diffuse alveolar hemorrhage have been described but they are rare. Secondary pulmonary hypertension from interstitial pneumonitis can occur.

APICAL FIBROCAVITARY DISEASE

Apical fibrocavitary lesions have been described in a very small number of patients with RA. A recent report suggested that this is a clinically distinct pattern of lung involvement in RA. Clinically, the lesions may suggest tuberculosis and look similar to the apical pulmonary lesions seen in ankylosing spondylitis. Pathologically, cavitary necrobiotic nodules (clinically unsuspected) and interstitial fibrosis are seen.

Other pulmonary conditions seen in patients with RA include malignancies, bronchiogenic carcinoma and lymphomas, and amyloid deposition that can present with interstitial infiltrates. Reduced respiratory muscle strength and endurance and a reduced aerobic capacity in RA patients recently have been reported. Finally, RA can involve structures that can affect the upper airway. Cricoarytenoid arthritis can produce laryngeal obstruction and stridor. In addition, C1–C2 subluxation, which can occur with neck hyperextension during oral endotracheal intubation, can produce quadriparesis.

1. Vourlekis JS, Brown KK. PCCU lesson 17, volume14—thoracic complications of RA. Available: http://www.chestnet.org/education/online/pccu/vol14
   Well-referenced recent review article. An excellent resource.

2. Dedhia HV, DiBartolomeo A. Rheumatoid arthritis. *Crit Care Clin*. 2002;18:841–854.

   A review article with an emphasis on ICU care and airway management.

3. Tanoue LT. Pulmonary manifestations of rheumatoid arthritis. *Clin Chest Med*. 1998;4:667.

   An excellent, concise well-referenced review article. A definitive source.

4. Anaya JM, et al. Pulmonary involvement in rheumatoid arthritis. *Semin Arthritis Rheum*. 1995;24:242.

   A comprehensive review article.

5. Helmers R, Galvin J, Hunninghake G. Pulmonary manifestations associated with rheumatoid arthritis. *Chest*. 1991;100:235.

   A concise, well-referenced review article.

6. Winterbauer RH, DePaso W, Lambert J. Pulmonary disease in rheumatoid arthritis patients. *J Respir Dis*. 1989;10:35.

   A clinically oriented review article.

7. Sahn SA. The pleura. *Am Rev Respir Dis*. 1988;138:184.

   State-of-the-art review of pleural effusion with a well-referenced section on rheumatoid pleural involvement. A definitive source.

8. Saag KG, et al. Rheumatoid arthritis lung disease. Determinants of radiographic and physiologic abnormalities. *Arthritis Rheum*. 1996;39:1711.

   Concludes that smoking is an independent predictor of radiographic and physiologic abnormalities suggestive of interstitial lung disease in RA.

9. Gabbay E, et al. Interstitial lung disease in recent onset rheumatoid arthritis. *Am J Respir Crit Care Med*. 1997;156:528.

10. Dawson JK, Fewins HE, Desmond J, et al. Predictors of progression of HRCT diagnosed fibrosing alveolitis in patients with RA. *Ann Rheum Dis*. 2002;61:517–521.

    They found a low diffusing capacity (<54% predicted) predicted progression.

11. Vassallo R, Matteson E, Thomas CF Jr. Clinical response of RA-associated pulmonary fibrosis to tumor necrosis factor-alpha inhibition. *Chest*. 2002;122:1093–1096.

    In this case report, infliximab treatments stabilized deteriorating pulmonary function and improved cough, dyspnea, and fatigue.

12. Oyama T, et al. Detection of interstitial pneumonitis in patients with rheumatoid arthritis by measuring circulating levels of KL-6, a human MUC1 mucin. *Lung*. 1997;175:379.

    This report associates active interstitial pneumonitis with an elevated serum KL-6 level. Potentially, a very useful test.

13. Ohnishi H, Yokoyama A, Kondo K, et al. Comparative study of KL-6, surfactant protein-A, surfactant protein-D, and monocyte chemoattractant protein-1 as serum markers for interstitial lung diseases. *Am J Respir Crit Care Med*. 2002;165:378–381.

    Of the markers studied, KL-6 is the best marker for interstitial lung disease. Twelve of the 33 patients with interstitial lung disease had collagen vascular diseases.

14. Hakala M. Poor prognosis in patients with rheumatoid arthritis hospitalized for interstitial lung fibrosis. *Chest*. 1988;93:114.

    A unique clinical analysis of one end of the spectrum of rheumatoid interstitial lung disease.

15. Kremer JM, et al. Clinical laboratory, radiographic, and histopathologic features of methotrexate-associated lung injury in patients with rheumatoid arthritis: a multicenter study with literature review. *Arthritis Rheum*. 1997;40:1829.

    An important review article.

16. Ohosonc Y, et al. Clinical characteristics of patients with rheumatoid arthritis and methotrexate induced pneumonitis. *J Rheumatol*. 1997;12:2299.

    This retrospective review defines risk factors for methotrexate pulmonary toxicity.

17. Dawson JK, Graham DR, Desmond J, et al. Investigation of the chronic pulmonary effects of low-dose methotrexate in patients with RA: a prospective study

incorporating HRCT scanning and pulmonary function tests. *Rheumatology* (Oxford). 2002;41:262–267.

18. Keane J, Gershon S, Wise RP, et al. Tuberculosis associated with infiximab, a tumor necrosis factoralpha-neutralizing agent. *N Engl J Med.* 2001;345:1098–1104.
    One must be aware of the potential for opportunistic infection with this drug. M. Tuberculosis *is the most common.*

19. Tomioka R, King Jr TE. Gold-induced pulmonary disease: clinical features, outcomes and differentiation from rheumatoid lung disease. *Am J Respir Crit Care Med.* 1997;155:1011.
    A clinically oriented article.

20. Perez T, Remy-Jardin M, Cortet B. Airways involvement in rheumatoid arthritis: clinical, functional and HRCT findings. *Am J Respir Crit Care Med.* 1998;157:1658.
    Study indicates that HRCT appears to be more sensitive than pulmonary function tests for detecting small airways disease.

21. Begin R, et al. Airways disease in a subset of non-smoking rheumatoid patients. *Am J Med.* 1983;72:743.
    Further evidence of the bronchiolitis of RA and its possible autoimmune basis.

22. Frank ST, et al. Pulmonary dysfunction in rheumatoid disease. *Chest.* 1973; 63:27.
    In this series, 41% had reduced diffusing capacity, including 50% of those with normal chest x-ray films.

23. Geddes DM, et al. Alpha-1-antitrypsin phenotypes in fibrosing alveolitis and rheumatoid arthritis. *Lancet.* 1977;2:1049.
    A highly significant increase in the frequency of MZ phenotype was found in patients with fibrosing alveolitis, both with and without RA—but not in patients with RA without lung involvement.

24. Geddes DM, et al. Progressive airway obliteration in adults and its association with rheumatoid disease. *Q J Med.* 1977;46:427.
    Six patients with RA and rapidly progressive obstructive airways disease are described; four were nonsmokers. Chest roentgenograms showed hyperinflation without infiltrates, and histologic examination revealed bronchiolitis obliterans.

25. Caplan A. Certain unusual radiological appearances in the chest of coal miners suffering from rheumatoid arthritis. *Thorax.* 1953;8:29.
    Initial description of rheumatoid pneumoconiosis.

26. Rubin EH, Gordon M, Thelmo WL. Nodular pleuropulmonary rheumatoid disease. *Am J Med.* 1967;42:567.
    A review of nonpneumoconiotic rheumatoid lung disease. Subpleural necrobiotic-type nodules and persistent bronchopleural fistula were seen.

27. Dawson JK, Goodson NG, Graham DR, et al. Raised pulmonary artery pressures measured with Doppler echocardiography in RA patients. *Rheumatology* (Oxford). 2000;39:1320–1325.
    Mild pulmonary hypertension was seen in 31% of RA patients.

28. Schwarz MI, et al. Isolated pulmonary capillaritis and diffuse alveolar hemorrhage in rheumatoid arthritis and mixed connective tissue disease. *Chest.* 1998;113:1609.
    First reported cases of diffuse alveolar hemorrhage in RA.

29. Morikawa J, et al. Pulmonary hypertension in a patient with rheumatoid arthritis. *Chest.* 1988;93:876.
    A case report and literature review of the rare association of pulmonary arteritis and RA.

30. Kay JM, Banik S. Unexplained pulmonary hypertension with pulmonary arteritis in rheumatoid disease. *Br J Dis Chest.* 1977;71:53.
    Describes a young woman with RA and pulmonary vasculitis, and reviews the related literature.

31. Yue CC. Apical fibro-cavitary lesions of the lung in rheumatoid arthritis: review of 2 cases and review of the literature. *Am J Med.* 1986;81:741.
    A good, clinically oriented report of this unusual condition.

32. Mellemkjaer L, et al. Rheumatoid arthritis and cancer risk. *Eur J Cancer.*
1996;324:1753.
   A positive association was seen between RA and non-Hodgkin's lymphoma,
   Hodgkin's disease, and lung cancer. There was a negative association between RA
   and colorectal cancer.
33. Cimen B, Deviren SD, Yorgacloglu ZR. Pulmonary function tests, aerobic capacity,
respiratory muscle strength, and endurance of patients with RA. *Clin Rheumatol.*
2001;20:168–173.
   Reduced respiratory muscle strength, endurance, and aerobic capacity was seen
   in this study of twenty-five RA patients with normal pulmonary function tests.
34. Lofgren RH, Montgomery WW. Incidence of laryngeal involvement in rheumatoid
arthritis. *N Engl J Med.* 1962;267:193.
   Describes features of cricoarytenoid involvement in RA.

96. THE LUNGS IN SYSTEMIC LUPUS ERYTHEMATOSUS PROGRESSIVE, SYSTEMIC SCLEROSIS AND ITS VARIANTS, POLYMYOSITIS, DERMATOMYOSITIS, AND MIXED CONNECTIVE TISSUE DISEASE

Asha Vyas Devereaux and Cecilia M. Smith

SYSTEMIC LUPUS ERYTHEMATOSUS

Systemic lupus erythematosus (SLE) commonly affects the lungs and pleura. Manifestations of SLE that directly affect the respiratory system include (1) pleuritis
with or without pleural effusions; (2) acute lupus pneumonitis; (3) chronic interstitial
pneumonitis and interstitial fibrosis; (4) hemorrhagic alveolitis with or without
hemoptysis; (5) bronchiolitis obliterans with organizing pneumonia (BOOP); (6)
diaphragm-respiratory muscle dysfunction; (7) upper airway dysfunction; and (8) pulmonary hypertension with or without thromboembolic disease. The indirect effects of
SLE on the lungs arise from predisposition to infection; in fact, pneumonia is the most
frequent cause of infiltrates in patients with lupus.
   Pleuritis and accompanying pleuritic chest pain, with or without effusions, is the
most common pulmonary manifestation of SLE, occurring in 50 to 75% of patients,
with a slightly higher male predominance. It can occur at any time during the clinical
course and is the initial manifestation in approximately one third of cases. The effusions are generally small and bilateral but can be massive, unilateral, or associated
with a pericardial effusion. The exudative fluid can be clear or serosanguinous and the
pH can be high or low; however, the glucose is usually greater than 56 mg/dL, which
is useful in distinguishing it from a rheumatoid effusion. Cell counts reveal predominantly polymorphonuclear cells. Total hemolytic complement and serum antinuclear
antibody (ANA) titers can be variable, but pleural fluid ANA titers greater than 1:320
strongly support the diagnosis of SLE pleuritis. Lupus erythematosus cells in the
pleural fluid are diagnostic. Although most pleural effusions resolve completely with
steroid therapy, some residual pleural thickening can persist.
   The incidence of interstitial pneumonitis in SLE is controversial, depending
whether clinical, pulmonary function testing, or histologic findings are used as the
criteria for diagnosis. Histologic changes display a spectrum similar to idiopathic interstitial pneumonitis, ranging from interstitial mononuclear infiltration to extensive
fibrosis. The presence of anti-Sm antibodies in the serum significantly correlates with
lung fibrosis. Clinically, acute lupus pneumonitis often presents with the sudden appearance of fever (as high as 104°F) and a nonproductive cough, which can progress

rapidly to frank respiratory failure. Histology reveals a florid mononuclear cell infiltrate, interstitial thickening, alveolitis, and vasculitis. Several series report findings of immune complexes and complement within the alveolar walls, the pulmonary arterioles, and small vessels.

In contrast to other collagen vascular diseases such as rheumatoid arthritis and scleroderma, chronic interstitial pneumonitis and interstitial fibrosis is uncommon in SLE. In one report, fibrosis was observed in fewer than 3% of patients with lupus. Patients with fibrosis tend to be older (45–50 years) and have had a prolonged duration of disease before the development of chronic lung disease. The histologic findings include evidence of (1) chronic or recurrent pneumonitis; (2) interstitial and alveolar fibrosis; and (3) immunoglobulin and complement deposition in the alveolar septae. The nail fold capillary density is a useful physical finding, because it correlates with the extent of gas exchange deficiency. Both acute and chronic lupus pneumonitis may clear radiographically. However, they can also progress to advanced interstitial fibrosis and honeycomb lung. Even after improvement in symptoms and radiographic appearance, decreased diffusing capacity of lung for carbon monoxide (DLCO), and restrictive defects in pulmonary function often persist.

Pulmonary alveolar hemorrhage is a relatively rare presenting feature of SLE. It occurs predominantly in women and is associated with the presence of lupus nephritis. In the correct setting, the combination of anemia and hypoxemia may suggest its presence. Mortality approaches 50% and is even higher in patients who have required mechanical ventilation, have received cyclophosphamide (perhaps indicating more advanced disease), or have a nosocomial infection. Pathology usually shows a small vessel capillaritis, arteriolitis, and venulitis. Immune complex deposition in a granular pattern distinguishes the pathology of diffuse alveolar hemorrhage (DAH) in SLE from Goodpasture's (linear distribution).

A relatively common histologic finding in open lung biopsy specimens is BOOP, which includes characteristic plugs of granulation tissue within small airways and alveolar ducts in conjunction with inflammatory changes of the bronchioles and pulmonary parenchyma. The usual associated clinical presentation is nonspecific and patients may show a restrictive ventilatory defect. Diagnosis requires open lung biopsy, and the pathologic changes tend to respond to steroid treatment.

Physiologic studies have recently disclosed the importance of diaphragmatic and respiratory muscle weakness as a cause of dyspnea and a restrictive ventilatory defect in some patients with SLE. A condition known as *shrinking lung syndrome* consists of dyspnea with chest radiograph findings of small lung volumes, elevated hemidiaphragms, and basilar atelectasis. Maximal inspiratory pressure and maximal expiratory pressure measurements demonstrate inspiratory and expiratory respiratory muscle weakness as the basis for the restrictive ventilatory defects. Comparing the movement of the two hemidiaphragms by fluoroscopy is not useful because both tend to be affected. Transdiaphragmatic pressure during active breathing, measured by esophageal and gastric balloons, confirms the presence of diaphragmatic weakness. Most patients do not have diffuse muscle weakness; therefore random muscle biopsy is of little utility. The pathogenesis remains unclear and the optimal therapy for this syndrome has not been established. Case reports show improvement in symptoms with β_2 agonists, steroids, or theophylline.

Although upper airway involvement is uncommon in SLE, hypopharyngeal ulceration, laryngeal inflammation, epiglottitis, and subglottic stenosis have been reported. These manifestations of SLE may result in complications following endotracheal intubation.

Pulmonary hypertension with cor pulmonale, which can be seen with or without associated pulmonary emboli, is significantly correlated with the antiphospholipid syndrome. In one series of 24 patients who had pulmonary hypertension, 68% had a lupus anticoagulant or anticardiolipin antibody. The cause of pulmonary hypertension in SLE is controversial, and can vary among patients. Possible causes include (1) small vessel arteriopathy; (2) chronic large vessel thromboembolic disease; and (3) secondary hypertension caused by end-stage parenchymal fibrosis. In many patients, the pathologic findings in the pulmonary vascular bed are indistinguishable from primary pulmonary hypertension. Raynaud's phenomenon is almost uniformly seen in cases not associated with parenchymal lung disease. Vasculitis and immune deposits are seen in SLE with or without the development of pulmonary hypertension. On the other hand, thromboembolism occurs in up to 25% of patients with SLE and is a major cause of death. Most patients with thromboembolism are treated with life-long anticoagulation. One case of successful thromboendarterectomy for chronic pulmonary thromboembolic disease in a patient with lupus was reported.

Acute reversible hypoxemia has been described in patients with lupus having normal chest radiographs and widened A–a oxygen gradients. Patients generally present with pleuritic chest pain, dyspnea, and chest discomfort. Vital capacity and DLCO are significantly reduced. The syndrome appears to respond to corticosteroids, which improve oxygenation. The cause may be transient, complement-mediated aggregation and neutrophil activation within the pulmonary vasculature. Active disease is associated with increased expression of E-selectin and vascular adhesion molecule-1 (VCAM-1), which may facilitate a leuco-occlusive vasculopathy in the lung.

Pulmonary function abnormalities are common, occurring in 70 to 80% of patients with SLE-associated lung disease even in the absence of symptoms and radiographic abnormalities. The most common abnormalities are decreased DLCO and reduced lung volumes. Airway obstruction is unusual. Hypoxemia at rest or with exercise is frequently present. Concomitant renal dysfunction is frequently seen with lupus-associated pulmonary disease.

The management of pulmonary involvement in SLE is generally supportive. Steroids appear to be the most useful drugs, with other agents such as cyclophosphamide and azathioprine added according to the severity of organ involvement. Even if the patient responds to therapy, pulmonary involvement is a poor prognostic sign; respiratory syndromes in SLE have been associated with a twofold increased risk of death at 1 year.

PROGRESSIVE SYSTEMIC SCLEROSIS

Progressive systemic sclerosis (PSS) or *systemic scleroderma* commonly affects the lung and pulmonary pathology is found in approximately 90% of patients at autopsy. The CREST syndrome consisting of (1) *c*alcinosis cutis; (2) *R*aynaud's phenomenon; (3) presence or absence of *e*sophageal dysfunction; (4) *s*clerodactyly; and (5) *t*elangiectasias was formerly considered a less progressive form of PSS. However, pulmonary vascular changes similar to those in PSS can be found, leading to pulmonary hypertension and cor pulmonale. Pulmonary function studies are abnormal in most patients; decreased DLCO is the most common finding, followed by reduced lung volumes and airway obstruction. Chest roentgenograms reveal interstitial infiltrates in approximately one third of patients. Isolated pulmonary hypertension without diffuse interstitial lung disease is more common in CREST than in typical PSS. In one study of 17 patients with the CREST syndrome, the incidence of pulmonary hypertension was 29%, and the development of lung carcinoma was 21%. For the remainder of this discussion, all forms of scleroderma are discussed as PSS.

The age distribution and gender predominance of pulmonary involvement reflect those of PSS in general: most patients are in the fourth to sixth decades with a 3:1 female predominance. The lung is the fourth most common organ involved in scleroderma, ranking behind skin, peripheral vascular, and esophageal disease. However, pulmonary complications are the most frequent cause of death, making early detection of lung involvement an important predictor of survival. The main processes encountered include (1) interstitial fibrosis; (2) pulmonary hypertension; (3) BOOP; (4) pleuritis; (5) aspiration pneumonitis; (6) respiratory muscle dysfunction (similar to SLE); and (7) predisposition to silica-associated pneumoconiosis, sarcoidosis, and bronchogenic carcinoma.

Although the lung is commonly affected, respiratory symptoms are rarely the presenting complaint. Dyspnea on exertion is the most common pulmonary symptom, followed by a nonproductive or minimally productive cough. Pleuritic chest pain and pleural effusions are rare. Lung examination reveals basilar inspiratory crackles. Signs of pulmonary hypertension may be present.

Approximately 74% of patients with scleroderma develop interstitial fibrosis, which pathologically resembles idiopathic pulmonary fibrosis (IPF). Recent evidence suggests a multifactorial complex pathologic process involving hyperproliferative lung fibroblasts from increased expression of transcription factor Sp1, endothelial injury, and impaired vasodilation. As fibrosis progresses, severe pulmonary architectural distortion occurs, which is associated with bronchiectasis and the formation of cystic air spaces of up to 1 to 2 cm in diameter in a subpleural distribution. Rupture of these cysts can result in spontaneous pneumothorax. Pulmonary hypertension can also develop in association with the interstitial lung process. Radiographic evidence of fine basilar reticular or reticulonodular changes is usually accompanied by restrictive pulmonary function defects. A reduced DLCO may be the first indication of pulmonary involvement and has been found to be quite sensitive. Further evaluation by lung scintigraphy may show a peripheral distribution of mismatch reflecting the microvascular pathology resulting in a reduced DLCO. In the absence of radiographic or ventilatory defects, significant dyspnea with a low DLCO suggests the presence of pulmonary vascular disease.

The incidence of pulmonary arterial hypertension (PAH) in scleroderma ranges from 6 to 60% depending on the study used to diagnose PAH. Additionally, the presence of autoantibodies to anti-topoisomerase 1 is associated with severe pulmonary vascular disease. The pathogenesis of PAH is presumed to be secondary to fibrosis and perivascular cellular infiltration with activated T cells in the pulmonary arteries leading to pulmonary hypertension and cor pulmonale. (Left ventricular failure, secondary to systemic hypertension or cardiomyopathy, is frequently coexistent). Isolated PAH has a worse prognosis than PAH secondary to fibrosis, with a 2-year survival of 40%. Oxygen, prostacyclin analog, and endothelin receptor antagonists (such as bosentan) have shown some effect on reducing pulmonary artery pressures, improving cardiac output and exercise capacity. Many authors advocate the addition of warfarin anticoagulation, based on its apparent efficacy in the treatment of primary pulmonary hypertension. BOOP is rare.

Pleuritis is present histologically in up to 85% of patients at autopsy, but is only symptomatic in 16% of patients with scleroderma. Clinically significant effusions are uncommon. Pleural effusions or pleural thickening occur as a result of scleroderma involving the pleura or secondary to congestive heart failure from cardiac involvement. Reexpansion of the lung after thoracentesis is usually slow because of decreased lung compliance and recurrence is common, often requiring pleurodesis.

Aspiration pneumonitis can occur because of esophageal dysfunction, which can contribute to the development of chronic pneumonitis. Respiratory muscle dysfunction without generalized weakness has been reported to occur, similar to the phenomenon described in SLE.

A twofold increased incidence of bronchogenic carcinoma has been observed with systemic sclerosis, relative to the normal population. Older patients, diffuse disease, presence of pulmonary fibrosis, and anti-topoisomerase 1 antibody were associated with an increase risk of cancer in scleroderma.

An association between sarcoidosis and scleroderma has been observed in clinical studies. Affected patients usually have a limited form of scleroderma, which typically precedes sarcoidosis by many years. Steroids are effective in treatment. In some instances, PSS is associated with silicosis and amyloidosis. These patients are described as having an acute onset of symptoms with predominance of pulmonary disease and, frequently, pleural effusion.

ANA typically of a speckled fluorescence is found in more than 90% of patients with scleroderma. Anti-DNA topoisomerase I (Scl-70), anti-U3 ribonucleoprotein (anti-U3-RNP), and anti-RNA polymerase I, II, and III antibodies are associated with diffuse scleroderma, whereas anticentromere antibodies (ACA) are associated with the CREST variant.

Patients who are ACA positive have been noted to have a decreased frequency of interstitial fibrosis and restrictive lung disease. On the other hand, anti–Scl-70 antibodies are associated with diffuse skin involvement, visceral organ involvement, interstitial lung disease, and a greater risk of cancer.

No therapeutic regimens exist to arrest or reverse the disease at an early stage. Most therapeutic trials have been uncontrolled and retrospective, involving patients at various stages of disease. However, a 1993 study of combined therapy with cyclophosphamide and low-dose prednisone reported an increase in forced vital capacity after 6 months of therapy with the improvement maintained at 12, 18, and 24 months. Similar results were reported in subsequent trials. Although the clinical data have limitations, the current recommendation for progressive interstitial disease is to begin alternate-day systemic corticosteroids (prednisone 0.5 mg/kg per day) for 3 months in conjunction with cyclophosphamide (1–2 mg/kg per day) or azathioprine (1–3 mg/kg per d) based on ideal body weight. This should then be followed by a gradual tapering of the steroid dose. In patients with indolent interstitial disease whose disease is stable, D-penicillamine (62.5 mg daily) or colchicine can be considered. Lung transplantation may be an option for limited scleroderma, if no other organ disease is present. Otherwise, treatment of pulmonary involvement in PSS is supportive.

POLYMYOSITIS

Polymyositis is an inflammatory, autoimmune myopathy characterized by proximal muscle weakness. Dermatomyositis is similar to polymyositis and additionally involves the skin with a characteristic heliotrope rash. Pulmonary involvement has been reported in up to 10% of patients and is a significant cause of mortality. Both conditions have a 2:1 female predominance with a peak incidence in the fifth and sixth decades. The syndromes associated with polymyositis and dermatomyositis can be loosely separated into the following categories: (1) adult polymyositis; (2) adult dermatomyositis; (3) childhood polymyositis or dermatomyositis; (4) polymyositis or dermatomyositis associated with malignancy; and (5) polymyositis or dermatomyositis associated with a preestablished collagen vascular disease.

The syndrome may affect the lung in any of the following ways: (1) primary interstitial pneumonitis with progression to fibrosis; (2) pulmonary hypertension secondary to interstitial lung disease or pulmonary vascular disease; (3) recurrent aspiration pneumonitis secondary to esophageal muscle dysmotility; (4) respiratory muscle weakness with resultant hypoventilation, atelectasis, and pneumonia; and (5) BOOP.

The pulmonary component of polymyositis or dermatomyositis can precede the muscle symptoms by years. When interstitial pneumonitis precedes muscle manifestations, the diagnosis can be missed because of the focus on the pulmonary disease. The presence of serum antibody to histidyl-tRNA-synthetase (anti–JO-1) significantly correlates with interstitial lung disease in up to 75% of patients. The discovery of this antibody in a patient with isolated pulmonary interstitial lung disease may be helpful in predicting the future development of polymyositis or dermatomyositis.

Two other forms of respiratory involvement can occur as complications of therapy: (1) opportunistic infection secondary to immunosuppressive drugs and (2) drug-induced lung changes secondary to cytotoxic therapy for the muscle component of the disease.

The pathologic findings differ between patients with acute, symptomatic interstitial lung disease and those with a more subacute or chronic presentation. In the acute presentation, patients may present with cough, fever, and dyspnea with or without skin or muscle findings. The chest radiographic study shows diffuse mixed alveolar interstitial infiltrates. The clinical course is similar to Hamman–Rich syndrome. Pathologic findings include an alveolitis, BOOP, or diffuse alveolar damage with focal alveolar hemorrhage. Small vessel vasculitis (pulmonary capillaritis) was recently reported in a several patients with polymyositis, where pulmonary and muscle symptoms presented simultaneously. With the chronic presentation, pathology usually is consistent with the usual interstitial pneumonitis. The pathogenesis of the muscle and pulmonary manifestations of the disease is thought to involve T-cell activation by muscle autoantigens, resulting in a release of IL-2 and γ-interferon. Subsequent promotion of macrophages and a newly recognized cytokine called *macrophage inflammatory protein* lead to eventual tissue injury.

Clinically, respiratory symptoms are absent in up to 40% of patients with roentgenographic or histologic pulmonary changes. When symptoms occur, patients may present with dyspnea, dysphagia, or a nonproductive cough. Examination of the lungs of patients with interstitial lung disease characteristically reveals fine, late inspiratory crackles (described as "Velcro-like") in a bibasilar distribution. Roentgenographically, the disease manifests as lower lobe reticulonodular infiltrates with an associated alveolar filling component in 20% of patients. Pleural involvement is rare. Pulmonary function studies typically show a restrictive pattern caused by either interstitial changes or respiratory muscle weakness. Commonly, a reduced DLCO is also found.

Routine laboratory findings are nonspecific. The sedimentation rate is usually elevated, whereas antinuclear antibodies and rheumatoid factor are negative. Serum levels of muscle enzymes (creatine kinase and aldolase) are elevated in most cases.

Response to therapy varies, depending on the histologic features. BOOP is most responsive to steroids, whereas diffuse alveolar damage has uniformly poor prognosis. Corticosteroids can be used alone, or in combination with cyclophosphamide or azathioprine for parenchymal lung disease.

MIXED TISSUE CONNECTIVE DISEASE

Mixed connective tissue disease (MCTD) has clinical and laboratory characteristics of SLE, polymyositis/dermatomyositis, and scleroderma. The distinguishing feature of MCTD is an antibody to extractable nuclear antigen (anti–nRNP-Ab) or ribonuclease-sensitive ribonucleoprotein (sn-RNP). Dilutions of sn-RNP greater than 1:10,000 is considered confirmatory of MCTD. Controversy continues regarding whether MCTD is a distinct entity from the other collagen vasculitides.

The incidence of pulmonary involvement in MCTD is approximately 85% ($n = 34$), of which 73% were asymptomatic. Pleural effusion (25–50%), interstitial pneumonitis, pulmonary vasculitis, pulmonary artery hypertension, pulmonary thromboembolic disease, aspiration pneumonia, and hypoventilatory failure can occur. Presenting symptoms include exertional dyspnea, nonproductive cough, pleuritic chest pain, and fever. Clubbing is not seen. Of the asymptomatic patients with MCTD, 75% have evidence of pulmonary involvement on chest radiograph study or pulmonary function studies. There is no significant HRCT finding that distinguishes MCTD from any of the other collagen vascular diseases, but interlobular septal thickening in the lower lobes predominate. A correlation with HLA-DR3 and interstitial pulmonary fibrosis has been observed in one small study.

Histopathology of the lung in interstitial lung disease associated with MCTD is similar to IPF. Additionally, a proliferative vasculopathy is associated with MCTD, characterized by intimal thickening with medial muscular hypertrophy of the pulmonary arteries and arterioles, which correlates with the presence of pulmonary hypertension.

Radiographically, bilateral basilar interstitial opacities, right ventricular hypertrophy, and pulmonary artery enlargement can be seen. Pulmonary function abnormalities include decreased DLCO (up to 67% of patients) and reduced lung volumes (50% of patients). Small airway obstruction is seen early and is an indication of functional impairment.

It had been reported that the pulmonary disease of MCTD is benign and responds to steroid therapy with improvement shown on the chest roentgenogram and pulmonary function studies. A few reports, however, describe progressive pulmonary disease and rapid deterioration despite steroid therapy. Renal disease and Raynaud's phenomenon is associated with a higher mortality rate. Some long-term follow-up studies show evolution of MCTD toward other connective tissue diseases (SLE, PSS, and rheumatoid arthritis). The overall prognosis is estimated to be similar to that seen in patients with SLE.

1. Prakash U. Respiratory complications in mixed connective tissue disease. *Clin Chest Med*. 1998;19:733.

    A comprehensive review of the pulmonary manifestations of MCTD, therapeutic options, and prognosis.
2. Schwarz M. The lung in polymyositis. *Clin Chest Med*. 1998;19:701.

    A clinicopathologic review of the pulmonary presentations of polymyositis.
3. Minai O, Dweik R, Arroliga A. Manifestations of scleroderma pulmonary disease. *Clin Chest Med*. 1998;19:713.

    A concise review of the lung's involvement in scleroderma, with emphasis on interstitial lung disease and pulmonary hypertension.

4. Murin S, Wiedemann H, Matthay R. Pulmonary manifestations of systemic lupus erythematosus. *Clin Chest Med.* 1998;19:641.
   An excellent and extensive review of the various forms of SLE-associated lung disease.
5. Bolster MB, Silver RM. Lung disease in systemic sclerosis (scleroderma). *Bailliere's Clin Rheumatol.* 1993;7:79.
   A review article on the pulmonary involvement of lung disease in scleroderma. Clinical, radiographic, and histopathologic aspects are discussed as well as treatment.
6. Lee P. Clinical aspects of systemic and localized sclerosis. *Curr Opin Rheumatol.* 1993;5:785.
   Discusses the risk factors (clinical and laboratory) associated with progressive disease, especially pulmonary, cardiac, and renal dysfunction.
7. Ginzler EM, Antoniadis I. Clinical manifestations of systemic lupus erythematosus, measures of disease activity, and longterm complications. *Curr Opin Rheumatol.* 1992;4:672.
   A review article of organ dysfunction and the association of SLE with the antiphospholipid antibody syndrome.
8. Mulherin D, Bresnihan B. Systemic lupus erythematosus. *Bailliere's Clin Rheum.* 1993;7:32.
   A review article describing the various pulmonary abnormalities associated with SLE, including drug-induced lupus.
9. Marie I, et al. Pulmonary involvement in polymyositis and in dermatomyositis. *J Rheumatol.* 1998;25:1336.
   A retrospective chart review of 55 patients was performed to assess the prevalence and characteristics of pulmonary involvement in polymyositis and dermatomyositis. Of the patients, 40% were found to have pulmonary disease, and the presence of anti–Jo-1 antibody correlated with lung disease.
10. Abu-Shakra M, Guillemin F, Lee P. Cancer in systemic sclerosis. *Arthritis Rheum.* 1993;36:460.
    A retrospective chart review of 248 patients was conducted to identify the types of cancer and risk factors. Lung and breast cancers occurred most frequently. Older age at diagnosis of scleroderma was a risk factor. Lung cancer was associated with the presence of pulmonary fibrosis.
11. Asherton RA, et al. Pulmonary hypertension in a lupus clinic: experience with 24 patients. *J Rheumatol.* 1990;17:1292.
    The frequency of antiphospholipid antibodies in 24 patients with pulmonary hypertension associated with connective tissue disease is discussed along with patient outcome; 68% of the patients had antiphospholipid antibodies.
12. Bernstein RM, et al. Anti-Jo-1 antibody: a marker for myositis with interstitial lung disease. *BMJ.* 1984;289:151.
    Anti–Jo-1 antibody is found in 25% of patients with myositis. Prevalence in patients with both myositis and interstitial lung fibrosis is 68% compared with 7.5% in those with myositis alone and 3% with interstitial lung fibrosis alone.
13. Groen H, et al. Pulmonary function in systemic lupus erythematosus is related to distinct clinical, serologic, and nailfold capillary patterns. *Am J Med.* 1992;93:619.
    Patients (n = 57) with SLE were studied to assess overlap with scleroderma in those patients with interstitial lung disease. Nailfold capillary abnormalities correlated with abnormal diffusing capacity.
14. Horn CA. Pulmonary hypertension and autoimmune disease. *Chest.* 1993;104:279.
    A case presentation followed by comments from three invited consultants regarding the relationship of pulmonary hypertension and autoimmune disease, medical management of pulmonary hypertension, and a discussion of transplantation.
15. Hsue YT, Paulus HE, Coulson WF. Bronchiolitis obliterans organizing pneumonia in polymyositis: a case report with long-term survival. *J Rheumatol.* 1993;20:877.
    A case report describing the outcome of long-term therapy with steroids and azathioprine.
16. Kostopoulos C, et al. Small airways dysfunction in systemic sclerosis: a controlled study. *Chest.* 1992;102:875.

Nonsmoking patients (n = 31) underwent pulmonary function studies. Of the 31, 7 had small airways disease. Based on this group of patients, small airways disease was described as uncharacteristic of scleroderma; but, when present, it did not correlate with the severity of the pulmonary involvement.

17. Marguerie C, et al. The clinical and immunogenetic features of patients with autoantibodies to the nucleolar antigen PM-Scl. *Medicine* (Baltimore). 1992;71:327.
    Describes the association of this autoantibody in 32 patients with overlap connective tissue disease. Significant renal and neurologic involvement was uncommon. Patients appeared to respond well to immunosuppressive therapy.

18. Silver RM, et al. Cyclophosphamide and low dose prednisone therapy in patients with systemic sclerosis (scleroderma) with interstitial lung disease. *J Rheumatol.* 1993;20:838.
    A report of 14 patients who received combined therapy. Improvement was seen by 6 months of therapy with significant changes in forced vital capacity. This improvement continued over time. No change in diffusing capacity occurred.

19. Tashkin DP, et al. Interrelationships between pulmonary and extrapulmonary involvement in systemic sclerosis. *Chest.* 1994;105:489.
    Nonsmoking patients (n = 62) with scleroderma were studied prospectively over 3 years to assess (1) the prognostic value of baseline lung function data; (2) the relationship between pulmonary involvement and other organs; and (3) the rate of change of lung function over time.

20. Wahl D, et al. Risk for venous thrombosis related to antiphospholipid antibodies in systemic lupus erythematosus—a meta-analysis. *Lupus.* 1997;6:467.
    A meta-analysis of 26 articles disclosed 2,249 patients with SLE tested for either lupus anticoagulant or anticardiolipin antibodies. A sixfold increased risk for venous thrombosis was found in patients with lupus anticoagulant versus a twofold increased risk in those with anticardiolipin antibody.

21. Diot E, et al. Is anti-topoisomerase 1 a serum marker of pulmonary involvement in systemic sclerosis? *Chest.* 1999;116:715.
    Patients (n = 48) with systemic sclerosis (20 with lung involvement and 28 without) were tested for anti-topoisomerase 1 activity. A significant association was noted with diffuse disease, pulmonary involvement, and the presence of anti-topoisomerase-1.

22. Tazelaar HD, et al. Interstitial lung disease in polymyositis and dermatomyositis. *Am Rev Respir Dis.* 1990;141:727.
    Describes 15 patients with autopsy or lung biopsy specimens, including correlation of histopathology with clinical, radiographic, and prognostic variables.

23. Wells AU, du Bois RM. Bronchiolitis in association with connective tissue disorders. *Clin Chest Med.* 1993;14:655.
    An overview of bronchiolitis associated with the different connective tissue diseases. The rare identification of bronchiolitis associated with connective tissue diseases may be secondary to the difficulty in diagnosing its presence.

24. Yousem SA. The pulmonary pathologic manifestations of the CREST syndrome. *Pathology.* 1990;21:467.
    Reports on the histopathologic changes seen in 17 patients with the CREST syndrome.

25. Grau J, et al. Interstitial lung disease related dermatomyositis. Comparative study with patients without lung involvement. *J Rheumatol.* 1996;23:1921.
    Of 104 patients with diagnosed dermatomyositis, 8 were prospectively identified over a 10-year period with associated lung disease. A significant association with anti–Jo-1 antibody was noted.

26. Zamora M, et al. Diffuse alveolar hemorrhage and systemic lupus erythematosus. *Medicine* (Baltimore). 1997;76:192.
    A retrospective review of all SLE admissions to a single hospital revealed a 3.7% incidence of alveolar hemorrhage in SLE, which was associated with a 50% mortality rate. Clinical presentation, histopathology, and outcomes are extensively reviewed.

27. Barile LA, et al. Pulmonary hemorrhage in systemic lupus erythematosus. *Lupus.* 1997;6:445.

A retrospective review of 34 patients with pulmonary hemorrhage secondary to SLE describes a 38% survival rate.

28. Elkaya O, et al. Restrictive lung disease due to diaphragmatic dysfunction in systemic lupus erythematosus. *Clin Exp Rheumatol.* 1992;10:267.

    Two patients are presented to highlight the association of dyspnea, restrictive lung function, and diaphragmatic dysfunction. Therapy is discussed.

29. Bridges AJ, et al. Bronchiolitis obliterans organizing pneumonia and scleroderma. *J Rheumatol.* 1992;19:1136.

    Reports on two patients with BOOP in association with scleroderma. The presentation and rapid response to steroid therapy are discussed.

30. Shinohara T, et al. Rapidly progressive interstitial lung disease associated with dermatomyositis responding to intravenous cyclophosphamide pulse therapy. *Intern Med.* 1997;36:519.

    A case report of a patient with dermatomyositis presenting with BOOP and interstitial fibrosis who developed respiratory failure on steroids and was successfully treated with cyclophosphamide.

31. Soubrier M, Dubost JJ, Piette JC. Shrinking lung syndrome in systemic lupus erythematosus: a report of three cases. *Rev Rhum Engl Ed.* 1995;62:395.

    Describes three patients with SLE with dyspnea and the common clinical findings of elevated diaphragm(s) and restrictive ventilatory defects. All responded to steroid therapy.

32. Fata F, et al. Bronchiolitis obliterans organizing pneumonia as the first manifestation of polymyositis. *South Med J.* 1997;90:227.

    The rare finding of BOOP preceding the clinical diagnosis of polymyositis is nicely discussed in this case report.

33. Friedman A, Targoff I, Arnett F. Interstitial lung disease with autoantibodies against aminoacyl-tRNA synthetase in absence of clinically apparent myositis. *Semin Arthritis Rheum.* 1996;26:459.

    An excellent discussion of the serologic, clinical, and functional presentation of 10 patients with isolated anti-synthetase antibodies and lung disease without myositis. The authors found that the lung disease is more responsive to therapy in such patients.

34. Mrowka C, Sieberth H. Detection of circulating adhesion molecules ICAM-1, VCAM-1, and E-selectin in Wegener's granulomatosis, systemic lupus erythematosus, and chronic renal failure. *Clin Nephrol.* 1995;43:288.

    Significant elevations in ICAM-1 and VCAM-1 were seen in the serum of 50 patients with SLE. The authors suggest a possible link with VCAM and the pathogenesis of vasculitis.

35. Eiser A, Shanies H. Treatment of lupus interstitial lung disease with intravenous cyclophosphamide. *Arthritis Rheum.* 1994;37:428.

    Reports the successful use of intravenous cyclophosphamide in two patients with SLE and interstitial lung disease.

36. Wilke RA, et al. Lupus-like autoimmune disease associated with silicosis. *Nephrol Dial Transplant.* 1996;11:1835.

    A case report of a patient with known silicosis presenting with renal failure and elevated ANA. Silicosis stimulating an autoimmune response is the theorized mechanism of disease.

37. Horiki T, et al. Fatal alveolar hemorrhage in a patient with mixed connective tissue disease presenting polymyositis features. *Intern Med.* 1998;37:554.

    A descriptive case report and review of the literature of alveolar hemorrhage in MCTD.

38. Saito Y, et al. Pulmonary involvement in mixed connective tissue disease: comparison with other collagen vascular diseases using high resolution CT. *J Comput Assist Tomogr.* 26(3):349–357.

    A retrospective review and comparison of CT findings in patients with MCTD, SLE, PM and DM.

39. Schwarz M, Brown K. Small vessel vasculitis of the lung. *Thorax* 2000;55:502–510.

    An up-to-date and concise review of small vessel vasculitis in a variety of pulmonary diseases including SLE.

40. Jimenez S, Derk C. Following the molecular pathways toward and understanding of the pathogenesis of systemic sclerosis. *Ann Intern Med.* 2004;140:37–50.

   An excellent discussion of the potential genetic and molecular mechanisms involved in the clinical and pathologic presentation of systemic sclerosis.

41. Flaherty K, et al. Fibroblastic foci in usual interstitial pneumonia, idiopathic versus collagen vascular disease. *Am J Respir Crit Care Med.* 2003;167:1410–1415.

   A retrospective review of 108 pathology specimens in patients diagnosed with UIP, 10 of which were CVD associated. The authors discovered a distinct decrease in the presence of fibroblastic foci (FF) as compared with idiopathic UIP and additionally noted that those with a low number of FF had an improved mortality.

42. Kono H, Inokuma S. Visualization and functional consequence of pulmonary vascular impairment in patients with rheumatic diseases. *Chest.* 2003;124:255–261.

   Seventy-two patients with collagen vascular disease underwent pulmonary function studies, DLCO and lung scintigraphy. The authors suggest that a peripheral distribution of V̇/Q̇ mismatch is consistent with the microvascular impairment that results in a reduced DLCO.

43. Rubin LJ, Badesch DB, Barst RJ, et al. Bosentan therapy for pulmonary arterial hypertension. *N Engl J Med.* 2002;346:896–903.

44. Hoeper MM. Pulmonary hypertension in collagen vascular disease. *Eur Respir J.* 2002;19:571–576.

97. PULMONARY LANGERHANS CELL HISTIOCYTOSIS

Gregory A. Ruff, David Bradshaw, and Cecilia M. Smith

Pulmonary Langerhans cell histiocytosis (PLCH) is a diffuse interstitial lung disease characterized histologically by a predominance of differentiated cells of the monocytes/macrophage lineage. PLCH, also known as histiocytosis X, is preferred over other names such as eosinophilic granuloma or Langerhans cell granulomatosis, both misnomers, because the pathologic lesions contain few if any eosinophils and do not form true granulomas. PLCH shares a spectrum of disease with Letterer–Siwe disease and Hand–Schüller–Christian disease. The latter two diseases have characteristic ages of onset (typically childhood), are more severe, and affect multiple organs including bone and occasionally soft tissues with an infiltration of the atypical histocytes. Although PLCH was initially described as a disease of bone, isolated lung disease and multisystem involvement are well described.

The incidence and prevalence of PLCH are unknown. However, it is uncommonly diagnosed, even at centers that specialize in diffuse interstitial pulmonary disease. PLCH may occur at any age. It has been reported as early as infancy (3 months of age) and up to the seventh decade; however, most are diagnosed in young adulthood. PLCH was previously believed to affect men more than women, but recent data support no gender predilection. Women tend to develop the disease at a later age than men. Caucasians appear to be affected more commonly than those of African and Asian descent. The most striking demographic feature of the disease is its strong association with current or past tobacco use. Fewer than 5% of patients are nonsmokers.

CLINICAL PRESENTATION

Although PLCH patients often present with pulmonary (cough, dyspnea, chest pain) or constitutional (fever, weight loss) symptoms, some present with asymptomatic radiographic findings. The most common finding in patients presenting with an abnormal radiograph is spontaneous pneumothorax. Hemoptysis may occasionally be reported but should prompt a search for opportunistic infections (especially *Aspergillus spp.*) or associated tumor. Painful bony lesions may precede lung involvement and may result in pathologic fracture as a presenting symptom. There are no findings on bone radiographs that are diagnostic. Diabetes insipidus secondary to hypothalamic involvement probably portends a poor prognosis. Airway involvement, pleural effusion, and lymphadenopathy are distinctly uncommon manifestations.

The physical examination is often normal. Crackles and finger clubbing are uncommon; however, in advanced disease, evidence of pulmonary hypertension with associated right heart failure may be present. Laboratory evaluation is typically normal. Peripheral eosinophilia is not associated with PLCH. Although spirometry and assessment of static lung volumes are often normal, obstructive or restrictive patterns may be seen and the diffusing capacity of the lung for carbon monoxide (D_{LCO}) is characteristically reduced. Resting room air blood gas measurements are typically normal until disease is advanced, but exercise testing may reveal gas exchange abnormalities as well as a reduction in maximum oxygen consumption and workload.

DIAGNOSIS

The diagnosis of PLCH is strongly suggested by typical findings on the chest radiograph and high-resolution computed tomography (CT) scan. Specifically, small (2–12 mm) stellate nodules, upper lobe reticuolnodular opacities, and cysts or honeycombing favoring the upper lung zones are strongly suggestive. The differential diagnosis of the radiologic findings might include lymphangioleiomyomatosis, tuberous sclerosis, hypersensitivity pneumonitis, chronic eosinophilic pneumonia, sarcoidosis, and end-stage idiopathic pulmonary fibrosis. In the appropriate clinical setting (i.e., young smokers), these findings may be pathognomonic. High-resolution CT scanning can detect disease not readily apparent on the chest radiograph and is extremely useful in monitoring disease progression and response to therapy. The radiographic findings have an upper lung zone predominance that characteristically spares the costophrenic angles. Patients with costophrenic angle involvement are more likely to experience disease progression and have an unfavorable prognosis.

The Langerhans' cell, the pathologic cell type involved in PLCH, is derived from the monocyte/macrophage lineage and is characterized by pale cytoplasm and a large nucleus with prominent nucleoli. Pentalaminar cytoplasmic inclusions seen on electron microscopy are known as Birbeck granules or X bodies, and are considered pathognomonic. Immunohistochemical stains are positive for S100 and CD1a. These cells are normally found scattered in the dermis, lung, pleura, and reticuloendothelial system. Small numbers may also be seen in the pulmonary parenchyma of patients with idiopathic pulmonary fibrosis. Immunostaining and identification of the S100 protein or CD1a receptor on pathologic specimens usually obviates the need for electron microscopy.

In a minority of patients with PLCH (15%), the diagnosis can be established on the basis of appropriate radiographic studies and the clinical history. In the absence of the classic findings, it is necessary to obtain tissue samples. Broncheoalveolar lavage (BAL) is usually insufficient, although recovery in the lavage fluid of more than 5% Langerhans cells is strongly suggestive. Transbronchial biopsy specimens may provide adequate tissue for analysis and is reported to be diagnostic in 10 to 40% of patients. However, the small sample size and potential for sampling error may yield false-negative results. Video-assisted thoracoscopic surgery or open lung biopsy provide larger specimens under direct visualization and are the most definitive diagnostic procedures.

Histopathologic specimens show an accumulation of the Langerhans' cell, tissue inflammation, fibrosis, and cystic spaces. Inflammatory lesions are centered around bronchioles, arterioles, and venules early in the disease course giving the characteristic stellate appearance. The cellular infiltrate consists of Langerhans' cells mixed with neutrophils, lymphocytes, and scattered eosinophils. Eosinophils are not a prominent component of the inflammatory process and well-formed granuloma are rare. Areas of desquamative interstitial pneumonia (pseudo-desquamative interstitial pneumonia) and respiratory bronchiolitis (smoker's bronchiolitis) may also be seen. End-stage fibrosis may occur. In these cases, the typical histopathology may no longer be present.

TREATMENT

Initial therapy should consist of smoking cessation; clinical and radiographic resolution have been well described with this intervention alone. Patients who continue to smoke can expect a gradual progression of disease. Corticosteroids and cytotoxic agents (vinblastine, methotrexate, cyclophosphamide, and chlorodeoxyadenosine) have failed to show any benefit in the therapy of pulmonary PLCH. Despite the lack of documented efficacy, systemic corticosteroids continue to be used in patients with progressive pulmonary disease, perhaps only because of the lack of any effective therapy. Radiation therapy is highly effective for isolated bone lesions, but has been disappointing with respect to pulmonary lesions. Recurrent pneumothorax has been effectively treated with medical and surgical pleurodesis. Lung transplantation has been successfully performed in patients with isolated end-stage lung disease, but PLCH has also been shown to recur in the transplanted lung.

The natural history of PLCH is extremely variable, with some patients experiencing complete remission and others progressing to end-stage lung disease. Median survival is reported to be 12 years from the time of diagnosis. Almost 50% of the deaths are from respiratory failure. Factors suggesting a worse prognosis include extremes of age at diagnosis, low FEV_1, and low DLCO at time of diagnosis, and presence of isolated lung disease. Patients with PLCH are at an increased risk of developing both malignant and nonmalignant tumors. These include bronchogenic carcinoma, pulmonary carcinoid tumors, as well as hematologic malignancies (both Hodgkins and non-Hodgkins lymphoma). Associated malignancy follows only respiratory failure as cause of death in patients with PLCH. Patients may also develop pulmonary hypertension out of proportion to the degree of pulmonary fibrosis and that may be responsive to systemic corticosteroids. Diabetes insipidus is usually responsive to chemotherapy, but patients may require long-term desmopressin replacement.

Detailed information for both patients and providers is available through the website of the Histiocytosis Association of America (www.histio.org).

1. Arico M, et al. Langerhans cell histiocytosis in adults. Report from the International Registry of the Histiocyte Society. *Eur J Cancer.* 2003;39:2341.
   One of the largest patient collections. Data on 274 patients from 13 countries. Paper presents demographic data, prognostic factors, and treatment. Highest mortality was reported in patients who had only localized pulmonary disease.
2. Chollet S, et al. Diagnosis of pulmonary histiocytosis X by immunodetection of Langerhans' cells in bronchoalveolar lavage fluid. *Am J Pathol.* 1984;115:225.
   Cells from BAL of 131 patients were analyzed for the presence of OKT6 reactive cells and Birbeck granules by electron microscopy. All 18 patients with pulmonary histiocytosis X had cells that stained for OKT3 and had granules present. Of the remaining patients (43 with sarcoidosis, 3 controls, and 61 of 67 with miscellaneous disorders) had less than 1% labeled cells (6 stained positively with OKT6 but did not contain the Birbeck granules). Histiocytosis X cells can be identified unequivocally only by transmission electron microscopy.
3. Sundar KM, et al. Pulmonary Langerhans cell histiocytosis: emerging concepts in pathobiology, radiology and clinical evolution of disease. *Chest.* 2003;123:1673.
   Excellent review with specific attention to etiopathologic basis of eosinophilic granuloma and radiologic modalities for monitoring disease.
4. Egan TM, et al. Single lung transplantation for eosinophilic granulomatosis. *South Med J.* 1992;85:551.
   A case report describing functional outcome of a 26-year-old woman who underwent single lung transplantation.
5. Vassallo R, et al. Clinical outcomes of pulmonary Langerhans'-cell histiocytosis in adults. *N Engl J Med.* 2002;346:484.
   Four-year follow up of a cohort of 102 patients. There were 33 deaths, 15 due to respiratory failure. Six hematologic cancers diagnosed. Survival significantly worse than predicted based on actuarial tables. Poor prognostic indicators included low FEV_1, high RV, and low DLCO.

6. Mendez JL, et al. Pneumothorax in pulmonary Langerhans' cell histiocytosis (PPLCH). *Chest.* 2004;125:1028.

   Retrospective review of 102 adults with pneumothorax in pulmonary Langerhans' cell histiocytosis assessing frequency, recurrence, and management of pneumothorax. Pneumothorax occurred in 16% and was recurrent in 63% of those patients. No pneumothoraces recurred after chest tube evacuation and pleurodesis.

7. Dacic S, et al. Genotypic analysis of pulmonary Langerhans' cell histiocytosis. *Human Pathol.* 2003;34:1345.

   Comparative genotypic analysis using loss of heterozygosity of tumor suppressor genes. Results indicated that the putative tumor suppressor genes may lie on chromosomes 9, 22, or both.

8. Lacronique J, et al. Chest radiological features of pulmonary histiocytosis X: a report based on 50 adult cases. *Thorax.* 1982;37:104.

   Classifies the radiographs of 50 adult patients, 44 of whom were men. Patients with both costophrenic angles clear never developed progressive disease.

9. Bernstrand C, et al. Pulmonary abnormalities at long-term follow-up of patients with Langerhans cell histiocytosis. *Med Pediatr Oncol.* 2001;36:459.

   Forty-one Swedish patients with 5 or more years of clinical follow up. Twenty-five percent had residual radiographic evidence of disease. Of those with abnormal radiographs, 20% were symptomatic. Smokers were much more likely to have persistently abnormal radiographs.

10. Housini I, et al. Transbronchial biopsy in patients with pulmonary eosinophilic granuloma. Comparison with findings on open lung biopsy. *Arch Pathol Lab Med.* 1994;118:523.

    Evaluates the yield of transbronchial biopsy in diagnosis of eosinophilic granuloma. Good specificity, but poor sensitivity because of sampling error associated with small tissue samples.

11. Powers MA, et al. Pulmonary eosinophilic granuloma. 25 year follow up. *Am Rev Respir Dis.* 1984;129:503.

    A 25-year follow up, through autopsy, of a patient with eosinophilic granuloma. Despite clinical stability, slow progression resulting in honeycomb lung and respiratory failure resulted.

12. Hamada K, et al. Pulmonary veno-occlusive disease in pulmonary Langerhans' cell granulomatosis. *Eur Respir J.* 2000;15:421.

    Unusual complication of eosinophilic granuloma. Pulmonary veno-occlusive disease discovered at autopsy despite corticosteroid therapy. Eosinophilic granuloma may be considered in the differential for pulmonary veno-occlusive disease.

13. Pomeranz SJ, Proto AV. Histiocytosis X: unusual-confusing features of eosinophilic granuloma. *Chest.* 1986;89:88.

    Seven cases of pulmonary histiocytosis X are discussed, highlighting the atypical chest x-ray findings.

14. Fartoukh M, et al. Severe pulmonary hypertension in histiocytosis X. *Am J Respir Crit Care Med.* 2000;161:216.

    Comparison of pulmonary hemodynamics in 21 patients with eosinophilic granuloma compared to 29 patients with other severe chronic lung disease. All patients with eosinophilic granuloma had pulmonary hypertension (mean PAP 59 ± 4 mm Hg), which was significantly worse than the control group. PaO_2 levels were similar in all groups. FEV_1 was worse in the control groups. When available, tissue analysis showed proliferative vasculopathy in the eosinophilic granuloma group, which appeared to worsen while parenchymal abnormalities remained stable. Suggests that pulmonary vasculopathy may be significant in the pathophysiology of eosinophilic granuloma.

15. Suzuki M, et al. Pulmonary Langerhans' cell histiocytosis presenting with an endobronchial lesion. *Intern Med.* 2004;43:227.

    Atypical presentation of eosinophilic granuloma. Case report of concomitant parenchymal and endobronchial evidence of eosinophilic granuloma, both of which spontaneously resolved.

16. Mogulkoc N, et al. Pulmonary Langerhans' cell histiocytosis: radiologic resolution following smoking cessation. *Chest.* 1999;115:1452.

Case report of two patients with clinical and radiologic resolution of eosinophilic granuloma following smoking cessation.

17. Howarth DM, et al. Langerhans cell histiocytosis: diagnosis, natural history, management, and outcome. *Cancer.* 1999;85:2278.
    Three hundred fourteen patients followed at Mayo clinic for <u>at least 4</u> years. Focuses on clinical features, treatment and outcome. There were 28 deaths. Patients with isolated bone lesions tended to have the most favorable prognosis. Multisystem involvement carried a 20% risk of progressive disease.

18. Tomashefski JF, Khiyami A, Kleinerman J. Neoplasms associated with pulmonary eosinophilic granuloma. *Arch Pathol Lab Med.* 1991;115:499.
    Describes the prevalence of pulmonary and extrapulmonary neoplasms seen in patients with pulmonary eosinophilic granuloma. Of 21 patients, 10 (48%) had benign (1 patient) or malignant (9 patients) neoplasms.

19. Travis WD, et al. Pulmonary Langerhans' cell granulomatosis (histiocytosis X): a clinicopathologic study of 48 cases. *Am J Surg Pathol.* 1993;17:971.
    A total of 48 patients with eosinophilic granuloma were studied to assess the usefulness of immunochemistry, electron microscopy, and high-resolution CT scan in diagnosing this disease. The combination of characteristic findings by high-resolution CT, in association with tissue biopsy findings, Birbeck granules by electron microscopy, or positive immunohistochemical staining for antibody to S-100 protein, supported the diagnosis.

20. Benyounes B, et al. Steroid-responsive pulmonary hypertension in a patient with Langerhans cell granulomatosis (histiocytosis X). *Chest.* 1996;110:284.
    Case report of a patient with precapillary pulmonary hypertension related to eosinophilic granuloma, which hemodynamically and clinically responded to therapy with systemic corticosteroids.

21. Brauner MW, et al. Pulmonary Langerhans' cell histiocytosis: evolution of lesions on CT scan. *Radiology.* 1997;204:497.
    Initial and final CT scans of 21 patients (11 with histologic diagnosis) with eosinophilic granuloma and CT evidence of pulmonary disease were compared retrospectively. Nodular opacities, thick-walled cysts, and ground-glass opacities underwent regression. Thin-walled cysts, linear opacities, and emphysematous lesions remained unchanged or progressed.

22. Crausman RS, et al. Pulmonary histiocytosis X: pulmonary function and exercise pathophysiology. *Am J Respir Crit Care Med.* 1996;153:426.
    Results of spirometry, lung volumes, and exercise physiology testing on 23 patients with eosinophilic granuloma. Half demonstrated restrictive physiology. Exercise performance was severely reduced with marked reductions in $\dot{V}_D/\dot{V}_T$ at rest and with exertion, suggesting pulmonary vascular dysfunction.

23. Gabbay E, et al. Recurrence of Langerhans' cell granulomatosis following lung transplantation. *Thorax.* 1998;53:322.
    A case report of pulmonary Langerhans' cell granulomatosis that recurred following lung transplantation and responded to cyclophosphamide.

98. NEUROFIBROMATOSIS, LYMPHANGIOMYOMATOSIS, AND TUBEROUS SCLEROSIS

John Scott Parrish, Tony S. Han, and Cecilia M. Smith

NEUROFIBROMATOSIS

Neurofibromatosis type 1 (NF1, von Recklinghausen's disease) is characterized by cutaneous neurofibromas, café-au-lait spots, Lisch nodules of the iris, and various other systemic manifestations. Von Recklinghausen's disease, an autosomal dominant disorder, appears in all races, with a prevalence of 1 of 3,000 live births. The *NF1* gene is located on chromosome 17. Interstitial pneumonitis occurs in 7 to 20% of adults with *NF1*. The onset of interstitial pneumonitis characteristically occurs in the third or fourth decade. The cause of the pneumonitis remains obscure. Pathologically, it is grossly and microscopically indistinguishable from idiopathic interstitial pneumonitis. The lung surface is often studded with bullae of varying sizes with a striking upper lobe predominance; a honeycombed appearance is common on sectioning. Histologic specimens show diffuse interstitial fibrosis and architectural disruption, with extensive alveolar destruction and cystic changes. Hyperplasia of neurolemma cells of intrapulmonary nerves has been described.

Dyspnea of insidious onset is often the presenting manifestation, although discovery in an asymptomatic individual through an incidental chest roentgenogram may occur. The chest film may initially reveal only accentuated interstitial markings or diffusely mottled, ill-defined infiltrates. The infiltrates usually progress over years to a coarse linear or reticulated pattern and bulla formation. Interstitial fibrosis is usually symmetric with a basal predominance. Bullae form the hallmark of neurofibromatosis; the most prominent are apical or subapical. In addition to the diffuse fibrobullous interstitial disease, other thoracic manifestations of this disease include paravertebral neurofibroma, lateral meningocele, kyphoscoliotic vertebral deformity, and cutaneous neurofibroma. Physiologic measurements reveal a combination of restrictive and obstructive defects, diminished carbon monoxide diffusing capacity (DLCO), and hypoxemia (initially limited to exercise).

The diagnosis is generally obvious because the neurocutaneous manifestations almost invariably precede the interstitial pneumonitis. Rarely, biopsy is necessary to exclude another infiltrative pulmonary process. The course is variable and often slowly progressive. Some patients develop progressive respiratory failure with pulmonary hypertension leading to death. No specific therapy currently exists for pulmonary fibrosis associated with NF.

Other thoracic manifestations include severe scoliosis and neurofibromas of the posterior or superior mediastinum. Neurofibromas arise from nerve sheaths in the sympathetic chain, vagus, and intercostal and intrapulmonary nerves. These tumors are commonly found adjacent to the spinal column. Neurogenic tumors involving the lung are rare, although multiple neurofibromas of varying size can occur. Hypoxemia can be caused by right-to-left shunts within these tumors. These tumors are usually benign, but malignant change can occur. The development of carcinoma can be a complication of the diffuse interstitial disease.

LYMPHANGIOLEIOMYOMATOSIS

Lymphangioleiomyomatosis or lymphangiomatosis (LAM) is a rare, progressive pulmonary disorder characterized by a hamartomatous proliferation of smooth muscle within the lungs. LAM frequently involves other organs (e.g., the kidneys, retroperitoneal lymph nodes, liver, uterus, and pancreas) in addition to the lungs. Renal angiomyolipomas have been reported in 15 to 60% of patients with LAM. The incidence of meningioma is increased in women with LAM.

Lymphangiomatosis occurs almost exclusively in women of childbearing age, in whom it can progress rapidly or slowly to respiratory failure and death. The cause of LAM is unknown. Its incidence in young women, exacerbations during pregnancy, and associated steroid receptors in the lung, coupled with the known effect of estrogen and progesterone on smooth muscle, suggest that hormonal interactions are important in its pathogenesis.

Pathologically, nodular and tortuous masses of smooth muscle cells without significant fibrosis are the hallmarks of LAM. Grossly, the pleura is thickened, and large thick-walled cystic airspaces give rise to a honeycombed appearance of the lungs. Hilar, mediastinal, and retroperitoneal lymph nodes are often enlarged and spongy, and the thoracic duct is distended with lymph. Chylothorax can be present because of lymphatic rupture. Microscopically, a striking nodular proliferation of smooth muscle is seen within the pleura and alveolar walls, as well as in and around the walls of bronchioles, venules, and lymphatics. These smooth muscle cells exhibit melanoma-related marker, HMB45 immunoreactivity, distinct from other smooth muscle proliferations. HMB45, a monoclonal antibody, also reacts with angiomyolipomas, clear cell tumors of the lung, and melanoma cells.

Bronchiolar obstruction from the smooth muscle proliferation leads to air trapping, resulting in destruction of alveolar septa and honeycombed cystic spaces, especially at the lung bases. Ultrastructural studies of lung biopsy specimens demonstrated degradation of elastic fibers in areas of smooth muscle accumulation, which can be a factor leading to the development of emphysematous changes. Venous obstruction results in dilation and rupture of venules, chronic low-grade hemorrhage, and, ultimately, hemosiderosis. Both estrogen and progesterone cell-surface receptors have been demonstrated in the lung.

Clinically, patients with LAM present most commonly with dyspnea (83%), pneumothorax (69%), and cough (66%). Other common signs and symptoms include chylothorax (23%), hemoptysis (20%), ascites (11%), pericardial effusion (6%), chyloptysis (3%), and chyluria (3%). With abdominal lymphatic obstruction, chylous ascites can develop. Occasionally, communications form between dilated retroperitoneal lymphatics and a kidney or ureter, resulting in chyluria. Patients presenting with angiomyolipoma and pulmonary symptoms should be evaluated for LAM by chest computed tomography (CT) scan, because the two are associated.

The physical examination frequently is not revealing until late in the clinical course, when end-inspiratory rales, diminished lower lobe breath sounds, scattered rhonchi, and signs of pleural effusion are present. An abrupt exacerbation of dyspnea may signal the development of pneumothorax. Clubbing is rare.

The chest roentgenogram initially may be normal, but later shows reticulonodular infiltration, with or without frank honeycombing. Occasionally, small cysts coalesce to form large blebs. This occurs predominantly at the lung bases. Unlike other forms of interstitial lung disease, in LAM the lungs often appear hyperinflated. CT scan is more useful than the chest film in assessing the presence and extent of cysts. CT demonstrates numerous small (2–20 mm) thin-walled cysts throughout both lungs. Greater morphologic and physiologic correlation is seen with the CT scan than with the chest radiograph.

Laboratory findings are nonspecific except for chyluria. Pulmonary function tests (PFTs) show mild to severe obstruction superimposed on a restrictive pattern. A bronchodilator response is present in 26% of patients. Hypoxemia (worsened by exertion), reduced flows and carbon monoxide diffusing capacity (DLCO), and progressive increase in plethysmographic lung volume are characteristic. Significant functional impairment usually precedes any radiographic abnormality (other than pneumothorax). Diminished exercise capacity is seen, and is most likely caused by ventilatory limitation. Serial exercise testing has been suggested as a means to monitor disease progression and to screen for exertional hypoxemia.

The radiographic distribution and character of the lesions are highly characteristic, but biopsy is necessary to confirm the diagnosis. Of 75 lung specimens obtained by transbronchial and open lung biopsy, only LAM showed HMB45-positive cells. It is suggested that if only a transbronchial biopsy is available, this marker can assist in confirming the diagnosis.

The differential diagnosis includes idiopathic interstitial pneumonitis, sarcoidosis, histiocytosis X, and pulmonary hemosiderosis. Low-grade sarcomas metastatic to the lung have been rarely misdiagnosed as LAM.

The mediastinal and pulmonary lymphangiomyomas are resistant to radiation therapy. Surgical or chemical obliteration (pleurodesis) of the pleural space may be necessary in patients with recurrent effusion or pneumothorax. Symptomatic therapy for bronchospasm or cor pulmonale may be required. Corticosteroids and cytotoxic agents appear to offer no benefit. Hormonal manipulation can affect muscle proliferation in this disease. Pregnancy and estrogen therapy can worsen the disease, and remission of the disease can occur after menopause. Oophorectomy or tamoxifen with progesterone therapy (or both) has been successful in some cases.

The most consistent improvement has occurred with oophorectomy and progesterone therapy. Functional impairment can be arrested, or even reversed, if such treatment is begun before destructive changes are advanced. It is unclear why some patients respond to hormonal manipulation and others do not. It may be that the presence of advanced disease limits response at the time therapy is instituted.

Lung transplantation is a viable alternative for patients with end-stage disease. Criteria for transplantation include (1) progression despite medical therapy; (2) severe functional defects (e.g., forced expiratory volume in 1 second/forced vital capacity [FEV_1/FVC] <50%, total lung capacity >130%, FEV_1 <30%); and (3) severe cystic disease on high-resolution CT (HRCT). Two-year survival is similar to outcomes observed following transplantation for other lung diseases. Recurrence of LAM in the transplanted lung has been reported.

Patients with extensive cystic changes and hyperinflation usually survive only 3 to 10 years following the onset of symptoms. A few with primarily mediastinal LAM with minimal parenchymal involvement survive longer.

TUBEROUS SCLEROSIS

Tuberous sclerosis is an autosomal dominant, hereditary, neurocutaneous disease. It has a broader systemic constellation of complications than LAM, but the pulmonary component of this disease appears identical to that in LAM. A controversy exists regarding whether LAM is a *forme fruste* of tuberous sclerosis.

Lung involvement in tuberous sclerosis is unusual, but occurs principally in young women of childbearing age; dyspnea rapidly worsens, and cor pulmonale develops within years of its onset. This differs from classic tuberous sclerosis, in which no gender predilection is seen. Pregnancy exacerbates both diseases. Both disorders are associated with renal angiofibrolipomatous tumors.

Tuberous sclerosis is a rare disease, occurring in 1 in 100,000 to 170,000 people in the general population. Two genes responsible for tuberous sclerosis (*TSC1, TSC2*) have been identified on chromosomes 9 and 16. The classic triad in this disease includes mental retardation, seizures, and dermal angiofibroma (adenoma sebaceum). The clinical features, however, can vary; for example, patient intelligence may be normal.

The primary features of tuberous sclerosis complex (TSC) have been described to be central nervous system (CNS) lesions of cortical and subependymal tubers, ungual fibromas, and facial angio-fibromas (sebaceous adenomas). Secondary lesions include Shagreen patches, cerebral tubers, retinal hamartomas, multiple renal tumors, sclerotic bone lesions, and cardiac rhabdomyomas.

Pulmonary involvement in tuberous sclerosis is rare, occurring in approximately 1 to 2% of patients. Pulmonary manifestations appear later than the cutaneous and neurologic ones. When pulmonary disease is manifested, it occurs most often in women of childbearing age without any CNS disease. When pulmonary disease is present, it usually dominates the clinical picture and can be the cause of death from either cor pulmonale or pneumothorax. (However, the most common cause of death is renal disease.) Lymph node involvement and chylous effusions are reported, but rarely. Pneumothorax and pulmonary insufficiency are common. Exertional dyspnea is the major symptom. Chronic cough and hemoptysis occur frequently. Lung histology, chest radiographic, and CT scan findings, pulmonary presentation, and clinical course are similar to LAM.

In suspected cases, thorough cutaneous and ophthalmologic examinations should be performed. The diagnostic workup should include cranial CT scan, renal ultrasound, and skeletal radiographs in addition to chest radiograph study, chest HRCT scan, and pulmonary physiology studies. A rare but early indicator of tuberous sclerosis is an unusual but characteristically expanded, dense rib deformity. These bony lesions can be mistaken for fibrous dysplasia or Paget's disease.

Estrogen receptors have been demonstrated in the lungs of patients with TSC. Tamoxifen and progesterone therapy have slowed the pulmonary disease in tuberous sclerosis, similar to descriptions for LAM. Genetic counseling is an important component in the management of patients with this disease.

1. Aberle DR, et al. Lymphangiomyomatosis: CT, chest radiographic, and functional correlations. *Radiology*. 1990;176:381.
   Reviews CT scan, chest radiographs, and PFT in eight patients with LAM. HRCT scan may be more sensitive than PFTs in the early detection of this disease.
2. Alper J, Kegel M. Skin signs in pulmonary disease. *Clin Chest Med*. 1987;8:299.
   A good overview chapter discussing neurofibromatosis and tuberous sclerosis as well as other diseases. Viewpoint is from skin signs but covers the general clinical presentation.
3. Berger U, et al. Pulmonary lymphangioleiomyomatosis and steroid receptors: an immunocytochemical study. *Am J Clin Pathol*. 1990;93:609.
   Describes the findings of estrogen, progesterone, or both receptors localized to the proliferative smooth muscle nodules and the interstitial tissue in the lung of two patients with LAM.
4. Boehler A, et al. Lung transplantation for lymphangioleiomyomatosis. *N Engl J Med*. 1996;335:1275.
   A retrospective study of 34 patients who underwent lung transplantation for end-stage LAM between 1983 and 1995. Actuarial survival rate was 69% at 1 year and 58% at 2 years.
5. Bonetti F, et al. Transbronchial biopsy in lymphangiomyomatosis of the lung: HMB45 for diagnosis. *Am J Surg Pathol*. 1993;17:1092.
   Describes the specificity of the melanoma-related marker HMB45 for smooth muscle in LAM. Various lung diseases were examined by staining transbronchial and open lung biopsy specimens, but only patients with LAM were positive for this marker.
6. Case Records of the Massachusetts General Hospital: Case 18-1994. A 37-year-old woman with pneumothorax. *N Engl J Med*. 1994;30:1300.
   A good discussion of the differential diagnosis of an abnormal roentgenograph associated with pneumothorax, including LAM and tuberous sclerosis.
7. Castro M, et al. Pulmonary tuberous sclerosis. *Chest*. 1995;107:189.
   Reviews the clinical presentations, chest radiographs, PFTs, and CT findings of nine patients with pulmonary involvement in TSC. Three of five patients treated with hormonal therapy had a clinical response. Discussion provides a thorough review of pulmonary tuberous sclerosis.
8. Chu SC, et al. Comprehensive evaluation of 35 patients with lymphangioleiomyomatosis. *Chest*. 1999;115:1041.
   Results of a prospective evaluation of patients with LAM who presented to the National Institutes of Health between 1995 and 1997.
9. Collins J. CT signs and patterns of lung disease. *Radiol Clin North Am*. 2001;39:1115–1135.
   A good review of CT appearance in LAM, TS, and other interstitial lung disease (ILD).
10. Costello LC, Hartman TE, Tyu JH. High Frequency of Pulmonary Lymphangioleiomyomatosis in women with tuberous sclerosis complex. *Mayo Clinic Proc*. 2000;75:591–594.

A retrospective cohort study demonstrating that the frequency of lung involvement (26%) in 78 women with TSC is substantially higher than previously suspected. This study supports routine screening Chest CT scans in women with TSC.

11. Crausman RS, et al. Lymphangioleiomyomatosis: the pathophysiology of diminished exercise capacity. *Am J Respir Crit Care Med.* 1996;153:1368.

    Sixteen patients with LAM underwent exercise testing. Poor exercise limitation was caused primarily by ventilatory limitation. Patients had ventilatory limitation because of airflow limitation and increased dead-space ventilation.

12. Fukuda Y, et al. Role of elastic fiber degradation in emphysema-like lesions of pulmonary lymphangiomyomatosis. *Hum Pathol.* 1990;21:1252.

    Describes electron microscopy and immunohistochemical analysis for elastin and a_1-antitrypsin on five open lung biopsy samples in a study of the structural remodeling of the lung in LAM.

13. Hancock E, Osborne J. Lymphangioleiomyomatosis: a review of the literature. *Respir Med.* 2002;96:1–6.

    A comprehensive review of LAM looking at clinical features and treatment of the disease.

14. Hoffman AD. Imaging of tuberous sclerosis lesions outside of the central nervous system. *Ann N Y Acad Sci.* 1991;615:94.

    Radiographic findings of the skeleton, lungs, heart, vascular system, kidneys, and liver in patients with tuberous sclerosis are discussed and illustrated with examples.

15. Johnson S. Lymphangioleiomyomatosis: clinical features, management and basic mechanisms. *Thorax.* 1999;54:254.

    A well-referenced(105 references) article containing an excellent review of the cell biology of LAM.

16. Johnson SR, Tattersfield AE. Decline in lung function in lymphangioleiomyomatosis—relation to menopause and progesterone treatment. *Am J Respir Crit Care Med.* 1999;160:628.

    Longitudinal PFT data were evaluated retrospectively for 43 patients with LAM in the United Kingdom. The decline in lung function in premenopausal and postmenopausal women and in those receiving progesterone therapy was compared with patients who had no hormone therapy. The study provides support for the suggestion that disease progression can be reduced by progesterone therapy.

17. Johnson SR, Tattersfield AE. Clinical experience of lymphangioleiomyomatosis in the UK. *Thorax.* 2000;55:1052–1057.

    A report on the experience of a large cohort of patients (50) in the UK that includes a discussion of the management of pneumothorax and LAM in pregnancy.

18. Kerr LA, et al. Renal angiomyolipoma in association with pulmonary lymphangioleiomyomatosis: forme fruste of tuberous sclerosis? *Urology.* 1993;41:440.

    The association and frequency of renal angiomyolipoma in 27 patients with LAM followed over a 13-year period; 7 had renal tumors, either unilaterally or bilaterally.

19. Lenoir S, et al. Pulmonary lymphangiomyomatosis and tuberous sclerosis: comparison of radiographic and thin-section CT findings. *Radiology.* 1990;175:329.

    Nine patients with LAM and two with tuberous sclerosis were evaluated by chest radiograph, HRCT scans, and PFTs. CT findings correlated better with diffusing capacity or DLCO than the chest films. CT scan was more sensitive and precise than chest roentgenograph at revealing the lung morphology.

20. Lie JT. Cardiac, pulmonary, and vascular involvement in tuberous sclerosis. *Ann N Y Acad Sci.* 1991;615:58.

    Describes the histopathology of tuberous sclerosis with photomicrographs with an extensive reference list.

21. Mahadeva R, Stewart S, Wallwork J. Metastatic endometrial stromal sarcoma masquerading as pulmonary lymphangioleiomyomatosis. *J Clin Pathol.* 1999;52:147.

    Case report of a 39-year-old woman who presented with bilateral pneumothoraces. Lung biopsy resulted in diagnosis of LAM. The patient was followed for 8 years. Autopsy revealed multiple pulmonary metastases from an endometrial stromal sarcoma.

22. Meyer FJ, et al. Bronchoalveolar lavage cytology in pulmonary fibrosis associated with neurofibromatosis. *Respir Med.* 1996;90:365.
      A case report describing bronchoalveolar lavage fluid findings of mild elevation of eosinophils and mast cells in a patient with pulmonary fibrosis associated with neurofibromatosis.

23. Moss J. Prevalence and clinical characteristics of lymphangioleiomyomatosis (LAM) in patients with tuberous sclerosis complex. *Am J Respir Crit Care Med.* 2001;164:669–671.
      Screening evaluation with CT showed an increased incidence of cystic lung disease in TSC patients, indicating early LAM may be asymptomatic with normal PFTs.

24. Moss J, DeCastro R, Patronas NJ, et al. Meningiomas in lymphangioleimyomatosis. *JAMA.* 2001;286:1879–1881.
      Screening study which demonstrated that women with LAM have a high prevalence of meningiomas. Because meningiomas have a reported mitogenic response to progesterone, the authors recommend that LAM patients be screened with CNS MRI prior to the initiation of therapy with progesterone.

25. Muller NL, Chiles C, Kullnig P. Pulmonary lymphangiomyomatosis: correlation of CT with radiographic and functional findings. *Radiology.* 1990;175:335.
      The CT scan's role in the diagnosis of LAM and assessment of severity of disease is presented. CT scan had a better correlation with gas exchange abnormalities than did chest radiograph.

26. NHLBI Workshop Summary. Report of workshop on lymphangioleiomyomatosis. National Heart, Lung, and Blood Institute. *Am J Respir Crit Care Med.* 1999;159:679–683.
      Workshop report documents the current understanding of the clinical features and molecular biology of LAM.

27. O'Donohue WJ, et al. Multiple pulmonary neurofibromas with hypoxemia. *Arch Intern Med.* 1986;146:1618.
      A case report describing hypoxemia caused by right-to-left shunting within intrapulmonary lesions.

28. Ohori NP, et al. Estrogen and progesterone receptors in lymphangioleiomyomatosis, epithelioid hemangioendothelioma, and sclerosing hemangioma of the lung. *Am J Clin Pathol.* 1991;96:529.
      This study reports no finding of estrogen and progesterone receptors in lung tissue of five patients with LAM as well as other diseases; these findings are contrary to the current viewpoint presented in the literature.

29. Popper HH, et al. Chromosome typing in lymphangioleiomatosis of the lung with and without tuberous sclerosis. *Eur Respir J.* 1993;6:753.
      Two cases, one with tuberous sclerosis and one with LAM, are discussed and compared. Chromosomal rearrangements were found in the peripheral blood lymphocytes in the patient with tuberous sclerosis, which were not demonstrated in the patient with LAM.

30. Popper HH, Juettner-Smolle FM, Pongratz MG. Micronodular hyperplasia of type II pneumocytes: a new lung lesion associated with tuberous sclerosis. *Histopathology.* 1991;18:347.
      A case report describing histologic, immunohistochemical, and electron microscopy findings in a woman with tuberous sclerosis. Describes alveolar lymphatic vessel and alveolar duct obstruction, resulting in emphysemalike changes.

31. Report of Workshop on Lymphangioleiomyomatosis. *Am J Respir Crit Care Med.* 1999;159:679–683.
      Reviews the differential diagnosis of LAM, smooth muscle abnormalities, tumor markers and the possible hormonal mechanisms in LAM. Offers recommendations for further directions in research.

32. Ryu JH, Doerr CH, Fisher SD, et al. Chylothorax in lymphangioleiomyomatosis. *Chest.* 2003;123:623–667.
      A retrospective review of 79 LAM patients, 8 of whom developed chylothorax. LAM patients with chylothorax had a variable clinical course. Management options for these patients with chylothorax are discussed.

33. Saleh HA, Beydoun R, Masood S. Cytology of malignant schwannoma metastatic to the lung: report of a case with diagnosis by fine needle aspiration biopsy. *Acta Cytol.* 1993;37:409.

   A case report describing the utility of fine-needle aspiration biopsy, S-100 staining, and electron microscopy to confirm the diagnosis of von Recklinghausen's disease.

34. Shepherd CW, et al. Causes of death in patients with tuberous sclerosis. *Mayo Clin Proc.* 1991;66:792.

   Of 355 patients studied with tuberous sclerosis, 49 had died, 9 from causes other than tuberous sclerosis. Of the remaining 40 patients, the most common cause of death was renal disease (11 of 40), followed by brain tumors (10 of 40); 4 of 40 patients died because of lung involvement.

35. Sullivan EJ. Lymphangioleiomyomatosis: a review. *Chest.* 1998;114:1689.

   An up-to-date comprehensive review of LAM (124 references).

36. Taveira-DaSilva AM, Stylianou MP, Hedin CJ, et al. Maximal oxygen uptake and severity of disease in lymphangioleiomyomatosis. *Am J Respir Crit Care Med.* 2003;168:1427–1431.

   Cardiopulmonary exercise testing (CPET) was performed in 217 LAM patients and exercise data was correlated with clinical markers of severity, CT scans, PFTs, and histology. In this study, CPET documented the presence of exercise-induced hypoxemia and assisted in the grading of disease severity and determination of supplemental oxygen requirements in LAM patients.

37. Taylor JR, et al. Lymphangioleiomyomatosis: clinical course in 32 patients. *N Engl J Med.* 1990;323:1254.

   An excellent review article. Mean survival for this group of patients was 10 years from onset of LAM.

38. Volpini E, et al. Pulmonary changes in a man affected by von Recklinghausen's disease. *Monaldi Arch Chest Dis.* 1996;51:123.

   Case reviews features of lung disease associated with NF1.

39. Yokoyama A, et al. Distal acinar emphysema and interstitial pneumonia in a patient with von Recklinghausen's disease: five year observation following quitting smoking. *Intern Med.* 1997;36:413.

   A case report documenting BAL fluid and transbronchial biopsy results in a smoker with pulmonary complications associated with von Recklinghausen's disease. Patient's symptoms and PFTs remained stable during 5-year observation following smoking cessation. Accompanying editorial by K. Miyamoto reviews pulmonary manifestations of neurofibromatosis type I.

99. PULMONARY ALVEOLAR PROTEINOSIS

Angela C. Wang

Pulmonary alveolar proteinosis (PAP) is a group of rare diseases characterized by the deposition within alveoli and airways of large amounts of eosinophilic material rich in lipids and protein, such as surfactant. PAP is now believed to involve defective surfactant catabolism in alveolar macrophages, either as a result of congential or acquired defects in surfactant production or abnormalities in granulocyte macrophage colony-stimulating factor (GM-CSF) signaling.

PATHOPHYSIOLOGY

Three clinically distinct forms of PAP exist: congenital, secondary, and acquired. Three main etiologies of secondary PAP have been identified: (1) lung infections, including *Pneumocystis carinii* pneumonia in patients with and without AIDS; (2) hematologic malignancies and other immune-altering conditions; and (3) exposure to inhaled chemicals and minerals. A number of toxic insults to the lung (silica, NO_2, ozone, and $ONOO^-$) can result in alveolar proteinosis. PAP has also been produced in laboratory animals by inhalation of inert dusts of extremely fine particulate matter.

Acquired PAP appears to result from the presence of autoantibodies that prevent binding of GM-CSF to its receptor. The peak age of onset is between 30 and 50 years; however, the disease has been described in all ages. In adults, the male to female ratio is approximately 3:1. Most patients are current or prior smokers. Although some patients are asymptomatic at the time of diagnosis, PAP most commonly presents insidiously with increasing dyspnea and cough. An abrupt onset can also occur usually in the setting of a concomitant respiratory infection. Sputum production is usually scant but on occasion has been described as containing small chunks of material. Other much less common symptoms include weight loss, weakness, chest pain, and hemoptysis. Physical findings, if present, are nonspecific. Fever usually implies superinfection, although a low-grade fever is occasionally present. Inspiratory crackles occur in up to 50% of patients; in severe cases, cyanosis and clubbing are observed.

The most common laboratory finding is a mildly elevated serum lactate dehydrogenase (LDH). The LDH may be used to follow disease activity and severity. Patients with severe disease may have secondary polycythemia. The leukocyte count is normal or slightly increased. Serum protein electrophoresis may reveal increased globulins. Serum levels of lung surfactant proteins A, B, and D have been found to be elevated in patients with PAP. Increased levels of these SP-A and SP-D proteins are also found in patients with idiopathic pulmonary fibrosis. In contrast, patients with interstitial pneumonia associated with various collagen-vascular diseases were found to have an elevated serum SP-D, but not SP-A. Elevated serum levels of carcinoembryonic antigen, cytokeratin 19 and mucin KL-6 have also been detected.

Pulmonary function tests may be normal but usually reveal a restrictive pattern with decreased static lung compliance and decreased carbon monoxide diffusing capacity (DLCO). Arterial blood gases demonstrate hypoxemia and a widened alveolar–arterial oxygen gradient. Chest radiographs typically show diffuse, finely nodular, soft infiltrates in a perihilar butterfly pattern, similar in appearance to pulmonary edema; however, other signs of left ventricular failure (cardiomegaly, Kerley B lines) are absent. A miliary, interstitial, or multinodular pattern and lobar consolidation can also be seen. Hilar adenopathy, pleural effusions, and cavitation are rare and suggest superimposed infection. Findings on high-resolution computed tomography (HRCT) scanning, although not pathognomonic, can be strongly suggestive of PAP and may demonstrate the extent and pattern of PAP more clearly than plain radiographs. The presence of the phospholipid or proteinaceous material within alveoli correlates with a ground glass appearance. Intralobular and interlobular septa are typically thickened, often in polygonal patterns, termed *crazy paving*.

DIAGNOSIS

The differential diagnosis includes any disease that can produce a diffuse acinar-filling pattern on chest roentgenogram, including cardiogenic and noncardiogenic pulmonary edema, toxic inhalations, pulmonary hemorrhage, viral pneumonia, and *P. carinii* infection. One of the clues to the diagnosis of PAP is the disparity between extensive radiographic abnormalities and the minimal clinical symptomatology. When chest roentgenograms reveal a predominant interstitial pattern, the diagnosis becomes more difficult. Although open lung biopsy has been thought of as the gold standard for diagnosing PAP, bronchoscopy with transbronchial biopsy and bronchoalveolar lavage (BAL) can establish the diagnosis in most cases when combined with clinical and radiographic findings. Typically, the BAL fluid in PAP appears opaque and milky. Microscopically, few alveolar macrophages are seen and these cells appear large and foamy. Increased lymphocytes may be seen. Large eosinophilic bodies appear amidst a background of periodic acid-Schiff positive granular debris. Using electron microscopy, this intra-alveolar material can be shown to contain numerous osmiophilic, fused membrane structures that are similar to lamellar bodies and tubular myelin. Both SP-A and SP-D levels are elevated in BAL fluid obtained from patients with acquired PAP and may prove helpful in distinguishing this disease from other diffuse lung disorders. Finally, a serologic test has been developed based on detecting the presence of neutralizing autoantibodies and appears very promising for the diagnosis of acquired PAP.

PROGNOSIS

The course of PAP is variable. Three categories of disease prognosis have been described: spontaneous improvement, stable but with persistent symptoms or progressive deterioration. A recent review found that approximately 8% fell into the first category. Another study demonstrated a 5-year survival rate of approximately 75%. The majority of deaths in the latter study were from respiratory failure from PAP, with about 20% from infection. Without lung transplantation, the prognosis in infants remains grave, with most deaths occurring between 3 and 6 months of age.

COMPLICATIONS

The major complication in PAP is infection. Bacterial, mycobacterial, and fungal infections have been reported frequently. Exacerbations of the disease often respond to antibiotics without a definite bacteriologic diagnosis. *Nocardia asteroides* and *Mycobacterium tuberculosis* have appeared most often in case reports. In one large series, *M. avium-intracellulare* was isolated from lavage fluid in 42% of cases. Consistent with the defect in host defense is the observation that infections in patients with PAP often occur outside the lung. Other complications include pulmonary fibrosis, cor pulmonale, and spontaneous pneumothorax.

TREATMENT

Treatment of secondary PAP focuses on the underlying condition (e.g., the inciting hematologic malignancy). Although lung transplantation has been performed for congenital cases of PAP, in general, treatment remains supportive. Whole-lung lavage is the only consistently successful treatment for acquired PAP; despite the lack of prospective, randomized trials, it is the standard of care. The possibility of spontaneous resolution of PAP has made clinical decision making regarding the need for and frequency of whole-lung lavage less clear. In one series from the Cleveland Clinic, 46% of patients followed over a prolonged period never required whole-lung lavage. Another 29% required repeated whole-lung lavage for recurring signs and symptoms of PAP. However, lavage may improve survival overall: in one group of 146 patients, mean survival ($\pm$ SD) at 5 years was $94 \pm 2\%$ with lavage versus $85 \pm 5\%$ without lavage. Because of the rarity of PAP, only a few referral centers have developed extensive experience in whole-lung lavage. In general, the indications for whole-lung lavage are dyspnea or hypoxemia. Radiographic evidence alone is probably not sufficient to warrant the procedure.

Pulmonary segmental flooding (lavage) by an endobronchial catheter or fiberoptic bronchoscope has been successful in clearing radiographic infiltrates. Placement of a Carlens tube allows ventilation of one lung with 100% oxygen, while the other lung is irrigated with 10 to 20 L of saline. If oxygen saturation does not reach satisfactory levels in 3 to 4 days, the procedure can be repeated. Improvement in gas exchange, pulmonary function tests, symptoms, and radiographic infiltrates occurs in approximately 80% of patients following lavage. Complications include hypotension during the irrigation phase and hypoxemia and carbon dioxide retention following lavage, caused by spillage into the ventilated lung or by ventilation-perfusion alterations in the lavaged and nonlavaged lungs.

Treatment for PAP has also included corticosteroids, supersaturated potassium iodide solution, and aerosolized and oral proteolytic agents. None of these treatments have been shown to be clearly beneficial and some may be detrimental. Although corticosteroids may be helpful in the treatment of acquired PAP as an autoimmune disease, they are relatively contraindicated because of the high incidence of associated infection. Similarly, the use of plasmapheresis to decrease circulating anti–GM-CSF levels has been described, but has not been properly tested in clinical trials. Several phase 2 trials involving GM-CSF therapy for the acquired form of PAP have been carried out or are ongoing at the time of this review. Although the mechanisms of effect remain unclear, results are promising. Lung transplantation has been considered an option for some patients, but its role in acquired PAP needs careful evaluation because the disease can recur. The possibility of bone marrow transplantation should be considered as potentially curative treatment for these patients.

1. Abraham J, McEuen D. Inorganic particulates associated with pulmonary alveolar proteinosis: SEM and x-ray microanalysis results. *Appl Pathol*. 1986;4:138.
   The lungs of 24 patients with PAP were studied with light microscopy, scanning electron microscopy, and radiographic analysis and found to have increased amounts of small inorganic particulate matter.
2. Altose M, Hicks R, Edwards M. Extracorporeal membrane oxygenation during bronchopulmonary lavage. *Arch Surg*. 1976;111:1148.
   Describes the technical aspects of membrane oxygenation with pulmonary lavage.
3. Bedrossian C. Alveolar proteinosis as a consequence of immunosuppression. *Hum Pathol*. 1980;2(Suppl):818A.
   Reviews the association with opportunistic infection and hematologic malignancies. Hypothesizes that PAP results from poor alveolar clearance in immunosuppressed patients.
4. Carnovale R, et al. Pulmonary alveolar proteinosis: its association with hematologic malignancy and lymphoma. *Radiology*. 1977;122:303.
   Describes five cases of PAP occurring in patients with hematologic malignancy or lymphoma. Speculates on possible mechanisms underlying this association.
5. Colon A, Lawrence R, Mills S. Childhood pulmonary alveolar proteinosis: report of a case and review of the literature. *Am J Dis Child*. 1971;121:481.
   The disease most often occurs in children younger than 1 year of age and has a more malignant course; 30% of the cases were associated with thymic alymphoplasia.
6. Corrin B, King E. Pathogenesis of experimental pulmonary alveolar proteinosis. *Thorax*. 1970;25:230.
   Rats exposed to aluminum powder or pure fine quartz developed pathologic changes identical to those of PAP.
7. deMello DE, Lin Z. Pulmonary alveolar proteinosis: a review. *Pediatr Pathol Mol Med*. 2001;20:413.
   Recent review focusing on congenital PAP.
8. Dranoff G, et al. Involvement of granulocyte-macrophage colony-stimulating factor in pulmonary homeostasis. *Science*. 1994;264:713.
   One of two original articles describing the development of PAP in GM-CSF–deficient mice.
9. Goldstein LS, et al. Pulmonary alveolar proteinosis: clinical features and outcomes. *Chest*. 1998;114:1357.
   A recent single-institution review of 24 patients referred to the Cleveland Clinic from 1965 to 1995 for whole-lung lavage. Confirms evolving diagnostic trend in which bronchoscopy is supplanting open lung biopsy as the initial diagnostic method for PAP. Also, suggests that BAL fluid may be diagnostic. Contains a nice summary of previously selected published studies in table form.
10. Hammon W, McCaffree R, Cucchiara A. A comparison of manual to mechanical chest percussion for clearance of alveolar material in patients with pulmonary alveolar proteinosis (phospholipidosis). *Chest*. 1993;103:1409.
    Manual chest percussion is superior to mechanical chest percussion or no percussion in clearance of alveolar material.
11. Kariman K, Kylstra J, Spock A. Pulmonary alveolar proteinosis: prospective clinical experience in 23 patients for 15 years. *Lung*. 1984;162:223.
    Of patients, 24% had spontaneous remission, 48% improved after lung lavage, and 13% did not improve after lung lavage.

12. Kavuru MS, Bonfield TL, Thomassen MJ. Plasmapheresis, GM-CSF, and alveolar proteinosis. *Am J Respir Crit Care Med.* 2003;167:1036.
    Case report of a patient with PAP successfully treated with plasmapheresis.
13. Kavuru MS, Sullivan EJ, Piccin R, et al. Exogenous granulocyte-macrophage colony-stimulating factor administration for pulmonary alveolar proteinosis. *Am J Respir Crit Care Med.* 2000;161:1143.
    Reports preliminary results for four patients treated in an open-label study of systemic GM-CSF.
14. Kitamura T, Uchida K, Tanaka N, et al. Serological diagnosis of idiopathic pulmonary alveolar proteinosis. *Am J Respir Crit Care Med.* 2000;162:658.
    Describes the development of a latex agglutination test for the serologic diagnosis of acquired PAP.
15. Masuda T, et al. Surfactant apoprotein-A concentration in sputum for diagnosis of pulmonary alveolar proteinosis. *Lancet.* 1991;337:580.
    References 11 and 12 describe a rapid technique of diagnosing PAP using monoclonal antibodies to surfactant protein A in the lavage fluid or sputum of patients with the disease.
16. Nhieu J, et al. Pulmonary alveolar proteinosis associated with *Pneumocystis carinii. Chest.* 1990;98:801.
    Analysis of BAL fluid from 26 patients with P. carinii pneumonia showed surfactantlike material consistent with PAP.
17. Parker LA, Novotny DB. Recurrent alveolar proteinosis following double lung transplantation. *Chest.* 1997;111:1457.
    A case report describing disease recurrence in a patient who underwent double lung transplantation for PAP.
18. Preger L. Pulmonary alveolar proteinosis. *Radiology.* 1969;92:1291.
    A review of the radiographic patterns of PAP.
19. Riker J, Wolinski H. Trypsin aerosol treatment of pulmonary alveolar proteinosis. *Am Rev Respir Dis.* 1973;108:108.
    A report of a patient who appeared to respond to aerosolized trypsin on three occasions.
20. Rosen S, Castleman B, Liebow A. Pulmonary alveolar proteinosis. *N Engl J Med.* 1958;258:1123.
    The classic article that first described this disease.
21. Selecky P, et al. The clinical and physiological effect of whole lung lavage in pulmonary alveolar proteinosis: a ten-year experience. *Ann Thorac Surg.* 1977;24:451.
    Describes the technique of massive pulmonary lavage and reviews the response of 18 patients; found that heparin or acetylcysteine is not needed in the lavage fluid.
22. Seymour JF, Presneill JJ, Schoch OD, et al. Therapeutic efficacy of granulocyte-macrophage colony-stimulating factor in patients with idiopathic acquired alveolar proteinosis. *Am J Respir Crit Care Med.* 2001;163:524.
    Fourteen patients treated with GM-CSF as an alternative to whole lung lavage.
23. Schoch OD, Schanz U, Koller M, et al. BAL findings in a patient with pulmonary alveolar proteinosis successfully treated with GM-CSF. *Thorax.* 2002;57:277.
    A case report describing the decrease in anti–GM-CSF antibody levels in a patient with PAP treated with systemic recombinant human GM-CSF.
24. Seymour JF, Presneill JJ. Pulmonary alveolar proteinosis: progress in the first 44 years. *Am J Respir Crit Care Med.* 2002;166:215–235.
    Analysis detailing the clinical presentation, demographics, and clinical course of 410 patients with PAP.
25. Singh G, et al. Pulmonary alveolar proteinosis: staining for surfactant apoprotein in alveolar proteinosis and in conditions simulating it. *Chest.* 1983;83:82.
    Intra-alveolar material in patients with primary PAP stained uniformly for surfactant-specific apoprotein, whereas the staining was focal in patients with secondary PAP.
26. Stanley E, et al. Granulocyte/macrophage colony-stimulating factor–deficient

mice show no major perturbation of hematopoiesis but develop a characteristic pulmonary pathology. *Proc Natl Acad Sci U S A*. 1994;91:5592.

Original article describing the unexpected development of a PAP-like disease in mice in which the GM-CSF gene was knocked out.

27. Trapnell BC, Whitsett JA, Nakata K. Pulmonary alveolar proteinosis. *N Engl J Med*. 2003;349:2527.

    Comprehensive review with emphasis on molecular mechanisms of disease and a detailed reference list.

28. Uchida K, Nakata K, Trapnell BC, et al. High-affinity autoantibodies specifically eliminate granulocyte-macrophage colony-stimulating factor activity in the lungs of patients with idiopathic pulmonary alveolar proteinosis. *Blood*. 2004;103:1089.

    Study demonstrating that anti–GM-CSF antibodies present in the lungs of patients with acquired PAP abrogate GM-CSF bioactivity.

29. Wasserman K, Mason GR. Pulmonary alveolar proteinosis. In: Murray JF, Nadel JA, eds. *Textbook of Respiratory Medicine,* 2nd ed. Philadelphia: WB Saunders; 1994:1933.

    A good, overall review with detailed description of whole-lung lavage.

30. Wang BM, et al. Diagnosing pulmonary alveolar proteinosis: a review and an update. *Chest*. 1997;111:460.

    An excellent review.

31. Witty L, Tapson V, Piantadosi A. Isolation of mycobacteria in patients with pulmonary alveolar proteinosis. *Medicine* (Baltimore). 1994;73:103.

    M. avium-intracellulare was isolated from the lavage fluid in 8 of 19 consecutive patients with PAP.

32. Xipell J, et al. Acute silicolipoproteinosis. *Thorax*. 1977;32:104.

    Presents a case of acute silicosis in which the lung showed areas of fibrotic nodules, interstitial fibrosis, and alveolar filling of a periodic acid-Schiff–positive material similar to that in PAP.

XI. NEOPLASTIC DISEASES

100. BRONCHIAL CARCINOIDS AND BENIGN NEOPLASMS OF THE LUNG

David H. Kupferberg

BRONCHIAL CARCINOIDS

Bronchial carcinoids and benign neoplasms of the lung account for less than 10% of all primary pulmonary neoplasms. They represent a clinical challenge because, when centrally located, they are often roentgenographically silent and may cause slowly progressive airflow obstruction, which can be confused with chronic airways disease.

When peripheral, these tumors are usually clinically silent but still pose the diagnostic challenge typical of any solitary pulmonary nodule. Carcinoid tumors are no longer classified along with benign bronchial adenomas, because they can behave like low-grade carcinomas. Hamartomas are the most common benign pulmonary neoplasms. Leiomyomas, true bronchial adenomas, lipomas, chondromas, fibromas, endometriosis, teratomas, and even rarer benign adenomas also occur.

Etiology

Bronchial carcinoids comprise the second largest group of lung tumors behind bronchogenic carcinomas and are responsible for approximately 0.5 to 2% of all bronchial tumors. They occur with a small increased frequency in women and with an earlier average age of onset (40 to 60 years old), as compared to noncarcinoid bronchogenic malignancies. Some studies suggest a greater incidence in Caucasians than in African Americans. There are some data to suggest that smoking may play a role in the pathogenesis of the atypical and more aggressive tumor subtypes.

Bronchopulmonary carcinoid tumors account for 25% of all carcinoid tumors. Most occur in the gastrointestinal tract. The bronchial type tends to develop centrally, in the large airways, within easy bronchoscopic visualization. Macroscopically, they can grow primarily either as a polypoid lesion or as a predominantly infiltrative process, with only minimal protrusion into the bronchial lumen (known as *iceberg tumor*). Growth is largely submucosal, and the surface epithelium is usually intact, although frequently metaplastic. Carcinoids have a wide histologic spectrum; most commonly, they appear as clumps of small, uniformly staining cells with a richly vascular stroma. Some form acini and produce mucin, however, and others appear highly malignant and may bear a striking resemblance to small-cell carcinoma. They can be classified along a spectrum as follows: (1) typical carcinoid with the best prognosis and bland-appearing histology; (2) atypical carcinoid with 2 to 10 mitoses per high power field and necrosis; (3) large-cell neuroendocrine carcinoma with a higher mitotic rate, greater atypia, and necrosis; and (4) small-cell carcinoma, the most aggressive. They appear to be derived from a precursor cell closely related to the Kulchitsky's cell of bronchial mucous glands and reveal neurosecretory granules on electron microscopy. Regional lymph nodes are involved approximately 10% of the time (more often in atypical carcinoid). The tumor is capable of elaborating a wide spectrum of neuroendocrine products. Careful interpretation of bronchoscopic biopsies is necessary, considering the similarities between small-cell carcinoma and carcinoid can be exaggerated in the setting of crush artifact and frozen sectioning. Atypical carcinoid may be misclassified with bronchoscopic biopsies because of difficulty with mitotic counts on limited sampling.

Clinical Presentation

The clinical manifestations of bronchial carcinoid tumors depend on the site of the tumor. Approximately 80% of bronchial carcinoids are central and can produce symptoms and signs of bronchial obstruction, including cough, fever, chest pain, and often a localized wheeze. Hemoptysis is present in approximately 50%, reflecting both their central origin and hypervascularity. Peripheral carcinoids most often are asymptomatic and are usually detected fortuitously by roentgenogram. Regional lymph node metastasis is present in approximately 10% of typical carcinoids at presentation, compared with 30 to 50% of atypical carcinoids.

Rarely, there are associated paraneoplastic findings. The most common is Cushing's syndrome, which can even predate visualization of a lung nodule. Acromegaly has also been reported with significantly elevated levels of growth hormone even without overt acromegalic features. The carcinoid syndrome occurs infrequently with an incidence as low as 0 to 3%. Production of high levels of 5-hydroxytryptamine and other substances (e.g., bradykinin, prostaglandins) enter the systemic circulation and cause flushing, wheezing, anxiety, vomiting, and hypotension. In addition, cardiac valvular damage can develop in the left heart in bronchial carcinoid syndrome, as opposed to the abdominal variety, in which it occurs on the right side. This syndrome always reflects metastasis of the carcinoid tumor, usually to the liver. Other neuroendocrine manifestations include the Zollinger–Ellison syndrome, hyperinsulinemia, and an association with multiple endocrine neoplasia type I.

The roentgenographic findings depend on the site of the tumor. Central tumors may cause bronchial obstruction and result in pneumonitis, atelectasis, bronchiectasis, and collapse. The partial collapse can result in hypoxic vasoconstriction and oligemia with expiratory gas trapping. Nonobstructive central and peripheral tumors may appear as a solitary pulmonary nodule, usually 4 cm or less in diameter, and are often slightly lobulated. Atypical carcinoids tend to be larger. Calcification may be present. Computed tomographic (CT) scanning is helpful in identifying endobronchial lesions as well as lymph node enlargement. Because carcinoid tumors tend to be highly vascular, there is marked enhancement with intravenous contrast. Newer localization modalities include radiolabeled somatostatin analog scintigraphy, which has been reported to find up to 85% of all primary and metastatic carcinoid lesions. Positron emission tomography (PET) scanning may yield false-negative results because of hypometabolic activity.

Pulmonary function testing is usually normal unless central obstruction occurs, in which case flow obstruction may be demonstrable. Serum or urine hormone levels can be elevated is association with the aforementioned neuroendocrine syndromes.

Diagnosis

Differential diagnosis includes all causes of solitary pulmonary nodules and obstructing airway lesions. The diagnosis of central tumors is usually made at bronchoscopy; the diagnosis of peripheral tumors often requires other methods (usually thoracotomy).

The hypervascularity of some tumors has raised concern about serious bleeding complications following bronchoscopic biopsy and transcutaneous needle aspiration. This has been tempered by a recent series demonstrating only a 2.5% incidence of significant hemorrhage with fewer than 1% requiring a transfusion or emergency surgery.

Treatment

Treatment for bronchial carcinoids is surgical. Lung-sparing procedures, which have been shown to yield similar survival results for typical carcinoids, should be attempted when possible. Lymph node dissection should be performed with atypical carcinoids or when higher grade lesions are suspected. Surgical treatment in those cases should be similar to resection of non–small-cell lung cancer with at least lobectomy. Lobectomy is often necessitated by bronchiectasis and parenchymal necrosis distal to an obstructive tumor. In such cases, the prognosis is excellent. There may be a role for Nd:YAG laser resection in typical carcinoid, particularly when patients are not good surgical candidates. Local recurrence rates are slightly higher. Survival rate in cases of nonmetastatic typical carcinoid is approximately 90%. Atypical carcinoid has a 5- and 10-year survival of 60% and 40%, respectively. Positive lymph nodes and larger tumor size correlate with poorer overall prognosis. Chemotherapy has limited benefit for metastatic disease when patients are unresponsive to other treatments and, overall, has limited use. Metastatic liver lesions have been treated successfully with hepatic artery embolization and local direct chemotherapeutic instillation. Interferon and octreotide have been reported to temporarily stabilize tumor growth, yet rarely produce any decrease in tumor size. Cushing's syndrome can be well controlled with octreotide with significant improvement in symptoms.

PULMONARY HAMARTOMAS
Etiology

Pulmonary hamartomas, the largest group of benign pulmonary neoplasms, occur more frequently in men than in women (3:1), with a peak incidence in the seventh decade. They are uncommon before age 30. Pathologically, they contain a mixture of tissues normally present in lung (i.e., smooth muscle, collagen, and rarely, cartilage); however, these components are totally disorganized. Ultrastructural studies indicate that pulmonary hamartomas represent a histologic spectrum of mesenchymal neoplasms derived from peribronchial connective tissue. Although pulmonary hamartomas can become extremely large, they remain benign.

Clinical Presentation

Hamartomas are clinically silent because of their peripheral location. Hemoptysis is rare. Roentgenographically, they appear as well-circumscribed, solitary pulmonary nodules, usually less than 4 cm in diameter; occasionally, they can be large, nearly filling the hemithorax. Calcification, resembling a kernel of popped popcorn, occurs in 5 to 15% of cases. CT scan of the lung may suggest the diagnosis. Multiple tumors rarely occur. Unless the roentgenogram and clinical course are classic, the diagnosis is made at thoracotomy because other methods usually fail to exclude carcinoma.

OTHER BENIGN NEOPLASMS

Infrequently, primary lung involvement may occur in other benign neoplasms. Signs and symptoms depend on the location, ranging from no clinical findings with peripheral lesions to cough, hemoptysis, or recurrent pneumonia from bronchial involvement. Roentgenographically, findings may be consistent with bronchial obstruction or only solitary or multiple nodules. True bronchial adenomas are benign tumors that arise from bronchial mucous glands and are quite rare. They can cause symptoms by obstructing airways. Leiomyomas arise from smooth muscle of the lung and are usually endobronchial. Most cases are asymptomatic. Women are affected more often than men, and the average age at presentation is 37. There appears to be a distinct entity in which multiple pulmonary fibroleiomyomas occur in women who have had uterine fibroids. Although such tumors are histologically and clinically benign, controversy exists regarding their in situ or metastatic origin. Lipomas are usually endobronchial (80%) and can occur on either side of the bronchial cartilage. They can change shape roentgenographically, as the individual assumes different positions. Chondromas are extremely rare. Unlike hamartomas, they derive exclusively from formed bronchial cartilage. Teratoma is a relatively common tumor of the mediastinum, but it is rarely found in lung tissue. Pulmonary teratomas may contain tissue from any germ layer. Roentgenographically, they may contain calcifications or even well-formed teeth. Expectoration of hair (trichoptysis) has been reported. Endometriosis can occur in the lung as a solitary nodule. The origin of this lung tumor is unclear; some consider it of metastatic origin, whereas others feel it arises from pleuripotential pulmonary tissue. Recurrent pneumothorax, particularly on the right side, or hemoptysis associated with menstruation should suggest the diagnosis.

1. Modlin IM, Sandor A. An analysis of 8305 cases of carcinoid tumors. *Cancer.* 1997;79:813.
   The largest epidemiologic combined series for patients between 1973 and 1991. An excellent review of carcinoid incidence and trends.
2. Godwin JD. Carcinoid tumors: an analysis of 2837 cases. *Cancer.* 1975;36:560.
   Found a 5-year survival for patients with bronchial carcinoids of 87%, which is higher than in most series.

3. Dusmet ME, McKneally MF. Pulmonary and thymic carcinoid tumors. *World J Surg*. 1996;20:168.

   A good review specifically related to bronchial carcinoid.
4. Fraser RS, et al, eds. *Fraser and Paré's Diagnosis of Diseases of the Chest*, 4th ed. Philadelphia: WB Saunders; 1999.

   A thorough, in-depth chapter with particular focus on pathology and histology.
5. Chughtai TS, et al. Bronchial carcinoid—twenty years' experience defines a selective approach. *Surgery*. 1997;122:801.

   A surgical review of 84 patients found a poor prognosis with atypical histology, lymph node metastases, or tumorlets. Overall, 93% and 82% 5- and 10-year survival, respectively. Advises lung sparing for patients at low risk.
6. Kulke MH, Mayer RJ. Carcinoid tumors. *N Engl J Med*. 1999;340:858.

   A comprehensive review of all carcinoid tumors, not only bronchial carcinoids. Best prognosis overall is with bronchial versus gastrointestinal carcinoid.
7. Cardillo G, et al. Bronchial carcinoid tumors: nodal status and long-term survival after resection. *Ann Thorac Surg*. 2004;77:1781.

   Makes the point that nodal status (N0 versus N1 and N2) and not tumor subtype predict survival.
8. Mak H, et al. Recurrent wheezing and massive atelectasis in an adolescent. *J Pediatr*. 1983;102:955.

   A case report of a 13-year-old boy with massive atelectasis and unilateral wheezing caused by bronchial carcinoid.
9. Onuki N, et al. Genetic changes in the spectrum of neuroendocrine lung tumors. *Cancer*. 1999;85:600.

   Describes molecular changes and mutations in DNA that support the notion of a disease continuum from typical carcinoid to small-cell carcinoma.
10. Schrevens L, et al. Clinical-radiological presentation and outcome of surgically treated pulmonary carcinoid tumors: a long-term single institution experience. *Lung Cancer*. 2004;43:39.

    Bronchoscopic biopsies cannot reliably make a diagnosis of atypical carcinoid and therefore detailed lymph node sampling is critical.
11. Kwekkeboom DJ, Krenning EP. Somatostatin receptor scintigraphy in patients with carcinoid tumors. *World J Surg*. 1996;20:157.

    Reports a sensitivity of 87% for finding carcinoid tumors when used with chest x-ray study and abdominal ultrasound. Found lesions in 11% of patients with normal radiography.
12. Churg A, Warnock ML. Pulmonary tumorlet: a form of peripheral carcinoid. *Cancer*. 1976;37:1469.

    These lesions are probably minute peripheral carcinoid tumors.
13. Condon VR, Phillips EW. Bronchial adenoma in children: a review of the literature and report of three cases. *AJR*. 1962;88:543.

    Bronchial adenoma should be included in the differential diagnosis of chronic cough, recurrent pneumonia, and atelectasis in children.
14. Di Bartolomeo M, et al. Clinical efficacy of octreotide in the treatment of metastatic neuroendocrine tumors: a study by the Italian Trials in Medical Oncology Group. *Cancer*. 1996;77:402.

    Octreotide controlled symptomatic and biochemical response with almost no response in tumor regression, which is similar to use of interferon.
15. Hage R, et al. Update in pulmonary carcinoid tumors: a review article. *Ann Surg Oncol*. 2003;10:697.

    Recent review with revised staging scheme, symptoms, and survival tables.
16. Carney JA, Aidan MD. Gastric stromal sarcoma, pulmonary chondroma, and extra-adrenal paraganglioma (Carney triad): natural history, adrenocortical component and possible familial occurrence. *Mayo Clin Proc*. 1999;74:543.

    Reviews 79 patients with Carney's triad, which includes pulmonary chondromas. Tumors can be separated by years (mean 8.4, longest 26).
17. Davies R. Recurrent spontaneous pneumothorax concomitant with menstruation. *Thorax*. 1968;23:370.

    A striking predilection for the right pleura is unexplained.

18. Ishida T, et al. Inflammatory pseudotumor of the lung in adults: radiographic and clinicopathological analysis. *Ann Thorac Surg*. 1989;48:90.
   Discusses patients with such tumors. Intraoperative gross appearance can resemble lung cancer, but this is a benign lesion.
19. White SH, et al. Leiomyomas of the lower respiratory tract. *Thorax*. 1985;40:306.
   Leiomyomas, which account for approximately 2% of benign tumors of the lower respiratory tract, are an incidental finding on a chest x-ray film. One third of patients are under the age of 20 years and 90% of pulmonary parenchymal leiomyoma occurs in women. Tracheal lesions may present as bronchial asthma.
20. Yellin A, Rosenman Y, Lieberman Y. Review of smooth muscle tumours of the lower respiratory tract. *Br J Dis Chest*. 1984;78:337.
   Case history and literature review. Advocates surgical resection of this lesion.
21. Dogan R, et al. Endobronchial lipoma. *Thorac Cardiovasc Surg*. 1988;36:241.
   This is an extremely rare benign tumor that can lead to bronchiectasis if undiagnosed. Bronchoscopic removal is possible.
22. Frist W, et al. Bronchial sleeve resection with and without pulmonary resection. *J Thorac Cardiovasc Surg*. 1987;93:350.
   Recommends sleeve resection "as the ideal form of incisional therapy for benign endobronchial tumors."
23. Gjevre JA, Myers JL, Prakash U. Pulmonary hamartomas. *Mayo Clin Proc*. 1996;71:14.
   A 17-year review of 215 patients, 98% asymptomatic.
24. Goodman ML, Laforet EG. Solitary primary chemodectomas of the lung. *Chest*. 1972;61:48.
   Chemodectoma may present as a coin lesion.
25. Nistal M, Hardisson D, Riestra ML. Multiple pulmonary leiomyomatous hamartomas associated with a bronchogenic cyst in a man. *Arch Pathol Lab Med*. 2003;53:485.
   Describes a case of occurring in a man.
26. Saltztein SL. Pulmonary malignant lymphomas and pseudolymphomas: classification, therapy, and prognosis. *Cancer*. 1963;16:928.
   Pseudolymphomas are characterized by presence of mature lymphocytes, true germinal centers, and lymph nodes free of lymphoma. (This is the classic article: pseudolymphomas are now referred to as "well-differentiated lymphocytic proliferation.")
27. Cassina PC, et al. Catamenial hemoptysis: diagnosis with MRI. *Chest*. 1997;111:1447.
   Diagnosis of pulmonary endometriosis by magnetic resonance imaging in a 24-year-old woman.
28. Sutedja TG, et al. Bronchoscopic therapy in patients with intraluminal typical bronchial carcinoid. *Chest*. 1995;107:556.
   A retrospective analysis of 11 patients with local typical carcinoid treated with Nd:YAG laser. Surgical resection showed no carcinoid tumor after laser treatment in six patients.
29. Cavaliere S, Foccoli P, Farina P. Nd:YAG laser bronchoscopy. *Chest*. 1988;94:115.
   A 5-year experience with 1,396 applications in 1,000 patients. This treatment was curative in almost all cases of benign tumor and in many carcinoid tumors as well. This should be considered in the approach to endobronchial benign tumors of the lung.
30. Kim TS, et al. Mucoepidermoid carcinoma of the tracheobronchial tree: radiographic and CT findings in 12 patients. *Radiology*. 1999;212:643.
   A radiologic review with findings suggestive of a endobronchial source of tumor.
31. Sibula JL. Endobronchial hamartomas. *Chest*. 1972;62:631.
   An infrequent presentation. Fever, wheezing, and hemoptysis can occur, in contrast with the asymptomatic presentation in parenchymal hamartomas.
32. Erasmus JJ, et al. Solitary pulmonary nodules: part I. Morphologic evaluation for differentiation of benign and malignant lesions. *Radiographics*. 2000;20:43.

Part I of 2-part series describing CT findings to help differentiate benign and malignant lesions, although indeterminate findings are often the case.

33. Gimenez A, et al. Unusual primary lung tumors: a radiologic-pathologic overview. *Radiographics.* 2002;22:601.
   A very nice CT and pathologic correlation for rare benign and malignant tumors.

101. LUNG CANCER: CLASSIFICATION, PATHOLOGY, AND EPIDEMIOLOGY

John E. Barkley

INCIDENCE

The incidence of lung cancer continues to increase worldwide. According to American Cancer Society estimates, there will be 171,900 new cases and 157,200 deaths from lung cancer in the U.S. in 2003. Recent data suggest that male death rates from lung cancer may have plateaued; however, the estimated 91,800 male deaths still exceeds the combined rates caused by prostate, colon, and pancreatic cancer. The incidence of lung cancer among women continues to increase and now accounts for 25% of all female cancer deaths; in contrast, breast cancer accounts for 15% of female cancer deaths. Over the past 20 years, the male preponderance of 5 to 7:1 has fallen to its current level of 1.2:1 because of the striking increase in lung cancer among women. Presumably, this changing pattern of disease is caused by the post–World War II increase in cigarette smoking in the general population, and in women in particular.

The term *lung cancer* comprises a number of specific malignancies (Table 101-1). Most classifications, including the one advanced by the World Health Organization and

Table 101-1. Histologic classification of malignant lung tumors

Squamous cell carcinoma (epidermoid carcinoma) variant
Spindle (squamous) carcinoma
Small-cell carcinoma
    Oat-cell type
    Intermediate cell type
    Combined oat-cell carcinoma
Adenocarcinoma
    Acinar adenocarcinoma
    Papillary adenocarcinoma
    Bronchoalveolar carcinoma
    Solid carcinoma with mucous formation
Large-cell carcinoma variants
    Giant-cell carcinoma
    Clear-cell carcinoma
Adenosquamous carcinoma
    Carcinoid tumor
    Bronchial gland carcinoma
Adenoid cystic carcinoma
    Mucoepidermoid carcinoma
    Others

divide lung cancer into four major types: squamous or epidermoid, adenocarcinoma, large-cell carcinoma, and small-cell carcinoma. With the exception of the small-cell type, these classifications are poorly predictive of tumor behavior. As a result, the clinician has been concerned primarily with the division of lung cancer into small-cell lung carcinoma (SCLC) and non-SCLC types.

For reasons that remain undefined, the incidence of squamous cell carcinoma has declined in the U.S. At the same time, there has been an increase in the incidence of adenocarcinoma, which is now the most common histologic subtype, accounting for 30 to 50% of primary lung cancers. In some series, bronchioloalveolar carcinoma is responsible for much of the increasing incidence of adenocarcinomas.

Squamous cell carcinoma arises from altered bronchial epithelium and is preceded by years of progressive mucosal changes that include squamous metaplasia, dysplasia, and carcinoma in situ. In its early stages of growth, the tumor may appear as a small, red, granular plaque or as a focus of leukoplakia. Later, it may appear as a large intrabronchial gray-white or yellow mass. Cavitation may occur in the lung distal to the obstructing mass. Microscopically, there are intercellular bridges connecting the abnormal neoplastic cells and abundant keratin formation. The latter may be considerably reduced or absent in the poorly differentiated subtypes. Squamous cell carcinomas comprise 50% of superior sulcus tumors (Pancoast's tumors) and are typically well differentiated.

CLASSIFICATION

Adenocarcinomas are classically peripheral tumors arising from the peripheral airways and alveoli; however, these tumors also may arise proximally from the epithelium or submucosal glands. When bronchial in origin, they are almost impossible to distinguish on a cytologic basis from metastatic pancreatic, renal, breast, and colonic adenocarcinoma. When peripheral, they may be similarly difficult to distinguish from metastatic adenocarcinoma or malignant mesothelioma. Peripheral adenocarcinomas are usually well-circumscribed, gray-white masses that rarely cavitate. Microscopically, there is a spectrum of well-developed to poorly developed cuboidal or columnar cells having microvilli and forming glandlike structures that may or may not produce mucin. In the bronchioloalveolar type, 40 to 50% of which secrete mucin, the cylindrical tumor cells grow along the wall of the alveoli.

SCLC begins as a submucosal disease and usually develops proximally as a large, bulky, soft, gray-white mass. When bronchial narrowing occurs, it commonly results from circumferential encasement by extraluminal tumor. Microscopically, small-cell carcinomas are composed of fusiform, round, or polygonal cells about twice the size of lymphocytes with inconspicuous nucleoli and modest amounts of cytoplasm. The presence of cytoplasmic dense-core granules has led to the concept that SCLC belongs in a group of tumors derived from neuroendocrine cells, responsible for the production and secretion of specific peptide products. Although SCLC is divided into oat-cell, intermediate cell, and combined cell patterns, it is unclear whether these subtypes differ in their natural history or response to therapy.

Large-cell carcinomas, like adenocarcinomas, are usually located peripherally. They may be quite large and not infrequently cavitate. Microscopically, they have large nuclei, prominent nucleoli, abundant cytoplasm, and distinct cytoplasmic membranes. Large-cell carcinomas lack evidence of either squamous or glandular differentiation; many may represent undifferentiated forms of adenocarcinoma or squamous cell carcinoma.

EPIDEMIOLOGY

Abundant epidemiologic data, as well as experimental animal data, point to the accoutrements of modern industrialized society as producing the major risks for lung cancer. Tobacco smoking appears to be the most important risk (and causal) factor, with the relative degree of risk, depending on the number of cigarettes smoked per day, duration of smoking in years, depth of inhalation, tar and nicotine content in the cigarettes smoked, and incompletely defined genetic factors. Prospective and retrospective studies have demonstrated an increased (8–20 times) death rate from lung cancer in smokers versus nonsmokers. Heavy smokers (>25 cigarettes/day) experience a risk that is 20 times that of nonsmokers. Carcinogenic risk in former smokers declines progressively for 15 years following smoking cessation, after which the risk approaches that of lifelong nonsmokers. The residual risk experienced by the former smoker is determined by his or her prior smoking history. In the group with the heaviest smoking history, the residual risk is probably never as low as that of a lifelong nonsmoker.

Although the exact risk of passive smoking remains controversial, current data suggest there is no zero-risk threshold for exposure and that a dose–response relationship exists between extent of exposure and risk. Estimates have ranged from 500 to 5,000 lung cancer-related deaths per year from passive smoking in the United States.

There are more than 2,000 chemicals in cigarette smoke; several of them are either direct carcinogens or cocarcinogens in animal (particularly hamster) models. In humans, smoking induces a spectrum of histologic changes in the bronchial epithelium that are not seen in nonsmokers. These changes include loss of bronchial cilia, basal epithelial hyperplasia, and nuclear abnormalities. The severity of such changes increases in heavy smokers and tends to be most severe in patients dying from lung cancer. Smoking-induced alterations in bronchial mucosa may resolve slowly in individuals who stop smoking.

Certain occupational factors may substantially increase the risk of lung cancer. An increased risk has been reported among workers in several industries, including metallurgy, mining, and manufacturing of industrial gases, pharmaceutical preparations, soaps and detergents, paints, inorganic pigments, and synthetic rubber. Specific pulmonary carcinogens include arsenic, asbestos, chloromethyl methyl ether, bis-chloromethyl ether, chromium, ionizing radiation, mustard gas, nickel, radon, and vinyl chloride. Many are additive or synergistic with cigarette smoke in the induction of pulmonary malignancies. Nonsmoking asbestos workers have a 5-fold increased risk of death from lung cancer, as compared with other nonsmoking workers. Asbestos workers who smoke one pack of cigarettes per day experience a 90-fold increased risk, as compared to unexposed nonsmokers.

The role of air pollution in carcinogenesis is uncertain. The incidence of lung cancer in urban residents is 1.2 to 2.3 times that of rural residents. The reducing types of pollutants (e.g., sulfur dioxide, carbonaceous particulate matter) are thought to be the major carcinogens; oxidants (e.g., hydrocarbons, nitrous oxides) are not considered important. Individuals with heavy exposure to motor vehicle emissions do not appear to have an increased incidence of lung cancer.

There may be significant individual susceptibility to lung cancer. Some studies suggest a familial predisposition; the incidence of lung cancer in close relatives appears to be two to three times that of the general population. There is also an association of lung cancer with certain diseases. Lung cancer may complicate pulmonary parenchymal diseases such as diffuse pulmonary fibrosis, sarcoidosis, and scleroderma. Up to 10% of patients with pulmonary fibrosis die from bronchogenic carcinoma. Emphysema and chronic bronchitis with airflow obstruction also represent independent risk factors for the development of lung cancer, even when age, gender, and smoking history have been controlled for.

Finally, certain dietary factors may modify the risk of lung cancer. Retrospective epidemiologic studies have demonstrated an inverse relationship between the risk of lung cancer and the intake of fruits and vegetables that contain β-carotene. High consumption of β-carotene, which is subsequently converted to retinol, has been associated with approximately a 50% reduction in the risk of lung cancer in comparison to low consumption. However, three prospective, randomized, controlled intervention trials found no benefit or increased incidence of death from bronchogenic carcinoma in those patients given beta carotene as a dietary supplement.

---

1. The Alpha–Tocopherol, Beta Carotene Cancer Prevention Study Group. The effect of vitamin E and beta carotene on the incidence of lung cancer and other cancers in men. *N Engl J Med*. 1994;330:1029.

In a randomized, double-blind, placebo-controlled trial the β-carotene arm had an 18% increased incidence of lung cancer.

2. Auerbach O, et al. Changes in bronchial epithelium in relation to lung cancer. *N Engl J Med.* 1961;265:267.

   One of the major pathologic studies supporting epidemiologic data linking cigarette smoking and the development of lung cancer.

3. Beckett WS. Epidemiology and etiology of lung cancer. *Clin Chest Med.* 1993;14:1.

   Comprehensive, well-referenced review of lung cancer epidemiology and etiology.

4. Cohen MH. Natural history of lung cancer. *Clin Chest Med.* 1982;3:229.

   Comprehensive, well-referenced review of the natural history of lung cancer.

5. Cone JE. Occupational lung cancer. *Occup Med.* 1987;2:273.

   Comprehensive review of the subject.

6. Hammond EC, Horn D. Smoking and death rates: report on 44 months follow-up of 187,783 men. *JAMA.* 1958;166:1294.

   Classic early epidemiologic paper linking cigarette smoking to an increased risk of death from lung and other cancers and from cardiovascular disease.

7. Hennekens CH, Buring JE, Manson JE, et al. Lack of effect of long-term supplementation with beta carotene on the incidence of malignant neoplasms and cardiovascular disease. *N Engl J Med.* 1996;334:1145.

   Randomized, double-blind, placebo-controlled trial found no difference in incidence or death rates from lung cancer with β-carotene supplementation.

8. Janerich DT, et al. Lung cancer and exposure to tobacco smoke in the household. *N Engl J Med.* 1990;323:632.

   Household exposure to 25 or more smoker-years in childhood and adolescence doubled the risk of lung cancer. Exposure to spousal smoking was not associated with an increased risk; neither was there evidence of an adverse effect from tobacco smoke exposure at work.

9. Knecht P, et al. Dietary antioxidants and the risk of lung cancer. *Am J Epidemiol.* 1991;134:471.

   The relationship between the intake of retinoids, carotenoids, vitamins E and C, and selenium and the subsequent risk of lung cancer was investigated in a large series of men followed up for 20 years.

10. Kung ITM, et al. Pulmonary scar cancer: a pathological reappraisal. *Am J Surg Pathol.* 1985;9:391.

    Article that questions the concept of "scar carcinoma."

11. American Cancer Society Statistics. Accessed December 6, 2003. Available: http://www.cancer.org/docroot/STT/stt_0.asp

    Excellent source for current cancer data and screening recommendations.

12. Omenn GS, Goodman GE, Thornquist MD, et al. Effects of a combination of beta carotene and vitamin A on lung cancer and cardiovascular disease. *N Engl J Med.* 1996;334:1150.

    Randomized, double-blind, placebo-controlled trial showed a 28% increased incidence of lung cancer in β-carotene arm and study was stopped 21 months earlier than planned.

13. *Smoking and Health: A Report of the Surgeon General* (Pub. no. [PHS] 79-50066). Washington, DC: U.S. Department of Health, Education, and Welfare; 1979.

    Reiteration of the 1964 report linking cigarette smoking to the development of lung cancer.

14. *The Health Consequences of Smoking: Cancer. A Report of the Surgeon General* (DHHS [PHS] 82-50179). Rockville, MD: U.S. Department of Health and Human Services; 1982.

    The most comprehensive review of the subject by the federal government's watch dog agency.

15. Tockman MS, Anthonisen NR, Wright EC, et al. Airways obstruction and the risk for lung cancer. *Ann Intern Med.* 1987;106:512.

    Comprehensive review of the subject.

16. World Health Organization. Histological typing of lung tumours, 2nd ed. *Am J Clin Pathol.* 1982;77:123.

    Histologic classification and description of benign and malignant lung cancers.

17. Travis WD. Pathology of lung cancer. *Clin Chest Med.* 2002;23:65.
    Excellent review of revised histologic classification system of lung neoplasms.
18. Yesner R. Classification of lung cancer histology. *N Engl J Med.* 1985;312:652.
    Report from a panel of lung cancer pathologists recommending the abandonment of subtyping small-cell carcinoma unless the tumor contains a prominent non–small-cell lung cancer component.

102. LUNG CANCER: CLINICAL PRESENTATION, DIAGNOSIS, STAGING, AND PROGNOSIS

John E. Barkley

CLINICAL PRESENTATION

Patients with bronchogenic carcinoma may present in a variety of ways, including (1) asymptomatic; (2) symptoms of local disease; (3) symptoms of metastatic disease; and (4) symptoms of paraneoplastic syndrome. The histologic type of lung cancer (non–small cell versus small cell), site of origin (central versus peripheral airways), the inherent biologic activity of the neoplasm, and comorbid conditions all determine how an individual patient presents.

Only 25 to 40% of patients present with early stage disease that is potentially resectable. Of these, perhaps 20% present with an incidental abnormality discovered on a chest radiograph. The remainder with early stage disease present with signs and symptoms of local tumor growth, including cough, dyspnea, wheezing, or hemoptysis. Additionally, patients may present with purulent sputum, fever, and chills from postobstructive pneumonia. More ominous signs and symptoms of local tumor growth include superior vena cava syndrome, Horner's syndrome, dysphagia, odynophagia, hoarseness, elevated hemidiaphragm from phrenic nerve impingement, dyspnea and chest pain from pleural effusion, and dyspnea and hemodynamic compromise from pericardial involvement.

Patients with metastatic disease usually have general symptoms of malaise and anorexia with or without weight loss. Other symptoms depend on the site(s) of metastases. The most common sites are supraclavicular and cervical lymph nodes, brain, bone, liver, and adrenal glands. However, no organ system is exempt from possible metastatic deposits.

Some patients present with signs or symptoms of a paraneoplastic syndrome. They can be divided into five categories: (1) endocrine-metabolic; (2) neuromuscular; (3) hematologic-vascular; (4) dermatologic; and (5) skeletal and connective tissue (see Chapter 105).

DIAGNOSIS AND STAGING

Clinical staging of lung cancer requires logical use of currently available diagnostic techniques. The approach should be to confirm that an intrathoracic lesion is a cancer, define its cell type, and accurately determine the extent of disease by the least invasive means available.

The first step in this diagnostic approach is to define the nature of the intrathoracic lesion as either malignant or benign. The relative difficulty of this first step differs for central (endobronchial) and peripheral lesions. For endoscopically visible central lesions, a positive tissue diagnosis can be made in essentially all cases by means of sputum and fiberoptic bronchoscopy. For peripheral lesions, bronchoscopic yield depends on the size of the lesion (the lowest yield occurring with lesions <2 cm) and its location. Overall yield for peripheral lesions is increased with a combination of washings, brushings, transbronchial biopsies, and a transbronchial needle aspiration. Transthoracic needle aspiration of peripheral lesions, especially when performed under computed tomographic (CT) guidance, can substantially increase yield. A negative bronchoscopic examination and needle aspiration, however, cannot absolutely exclude the possibility of cancer. Unless a specific diagnosis is obtained, a thoracotomy or a period of careful observation in higher risk surgical patients is indicated.

For non–small cell lung cancer the international system for staging lung cancer is used (Table 102-1). Several classification changes were made in the most recent revision in 1997: (1) noninvasive tumors (TIS) are stage 0; (2) T3 tumors invade structures but can be resected; (3) T4 tumors now include those primary tumors with satellite

Table 102-1. Staging of non–small-cell lung cancer—TNM definitions

Primary Tumor (T)

TX	Occult carcinoma
T0	No evidence of primary tumor
Tis	Carcinoma in situ
T1	Tumor ≤3 cm in greatest dimension, surrounded by lung or visceral pleura, and without bronchoscopic evidence of invasion proximal to a lobar bronchus (i.e., not main bronchus)
T2	A tumor >3 cm in greatest dimension, or a tumor of any size that either invades the visceral pleura or has associated atelectasis or obstructive pneumonitis that extends to the hilar region; at bronchoscopy, proximal extent of demonstrable tumor must be within a lobar bronchus or at least 2 cm distal to the main carina; any associated atelectasis or obstructive pneumonitis must involve less than an entire lung
T3	A tumor of any size with direct extension into the chest wall (including superior sulcus tumors), diaphragm, or mediastinal pleura or pericardium without involving the heart, great vessels, trachea, esophagus, or vertebral bodies; or a tumor in the main bronchus within 2 cm of main carina without involving it
T4	A tumor of any size with invasion of the mediastinum or involving the heart, great vessels, trachea, esophagus, vertebral bodies, or main carina; or with the presence of malignant pleural effusion, satellite nodule in the same lobe

Nodal Involvement (N)

NX	Occult carcinoma
N0	No regional lymph node metastasis
N1	Metastasis of lymph nodes in peribronchial or ipsilateral hilar region, or both, including direct extension
N2	Metastatic involvement of ipsilateral mediastinal lymph nodes and/or subcarinal lymph nodes
N3	Metastatic involvement of contralateral mediastinal lymph nodes, contralateral hilar lymph nodes, or ipsilateral or contralateral scalene or supraclavicular lymph nodes

Distant Metastatic Involvement (M)

M0	No (known) distant metastatic involvement
M1	Distant metastatic disease involvement (specify site(s)); tumor nodule(s) in the ipsilateral lung nonprimary tumor-bearing lobe

lesions in the same lobe; (4) satellite nodules in the ipsilateral lung but different lobe represent M1 disease; (5) stage I and II are now IA/IB and IIA/IIB based on size of the primary tumor and presence or absence of N1 nodes; and (6) T3N0M0 lesions are now classified as stage IIB.

To define the T characteristics of a lesion, chest radiograph, CT scanning, positron emission tomography (PET), magnetic resonance imaging (MRI), and bronchoscopy may all be helpful. MRI may be particularly useful in assessing patients with possible T3 or T4 lesions.

To accurately define the N (nodal) status of a lesion, some combination of chest radiography, CT scan, PET, transbronchial needle aspiration, ultrasound-guided transesophageal or transbronchial needle aspiration, mediastinoscopy, mediastinotomy, thoracoscopy, and thoracotomy is required.

There is now general agreement that nodal enlargement identified by CT requires tissue confirmation of metastasis by mediastinoscopy or alternate biopsy technique, except when gross mediastinal invasion by tumor (T4) is present. A patient should not be denied potentially curative surgery based solely on radiographic criteria. Emphasizing this point, a recent study demonstrated that 36% of lymph nodes measuring 2 to 4 cm in short-axis diameter on CT did not contain metastases at the time of surgery. CT scanning is also useful in identifying the site(s) of mediastinal node enlargement, especially those that may not be accessible to standard mediastinoscopy (aortopulmonary nodes, anterior mediastinal nodes, paraesophageal nodes, and inferior pulmonary ligament nodes). Also, extension of the CT examination to include the adrenal glands and liver may often detect occult metastatic disease. There is considerably less agreement on the need for mediastinoscopy in patients with normal lymph nodes on CT. Some authors suggest that patients with T1 tumors and mediastinal nodes with a short-axis diameter of 10 mm or less can proceed directly to thoracotomy without first undergoing mediastinoscopy. Others disagree, citing a significant incidence of intranodal tumor in normal-sized lymph nodes. The role of MRI scanning remains limited because of its poorer spatial resolution compared to CT, expense, and limited ability to detect calcification.

Previously, radiographic imaging was limited to anatomic considerations only. The advent of PET allows assessment of the metabolic activity of lesions, with malignant lesions tending to be hypermetabolic. Several recent studies demonstrated the superiority of PET over CT scanning in the noninvasive staging of bronchogenic carcinoma. The major current limitation of PET is its lack of widespread availability. Single-photon emission CT (SPECT) is widely available and has led to investigations of alternative agents to noninvasively detect bronchogenic carcinoma. Preliminary evidence suggests that the somatostatin analog depreotide combined with [99m]-technetium is equivalent to PET imaging in evaluating solitary pulmonary nodules. More investigation is needed to determine the role of SPECT imaging in evaluating local/regional and distant disease in bronchogenic carcinoma.

Several series have demonstrated the ability of transbronchial needle aspiration (TBNA) to sample mediastinal nodes. False-positive aspirates, although rare, have been reported, and contamination should be suspected if TBNA contains a number of columnar epithelial cells and a paucity of lymphocytes and malignant cells, or if the aspirate is performed adjacent to a parenchymal mass that abuts the mediastinum. Whether a positive aspirate from an enlarged mediastinal node has the same prognostic and therapeutic implications as a positive aspirate from a normal-sized lymph node is unknown.

To define the M (metastasis) characteristics of a lesion, a thorough history and physical examination, chemistry panel, liver function tests, chest radiograph, and CT scan of the chest (to include the liver and adrenal glands) are recommended. Other diagnostic workup should be guided by the initial evaluation. Specifically, routine bone scanning and cranial CT scanning is not recommended. It should be pointed out that some authorities recommend cranial CT scanning in patients with known adenocarcinoma because of the 5 to 10% risk of asymptomatic metastatic disease. Finally, initial experience with whole body PET indicates that unsuspected metastatic disease may be found in 11 to 29% of patients. This is independent of

Table 102-2. New international revised stage grouping

Stage	T N M Subset
0	Carcinoma in situ
IA	T1N0M0
IB	T2N0M0
IIA	T1N1M0
IIB	T2N1M0
	T3N0M0
IIIA	T3N1M0
	T1N2M0
	T2N2M0
	T3N2M0
IIIB	T4N0M0
	T4N1M0
	T4N2M0
	T1N3M0
	T2N3M0
	T3N3M0
	T4N3M0
IV	Any T Any N M1

the central nervous system, which is not well imaged with PET. The role of PET in the routine assessment of patients with bronchogenic carcinoma continues to be evaluated.

Stages of lung cancer are defined by combining the TNM components (Table 102-2). Stage I includes those patients with no lymph node involvement (N0) and no invasion of structures. Stage II includes patients with hilar (N1) lymph node metastases and those patients with chest wall invasion and no lymph node involvement T3N0 (stage IIB). Stage III is divided into those with potentially resectable disease (IIIA) and those with unresectable disease (IIIB). Stage IV disease is confined to those patients with metastasis to distant sites.

With advances in understanding the biology of lung cancer and more effective therapeutic interventions, the staging system continues to be refined. Critical to these advances is accurately staging patients using the current system. Perhaps the most important part of accurate classification is determination of the N (nodal) status. Routine use of the American Joint Committee on Cancer (AJCC) regional lymph node map allows for uniformity in reporting patient data.

PROGNOSIS

Survival is most strongly correlated with the stage of disease at presentation. With surgery the 5-year survival for stage IA, IB, and IIA/IIB disease is approximately 70 to 80%, 50 to 60%, and 35 to 50%, respectively. Stage III patients have 5-year survival ranging from less than 5 to 25 or 30%, depending on the particular TNM status and treatment modalities employed (see Chapter 104). Patients with stage IV disease have a 1-year survival of 10 to 20% and 5-year survival of less than 5%. Occasionally, patients with stage IV disease who respond well to chemotherapy may survive 2 to 3 years or longer.

In addition to stage at presentation, the patient's performance status at diagnosis is extremely important prognostically. Finally, several histopathologic markers and molecular biologic characteristics have been found to correlate with survival and may ultimately become incorporated into the staging system.

Small-cell lung cancer is divided into limited and extensive stage disease. Limited stage is defined as disease limited to one hemithorax with or without ipsilateral supraclavicular lymph node involvement. Extensive stage disease is everything else. Without treatment, survival is 6 to 12 weeks in extensive stage disease and 3 to 6 months in patients with limited stage disease. With modern treatment, median survival is approximately 9 months and 20 months in extensive and limited stage patients, respectively. Five-year survival is less than 5% and 10 to 20%, respectively.

---

1. Adjei AA, Marks RS, Bonner JA. Current guidelines for the management of small cell lung cancer. *Mayo Clin Proc*. 1999;74:899.
   Excellent, concise review of the evaluation and treatment of patients with small-cell lung cancer.
2. American Thoracic Society/European Respiratory Society. Pretreatment evaluation of non-small cell lung cancer. *Am J Respir Crit Care Med*. 1997;156:320.
   Excellent review of current literature on the evaluation of patients with non–small cell lung cancer.
3. Coughlin M, et al. Role of mediastinoscopy in pretreatment of patients with primary lung cancer. *Ann Thorac Surg*. 1985;40:556.
   Demonstrates that mediastinoscopy is both sensitive and specific for nodes in the superior mediastinum. Chest roentgenography was poorly predictive of mediastinal involvement.
4. Dales RE, et al. Computed tomography to stage lung cancer: approaching a controversy using meta-analysis. *Am Rev Respir Dis*. 1990;141:1096.
   Confirms the need for surgical evaluation based on a 20% false-positive and 20% false-negative rate of CT scanning.
5. Dasgupta A, Mehta AC. Transbronchial needle aspiration: an underused diagnostic technique. *Clin Chest Med*. 1999;20:39.
   Excellent review of the role of transbronchial needle aspiration in lung cancer. Excellent bibliography.
6. Detterbeck FC. Pancoast (superior sulcus) tumors. *Ann Thorac Surg*. 1997; 63:1810.
   Excellent review with good bibliography.
7. Kwiatkowski DJ, Harpole DH, Godleski J, et al. Molecular pathologic substaging in 244 stage I non–small cell lung cancer patients: clinical implications. *J Clin Oncol*. 1998;16:2468.
   Retrospective study which gives a "view to the future" in staging using molecular markers. Excellent bibliography.
8. Martini N, et al. The role of surgery in N2 lung cancer. *Surg Clin North Am*. 1987;67:1037.
   Discusses the role of surgery in N2 disease, including factors that positively and negatively influence survival.
9. McLoud TC, Bourgouin PM, Greenberg RW, et al. Bronchogenic carcinoma: analysis of staging in the mediastinum with CT by correlative lymph node imaging and sampling. *Radiology*. 1992;182:319.
   Using lymph node size greater than 10 mm (short-axis diameter), CT scanning had sensitivity and specificity of 64% and 62%, respectively.
10. Mountain CF. Revisions in the International System for Staging Lung Cancer. *Chest*. 1997;111:1710.
    Revised AJCC staging system for non–small cell lung cancer.
11. Mountain CF, Dresler CM. Regional lymph node classification for lung cancer staging. *Chest*. 1997;111:1718.
    Revised AJCC staging system for non–small cell lung cancer. Updated mediastinal lymph node map.
12. Patterson GA, et al. Significance of metastatic disease in subaortic lymph nodes. *Ann Thorac Surg*. 1987;43:155.
    Patients with left upper lobe or left main stem tumors and subaortic (AJCC station 5) lymph node involvement as only site of metastasis had 5-year survival of 28%.

13. Pearson FG, et al. Significance of positive superior mediastinal nodes identified at mediastinoscopy in patients with resectable lung cancer. *J Thorac Cardiovasc Surg.* 1982;83:11.

    The survival rate was significantly worse when N2 disease was established at mediastinoscopy than when it was established at thoracotomy following a negative mediastinoscopy.

14. Salazar AM, Westcott JL. The role of transthoracic needle biopsy for the diagnosis and staging of lung cancer. *Clin Chest Med.* 1993;14:99.

    Comprehensive, well-referenced review of percutaneous transthoracic needle biopsy.

15. Salerno CT, Frizelle S, Niehans GA, et al. Detection of occult micrometastases in non-small cell lung carcinoma by reverse transcriptase-polymerase chain reaction. *Chest.* 1998;113:1526.

    Using reverse transcriptase-polymerase chain reaction occult metastatic disease was found in 38% of hilar and mediastinal lymphs nodes negative by hematoxylin and eosin staining.

16. Seely JM, Mayo JR, Miller RR, et al. T1 lung cancer: prevalence of mediastinal nodal metastases and diagnostic accuracy of CT. *Radiology.* 1993;186:129.

    Of 104 patients, 21% with T1 lesions had mediastinal nodal metastases.

17. The Lung Cancer Study Group. Should subcarinal lymph nodes be routinely examined in patients with non-small cell lung cancer? *J Thorac Cardiovasc Surg.* 1988;95:883.

    The results of this study confirm previously reported observations that having multiple levels of mediastinal lymph node metastases adversely affects prognosis.

18. Vansteenkiste JF, Stroobants SG, DeLeyn PR, et al. Lymph node staging in non-small cell lung cancer with FDG-PET scan: a prospective study on 690 lymph node stations from 68 patients. *J Clin Oncol.* 1998;16:2142.

    Combination of PET and CT scanning dramatically improved the accuracy of staging the mediastinum.

19. Silvestri GA, Tanoue LT, Margolis ML, et al. The noninvasive staging of non-small cell lung cancer: the guidelines. *Chest.* 2003;123:147S.

    American College of Chest Physicians evidence-based guidelines for noninvasive staging of bronchogenic carcinoma.

20. Detterbeck FC, DeCamp MM, Kohman LJ, et al. Invasive staging: the guidelines. *Chest.* 2003;123:167S.

    American College of Chest Physicians evidence-based guidelines for invasive staging of bronchogenic carcinoma.

21. Gould MK, Kuschner WG, Rydzak CE, et al. Test performance of positron emission tomography and computed tomography for mediastinal staging in patients with non-small cell lung cancer: a meta-analysis. *Ann Intern Med.* 2003;139:879.

    Excellent review of the literature on noninvasive staging of lung cancer with PET and CT scanning.

22. Blum J, Handmaker H, Lister-James J, et al. A multicenter trial with a somatostatin analog [99m]-Tc in the evaluation of solitary pulmonary nodules. *Chest.* 2000;117:1232.

103. LUNG CANCER SCREENING

David M. Burns

Lung cancer is responsible for the highest proportion of cancer deaths in the United States. Surgical resection of early stage neoplasm is the only treatment that consistently results in high rates of long-term survival. The combination of a high frequency of lung cancer in cigarette smokers and the ability to cure early stage disease would seem to be ideal prerequisites for a screening program. In the 1970s, several randomized controlled trials investigated lung cancer screening using chest radiographs and sputum cytology. These trials demonstrated that lung cancer could be detected earlier (i.e., before symptoms), at a smaller size, and at a more resectable stage. Patients with screen-detected lung cancers had longer 5-year survival and a lower case fatality (the fraction of those who develop a disease who die of that disease) rate. However, screening did not reduce lung cancer mortality rates in the screened group as compared to the control population, and screening for lung cancer with chest radiographs and sputum cytology was abandoned. Although most organizations recommended against chest radiographic screening, the disconnect between the ability to detect lung cancer earlier and the absence of a mortality benefit remains unsettling, and the limitations of these earlier studies raised concern about their use as the basis of public policy for lung cancer screening.

Radiographic chest imaging has advanced substantially since the 1970s. Current scanners can detect lesions in the 2- to 3-mm range using a single-breath spiral computed tomography (CT) scan, in contrast to the 1- to 1.5-cm range for chest roentgenography. Several large observational studies have demonstrated that annual CT screening of high-risk populations yields a substantial number of asymptomatic lung cancers, most at an early stage. These advances have rekindled enthusiasm for lung cancer screening based on the compelling logic that finding high rates of early stage lung cancer in a high-risk population should reduce lung cancer mortality. This enthusiasm for screening also has stimulated considerable opposition to implementing screening in the absence of evidence from randomized trials with mortality endpoints. Screening opponents point to the experience with chest radiographs as a cautionary tale, and insist that randomized trial data are essential no matter how encouraging may be observational data.

Currently, the National Cancer Institute (NCI) and the American College of Radiology Imaging Network are conducting a randomized trial of CT screening with lung cancer mortality as the endpoint, and it is likely that most organizations that issue screening guidelines will await these results before developing recommendations. This leaves the physician in the difficult position of making recommendations to individual patients based on judgments from imperfect, existing evidence. While awaiting national guidelines, it is useful to examine current evidence supporting both claims and concerns about screening.

Lung cancer detected from symptoms carries an abysmal 15% 5-year survival, largely because diagnosis is made at an advanced stage. In contrast, early stage lung cancer treated with surgical resection has a 5-year survival of approximately 80% when detected in the absence of a screening program.

There is general agreement that (1) CT can detect smaller lesions than a chest radiograph and identifies more lung cancers in a population receiving both procedures and (2) screening a high-risk population such as long-term cigarette smokers identifies asymptomatic individuals with lung cancer by conventional pathologic criteria and shifts the distribution of screen-detected lung cancers in the direction of early stage disease. Beyond these areas of consensus, concerns about the value of screening may be characterized by the following series of questions.

WILL SCREENING CAUSE MORE HARM THAN THE GOOD PRODUCED BY EARLY DETECTION?

Screening by itself confers no survival advantage unless it is accompanied by improved diagnosis and subsequent treatment. As a corollary, diagnostic evaluation, particularly with invasive procedures, for screen-detected lesions that turn out to be benign creates the possibility of harm from a screening program that must be weighed against potential benefits. Therefore, how a positive finding on CT is evaluated and treated is essential in determining both the potential benefits and risks of CT screening.

The frequency of a positive finding on the initial CT for screened populations ranges from 20 to 50%, depending on the population and geographic location. Higher rates have been reported when a positive finding is defined as any abnormality rather than one that requires an evaluation different from that for individuals with a negative scan (i.e., a scan at the next annual interval). The vast majority of scan abnormalities represent benign disease rather than lung cancer. Some studies, most notably those conducted at the Mayo Clinic, have reported very high rates of positive scans partially because of the high prevalence of histoplasmosis in the population scanned. However, over one half of these positive scans found lesions less than 5 mm in diameter and the recommended follow-up for these small lesions was the same annual scan recommended for those with normal scans. The frequency of a new positive lesion on a repeat annual scan is much lower, in the range of 2 to 10%.

This high rate of positive scans creates the potential for large numbers of diagnostic procedures, including invasive ones, for benign disease. The problem is not unique to screening; chest CT is used commonly in clinical medicine and the question of what to do with small, incidental lesions found on CT is one for which most clinical programs have already developed operational answers. Most screening programs have taken this a step further by developing guidelines for evaluating positive scans. These guidelines recommend follow-up scans to evaluate growth, treatment of some lesions with antibiotics, and further diagnostic evaluations depending on the size and characteristics of the lesion. As a result of these protocols, the fear that screening would result in large numbers of unnecessary invasive procedures has not become a reality. All programs reporting results to date have documented very low rates of invasive procedures for benign disease. Even the large NCI trial of CT screening, which relied on each patient's treating physician to manage a positive scan, reported a rate of benign disease at surgical intervention well below 50%, a rate commonly reported for resection of solitary pulmonary nodules. The best programs report 80 to 90% lung cancers on surgical resection. Although follow-up scans to evaluate growth may increase the costs of screening, they carry very low risk for the patient. It is now clear that the vast majority of benign lesions found on scans do not have to lead to surgical intervention. However, a carefully thought out approach to positive lesions is essential in any screening program, and screening should only be conducted in settings where such an approach is utilized. As the experience with evaluating and following nodules increases, it is likely that the rate of surgical intervention for benign disease will continue to decline.

DOES FINDING SMALL LESIONS WITH SCREENING ALTER LUNG CANCER OUTCOMES?

There is agreement that screening programs find lung cancer earlier than symptom-detected disease in the absence of screening. Data from screening trials demonstrate a much higher proportion of early stage disease in the cancers detected. Early stage lung cancer discovered in the absence of screening trials has an excellent survival with surgical resection. For many, these observations offer a compelling justification for screening high-risk patients as the only viable approach to ensuring that lung cancers is detected at a stage where curative treatment is an option. Others argue that data derived from lung cancer detection in the absence of organized screening cannot be used to predict the results of screening asymptomatic individuals. Several biases do exist with screening. If lung cancers are identified earlier, they would be expected to be associated with longer survival after diagnosis simply because of earlier detection (lead-time bias), even if there is no impact on ultimate outcome. In addition, screening would be expected to detect more slowly growing lesions, particularly in the first screen, and these slow growing cancers would be expected to have a better prognosis and be at an earlier stage at diagnosis than rapidly growing lesions that present with symptoms. These biases are well recognized in all screening programs, but they are not the major points of contention about lung cancer screening. The arguments that finding early stage disease in screening programs may not alter disease outcomes are based on two concerns.

First, finding earlier or smaller lesions by screening may not change disease outcomes. This argument suggests that at the time of diagnosis those lung cancers that are going to metastasize have already disseminated, and those which have not yet disseminated at diagnosis are far less likely to do so in the future. The improved survival with stage I lung cancers is then because of their inherent biology rather than earlier detection. Therefore, earlier detection does not alter outcome because those biologically aggressive cancers already have disseminated prior to detection. This hypothesis is supported by observations from a single group that reported no difference in survival based on size at time of diagnosis for stage I lung cancers. Subsequent studies from several other groups, including the population-based Surveillance, Epidemiology and End Results (SEER) registry, have demonstrated a clear relationship between smaller size at diagnosis and improved survival. It should be noted that the survival for all groups in the initial study was over 80%, limiting the ability of the evaluation to find an improvement in survival. Data also now exist to directly examine this question. If the hypothesis that cancer outcomes are predetermined at diagnosis is true, then screen-detected lung cancers should have outcomes similar to those diagnosed without screening, even though there is a shift to earlier stage cancer. A corollary would be that stage I lung cancers diagnosed with screening would have worse outcomes than those reported in the literature for detection in the absence of screening. Data from the existing observational screening studies demonstrate that outcomes for lung cancer detected by screening are far better than the experience for lung cancers detected in the absence of screening, and screen-detected stage I lung cancers have survivals similar to those published for disease detected in the absence of screening. Clearly, early detection and treatment can alter outcomes for lung cancer and lung cancers are not biologically predetermined for their outcomes at diagnosis.

A second concern suggests that many lung cancers detected in screening trials are growing so slowly or are so biologically inert that they would rarely result in death, and, therefore, lung cancer is being overdiagnosed in screening trials. The term *overdiagnosis* is often used without precise definition, leading to some confusion. It is useful to consider overdiagnosis using three different definitions to reduce the miscommunication about screening.

The first use of *overdiagnosis* is for those lung cancers identified by screening where the individual would have died from other causes before the biologically malignant cancer would have been diagnosed based on symptoms (e.g., death in a traffic accident shortly after the screening diagnosis). Most agree that this form of overdiagnosis is present in all screening studies, but that its effect in lung cancer screening is modest because of the aggressive nature of this malignant disease.

A second form of overdiagnosis relates to the identification of abnormalities on CT that are of questionable biologic malignancy. These lesions appear as nonsolid or "ground-glass" consistency on the scan and may have pathologic morphology that varies from atypical adenomatous hyperplasia through low-grade bronchoalveolar carcinoma. When these lesions contain no "solid" elements on CT, they have been observed to be stable for long periods of time, raising a question as to whether they should appropriately be classified as lung cancers. Once these lesions develop solid elements, they commonly have morphology that is more malignant in form and often are both classified as, and have a clinical pattern consistent with, adenocarcinoma. These lesions raise important questions about their management and whether they should be counted as cancers. Although the combination of radiologic and pathologic morphology allows them to be identified in screening programs, they are not usually considered as lung cancers in the studies.

The last form of overdiagnosis is the most controversial. It is a lung nodule that pathologic examination identifies as a typical lung cancer by all morphologic characteristics, but that has a clinical course more consistent with benign disease with very slow or nonexistent growth and without metastatic spread. Concern about this form of overdiagnosis for lung cancer was generated by demonstration that the group screened with chest radiographs in the Mayo Clinic screening trial three decades ago had a 30% higher rate of lung cancer incidence when compared to the control population. The long follow-up and the similar lung cancer death (as opposed to the higher incidence) rates between the two study populations led to concern that biologically benign disease was being identified as lung cancer in screening. Retrospective review of the pathology found that screening-diagnosed tumors were malignant by standard current pathologic criteria and it was suggested that some of these cancers were biologically benign, similar to the overdiagnosis identified for prostate cancer. Although this is a theoretical concern, there is substantial evidence that it is not a real phenomenon. Not all early stage lung cancers are surgically resected, either because of medical contraindications or by patient choice. If a substantial fraction of lung cancers are biologically benign, then that fraction should have prolonged survival even without treatment. However, in multiple examinations of populations with stage I lung cancers that were not surgically resected, the outcomes are uniformly grim. In the population followed in the early Mayo Clinic trial that generated the concern about overdiagnosis, the 5-year survival for lung cancers not undergoing resection was 2% and all were dead by 6 years. The poor outcome for lung cancers not surgically resected has also been demonstrated for both screen-detected as well as symptom-detected disease. Although rare lung cancer may have a relatively slow-growing or apparently benign course, there is little evidence that this occurs with sufficient frequency to be of concern in the management of early stage lung cancers.

DOES SCREENING FOR LUNG CANCER INHIBIT SMOKING CESSATION?

There has been concern that providing smokers with a negative screening result might provide reassurance and reduce their interest in quitting, or that smokers would view screening as an alternative to cessation that would allow them to continue smoking but still have their cancers detected at a curable stage. There is no evidence to support this concern, and two independent screening programs have demonstrated high rates of cessation in screened patients who simultaneously receive cessation advice and assistance. Current evidence does suggest that screening represents an opportunity to reach smokers when they are receptive to smoking cessation interventions. Therefore, screening should be viewed as an adjunct, rather than an alternative, to cessation.

DOES LUNG CANCER SCREENING REDUCE LUNG CANCER MORTALITY RATES?

To date there are no studies comparing populations randomized to receive screening with CT or a control condition not including CT screening. Many insist that the only valid evaluation of an intervention is a randomized controlled trial with a mortality endpoint and they point to the experience with chest radiograph screening as a caution to making decisions without this evidence. It is also likely that agencies that provide clinical or reimbursement guidelines will wait for such a trial. Others argue that a delay in offering screening to high-risk populations will result in preventable deaths in view of the clear evidence that screening can produce a stage shift in diagnosis toward early stage lung cancers with excellent survival. In the absence of clear national standards on lung cancer screening, it is the responsibility of individual clinicians to review the evidence and determine what advice to offer their patients.

---

1. Cox LS, Clark MM, Jett JR, et al. Change in smoking status after spiral chest computed tomography scan screening. *Cancer*. 2003;98:2495–2501.
   A demonstration that smoking cessation programs can be very effective when implemented in conjunction with lung cancer screening programs. This clearly demonstrates that smokers do not see screening as an alternative to cessation, and that screening represents an opportunity to deliver cessation assistance to a receptive population.

2. Crestanello JA, Allen MS, Jett JR, et al. Thoracic surgical operations in patients enrolled in a computed tomographic screening trial. *J Thorac Cardiovasc Surg.* 2004;129:254–259.

   The Mayo Clinic experience with the need for, and yield of, surgical interventions resulting from a lung cancer screening program using CT under conditions where a very high prevalence of abnormal scans exists. Ten of 55 surgical interventions yielded benign diagnoses with the remaining 45 yielding a cancer diagnosis.

3. Diederich S, Thomas M, Semik M, et al. Screening for early lung cancer with low-dose spiral computed tomography: results of annual follow-up examinations in asymptomatic smokers. *Eur Radiol.* 2004;14:691–702.

   The experience with a screening program delivered in Germany, which found that 70% of the cancers detected by screening were in stage I.

4. Flehinger BJ, Kimmel M, Melamed MR. The effect of surgical treatment on survival from early lung cancer: implications for screening. *Chest.* 1992;101:1013–1018.

   A demonstration of the extremely poor survival among early stage lung cancer in the absence of surgical therapy.

5. Gohagan J, Marcus P, Fagerstrom R, et al, for the Writing Committee, Lung Screening Study Research Group. Baseline findings of a randomized feasibility trial of lung cancer screening with spiral CT scan vs chest radiograph: the Lung Screening Study of the National Cancer Institute. *Chest.* 2004;126:114–121.

   This paper presents the initial results of the NCI randomized trial of screening for lung cancer with chest CT. Thirty lung cancers (10% of those screened) were found in the CT screened group in contrast to seven in the chest radiograph group. Thirty of the 56 individuals who underwent any invasive procedure (bronchoscopy, lung biopsy, or resection) were diagnosed with lung cancer in contrast to 7 of 15 for the chest radiograph group.

6. Henschke CI, Yankelevitz DF, Smith JP, et al. Screening for lung cancer: the Early Cancer Action Approach. *Lung Cancer.* 2002;35:143–148.

   A detailed description of the screening and follow-up protocols used by the Early Lung Cancer Action Program.

7. Henschke CI, Naidich DP, Yankelevitz DF, et al. Early Lung Cancer Action Project: initial findings on repeat screenings. *Cancer.* 2001;92:153–159.

   Results of the annual repeat scans by the Early Lung Cancer Action Project group, which found 2.5% of scans had new nodules. Only 8 of the 30 new nodules required invasive evaluation, and 7 of these were cancers, 5 of which were stage IA.

8. Henschke CI, McCauley DI, Yankelevitz DF, et al. Early Lung Cancer Action Project: overall design and findings from baseline screening. *Lancet.* 1999;354:99–105.

   The first study in a U.S. population that demonstrated 23 of 27 lung cancers diagnosed by CT screening were in stage I. Of the 28 lesions requiring biopsy, only 1 did not yield a malignant diagnosis. This is the paper that generated much of the current interest in CT screening for lung cancer.

9. Marcus PM, Bergstralh EJ, Fagerstrom RM, et al. Lung cancer mortality in the Mayo Lung Project: impact of extended follow-up. *J Natl Cancer Inst.* 2000;92:1308–1316.

   A detailed examination of long-term follow-up of the Mayo Clinic trial of chest radiograph screening for lung cancer. It demonstrates a 30% increase in lung cancer diagnosis among the screened group in comparison with the controls with no difference in lung cancer mortality. It concludes that the most likely explanation for this result is a high rate of diagnosis as lung cancer of lesions that would not go on to cause death from lung cancer if untreated. This is the principal set of analyses that has raised the question of overdiagnosis in lung cancer screening.

10. Ostroff JS, Buckshee N, Mancuso CA, et al. Smoking cessation following CT screening for early detection of lung cancer. *Prev Med.* 2001;33:613–621.

    A demonstration that smoking cessation programs can be very effective when implemented in conjunction with lung cancer screening programs.

11. Pastorino U, Bellomi M, Landoni C, et al. Early lung-cancer detection with spiral CT and positron emission tomography in heavy smokers: 2-year results. *Lancet.* 2003;362:593–597.

An Italian experience with CT screening that found 55% of cancers were stage I with the initial screen and 100% of the cancers identified in the first follow-up scans were stage I.

12. Patz EF Jr, Goodman PC, Bepler G. Screening for lung cancer. *N Engl J Med.* 2000;343:1627–1633.

A clear presentation of the different biases that can influence outcome measurements in screening trials.

13. Sobue T, Moriyama N, Kaneko M, et al. Screening for lung cancer with low-dose helical computed tomography: anti-lung cancer association project. *J Clin Oncol.* 2002;20:911–920.

Eighty-two percent of the lung cancers identified by CT screening in Japan were stage IA and the 5-year survival was 76.2% for all cancers without regard to stage at diagnosis in the initial scan and 5-year survival was 64.9% for those diagnosed by follow-up scan. Survival for stage I disease was even higher. The outcomes for cancers diagnosed through a screening program are dramatically better than those for cancers diagnosed in the absence of screening.

14. Sone S, Li F, Yang ZG, et al. Results of three-year mass screening programme for lung cancer using mobile low-dose spiral computed tomography scanner. *Br J Cancer.* 2001;84:25–32.

Eighty-eight percent of the cancers identified were stage IA.

15. Sone S, Takashima S, Li F, et al. Mass screening for lung cancer with mobile spiral computed tomography scanner. *Lancet.* 1998;351:1242–1245.

A clear demonstration of the relative sensitivity of chest radiography, sputum cytology, and chest CT for diagnosis of lung cancer in the same population.

16. Strauss GM. The Mayo Lung Cohort: a regression analysis focusing on lung cancer incidence and mortality. *J Clin Oncol.* 2002;20:1973–1983.

A careful reexamination of the limitations of the existing studies, particularly the Mayo Clinic study, with a presentation of the arguments for screening.

17. Swensen SJ, Jett JR, Hartman TE, et al. Lung cancer screening with CT: Mayo Clinic experience. *Radiology.* 2003;226:756–761.

The Mayo clinic experience with repeat scans following a baseline scan. Eleven cancers were diagnosed with 6 in stage I. After 3 years, 8 of 39 surgical interventions were for benign disease.

18. Swensen SJ, Jett JR, Sloan JA, et al. Screening for lung cancer with low-dose spiral computed tomography. *Am J Respir Crit Care Med.* 2002;165:508–513.

Presentation of the initial screening results by the Mayo Clinic. Only 12 of the 21 non–small-cell cancers detected by screening were stage IA at diagnosis.

19. U.S. Preventive Services Task Force. Lung cancer screening: recommendation statement. *Ann Intern Med.* 2004;140:738–739.

A recent revision of the screening recommendations for lung cancer, which changes from a recommendation against screening to a statement that the evidence is not sufficient to recommend either for or against screening with either chest radiographs or chest CT.

20. Wisnivesky JP, Yankelevitz D, Henschke CI. The effect of tumor size on curability of stage I non-small cell lung cancers. *Chest.* 2004;126:761–765.

A careful examination of the SEER data demonstrating improved 12 year survival with stage 1 lung cancers with smaller tumor size at surgery. Size of the lesion does matter, even in stage 1 lesions.

104. LUNG CANCER: TREATMENT

John E. Barkley

The prognosis for patients diagnosed with lung cancer remains poor. However, this disease remains a major focus of research, and some exciting developments offer hope. Specific treatment recommendations are guided by (1) the histologic type of tumor (small-cell versus non–small-cell); (2) the stage of disease; and (3) the patient's performance status. Optimal evaluation and management require a multidisciplinary team from pulmonary medicine, thoracic surgery, medical oncology, radiation oncology, radiology, pathology, and nursing.

The initial goal in managing patients with non–small-cell lung cancer (non-SCLC) is to determine (1) whether the patient is operable, namely, will the patient survive surgery with an acceptable risk for morbidity and mortality, and (b) whether the cancer is resectable, namely, can the lesion be removed technically and will surgery improve prognosis.

OPERABILITY

A patient's operability is usually assessed by routine cardiovascular evaluation, simple spirometry, and arterial blood gases. If pulmonary reserve is marginal, we obtain DLCO, quantitative ventilation–perfusion ($\dot{V}/\dot{Q}$) scanning and formal cardiopulmonary exercise testing. $\dot{V}/\dot{Q}$ scanning can be helpful in predicting postoperative pulmonary function. A predicted postoperative FEV_1 or DLCO of less than 40% suggests an increased risk of postoperative morbidity and mortality. Patients with a marginal FEV_1 may not lose lung function if the lobar bronchus (and artery) to be resected is already obstructed and not participating in gas exchange (or perfusion). Cardiopulmonary exercise testing allows the determination of a patient's maximal oxygen consumption ($\dot{V}o_{2max}$) that can be used for further risk stratification. Patients with a $\dot{V}o_{2max}$ <10 mL/kg per minute should not be operated on, whereas those with $\dot{V}o_{2max}$ of 15 mL O_2/kg per minute or higher should do well. Unfortunately, no single test can accurately predict postoperative functional outcome and each patient must be considered individually. Patients with marginal lung function may benefit from preoperative pulmonary rehabilitation as well. Finally, the role of lung volume reduction surgery to improve lung function (and, therefore, decrease operative risk) in patients with lung cancer and advanced emphysema remains controversial.

RESECTABILITY

The resectability of a lung cancer is determined by clinical staging of the disease. Both stage I and II disease are resectable by definition and should be treated with surgery whenever possible. Despite recent refinements in lung cancer staging, stage III is composed of a heterogeneous group of patients with widely varying 5-year survival following surgical resection alone. Patients with bulky, multistation N2 disease do poorly with surgery alone and should not undergo primary surgical resection; however, patients with a negative mediastinoscopic examination and single-station, microscopic mediastinal nodal metastatic disease discovered at thoracotomy may have a 25 to 30% 5-year survival with surgery alone. Patients with stage IIIB (N3 or T4) or stage IV disease usually should not undergo resection, but in rare circumstances are candidates for surgical therapy with curative intent.

CHEMOTHERAPY AND RADIOTHERAPY

Chemotherapy and radiotherapy for non-SCLC can be used preoperatively (neoadjuvant therapy), postoperatively (adjuvant therapy), and separately (sequential) or together (concurrent) as definitive therapy.

Neoadjuvant therapy is an area of active investigation in stage I, II, and III disease. Phase II data indicate the feasibility of this approach in stage I to III disease. However, limited compelling phase III data are available at this time. Although many clinicians use neoadjuvant chemotherapy routinely, toxicity can be significant and its use outside of the protocol setting cannot currently be recommended.

Adjuvant therapy in patients with completely resected stages I, II, and III disease has been studied. Adjuvant chemotherapy does prolong disease-free survival; one phase III study recently demonstrated 4% improvement in overall survival. The role of adjuvant chemotherapy remains controversial. Adjuvant radiotherapy, which has recently been reviewed, may be detrimental in patients with early stage non-SCLC (stage I and II). Adjuvant radiotherapy in resected stage III disease decreases the local recurrence rate and may improve long-term survival.

For most patients with stage IIIA (N2) and IIIB disease, a combined or multimodality approach should be considered. With radiotherapy alone 5-year survival is less than 10%. By adding induction chemotherapy prior to radiotherapy, long-term survival increases to 17%. Patients with minimal weight loss and good performance status should be considered for combined modality therapy.

STAGE IV DISEASE

Stage IV non-SCLC is almost always incurable, but patients may benefit significantly from systemic chemotherapy. Several studies have documented 40 to 60% 1-year survival in patients with stage IV disease and good performance status. Several novel chemotherapeutic agents are now available and offer the possibility of improved survival with less toxicity. Recently, the first molecularly targeted agent in non-SCLC was approved for patients with advanced stage disease who have progressive disease after platinum-based and docetaxel therapy.

SMALL-CELL CARCINOMA

Without treatment, SCLC is rapidly fatal. Patients with limited stage disease have an average survival of approximately 20 months when treated with concurrent chemotherapy and radiotherapy. The 2-year survival approaches 45% with 5-year survival of 15 to 20%. Patients achieving complete remission should be considered for prophylactic cranial irradiation (PCI) because metastases to the central nervous system (CNS) are a common site of relapse. The risk of this devastating complication can be reduced from 30 to 10% with PCI. A recent meta-analysis examining PCI reported a survival advantage as well. Late CNS toxicity has been reported and is often cited as a reason not to use PCI. Extensive stage SCLC is fatal in 1 to 3 months without treatment. With combination chemotherapy, average survival increases to 9 to 12 months. Radiotherapy for extensive stage disease is generally reserved for palliation of symptomatic metastatic disease not responding to chemotherapy or at the time of relapse.

The role of surgery in SCLC remains controversial. Typically, patients are found to have SCLC during thoracotomy for a solitary pulmonary nodule. Survival in this setting approaches 50%. Although no randomized trials have been performed, the general consensus is to treat these rare patients with adjuvant chemotherapy.

PALLIATIVE TREATMENT

The palliation of patients with unresectable, inoperable, or recurrent disease can involve multiple modalities. More active systemic chemotherapeutic agents are being developed and offer a real opportunity for improving survival without significant toxicity. Radiation therapy is effective at palliating metastatic disease that produces symptoms of pain, cough, hemoptysis, superior vena cava obstruction, and atelectasis. CNS disease can often be palliated with radiation as well. Central airway obstruction in lung cancer is common and can be devastating. Both flexible and rigid bronchoscopy can be invaluable in assisting these patients. Endobronchial stenting, laser therapy, endobronchial radiation therapy (brachytherapy), electrocautery, cryotherapy, balloon dilatation, and photodynamic therapy can all be useful in restoring patency of the central airways and improving the patient's quality of life.

1. Adjei AA, Marks RS, Bonner JA. Current guidelines for the management of small cell lung cancer. *Mayo Clin Proc.* 1999;74:809.

An excellent, concise review of the evaluation and treatment of patients with SCLC.

2. Auperin A, et al. Prophylactic cranial irradiation for patients with small cell lung cancer in complete remission. Prophylactic cranial irradiation overview collaborative group. *N Engl J Med.* 1999;341:476.

   A meta-analysis demonstrating improved survival in patients with SCLC in complete remission treated with PCI.

3. Brutinel WM, et al. A two-year experience with neodymium-YAG laser in endobronchial obstruction. *Chest.* 1987;91:159.

   Treatment with laser therapy is most successful when the lesions are short in length, when the distal bronchi are free of tumor, and when functional lung tissue is distal to the tumor.

4. Cavaliere S, et al. Nd:YAG laser bronchoscopy: a five-year experience with 1396 applications in 1000 patients. *Chest.* 1988;94:15.

   Describes the authors' experience using Nd:YAG laser bronchoscopy in obstructive lesions of the tracheobronchial tree, including 649 patients with malignant tumors. In 92% of patients, a normal airway lumen or a significant improvement in ventilation was achieved.

5. Dillman RO, et al. Improved survival in stage III non-small-cell lung cancer; seven-year follow-up of Cancer and Leukemia Group B (CALGB) 8433 trial. *J Natl Cancer Inst.* 1996;88:1210.

   Initial randomized trial demonstrating improvement in 5-year survival with chemotherapy and radiotherapy versus radiotherapy alone, 17% and 6%, respectively.

6. Dumon JF. A dedicated tracheobronchial stent. *Chest.* 1990;97:328.

   Discusses the use of a dedicated tracheobronchial prosthesis in the treatment of 66 patients with extrinsic compression of the major airways.

7. The International Adjuvant Lung Cancer Trial Collaborative Group. Cisplatin-based adjuvant chemotherapy with completely resected non-small lung cancer. *N Engl J Med.* 2004;350:351.

   IALT is the first positive adjuvant trial published

8. Johnson BE, et al. Neurologic, neuropsychiatric, and computed cranial tomography scan abnormalities in 2 to 10 year survivors of small-cell lung cancer. *J Clin Oncol.* 1985;3:1659.

   Neurologic abnormalities are more prominent in patients administered high-dose chemotherapy during cranial irradiation or treated with large radiation fractions.

9. Johnston MR. Selecting patients with lung cancer for surgical therapy. *Semin Oncol.* 1988;15:246.

   Describes selection of patients with lung cancer for surgical therapy.

10. Kris MA, et al. Efficacy of gefitinib, an inhibitor of the epidermal growth factor receptor tyrosine kinase, in symptomatic patients with non-small cell lung cancer. *JAMA.* 2003;290:2149.

    Phase II data describing first molecularly targeted agent for non-SCLC. A well-referenced, comprehensive review of the surgical approach to lung cancer.

11. Lischner M, et al. Late neurological complications after prophylactic cranial irradiation in patients with small-cell lung cancer: the Toronto experience. *J Clin Oncol.* 1990;8:215.

    Describes late neurologic complications following PCI.

12. Lung Cancer Study Group. Effect of postoperative mediastinal radiation on completely resected stage II and stage III epidermoid cancer of the lung. *N Engl J Med.* 1986;315:137.

    Findings were a decreased incidence of local recurrence, but no improvement in survival with postoperative radiation therapy.

13. Lung Cancer Study Group. Surgical adjuvant therapy for stage II and stage III adenocarcinoma and large-cell undifferentiated carcinoma. *J Clin Oncol.* 1986;4:710.

    Adjuvant chemotherapy prolonged disease-free but not long-term survival. Median survival was extended but did not reach statistical significance.

14. Lung Cancer Study Group. The benefit of adjuvant treatment for resected locally advanced non-small cell lung cancer. *J Clin Oncol.* 1988;6:9.

    Cyclophosphamide, adriamycin, and cisplatin chemotherapy improved disease-free survival but not overall survival.

15. Machtay M, et al. Two commonly used neoadjuvant chemoradiotherapy regimens for locally advanced stage III non-small cell lung carcinoma: long-term results and associations with pathologic response. *J Thorac Cardiovasc Surg.* 2004;127: 108.

    Results of neoadjuvant therapy for non-SCLC

16. Mentzer SJ, Swanson SJ. Treatment of patients with lung cancer and severe emphysema. *Chest.* 1999;116:477S.

    A concise review of the role of lung volume reduction surgery and pulmonary rehabilitation in patients with resectable bronchogenic carcinoma.

17. Murren JR, et al. Critical analysis of neoadjuvant therapy for stage IIIa non-small cell lung cancer. *Am Rev Respir Dis.* 1991;143:889.

    A comprehensive review of the role of neoadjuvant chemotherapy in lung cancer.

18. Osterlind K, et al. Treatment policy of surgery in small cell carcinoma of the lung: retrospective analysis of a series of 874 consecutive patients. *Thorax.* 1985;40: 272.

    A treatment policy of surgery for limited SCLC did not lead to better overall results than treatment with chemotherapy and radiotherapy alone.

19. Post Meta-analysis Trialists Group. Post-operative radiotherapy in non–small-cell lung cancer: systematic review and meta-analysis of individual patient data from nine randomised controlled trials. *Lancet.* 1998;352:257.

    A large meta-analysis calling into question routine postoperative (adjuvant) radiotherapy in patients with completely resected non-SCLC. An increased mortality rate was seen in patients with stage I and II cancer who received adjuvant radiotherapy.

20. Ramanathan RK, Belani CP. Chemotherapy for advanced non-small cell lung cancer: past, present and future. *Semin Oncol.* 1997;24:440.

    A good review with excellent references. Entire issue devoted to lung cancer.

21. Reilly Jr JJ. Evidence-based preoperative evaluation of candidates for thoracotomy. *Chest.* 1999;116:477S.

    An excellent review of preoperative assessment of patients with bronchogenic carcinoma being evaluated for resection.

22. Rosell R, et al. A randomized trial comparing pre-operative chemotherapy plus surgery with surgery alone in patients with non-small-cell lung cancer. *N Engl J Med.* 1994;330:153.

    Patients receiving neoadjuvant chemotherapy did much better than those treated with surgery alone.

23. Roth JA, et al. A randomized trial comparing perioperative chemotherapy and surgery with surgery alone in resectable stage IIIA non–small-cell lung cancer. *J Natl Cancer Inst.* 1994;86:673.

    Patients receiving neoadjuvant chemotherapy did much better than patients treated initially with surgery alone.

24. Spira A, Ettinger DA. Multimodality management of lung cancer. *N Engl J Med.* 2004:350:379.

    Excellent review of the treatment of both SCLC and non-SCLC.

25. Turrisi AT, et al. Twice daily compared with once daily thoracic radiotherapy in limited small-cell lung cancer treated concurrently with cisplatin and etoposide. *N Engl J Med.* 1999;340:265.

    Four cycles of chemotherapy with concurrent radiotherapy initiated with cycle 1 of chemotherapy led to 2-year and 5-year survival rates of 44% and 23%, respectively.

105. EXTRATHORACIC AND ENDOCRINE MANIFESTATIONS OF LUNG CANCER

Shari A. Brazinsky and Deborah Shure

The extrathoracic manifestations of bronchogenic carcinoma can be categorized into those related to local spread, those related to metastases, and those that are independent of cancer spread, namely, the paraneoplastic syndromes.

MANIFESTATIONS OF LOCAL SPREAD

Local spread, which causes extrathoracic manifestations, is most often caused by superior sulcus tumors involving the eighth cervical and first thoracic nerves. Patients complain of pain in the shoulder and along the ulnar distribution of the arm. Paravertebral involvement of the sympathetic chain can cause a Horner's syndrome. Tumor also can involve the recurrent laryngeal nerve and produce hoarseness. Superior vena cava syndrome is caused by tumor compression anywhere along the course of this vessel. Other extrathoracic symptoms may result from spread into the mediastinum, with involvement of the heart and esophagus.

METASTATIC DISEASE

Although metastatic disease is common in patients dying of lung cancer (96%), symptomatic disease is less frequent. Metastases are most common in lymph nodes (70%), liver (39%), brain (30%), adrenals (25%), bone (20%), and kidneys (18%), although they can involve any organ or tissue. Lymph node, adrenal, and renal metastases are rarely symptomatic. Bony metastases can produce local pain and even spinal cord compression if the vertebral bodies are involved. The diagnosis and treatment of spinal cord compression is a medical emergency and should always be considered in this setting, particularly if neurologic symptoms are present. Liver involvement is generally asymptomatic but can cause abdominal discomfort. Brain metastases can mimic cerebrovascular disease or primary intracranial neoplasm.

PARANEOPLASTIC SYNDROMES

The paraneoplastic syndromes can be characterized as (1) constitutional, (2) hematologic, (3) skeletal, (4) neuromuscular, (5) cutaneous, (6) vasculitic, and (7) endocrine. The most common constitutional syndromes are weight loss, anorexia, and fatigue. Tumor size alone does not explain the presence or magnitude of symptoms and their cause(s) is unknown. Cachexia is a significant prognostic factor in the course of lung cancer. Recent studies suggest that splenic cytokines such as tumor necrosis factor influence cachexia, as well as tumor growth. Megestrol acetate, a synthetic progestin, has been found to improve well-being, as well as allow weight gain, in many types of lung cancer.

Normochromic, normocytic anemia occurs in less than 10% of patients with bronchogenic carcinoma and is unrelated to marrow infiltration or therapy. A number of coagulopathies are associated with lung cancer. They include migratory thrombophlebitis (Trousseau's syndrome), disseminated intravascular coagulation, chronic hemorrhagic diathesis, nonbacterial thrombotic endocarditis, and arterial embolization. Trousseau's syndrome often involves unusual sites such as the upper extremities or the vena cava and is frequently unresponsive to anticoagulant therapy. Non-small-cell carcinomas have also been associated with tumor-related leukocytosis, which is cytokine mediated and carries an ominous prognosis.

Hypertrophic pulmonary osteoarthropathy occurs in 4 to 12% of patients with lung cancer, most commonly with epidermoid carcinoma and only rarely with small-cell carcinoma (5%). It consists of periosteal new bone formation in the long bones, with digital clubbing and symmetric arthritis. Vasomotor instability is often present with episodic blanching, swelling, and diaphoresis of the hands and feet. The ankles, wrists, and long bones can be very painful and tender. Although new bone growth is present, the syndrome does not seem to be caused by ectopic human growth hormone production, but it may be mediated by autonomic reflexes. It usually regresses after tumor removal, vagotomy, or thoracotomy without tumor resection. Prognosis does not appear to be altered if this syndrome is present, and tumor recurrence is frequently accompanied by recurrent osteopulmonary arthropathy. Unilateral facial pain and cluster headaches can be referred pain, or caused by hypertrophic osteopathy or paraneoplastic circulating humoral factors. Pain can be relieved by radiotherapy or tumor resection with vagotomy.

An increasing number of neuromuscular syndromes have been associated with bronchogenic carcinoma, most commonly small-cell carcinoma. These syndromes may precede the clinical appearance of the tumor by months to years. The most potentially devastating are cerebral encephalopathy and cortical cerebellar degeneration, both of which can occur precipitously. Peripheral neuropathies, usually sensorimotor and often presenting as pain and paraesthesias of the lower extremities, occur in up to 15% of patients with lung cancer. This can be followed by the gradual onset of a neuropathic arthropathy. A myasthenia (Eaton–Lambert) syndrome occurs in 6% of patients with small-cell carcinoma and differs from myasthenia gravis primarily by an increase in the muscle action potential on repetitive stimulation and the lack of improvement in muscle strength with anticholinesterases. Symmetric proximal muscle neuromyopathy associated with muscle wasting is also common. Non–small-cell tumors have been reported with a paraneoplastic necrotizing myopathy. Paraneoplastic encephalomyelitis, frequently associated with small-cell carcinoma, is characterized by inflammatory infiltrates and neuronal loss. A rapidly progressive binocular vision loss, termed *cancer-associated retinopathy*, has been described in patients with small-cell carcinoma. Also associated with small-cell carcinoma is an adult-onset opsoclonus-myoclonus syndrome. There is no specific immunoreactivity, and the paraneoplastic variety has a worse prognosis than if idiopathic. If the tumor is treated effectively, significant neurologic recovery is noted.

The cause of these neuromuscular paraneoplastic syndromes is generally not known. Evidence has been found, however, for an autoimmune basis for several of these syndromes. In these cases, antibodies have been found that cross-react with tumor and normal tissue antigens. In Eaton–Lambert syndrome, the antibodies cross-react with presynaptic voltage-gated calcium channels at the neuromuscular junction. In cancer-associated retinopathy, antibodies to a tumor antigen cross-react with a subset of retinal ganglion cells (to the photoreceptor protein recoverin). Prednisone therapy has been reported to reduce antibody titers and stabilize visual fields. A heterogeneous group of cases including of paraneoplastic encephalomyelitis, cerebellar degeneration, Eaton–Lambert myasthenic syndrome, and sensory neuronopathy with small-cell carcinoma associated with a specific antibody in the serum or cerebral spinal fluid, is considered part of the anti-Hu syndrome (bearing the name of the first patient in whom the antibody was discovered). These include the presence of high titers of Hu antibody associated with more severe cerebellar degeneration than in the subset without the antibody. An anti-Purkinje cell antibody has also been found in some patients with paraneoplastic cerebellar degeneration. In patients with lung cancer, however, the antibody is rarely found, and the clinical picture is less severe and slower to develop than when the syndrome is associated with other types of cancer. Lower motor neuron disease as a paraneoplastic syndrome has also been seen with anti-Hu antibody. Some studies have found more than one antibody present in patients with paraneoplastic syndrome, raising the possibility of multimodal autoantibody production. Such autoantibodies are found to be associated with other paraneoplastic syndromes. Gastrointestinal motor dysfunction is now known to be associated with small-cell carcinoma (with multiple paraneoplastic autoantibodies) and can precede the recognition of tumor by months to years. Dysfunction includes delayed gastric emptying, esophageal dysmotility, and abnormal autonomic reflexes.

Cutaneous manifestations include features of dermatomyositis, hyperpigmentation caused by ectopic production of melanocyte-stimulating hormone, and acanthosis nigricans. The last is a hyperkeratotic, hyperpigmented dermatosis with small papillomatous lesions giving the skin a velvety texture. It is symmetric and prominent in skin folds. When it occurs after age 40, it is almost always associated with cancer (90% intra-abdominal, 5% lung). Dermatomyositis has been associated with an autoantibody to a nuclear complex of unknown function. Other rare manifestations include erythema gyratum (thickened, bandlike urticarial plaques imparting a "knotty pine" appearance) with small-cell carcinoma, universal hypertrichosis lanuginosa with epidermoid carcinoma, and rapidly progressive digital necrosis with small-cell carcinoma. Recently, benign dermatosis granuloma annulare, interstitial granulomatous dermatitis, tripe palms, and subacute cutaneous lupus erythematosus were reported as being temporally associated with carcinoma of the lung, and regressed with successful treatment of the malignancy.

Non–small-cell carcinomas have been associated with cutaneous vasculitis and purpura rheumatica. Disseminated vasculitis has now been reported with small-cell carcinoma of the lung. A nonsystemic subacute vasculitic neuropathy called *paraneoplastic vasculitic neuropathy* has been described with small-cell carcinoma of the lung. The neuropathy, which varies from a mononeuropathy multiplex to a symmetric polyneuropathy, is associated with an elevated erythrocyte sedimentation rate and high cerebrospinal fluid protein count. Both chemotherapy and immunotherapy for vasculitis are effective in this disorder.

Many endocrine and metabolic syndromes are associated with bronchogenic carcinoma; they are primarily, but not exclusively, associated with small-cell carcinoma. It is theorized that lung cells embryologically derived from neural crest cells with the ability for amine precursor uptake and decarboxylation undergo malignant derepression and secrete one or more peptide hormones. Overt clinical syndromes appear in approximately 10% of patients with lung cancer, although subclinical hormone production is more common. The hormones produced are peptides and include adrenocorticotropic hormone (ACTH), melanocyte-stimulating hormone, parathyroid hormone, antidiuretic hormone (ADH), human chorionic gonadotropin, prolactin, serotonin, insulin, glucagon, corticotropin-releasing factor, and calcitonin. Most is known about ectopic ACTH, parathyroid hormone, and ADH.

Probably the most commonly produced ectopic hormone is ACTH (50% of patients with small-cell carcinoma), although Cushing's syndrome is rare with bronchogenic carcinoma. Tumors appear to elaborate both active ACTH (in small amounts) and an immunoreactive, but biologically weak big ACTH, which can be a precursor molecule. Big ACTH was evaluated as a marker for lung cancer, because it is present in more than 80% of all patients who have lung cancer. It is not, however, specific, because it also occurs in a significant number of patients with chronic obstructive pulmonary disease. When Cushing's syndrome does occur in association with tumor ACTH secretion, it is a virulent disease with poor prognosis. Ketoconazole, an inhibitor of adrenal steroid synthesis secondary to its inhibitory effects on the cytochrome P-450 enzyme system, has been reported to significantly suppress serum cortisol levels in a patient with Cushing's syndrome caused by small-cell carcinoma.

Hypercalcemia occurs in at least 12% of patients with lung cancer, mainly with epidermoid carcinomas. Although small-cell carcinoma frequently metastasizes to bone, it rarely causes hypercalcemia. Ectopic parathyroid hormone production is one cause of hypercalcemia that usually responds to therapy. Some cases may be caused by tumor-secreted prostaglandin E. The hypercalcemia in these patients can be suppressed by aspirin or indomethacin. Other cases may be caused by tumor production of a peptide with significant structural homology to parathyroid hormone, but without immunologic cross-reactivity.

The syndrome of inappropriate ADH (SIADH) results from ectopic ADH secretion. It occurs in 11% of patients with small-cell carcinoma and, although hyponatremia can be severe, symptoms occur in only about 25% of patients with tumor-induced SIADH. It usually resolves within 3 weeks of the initiation of chemotherapy. Occasionally, severe SIADH can occur in the first 5 days following the start of chemotherapy; thus, patients should be monitored carefully during this time. Preliminary studies have used ^{131}I-labeled antibodies against vasopressin-associated neurophysin to localize tumors using radioimaging.

Other causes of hyponatremia associated with lung cancer are much less common. Renal tubular dysfunction in association with glycosuria and aminoaciduria has been reported, as has sodium loss associated with massive bronchorrhea in bronchoalveolar cell carcinoma. In addition, some hyponatremic patients with lung cancer who have normal levels of ADH have been found to have increased messenger RNA levels for atrial natriuretic factor as a possible mechanism for their deranged sodium homeostasis.

Gonadotropin production occurs predominantly with large-cell carcinoma and can cause gynecomastia, which can be unilateral. Gynecomastia in a man should be evaluated with hCG testing. Prolactin production by anaplastic tumors can cause lactation in women. Rarely, epidermoid carcinomas have been associated with the production of vasoactive intestinal peptides, resulting in a syndrome of watery diarrhea, hypokalemia, and achlorhydria. In addition, bronchogenic carcinomas have been found to produce small, biologically active amines or peptides, including serotonin, histamine, and a substance resembling eosinophilic chemotactic factor of anaphylaxis.

Currently, most of these hormones represent curiosities. In the future, some may become useful markers of disease or response to therapy, and the mechanisms of their production may provide insights into the behavior of carcinoma.

A retrospective study of 40 years of reports in the literature found that 13% of patients with resectable non–small-cell lung cancer had a paraneoplastic syndrome. The authors suggested that recent onset arthritis and arthralgias, without other explanations, should be considered as early clues to possible lung cancer. Positron emission tomography (PET) appears to be useful in localizing (particularly small-cell) carcinoma in patients presenting with paraneoplastic syndromes. Increasing recognition of new paraneoplastic syndromes, many of which are felt to be immunologically mediated, has been accompanied by frequently disappointing trials of therapy with steroids, immunoglobulins, and plasmapheresis. Ongoing study of immunoadsorption with protein A for paraneoplastic neurologic syndromes has shown some initial success and merits further trials.

---

1. Antoine JC, Absi L, Honnorat J, et al. Antiamphiphysin antibodies are associated with various paraneoplastic neurological syndromes and tumors. *Arch Neurol.* 1999;56:172.
   These antibodies, which are not specific for one tumor type or one neurologic syndrome, can be part of a multimodal autoantibody production.
2. Bataller L, Graus F, Sarz A, et al. Clinical outcome in adult onset idiopathic or paraneoplastic opsoclonus-myoclonus. *Brain.* 2001;124(Pt 2):437.
   A comparison of patients with idiopathic and paraneoplastic presentations of this rare syndrome with very different outcomes.
3. Batchelor TT, Platten M, Hochberg FH. Immunoadsorption therapy for paraneoplastic syndromes. *J Neurooncol.* 1998;40:131.
   A report of 13 patients treated with protein A immunoadsorption with promising results (75% with complete or partial response).
4. Beck C, Burger HG. Evidence for the presence of immunoreactive growth hormone in cancers of the lung and stomach. *Cancer.* 1972;30:75.
   Growth hormone was found in 7 of 18 lung tumors. The patients were not symptomatic.
5. Campanella N, Moraca A, Pergolini M, et al. Paraneoplastic syndromes in 68 cases of resectable non-small cell carcinoma: can they help in early detection? *Med Oncol.* 1999;16:129.
   Compilation of prior publications suggesting that recent onset of unexplained arthralgias and arthritis could be early clues of lung cancer.
6. Chester KA, Lang B, Gill J, et al. Lambert–Eaton syndrome antibodies: reaction with membranes from a small cell lung cancer xenograft. *J Neuroimmunol.* 1988;18:97.
   Reviews evidence for an IgG-mediated reduction in the number of presynaptic voltage-gated calcium channels at neuromuscular junctions in Eaton–Lambert syndrome.

7. Crotty E, Patz EF Jr. FDG-PET imaging in patients with paraneoplastic syndromes and suspected small cell lung cancer. *J Thoracic Imaging.* 2001;16:89–93.
   New imaging techniques help to locate tumors in suspected paraneoplastic syndromes.

8. Dimopoulos MA, Fernandez JF, Samaan NA, et al. Paraneoplastic Cushing's syndrome as an adverse prognostic factor in patients who die early with small cell lung cancer. *Cancer.* 1992;69:66.
   Of patients with Cushing's syndrome, 82% died within 14 days of initiation of chemotherapy compared with 25% of the control patients. Median survival was halved, and 45% of the deaths were caused by opportunistic infection in the patients with Cushing's syndrome. Biochemical control of Cushing's syndrome before initiation of chemotherapy may ameliorate the poor prognosis.

9. Gewirtz G, Yalow RS. Ectopic ACTH production in carcinoma of the lung. *J Clin Invest.* 1974;53:1022.
   "Big" ACTH was found in primary tumor and metastases in all types of lung cancer examined.

10. Grunwald GB, Kornguth SE, Towfighi J, et al. Autoimmune basis for visual paraneoplastic syndrome in patients with small cell lung carcinoma. *Cancer.* 1987;60:780.
    Describes the visual paraneoplastic syndrome and the antibodies to tumor antigens that cross-react with the subset of retinal ganglions involved in the syndrome.

11. Heckmayr M, Gatzemeier U. Treatment of cancer weight loss in patients with advanced lung cancer. *Oncology.* 1992;49(Suppl 2):32.
    Megestrol acetate is an effective therapy for weight gain and well-being of patients with lung cancer cachexia.

12. Hoffman DM, Brigham B. The use of ketoconazole in ectopic adrenocorticotropic hormone syndrome. *Cancer.* 1991;67:1447.
    Ketoconazole therapy resulted in significant suppression of serum cortisol levels.

13. Holling H, Brody R, Boland H. Pulmonary hypertrophic osteoarthropathy. *Lancet.* 1961;2:1269.
    An old, but excellent, review of the clinical features of this paraneoplastic syndrome.

14. Kasuga I, Makino S, Kiyokawa H, et al. Tumor-related leukocytosis is linked with poor prognosis in patients with lung carcinoma. *Cancer.* 2001;92:2399.
    Reports of a paraneoplastic syndrome associated with large cell carcinomas and mediated by hematopoietic cytokines.

15. Keltner JL, Thirkill CE, Tyler CE, et al. Management and monitoring of cancer-associated retinopathy. *Arch Ophthalmol.* 1992;110:48.
    Discusses the efficacy of prednisone to stabilize visual fields in cancer-associated retinopathy. Includes a case report where antibody titers were followed to make clinical decisions regarding institution of steroid therapy.

16. Lee HR, Lennon VA, Camilleri M, et al. Paraneoplastic gastrointestinal motor dysfunction: clinical and laboratory characteristics. *Am J Gastroenterol.* 2001;96:373–379.
    Gastrointestinal symptoms preceded the diagnosis of small-cell carcinoma, and was associated with anti-Hu and other paraneoplastic autoantibodies.

17. Levin KH. Paraneoplastic neuromuscular syndromes. *Neurol Clin.* 1997;15:597.
    A good review of neuromuscular paraneoplastic syndromes.

18. Levin MI, Mozaffar T, Al-Lozi MT, et al. Paraneoplastic necrotizing myopathy: clinical and pathological features. *Neurology.* 1998;50:764.
    Describes a rapidly progressive, symmetric, proximal muscle weakness associated with non–small-cell carcinoma.

19. List AF, Hainsworth JD, Davis BW, et al. The syndrome of inappropriate secretion of antidiuretic hormone (SIADH) in small cell lung cancer. *J Clin Oncol.* 1986;4:1191.
    A comprehensive review of the clinical aspects of this syndrome in lung cancer.

20. Merrill WW, Bondy PK. Production of biochemical marker substances by bronchogenic carcinomas. *Clin Chest Med.* 1982;3:307.
    A good review with extensive references.

21. Miller FW. Myositis-specific autoantibodies. *JAMA*. 1993;270:1846.
    Divides myositis into groups based on autoantibodies that have clinical and prognostic significance.
22. Marchioli CC, Graziano SL. Paraneoplastic syndromes associated with small cell lung cancer. *Chest Surg Clin North Am*. 1997;7:65.
    An excellent general review of the topic.
23. Mason WP, Graus F, Lang B, et al. Small-cell lung cancer, paraneoplastic cerebellar degeneration and the Eaton–Lambert myasthenic syndrome. *Brain*. 1997;120:1279.
    A more detailed discussion of the anti-Hu syndrome and neuromuscular paraneoplastic syndromes.
24. Matsubara S, Yamaji Y, Fujita T, et al. Cancer-associated retinopathy syndrome: a case of small cell lung cancer expressing recoverin immunoreactivity. *Lung Cancer*. 1996;14:265.
    The presence of recoverin immunoreactivity supports that cancer-retina immunologic cross-reaction leads to visual loss.
25. Mortin D, Itabashi H, Grimes D. Nonmetastatic neurologic complications of bronchogenic carcinoma: the carcinomatous myopathies. *J Thorac Cardiovasc Surg*. 1966;51:14.
    Chest radiographs were normal in one third of the patients presenting with this syndrome. It was more common in small-cell carcinoma (2.5:1).
26. Moses AM, Scheinman SJ. Ectopic secretion of neurohypophyseal peptides in patients with malignancy. *Endocrinol Metab Clin North Am*. 1991;20:489.
    A good review of SIADH, including pathogenesis and therapy.
27. Oh SJ. Paraneoplastic vasculitis of the peripheral nervous system. *Neurol Clin*. 1997;15:849.
    Discusses potentially treatable neuropathy associated with small-cell cancer of the lung.
28. Patel AM, Davila DG, Peters SG. Paraneoplastic syndromes associated with lung cancer. *Mayo Clin Proc*. 1993;68:278.
    An excellent general review including mechanisms, diagnosis, and treatment.
29. Richardson GE, Johnson BE. Paraneoplastic syndromes in lung cancer. *Curr Opin Oncol*. 1992;4:323.
    Reviews recent literature on humoral hypercalcemia, autoimmune paraneoplastic syndromes, and cancer cachexia.
30. Rosen SW, Becker CE, Schlaff S, et al. Ectopic gonadotropin production before clinical recognition of bronchogenic carcinoma. *N Engl J Med*. 1968;279:640.
    Gynecomastia appeared 1 year before the discovery of the carcinoma.
31. Sack G, Levin J, Bell W. Trousseau's syndrome and other manifestations of chronic disseminated coagulopathy in patients with neoplasm. *Medicine* (Baltimore). 1977;56:1.
    In this review of 182 cases, 20% were associated with lung cancer, second only to pancreatic carcinoma (24%).
32. Sarlani E, Schwartz AH, Greenspan JD, et al. Facial pain as first manifestation of lung cancer: a case of lung cancer-related cluster headache and a review of the literature. *J Orofac Pain*. 2003;17:262–267.
    A summary of 32 cases of facial pain suggesting that with atypical or refractory facial pain, should include lung cancer in the possible etiologies.
33. Schiller JH, Jones JC. Paraneoplastic syndromes associated with lung cancer. *Curr Opin Oncol*. 1993;5:335.
    Reviews recent advances in the diagnosis and treatment of endocrinologic and neurologic manifestations of lung cancer syndromes.
34. Seyberth HW, Segre GV, Morgan JL, et al. Prostaglandins as mediators of hypercalcemia associated with certain types of cancer. *N Engl J Med*. 1975;293:1278.
    An increased urinary level of a prostaglandin metabolite was associated with hypercalcemia that was reversed by prostaglandin inhibitors.
35. Silva OL, Becker KL, Primack A, et al. Ectopic secretion of calcitonin by oat-cell carcinoma. *N Engl J Med*. 1974;290:1122.
    The patients were not symptomatic, and their calcium levels were normal.

36. Yatura S, Harrara E, Nopajaroonsri C, et al. Gynecomastia attributable to human chorionic gonadotropin-secreting giant cell carcinoma of lung. *Endocr Pract.* 2003;9:233–235.
    hCG-secreting carcinoma can present as painful gynecomastia, which responds to treatment of the tumor.

106. SOLITARY PULMONARY NODULE

Henri G. Colt

A *solitary pulmonary nodule* (SPN) is a well-circumscribed spherical lesion completely surrounded by aerated lung and not associated with atelectasis or adenopathy. Often inappropriately referred to as *coin lesions,* SPNs are not pleural or mediastinal based. Although no consensus exists as to the upper limit of size, most authors agree that true SPNs are less than 3 cm in diameter, differentiating SPN from a solitary mass lesion, which has a greater likelihood of being malignant. At present, it is felt that 1 out of every 500 chest radiographs demonstrates a lung nodule, and more than 150,000 patients per year in the United States see physicians because of incidental findings of lung nodules on imaging studies. Much effort, therefore, has been spent trying to determine which SPNs can be safely observed and which require diagnostic interventions or thoracotomy with resection.

ETIOLOGY AND PATHOPHYSIOLOGY

Cancer or granulomatous disease (e.g., tuberculosis, coccidioidomycosis, and histoplasmosis) cause most SPNs. Bronchogenic carcinoma presents as SPN in 10 to 20% of instances. Most of these are adenocarcinomas, although squamous cell carcinoma, bronchioalveolar cell carcinoma, carcinoid tumors, and even small-cell carcinomas can also present as SPNs. Approximately 5% of SPNs represent metastases from cancer in other organs including colon, breast, kidney, testicle, bone sarcoma, or malignant melanoma. These findings have prompted the "when in doubt, cut it out" approach to SPNs and underscore the importance of prompt evaluation and management, especially in patients with risk factors (e.g., smoking) or a previous history of cancer.

Benign SPNs are usually granulomatous from tuberculous or fungal infection. *Pneumocystis carinii* infection can also appear nodular, as can viral infections (e.g., cytomegalovirus). Less common causes include resolving pneumonia, pulmonary infarction, lung abscess, hamartomas, Kaposi sarcoma, pulmonary arteriovenous malformation, pulmonary contusion, pulmonary sequestration, Wegener's granulomatosis, mucoid impaction, and bronchogenic cysts. Although more than 50% of SPNs are benign, the watchful waiting approach is usually not adopted before completing careful examination of imaging studies and analysis of the nodule's probability for malignancy. Bronchoscopic or percutaneous diagnostic procedures are usually indicated, especially if the likelihood of neoplasm is high and results will affect management. Patients must be encouraged to participate in the decision-making process.

CLINICAL PRESENTATION

Four clinical features are usually cited that increase the likelihood that a SPN is benign: (1) absence of growth of the nodule over a 2-year period; (2) absence of risk factors for cancer; (3) presence of calcium in characteristic patterns on imaging studies; and (4) age less than 35 years. Nonsmoking, younger patients living in areas endemic for fungal disease are more likely to have benign nodules. Risks for malignancy increase with age, smoking history, and nodule size, although the probability for malignancy cannot be accurately based on any single characteristic. A careful history and physical examination are essential and should include smoking and occupational history, history of cancer, and careful inquiry regarding the patient's known place of residence and travel (especially to areas endemic for histoplasmosis or coccidioidomycosis). Unexplained hypoxemia may suggest arteriovenous malformation. Pulmonary function studies are useful to assess the potential risk of thoracotomy. Sputum cytology is usually not helpful. Skin tests and serologies can be helpful if tuberculosis or fungal diseases are suspected, especially in endemic areas.

DIAGNOSIS

Initial assessment of an SPN is usually made with a posteroanterior and lateral chest radiograph. Unfortunately, the shape, location, and margins of the lesion or the presence of cavitation are unreliable for differentiating malignant from benign SPNs. Lobulation and larger size tend to be associated with malignancy, although these characteristics are not definitive. Only two features—calcification and growth rate—can be used with some degree of confidence to predict a benign lesion. An SPN can be assumed to be benign if calcifications fit one of four distinct patterns: (1) central calcification; (2) ring or halo pattern; (3) diffusely speckled calcification; or (4) dense, irregular pattern termed *popcorn calcification*. Comparison of recent chest radiographs with previous ones is necessary and very helpful. Up to 10% of SPNs may be seen only or better on the lateral view. Fluoroscopy can be used to differentiate SPN from other opacities (e.g., a nipple shadow). Computed tomography (CT) scans, particularly thin-section studies, have been shown to be cost effective and have greater sensitivity than conventional tomography. CT scanning has become commonplace in the routine evaluation of SPNs. In fact, SPNs are often detected when patients undergo CT scanning for other purposes such as evaluation of an illness, a staging procedure, or a screening test as part of a routine health examination. If no calcifications are seen on CT, nodule density compared with a densitometry phantom (density ~185 Hounsfield units) may help to detect calcifications in otherwise indeterminate nodules. For example, up to 25% of hamartomas have CT evidence of calcification. In addition, many hamartomas are partially composed of CT-visible fat-density tissue. Small, eccentric calcifications within a SPN do not ensure benignity because this pattern can be found in scar carcinoma.

If malignancy is suspected, the CT scan assists in staging the mediastinum and upper abdomen. CT is more sensitive than chest radiography and may identify multiple pulmonary nodules when only one is suspected. Chest CT, therefore, should be performed in patients with an SPN who are candidates for cancer resection, particularly if resection of known metastatic nodules is being considered. Low-dose spiral or helical CT (single breath hold, entire lung volume scanning) techniques provide an opportunity to diagnose lung cancer at an early stage. Nodules that resolve with or without antibiotics and nodules less than 5 mm in diameter are more likely to be benign. It is also noteworthy, however, that nodules with doubling times of 6 to 12 weeks can be detected by volumetric assessments even when a change in size is not apparent on standard CT. The potential of using spiral CT in addition to sputum cytology for early lung cancer screening is still debated. Another exciting diagnostic modality is dynamic positron emission tomography (PET). At least one meta-analysis has shown that sensitivity and specificities of this noninvasive diagnostic modality in detecting malignancy are approximately 97% and 78%, respectively. Differentiation of benign from malignant lesions is achieved by qualitative or quantitative analysis of glucose metabolism of tissues. Results depend, however, on the generation of scanner used. Performance of scanners appears to be similar for nodules measuring at least 10 mm in diameter. The clinical utility of Fluorodeoxyglucose-Positron Emission Tomography (FDG-PET) is unclear. For low-risk patients with SPN, normal (no uptake) PET has a high negative predictive value. For patients with an SPN who are marginal surgical candidates, a negative PET warrants repeat CT scanning again in 3 months. Most noteworthy, however, is that FDG-PET is more accurate than CT in detecting regional lymph node metastases, which may occur in 21% of stage T1 lung cancer!

Tissue diagnosis usually requires flexible bronchoscopy or percutaneous procedures. Bronchoscopy with washings, brushings, and biopsy under fluoroscopic guidance has a yield of 40 to 80%, and complications are infrequent (<2%). Yield decreases when nodules are less than 2 cm in diameter. A *positive bronchus* sign (evidence of a bronchus leading to the nodule) seen on CT scan may indicate a higher diagnostic yield for bronchoscopy. Bronchoscopy also allows airway inspection and detection of otherwise unrecognizable endobronchial disease. Yield is increased by using transbronchial needle aspiration (TBNA). Bronchoscopy for biopsy of the nodule is usually not indicated if nodules are less than 2 cm in diameter.

Percutaneous procedures include transthoracic needle aspiration (TTNA) under fluoroscopic, ultrasound, or CT guidance. Yield is greater (80–95%), but so are complications (pneumothorax in 25%). Also, false-negative results can occur in up to 30% of cases. A central location and lung hyperinflation increase the risk of pneumothorax. TTNA is particularly helpful in smaller peripheral nodules that are more difficult to reach by bronchoscopy and with a strong suggestion of a granulomatous cause. A nonspecific or nondiagnostic (normal) TTNA requires careful clinical and radiographic follow-up, and does not preclude surgical resection. If a malignancy is diagnosed by TTNA, bronchoscopy should probably be performed to evaluate the central airways and to sample mediastinal nodes, especially if the chest radiograph or CT scan suggests enlarged lymph nodes, Tumor can be diagnosed in up to 50% of enlarged nodes by bronchoscopic needle aspiration, thereby sparing some patients a thoracotomy. Overall, many experts believe that bronchoscopic needle aspiration is underutilized, probably because of insufficient exposure to the procedure during pulmonary specialty training.

MANAGEMENT

Management goals in patients with SPN include limiting the number of unnecessary thoracotomies for benign disease and expediting potential curative lung resection in patients with malignancy. Much controversy persists, however, regarding optimal diagnostic evaluation. Some decision analysis studies suggest watchful waiting when the probability for malignancy is less than 5% or the risk of surgery is high. Again, the importance of risk factors (e.g., smoking or asbestos exposure) or the presence of systemic symptoms possibly related to cancer (e.g., weight loss, hemoptysis, new cough, or change in the pattern of chronic cough) must be emphasized. Although specific symptoms may not be caused by the SPN per se, radiographically occult processes may be discovered. A careful physical examination to exclude melanoma or testicular carcinoma is important before adopting a conservative approach. When the watchful waiting approach is advocated, repeat chest radiographs should probably be obtained at least every 2 to 3 months for the first year. Increasingly, experts recommend repeat CT scanning rather than chest radiographs for patient follow-up.

Although survival appears inversely proportional to nodule size, no studies have demonstrated decreased survival with a few months of careful observation. Therefore, management decisions can probably be safely postponed until old radiographs or CT scans are obtained for review. Patients with recent chest-wall trauma or pneumonia may warrant a few weeks of observation to see if lesions resolve. If a lesion has been stable for 2 or more years, further diagnostic evaluation probably can be avoided unless the patient is symptomatic. If patients have an SPN, are marginal surgical candidates, and the nodule is unchanged on chest radiograph or CT, and PET is negative, follow-up CT scanning might still be warranted at 3, 6, 9, 12, and 24 months.

Moving from a watchful waiting approach toward intervention is often based on change in appearance or growth of the SPN. The growth rate of a SPN can be determined by measuring its doubling time (DT), which refers to doubling of volume, not diameter. DT is derived from the formula for a sphere: $V = 4\ r^3$, where V = volume and r = radius. A very slow (>2 years) or very fast (<7 days) DT suggests benignity. Growth assessment, however, is difficult. For example, a 1-cm nodule that doubles in volume only increases 26% in diameter.

Immediate thoracotomy for a SPN has been advocated as an alternative approach, although there is some risk in resecting a SPN with surgical mortality reported as high as 4% in patients at higher risk. In carefully selected patients, video-assisted thoracoscopic surgery (VATS) may be used, but this technique precludes precise manual palpation of lung parenchyma and nodules not seen on CT scan can be missed. In some instances, CT or ultrasound guidance is used to insert a guidewire to facilitate thoracoscopic detection. When compared with bronchoscopy or percutaneous needle aspiration, thoracoscopy is virtually 100% sensitive and 100% specific, offering an excellent, albeit expensive alternative. Additional prospective studies comparing thoracoscopic wedge resection with standard resection by thoracotomy for cure of bronchogenic carcinoma are necessary before VATS is adopted generally for more than diagnosis. Nevertheless, many agree that, in experienced hands, VATS is associated with less postoperative pain than traditional thoracotomy. Also, stapled lobectomy for curative resection is possible and easily combined with lymph node sampling. All pulmonary resections for lung cancer must include a systematic lymph node dissection.

Three clinical situations demand special consideration. First, in patients without tissue diagnosis after bronchoscopy and TTNA, cancer cannot be excluded, and it is probably best to proceed to resection. The impact of a negative FDG-PET scan in this setting was described previously. If surgical risk is high or the suspicion of malignancy is low, lesions can be followed by serial chest radiographs at least every 2 to 3 months for 1 year and every 4 to 6 months for the second year (although experts increasingly recommend serial CT scans at 3, 6, 9, 12, and 24 months) or longer until any suspicion that the nodule is a slow-growing malignancy has been alleviated. Informing patients and families of all diagnostic and therapeutic options and encouraging their participation in the clinical decision-making process are essential.

The second special situation is when a biopsy or needle aspiration of an SPN reveals small-cell carcinoma. Although uncommon, small-cell carcinomas presenting as an SPN appear to have a better prognosis than the standard type. Stage I tumors have had a 5-year survival rate of 35% when treated by resection alone. Before surgical resection, however, the possibility of distant metastasis must be excluded. Postoperative adjuvant chemotherapy has also been advocated.

The third special situation is when a SPN occurs in a patient with a history of malignancy. Tissue diagnosis is usually required because conclusive evidence of metastatic disease dictates further therapy. Pulmonary metastatectomy favorably influences survival, especially in patients with soft tissue sarcoma or melanoma. In patients with a history of cancer, an SPN should never be presumed to be metastatic. Indeed, there is a 50% likelihood that a new SPN is either benign or a different, treatable primary malignancy. Metastatic disease is more likely if (1) the known primary tumor is an adenocarcinoma; (2) the lung lesion appears within 12 months after treatment of the primary tumor; (3) the patient is young and a nonsmoker; and (4) the primary tumor was associated with metastatic lymphadenopathy. In the absence of known extrapulmonary malignancy, the SPN proves to be a metastasis in fewer than 5% of cases.

PROGNOSIS

Patients undergoing pulmonary metastatectomy have a 5-year survival rate of 20 to 30%, as long as the primary tumor has been controlled and no other evidence is seen of other metastases. The prognosis of bronchogenic carcinoma presenting as an SPN, particularly T1N0M0 disease, is very good, justifying a vigorous diagnostic approach in patients at high risk.

1. Baaklini WA, Reinoso MA, Gorin AB, et al. Diagnostic yield of fiberoptic bronchoscopy in evaluating solitary pulmonary nodules. *Chest.* 2000;117:1049–1054.
   Yield decreases with nodules of decreasing size.
2. Batra P, Brown K, Aberle DR, et al. Imaging techniques in the evaluation of pulmonary parenchymal neoplasms. *Chest.* 1992;101:239.
   A summary of the current roles of chest radiographs, CT scans, and magnetic resonance imaging in the evaluation of pulmonary opacities.
3. Collard JM, Reymond MA. Video-assisted thoracic surgery (VATS) for cancer. Risk of parietal seeding and of early local recurrence. *Int Surg.* 1996;81:343.
   Special precautions should be used (such as enveloping specimens in an endobag) before removal through the intercostal tissues.
4. Cummings SR. Estimating the probability of malignancy in solitary pulmonary nodules: Bayesian approach. *Am Rev Respir Dis.* 1986;134:449.

Provides a table of likelihood ratios and a formula to determine the risk of cancer in an individual patient. This information may be useful in deciding on a conservative or aggressive approach to diagnosis.

5. Cummings SR, Lillington GA, Richard RJ, et al. Managing solitary pulmonary nodules: the choice of strategy is a "close call." *Am Rev Respir Dis.* 1986;134:453.

    Decision analysis is applied to the evaluation of SPNs, taking into consideration risks of procedure, treatment, and delayed treatment. The authors suggest that patients should play an active role in the decision-making process.

6. Goldberg SK, Walkenstein MD, Steinbach A, et al. The role of staging bronchoscopy and the pre-operative assessment of a solitary pulmonary nodule. *Chest.* 1993;104:94.

    A retrospective review of 33 cases. No evidence of endobronchial disease was seen in 23 patients with malignant, asymptomatic SPNs. The authors advocate abandonment of routine staging fiberoptic bronchoscopy in patients with indeterminate SPNs.

7. Gould MK, Maclean CC, Kuschner WG, et al. Accuracy of positron emission tomography for diagnosis of pulmonary nodules and mass lesions. *JAMA.* 2001;285:914–924.

    Essential meta-analysis of data sources from 1966–200 using MEDLINE and CANCERLIT to estimate diagnostic accuracy of FDG-PET for malignant focal pulmonary nodules.

8. Gupta N, Gill H, Graeber G, et al. Dynamic positron emission tomography with F-18 fluorodeoxyglucose imaging in differentiation of benign from malignant lung/mediastinal lesions. *Chest.* 1998;114:1105.

    Distinct time–activity curve patterns were identified in malignant and benign lesions. Continued uptake is noted in malignant lesions, suggesting a role for PET scanning in patients with equivocal findings on other imaging studies.

9. Henschke CI, McCauley DJ, Yankelevitz DF, et al. Early Lung Cancer Action Project: overall design and findings from baseline screening. *Lancet.* 1999;354:99.

    Using helical CT scanning in a prospective study of 1,000 smokers, investigators detected noncalcified nodules in 233 (23%); 27 of these (12%) were subsequently found to have lung cancer. Only 7 of these 27 cancers were visible on chest radiographs.

10. Huston J III, Muhm JR. Solitary pulmonary nodules: evaluation with a CT reference phantom. *Radiology.* 1989;170:653.

    Describes techniques and use of reference phantoms.

11. Khan JH, McElhinney DB, Rahman SB, et al. Pulmonary metastases of endocrine origin: the role of surgery. *Chest.* 1998;114:526.

    Patients with carcinoid, thyroid, pheochromocytoma, and parathyroid tumors with pulmonary metastases should undergo surgical resection in cases of good control of the primary tumor, no evidence of extrathoracic disease, and satisfactory lung function.

12. Lewis RJ, Caccavale RJ, Sisler GE, et al. One hundred video-assisted thoracic surgical simultaneously stapled lobectomies without rib spreading. *Ann Thorac Surg.* 1997;63:1415.

    For lesions ranging from 1.5 to 8 cm, stapled lobectomy through VATS had results similar to those obtained from open surgical techniques. Hospitalization was less than 3 days on average.

13. Levine MS, Weiss JM, Harrell JH, et al. Transthoracic needle aspiration biopsy following negative fiberoptic bronchoscopy in solitary pulmonary nodules. *Chest.* 1988;93:1152.

    Authors suggest that nondiagnostic TTNA is more likely to occur with a benign rather than a malignant SPN and state that this procedure cannot be the decisive factor in opting for or against definitive resection.

14. Libby DM, Smith JP, Altorki NK, et al. Managing the small pulmonary nodule discovered by CT. *Chest.* 2004;125:1522–1529.

    Prospective, noncomparative study of smokers without prior malignancy also includes a review of the literature of CT screening and lung cancer.

15. Lillington GA. Management of solitary pulmonary nodules. *Dis Mon.* 1991;37:274.

A careful review of SPNs, with a description of several decision analysis studies suggesting the importance of patients' wishes regarding management strategies.

16. O'Keefe ME Jr, Good CA, McDonald JR, et al. Calcification in solitary nodules of the lung. *AJR*. 1957;77:1023.

    Benign patterns of calcification are described. Eccentric calcifications can occur in malignant lesions.

17. Mack MJ, Hazelrigg SR, Landreneau RJ, et al. Thoracoscopy for the diagnosis of the indeterminate solitary pulmonary nodule. *Ann Thorac Surg*. 1993;56:825.

    A multi-institutional review of 242 patients with SPNs undergoing thoracoscopic excisional biopsy as the primary diagnostic method. A definite diagnosis was obtained in all patients. A fine discussion follows the references, bringing to light several areas of controversy regarding this procedure.

18. McCormack PM, Ginsberg KB, Bains MS, et al. Accuracy of lung imaging in metastases with implications for the role of thoracoscopy. *Ann Thorac Surg*. 1993;56:863.

    A retrospective study in which CT scans differed from pathologic findings in 42% of patients (18 patients had more cancers than CT reported). Because thoracoscopy does not allow manual palpation of the lung to locate lesions not seen on the lung surface, the validity of using thoracoscopic resection as a definitive procedure is questioned.

19. Naidich DP, Sussman R, Kutcher WL, et al. Solitary pulmonary nodules: CT-bronchoscopic correlation. *Chest*. 1988;93:595.

    A retrospective review of 65 patients undergoing thin-section CT scanning, which reports the value of a positive bronchus sign. Of the patients with positive bronchus sign, 60% were diagnosed bronchoscopically.

20. Swensen SJ. An integrated approach to evaluation of a solitary pulmonary nodule. *Mayo Clin Proc*. 1990;65:173.

    A fine review that also addresses TNM staging. Many references are provided.

21. Reichenberger F, Weber J, Tamm M, et al. The value of transbronchial needle aspiration in the diagnosis of peripheral pulmonary lesions. *Chest*. 1999;116:704.

    In this retrospective study of 172 patients (126 with malignant disease), TBNA increased the diagnostic yield of bronchoscopy from 35% to 51%.

22. Tan BB, Flaherty KR, Kazerooni EA, et al. The solitary pulmonary nodule. *Chest*. 2003;123:89S–96S.

    Includes recommendations for imaging modalities and obtaining tissue preoperatively based on review of current literature.

23. Tschernko EM, Hofer S, Bieglmayes C, et al. Early postoperative stress: video assisted wedge resection/lobectomy vs conventional axillary thoracotomy. *Chest*. 1996;109:1636.

    In this study of 22 patients undergoing VATS and 25 undergoing axillary thoracotomy for pulmonary nodule, less postoperative pain and better oxygenation were noted in the VATS group.

---

107. MEDIASTINAL MASS

Stephen P. Bradley

PATHOPHYSIOLOGY

A variety of benign and malignant processes can present as a mediastinal mass. The differential diagnosis requires knowledge of normal mediastinal anatomy. The mediastinum can be divided into three compartments based on the lateral chest radiograph. The *anterior mediastinum* is bounded by the thoracic inlet superiorly, the sternum anteriorly, and the anterior pericardium posteriorly. It contains the upper esophagus and trachea, thymus, aortic arch, adipose tissue, and lymphatics. The *middle* or *visceral mediastinum* holds the pericardium and its contents, the low trachea, carina, main bronchi, and associated lymph nodes. The *posterior mediastinum* reaches from the posterior pericardium to the anterior vertebral column and posterior ribs, including the paravertebral gutters. It contains the esophagus, descending aorta, sympathetic ganglia, and peripheral nerves.

DIAGNOSIS

The differential diagnosis is based primarily on the location of the mediastinal mass. Approximately one half of mediastinal masses arise in the anterior compartment. These include thymomas, germ-cell neoplasms, lymphomas; cysts of pericardial, bronchogenic, or thymic origin; and intrathoracic goiters. Much less common are mesenchymal tumors (lipomas, fibromas, lymphangiomas, hemangiomas, cystic hygromas, and their malignant counterparts), carcinoma of unknown primary, and angiofollicular lymphoid hyperplasia (Castleman's disease).

ETIOLOGY

Mass lesions of the middle mediastinum (18–25% of total) include pericardial, bronchogenic, or enteric cysts; lymphomas, granulomatous lesions (tuberculosis, sarcoidosis, or histoplasmosis); carcinoma; and mesenchymal tumors. Metastatic carcinoma to the middle mediastinum is frequent, but in almost all cases the site of the primary tumor is apparent.

Of the 23 to 27% of mediastinal masses that arise in the posterior compartment, approximately three fourths are neural in origin. Other mass lesions of the posterior mediastinum include cysts, alimentary tract duplications, intrathoracic thyroid, pheochromocytomas, and ectopic thymus.

The most common mediastinal tumors vary from series to series. In children, neural tumors lead in frequency (33%), followed by lymphomas (14%), teratomas (10%), thymic masses (8.5%), bronchogenic cysts (7.5%), enteric cysts (7.0%), angiomatous tumors (6.8%), and inflammatory nodal masses (4.4%). The frequency of malignancy in mediastinal mass lesions in children (up to age 16) is approximately 50%.

Large series involving mostly adult patients report widely varying frequencies of different mediastinal lesions. By combining 13 reported studies involving 2,399 patients, the following mean (and range) percentage rates for mediastinal lesions are derived: neurogenic tumors, 20.7% (14–36%); thymoma, 19.1% (10–27%); cyst, 18.3% (0–26%); lymphoma, 12.5% (5–23%); germ cell neoplasm, 10.0% (5–29%); endocrine tumor, 6.4% (0–23%); mesenchymal tumor, 6.0% (0–11%); primary carcinoma, 4.6% (0–23%); and miscellaneous masses, 2.4% (1–14%).

CLINICAL PRESENTATION

Approximately one half of mediastinal masses are discovered incidentally on chest roentgenogram. Malignant lesions of all types are much more likely to be symptomatic on presentation than benign lesions. Signs and symptoms, which usually result from a mass effect on surrounding structures, include dyspnea, cough, wheezing, hemoptysis, chest pain, dysphagia, superior vena cava syndrome, and Horner's syndrome. Neural tumors with an intraspinal component (dumbbell tumors) can cause cord compression. Lymphoma may present with fever, weight loss or night sweats.

The appearance of a mediastinal mass on posteroanterior and lateral chest roentgenograms can narrow the differential diagnosis by localizing the lesion to a certain mediastinal compartment. Computed tomography (CT) is useful in more precisely localizing and defining the extent of the mass and can help determine the best approach for biopsy. With some masses (e.g., intrathoracic goiter and mature teratomas), a confident diagnosis can be made based on CT findings. When intravenous contrast is used, CT scanning can distinguish vascular lesions (e.g., congenital vascular rings, enlarged pulmonary arteries, double vena cavae, and aortic aneurysms) that can mimic mediastinal masses. Other masqueraders that can usually be ruled out by CT include diaphragmatic hernias, anterior meningoceles, and pulmonary lobar sequestration. The primary role of magnetic resonance imaging (MRI) has been as a problem-solving device, especially when results of CT have been equivocal. Advantages of MRI include the lack of ionizing radiation, the ability to image in virtually any plane (useful when imaging masses in the aorticopulmonary window and paraspinal areas), and the ability to differentiate blood vessels from soft tissues without the use of intravenous contrast. In addition, MRI is the technique of choice in evaluating posterior mediastinal masses thought to be neurogenic because it can determine whether there is extension into the spinal canal, precluding the need for a myelogram. ^{123}I thyroid scintigraphy is useful in defining the nature and extent of substernal thyroid tissue. A positive gallium scan suggests that a mediastinal mass is caused by lymphoma or seminoma. PET-FDG scanning is also usually positive in metabolically active malignancies (lymphoma, seminoma), but is less likely to be positive with slowly growing malignancies (thymoma). In addition, false-positive results of Fluorodeoxyglucose-Positron Emission Tomography (FDG-PET) scanning may be seen in granulomatous diseases.

DIAGNOSIS

The radiographic appearance of a mediastinal mass rarely provides a diagnosis. Testing for serum β-human chorionic gonadotropin (hCG) and α-fetoprotein (AFP) is indicated for anterior mediastinal masses in young men in whom germ cell tumors are most common. Anti-acetylcholinesterase receptor antibodies should be measured when thymoma is suspected. The results of transthoracic fine-needle aspiration vary between series. The sensitivity for diagnosing malignancy is reported to be as high as 90%, but a precise tissue diagnosis is made in only 60 to 80% of patients. The diagnosis of lymphoma and thymoma can be particularly difficult on fine-needle aspiration specimens. Cervical mediastinoscopy (for anterior mediastinal masses) and anterior thoracotomy (for masses in the aorticopulmonary window) can often provide sufficient tissue for a specific diagnosis. Bronchoscopy with transcarinal needle aspiration may lead to a diagnosis of a subcarinal mass; ultrasound-guided bronchoscopic biopsy of an anterior and middle mediastinal mass also has been reported to be helpful in obtaining a diagnosis.

The purpose of biopsy is to provide a diagnosis (e.g., lymphoma, seminoma, or metastatic carcinoma) for which resection is not the primary treatment modality. In the remaining patients, diagnosis is made at exploratory thoracotomy, thoracoscopy (video-assisted thoracic surgery), or median sternotomy. Caution must be used when subjecting patients with large mediastinal masses to general anesthesia. These patients are at risk of developing airway compromise because of tracheobronchial compression. The greatest risk is in children, in whom the degree of respiratory symptoms is not a reliable predictor of the degree of tracheobronchial compromise. For patients in whom preoperative CT scan demonstrates greater than one third compression of the airway, it may be necessary to avoid the supine position, use spontaneous ventilation, and occasionally perform cardiopulmonary bypass.

Between 20 and 30% of neural tumors are malignant; three fourths of these occur in children. Thus, adult neural tumors are almost all benign. In adults, the most common neural tumors are schwannomas (neurilemomas), which arise from the Schwann's cells that sheath nerve cell axons, and neurofibromas, which arise from nerve sheath fibrous tissue. Rarely, malignant degeneration of both schwannomas and neurofibromas can occur; prior irradiation or neurofibromatosis each increases that risk. In contrast, most (50–60%) neural tumors in children are malignant. Neuroblastomas, arising from peripheral nerve cells, are the most frequent mediastinal tumor in children. These highly aggressive tumors are usually diagnosed in children before age 3. Ganglioneuromas (benign) and ganglioneuroblastomas (malignant) arising from sympathetic ganglia are also common in children. More than 50% of neural tumors are found incidentally on chest radiograph. Rib and vertebral changes seen on x-ray film may be caused by pressure phenomena and do not necessarily connote malignancy. Benign neural tumors are treated definitively by surgical excision; dumbbell tumors require combined thoracotomy and laminectomy as a one-step operation. Postoperative radiation therapy is given for malignant lesions.

Mediastinal developmental cysts are nearly always benign and, except in infants and young children, are usually asymptomatic at presentation. Bronchial cysts are most often found in the middle mediastinum near the tracheal bifurcation but can be found in all three compartments. They rarely communicate with the tracheobronchial tree.

Pericardial cysts typically occur in the anterior cardiophrenic angle, most often on the right. A small minority communicate with the pericardial space. Esophageal cysts, the least common, are found in either the posterior or middle mediastinum. Because two thirds of patients with foregut (bronchial and esophageal) cysts eventually develop symptoms, treatment is usually recommended. Simple aspiration of the cyst may lead to resolution; surgical resection is definitive therapy. Pericardial cysts rarely become symptomatic and can be managed expectantly.

Thymomas are the most common anterior mediastinal mass. Four cell types are seen: lymphocytic, epithelial, spindle, and mixed. All thymomas are considered to be malignant neoplasms because of their tendency to invade local structures. The majority (55–65% of total) are found at surgery to be contained within a thick fibrous capsule; surgical removal is considered curative, although 2 to 12% recur, necessitating long-term radiographic follow-up. Invasive thymomas are defined by invasion through the capsule and typically spread locally. Therapy consists of surgical excision (if possible) and postoperative radiation therapy. Prolonged survival in patients with locally advanced disease has been described, emphasizing the indolent nature of these tumors. Parathymic syndromes occur in up to 50% of patients with benign or invasive thymoma. Myasthenia gravis occurs in 30 to 50% of all thymomas (15% of patients with myasthenia gravis have thymoma); resolution after thymectomy occurs in approximately 25% of patients, particularly in young women. Thymomas have also been associated with pure red cell aplasia (5% of patients) and hypogammaglobulinemia (10%). Thymic carcinoma (distinguished by cellular atypia, early local invasion, and distant metastases), thymic carcinoid, thymolipoma, and thymic cysts are uncommon causes of anterior mediastinal masses.

Of patients with lymphoma, 5 to 10% present with primary mediastinal masses. These patients often have massive mediastinal adenopathy; they are treated with combined radiation therapy and chemotherapy, thereby obviating the need for staging laparotomy and the risk of airway compromise. Survival rates of up to 75% are reported in mediastinal Hodgkin's disease treated with chemotherapy with or without radiation therapy. Non-Hodgkin's lymphoma (lymphocytic, histiocytic, mixed) is associated with a poorer prognosis, despite the use of aggressive chemotherapeutic regimens. Gallium and PET-FDG scanning are useful in following response to treatment of lymphoma because they distinguish residual disease from scar tissue.

The anterior mediastinum is the most common extragonadal site for *germ cell neoplasms*, which typically present in the third decade of life. They can be divided into dermoids (only an epithelial layer present) and teratoids (all three germ layers present). Of dermoids, 10 to 15% are malignant, as are 15 to 40% of teratomas. Dermoids are usually cystic; teratomas can be cystic (usually benign) or solid (usually malignant). Surgical excision is curative for benign germ cell tumors. More than 90% of malignant teratomas (seminoma, teratocarcinoma, embryonal cell carcinoma, entodermal sinus tumors) occur in men. Choriocarcinomas are associated with gynecomastia in at least half of cases and with tumor production of hCG in 100% of cases, whereas AFP is present in 97% of entodermal sinus (yolk sac) tumors. Low levels of hCG are produced by approximately 10% of seminomas. Results of therapy for seminoma have improved significantly with the use of aggressive combination chemotherapy followed by surgical excision of residual tumor; the prognosis for nonseminomatous germ cell tumors remains poor.

A syndrome of poorly differentiated carcinoma occurring in young men with mediastinal masses has been described. Serum assays for hCG and AFP are often negative; however, further evaluation has revealed that a subset of these patients have extragonadal germ cell tumors and respond to appropriate chemotherapy.

---

1. Abebonojo SA, Nicola ML. Teratoid tumors of the mediastinum. *Am Surg.* 1976; 42:361.

A clear summary of different elements within the classification of teratoid tumors of the mediastinum.

2. Besznyak I, Sebesteny M, Kurchar F. Primary mediastinal seminoma. *J Thorac Cardiovasc Surg*. 1973;65:930.

   A literature review of all mediastinal seminomas reported up to 1973.

3. Cohen AJ, Thompson L, Edwards FH, et al. Primary cysts and tumors of the mediastinum. *Ann Thorac Surg* 1991;51:378.

   A large series over 45 years, emphasizes the change in preoperative evaluation and operative approach over that time.

4. Hyson EA, Ravin CE. Radiographic features of mediastinal anatomy. *Chest*. 1979;75:609.

   Describes normal mediastinal structures visible on posteroanterior and lateral chest films.

5. Richardson RL, Schoumacher RA, Fer MF, et al. The unrecognized extragonadal germ-cell cancer syndrome. *Ann Intern Med*. 1981;94:181.

   Describes a syndrome of mediastinal masses occurring principally in young men. Patients are frequently diagnosed initially as having undifferentiated carcinoma, but further evaluation, including tumor markers, reveals the correct diagnosis.

6. Strollo DC, Rosado de Christenson ML, Jett JR. Primary mediastinal tumors. Part 1: tumors of the anterior mediastinum. *Chest*. 1997;112:511.

   An excellent review of the presentation, prognosis, and management of both common and uncommon anterior mediastinal masses.

7. Strollo DC, Rosado de Christenson ML, Jett JR. Primary mediastinal tumors. Part 2: tumors of the posterior mediastinum. *Chest*. 1997;112:1344.

   An excellent review.

8. Azizkhan RG, Dudgeon DL, Buck JR, et al. Life-threatening airway obstruction as a complication to the management of mediastinal masses in children. *J Pediatr Surg*. 1985;20:816.

   Discusses the value of a CT scan to evaluate tracheobronchial compression in children with mediastinal masses and predicts the risk for total airway obstruction during general anesthesia.

9. Maggi G, Giaccone G, Donadio M, et al. Thymomas. A review of 169 cases, with particular reference to results of surgical treatment. *Cancer*. 1986;58:765.

   A large series emphasizing the importance of tumor invasiveness and degree of excision on prognosis.

10. Batra P, Brown K, Steckel R. Diagnostic imaging techniques in mediastinal malignancies. *Am J Surg*. 1988;156:4.

    Emphasizes the importance of CT in the assessment of mediastinal malignancies. Also has a good discussion of each tumor type.

11. Conkle DM, Adkins Jr RB. Primary malignant tumors of the mediastinum. *Ann Thorac Surg*. 1972;14:553.

    A large experience with malignant mediastinal masses; notes high incidence of symptoms and poor prognosis associated with malignant lesions.

12. Davis RD Jr, Oldham HN Jr, Sabiston DC Jr, et al. Primary cysts and neoplasms of the mediastinum: recent changes in clinical presentation, methods of diagnosis, management, and results. *Ann Thorac Surg*. 1987;44:229.

    A large series spanning 56 years. Emphasizes improved preoperative diagnosis of all lesions and improved survival in patients with Hodgkin's disease and germ cell tumors in recent years.

13. Morrissey HA, Adams H, Gibbs AR, et al. Percutaneous needle biopsy of the mediastinum: review of 94 procedures. *Thorax*. 1993;48:632.

    Fine-needle aspiration is less accurate in diagnosing thymoma, lymphoma, and neural tumors than carcinomatous lesions.

14. Pokorny WJ, Sherman JO. Mediastinal masses in infants and children. *J Thorac Cardiovasc Surg*. 1974;68:869.

    A general review of pediatric cases. More than 50% of patients in this series had malignant lesions.

15. Rubush JL, Gardner IR, Boyd WC, et al. Mediastinal tumors: review of 186 cases. *J Thorac Cardiovasc Surg*. 1973;65:216.

    A fine review of the distribution of mediastinal masses in a general hospital population. Excellent comparative tables review different series from the literature.

16. Salyer DC, Salyer WR, Eggleston JC. Benign developmental cysts of the mediastinum. *Arch Pathol Lab Med*. 1977;101:136.

   A summary of bronchogenic, esophageal, pericardial, and gastroenteric cysts.

17. Weinreb JC, Naidich DP. Thoracic magnetic resonance imaging. *Clin Chest Med*. 1991;12:33.

   Reviews imaging techniques, strengths, and weaknesses of MRI in evaluating thoracic lesions.

18. Suster S, Rosai J. Thymic carcinoma. A clinicopathologic study of 60 cases. *Cancer*. 1991;67:1025.

   In contrast with thymoma, morphologic features (as well as invasiveness) determine prognosis.

19. Akwari OE, Payne WS, Onofrio BM, et al. Dumbbell neurogenic tumors of the mediastinum. Diagnosis and management. *Mayo Clin Proc*. 1978;53:353.

   A large series emphasizing the importance of a combined thoracic surgical and neurosurgical approach to dumbbell tumors.

20. Ribet ME, Cardot GR. Neurogenic tumors of the thorax. *Ann Thorac Surg*. 1994;58:1091.

   Includes both children and adults. Compared with adults, children more often are symptomatic at presentation, have nerve cell (versus nerve sheath) tumors, and have a higher incidence of malignancy.

21. Bukowski RM, Wolf M, Kulander BG, et al. Alternating combination chemotherapy in patients with extra-gonadal germ cell tumors. *Cancer*. 1993;71:2631.

   Aggressive chemotherapy followed by surgical excision of residual tumor resulted in 60% 4-year survival in patients who presented with mediastinal masses.

22. Wychulis AR, Payne WS, Clagett OT, et al. Surgical treatment of mediastinal tumors: a 40-year experience. *J Thorac Cardiovasc Surg*. 1971;62:379.

   From a 40-year Mayo Clinic experience, this is a very representative series with attention to differential diagnoses and therapeutic approaches.

23. Bower RJ, Kiesewetter WB. Mediastinal masses in infants and children. *Arch Surg*. 1977;112:1003.

   Describes a pediatric patient population from a general children's hospital. Frequency of neural tumors emphasized.

24. Cameron TB, et al. Neoplasms of the mediastinum. In: DeVito, Hellman, Rosenberg, eds. *Principles and Practice of Oncology*, 6th ed. Philadelphia: Lippincott Williams & Wilkins; 2000;1024.

   Contains a complete list of the paraneoplastic syndromes associated with thymoma.

25. Newman JS, Francis IR, Kaminski MS, et al. Imaging of lymphoma with PET with 2-(F-18)-fluoro-2-deoxy-D-glucose: correlation with CT. *Radiology*. 1994;190:111.

   Describes the excellent accuracy of PET-FDG scanning in patients with low- and intermediate-grade thoracoabcominal lymphomas.

26. Ferguson MK, Lee E, Skinner DB, et al. Selective operative approach for diagnosis and treatment of anterior mediastinal masses. *Ann Thorac Surg*. 1987;44:583–586.

   Gallium scans were found to be positive in patients with lymphoma and seminoma. The authors found that a positive gallium scan followed by mediastinoscopy to establish diagnosis avoids unnecessary thoracotomy in these patients.

108. NEOPLASTIC DISEASE OF THE PLEURA

Henri G. Colt

ETIOLOGY AND PATHOPHYSIOLOGY

Neoplastic disease of the pleura can be primary, arising from the cellular elements of the pleural surface (e.g., mesothelial tissue), or metastatic, arising from either thoracic or extrathoracic sites. Metastatic pleural tumors comprise most pleural neoplasms, histologically resemble the primary tumor, and are usually associated with a roentgenographically apparent effusion or pleural thickening.

Primary tumors of the pleura are rare and are classified as benign mesotheliomas (i.e., solitary or localized fibrous) or diffuse malignant mesotheliomas. Solitary fibrous tumors of the pleura occur equally in men and women with a peak incidence in the fourth to sixth decades. The tumor is grossly well encapsulated and histologically composed of fibrous elements. The cause is unknown, but similar lesions have been reported as postinflammatory tumors of the pleura, leading to speculation that they are part of a spectrum of mesothelial cell response to a variety of stimuli. Immunohistochemical, ultrastructural, and tissue culture studies previously were felt to support a mesenchymal origin, but most agree now that these tumors are derived from fibroblasts and have the potential for multidirectional differentiation. Tobacco smoking and exposure to asbestos do not appear to increase the risk for any of these tumors.

The pathogenesis of metastatic malignant pleural disease is unclear. Metastatic tumor deposits without pleural effusion are frequently noted at postmortem examinations in patients dying from malignancy; unless extensive, they are clinically undetectable on radiographs or CT scans, although pleural thickening may be noted. These deposits are felt to result from hematogenous spread. The lack of accompanying effusion has prompted some authors to emphasize the role of lymphatic obstruction in the pathogenesis of malignant effusion. In fact, a frequent finding during thoracoscopic inspection of the parietal pleura is swollen lymphatics, particularly along the posterior and inferior costal parietal pleura.

CLINICAL PRESENTATION

Clinically, 30 to 40% of patients with these tumors are asymptomatic at the time of diagnosis; others complain of chest pain, cough, dyspnea, and weight loss in decreasing frequency. The tumors can reach an enormous size. They can be attached to the pleura by a pedicle and lead to a sensation of something moving about in the chest after a positional change. Rarely, they cause lobar collapse or superior vena caval obstruction. Other times, they present as wide-based parietal pleural abnormalities noted on chest radiographs or computed tomography (CT) scans. Infrequently, tumors involve the visceral pleural surface, presenting radiographically as solitary pulmonary nodules.

The physical examination is usually unrewarding but may show evidence of pleural effusion, clubbing (<20%), or osteoarthropathy or arthropathy (<15%), simulating rheumatoid arthritis. The chest roentgenogram usually reveals a localized mass; pleural effusion occurs in fewer than 15% of cases. In some large tumors, hypoglycemia has been reported. Although needle biopsy, pleural fluid cytology, or pleural biopsy may suggest the diagnosis, the definitive diagnosis of solitary fibrous tumors of the pleura usually requires thoracoscopy or thoracotomy. Preoperative differential diagnoses include malignant mesothelioma, metastatic carcinoma, sarcomas, and bizarre pseudotumors related to the organization of a pleural exudate. Surgical resection is usually curative but can be difficult in cases of gross invasion of contiguous vascular, neural, or mediastinal structures. Recurrences may not appear for years following initial resection. Often, the arthropathy disappears with tumor resection but can recur with regrowth. It can then be relieved by further resection.

DIAGNOSIS AND TREATMENT

The most common primary pleural neoplasm is a mesothelioma. It must be distinguished from other neoplasms, such as soft tissue sarcoma and leukemia or lymphoma involving the pleura. Mesothelioma is rare, accounting for less than 1% of all cancer deaths in the general population; however, its incidence is rising because of (1) the delayed effects of an increase in the occupational exposure to asbestos; (2) increased awareness by pathologists of this disease; and (3) more accurate diagnostic methods, such as electron microscopy and immunohistochemistry. Today, it is felt that approximately 2,000 cases are diagnosed yearly in the United States.

Malignant mesotheliomas also occur as primary tumors of the peritoneum and tunica vaginalis of the testes; simultaneous occurrence of pleural mesothelioma with mesothelioma at these other sites has not been described, although patients may have both pleural and peritoneal involvement during the course of their illness. Pathologically, this tumor appears early as single or multiple, small, white or gray lesions; later it may produce a thick, gelatinous, gray–pink sheath enveloping the affected lung. It is noteworthy that thoracoscopic appearance can be misleading. Parietal pleura can appear normal, as is often the case in stage 1A malignant mesothelioma, or appear as a conglomeration of small or large nodules involving parietal, visceral, or both pleural surfaces.

Histologically, tumors are composed of epithelial and mesenchymal (fibrosarcomatous) elements and are classified as epithelial (54%), fibrosarcomatous (21%), or mixed (25%). Epithelial mesotheliomas are the most frequently diagnosed histologic type. Seven types of epithelial mesotheliomas are seen, the most common of which is the tubulopapillary pattern. Sarcomatoid mesotheliomas, which account for approximately 20% of mesotheliomas, are usually positive on keratin staining, unlike most sarcomas. Of epithelial mesotheliomas, 20% produce hyaluronic acid, which can be identified by specific stains. The presence of hyaluronic acid contributes to the increased viscosity often noted in pleural fluid from patients with mesothelioma. Carcinoembryonic antigen (CEA) has been reported as negative in 88% of mesotheliomas. This immunostaining procedure can be helpful in excluding mesothelioma from the diagnosis. Immunohistochemical and ultrastructural analysis of pleural neoplasms can lead to an accurate diagnosis of mesothelioma in most cases, although a careful review of an entire battery of tests often including CEA, *Leu*-M1, and mucicarmine staining, is necessary. Electron microscopy can be helpful when abnormalities such as long, slender microvilli are noted. On rare occasions, diagnosis can only be made retrospectively, after review of the exposure history, clinical history, immunohistochemical stains and ultrastructural analyses, clinical and radiographic progressions of disease (usually one of gradual entrapment of the lung with associated pleural thickening, and dyspnea), and autopsy findings. Increasingly, magnetic resonance imaging and CT scans are used to help accurately stage patients.

The staging system of the International Mesothelioma Interest Group is generally used. Although the pathogenesis of malignant mesothelioma is unclear, asbestos is the single most important causative agent. This conclusion is based on (1) retrospective studies showing a strikingly higher incidence (300×) of malignant mesothelioma among asbestos workers; (2) studies showing a significantly higher incidence of asbestos exposure among new mesothelioma cases versus controls; and (3) direct measurements of significantly increased asbestos fiber content of the lungs of patients with mesothelioma (95%) with respect to controls. A threshold amount of asbestos exposure necessary to induce mesothelioma is unknown but presumed. Cigarette smoking is not a risk factor for malignant mesothelioma, but the addition of smoking to asbestos exposure significantly increases risk for lung cancer. New histologic, biologic, and cellular prognostic factors have been identified. Some of these include microvessel density of tumor specimens, overexpression of COX-2, levels of MIB-1, and the still controversial role for Simian SV40 virus (a DNA virus shown to induce mesothelioma in up 100% of hamsters after intrapleural injection).

Asbestos exposure can occur occupationally, as in textile, shipyard, mining, insulation, and construction industries, or it can occur environmentally, as with persons living near asbestos mines and mills. Significant exposure can also occur when family members of asbestos workers handle the workers' clothing (paraoccupational). Thus, the level of exposure may seem inconsequential and the fiber burden may be less than expected to cause asbestosis. Fiber size can be important in that fibers that are long and thin have been found to be more tumorigenic than shorter, thicker fibers, although all types of asbestos can induce mesotheliomas. The various types of asbestos vary in tumorigenicity. Fibers with the longest length:diameter ratio are the most carcinogenic. It appears that amphiboles, particularly crocidolite (but also amosite, anthrophyllite, tremolite, and actinolite), are more frequently associated with malignancy than serpentine fibers such as chrysotile asbestos.

A direct relationship exists between intensity and duration of exposure with tumor incidence. Intensity of exposure is related inversely to time of presentation. The mean time between exposure and presentation (latency period) is approximately 29 years for factory workers and 48 years for those exposed environmentally. Asbestos fibers are inhaled and deposited at the level of smaller bronchioles and alveoli, where they are ingested by pulmonary alveolar macrophages and coated with a ferrous proteinaceous material. Asbestos fibers are believed to be both promoters and initiators of malignant transformation. Once inhaled, asbestos fibers cannot be destroyed or removed; thus, the lifetime risk for mesothelioma increases over time.

Other nonasbestos causes of mesothelioma are also seen, including naturally occurring fibrous silicate minerals called *erionite*, a fibrous zeolite. Individuals living in small villages in central Turkey where this mineral was used in building materials have had the highest incidence of mesothelioma in the world. Most artificial fibers (e.g., ceramic fibers, glass wool, and rock wool) have not been shown to cause mesothelioma.

In contrast to patients with solitary fibrous tumors of the pleura, almost all patients with malignant mesothelioma are symptomatic at the time of diagnosis, although presentation as an incidental radiographic finding of pleural effusion is increasingly common. Chest pain (43%) of a constant gnawing character is a frequent complaint. Occasionally positional, it is rarely pleuritic in nature. Dyspnea is another frequent symptom (27%), with or without chest pain at presentation. Cough (19%), weight loss (13%), and fever (7%) also occur. Weight loss is a poor prognostic sign.

The physical examination frequently reveals evidence of pleural effusion. Clubbing is infrequent (<5%). Auscultation of the chest may reveal decreased breath sounds unilaterally, coarse crackles, squeaks, or pleuropericardial rubs. Horner's syndrome, hoarseness, or tumor extending through the chest wall in the tract of a previous needle tract or incision site are infrequently noted today. The chest roentgenogram typically reveals either a unilateral pleural effusion, pleural nodularity or thickening, or a localized mass lesion. A massive effusion without mediastinal shift away from the side of the fluid collection should raise suspicions for mesothelioma, especially with a history of asbestos exposure. Rib destruction may be present adjacent to the pleural lesion. Interstitial fibrotic changes or diaphragmatic pleural calcifications suggest prior asbestos exposure and are not indicative of malignant pleural mesothelioma. CT scan may demonstrate pleural calcifications, a distinct pleural mass, invasion of contiguous structures, or abdominal extension not otherwise apparent radiographically.

The tissue diagnosis of malignant mesothelioma can be difficult. Sputum cytology is negative, and bronchoscopy usually reveals no endobronchial lesions, although extrinsic bronchial compression caused by mediastinal pleural thickening, a large pleural effusion, or entrapped lung with volume loss is observed occasionally. The pleural fluid from a thoracentesis is usually straw colored but can be serosanguinous or bloody in 30 to 50% of cases. Typically, the protein level is elevated, ranging from 3.5 to 5.5 g/dL and lactic acid dehydrogenase is high. An elevated concentration of hyaluronic acid has been observed by some investigators; however, it appears to be neither specific nor sensitive for the diagnosis of mesothelioma. The value of pleural fluid cytology is controversial, although many experts believe that cytology is of limited value because benign and malignant mesothelial cells closely resemble each other.

Closed pleural biopsy using a Cope, Abrams, or Trucut biopsy needle may confirm the diagnosis, but usually provides insufficient tissue for a pathologic conclusion. Thoracoscopy, on the other hand, allows complete evacuation of pleural effusion, thorough examination of parietal and visceral pleural surfaces, assessment of lung expandability, and visually guided biopsy of both normal and abnormal appearing areas of the costal and diaphragmatic parietal pleura. Procedures are almost always diagnostic. In addition, if intrapleural chemotherapy is not planned, patients can simultaneously undergo thoracoscopic talc pleurodesis, which is successful in preventing fluid reaccumulation in more than 80% of instances. Rarely, open thoracotomy is necessary for definitive diagnosis, but should probably not be performed unless an open parietal pleural biopsy has been unsuccessful. Sometimes, even after the removal of substantial tissue mass, the pathologist has great difficulty in making a diagnosis.

Major differential diagnoses include adenocarcinoma of the lung, bronchoalveolar cell carcinoma, and metastatic pleural tumors (especially from the pancreas, gastrointestinal tract, and ovary). Of course, mesothelial cell proliferation from a benign inflammatory process also needs to be excluded. The histologic distinction for metastatic adenocarcinoma, at times, is so difficult that diagnosis is based on exclusion of another primary tumor, as well as the gross appearance of the pleural tumor at thoracoscopy or surgery. Electron microscopy can be useful, particularly in excluding bronchoalveolar cell carcinoma and adenocarcinoma from the lung, breast, and upper gastrointestinal tract.

Malignant mesothelioma is an unrelenting, progressively fatal disease. Aggressive surgical resection, radiation therapy, and chemotherapy have all yielded poor results. Newer regimens using combined treatment modalities are under evaluation but have yet to alter the grim prognosis. Novel gene therapy protocols, although initially promising, are still in the experimental stage and have not been shown to alter outcome significantly.

As disease progresses, patients may present with obstruction of the superior or inferior vena cava (or both) or pericardial involvement. Involvement of the soft tissues of the chest cage, ipsilateral lung, contralateral pleura, supraclavicular nodes, and peritoneal cavity is also seen. Distant metastases to bone, liver, or brain rarely occur. The average survival time in most series of mesothelioma is 6 to 12 months after diagnosis and 8 to 14 months after the onset of symptoms.

Metastatic pleural involvement (increasingly referred to as *pleural carcinomatosis*) is the most common form of neoplastic pleural disease. It usually presents as a pleural effusion that can be pathogenically related to visceral or parietal pleural implants, peripheral or mediastinal lymphatic and venous obstruction, thoracic duct obstruction, or a combination of these mechanisms. Tumor lymphatic obstruction, thoracic duct invasion, or both can also result in chylothorax. It is noteworthy that chylothorax is not necessarily milky in appearance. Metastatic pleural carcinomatosis is responsible for 50% of all pleural effusions. The most common neoplastic sources are primary lung (33%), especially adenocarcinoma and undifferentiated cell, breast (21%), and stomach (7%). Other less common primary tumors are those of the ovary, pancreas, liver, kidney, uterus, adrenal glands, testis, larynx, and thyroid. In addition, benign pelvic tumors can be associated with a pleural effusion and ascites (Meigs–Salmon syndrome) that subside following tumor resection.

The clinical manifestations of metastatic pleural tumors relate to the primary neoplastic process and the size of the effusion. Dyspnea can be severe if a large amount of fluid accumulates. Roentgenographically, the findings of mediastinal shift toward the side of the pleural effusion (implying atelectasis), an underlying parenchymal or mediastinal mass, or rib erosions suggest a malignant cause. In many of these cases, flexible bronchoscopy is warranted to exclude bronchial obstruction before performing thoracoscopy or chest tube insertion. The diagnosis of pleural carcinomatosis can be based on evaluation of the pleural fluid, pathologic evaluation of biopsied specimens, or both. Characteristically, the fluid is an exudate and is often blood tinged. In long-standing effusions, the glucose can be low and the pH less than 7.35. The white cell count is typically low and predominantly lymphocytic. Cytologic examination can identify the primary site in up to 70% of cases. Not surprisingly, repeated thoracenteses increase the yield, as the pleural fluid malignant cell burden can increase over time, and as the malignant disease itself progresses.

Closed-needle pleural biopsy yields a diagnosis in up to 50% of cases and, when combined with cytology, in close to 90%. Thoracoscopy almost always makes the diagnosis (the only false-negative findings being in patients with early malignant mesothelioma), and provide an opportunity of thoracoscopic pleurodesis in case of rapidly recurrent pleural effusions. This procedure can be performed using local or general anesthesia. It can be performed in a fully equipped endoscopy suite where patients are sedated but not intubated (recently referred to as *medical thoracoscopy*), or it can be performed in the operating room using single- or double-lumen endotracheal tubes and general anesthesia (video-assisted thoracic surgery).

The treatment and prognosis of malignant pleural disease are those of the primary tumor. Symptomatic treatment of recurrent effusions has included intrapleural instillation of sclerosing agents, such as quinacrine, *Corynebacterium parvum,* nitrogen mustard, talc, mitoxantrone, tetracycline (no longer commercially available), and pleural abrasion or pleurectomy during thoracoscopy or thoracotomy. Bleomycin has also been used but is less effective (<60% success in most studies) and far more costly. Doxycycline and minocycline are available now to replace tetracycline, but the success rates using these agents, similar to the success rate of tetracycline, are at best 72% and 86%, respectively.

Asbestos-free, sterile talc powder (also commercially available in an aerosol can) is the most effective and least expensive pleurodesis agent available. Talc pleurodesis can be achieved during thoracoscopy, at which time fluid is evacuated, talc is sprayed over all visceral and parietal pleural surfaces, and a chest tube is inserted to keep the pleural space dry and enhance complete lung expansion. Hospitalization is usually required for approximately 5 days. Talc pleurodesis can also be achieved using talc slurry (a mixture of talc powder and normal saline solution) instilled into the pleural cavity through a previously placed large-bore chest tube. The precise role for talc slurry versus thoracoscopic talc powder pleurodesis remains to be defined.

1. Ayres JG, Crocker JG, Skilbeck NQ. Differentiation of malignant from normal reactive mesothelial cells by the argyrophil technique for nucleolar organizer region associated proteins. *Thorax.* 1988;43:366.
   The argyrophilic technique separates reactive pleural disease from mesothelioma with a high degree of confidence.
2. Baas P. Predictive and prognostic factors in malignant pleural mesothelioma. *Curr Opin Oncol.* 2003;15:127–130.
   A recent review of established prognostic factors as well as a summary of recent developments in molecular biology and potential place for SV40.
3. Berghmans T, Paesmans M, Lalami Y, et al. Activity of chemotherapy and immunotherapy on malignant mesothelioma: a systematic review of the literature with meta-analysis. *Lung Cancer.* 2002;38:111–121.
   Concluding that the most effective single agent for chemotherapeutic treatment of malignant mesothelioma remains cisplatin, and proposing that the combination cisplatin and doxorubicin be used as control arm of future randomized clinical trials.
4. Boutin C, Rey F, Viallat JR. Prevention of malignant seeding after invasive diagnostic procedures in patients with pleural mesothelioma. A randomized trial of local radiotherapy. *Chest.* 1995;108:754.
   Tumor growth through thoracoscopic access sites is prevented by 21 Gy delivered over a small surface.
5. Britton M. The epidemiology of mesothelioma. *Semin Oncol.* 2002;29:18–25.
   A nice review of the fiber controversy surrounding mesothelioma.
6. Cantao A, et al. Videothoracoscopy in the diagnosis and treatment of malignant pleural mesothelioma with associated pleural effusions. *Thorac Cardiovasc Surg.* 1997;45:16.
   Thoracosocpy has a definite role and also allows early pleurodesis.
7. Canto AA. Diagnostic results in secondary malignant pleural effusions. *Pneumologie.* 1989;43:58.
   Results of 365 thoracoscopies, describing the location and overall appearance of pleural tumors.

8. Colt HG. Mesothelioma: epidemiology, presentation, and diagnosis. *Semin Respir Crit Care Med*. 1997;18:353.

   A recent and concise review of many issues, including fibers, latency periods, and risk factors.

9. Colt HG. Thoracoscopic management of malignant pleural effusions. *Clin Chest Med*. 1995;16:505.

   A detailed review of diagnostic and treatment roles as well as techniques of this minimally invasive procedure that is increasingly used in patients with pleural disease.

10. Danby CA, Adebonojo SA, Moritz DM. Video-assisted talc pleurodesis for malignant pleural effusions utilizing local anesthesia and IV sedation. *Chest*. 1998;113:739.

    This procedure can be done safely under local anesthesia only, eliminating costly operating room stays.

11. Eibel R, Tuengerthal S, Schoenberg SO. The role of new imaging techniques in diagnosis and staging of malignant pleural mesothelioma. *Curr Opin Oncol*. 2003;15:131–138.

    A description of the most recently developed staging system from the International Mesothelioma Interest Group in addition to a careful description of the utility of contrast-enhanced magnetic resonance imaging as well as advantages and disadvantages of positive emission tomography in this patient population.

12. England DM, Hochholzer L, McCarthy MJ. Localized benign and malignant fibrous tumors of the pleura: a clinicopathologic review of 223 cases. *Am J Surg Pathol*. 1993;17:876.

    In this study, 223 tumors of the pleura were reviewed: 141 benign, 82 malignant. The presenting symptoms were chest pain, dyspnea, and cough. One fourth of the patients had hypoglycemia, clubbing, or a pleural effusion. Two thirds of tumors involved the visceral pleura. Neoplasms were seen in atypical sites, such as fissure and inverted into the peripheral lung. Of the malignant tumors, 45% were cured by surgical excision. These lesions primarily were pedunculated or well circumscribed. Resectability, therefore, is the single most important indicator of clinical outcome.

13. Foresti V, et al. Malignant pleural effusions: meaning of pleural fluid pH determination. *Oncology*. 1990;47:62.

    The pH and glucose concentrations in the pleural fluid of patients with malignant effusions are frequently low. Survival and response to pleurodesis is the same in patients with low pH malignant effusions as in patients with normal pH malignant effusions.

14. Harvey JC, Erdman CB, Beattie EJ. Early experience with videothoracoscopic hydrodissection pleurectomy in the treatment of malignant pleural effusion. *J Surg Oncol*. 1995;59:243.

    Pleurectomy, although seldom performed in the United States for patients with pleural carcinomatosis, is possible and can be performed safely. Most experts agree, however, that chemical or talc pleurodesis is preferable to pleurectomy in patients with advanced neoplastic disease.

15. International Mesothelioma Interest Group. A proposed new international TNM staging system for malignant mesothelioma. *Chest*. 1995;108:1122.

    Reviews and describes previously used staging systems and proposes a new classification system that might provide a framework for analyzing results of prospective clinical trials.

16. Marchevsky AM, Wick MR. Current controversies regarding the role of asbestos exposure in the causation of malignant mesothelioma: the need for an evidence-based approach to develop medicolegal guidelines. *Ann Diagn Pathol*. 2003;7:321–332.

    A recent and well-written review of the asbestos controversy as causation of mesothelioma.

17. Martensson G. Prediction of the diagnostic utility of thoracoscopy in pleural effusion. *Pneumologie*. 1989;43:72.

    Thoracoscopy is the method of choice for evaluating patients with possible primary pleural malignancies.

18. Mitchell JD. Solitary fibrous tumor of the pleura. *Semin Thorac Cardiovasc Surg.* 2003;15:305–309.

    A review of the clinical presentation, imaging aspects, and surgical treatment of these benign tumors derived from mesenchymal cells.

19. Mohanty SK, Dey P. Serous effusions: diagnosis of malignancy beyond cytomorphology. An analytic review. *Postgrad Med J.* 2003;79:569–582.

    An interesting overview of newer cytopathology techniques for differential diagnosis of pleural carcinomatosis, including flow cytometry, immunofluorescence, telomerase activity, PCR, and oncogene products.

20. Ordonez NG. The immunohistochemical diagnosis of mesothelioma: differentiation of mesothelioma and lung adenocarcinoma. *Am J Surg Pathol.* 1989;13:276.

    Immunostaining for both CEA and one or more of TAG-72 (B72.3), Leu-M1, SC, CA19-9, and SP1 increased sensitivity in differentiating mesothelioma from the adenocarcinoma.

21. Pettersson T, et al. Concentration of hyaluronic acid and pleural fluid as a diagnostic aid for malignant mesothelioma. *Chest.* 1988;94:1037.

    Pleural effusions associated with mesothelioma have a high concentration of hyaluronic acid in the pleural fluid and a low concentration of CEA.

22. Powers A, Carbone M. The role of environmental carcinogens, viruses, and genetic predisposition in the pathogenesis of mesothelioma. *Cancer Biol Ther.* 2002;1:348–353.

    Focus on potential new research fronts including simian virus 40 and other genetic factors.

23. Renshaw AA, et al. The role of cytologic evaluation of pleural fluid in the diagnosis of malignant mesothelioma. *Chest.* 1997;111:106.

    Fluid cytology may be more helpful than previously thought.

24. Rodriguez-Panadero F, Borderas NF, Lopez MJ. Pleural metastatic tumors and effusions: frequency in pathogenic mechanisms in a post-mortem series. *Eur Respir J.* 1989;2:366.

    Reviews 191 patients with one or more malignant tumors.

25. Rubins JB, et al. Lovastatin induces apoptosis in malignant mesothelioma cells. *Am J Respir Crit Care Med.* 1998;157:1616.

    Mesothelial cell viability was decreased in a dose-dependent manner by lovastatin, probably by inhibition of mevalonate synthesis. This article expands on the concept of potential adjunctive treatment of patients with this deadly disease.

26. Ruffie P, Lehmann M, Galateau-Salle F, et al. Malignant mesothelioma. *Br J Cancer* 2001;84(Suppl 2):49–50.

    A neat, concise review of diagnostic criteria, immunohistochemistry, therapeutic recommendations (early pleurodesis unless intracavitary treatment is planned), and prognosis.

27. Rusch VW. Treatment of malignant pleural mesothelioma. *Semin Respir Crit Care Med.* 1997;18:363.

    A well-written, recent review of surgical and medical treatment modalities.

28. Rusch VW. Pleural mesothelioma: the role of extrapleural pneumonectomy in malignant pleural mesothelioma. A Lung Cancer Study Group trial. *J Thorac Cardiovasc Surg.* 1991;102:1.

    Of 83 patients with this condition, 20 underwent extrapleural pneumonectomy; 3 died postoperatively. Recurrence-free survival, but not overall survival, was significantly improved with surgery.

29. Sterman DH, Kaiser LR, Abelda SM. Advances in the treatment of malignant pleural mesothelioma. *Chest.* 1999;116:504.

    Another recent review of treatment modalities that also includes a discussion of emerging immunotherapy and gene therapy approaches, including intratumoral therapy, and tumor vaccines.

30. Tomek S, Emri S, Krejcy K, et al. Chemotherapy for malignant pleural mesothelioma: past results and recent developments. *Br J Cancer.* 2003;88:167–174.

    A nice summary of previously conducted clinical trials and results suggesting favorable effects of antimetabolites such as pemetrexed in combination with platinum compounds.

31. Van Ruth S, Bass P, Zoetmulder FA. Surgical treatment of malignant pleural mesothelioma. *Chest*. 2003;123:551–561.

   A concise review of the questionable survival benefits for patients undergoing surgical resection, including a discussion of intracavitary therapies.

32. Walker-Renard P. Chemical pleurodesis for malignant pleural effusions. *Ann Intern Med*. 1994;120:56.

   An excellent recent review of agents used for chemical pleurodesis.

SUBJECT INDEX

Pages followed by *f* indicate figures; pages followed by *t* indicate tables.